Techniques of Scientific Computing (Part 1)
Numerical Methods for Solids (Part 1)
Solution of Equations in $\mathbb{R}^n$ (Part 2)

Handbook of Numerical Analysis

General Editors:

P.G. Ciarlet

*Analyse Numérique, Tour 55–65
Université Pierre et Marie Curie
4 Place Jussieu
75005 PARIS, France*

J.L. Lions

*Collège de France
Place Marcelin Berthelot
75005 PARIS, France*

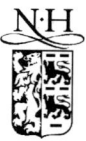

NORTH-HOLLAND
AMSTERDAM · LONDON · NEW YORK · TOKYO

Volume III

Techniques of Scientific Computing (Part 1)

Numerical Methods for Solids (Part 1)

Solution of Equations in $\mathbb{R}^n$ (Part 2)

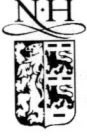

1994
NORTH-HOLLAND
AMSTERDAM · LONDON · NEW YORK · TOKYO

ELSEVIER SCIENCE B.V.
Sara Burgerhartstraat 25
P.O. Box 211, 1000 AE Amsterdam, The Netherlands

LIBRARY OF CONGRESS CATALOGING-IN-PUBLICATION DATA
(Revised for Vol. 3)

Handbook of numerical analysis.

Includes bibliographical references and indexes.
Contents: v. 1. Finite difference methods (pt. 1);
Solutions of equations in $\mathbb{R}^n$ (pt. 1)–v. 2. Finite
element methods (pt. 1)–v. 3. Techniques of scientific
computing (pt. 1); Numerical methods for solids (pt. 1);
Solutions of equations in $\mathbb{R}^n$ (pt. 2)
1. Numerical analysis. I. Ciarlet, Philippe G.
II. Lions, Jacques Louis.
QA297.H287 1989   519.4   89-23314
ISBN 0-444-70366-7 (v. 1)
ISBN 0-444-70365-9 (v. 2)

ISBN: 0 444 89928 6

© 1994 ELSEVIER SCIENCE B.V. All rights reserved.

No part of this publication may be reproduced, stored in a retrieval system or transmitted in any form or by any means, electronic, mechanical, photocopying, recording or otherwise, without the prior written permission of the publisher, Elsevier Science B.V., Copyright & Permissions Department, P.O. Box 521, 1000 AM Amsterdam, The Netherlands.

Special regulations for readers in the U.S.A. – This publication has been registered with the Copyright Clearance Center Inc. (CCC), Salem, Massachusetts. Information can be obtained from the CCC about conditions under which photocopies of parts of this publication may be made in the U.S.A. All other copyright questions, including photocopying outside of the U.S.A., should be referred to the copyright owner, Elsevier Science B.V.

No responsibility is assumed by the publisher for any injury and/or damage to persons or property as a matter of products liability, negligence or otherwise, or from any use or operation of any methods, products, instructions or ideas contained in the material herein.

This book is printed on acid-free paper.

Printed in The Netherlands

General Preface

During the past decades, giant needs for ever more sophisticated mathematical models and increasingly complex and extensive computer simulations have arisen. In this fashion, two indissociable activities, *mathematical modeling* and *computer simulation*, have gained a major status in all aspects of science, technology, and industry.

In order that these two sciences be established on the safest possible grounds, mathematical rigor is indispensable. For this reason, two companion sciences, *Numerical Analysis* and *Scientific Software*, have emerged as essential steps for validating the mathematical models and the computer simulations that are based on them.

Numerical Analysis is here understood as the part of *Mathematics* that describes and analyzes all the numerical schemes that are used on computers; its objective consists in obtaining a clear, precise, and faithful, representation of all the "information" contained in a mathematical model; as such, it is the natural extension of more classical tools, such as analytic solutions, special transforms, functional analysis, as well as stability and asymptotic analysis.

The various volumes comprising the *Handbook of Numerical Analysis* will thoroughly cover all the major aspects of Numerical Analysis, by presenting accessible and in-depth surveys, which include the most recent trends.

More precisely, the Handbook will cover the *basic methods of Numerical Analysis*, gathered under the following general headings:

- Solution of Equations in $\mathbb{R}^n$,
- Finite Difference Methods,
- Finite Element Methods,
- Techniques of Scientific Computing,
- Optimization Theory and Systems Science.

It will also cover the *numerical solution of actual problems of contemporary interest in Applied Mathematics*, gathered under the following general headings:

- Numerical Methods for Fluids,
- Numerical Methods for Solids,
- Specific Applications.

"Specific Applications" include: Meteorology, Seismology, Petroleum Mechanics, Celestial Mechanics, etc.

Each heading is covered by several *articles*, each of which being devoted to a specialized, but to some extent "independent", topic. Each article contains a thorough description and a mathematical analysis of the various methods in actual use, whose practical performances may be illustrated by significant numerical examples.

Since the Handbook is basically expository in nature, only the most basic results are usually proved in detail, while less important, or technical, results may be only stated or commented upon (in which case specific references for their proofs are systematically provided). In the same spirit, only a "selective" bibliography is appended whenever the roughest counts indicate that the reference list of an article should comprise several thousand items if it were to be exhaustive.

Volumes are numbered by capital Roman numerals (as Vol. I, Vol. II, etc.), according to their *chronological appearance*.

Since all the articles pertaining to a given *heading* may not be simultaneously available at a given time, a given heading usually appears in more than one volume; for instance, if articles devoted to the heading "Solution of Equations in $\mathbb{R}^n$" appear in Volumes I and III, these volumes will include "Solution of Equations in $\mathbb{R}^n$ (Part 1)" and "Solution of Equations in $\mathbb{R}^n$ (Part 2)" in their respective titles. Naturally, all the headings dealt with within a given volume appear in its title; for instance, the complete title of Volume I is "Finite Difference Methods (Part 1)—Solution of Equations in $\mathbb{R}^n$ (Part 1)".

Each article is subdivided into *sections*, which are numbered consecutively throughout the article by *Arabic numerals*, as Section 1, Section 2, ..., Section 14, etc. Within a given section, *formulas, theorems, remarks, and figures*, have their own independent numberings; for instance, with Section 14, formulas are numbered consecutively as (14.1), (14.2), etc., theorems are numbered consecutively as Theorem 14.1, Theorem 14.2, etc. For the sake of clarity, the article is also subdivided into *chapters*, numbered consecutively throughout the article by *capital Roman numerals*; for instance, Chapter I comprises Sections 1 to 9, Chapter II comprises Sections 10 to 16, etc.

P.G. CIARLET
J.L. LIONS
May 1989

Contents of Volume III

GENERAL PREFACE v

TECHNIQUES OF SCIENTIFIC COMPUTING (PART 1)

    Historical Perspective on Interpolation, Approximation and
        Quadrature, *C. Brezinski*   3
    Padé Approximations, *C. Brezinski and J. Van Iseghem*   47
    Approximation and Interpolation Theory, *Bl. Sendov and*
        A. Andreev   223

NUMERICAL METHODS FOR SOLIDS (PART 1)

    Numerical Methods for Nonlinear Three-Dimensional Elasticity,
        P. Le Tallec   465

SOLUTION OF EQUATIONS IN $\mathbb{R}^n$ (PART 2)

    Numerical Solution of Polynomial Equations, *Bl. Sendov,*
        A. Andreev and N. Kjurkchiev   625

Contents of the Handbook

VOLUME I

FINITE DIFFERENCE METHODS (PART 1)

Introduction, *G.I. Marchuk*	3
Finite Difference Methods for Linear Parabolic Equations, *V. Thomée*	5
Splitting and Alternating Direction Methods, *G.I. Marchuk*	197

SOLUTION OF EQUATIONS IN $\mathbb{R}^n$ (PART 1)

Least Squares Methods, *Å. Björck*	465

VOLUME II

FINITE ELEMENT METHODS (PART 1)

Finite Elements: An Introduction, *J.T. Oden*	3
Basic Error Estimates for Elliptic Problems, *P.G. Ciarlet*	17
Local Behavior in Finite Element Methods, *L.B. Wahlbin*	353
Mixed and Hybrid Methods, *J.E. Roberts and J.-M. Thomas*	523
Eigenvalue Problems, *I. Babuška and J. Osborn*	641
Evolution Problems, *H. Fujita and T. Suzuki*	789

VOLUME III

TECHNIQUES OF SCIENTIFIC COMPUTING (PART 1)

Historical Perspective on Interpolation, Approximation and Quadrature, *C. Brezinski*	3
Padé Approximations, *C. Brezinski and J. Van Iseghem*	47
Approximation and Interpolation Theory, *Bl. Sendov and A. Andreev*	223

NUMERICAL METHODS FOR SOLIDS (PART 1)

Numerical Methods for Nonlinear Three-Dimensional Elasticity, *P. Le Tallec*	465

SOLUTION OF EQUATIONS IN $\mathbb{R}^n$ (PART 2)

    Numerical Solution of Polynomial Equations, *Bl. Sendov, A. Andreev and N. Kjurkchiev*   625

Techniques of Scientific Computing (Part 1)

Historical Perspective on Interpolation, Approximation and Quadrature

Claude Brezinski

Laboratoire d'Analyse Numérique et d'Optimisation UFR d'IEEA - M3
Université des Sciences et Technologies de Lille
F-59655 Villeneuve d'Ascq Cedex, France

Contents

CHAPTER I. Interpolation — 7

  1. Polynomial interpolation — 7
  2. Padé approximation — 9
  3. Rational interpolation — 11
  4. Spline interpolation — 12
  5. Multivariate interpolation — 14
  6. The general interpolation problem — 15

CHAPTER II. Approximation — 17

  7. Linear approximation — 18
  8. Nonlinear approximation — 21
  9. Multivariate approximation — 23

CHAPTER III. Numerical Quadrature — 25

  10. Newton–Cotes formulae — 26
  11. Gaussian quadratures — 29
  12. Cubatures — 32

REFERENCES — 33

SUBJECT INDEX — 45

CHAPTER I

Interpolation

One of the easiest procedures for approximating a function f is by interpolation. The values y_i of f at several distinct points $x_0, x_1, \ldots, x_n$ being known, it consists in determining the free parameters $a_0, a_1, \ldots, a_n$ of a function F of a given form in order that the interpolation conditions

$$F(x_i) = y_i = f(x_i)$$

are satisfied for $i = 0, \ldots, n$.

If the first derivatives of f at some of the points x_i are also known, one can also try to determine the free parameters in F such that

$$F^{(j)}(x_i) = f^{(j)}(x_i) \tag{0.1}$$

for $i = 0, \ldots, k$ and $j = 0, \ldots, k_i$ with $\sum_{i=0}^{k}(k_i + 1) = n + 1$.

1. Polynomial interpolation

Obviously, the easiest functions F to use are polynomials. Interpolation, a vocable due to John WALLIS [1656] (1616–1703), has a long history which was initiated, after an early attempt by Thomas HARRIOT [1611] (1560–1621), by Henry BRIGGS (1561–1630) when constructing his table of logarithms. His method, described in his book *Arithmetica Logarithmica* [1624], assumed that the interpolation points are equidistant and used first and second order *finite differences*, $\Delta y_i = y_{i+1} - y_i$ and $\Delta^2 y_i = \Delta y_{i+1} - \Delta y_i = y_{i+2} - 2y_{i+1} + y_i$ but no proof or suggestion of how he obtained his method was given. It corresponds to interpolation by a polynomial of degree two. A scheme for quadratic interpolation was also used much earlier by the great Arabic mathematician Al-Birûni (973–1048) and certainly by many of his followers.

Interpolation by a polynomial with an arbitrary degree (still for equidistant points), known as the *Gregory–Newton formula*, was discussed by James GREGORY (1638-1675) in a letter to John COLLINS (1625–1683) of November 23, 1670 and by Isaac NEWTON (1642–1727) in Lemma 5 of Book III of his *Principia Mathematica* [1687], but the formula was known to him at least since 1676 as pointed out by FRASER [1927]. Then, Newton extended it to the case of arbitrary interpolation points using *divided differences*, a term first used by Augustus DE MORGAN (1806–1871) in his book *Differential and Integral Calculus*

([1842], p. 550) (André Marie AMPÈRE [1825–1826] (1775–1836) used the name *interpolatory functions*). The formula was written into a more suitable form by Roger COTES [1708] (1682–1712). The other interpolation formulae named after Gauss, Stirling and Bessel were already known to Newton. It seems that Gottfried Wilhelm LEIBNIZ (1646–1716) also obtained similar results independently around 1672 (see HOFMANN [1974]). Interpolation in the points of a geometric progression leads to a simplification similar to the case of an arithmetical progression. This problem was first studied by James STIRLING [1730] (1692–1770). Then Karl Heinrich SCHELLBACH [1864] (1805–1892) put Stirling's result into an elegant algorithmic form. The process was then rediscovered by Carl RUNGE [1891] (1856–1927) (see SCHOENBERG [1981] for an extensive study).

Let us mention that interpolation, nowadays presented as a purely numerical method, had great importance in the development of calculus since Newton's formula was used independently by Gregory and Newton to derive the binomial theorem. It was also used by Brook TAYLOR [1715] (1685–1731) for obtaining the expansion of a function into an infinite series but it seems that Gregory also discovered it 44 years earlier.

The work of Briggs was first appreciated by Joseph Louis LAGRANGE [1783] (1736–1813) who wrote on the subject while he was in Berlin. In 1794, he gave his famous interpolation formula which he attributed to Newton but some commentators claim that it goes back to Leonhard EULER [1775] (1707–1783) or to Edward WARING [1779] (c. 1736–1798). Lagrange's formula can be found in his *Leçons Elémentaires sur les Mathématiques* given at the Ecole Normale in Paris (see LAGRANGE [1795] and Oeuvres, vol. 7, p. 286). The classical error formula for the Lagrange interpolation polynomial was first given by Augustin Louis CAUCHY [1840] (1789–1857). Its proof was then simplified by Angelo GENOCCHI [1878, 1880–1881] (1817–1889), Hermann Amandus SCHWARZ [1881–1882] (1843–1921) and Thomas Jan STIELTJES [1882] (1858–1894) who proved it from its integral representation given by Charles HERMITE [1878] (1822–1901). Finally the modern proof of the error was given by Giuseppe PEANO [1918] (1858–1932).

The interpolation polynomials at $x_i, \ldots, x_{i+k}$ can be recursively computed for varying i and k by using an algorithm first due to Alexander Craig AITKEN [1932] (1895–1967) and improved by Eric Harold NEVILLE [1934] (1889–1961) two years later. This is the *Neville–Aitken scheme* which was extended by Günter MÜLBACH [1973] for interpolation by any family of functions forming a *Chebyshev system*. These two formulae lead respectively to *Richardson's process* and the *E-algorithm* for convergence acceleration by extrapolation (see BREZINSKI and REDIVO ZAGLIA [1991]).

The interpolation problem (0.1) was treated in its full generality by HERMITE [1878]. It is now called the *Hermite interpolation problem*. As already mentioned, Hermite gave an integral representation of the error which was put into usual form by STIELTJES [1882]. Interpolation with some nonnecessarily consecutive derivatives imposed is called *Hermite–Birkhoff interpolation*. It is extensively treated by LORENTZ, JETTER and RIEMENSCHNEIDER [1983], where a history of interpolation and approximation since 1960 can also be found.

The first examples of the nonconvergence of a sequence of interpolation polynomials when the interpolation points are equidistant in an interval, are due to Charles MÉRAY [1884, 1896] (1835–1911), RUNGE [1901] and Emile BOREL [1897] (1871–1956) around 1900. The problem was then studied theoretically by Georg FABER [1914] and Sergey Natanovich BERNSTEIN [1914] (1880–1968) who proved simultaneously that when any family of interpolation points is given in a closed interval, it is always possible to find a continuous function such that the sequence of interpolation polynomials at these points does not converge uniformly to it. As proved by Geza GRÜNWALD [1935] (1910–1942) and József MARCINKIEWICZ [1935] (1910–1940), divergence can occur even if the interpolation points are the zeros of the Chebyshev polynomials. Cases of convergence were studied by Lipót FEJÉR [1931] (1880–1959) and James Alexander SHOHAT [1933] (1886–1944). The case of Hermite interpolation was also treated by Fejér. When the interpolation points are the zeros of orthogonal polynomials, then convergence in the L^2 sense occurs as proved by ERDÖS and TURÁN [1937]. All these results can be found in FELDHEIM [1939].

2. Padé approximation

Let us consider the interpolation conditions (0.1) where F is a rational fraction with a numerator of degree p and a denominator of degree q. We also take $k = 0, x_0 = 0$ and $k_0 = p + q$. Thus we are looking for a rational fraction whose series expansion in ascending powers of the variable agrees with a given power series up to and including the term of degree $p + q$. Such a rational function is called a *Padé approximant*. Padé approximants have quite a long history since they are connected to *continued fractions*, a concept which can be traced back to Euclid's algorithm for the greatest common divisor.

Padé approximants were discovered independently by two prominent mathematicians of the 18th century. The first is Johann Heinrich LAMBERT [1758] (1728–1777) who gave their direct derivation. He considered the series (in his notation)

$$x = \frac{v^2}{2!} - \frac{v^4}{4!} + \frac{v^6}{6!} - \frac{v^8}{8!} + \cdots,$$

which he multiplied by $1 + mv^2 + nv^4$ and then chose m and n so that the terms of degrees 6 and 8 disappear. He obtained

$$x = \frac{7560v^2 - 300v^4}{15120 + 660v^2 + 13v^4} + O(v^{10}).$$

Since the degree of approximation is the sum of the degrees of the numerator and the denominator it is, by definition, a Padé approximant of the series x.

The second discoverer of Padé approximants was LAGRANGE [1776] who wrote a paper where he developed a general method for obtaining the solution of a differential equation as a continued fraction. Since continued fractions were not easy to manipulate, he reduced their *successive convergents* to ordinary fractions by using the recurrence relations proved by WALLIS [1656] in his book *Arithmetica Infinitorum* and he added that these fractions are exact up to the term that is the product of the two highest terms in the numerator and in the denominator. This is exactly the definition of Padé approximants.

In fact, some examples of Padé approximants had already been obtained by several mathematicians but they were not aware of their fundamental property to match the original series as far as possible and, thus, they could not be credited for their discovery. For instance, Euler transformed many power series into continued fractions by a process similar to Euclid's algorithm for the greatest common divisor and the convergents of these continued fractions are Padé approximants under some conditions which were analyzed by BREZINSKI [1985].

The determinantal formula for Padé approximants was obtained by Carl Gustav Jacob JACOBI [1845] (1804–1851) from that for interpolation rational fractions given by CAUCHY [1821]. Recurrence relations between three adjacent Padé approximants (that is, approximants with a difference of at most one unit in the degrees of the numerators and the denominators) were proved by Georg Ferdinand FROBENIUS [1881] (1849–1917). The name of many other well known mathematicians is attached to Padé approximants. The interested reader is referred to BREZINSKI [1991] for an extensive history. We shall only mention here Charles HERMITE [1873] who proved, using a generalization of Padé approximants, that the number e is transcendental. His proof was extended by Carl Louis Ferdinand LINDEMANN [1882] (1852–1939) who proved the transcendence of π thus ending the problem of the quadrature of the circle, an open question for more than 2000 years, with a negative answer.

Let us now come to Henri Eugène PADÉ. He was born in Abbeville (France) on December 17, 1863. In 1883, he entered the Ecole Normale Supérieure and obtained his Agrégation de Mathématiques in 1886. After teaching in several secondary schools, he went to Leipzig and Göttingen. On June 21, 1892 he defended, under the supervision of Hermite, a thesis entitled *Sur la représentation approchée d'une fonction par des fractions rationnelles* (see PADÉ [1892]). This was the first systematic study of Padé approximants and he arranged them in a double entry table now called the *Padé table*. Then he taught in Lille, first in a secondary school and then at the University as an Associate Professor. He went to Poitiers where he became Full Professor in 1902. Then he moved to Bordeaux and was awarded the *Grand Prix des Sciences Mathématiques* of the French Academy of Sciences in 1906. After that, he almost stopped doing research since he was successively appointed as Rector of the Academies of Besançon, Dijon and Aix-en-Provence where he died in 1953. More details about his life and works can be found in PADÉ [1984].

Important results on Padé approximants are due to Robert Fernand Bernard DE MONTESSUS DE BALLORE [1902] (1870–1937) who gave a convergence theorem for meromorphic functions with a finite number of poles in a disc and no other singularity. This result was extended by Rowland WILSON [1927]. After this date, Padé approximants remained almost forgotten until they were rediscovered around 1960 by physicists who used them for solving many problems where the solution is obtained as a formal power series expansion. Since then, they have been applied in various branches of mathematics and applied sciences and they have been generalized in several directions.

To conclude, let us mention that Gaspard Riche DE PRONY [1795] (1755–1839) gave a method for interpolation by a sum of exponential functions and that his method is closely related to Padé approximation.

Padé approximation for multivariate series leads to several generalizations. The first problem concerns the representation of a polynomial in several variables. The powers of the various variables must belong to some lattice in $\mathbb{N}^n$ where n is the number of variables. Thus one has to choose one lattice for the numerator of the appproximant, another one for its denominator and one more for the powers of the series expansion of the approximant which have to be identified to those of the series. Of course one must have as many equations as unknowns. A general study on the relations between these lattices was conducted by LEVIN [1976]. The first approximants in two variables to be introduced were those of CHISHOLM [1973]. In these approximants, the number of equations is too small and Chisholm added some supplementary equations thus destroying the *consistency principle* which states that if the series to be approximated is a rational function, then it must be exactly recovered by Padé approximants. Another type of approximants, corresponding to a rectangular lattice for the powers of the two variables, was studied by BREZINSKI [1978]. The same idea was used by ARIOKA [1987] but for a triangular lattice and the Kergin interpolation polynomial. The approach of CUYT [1984] makes use of homogeneous approximants. Since Padé approximants in one variable are related to polynomial interpolation, it is possible to study the multivariate case from this starting point. This was the approach of SABLONNIÈRE [1983], who used the Hakopian interpolation polynomial, and that of KIDA [1990]. A completely different approach was followed by CHAFFY [1984] who constructed the Padé approximant with respect to the first variable and then the Padé approximant of this first approximant with respect to the second variable. Homogeneous Padé approximants in two variables, leading to an interesting theory of orthogonal polynomials in two variables, were recently constructed by BENOUAHMANE [1991].

Padé approximation is the subject of the article by BREZINSKI and VAN ISEGHEM [1993] in this volume.

3. Rational interpolation

After the first attempts due to Cauchy and Jacobi, PADÉ [1900] treated the problem of interpolation by a rational fraction. He arranged these fractions in a table similar to his Padé table and gave the recurrence relations satisfied by the numerators and the denominators of three adjacent fractions. However, his work was quite restrictive.

A method for constructing interpolating rational fractions as the successive convergents of a continued fraction was given by Thorvald Nicolai THIELE [1906] (1838–1910). First he defined the *reciprocal differences* and then used them for developing a function into a continued fraction, a formula quite similar to Newton's, which makes use of divided differences. Since this formula terminates if the function is a rational function, it can be compared to the Taylor's expansion which terminates if the function is a polynomial. These results were extended by Niels Erik NÖRLUND [1911] (1885–1981) who studied their convergence.

For recent developments of this question, including rational Hermite interpolation and the case of functions of several variables, see CUYT and WUYTACK [1987] and CUYT [1992]. The Cauchy interpolation problem was extensively studied by DONOGHUE [1974].

4. Spline interpolation

Cardinal interpolation refers to interpolation at the integer points on the real line. The first survey on this question goes back at least to the book by WHITTAKER [1935]. The subject is also connected to *cardinal series* as explained by HIGGINS [1985]. On the other hand, *spline interpolation* consists of piecewise polynomial interpolation. Thus, a spline function is a *piecewise polynomial* whose values and the values of some of its first derivatives coincide at the interpolation points. Although the subject had been studied as early as 1906 by George David BIRKHOFF [1906] (1884–1944), its development really starts in 1946 with a paper by Isaac Jacob SCHOENBERG [1946] (1903–1990). As he reported himself in SCHOENBERG [1988], he was working, during the war, at the Ballistics Research Laboratory in Aberdeen, Maryland, USA. Once he had to smooth data by analytic functions for computing trajectories of projectiles. He solved this problem by what he later called *cardinal splines*. Splines constructed on equidistant nodes were already used before that time by RUNGE [1901] (quadratic splines) and by QUADE and COLLATZ [1938] (arbitrary degree) for the approximation of the Fourier coefficients of periodic functions but not for their approximation. This is the first study where periodic polynomial splines for equidistant nodes are used (see also EAGLE [1928]). SCHOENBERG [1946] relied his work on the *osculatory interpolation problem* studied, in particular, by GREVILLE [1944].

With the exception of a paper by GOLOMB and WEINBERGER [1958] dealing with the optimal approximation of continuous linear functionals, the history of splines can be divided into two different periods as stated by LAURENT [1972]. Before 1964, papers were mostly devoted to properties of piecewise polynomials while, after that date, the introduction of functional analysis allowed generalizations in Hilbert spaces to be obtained and their minimization properties studied.

Spline functions have many applications in computer aided design. As recorded by FARIN [1991], the story began when the French automobile company Citroën asked Paul DE CASTELJAU in 1958 to develop a system for helping engineers to design cars. De Casteljau had the idea of using Bernstein polynomials for this purpose but, due to secrecy, he was not allowed to publish his results. However, the secret was not total since, in the early sixties, Pierre BÉZIER, an engineer at Renault, heard that Citroën was developing such a project and he initiated a new approach to curves and surfaces approximation, consisting of piecewise polynomials controlled by polygonal lines. Such curves and surfaces are now known as *Bézier curves* and *surfaces*. It was FORREST [1972] who proved, while translating the book of BÉZIER [1972], that both approaches were identical since Bézier curves and surfaces can be formulated in terms of Bernstein polynomials.

An important class of spline functions (because of their small support) is that of *B-splines* which originated with SCHOENBERG [1946]. However, these splines became only widely used after a recurrence relation for their computation was obtained by COX [1972] and DE BOOR [1972]. Their algorithm provides the best means for computing their values at a given point. For a standard reference on the subject and other questions about splines, see DE BOOR [1978].

The case of two variables began to be treated in the late sixties by a tensor product approach. However, many curves and surfaces are badly represented by polynomials and need the introduction of rational curves and surfaces. The first results in this direction used weighted points but their applications were limited. This is the reason why FIOROT and JEANNIN [1989] introduced the notion of massic vectors instead of control points.

Radial basis functions can be considered as a generalization of splines to several dimensions. The usual linear spline function of one variable interpolating a function f at the points $x_0 < x_1 < \cdots < x_n$ can be considered as the function

$$F(x) = \sum_{i=0}^{n} \lambda_i |x - x_i|,$$

where the coefficients λ_i are defined by the interpolation conditions. In the univariate case, these two approaches are equivalent and they obviously suggest an extension to the multivariate case by replacing the absolute value in the preceding expression by the Euclidean norm. Thus F becomes a linear combination of translates of a function which is spherically symmetric about the origin, a characteristic of radial basis function approximation. In order to similarly generalize higher degree spline functions to the multivariate case, one has to consider the more general form

$$F(x) = \sum_{i=0}^{n} \lambda_i \Phi(\|x - x_i\|),$$

where Φ is some given function. A general exposition of this subject can be found in LIGHT [1992] and POWELL [1992].

Another alternative, now very much in favor, is the use of *wavelets* (see MEYER [1990] and DAUBECHIES [1992]).

5. Multivariate interpolation

The difficulty with multivariate interpolation comes from the nonexistence of Chebyshev systems in $\mathbb{R}^k$ for $k > 1$. Thus the *unisolvence* of the interpolation problem depends on the relative locations of the interpolation points. Then, the second difficulty arises from the generalization of divided differences to several variables (see THACHER and MILNE [1960], GUENTHER and ROETMAN [1970]). It seems that the first attempts to study multivariate polynomial interpolation are due to NARUMI [1920], NEDER [1926] and STEFFENSEN [1927].

In the sixties, this problem became very tractable thanks to the development of the *finite element method* for the numerical solution of partial differential equations. This question was extensively studied by CIARLET and RAVIART [1972], NICOLAIDES [1972], CHUNG and YAO [1977] and CIARLET [1978, 1991].

As pointed out by CIARLET and RAVIART [1972], there are basically two different types of approach to the interpolation problem in several variables. The first is the classical approach consisting of prescribing some points in the domain and the values of the function at these points and then looking for the (Lagrange or Hermite) interpolation polynomial. Generally, the error bounds are obtained as the sup-norm of some higher-order derivatives of the function. This question was studied in detail in his thesis by Christian COATMÉLEC [1966] using the analytic extension of differentiable functions defined on closed sets due to Hassler WHITNEY [1934] (1907–1989). Most of the time, the Cartesian coordinates are used, which limits both the theoretical results that can be proved and the examples that can be treated. A coordinate-free approach was used by CIARLET and WAGSCHAL [1971] and by COATMÉLEC [1966]. Let us mention that COATMÉLEC [1966] also defined *pseudo-splines* on simplices analogous to those of SCHOENBERG [1958] and gave convergence theorems.

The second approach studied by CIARLET and RAVIART [1972] consists of approximating the function in the Sobolev space

$$W^{k+1,p}(\Omega) = \{v \in L^p(\Omega): \partial^\alpha v \in L^p(\Omega) \text{ for all } |\alpha| \leq k+1\}$$

with the sole assumption that some polynomials remain invariant in the approximation procedure. Such an approximation is not necessarily defined as an interpolation problem but it contains Lagrange and Hermite interpolation as special cases. Error estimates depend upon the geometry of the domain. For the historical development of these questions, see the article by ODEN [1991].

Schemes, generalizing those of Lagrange, Newton and Neville–Aitken were obtained by GASCA and LOPEZ CARMONA [1982], GASCA and MAETZU [1982], GASCA and LEBRON [1983, 1987], GASCA and RAMIREZ [1984]. Their approach can yield either Lagrange or Hermite interpolation. Hermite interpolation was first studied by BUSCH [1985]. An overview of these topics can be found in GASCA [1990].

The problem of interpolation on subsets of grids was solved by Helmut WERNER [1980] (1931–1985). The work of HAKOPIAN [1982] must also be quoted. Hermite–Birkhoff interpolation in several variables was treated by GASCA and MAEZTU [1982]; see LORENTZ [1991] for a review.

6. The general interpolation problem

Let E be a vector space of dimension $n+1$. The general interpolation problem consists of finding $F \in E$ such that

$$L_i(F) = y_i \quad \text{for } i = 0, \ldots, n,$$

where the L_i are linear functionals on E. If $e_0, e_1, \ldots, e_n$ form a basis of E, then F can be written as $F = a_0 e_0 + \cdots + a_n e_n$ and the preceding interpolation conditions lead to

$$a_0 L_i(e_0) + \cdots + a_n L_i(e_n) = y_i \quad \text{for } i = 0, \ldots, n,$$

which is a system of $n+1$ equations in the $n+1$ unknowns $a_0, \ldots, a_n$. This formalism, proposed by DAVIS [1963], is the most general one and it includes, as particular cases, all the examples mentioned above. The corresponding algorithms were recently developed on the basis of *biorthogonality* by BREZINSKI [1992]. Biorthogonality has many applications in numerical analysis including Lánczos and other projection methods for solving systems of linear equations, generalizations of Padé approximants, sequence transformations, biorthogonal polynomials and least squares.

As already mentioned, a recursive scheme for interpolation by a linear combination of functions forming a complete Chebyshev system is due to MÜHLBACH [1973]. It is a generalization of the Neville–Aitken scheme. An important particular case, which is not treated here, is interpolation by a linear combination of trigonometric functions.

CHAPTER II

Approximation

Interpolation could obviously be used for approximating a given continuous function f. However it presents some difficulties because of its nonconvergence even in the polynomial case. Contrary to these negative results, the theorem proved by WEIERSTRASS [1885] is quite remarkable since it states that a sequence of polynomials converging uniformly to f on a closed bounded interval exists. However, these polynomials cannot be obtained by interpolation at a fixed set of points. In his proof, Carl Theodor WEIERSTRASS [1885] (1815–1897) made use of the theory of analytic functions. The proofs of Emile PICARD [1891] (1856–1941), Vito VOLTERRA [1897] (1860–1940) and Mathias LERCH [1903] (1860–1922) are based on Fourier expansions. More elementary proofs were given by RUNGE [1885a, 1885b], Henri LEBESGUE [1898] (1875–1941) and Gösta MITTAG-LEFFLER [1900] (1846–1927). The proof of BERNSTEIN [1912] is a constructive one where the *Bernstein polynomials*, uniformly converging to the function to be approximated, were introduced. The result of WEIERSTRASS [1885] was generalized to a compact set (instead of an interval) by Marshall Harvey STONE [1948] (1903–1989) and by Chaim MÜNTZ [1914] who considered an approximating function of the form

$$F(x) = \sum_{i=0}^{n} a_i x^{\lambda_i},$$

where $0 = \lambda_0 < \lambda_1 < \cdots < \lambda_i < \lambda_{i+1} < \cdots$.

When trying to approximate a given function, one is facing two choices:
(i) the form of the approximating function F, and
(ii) the distance (the norm) to be used.

Then various problems about the solution have to be solved: existence and uniqueness, characterization and other properties such as convergence and effective construction.

Let us recall that the L_p-norm of the function f on $[a, b]$ is defined by

$$L_p(f) = \left[\int_a^b |f(x)|^p \, dx \right]^{1/p}$$

and that the Chebyshev (or uniform) norm is defined by
$$L_\infty(f) = \sup_{a \leqslant x \leqslant b} |f(x)|.$$
The *best approximation problem* consists of finding F in some set of functions such that $L_p(f - F)$ is a minimum.

In the case where F is a polynomial, the Chebyshev norm was used for the first time by Pierre Simon DE LAPLACE [1799] (1749–1827) in Section 39 of Volume III of his *Mécanique Céleste* for approximating the solution of an inconsistent system of linear equations. He gave a method for obtaining the solution but it was completely impracticable for hand computations. In 1806, in an appendix to his *Nouvelles Méthodes pour la Détermination des Orbites des Comètes*, Adrien Marie LEGENDRE [1806] (1752–1833) took over the same problem but with the L_2-norm thus discovering least squares approximation. L_1-approximation was studied by Andrei Andreievich MARKOV [1898] (1856–1922) but the corresponding computational technique was only obtained much later by Norbert WIENER [1933] (1894–1964).

We shall now review some of these topics in more detail.

7. Linear approximation

By linear approximation, it is meant that the approximating function F has the form
$$F(x) = \sum_{i=0}^{n} a_i g_i(x),$$
where the g_i's are given functions.

Obviously the easiest case corresponds to polynomials, that is $g_i(x) = x^i$. The first systematic and extensive study of this case is due to Pafnouty Lvovitch CHEBYSHEV (1821–1894) who devoted 40 years to it. In his first paper (CHEBYSHEV [1854]), he was looking for "approximation methods which could provide the maximum of accuracy for all the values of the variable within two given limits". As he mentioned, the problem was considered before him by Jean Victor PONCELET [1835] (1788–1867) for approximating square roots by linear functions.

If $f(x) = x^n$ and $F(x) = a_0 + \cdots + a_{n-1} x^{n-1}$, the solution leads to the well-known *Chebyshev polynomials* of the first kind defined on the interval $[-1, +1]$ by
$$T_n(x) = \cos(n \arccos x).$$
They form a family of *orthogonal polynomials* with respect to the *weight function*
$$\Omega(x) = (1 - x^2)^{-1/2},$$
that is, they satisfy the orthogonality condition
$$\int_{-1}^{1} T_n(x) T_k(x) \Omega(x) \, dx = 0 \quad \text{if } n \neq k.$$

CHEBYSHEV [1854] assumed without proof the existence of the best uniform approximation polynomial. A characterization theorem was given by KIRCHBERGER [1902] but the actual proof of existence is due to BOREL [1905]. In the same book, BOREL [1905] also proved the uniqueness of the best uniform approximation polynomial (p. 85), the continuity of the operator of best approximation (p. 89) and he gave the *alternation theorem* stating that the error of the best uniform approximation polynomial of degree n achieves its maximum value in at least $n + 1$ points with alternating signs. Obviously, this result means that the best uniform approximation polynomial interpolates the function f in at least n points. This question of approximation with nodes was later studied by PASZKOWSKI [1955, 1956, 1957].

Explicit expressions for the error when approximating by a polynomial of degree at most n on $n+2$ points were given by Charles DE LA VALLÉE POUSSIN [1911b] (1866–1962).

An always converging algorithm for constructing the best uniform approximation polynomial of a continuous function was given by Georg PÓLYA [1913] (1887–1985). Let us mention that a method for approximating a continuous function f by a polynomial of the form

$$F(x) = \sum_{k=0}^{n} f(k/n) \Phi_{nk}(x),$$

where the Φ are some given functions, was already given by BOREL ([1905], p. 80). The proof of BERNSTEIN [1912] of the theorem of WEIERSTRASS [1885] follows this idea and it corresponds to the choice

$$\Phi_{nk}(x) = C_n^k x^k (1-x)^{n-k}.$$

The general theory of such operators is due to FAVARD [1944].

Results on the rate of convergence of the error of best uniform polynomial approximation, depending on properties of the function to be approximated, were given by Dunham JACKSON (1888–1946) in his *Dissertation* [1911]. Such results are now known as *Jackson-type theorems*. The geometric character of the convergence for functions analytic on $]a, b[$ (a necessary and sufficient condition) was proved by BERNSTEIN [1912].

It was proved by PÁL [1914] that every continuous function on $[a, b]$ with $0 < a < b < 1$ can be uniformly approximated by polynomials with integer coefficients.

Uniform approximation by a general linear family of functions was studied by CHEBYSHEV [1859]. The alternation theorem for an arbitrary linear family satisfying the *Haar condition* is due to John Wesley YOUNG [1907] (1879–1932) (a result often incorrectly attributed to BERNSTEIN [1926]). General results on systems of functions satisfying the Haar condition were given by BERNSTEIN [1926], LAASONEN [1949], Mark Grigorievich KREIN [1951] (1907–1989) and REMES [1957]. Haar's theorem is due to Alfred HAAR [1918] (1885–1933) but it was used before by DE LA VALLÉE POUSSIN [1911a]. The complex case was treated by Andrei Nikolaevich KOLMOGOROV [1948] (1903–1987). The necessary and sufficient condition that the set of best approximations has dimension less than or equal to n was given by RUBINSTEIN [1955].

Exchange algorithms for constructing the best uniform approximation by a linear family were obtained by REMES [1935]. What is now known as Remes' second algorithm was in fact given in REMES [1934]. This algorithm converges quadratically under certain conditions as proved by VEIDINGER [1960]. The convergence of Remes' algorithm without the Haar condition was studied by CARASSO [1972].

Approximation by polynomials in the complex domain is quite different from the real case. Uniqueness in the complex case was studied by Leonida TONELLI [1908] (1885–1946) who also treated the case of several variables. Weierstrass' theorem was extended by Joseph Leonard WALSH [1926] (1895–1973) who devoted a monograph to this problem (see WALSH [1935a]). The main questions treated in this monograph are the relations between the geometric degree of the convergence and the regions of analyticity of the function to be approximated and the regions of uniform convergence. The question of the relations of the behavior of the function on the boundary of the region of convergence and the degree of convergence on a given set was treated by SEWELL [1942]. For a review on the asymptotic behavior of best approximations to analytic functions on the unit disk, see HENRICI [1983] (1923–1987).

Since the best approximation polynomial in the Chebyshev sense can be difficult to obtain in practice, HORNECKER [1958] studied how to obtain *near-best approximants*. His method can be extended to the rational case; see HORNECKER [1959].

Convergence in the mean with the weight function Ω, that is for the norm

$$\|f\| = \left(\int_a^b f^2(x) \Omega(x) \, \mathrm{d}x \right)^{1/2},$$

leads to orthogonal systems of functions ω_k (a particular case being orthogonal polynomials) and to Fourier's expansion with respect to the ω_k. The minimum property of Fourier expansions was given by TOEPLER [1876]. The linear independence of a system of functions was studied by Jorgen Pedersen GRAM [1883] (1850–1916) and the orthogonalization with respect to Ω of such a family by Erhard SCHMIDT [1907] (1876–1959). Orthogonalization of the family $\omega_k(x) = x^k$ by the *Gram–Schmidt process* leads to families of orthogonal polynomials. As explained in BREZINSKI [1991], these polynomials were in fact introduced via the theory of continued fractions. It is not our purpose here to study their history but let us give a few facts about them. The *Christoffel–Darboux formula* was first proved by Elwin Bruno CHRISTOFFEL [1858] (1829–1900) for the case of Legendre polynomials and then generalized to arbitrary weight functions by Gaston DARBOUX [1878] (1842–1917). Legendre polynomials were introduced by LEGENDRE [1785] and Olinde RODRIGUES [1816] (1794–1851) expressed them as the nth derivatives of $(x^2 - 1)^n$. In fact, Legendre polynomials are the denominators of the successive convergents of the continued fraction for

$$\ln \frac{x+1}{x-1}$$

and, thus, they satisfy a three-term recurrence relationship. The property of their zeros to be real, distinct and in $[-1,+1]$ can be directly derived from the Rodrigues formula. It was proved by FAVARD [1935] that every family of polynomials satisfying a three-term recurrence relation is, under a mild condition, a family of orthogonal polynomials. Orthogonal polynomials of a discrete variable are useful in approximation problems where the function is only known at some points as described by NIKIFOROV, SUSLOV and UVAROV [1991].

Given a sequence (c_n) of numbers, the *problem of moments* consists of finding Ω such that

$$c_n = \int_a^b x^n \Omega(x) \, dx \quad \text{for } n = 0, 1, \ldots .$$

This is an important problem, studied by many mathematicians around 1920–1922 (see BREZINSKI [1991], p. 288), and it gave rise to the spectral theory of operators and to Riesz theorem about the representation of linear functionals.

Orthogonal polynomials with respect to a general linear functional, no longer necessarily represented as a definite integral with respect to a weight function, is nowadays very much in favor; see BREZINSKI [1980] and MARONI [1991]. They have applications in Padé approximation and in recursive algorithms (such as the biconjugate gradient method) for implementing Lánczos method for solving systems of linear equations and its extensions to nonlinear systems; see BREZINSKI and SADOK [1993].

Extensive tabulations of best approximations to elementary functions can be found in HASTINGS [1955], ABRAMOWITZ and STEGUN [1964], HART, CHENEY, LAWSON, MAEHLY, MESZTENYI, RICE, THACHER JR. and WITZGALL [1965], and SPANIER and OLDHAM [1987].

More results and historical references are given in NATANSON [1964] and CHENEY [1966].

8. Nonlinear approximation

The simplest case of approximation by a nonlinear family is approximation by rational functions. The subject was first discussed by CHEBYSHEV [1859] who proved that the error of best approximation must reach its maximum value in at least n points but he did not prove the alternation in the signs. Egor Ivanovich ZOLOTAREFF [1878] (1847–1878) gave formulae for the best rational approximations to $x^{1/2}$ on a positive interval. The existence of best rational approximation was studied by WALSH [1931]. A characterization theorem was obtained by Naoum Ilich ACHIESER [1930] (1901–1980) together with the alternation theorem. Then, he proved the uniqueness in ACHIESER [1947]. A complete exposition of the theory can be found in WALSH [1935b]. It is based on Montel's theory of normal families and on Carathéodory's theory of conformal mapping of variable regions and it discusses the possibility of approximation by polynomials and rational functions, the degree of convergence and overconvergence (a concept that cannot be explained here), best rational approximation with pre-assigned nodes and extremal problems for analytic functions. Several other topics on polynomial approximation are also included. Almost 30 years later, WALSH [1964] proved that the best uniform rational approximant on a disk of radius ε tends to the Padé approximant when ε tends to zero.

The first result on the continuity for ordinary rational approximation appears in MAEHLY and WITZGALL [1960] and it was completed by CHENEY and LOEB [1964]. Stability and existence was treated by GOLDSTEIN [1963]. For a review on the characterization of best or local best complex rational approximations, consult GUTKNECHT [1983a].

The difficulties encountered in the construction of best uniform rational approximations come from their nonlinearity, their possible nonexistence and the degeneracy problem. However two algorithms have interesting properties: Remes algorithm and the differential correction algorithm. There exist several extensions of Remes algorithm to the case of rational functions but the algorithm obtained by WERNER [1962] works in most situations and it has a quadratic convergence as in the polynomial case. The *differential correction algorithm* was proposed by CHENEY and LOEB [1961] and modified in CHENEY and LOEB [1962]. It has global convergence properties and is more robust than the Remes algorithm although its convergence is slower.

Three algorithms for adjusting the coefficients of a continued fraction and thus, for obtaining convergents which are *nearly best uniform rational approximations* were given by MAEHLY [1960]. They all have the same advantages but also the same drawbacks, namely that the computations of the corrections for the coefficients are quite simple and stable but a *true* Chebyshev approximation is obtained only if the interval of approximation is very small. As already mentioned, some other procedures for constructing nearly best uniform rational approximations are due to HORNECKER [1959, 1961]. The *Carathéodory–Fejér* method allows the construction of near-best Chebyshev approximations of rational functions analytic on a disk by functions of the same type but with a lower order (see GUTKNECHT [1983b]). For this type of approximation, the error curves are nearly circular (see TREFETHEN [1983]).

An important result was obtained by NEWMAN [1964] who showed that $|x|$ is much better approximated uniformly on $[-1, +1]$ by rational functions than by polynomials. This result stimulated many research on best rational approximation. In particular, an interesting and important problem is the approximation of the exponential function. The asymptotic behavior of the error of the best uniform rational approximation of e^x on $[-1, +1]$ was conjectured by MEINARDUS [1967] and the proof was given by BRAESS [1984]. The uniform approximation of e^{-x} on $[0, \infty)$ is connected with *A-stable methods* for integrating *stiff* differential equations. Many papers have appeared on this question. They are reviewed in

PETRUSHEV and POPOV [1987].

Rational approximation is subject to interesting phenomena described by VARGA [1982]: there exist real continuous functions f on $[-1, +1]$ for which (i) complex best uniform rational approximation to f is better than real best uniform rational approximation of the same degree, and (ii) complex best uniform rational approximation is not unique.

Recently there has been a renewal of interest in various conjectures concerning some approximation problems. They lead to intensive computations that are reported in VARGA [1990].

Approximation by general rational functions of the form

$$F(x) = \frac{\sum_{i=0}^{n} a_i f_i(x)}{\sum_{i=0}^{m} b_i g_i(x)}$$

is a much more difficult problem. The question of existence was treated by Lothar COLLATZ [1960] (1910–1990), by BOEHM [1964] in his thesis and by others. The characterization and uniqueness were studied by RICE [1961].

The first results on Chebyshev approximation by

$$F(x) = \sum_{i=0}^{n} a_i e^{t_i x},$$

where the a_i and the t_i have to be determined, were obtained by RICE [1960] for $n = 1$ and two years later for the general case by RICE [1962] again. The fundamental concept in the theory is that of *varisolvence* introduced by RICE [1960] but, as showed by BRAESS [1967], a best approximation is not always unique and varisolvence does not provide a complete theory.

The case of approximation by a γ-polynomial of the form

$$F(x) = \sum_{i=0}^{n} a_i \gamma(t_i, x)$$

was treated by HOBBY and RICE [1967]. Approximation by spline functions with free nodes is quite similar to approximation by γ-polynomials. The case of nodes with prescribed multiplicities and the L_p-case have also been studied; see BRAESS [1986] for a review.

For a modern exposition of nonlinear approximation, consult RICE [1969], BRAESS [1986] and PETRUSHEV and POPOV [1987].

9. Multivariate approximation

Let us begin by saying that the theorem of WEIERSTRASS [1885] was extended to several variables by PICARD [1891] and that the uniqueness for linear functions of two variables is due to COLLATZ [1956].

There are many differences between univariate and multivariate approximation. An important result of MAIRHUBER [1956] states that the space of continuous real-valued functions on a compact Hausdorff space S contains a Haar subspace of dimension equal to or greater than 2 if S is homeomorphic to a subset of the circumference of a circle.

Another difference is the occurrence of infinite-dimensional subspaces for the approximants and unusual Banach spaces and norms. Moreover, the geometry of the domain of approximation plays a crucial rôle.

Linear projection operators are very useful since they allow multivariate approximants to be built from univariate functions by means of tensor products as described by LIGHT and CHENEY [1985].

Finally, the question of the existence of best approximations, called *proximinality*, becomes a difficult question in multivariate approximation.

All these questions are reviewed in detail by CHENEY [1986].

Since there are no Chebyshev sets of functions of several variables, there is no way of extending the L_∞-theory while there is no difficulty in extending the L_2-theory. In particular, since the best Chebyshev approximation is not always unique, one has to select the best approximant among the best ones which led RICE [1963] to the definition of *strict* approximation of functions defined on a finite set. As proved by DESCLOUX [1963] this strict approximation is the limit when p tends to infinity of the best approximation in L_p.

An algorithm for the computation of the best Chebyshev approximation is due to DESCLOUX [1961] and one for the strict approximation was given by RICE [1963]. Remes' algorithm was extended to the multivariate case by STIEFEL [1959] and to an arbitrary vector space by LAURENT [1967a] who proved its convergence. Characterization theorems were also given by LAURENT [1967b]. A complete theory of approximation in a Hilbert space can be found in the book by LAURENT [1972].

Bernstein-type polynomial operators for integrable functions on a simplex were introduced by DERRIENNIC [1985]. They are an extension of those of DURRMEYER [1978] for the one-dimensional case.

A more recent approach to the problem of multivariate approximation consists of using wavelets. Wavelets, which mimic an orthonormal basis for $L^2(\mathbb{R}^n)$, combine the advantages of trigonometric families (which are well localized in frequency but not in space) and of Haar's families (which are exactly the contrary). It is a subject currently in full expansion (see MEYER [1990] and DAUBECHIES [1992]).

Obviously, due to the enormous literature on approximation theory, many topics are missing in this section. For a broad survey about approximation theory and for the more recent notions of widths, ε-entropy and optimal recovery, see TIKHOMIROV [1990].

CHAPTER III

Numerical Quadrature

A *numerical quadrature formula* is a formula for obtaining an approximate numerical value of a definite integral

$$I(f) = \int_a^b f(x)\,dx.$$

For reasons that will appear later, one can also try to compute an integral of the form

$$I(f) = \int_a^b f(x)\Omega(x)\,dx,$$

where the weight function Ω does not vanish in the open interval $]a,b[$ and is integrable in $[a,b]$.

Quadrature methods are very old and they appear in the records of many ancient civilizations since they are in fact related to the geometrical problem of the determination of areas. In particular, the work of Archimedes (287–212 B.C.) on the computation of the area of a circle and the determination of the value of π is well known. We shall not develop these questions here.

The basic idea of quadrature methods is to replace the function f by an interpolation polynomial P_{n-1} of degree $n-1$ and to integrate it. Doing so, we obtain an approximate value $I_n(f)$ of $I(f)$ under the form

$$I_n(f) = \sum_{i=1}^n A_i^{(n)} f(x_i),$$

where the x_i are the interpolation points. They are called the *nodes* of the quadrature formula and they can depend on n. The numbers $A_i^{(n)}$ are called the *weights* of the formula. For obvious reasons, such a quadrature formula is called *interpolatory* and it is exact on $\mathbb{P}_{n-1}$, the vector space of polynomials of degree at most $n-1$. According to a terminology due to Rodolphe RADAU [1880] (1835–1911), the formula is said to have a *degree of exactness* equal to $n-1$.

The nodes x_i can be chosen arbitrarily. If, for simplicity, they are taken equidistant in $[a,b]$, the corresponding quadrature formula is named after Newton and Cotes. If they are taken in an *optimal* way (that is to achieve the highest possible degree of exactness), the quadrature formula is named after Gauss.

10. Newton–Cotes formulae

It seems that Bonaventura CAVALIERI [1639] (1598–1647) was the first to propose a formula for numerical integration. Using a geometrical approach based on his *method of indivisibles*, he found what is now called *Simpson's formula*. In fact, this rule was given by James GREGORY in his *Exercitationes Geometricae* [1668]. Moreover, in a letter to Collins dated November 23, 1670, he proposed the *Gregory quadrature formula*.

In his book *Arithmetica Infinitorum* [1656], John WALLIS (1616–1703) was interested in the computation of

$$\pi/4 = \int_0^1 (1-x^2)^{1/2} \, dx.$$

Starting from the values of

$$\int_0^1 (1-x^p)^q$$

for some p and q and using what he called *continuity principles*, which are in fact equivalent to an interpolation process, he proved that (using his notations)

$$\Box = 4/\pi = \frac{3 \cdot 3 \cdot 5 \cdot 5 \cdot 7 \cdot 7 \cdots}{2 \cdot 4 \cdot 4 \cdot 6 \cdot 6 \cdot 8 \cdots}.$$

This infinite product for $\Box = 4/\pi$ has a great historical importance since Wallis asked Lord William BROUNCKER (1620–1684), the founder and first President of the Royal Society, "to show in what form that quantity $\Box$ could be most conveniently designated". Brouncker came up with his celebrated continued fraction

$$\Box = 4/\pi = 1 + \frac{1}{\lvert 2} + \frac{9}{\lvert 2} + \frac{25}{\lvert 2} + \frac{49}{\lvert 2} + \cdots.$$

Let us recall that WALLIS [1656] was the first (at least in Europe) to prove the three-term recurrence relation for the numerators and denominators of the convergents of a continued fraction (BREZINSKI [1991]) and he also introduced the symbol ∞ for *infinity* (see SCOTT [1981]).

Simpson's formula also appeared in NEWTON's book, *Principia Mathematica* [1687]. He wrote "... the area under the curve can be found, since the quadrature of a parabolic curve can be effected". As an example he gave, without proof, the area under a polynomial of degree 3 passing through four equidistant points as

$$\frac{A+3B}{8}R,$$

where A is the sum of the first and last ordinates, B the sum of the second and penultimate ones and R the step-size.

In the *Opusculae* published with his *Harmonia Mensurarum* [1722], COTES took up Newton's work and gave the quadrature formulae up to 11 points of interpolation. He said that he already gave them in his lessons in 1709, not being aware of Newton's results which only came to his knowledge in 1711 in a letter from the editor William JONES (1675–1749). Cotes gave no hint of his procedure for obtaining his formulae but it is obvious that he obtained them by integrating Newton's interpolation polynomial. These formulae are now called *Newton–Cotes quadrature formulae* and the weights are called the *Cotes numbers*. The case $n = 1$ is the *trapezoidal rule* and the case $n = 2$ is usually called *Simpson's rule* because George ATWOOD [1798] (1745–1807) said that it was obtained by Thomas SIMPSON (1710–1761) "from the properties of the conic parabola".

Cotes work was published in 1722, 6 years after his death. In the meantime, James STIRLING [1718] (1692–1770) presented a paper to the Royal Society, where he obtained the same formulae but only for even values of n up to 10. As an example, he integrated $(1 + x^2)^{-1}$ between 0 and 1 using the 9-point formula and he found 0.785398187 instead of $\pi/4 = 0.78539816\ldots$. He says:

> "I had computed these tables further, but the expressions for eleven or more ordinates are useless by reason of the immense greatness of the numeral coefficients; but if nine ordinates do not give the area sufficiently accurate, divide the base into two or more parts, and by this the area is divided into as many parts; then if you seek each of them separately by nine ordinates, you will have the whole area as accurate as you will."

This is exactly the definition of a *composite quadrature rule*.

SIMPSON [1743] gave the rules up to $n = 6$. He seems to have been the first to suggest a repeated application of the rule for $n = 2$ in the case of an arbitrary number of subintervals. This method is now known as *Simpson's rule*.

The usual procedure for computing Cotes numbers (which can be made independent of the step-size and the origin) is to write down the interpolation polynomial in terms of the powers of the forward difference operator Δ. This was the method followed by George BOOLE [1860] (1815–1864) up to the degree 6 and by WEDDLE [1854] up to 8. However, the general expression of the weights as integrals of the Lagrange's basis was only given by Joseph BERTRAND [1870] (1822–1900) in his book.

Let us now come to the *Euler–Maclaurin formula*, given by Colin MACLAURIN [1742] (1698–1746) in his book *A Treatise of Fluxions*. It can be found in Chapter X of Book I, pp. 293ff, but the proof and many examples are given in Chapter V of Book II, pp. 672ff. He said that "this method was given by Dr. Taylor, method. increm.". However, his name remained attached to the result because it was a fundamental tool for him and not just a simple corollary of Taylor's result. In a footnote (Book II, p. 651), Maclaurin remarks:

> "I take this opportunity to mention, that having occasionally shown in 1737, the 292, 293 pages of this treatise (after they were printed) to Mr. Stirling, he took notice that a theorem similar to the first of these described in art. 352 had been communicated to him by Mr. Euler."

The formula was thus discovered independently by EULER [1738]. The formulae of Gregory and Euler–Maclaurin can be obtained one from each other by replacing the differences by the derivatives.

For a detailed history of these questions, see JOHNSON [1915], GOLDSTINE [1977], and GOWING [1983].

The general convergence theorem states that a necessary and sufficient condition for a quadrature formula to be convergent for every continuous function in $[a, b]$ is that it converges for polynomials and that it exists M such that for all n, $\sum_{i=1}^{n} |A_i^{(n)}| \leqslant M$. The sufficiency was proved by Vladimir Andreevich STEKLOV [1916] (1864–1926) while the necessity is due to Georg PÓLYA [1933] (1887–1985). Thus interpolatory quadratures with positive weights are convergent since they integrate exactly polynomials of degree zero at least. Lipót FEJÉR [1933] (1880–1959) proved that this is the case when the nodes are the zeros of the Chebyshev polynomials of the first or second kind. R.O. KUZMIN [1931] (1891–1949) showed that, for equidistant nodes, the condition is not satisfied for a function continuous or even analytical in $]0, 1[$. He gave asymptotic formulae for the $A_i^{(n)}$'s and proved that $|A_i^{(n)}|$ becomes arbitrarily large when n tends to infinity.

CHEBYSHEV [1874] became interested in finding A and the x_i such that the quadrature formula

$$\int_{-1}^{1} f(x) \, dx \simeq A \sum_{i=1}^{n} f(x_i)$$

is exact on $\mathbb{P}_n$, the vector space of polynomials of degree at most n. He gave the solution for $n \leqslant 7$ but, for $n = 8$, imaginary values are obtained for the nodes. BERNSTEIN [1937, 1938] proved that the problem is not solvable, because of complex nodes, for $n \geqslant 9$.

The trapezoidal rule is convergent for every continuous function f in $[a, b]$. However its convergence can be quite slow and the idea came to accelerate it. The error of the trapezoidal rule is given, for a sufficiently differentiable function, by the Euler–Maclaurin expansion. William Fleetwood SHEPPARD [1900] (1863–1936) used the trapezoidal rule with the step-sizes $h_n = r_n h, 1 = r_0 < r_1 < r_2 < \cdots$, in order to eliminate the successive terms in this expansion. Lewis Fry RICHARDSON [1910] (1881–1953) used a linear combination of the results obtained with h and $2h$ for eliminating the first term of the error. He called this procedure the *deferred approach to the limit* or h^2-*extrapolation*. ROMBERG [1955] was the first to use an iterative scheme for eliminating the successive terms in the Euler–Maclaurin expansion for the error of the trapezoidal rule. His method became widely known when BAUER [1961] gave a rigorous error analysis of the process. The convergence of the *Richardson extrapolation method* was studied by LAURENT [1963] who proved that the sequence of step-sizes must satisfy the α-condition, namely that it exists α such that for all n

$$h_n/h_{n+1} \geqslant \alpha > 1.$$

Later, *Romberg's method* was extended to several cases where the function f or its derivatives present some discontinuities in the interval of integration and, thus, the Euler–Maclaurin expansion no longer holds; see HÅVIE [1979] for a synthesis.

11. Gaussian quadratures

An important question is the following: if we let the nodes vary freely and then compute the weights, what is the maximum degree of exactness that can be achieved and how can these optimal nodes be obtained? On September 16, 1814, Carl Friedrich GAUSS [1814] (1777–1855) presented a paper to the Göttingen Society where he raised this question and solved it by means of the continued fraction for the hypergeometric series he obtained in GAUSS [1812]. A particular case of Gauss' continued fraction for the ratio of two hypergeometric series gives

$$\ln \frac{z+1}{z-1} = \int_{-1}^{1} \frac{dx}{z-x} = \frac{2 \rfloor}{z} - \frac{1/3 \rfloor}{z} - \cdots = 2 \left[\frac{1}{z} + \frac{1}{3z^3} + \cdots \right].$$

The nth convergent of this continued fraction, which is a rational fraction with a numerator of degree $n-1$ in z and a denominator of degree n, has a power series expansion in $1/z$ which agrees with that of the function up to the term of degree $2n$ inclusively and, thus, it is the $[n - 1/n]$ Padé approximant of the function. Then Gauss decomposed this Padé approximant in partial fractions and took the residues and the poles as the weights and the nodes of his quadrature formula (since the denominators are the Legendre polynomials, the nodes are their zeros). Because of the *accuracy-through-order* property of Padé approximants, this quadrature formula has a degree of exactness equal to $2n - 1$. Gauss also gave an integral formula for the weights.

Carl Gustav Jacob JACOBI [1826] (1804–1851) took up the work of Gauss and the central concept of orthogonality emerged. He proved that, for any k, the quadrature has degree of exactness $n + k - 1$ if and only if it is an interpolatory quadrature formula and

$$\int_a^b v_n(x) p(x) \, dx = 0, \quad \forall p \in \mathbb{P}_{k-1},$$

where $v_n(x) = (x - x_1) \cdots (x - x_n), x_1, \ldots, x_n$ being the nodes of the formula. Thus, each additional degree of exactness requires the orthogonality of v_n to one additional power of x. Since v_n cannot be orthogonal to itself, then k could be at most equal to n and it follows that the maximum degree of exactness that can be achieved is $2n - 1$. In that case, v_n is the Legendre polynomial of degree n if $[a, b]$ is $[-1, +1]$. Then Jacobi obtained the *Rodrigues formula* and concluded that the nodes are real, simple and in $[-1, +1]$.

CHRISTOFFEL [1858] considered the same problem again although his work extends easily to an arbitrary weight function Ω. He fixed some of the nodes of the quadrature formula outside the open interval of integration and determined the remaining nodes in order to attain the maximal degree of exactness. This corresponds to orthogonality with respect to a polynomial weight function with a constant sign in the interval. He gave a formula for the weights in the Legendre case. The case where only two nodes are fixed at a and b, was already treated by Rehuel LOBATTO [1852] (1797–1866). It leads to the *Gauss–Lobatto formulae*. The formulae with only one fixed node, a or b, were then discussed by RADAU [1880] and are called *Gauss–Radau formulae*.

Various weight functions began to be studied around 1864 by different mathematicians and, among them, Gustav MEHLER [1864] (1835–1895). In particular, he studied the weight function $(1-x)^\alpha(1+x)^\beta$. This is the *Gauss–Jacobi quadrature formula* since the corresponding orthogonal polynomials are those studied by JACOBI [1859].

Constantin POSSÉ [1875] (1847–1928) proved that the only formula whose weights are all equal is that corresponding to the weight $(1 - x^2)^{1/2}$ which leads to Chebyshev polynomials. In that case, the weights and nodes can be explicitly obtained in terms of trigonometrical functions as proved by Possé in the same paper and independently by STIELTJES [1884]. The reciprocal of Possé's result was proved by GERONIMUS [1944].

The case of infinite intervals was first considered by RADAU [1883] for the weight e^{-x} on $[0, \infty)$ and by GOURIER [1883] for $e^{-x^2/2}$ on $(-\infty, \infty)$. The former case leads to the polynomials named after Edmond LAGUERRE [1879] (1834–1886) and the later to those of HERMITE [1864]. As pointed out by GAUTSCHI [1981], these names are not fully justified historically.

The case of an arbitrary weight function was first studied in its full generality by POSSÉ [1875] and CHRISTOFFEL [1877]. In particular, Christoffel treated the case of an arbitrary weight function and proved the Christoffel–Darboux formula.

Another approach to Gauss formula is due to MARKOV [1885] via Hermite interpolation. It has the advantage of giving an explicit expression for the error of the quadrature formula. A representation of the error as a Peano kernel can also be given. The error can be expanded as a Euler–Maclaurin type formula as done by BILHARZ [1951] for the Gauss–Legendre formula and KRYLOV ([1959], Chapter 11, Section 3) for an arbitrary weight. If the function to be integrated is holomorphic, a representation of the error as a contour integral was given by DARBOUX [1878] and by Heinrich Eduard HEINE [1881] (1821–1881). Strict error bounds can then be obtained. Let us mention that bounds for the error can also be obtained by using Hilbert space methods, an idea introduced by DAVIS [1953], or by using best uniform polynomial approximation as done by BERNSTEIN [1918].

The convergence of Gaussian quadrature methods was first studied by STIELTJES [1884] who proved the convergence for every function integrable in the Riemann–Stieltjes sense. When the interval of integration is finite, it follows, from the general result of Steklov and Pólya on interpolatory quadratures, that Gaussian rules are convergent for every continuous function. The case of an infinite interval of integration is more difficult since it is related to the determinacy of the moment problem. In particular, this determinacy implies the convergence for the function $f(x) = (z-x)^{-1}$ with $z \notin [0, \infty)$. Other functions were treated by James Victor USPENSKY [1916, 1928] (1883–1947), James SHOHAT [1927] (1886–1944), JOURAVSKY [1928] and by SHOHAT and TAMARKIN [1943] in their book. See FELDHEIM [1939] for a review.

Gaussian quadrature rules with multiple nodes having the same multiplicity r were first considered by TURÁN [1950] (1910–1976). They correspond to Hermite interpolation instead of Lagrange's. They lead to a new type of orthogonality, called r-orthogonality, where it is the rth power of v_n which must be orthogonal to all polynomials of degree at most $n-1$. Such an orthogonality can only hold if r is odd, that is $r = 2s+1, s \geqslant 0$. The degree of exactness becomes $rn+n-1$. Most of the properties of Gaussian quadratures are still valid but not the positivity of the weights. In the case of the Chebyshev weight function, it was proved by BERNSTEIN [1930] that the zeros of the Chebyshev polynomials are the optimal nodes for Turán rules. The remaining term was studied by IONESCU [1967] and OSSICINI [1968].

For a detailed history, see RUNGE and WILLERS [1915] and GAUTSCHI [1981].

It is possible to estimate the error for an n-point quadrature method by comparison with a more precise one. The difference between both results usually provides a good estimation for the error on the less precise method. KRONROD [1964, 1965] used this idea for estimating the error for an n-point Gaussian quadrature method. For that purpose, he wanted to use a $(2n+1)$-point formula of higher degree of exactness. Obviously it is possible to choose it as a Gaussian quadrature formula. However, the drawback is that the values of the function to be integrated have to be computed at $2n+1$ new points. Thus Kronrod had the idea of taking the n points of the Gaussian formula already used, and to add $n+1$ new points. In order to achieve the best possible result, these $n+1$ points have to be chosen in an optimal way. Doing so, he obtained a formula with a degree of exactness $3n+1$. These new nodes are the zeros of the *Stieltjes polynomials* since they were introduced by Stieltjes in his very last letter to Hermite dated November 8, 1894, less than 2 months before his death (see BAILLAUD and BOURGET [1905]). Of course, these new nodes can only be used if they are real, distinct, in the interval of integration and distinct from the n nodes of the Gaussian quadrature formula. This question has been the subject of an extensive literature, that has been reviewed in GAUTSCHI [1988]. The same idea has been used for estimating the error in Padé approximation, which can be viewed as a formal Gaussian quadrature process (see BREZINSKI [1988]).

12. Cubatures

Numerical procedures for approximating multiple integrals are called *cubatures*. The difficulties of evaluating multiple integrals come from the infinite number of different types of regions and the behavior of functions of several variables, which can be much more complicated than that of functions of a single variable.

As mentioned by COOLS [1992], the first cubature formulae were proposed by James Clerk MAXWELL [1877] (1831–1879). He constructed a formula of degree 7 (that is exact for polynomials of degree at most 7 in the variables) with 13 nodes for the square $[-1, +1]^2$ and another one of degree 7 with 27 nodes for the cube $[-1, +1]^3$. He obtained the nodes and the weights by solving the corresponding system of nonlinear equations. However, for the first formula, he found one negative weight and the formula for the cube contained several nodes outside the domain.

The first mathematician to investigate the connection between orthogonal polynomials in two variables and cubatures was Paul APPELL [1890] (1855–1930). Other results are due to Johann RADON [1948] (1887–1956) who constructed formulae for the square, the circle and the triangle using orthogonal polynomials. Cubature formulae on the sphere were studied by S.L. SOBOLEV [1962a–c] (1909–1989).

The difficulties encountered with nonstandard types of regions and the necessity of economizing the number of function evaluations led to the introduction of *Monte Carlo methods* whose idea is due to Stanislaw ULAM (1909–1984), Nick METROPOLIS and John VON NEUMANN (1903–1957) in 1945. It is an acceptance-rejection process based on pseudo-random numbers (see METROPOLIS and ULAM [1949]). In 1944/45, physicists were involved in the *Manhattan Project* and they had no time to spend on theoretical work. Thus, the idea was to perform an enormous number of simulations on the computer for obtaining an approximate value of the exact result. The history of Monte-Carlo methods is given by METROPOLIS [1989] and ECKHARDT [1989].

For some sets of points, an extension of the Euler–Maclaurin formula and extensions of Romberg's extrapolation method have been obtained (see LYNESS [1986] for a review).

An overview of the results on cubature formulae is given by STROUD [1971] and in DAVIS and RABINOWITZ [1984]. Recent developments on the subject can be found in KEAST and FAIRWEATHER [1987] and ESPELID and GENZ [1992].

Most of the mathematical questions about interpolation, approximation and numerical quadrature are extensively developed in the article by SENDOV and ANDREEV [1994] in this volume.

References

ABRAMOWITZ, M. and I.A. STEGUN, eds. (1964), *Handbook of Mathematical Functions with Formulas, Graphs, and Mathematical Tables*, N.B.S. Applied Math. Series **55** (Natl. Bur. of Standards).
ACHIESER, N.I. (1930), On extremal properties of certain rational functions, *Dokl. Akad. Nauk SSSR* **18**, 495–499 (in Russian).
ACHIESER, N.I. (1947), *Lectures on the Theory of Approximation*, (Gostekhizdat, Moscow) (in Russian).
AITKEN, A.C. (1932), On interpolation by proportional parts, without use of differences, *Proc. Edinburgh Math. Soc.* **3**, 56–76.
AMPÈRE, A.M. (1825–1826), Essai sur un nouveau mode d'exposition des principes du calcul différentiel, du calcul aux différences, et de l'interpolation des suites considérées comme dérivant d'une source commune, *Ann. Math. Pures Appl.* **16**, 329–349.
APPELL, P. (1890), Sur une classe de polynômes à deux variables et le calcul approché des intégrales doubles, *Ann. Fac. Sci. Toulouse* **4**, H1–H20.
ARIOKA, S. (1987), Padé-type approximants in multivariables, *Appl. Numer. Math.* **3**, 497–511.
ATWOOD, G. (1798), Disquisition on the stability of ships, *Philos. Trans.* **88**, 260.
BAILLAUD, B. and H. BOURGET (1905), *Correspondance d'Hermite et de Stieltjes* (Gauthier-Villars, Paris).
BAUER, F.L. (1961), La méthode d'intégration numérique de Romberg, in: *Colloque sur l'Analyse Numérique*, (Librairie Universitaire, Louvain), 119–129.
BENOUAHMANE, B. (1991), Approximants de Padé "homogènes" et polynômes orthogonaux à deux variables, *Rend. Mat. (7)* **11**, 673–689.
BERNSTEIN, S.N. (1912), Sur la valeur asymptotique de la meilleure approximation des fonctions analytiques, *C. R. Acad. Sci. Paris* **155**, 1062–1065.
BERNSTEIN, S.N. (1914), Quelques remarques sur l'interpolation, *Comm. Soc. Math. Kharkoff (2)* **14**.
BERNSTEIN, S.N. (1918), Quelques remarques sur l'interpolation, *Math. Ann.* **79**, 1–12.
BERNSTEIN, S.N. (1926), *Leçons sur les Propriétés Extrémales et la Meilleure Approximation des Fonctions Analytiques d'une Variable Réelle* (Gauthier-Villars, Paris).
BERNSTEIN, S.N. (1930), Sur les polynômes orthogonaux relatifs à un segment fini, *J. Math. Pures Appl. (9)* **9**, 127–177.
BERNSTEIN, S.N. (1937), On the quadrature formulas of Cotes and Chebyshev, *Dokl. Akad. Nauk SSSR* (in Russian).
BERNSTEIN, S.N. (1938), Sur un système d'équations indéterminées, *J. Math. Pures Appl. (9)* **17**, 179–186.
BERTRAND, J. (1870), *Traité de Calcul Différentiel et de Calcul Intégral* (Gauthiers-Villars, Paris).
BÉZIER, P. (1972), *Numerical Control: Mathematics and Applications* (Wiley, New York).
BILHARZ, H. (1951), Über die Gaußsche Methode zur angenäherten Berechnung bestimmter Integrale, *Math. Nachr.* **6**, 171–192.
BIRKHOFF, G.D. (1906), General mean value and remainder theorems with applications to mechanical differentiation and quadrature, *Trans. Amer. Math. Soc.* **7**, 107–136.

BOEHM, B.W. (1964), Existence, Characterization, and Convergence of Best Rational Tchebycheff Approximations, Ph.D. Thesis, University of California, Los Angeles.
BOOLE, G. (1860), *A Treatise on the Calculus of Finite Differences* (Cambridge).
BOREL, E. (1897), Sur l'interpolation, *C. R. Acad. Sci. Paris* **104**, 673–676.
BOREL, E. (1905), *Leçons sur les Fonctions de Variables réelles* (Gauthier-Villars, Paris).
BRAESS, D. (1967), Approximation mit Exponentialsummen, *Computing* **2**, 309–321.
BRAESS, D. (1984), On the conjecture of Meinardus on rational approximation of e^x, II, *J. Approx. Theory* **40**, 375–379.
BRAESS, D. (1986), *Nonlinear Approximation Theory* (Springer, Berlin).
BREZINSKI, C. (1978), Padé-type approximants for double power series, *J. Indian Math. Soc.* **42**, 267–282.
BREZINSKI, C. (1980), *Padé-type Approximation and General Orthogonal Polynomials*, ISNM, Vol. 50 (Birkhäuser, Basel).
BREZINSKI, C. (1985), The birth and early developments of Padé approximants, in: G.M. RASSIAS and T.M. RASSIAS, eds., *Differential Geometry, Calculus of Variations, and their Applications* (Marcel Dekker, New York) 105–121.
BREZINSKI, C. (1988), Error estimate in Padé approximation, in: M. ALFARO, J.S. DEHESA, F.J. MARCELLAN, J.L. RUBIO DE FRANCIA and J. VINUESA, eds., *Orthogonal Polynomials and their Applications*, Lecture Notes in Mathematics **1329** (Springer, Berlin) 1–19.
BREZINSKI, C. (1991), *History of Continued Fractions and Padé Approximants* (Springer-Verlag, Berlin).
BREZINSKI, C. (1992), *Biorthogonality and its Applications to Numerical Analysis* (Marcel Dekker, New York).
BREZINSKI, C. and M. REDIVO ZAGLIA (1991), *Extrapolation Methods. Theory and Practice* (North-Holland, Amsterdam).
BREZINSKI, C. and H. SADOK (1993), Lanczos type algorithms for solving systems of linear equations, *Appl. Numer. Math.* **11**, 443–473.
BREZINSKI, C. and J. VAN ISEGHEM (1994), Padé approximations, in: P.G. CIARLET and J.L. LIONS, eds., *Handbook of Numerical Analysis*, Vol. III: Techniques of Scientific Computing (Part 1), Solutions of Equations in $\mathbb{R}^n$ (Part 2), Numerical Methods for Solids (Part 1) (North-Holland, Amsterdam).
BRIGGS, H. (1624), *Arithmetica Logarithmica* (London).
BUSCH, J.R. (1985), Osculatory interpolation in $\mathbb{R}^t$, *SIAM J. Numer. Anal.* **22**, 107–113.
CARASSO, C. (1972), Etude de l'algorithme de Rémès en l'abscence de condition de Haar, *Numer. Math.* **20**, 165–178.
CAUCHY, A.L. (1821), *Cours d'Analyse*, Vol. 1 (L'Imprimerie Royale, Paris).
CAUCHY, A.L. (1840), Sur les fonctions interpolaires, *C. R. Acad. Sci. Paris* **11**, 775–789.
CAVALIERI, B. (1639), *Centuria di varii Problemi per Dimostrare...* (Monti and Zenero, Bologna).
CHAFFY, C. (1984), A homogeneous process for Padé approximants in two variables, *Numer. Math.* **45**, 149–164.
CHEBYSHEV, P.L. (1854), Théorie des mécanismes connus sous le nom de parallélogrammes, *Mém. présentés à l'Acad. Sci. St. Pétersbourg par divers Savants* **7**, 539–568.
CHEBYSHEV, P.L. (1859), Sur les questions de minima qui se rattachent à la représentation approximative des fonctions, *Mém. Acad. Imp. Sci. St. Pétersbourg, sér. 6, Sci. Math. Phys.* **7**, 199–291.
CHEBYSHEV, P.L. (1874), Sur les quadratures, *J. Math. Pures Appl. (2)* **19**, 19–34.
CHENEY, E.W. (1966), *Introduction to Approximation Theory* (McGraw-Hill, New York).
CHENEY, E.W. (1986), *Multivariate Approximation Theory: Selected Topics* (SIAM, Philadelphia).
CHENEY, E.W. and H.L. LOEB (1961), Two new algorithms for rational approximation, *Numer. Math.* **3**, 72–75.
CHENEY, E.W. and H.L. LOEB (1962), On rational Chebyshev approximation, *Numer. Math.* **4**, 124–127.
CHENEY, E.W. and H.L. LOEB (1964), Generalized rational approximations, *SIAM J. Numer. Anal.* **1**, 11–25.

CHISHOLM, J.S.R. (1973), Rational approximants defined from double power series, *Math. Comput.* **27**, 841–848.
CHRISTOFFEL, E.B. (1858), Über die Gauss'sche Quadratur und eine Verallgemeinerung derselben, *J. Reine Angew. Math.* **55**, 61–82.
CHRISTOFFEL, E.B. (1877), Sur une classe particulière de fonctions entières et de fractions continues, *Ann. Mat. Pura Appl. (2)* **8**, 1–10.
CHUNG, K.C. and T.H. YAO (1977), On lattices admitting unique Lagrange interpolation, *SIAM J. Numer. Anal.* **14**, 735–743.
CIARLET, P.G. (1978), *The Finite Element Method for Elliptic Problems* (North-Holland, Amsterdam).
CIARLET, P.G. (1991), Basic error estimates for elliptic problems, in: P.G. CIARLET and J.L. LIONS, eds., *Handbook of Numerical Analysis*, Vol. II: Finite Element Methods (Part 1) (North-Holland, Amsterdam) 17–351.
CIARLET, P.G. and P.A. RAVIART (1972), General Lagrange and Hermite interpolation in $\mathbb{R}^N$ with applications to finite element methods, *Arch. Rat. Mech. Anal.* **46**, 177–199.
CIARLET, P.G. and C. WAGSCHAL (1971), Multipoint Taylor formulas and applications to the finite element method, *Numer. Math.* **17**, 84–100.
COATMÉLEC, C. (1966), Approximation et interpolation des fonctions différentiables de plusieurs variables, *Ann. Scient. École Norm. Sup. (3)* **83**, 271–341.
COLLATZ, L. (1956), Approximation von Funktionen bei einer und bei mehreren unabhängigen Veränderlichen, *Z. Angew. Math. Mech.* **36**, 198–211.
COLLATZ, L. (1960), Tschebyscheffsche Annäherung mit rationalen Funktionen, *Abh. Math. Sem. Hamburg* **24**, 70–78.
COOLS, R. (1992), A survey of methods for constructing cubature formulae, in: T.O. ESPELID and A. GENZ, eds., *Numerical Integration* (Kluwer, Dordrecht) 1–24.
COTES, R. (1708), *De Methodo Differentiali Newtoniana*.
COTES, R. (1722), *Harmonia Mensurarum* (R. Smith, Cambridge).
COX, M.G. (1972), The numerical evaluation of B-splines, *J. Inst. Math. Appl.* **10**, 134–149.
CUYT, A. (1984), *Abstract Padé Approximants for Operators: Theory and Applications*, Lecture Notes in Mathematics **1065** (Springer, Berlin).
CUYT, A. (1992), Rational Hermite interpolation in one and more variables, in: S.P. SINGH, ed., *Approximation Theory, Spline Functions and Applications* (Kluwer, Dordrecht) 69–103.
CUYT, A. and L. WUYTACK (1987), *Nonlinear Methods in Numerical Analysis* (North-Holland, Amsterdam).
DARBOUX, G. (1878), Mémoire sur l'approximation de très grands nombres et sur une classe étendue de développements en série, *J. Math. Pures Appl.* **4**, 5–57.
DAUBECHIES, I. (1992), *Ten Lectures on Wavelets* (SIAM, Philadelphia).
DAVIS, P.J. (1953), Errors of numerical approximation for analytic functions, *J. Rat. Mech. Anal.* **2**, 303–313.
DAVIS, P.J. (1963), *Interpolation and Approximation* (Blaisdell, Waltham).
DAVIS, P.J. and P. RABINOWITZ (1984), *Methods of Numerical Integration* (Academic Press, New York).
DE BOOR, C. (1972), On calculating with B-splines, *J. Approx. Theory* **6**, 50–62.
DE BOOR, C. (1978), *A Practical Guide to Splines* (Springer, New York).
DE LAPLACE, P.S. (1799), *Mécanique Céleste* (Duprat, Paris).
DE LA VALLÉE POUSSIN, C. (1911a), Sur les polynômes d'approximation et la représentation approchée d'un angle, *Bull. Cl. Sci. Acad. R. Belg.* **12**, 808–844.
DE LA VALLÉE POUSSIN, C. (1911b), Sur la méthode de l'approximation minimum, *Ann. Soc. Sci. Brux., Ser. II, Mémoires* **35**, 1–16.
DE MONTESSUS DE BALLORE, R. (1902), Sur les fractions continues algébriques, *Bull. Soc. Math. France* **30**, 28–36.
DE MORGAN, A. (1842), *The Differential and Integral Calculus* (London).
DE PRONY, G.R. (1795), Essai expérimental et analytique, *J. École Polytechnique* **1** (2), 24–76.

DERRIENNIC, M.M. (1985), On multivariate approximation by Bernstein-type polynomials, *J. Approx. Theory* **45**, 155–166.

DESCLOUX, J. (1961), Dégénérescence dans les approximations de Tschebycheff linéaires et discrètes, *Numer. Math.* **3**, 180–187.

DESCLOUX, J. (1963), Approximation in L_p and Tchebycheff approximation, *SIAM J. Appl. Math.* **11**, 1017–1026.

DONOGHUE JR., W.F. (1974), *Monotone Matrix Functions and Analytic Continuation* (Springer, Berlin).

DURRMEYER, J.L. (1978), Une Formule d'Inversion de la Transformée de Laplace. Applications à la Théorie des Moments, 3rd Cycle Thesis, Université de Rennes, France.

EAGLE, A. (1928), On the relation between Fourier constants of a periodic function and the coefficients determined by harmonic analysis, *Philos. Mag.* **5**, 113–132.

ECKHARDT, R. (1989), Stan Ulam, John von Neumann, and the Monte Carlo method, in: N. GRANT COOPER, ed., *From Cardinals to Chaos* (Cambridge University Press, Cambridge) 131–137.

ERDÖS, P. and P. TURÁN (1937), On interpolation, I. Quadrature- and mean-convergence in the Lagrange interpolation, *Ann. Math.* **38**, 142–155.

ESPELID, T.O. and A. GENZ, eds., (1992), *Numerical Integration. Recent Developments, Software and Applications* (Kluwer, Dordrecht).

EULER, L. (1738), Methodus generalis summandi progressiones, *Comm. Acad. Imp. Petrop.* **6**, 68–97.

EULER, L. (1775), De eximio usu methodi interpolationum in serierum doctrina.

FABER, G. (1914), Über die interpolatorische Darstellung stetiger Funktionen, *Jahresber. Dtsch. Math.-Ver.* **23**, 192–210.

FARIN, G. (1991), Splines in CAD/CAM, *Surv. Math. Ind.* **1**, 39–73.

FAVARD, J. (1935), Sur les polynômes de Tchebicheff, *C. R. Acad. Sci. Paris* **200**, 2052–2053.

FAVARD, J. (1944), Sur les multiplicateurs d'interpolation, *J. Math. Pures Appl.* **23**, 219–247.

FEJÉR, L. (1931), Les points conjugués dans l'interpolation de Lagrange, *Math. és Term.-tud. Ért.* **48**, 631–643, (in Hungarian).

FEJÉR, L. (1933), Mechanische Quadraturen mit positiven Cotesschen Zahlen, *Math. Z.* **37**, 287–309.

FELDHEIM, E. (1939), *Théorie de la Convergence des Procédés d'Interpolation et de Quadrature Numérique*, Mémorial des Sciences Mathématiques, Fascicule XCV (Gauthier-Villars, Paris).

FIOROT, J.C. and P. JEANNIN (1989), *Courbes et Surfaces Rationnelles. Applications à la CAO* (Masson, Paris).

FORREST, A.R. (1972), Interactive interpolation and approximation by Bézier polynomials, *Comput. J.* **15**, 71–79.

FRASER, D.C. (1927), Newton and interpolation, in: W.J. GREENSTREET, ed., *I. Newton, a Memorial Volume* (G. Bell, London) 45–69.

FROBENIUS, G. (1881), Über Relationen zwischen den Näherungsbrüchen von Potenzreihen, *J. Reine Angew. Math.* **90**, 1–17.

GASCA, M. (1990), Multivariate polynomial interpolation, in: W. DAHMEN, M. GASCA and C.A. MICCHELLI, eds., *Computation of Curves and Surfaces* (Kluwer, Dordrecht) 215–236.

GASCA, M. and E. LEBRON (1983), A note on recurrence interpolation formulae for certain sets of points in $\mathbb{R}^k$, in: L. COLLATZ, G. MEINARDUS and H. WERNER, eds., *Numerical Methods of Approximation Theory*, Vol. 7 (Birkhäuser, Basel) 77–85.

GASCA, M. and E. LEBRON (1987), On Aitken–Neville formulae for multivariate interpolation, in: E.L. ORTIZ, ed., *Numerical Approximation of Partial Differential Equations* (North-Holland, Amsterdam) 133–140.

GASCA, M. and A. LOPEZ CARMONA (1982), A general recurrence interpolation formula and its applications to multivariate interpolation, *J. Approx. Theory* **34**, 361–374.

GASCA, M. and J.I. MAETZU (1982), On Lagrange and Hermite interpolation problems in $\mathbb{R}^k$, *Numer. Math.* **39**, 1–14.

GASCA, M. and V. RAMIREZ (1984), Interpolation systems in $\mathbb{R}^k$, *J. Approx. Theory* **42**, 36–51.

GAUSS, C.F. (1812), Disquisitiones generales circa seriem infinitam $1 + ((\alpha\beta)/(1\gamma))x + \cdots$, *Comm. Soc. R. Sci. Gott. Recens.* **2**, 1–46.

GAUSS, C.F. (1814), Methodus nova integralium valores per approximationem inveniendi, *Comm. Soc. R. Sci. Gott. Recens.* **3**, 39–76.
GAUTSCHI, W. (1981), A survey of Gauss-Christoffel quadrature formulae, in: P.L. BUTZER and F. FEHÉR, eds., *E.B. Christoffel, the Influence of his Work on Mathematics and the Physical Sciences* (Birkhäuser, Basel) 72–147.
GAUTSCHI, W. (1988), Gauss-Kronrod quadrature - A survey, in: G.V. MILOVANOVIĆ, ed., *Numerical Methods and Approximation Theory, III* (Faculty of Electronic Engineering, University of Niš, Niš) 39–66.
GENOCCHI, A. (1878), Sur la formule sommatoire de Maclaurin et les fonctions interpolaires, *C. R. Acad. Sci. Paris* **86**, 466–469.
GENOCCHI, A. (1880–1881), Sopra una proprietà delle funzioni interpolatori, *Atti Accad. Sci. Torino* **16**, 269–275.
GERONIMUS, J.L. (1944), On Gauss' and Tchebysheff's quadrature formulas, *Bull. Amer. Math. Soc.* **50**, 217–221.
GOLDSTEIN, A.A. (1963), On the stability of rational approximation, *Numer. Math.* **5**, 431–438.
GOLDSTINE, H.H. (1977), *A History of Numerical Analysis from the 16th through the 19th Century* (Springer, New York).
GOLOMB, M. and H. WEINBERGER (1958), Optimal approximation and error bounds, in: R. LANGER, ed., *On Numerical Approximation* (University of Wisconsin) 117–190.
GOURIER, G. (1883), Sur une méthode capable de fournir une valeur approchée de l'intégrale $\int_{-\infty}^{+\infty} F(x)\, dx$, *C. R. Acad. Sci. Paris* **97**, 79–82.
GOWING, R. (1983), *Roger Cotes, Natural Philosopher* (Cambridge University Press, Cambridge).
GRAM, J.P. (1883), Über die Entwicklung reeller Funktionen in Reihen mittels der Methode der kleinsten Quadrate, *J. Reine Angew. Math.* **94**, 41–73.
GREGORY, J. (1668), *Exercitationes Geometricae* (London).
GREVILLE, T.N.E. (1944), The general theory of osculatory interpolation, *Trans. Actuarial Soc. Amer.* **45**, 202–265.
GRÜNWALD, G. (1935), Sur les phénomènes de divergence des polynômes d'interpolation de Lagrange, *Math. Fiz. Lapok* **42** (in Hungarian).
GUENTHER, R.B. and E.L. ROETMAN (1970), Some observations on interpolation in higher dimensions, *Math. Comput.* **24**, 517–521.
GUTKNECHT, M.H. (1983a), On complex rational approximation, part I: The characterization problem, in: H. WERNER, L. WUYTACK, E. NG and H.J. BÜNGER, eds., *Computational Aspects of Complex Analysis* (Reidel, Dordrecht) 79–101.
GUTKNECHT, M.H. (1983b), On complex rational approximation, part II: The Carathéodory-Fejér method, in: H. WERNER, L. WUYTACK, E. NG and H.J. BÜNGER, eds., *Computational Aspects of Complex Analysis* (Reidel, Dordrecht) 103–132.
HAAR, A. (1918), Die Minkowskische Geometrie und die Annäherung an stetige Funktionen, *Math. Ann.* **78**, 294–311.
HAKOPIAN, H.A. (1982), Multivariate divided differences and multivariate interpolation of Lagrange and Hermite type, *J. Approx. Theory* **34**, 286–305.
HARRIOT, T. (1611), *De Numeris Triangularibus et inde de Progressionibus Arithmeticis Magisteria magna*.
HART, J.F., E.W. CHENEY, C.L. LAWSON, H.J. MAEHLY, C.K. MESZTENYI, J.R. RICE, H.G. THACHER JR., and C. WITZGALL (1965), *Handbook of Computer Approximations* (Wiley, New York).
HASTINGS, C. (1955), *Approximations for Digital Computers* (Princeton University Press, Princeton).
HÅVIE, T. (1979), Generalized Neville type extrapolation schemes, *BIT* **19**, 204–213.
HEINE, H.E. (1881), *Anwendungen der Kugelfunktionen und der verwandten Funktionen*, 2nd ed. (Reimer, Berlin).
HENRICI, P. (1983), Topics in computational complex analysis, part III: The asymptotic behavior of best approximations to analytic functions on the unit disk, in: H. WERNER, L. WUYTACK, E. NG and H.J. BÜNGER, eds., *Computational Aspects of Complex Analysis* (Reidel, Dordrecht) 169–191.
HERMITE, C. (1864), Sur un nouveau mode de développement en série des fonctions, *C. R. Acad. Sci. Paris* **58**, 93–100, 266–273.

HERMITE, C. (1873), Sur la fonction exponentielle, *C. R. Acad. Sci. Paris* **77**, 18–24, 74–79, 226–233, 285–293.

HERMITE, C. (1878), Sur la formule d'interpolation de Lagrange, *J. Reine Angew. Math.* **84**, 70–79.

HIGGINS, J.R. (1985), Five short stories about the cardinal series, *Bull. Amer. Math. Soc.* **12**, 45–89.

HOBBY, C.R. and J.R. RICE (1967), Approximation from a curve of functions, *Arch. Rat. Mech. Anal.* **27**, 91–106.

HOFMANN, J.E. (1974), *Leibniz in Paris, 1672–1676* (Cambridge University Press, Cambridge).

HORNECKER, G. (1958), Evaluation approchée de la meilleure approximation polynomiale d'ordre n de $f(x)$ sur un segment fini $[a,b]$, *Chiffres* **1**, 157–169.

HORNECKER, G. (1959), Approximations rationnelles voisines de la meilleure approximation au sens de Tchebycheff, *C. R. Acad. Sci. Paris* **249**, 939–941.

HORNECKER, G. (1961), Méthodes pratiques pour la détermination approchée de la meilleure approximation polynomiale ou rationnelle, *Chiffres* **3**, 193–228.

IONESCU, D.V. (1967), Restes des formules de quadratures de Gauss et de Turán, *Acta Math. Acad. Sci. Hungar* **18**, 283–295.

JACOBI, C.G.J. (1826), Ueber Gauss neue Methode, die Werthe der Integrale näherungsweise zu finden, *J. Reine Angew. Math.* **1**, 301–308.

JACOBI, C.G.J. (1845), Über die Darstellung einer Reihe gegebener Werthe durch eine gebrochen rationale Funktion, *J. Reine Angew. Math.* **30**, 127–156.

JACOBI, C.G.J. (1859), Untersuchungen über die Differentialgleichung der hypergeometrische Reihe, *J. Reine Angew. Math.* **56**, 149–165.

JACKSON, D. (1911), Über die Genauigkeit der Annäherung Stetiger Funktionen durch Ganze Rationale Funktionen, Dissertation, Göttingen, Germany.

JOHNSON, W.W. (1915), On Cotesian numbers: their history, computation, and values to $n = 20$, *Quart. J. Pure Appl. Math.* **46**, 52–65.

JOURAVSKY, A. (1928), Sur la convergence des formules des quadratures mécaniques dans un intervalle infini, *J. Soc. Phys.-Math. Leningrad* **2**, 31–52.

KEAST, P. and G. FAIRWEATHER, eds. (1987), *Numerical Integration* (Reidel, Dordrecht).

KIDA, S. (1990), Padé-type and Padé approximations in several variables, *Appl. Numer. Math.* **5**, 371–391, 393–404.

KIRCHBERGER, P. (1902), Über Tchebychefsche Annäherungsmethoden, Dissertation, Göttingen, Germany.

KOLMOGOROV, A.N. (1948), A remark on the polynomials of P.L. Chebyshev deviating the least from a given function, *Usp. Math. Nauk* **3**, 216–221 (in Russian).

KREIN, M.G. (1951), The ideas of P.L. Chebyshev and A.A. Markov in the theory of limiting values of integrals and their further development, *Usp. Math. Nauk SSSR* **6**, 3–120, *Amer. Math. Soc. Transl. (II)* **12** (1959), 1–122.

KRONROD, A.S. (1964), Integration with control of accuracy, *Dokl. Akad. Nauk SSSR* **154**, 283–286 (in Russian).

KRONROD, A.S. (1965), *Nodes and Weights for Quadrature Formulae. Sixteen-place Tables* (Consultants Bureau, New York).

KRYLOV, V.I. (1959), *Approximate Calculation of Integrals* (Izdat. Fiz.-Mat. Lit., Moscow) (in Russian).

KUZMIN, R.O. (1931), On the theory of mechanical quadratures, *Bull. Polyt. Inst. Leningrad, Dept. of Tech. Sci., and Math.* (in Russian).

LAGRANGE, J.L. (1776), Sur l'usage des fractions continues dans le calcul intégral, *Nouv. Mém. Acad. Sci. Berlin* **7**, 236–264.

LAGRANGE, J.L. (1783), Sur une méthode particulière d'approximation et d'interpolation, *Nouv. Mém. Acad. Sci. Berlin* **38**, 279–289.

LAGRANGE, J.L. (1795), *Leçons Elémentaires sur les Mathématiques* (Paris).

LAGUERRE, E.N. (1879), Sur l'intégrale $\int_x^\infty e^{-x}\,dx/x$, *Bull. Soc. Math. France* **7**, 72–81.

LAMBERT, J.H. (1758), Observationes variae in mathesin puram, *Acta Helvetica* **3**, 128–168.

LAASONEN, P. (1949), Einige Sätze über Tschebyscheffsche Funktionensysteme, *Ann. Acad. Scient. Fennicae* **52**, 123–199.

LAURENT, P.J. (1963), Un théorème de convergence pour le procédé d'extrapolation de Richardson, *C. R. Acad. Sci. Paris* **256**, 1435–1437.
LAURENT, P.J. (1967a), Généralisation de l'algorithme de Rémès pour l'obtention d'une meilleure approximation dans un espace normé, *C. R. Acad. Sci. Paris* **264**, 22–24.
LAURENT, P.J. (1967b), Théorèmes de caractérisation d'une meilleure approximation dans un espace normé et généralisation de l'algorithme de Rémès, *Numer. Math.* **10**, 190–208.
LAURENT, P.J. (1972), *Approximation et Optimisation* (Hermann, Paris).
LEBESGUE, H. (1898), Sur l'approximation des fonctions, *Bull. Sc. Math.* **22**, 278–287.
LEGENDRE, A.M. (1785), Recherche sur l'attraction des sphéroïdes homogènes, *Mém. Math. Phys. Présentés à l'Acad. des Sci.* **10**, 411–434.
LEGENDRE, A.M. (1806), *Nouvelles Méthodes pour la Détermination des Orbites des Comètes* (Courcier, Paris).
LERCH, M. (1903), Sur un point de la théorie des fonctions génératrices d'Abel, *Acta Math.* **27**, 339–352.
LEVIN, D. (1976), General order Padé-type approximants defined from double power series, *J. Inst. Math. Applics* **18**, 1–8.
LIGHT, W.A. (1992), Some aspects of radial basis function approximation, in: S.P. SINGH, ed., *Approximation Theory, Spline Functions and Applications* (Kluwer, Dordrecht) 163–190.
LIGHT, W.A. and CHENEY, E.W. (1985), *Approximation Theory in Tensor Product Spaces*, Lecture Notes in Mathematics **1169** (Springer, Berlin).
LINDEMANN, F. (1882), Ueber die Zahl π, *Math. Ann.* **20**, 213–225.
LOBATTO, R. (1852), *Lessen over de Differentiaal- en Integraal-Rekening, II: Integraal-Rekening* (Van Cleef, The Hague).
LORENTZ, G.G., K. JETTER, and S.D. RIEMENSCHNEIDER (1983), *Birkhoff Interpolation* (Addison-Wesley, Reading, MA).
LORENTZ, R.A. (1991), A survey of bivariate Birkhoff interpolation, in: C.K. CHUI, ed., *Approximation Theory and Functional Analysis* (Academic Press, New York) 81–111.
LYNESS, J. (1986), Numerical integration, part A: extrapolation methods for multi-dimensional quadrature, in: J.L. MOHAMED and J. WALSH, eds., *Numerical Algorithms* (Clarendon Press, Oxford) 105–124.
MACLAURIN, C. (1742), *A Treatise of Fluxions* (Edinburgh).
MAEHLY, H.J. (1960), Methods for fitting rational approximations, *ACM J.* **7**, 150–162; **10** (1963) 257–277.
MAEHLY, H.J. and C. WITZGALL (1960), Tschebyscheff-Approximationen in kleinen Intervallen, *Numer. Math.* **2**, 142–150, 293–307.
MAIRHUBER, J.C. (1956), On Harr's theorem concerning Chebyshev approximation problems having unique solutions, *Proc. Amer. Math. Soc.* **7**, 609–615.
MARCINKIEWICZ, J. (1935), Sur les polynômes d'interpolation, *Wiadom. Mat.* **39**, 85–115 (in Polish).
MARKOV, A.A. (1885), Sur la méthode de Gauss pour le calcul approché des intégrales, *Math. Ann.* **25**, 427–432.
MARKOV, A.A. (1898), Recherches sur les valeurs extrêmes des intégrales et sur l'interpolation, *Zap. Imp. Akad. Nauk. St. Petersburg (8)* **6**, French transl., *Acta Math.* **28** (1904) 243–301.
MARONI, P. (1991), Une théorie algébrique des polynômes orthogonaux. Application aux polynômes orthogonaux semi-classiques, in: C. BREZINSKI, A. DRAUX, A.P. MAGNUS, P. MARONI and A. ROUVEAUX, eds., *Orthogonal Polynomials and their Applications* (Baltzer, Basel) 95–130.
MAXWELL, J.C. (1877), On approximate multiple integration between limits of summation, *Proc. Cambridge Philos. Soc.* **3**, 39–47.
MEHLER, F.G. (1864), Bemerkungen zur Theorie der mechanischen Quadraturen, *J. Reine Angew. Math.* **63**, 152–157.
MEINARDUS, G. (1967), *Approximation of Functions: Theory and Numerical Methods* (Springer, Berlin).
MÉRAY, C. (1884), Observations sur la légitimité de l'interpolation, *Ann. École Norm. Sup.* **2**, 165–176.
MÉRAY, C. (1896), Nouveaux exemples d'interpolation illusoires, *Bull. Sci. Math.* **20**, 266–271.

METROPOLIS, N. (1989), The beginning of the Monte Carlo method, in: N. GRANT COOPER, ed., *From Cardinals to Chaos* (Cambridge University Press, Cambridge) 125–130.

METROPOLIS, N. and S. ULAM (1949), The Monte Carlo method, *J. Amer. Stat. Assoc.* **44**, 335–341.

MEYER, Y. (1990), *Ondelettes* (Hermann, Paris).

MITTAG-LEFFLER, G. (1900), Sur la représentation analytique des fonctions d'une variable réelle, *Rend. Circ. Mat. Palermo* **14**, 217–224.

MÜHLBACH, G. (1973), A recurrence formula for generalized divided differences and some applications, *J. Approx. Theory* **9**, 165–172.

MÜNTZ, C.H. (1914), Über den Approximationssatz von Weierstrass, *H.A. Schwarz Festschrift, Math. Abh. Berlin*, 303–312.

NARUMI, S. (1920), Some formulas in the theory of interpolation of many independent variables, *Tôhoku Math. J.* **18**, 309–321.

NATANSON, I.P. (1964), *Constructive Function Theory*, 3 vols. (Ungar, New York).

NEDER, L. (1926), Interpolations Formeln für Funktionen mehrerer Argumenten, *Skandinav. Aktuariet*.

NEVILLE, E.H. (1934), Iterative interpolation, *J. Indian Math. Soc.* **20**, 87–120.

NEWMAN, D.J. (1964), Rational approximation to $|x|$, *Michigan Math. J.* **11**, 11–14.

NEWTON, I. (1687), *Philosophiae Naturalis Principia Mathematica* (London).

NICOLAIDES, R.A. (1972), On a class of finite elements generated by Lagrange interpolation, *SIAM J. Numer. Anal.* **9**, 435–445.

NIKIFOROV, A.F., S.K. SUSLOV, and V.B. UVAROV (1991), *Classical Orthogonal Polynomials of a Discrete Variable* (Springer, Berlin).

NÖRLUND, N.E. (1911), Fractions continues et différences réciproques, *Acta Math.* **34**, 1–108.

ODEN, J.T. (1991), Finite elements: an introduction, in: P.G. CIARLET and J.L. LIONS, eds., *Handbook of Numerical Analysis*, Vol. II, Finite Element Methods (Part 1) (North-Holland, Amsterdam) 3–15.

OSSICINI, A. (1968), Le funzioni di influenza nel problema di Gauss sulle formule di quadratura, *Matematiche (Catania)* **23**, 7–30.

PADÉ, H. (1892), Sur la représentation approchée d'une fonction par des fractions rationnelles, *Ann. Sci. École Norm. Sup.* **9**, 1–93.

PADÉ, H. (1900), Sur l'extension des propriétés des réduites d'une fonction aux fractions d'interpolation de Cauchy, *C. R. Acad. Sci. Paris* **130**, 697–700.

PADÉ, H. (1984), in: C. BREZINSKI, ed., *Oeuvres* (Librairie Scientifique et Technique A. Blanchard, Paris).

PÁL, J. (1914), Zwei kleine Bemerkungen, *Tôhoku Math. J.* **6**, 42–43.

PASZKOWSKI, S. (1955), Sur l'approximation uniforme avec des noeuds, *Ann. Pol. Math.* **2**, 129–146.

PASZKOWSKI, S. (1956), On the Weierstrass approximation theorem, *Colloq. Math.* **4**, 206–210.

PASZKOWSKI, S. (1957), On approximation with nodes, *Rozpr. Mat.* **14**.

PEANO, G. (1918), Resto nelle formule di interpolazione, in: *Scritti Matematici Offerti ad Enrico d'Ovidio* (Bocca, Torino) 333–335.

PETRUSHEV, P.P. and V.A. POPOV (1987), *Rational Approximation of Real Functions* (Cambridge University Press, Cambridge).

PICARD, E. (1891), Sur la représentation approchée des fonctions, *C. R. Acad. Sci. Paris* **112**, 183–186.

PÓLYA, G. (1913), Sur un algorithme toujours convergent pour obtenir les polynômes de meilleures approximation de Tchebycheff pour une fonction continue quelconque, *C. R. Acad. Sci. Paris* **157**, 840–843.

PÓLYA, G. (1933), Über die Konvergenz von Quadraturverfahren, *Math. Z.* **37**, 264–286.

PONCELET, J.V. (1835), Sur la valeur approchée linéaire et rationnelle des radicaux de la forme $\sqrt{(a^2 + b^2)}$, $\sqrt{(a^2 - b^2)}$, etc., *J. Reine Angew. Math.* **13**, 277–291.

POSSÉ, C. (1875), Sur les quadratures, *Nouv. Ann. Math. (2)* **14**, 49–62.

POWELL, M.J.D. (1992), The theory of radial basis function approximation in 1990, in: W. LIGHT, ed., *Advances in Numerical Analysis*. Vol. II: Wavelets, Subdivision Algorithms, and Radial Basis Functions (Clarendon Press, Oxford) 105–210.

QUADE, W. and COLLATZ, L. (1938), Zur Interpolationstheorie der reellen periodischen Funktionen, *Proc. Preuss. Akad. Wiss. (Math.-Phys. Kl.)* **30**, 383–429.

RADAU, R. (1880), Etude sur les formules d'approximation qui servent à calculer la valeur numérique d'une intégrale définie, *J. Math. Pures Appl. (3)* **6**, 283–336.

RADAU, R. (1883), Remarque sur le calcul d'une intégrale définie, *C. R. Acad. Sci. Paris* **97**, 157–158.

RADON, J. (1948), Zur mechanischen Kubatur, *Monatsh. Math.* **52**, 286–300.

REMES, E. YA. (1934), Sur le calcul effectif des polynômes d'approximation de Tchebichef, *C. R. Acad. Sci. Paris* **199**, 337–340.

REMES, E. YA. (1935), *On the Best Approximation of Functions in the Tchebycheff Sense* (Kiev) (in Ukrainian).

REMES, E. YA. (1957), *General Computational Methods of Tchebycheff Approximation*, AECT no. **4491**, (Kiev) (in Russian).

RICE, J.R. (1960), Chebyshev approximation by $ab^x + c$, *J. Soc. Ind. Appl. Math.* **8**, 691–702.

RICE, J.R. (1961), Tchebycheff approximations by functions unisolvent of variable degree, *Trans. Amer. Math. Soc.* **99**, 298–302.

RICE, J.R. (1962), Chebyshev approximation by exponentials, *J. Soc. Ind. Appl. Math.* **10**, 149–161.

RICE, J.R. (1963), Tchebycheff approximation in several variables, *Trans. Amer. Math. Soc.* **109**, 444–466.

RICE, J.R. (1969), *The Approximation of Functions. Vol. 2: Nonlinear and Multivariate Theory* (Addison-Wesley, Reading, MA).

RICHARDSON, L.F. (1910), The approximate arithmetic solution by finite differences of physical problems involving differential equations, with an application to the stress in a masonry dam, *Phil. Trans. Roy. Soc. London, Ser. A* **210**, 307–357.

RODRIGUES, O. (1816), Mémoire sur l'attraction des sphéroïdes, *Correspondance sur l'École Polytechnique* **3**, 361–385.

ROMBERG, W. (1955), Vereinfachte numerische Integration, *Kgl. Norske Vid. Selsk. Forsk.* **28**, 30–36.

RUBINSTEIN, G.S. (1955), A method of studying convex sets, *Dokl. Akad. Nauk SSSR* **102**, 451–454 (in Russian).

RUNGE, C. (1885a), Zur Theorie der eindeutigen analytischen Funktionen, *Acta Math.* **6**, 229–245.

RUNGE, C. (1885b), Über die Darstellung willkürlicher Funktionen, *Acta Math.* **7**, 387–392.

RUNGE, C. (1891), Über eine numerische Berechnung der Argumente der cyclischen, hyperbolischen und logarithmischen Funktionen, *Acta Math.* **15**, 221–247.

RUNGE, C. (1901), Über empirische Funktionen und die Interpolation zwischen äquidistanten Ordinaten, *Z. Angew. Math. Phys.* **46**, 224–243.

RUNGE, C. and WILLERS, F.A. (1915), Numerische und graphische Integration, in: *Encyklopädie der mathematischen Wissenschaften*, Vol. 2, Sec. 3, Heft 2 (Teubner, Leipzig) 47–176.

SABLONNIÈRE, P. (1983), A new family of Padé-type approximants in $\mathbb{R}^n$, *J. Comput. Appl. Math.* **9**, 347–359.

SCHELLBACH, K.H. (1864), *Die Lehre von den elliptischen Integralen und den Theta-Funktionen* (Berlin).

SCHMIDT, E. (1907), Zur Theorie der linearen und nichtlinearen Integralgleichungen, I Theil: Entwicklung willkürlicher Funktionen nach Systemen vorgeschriebenen, *Math. Ann.* **63**, 433–476.

SCHOENBERG, I.J. (1946), Contributions to the problem of approximation of equidistant data by analytic functions, *Quart. Appl. Math.* **4**, 45–99, 112–141.

SCHOENBERG, I.J. (1958), Spline functions, convex curves, and mechanical quadratures, *Bull. Amer. Math. Soc.* **64**, 352–357.

SCHOENBERG, I.J. (1981), On polynomial interpolation at the points of a geometric progression, *Proc. Roy. Soc. Edinburgh* **90A**, 195–207.

SCHOENBERG, I.J. (1988), A brief account of my life and work, in: C. DE BOOR, ed., *I.J. Schoenberg Selected Papers*, Vol. **1** (Birkhäuser, Basel) 1–10.

SCHWARZ, H.A. (1881–1882), Démonstration élémentaire d'une propriété fondamentale des fonctions interpolaires, *Atti Accad. Sci. Torino* **17**, 740–742.

SCOTT, J.F. (1981), *The Mathematical Work of John Wallis* (Chelsea, New York).

SENDOV, B.H. and ANDREEV, A.S. (1994), Approximation and interpolation theory, in: P.G. CIARLET and J.L. LIONS, eds., *Handbook of Numerical Analysis*, Vol. III: Techniques of Scientific Computing (Part 1), Solutions of Equations in $\mathbb{R}^n$ (Part 2), Numerical Methods for Solids (Part 1) (North-Holland, Amsterdam).
SEWELL, W.E. (1942), *Degree of Approximation by Polynomials in the Complex Domain* (Princeton University Press, Princeton).
SHEPPARD, W.F. (1900), Some quadrature formulas, *Proc. London Math. Soc.* **32**, 258–277.
SHOHAT, J.A. (1927), Sur les quadratures mécaniques et sur les zéros des polynômes de Tchebycheff dans un intervalle infini, *C. R. Acad. Sci. Paris* **185**, 597–598.
SHOHAT, J.A. (1933), On interpolation, *Ann. Math., Ser. 2*, **34**, 130–146.
SHOHAT, J.A. and TAMARKIN, J.D. (1943), *The Problem of Moments* (Amer. Math. Soc., New York).
SIMPSON, T. (1743), *Mathematical Dissertations on a Variety of Physical and Analytical Subjects* (London).
SOBOLEV, S.L. (1962a), Cubature formulas on the sphere invariant under finite groups of rotations, *Soviet Math. Dokl.* **3**, 1307–1310.
SOBOLEV, S.L. (1962b), The formulas of mechanical cubature on the surface of a sphere, *Sibirsk. Mat. Z.* **3**, 769–796.
SOBOLEV, S.L. (1962c), The number of nodes in cubature formulas on the sphere, *Soviet Math. Dokl.* **3**, 1391–1394.
SPANIER, J. and K.B. OLDHAM (1987), *An Atlas of Functions* (Hemisphere, Washington).
STEFFENSEN, J.F. (1927), *Interpolation* (Chelsea, New York).
STEKLOV, V.A. (1916), On the approximate calculation of definite integrals by means of formulae of mechanical quadrature, *Izv. Akad. Nauk SSSR (6)* **10**, 169–186 (in Russian).
STIEFEL, E.L. (1959), Über diskrete und lineare Tscheyscheff-Approximationen, *Numer. Math.* **2**, 1–28.
STIELTJES, T.J. (1882), Over Lagrange's interpolatie-formule, *Akad. Versl. en Meded. Amsterdam* **17**, 239–254.
STIELTJES, T.J. (1884), Notes sur quelques formules pour l'évaluation de certaines intégrales, *Bull. Astr. Paris* **1**, 568–569.
STIRLING, J. (1718), Methodus differentialis Newtoniana illustrata, *Phil. Trans. Roy. Soc.* **30**, 1050–1070.
STIRLING, J. (1730), *Methodus differentialis: sive Tractatus de Summatione et Interpolatione Serierum infinitarum* (London).
STONE, M.H. (1948), The generalized Weierstrass approximation theorem, *Math. Mag.* **21**, 167–184, 237–254.
STROUD, A.H. (1971), *Approximate Calculation of Multiple Integrals* (Prentice-Hall, Englewood Cliffs, NJ).
TAYLOR, B. (1715), *Methodus Incrementorum Directa et Inverta* (London).
THACHER JR., H.C. and MILNE, W.E. (1960), Interpolation in several variables, *J. SIAM* **8**, 33–42.
THIELE, T.N. (1906), Différences réciproques, *Overs. Danske Vids. Selsk. Forhandl. (Sitzber. Akad. Kopenhagen)* 153–171.
TIKHOMIROV, V.M. (1990), Approximation theory, in: R.V. GAMKRELIDZE, ed., *Analysis II* (Springer, Berlin) 93–243.
TOEPLER, A. (1876), Notiz über eine bemerkenswerte Eigenschaft der periodischen Reihen, *Wiener Akad. Anz.*, 205–209.
TONELLI, L. (1908), I polinomi d'approssimazione di Tchebychev, *Ann. Mat. Pura Appl.* **15**, 47–119.
TREFETHEN, L.N. (1983), Chebyshev approximation on the unit disk, in: H. WERNER, L. WUYTACK, E. NG and H.J. BÜNGER, eds., *Computational Aspects of Complex Analysis* (Reidel, Dordrecht) 309–323.
TURÁN, P. (1950), On the theory of the mechanical quadrature, *Acta Sci. Math. Szeged* **12**, 30–37.
USPENSKY, J.V. (1916), On the convergence of mechanical quadratures between infinite limits (in Russian), *Dokl. Akad. Nauk SSSR* **10**, 851–866.
USPENSKY, J.V. (1928), On the convergence of quadrature formulas related to an infinite interval, *Trans. Amer. Math. Soc.* **30**, 542–559.

VARGA, R.S. (1982), *Topics in Polynomial and Rational Interpolation and Approximation* (Les Presses de l'Université de Montréal, Montreal).
VARGA, R.S. (1990), *Scientific Computation on Mathematical Problems and Conjectures* (SIAM, Philadelphia).
VEIDINGER, L. (1960), On the numerical determination of the best approximations in the Chebyshev sense, *Numer. Math.* **2**, 99–105.
VOLTERRA, V. (1897), Sul principio di Dirichlet, *Rend. Circ. Mat. Palermo* **11**, 83–86.
WALLIS, J. (1656), *Arithmetica Infinitorum* (Oxford).
WALSH, J.L. (1926), Über die Entwicklung einer analytischen Funktion nach Polynomen, *Math. Ann.* **96**, 430–436.
WALSH, J.L. (1931), The existence of rational functions of best approximation, *Trans. Amer. Math. Soc.* **33**, 668–689.
WALSH, J.L. (1935a), *Approximation by Polynomials in the Complex Domain*, Mémorial des Sciences Mathématiques, Fascicule LXXIII (Gauthier-Villars, Paris).
WALSH, J.L. (1935b), *Interpolation and Approximation by Rational Functions in the Complex Domain* (Amer. Math. Soc., Providence, RI).
WALSH, J.L. (1964), Padé approximants as limits of rational functions of best approximation, *J. Math. Mech.* **13**, 305–312.
WARING, E. (1779), Problems concerning interpolations, *Phil. Trans.* **69**, 59–67.
WEDDLE, T. (1854), On a new and simple rule for approximating to the area of a figure by means of seven equidistant ordinates, *Cambridge and Dublin Math. J.* **9**, 79–80.
WEIERSTRASS, K. (1885), Über die analytische Darstellbarkeit sogenannter willkürlicher Funktionen einer reellen Veränderlichen, *Sitz.-Ber. Akad. Wiss. Berlin*, 633–639, 789–805.
WERNER, H. (1962), Tschebyscheff-Approximation im Bereich der rationalen Funktionen bei Vorliegen einer guten Ausgangsnäherung, *Arch. Rat. Mech. Anal.* **10**, 205–219.
WERNER, H. (1980), Remarks on Newton type multivariate interpolation for subsets of grids, *Computing* **25**, 181–191.
WHITNEY, H. (1934), Analytic extensions of differentiable functions defined in closed sets, *Trans. Amer. Math. Soc.* **36**, 63–89.
WHITTAKER, J.M. (1935), *Interpolatory Function Theory* (Cambridge University Press, Cambridge).
WIENER, N. (1933), *The Fourier Integral and Certain of its Applications* (Cambridge University Press, Cambridge).
WILSON, R. (1927), Divergent continued fractions and polar singularities, *Proc. London Math. Soc.* **26**, 159–168; **27** (1928) 497–512; **28** (1928) 128–144.
YOUNG, J.W. (1907), General theory of approximation by functions involving a given number of arbitrary parameters, *Trans. Amer. Math. Soc.* **8**, 331–344.
ZOLOTAREFF, E.I. (1878), Sur l'application des fonctions elliptiques aux questions de maxima et de minima, *Bull. Acad. Sci. St. Pétersbourg* **24**, 305–310.

Subject Index

A-stable methods, 22
Alternation theorem, 19
Approximation, 17

B-splines, 13
Bernstein polynomials, 12, 17
Best approximation in L_p, 24
Best approximation problem, 18
Best rational approximation, 21
Best uniform approximation, 19
Best uniform polynomial approximation, 31
Bézier curves and surfaces, 13
Binomial theorem, 8
Biorthogonality, 15

Carathéodory–Fejér method, 22
Cardinal interpolation, 12
Cardinal series, 12
Cardinal splines, 12
Cauchy interpolation problem, 12
Chebyshev approximation, 23, 24
Chebyshev norm, 18
Chebyshev polynomials, 18, 31
Chebyshev system, 8, 15
Christoffel–Darboux formula, 20, 30
Composite quadrature rule, 27
Computer aided design, 12
Conformal mapping, 22
Consistency principle, 11
Continued fraction, 9, 12, 20, 22, 26, 29
Continuity principles, 26
Cotes numbers, 27
Cubatures, 32

Deferred approach to the limit, 28
Degree of exactness, 25
Differential correction algorithm, 22
Divided differences, 7, 14

E-algorithm, 8

Euclid's algorithm, 9, 10
Euler–Maclaurin formula, 27, 28, 30, 32
Exchange algorithms, 20
Exponential function, 22

Finite differences, 7
Finite element method, 14
Fourier expansion, 20
Fourier's expansion, 17

γ-polynomial, 23
Gauss–Jacobi quadrature formula, 30
Gauss–Lobatto formulae, 30
Gauss–Radau formulae, 30
Gaussian quadratures, 29
General interpolation problem, 15
Gram–Schmidt process, 20
Greatest common divisor, 9, 10
Gregory quadrature formula, 26
Gregory–Newton formula, 7

h^2-extrapolation, 28
Haar condition, 19
Hakopian interpolation polynomial, 11
Hermite interpolation, 14, 30
Hermite interpolation problem, 8
Hermite–Birkhoff interpolation, 8, 14
Homogeneous approximants, 11
Homogeneous Padé approximants, 11

Infinity, 26
Interpolation, 7
Interpolatory, 25
Interpolatory functions, 8
Interpolatory quadratures, 28

Jackson-type theorems, 19

Kergin interpolation polynomial, 11
Kronrod quadratures, 31

L_1-approximation, 18
Lagrange interpolation, 8, 14
Lánczos method, 15, 21
Least squares, 15
Least squares approximation, 18
Legendre polynomials, 20, 29, 30
Linear approximation, 18
L_p-norm, 17

Massic vectors, 13
Meromorphic functions, 10
Method of indivisibles, 26
Monte Carlo methods, 32
Multivariate approximation, 23
Multivariate interpolation, 14

Near-best approximants, 20
Nearly best uniform rational approximations, 22
Neville–Aitken scheme, 8, 14, 15
Newton–Cotes formulae, 26
Newton–Cotes quadrature formulae, 27
Nodes, 25
Nonlinear approximation, 21
Normal families, 22
Numerical quadrature, 25
Numerical quadrature formula, 25

Orthogonal polynomials, 18, 21, 32
Orthogonality, 29
Orthogonalization, 20
Osculatory interpolation problem, 12

Padé approximant, 9, 22, 29
Padé approximation, 9, 21, 31
Padé table, 10
Piecewise polynomial, 12
Polynomial interpolation, 7
Problem of moments, 21
Proximinality, 24
Pseudo-splines, 14

Quadrature of the circle, 10

r-orthogonality, 31
Radial basis functions, 13
Rational curves and surfaces, 13
Rational functions, 21
Rational Hermite interpolation, 12
Rational interpolation, 11
Reciprocal differences, 12
Recurrence relation, 10, 21, 26
Remes algorithm, 20, 22, 24
Richardson extrapolation method, 29
Richardson's process, 8
Rodrigues formula, 21, 30
Romberg's extrapolation method, 32
Romberg's method, 29

Simpson's formula, 26
Simpson's rule, 27
Spline functions, 23
Spline interpolation, 12
Stieltjes polynomials, 31
Stiff differential equations, 22
Strict approximation, 24
Successive convergents, 9

Tensor product, 13
Transcendence, 10
Trapezoidal rule, 27, 28
Turán quadratures, 31

Uniform norm, 18
Unisolvence, 14

Varisolvence, 23

Wavelets, 13, 24
Weierstrass theorem, 17, 19, 23
Weight function, 18
Weights, 25

Padé Approximations

Claude Brezinski

Laboratoire d'Analyse Numérique et d'Optimisation UFR d'IEEA - M3
Université des Sciences et Technologies de Lille
F-59655 Villeneuve d'Asq Cedex, France

Jeannette Van Iseghem

UFR de Mathématiques Pures et Appliquées
Université des Sciences et Technologies de Lille
F-59655 Villeneuve d'Asq Cedex, France

HANDBOOK OF NUMERICAL ANALYSIS, VOL. III
Techniques of Scientific Computing (Part 1)
Numerical Methods for Solids (Part 1)
Solutions of Equations in $\mathbb{R}^n$ (Part 2)
Edited by P.G. Ciarlet and J.L. Lions
© 1994 Elsevier Science B.V. All rights reserved

Contents

PREFACE	51
CHAPTER I. Algebraic Theory	53
1. Introduction	53
2. Definitions	55
3. Algebraic properties	61
4. Formal orthogonal polynomials	64
5. Adjacent families of orthogonal polynomials	68
6. Recursive computation of Padé approximants	71
7. The ε-algorithm	74
8. Continued fractions	75
9. Error estimation	77
10. Duality	85
11. The method of moments	88
CHAPTER II. Convergence	93
12. Introduction to the convergence problem	93
13. Meromorphic functions	99
14. Functions with smooth Taylor series coefficients. Entire functions	106
15. Stieltjes series	110
16. Pólya frequency series	120
17. Convergence in capacity	121
18. Inverse problem	126
CHAPTER III. Generalizations	131
19. Padé-type approximants	131
20. Partial Padé approximants	140
21. Multipoint Padé approximants	151
22. Cauchy-type approximants	157
23. Series of functions	161
24. Padé–Hermite approximants	167
25. Vector Padé approximants	169
26. The noncommutative case	176
27. Multivariate approximants	180
CHAPTER IV. Applications	193
28. The exponential function	193
29. A-acceptable approximations to the exponential function	195
30. Borel transform	198
31. z-transform	200
32. Laplace transform inversion	203

REFERENCES 213

SUBJECT INDEX 221

Preface

The subject of approximation by Padé approximants has a long history since it is connected to continued fractions which, for example, form the basis of Euclid's algorithm for the g.c.d. of two numbers. It is also an important subject in itself which had a great influence in number theory (the proofs for the transcendence of the numbers e and π), in set theory (Cantor's proof that $\mathbb{R}$ and $\mathbb{R}^2$ have the same cardinality), in the construction, by Hilbert from Stieltjes' ideas, of the spectral theory of operators, in numerical analysis and in applied mathematics for the computation of special functions, etc. ... The usefulness of Padé approximants was rediscovered some decades ago when physicists realized that they were very attractive in the solution of problems involving convergent and divergent power, they were found to be connected with A-stable methods for integrating partial differential equations and useful for the computation of special functions.

There is actually a growing interest in the subject as proved by the many international conferences held, by the literature which contains more than 6000 items and by the numerous applications ranging from various topics in physics and chemistry to signal processing, astronomy, computer arithmetic, stochastic processes, statistics, numerical analysis, number theory, electronics, among others.

Padé approximants are also closely related to many other important questions as continued fractions, orthogonal polynomials and biorthogonality, and projection methods for the solution of systems of linear and nonlinear equations. Padé approximation has already been the subject of several books. Thus, it was not our purpose here to mimic them more or less well or to try to be complete. Our aim was to give the reader a good idea of the field and its last developments and applications, to provide him with the necessary tools for going deeper into it and to refer him to the existing literature. No special background is required except, may be, some knowledge of complex analysis which can be minimized by skipping over the proofs of some results.

CHAPTER I

Algebraic Theory

1. Introduction

Let f be a formal power series. A Padé approximant of f is a rational function whose numerator and denominator are chosen so that its power series expansion (which is obtained by dividing the numerator by the denominator) agrees with f, as far as possible, that is at least up to the term whose degree equals the sum of the degrees of the numerator and the denominator of the rational function.

Such approximants have a long history and they played an important rôle in the solution of many problems such as the transcendence of the numbers e and π and gave birth to some fundamental ideas in mathematics such as the spectral theory of operators. They are also closely connected with continued fractions; see BREZINSKI [1990c, 1991b]. Twenty years ago, Padé approximants were rediscovered by physicists and they proved to be a very efficient tool not only able to improve existing methods but also worthwhile for extracting important information from power series and thus leading to new possibilities which were not open before. Let us give some examples and begin by a purely mathematical one. We shall consider the series

$$f(z) = z - z^2/2 + z^3/3 - z^4/4 + \cdots$$

which is known to converge to $\ln(1+z)$ for $|z| \leqslant 1$, $z \neq -1$. Thus the simplest process for obtaining an approximate value of $\ln(1+z)$ is to sum the series up to a certain term. Let us denote by $S_k(z)$ the partial sum of f up to the term of degree k inclusively and let $[p/q]_f(z)$ be the Padé approximant of f whose numerator and denominator have the respective degrees p and q at most. As we shall see below, the computation of this Padé approximant needs the knowledge of the coefficients of f up to that of the power $p+q$. For $z=1$ we have $\ln 2 = 0.6931471805599453\ldots$ and we obtain the numerical results displayed in Table 1.1. For $z=2$, the series diverges and we have $\ln 3 = 1.098612288668110\ldots$ and the results are given in Table 1.2.

Let us now give an example from physics. It is taken from BENDER and ORSZAG [1978].

We consider Schrödinger's equation

$$\left[-\frac{d^2}{dx^2} + V(x) + W(x)\right]\varphi(x) = E\varphi(x)$$

TABLE 1.1.

k	$S_{2k}(1)$	$[k/k]_f(1)$
1	0.830	0.7
2	0.783	0.6933
3	0.759	0.693152
4	0.745	0.69314733
5	0.736	0.6931471849
6	0.730	0.69314718068
7	0.725	0.693147180563
8	0.721	0.69314718056000
9	0.718	0.6931471805599485
10	0.716	0.6931471805599454

TABLE 1.2.

k	$S_{2k}(2)$	$[k/k]_f(2)$
1	0.260×10^1	1.14
2	0.506×10^1	1.101
3	0.126×10^2	1.0988
4	0.375×10^2	1.098625
5	0.121×10^3	1.0986132
6	0.410×10^3	1.09861235
7	0.142×10^4	1.098612293
8	0.504×10^4	1.0986122890
9	0.181×10^5	1.098612288692
10	0.655×10^5	1.0986122886698

with the boundary condition

$$\lim_{|x| \to \infty} \varphi(x) = 0.$$

We are looking for the eigenfunctions φ and the eigenvalues E (energy) of this equation when V and W are continuous functions and when V and $V + W$ (the potential) tend to infinity when $|x|$ tends to infinity. It is possible to prove that, under the preceding assumptions, this problem has a nontrivial solution for some values of E. However, if the potential has a complicated expression, the solutions cannot be expressed in closed form. In that case a solution (E_0, φ_0) of the problem without W is first obtained and then the perturbed problem

$$\left[-\frac{d^2}{dx^2} + V(x) + \varepsilon W(x) \right] \varphi(x) = E\varphi(x)$$

is solved under the form

$$E = \sum_{n=0}^{\infty} E_n \varepsilon^n,$$

$$\varphi(x) = \sum_{n=0}^{\infty} \varphi_n(x) \varepsilon^n.$$

Replacing, in the perturbed Schrödinger's equation, gives recurrence relations for computing the E_n's and the φ_n's. If $V(x) = x^2/4$, the solutions of the equation without W are

$$E_0 = k + 1/2, \quad k = 0, 1, \ldots,$$

$$\varphi_0(x) = e^{-x^2/4} H_k(x), \quad k = 0, 1, \ldots,$$

where H_k is the Hermite polynomial of degree k. If $W(x) = x^4/4$, we find for the smallest eigenvalue ($k = 0$) the series

$$E = \frac{1}{2} + \frac{3}{4}\varepsilon - \frac{21}{8}\varepsilon^2 + \frac{333}{16}\varepsilon^3 - \cdots$$

which has a zero radius of convergence. The perturbed problem is singular and its solution is an asymptotic series. However, it is a Stieltjes series (see Section 15) whose sum can be computed by Padé approximants. We obtain

$$[1/1] = \frac{0.5 + 2.5\varepsilon}{1 + 3.5\varepsilon} \qquad [0/2] = \frac{0.5}{1 - 1.5\varepsilon + 7.5\varepsilon^2}$$

$$[1/2] = \frac{0.5 + 4.05\varepsilon}{1 + 6.6\varepsilon - 4.65\varepsilon^2} \qquad [0/3] = \frac{0.5}{1 - 1.5\varepsilon + 7.5\varepsilon^2 - 60.75\varepsilon^3}.$$

For other examples from physics the interested reader is referred to the very complete book of BAKER and GRAVES-MORRIS [1981], to the work of A.P. MAGNUS [1988] and to GUTTMANN [1989]. Applications to numerical analysis, by the bias of continued fractions, are described by JONES and THRON [1988].

2. Definitions

We shall now give the exact definition of Padé approximants. In fact we shall give two approaches to the subject: a direct one which is sufficient to understand it and a more complicated one which leads to a better grasp of its numerous relations with the theory of formal orthogonal polynomials and will serve as a basic tool for developing recurrence relations for the computation of Padé approximants, for estimating the error, and for the various generalizations of Padé approximation which will be discussed later.

Let f be a formal power series with complex coefficients

$$f(z) = c_0 + c_1 z + c_2 z^2 + c_3 z^3 + \cdots.$$

DEFINITION 2.1. The *Padé approximant* $[p/q]_f(z)$ is a rational function $N(z)/D(z)$ such that

degree $N \leq p$,
degree $D \leq q$,
$N(z) - f(z)D(z) = O(z^{p+q+1})$ $(z \to 0)$.

Let us write

$N(z) = a_0 + a_1 z + \cdots + a_p z^p$
$D(z) = b_0 + b_1 z + \cdots + b_q z^q$.

Then the conditions of Definition 2.1 lead to
$a_0 = c_0 b_0$,
$a_1 = c_1 b_0 + c_0 b_1$,
$\vdots$
$a_p = c_p b_0 + c_{p-1} b_1 + \cdots + c_{p-q} b_q$,
$0 = c_{p+1} b_0 + c_p b_1 + \cdots + c_{p-q+1} b_q$,
$\vdots$
$0 = c_{p+q} b_0 + c_{p+q-1} b_1 + \cdots + c_p b_q$

with the convention that $c_i = 0$ for $i < 0$.

The last q equations contain $q+1$ unknowns $b_0, \ldots, b_q$ and, thus, this system has a nontrivial solution. Knowing the b_i's, the first $p+1$ equations directly give the a_i's.

Two solutions of the problem lead to the same rational function since $N_1(z) - f(z)D_1(z) = O(z^{p+q+1})$ and $N_2(z) - f(z)D_2(z) = O(z^{p+q+1})$ imply $N_1(z)D_2(z) - D_1(z)N_2(z) = O(z^{p+q+1})$. But the degree of $N_1 D_2 - D_1 N_2$ is at most $p+q$ and thus $N_1(z)D_2(z)$ is identical to $D_1(z)N_2(z)$. N and D can have a common factor. In particular if z^k is a factor of D, it is also a factor of N, as can be seen from the previous system, and thus $N(z)/D(z)$ cannot have a pole at the origin. Dividing by the highest power k in z contained in D, gives a solution with $D(0) \neq 0$ and

degree $N \leq p - k$,
degree $D \leq q - k$,
$N(z) - f(z)D(z) = O(z^{p+q+1-k})$,

and we have

THEOREM 2.1. *Let $R(z) = N(z)/D(z)$ be an irreducible rational function with*

degree $N = p - k$,
degree $D = q - k$,
$N(z) - f(z)D(z) = O(z^{p+q+1-k})$ $(k \geq 0)$.

Then for $i, j = 0, \ldots, k$

$$[p - k + i/q - k + j]_f(z) \equiv R(z)$$

and no other Padé approximant is identical to R if k is maximum.

PROOF (WALL [1948]). For $i, j = 0, \ldots, k$ we have

$$(p - k + i) + (q - k + j) + 1 \leqslant p + q + 1.$$

Thus the result follows from the definition of Padé approximants and their uniqueness. This identity between Padé approximants can hold for all i and j (see Property 3.4) and, in that case, f is a rational function with a numerator of degree $p - k$ and a denominator of degree $q - k$ or there may be a largest k for which it holds and, in that case, no other Padé approximant is identical to R. □

Usually the Padé approximants are arranged in a double entry table known as the Padé table

[0/0] [0/1] [0/2] ...
[1/0] [1/1] [1/2] ...
[2/0] [2/1] [2/2] ...
  ⋮   ⋮   ⋮   ⋱

Theorem 2.1, which was proved by Henri Padé in 1892 (see PADÉ [1984]), shows that identical Padé approximants can only occur in square blocks of the table, a property known as the block structure of the Padé table. If the Padé table does not contain blocks, it is said to be normal, otherwise it is called nonnormal. This block structure corresponds in fact to the block structure of the table of formal orthogonal polynomials (see Section 4) which itself mimics the block structure of the table of Hankel determinants (see Section 5). On these questions see GRAGG [1972], DE BRUIN and VAN ROSSUM [1975] and GILEWICZ [1978]. Other algebraic properties of Padé approximants will be given in Section 3.

Let us now come to the second approach to the subject. Let c be the linear functional on the space of complex polynomials defined by

$$c(x^i) = c_i.$$

The functional c can be extended to the space of formal power series, thus leading to formal (that is term-by-term) identities. Our second approach is based on the following obvious formal identity which is given as a theorem since it is fundamental.

THEOREM 2.2.

$$f(z) = c\left(\frac{1}{1 - xz}\right).$$

PROOF.

$$\begin{aligned}c((1-xz)^{-1}) &= c(1+xz+x^2z^2+\cdots)\\ &= c(1)+c(x)z+c(x^2)z^2+\cdots\\ &= c_0+c_1z+c_2z^2+\cdots\\ &= f(z).\end{aligned}$$ □

The problem of approximating $f(z)$ is classical in numerical analysis. For example if an approximation of

$$I = \int_a^b g(x)w(x)\,dx$$

is wanted, one can replace $g(x)$ by an interpolation polynomial and integrate it. This procedure leads to a so-called interpolatory quadrature formula which is exact on the space of polynomials of degree at most $k-1$ if k interpolation points are used. If these interpolation points are the zeros of the polynomial of degree k belonging to the family of orthogonal polynomials on $[a,b]$ with respect to w, the quadrature formula, called a Gaussian quadrature formula, becomes exact on the space of polynomials of degree at most $2k-1$ (instead of $k-1$). Thus, in order to obtain an approximation of $f(z)$, let us replace $1/(1-xz)$ by its (Hermite) interpolation polynomial and then apply the functional c (which is analogous to integration). We have

THEOREM 2.3. *Let $v_k(x) = (x-x_1)^{k_1}\cdots(x-x_n)^{k_n}$ where $x_1,\ldots,x_n$ are distinct points in the complex plane and $k = k_1+\cdots+k_n$. The polynomial*

$$R_k(x) = \frac{1}{1-xz}\left(1-\frac{v_k(x)}{v_k(z^{-1})}\right)$$

is the Hermite interpolation polynomial of degree $k-1$ of $(1-xz)^{-1}$, that is the polynomial such that

$$R_k^{(j)}(x_i) = \left.\frac{d^j}{dx^j}(1-xz)^{-1}\right|_{x=x_i}$$

for $i=1,\ldots,n$ and $j=0,\ldots,k_i-1$.

PROOF. Let us first prove that R_k is a polynomial of degree exactly $k-1$ in x. We set

$$v_k(x) = a_0+\cdots+a_kx^k,\quad\text{where } a_k\neq 0.$$

Then

$$\begin{aligned}v_k(z^{-1})-v_k(x) &= a_1(z^{-1}-x)+\cdots+a_k(z^{-k}-x^k)\\ &= a_1z^{-1}(1-xz)+\cdots+a_kz^{-k}(1-x^kz^k).\end{aligned}$$

Thus

$$\frac{v_k(z^{-1}) - v_k(x)}{1 - xz} = a_1 z^{-1} + a_2 z^{-2}(1 + xz) + \cdots + a_k z^{-k}(1 + xz + \cdots + x^{k-1} z^{k-1})$$

which shows that R_k is a polynomial of degree $k - 1$ in x since $a_k \neq 0$.

Let us now prove that R_k satisfies the interpolation conditions stated in the theorem. We have

$$R_k^{(j)}(x) = \frac{d^j}{dx^j}(1 - xz)^{-1} - \frac{1}{v_k(z^{-1})} \frac{d^j}{dx^j} v_k(x)(1 - xz)^{-1}.$$

Since $v_k^{(j)}(x_i) = 0$ for $i = 1, \ldots, n$ and $j = 0, \ldots, k_i - 1$ then

$$\frac{d^j}{dx^j}\left(\frac{v_k(x)}{1 - xz}\right)_{x = x_i} = 0$$

and the result follows. □

The proof of this result was given by BREZINSKI [1983a]. Let us now apply the functional c to R_k in order to obtain an approximation of $f(z)$. We have

$$c(R_k(x)) = \frac{1}{v_k(z^{-1})} c\left(\frac{v_k(z^{-1}) - v_k(x)}{1 - xz}\right).$$

Setting

$$w_k(z) = c\left(\frac{v_k(z) - v_k(x)}{z - x}\right)$$

where c acts on x and z is a parameter, it is easy to see that w_k is a polynomial of degree $k - 1$ in z and that

$$c(R_k(x)) = \tilde{w}_k(z)/\tilde{v}_k(z)$$

where $\tilde{w}_k(z) = z^{k-1} w_k(z^{-1})$ and $\tilde{v}_k(z) = z^k v_k(z^{-1})$. Thus $c(R_k(x))$ is a rational function whose numerator has degree at most $k - 1$ and whose denominator has degree at most k. Moreover

$$c(R_k(x)) = c\left(\frac{1}{1 - xz}\right) - \frac{z^k}{\tilde{v}_k(z)} c\left(\frac{v_k(x)}{1 - xz}\right)$$
$$= f(z) + O(z^k).$$

This property is quite similar to the property of interpolatory quadrature formulae to be exact on the space of polynomials of degree at most $k - 1$. thus $c(R_k(x))$ appears as a generalization of such formulae for the function $(1 - xz)^{-1}$.

Such rational functions, whose poles (the zeros of $\tilde{v}_k$) are arbitrarily chosen, are called Padé-type approximants of f. They will be denoted by $(p/q)_f(z)$. They generalize the Padé approximants of Definition 2.1; they have very interesting properties and will be studied in detail in Section 19. From the above formula for the error, we have

$$c(R_k(x)) = f(z) - \frac{z^k}{\tilde{v}_k(z)} c\left[v_k(x)\left(1 + xz + \cdots + x^{k-1}z^{k-1} + \frac{x^k z^k}{1 - xz}\right)\right].$$

The polynomial v_k, called the generating polynomial of the Padé-type approximant $(k - 1/k)$, can be arbitrarily chosen and we have k degrees of freedom (its k zeros or k among its $k + 1$ coefficients since the numerator and the denominator of a rational function are uniquely defined apart from a multiplying factor). Thus, let us take v_k such that

$$c(x^i v_k(x)) = 0 \quad \text{for } i = 0, \ldots, k - 1.$$

In that case we shall have

$$c(R_k(x)) = f(z) + O(z^{2k}).$$

But $2k = (k - 1) + k + 1$ which shows that $c(R_k(x))$ matches the original series f up to the degree of the numerator plus the degree of the denominator. Thus $c(R_k(x))$ is the Padé approximant $[k - 1/k]$ of f. It can be understood as a generalization of Gaussian quadrature formulae for the function $(1 - xz)^{-1}$ since it is exact on the space of polynomials of degree at most $2k - 1$.

The relations $c(x^i v_k(x)) = 0$ for $i = 0, \ldots, k - 1$ show that v_k is the polynomial of degree k belonging to the family of (formal) orthogonal polynomials with respect to the functional c. In that case v_k will be denoted by P_k. Thus formal orthogonal polynomials appear in a very natural way in the theory of Padé approximants. They form the basis of their algebraic study and lead to recurrence relationships for their computation. These questions will be studied in Section 6.

Moreover, by construction, we have the following error formula

$$f(z) - [k - 1/k]_f(z) = \frac{z^{2k}}{\tilde{P}_k(z)} c\left(\frac{x^k P_k(x)}{1 - xz}\right).$$

But $(P_k(x) - P_k(z^{-1}))/(1 - xz)$ is a polynomial of degree $k - 1$ in x and, due to the orthogonality relations of P_k

$$c\left(\frac{P_k(x) - P_k(z^{-1})}{1 - xz} P_k(x)\right) = 0 = c\left(\frac{P_k^2(x)}{1 - xz}\right) - P_k(z^{-1}) c\left(\frac{P_k(x)}{1 - xz}\right)$$

and thus

$$f(z) - [k - 1/k]_f(z) = \frac{z^{2k}}{\tilde{P}_k^2(z)} c\left(\frac{P_k^2(x)}{1 - xz}\right).$$

These expressions will be useful later for estimating the error in Padé approximation (Section 9). It is easy to see that

$$f(z) - [k-1/k]_f(z) = \frac{z^{2k}}{\tilde{P}_k(z)} \sum_{i=0}^{\infty} d_{i+k} z^i$$

with $d_i = c(x^i P_k(x)) = b_0 c_i + b_1 c_{i+1} + \cdots + b_k c_{i+k}$ and $P_k(x) = b_0 + \cdots + b_k x^k$.
Obviously, by the orthogonality property of P_k, $d_i = 0$ for $i = 0, \ldots, k-1$.

3. Algebraic properties

In this section we shall give some algebraic properties of Padé approximants. The first one is a determinantal formula which was obtained by Jacobi in 1846 using a determinantal formula due to Cauchy for interpolating rational functions. We set

$$f_k(z) = \sum_{i=0}^{k} c_i z^i \quad \text{for } k \geq 0$$
$$= 0 \quad \text{for } k < 0.$$

Then, it follows that

$$[p/q]_f(z) = \frac{\begin{vmatrix} z^q f_{p-q}(z) & z^{q-1} f_{p-q+1}(z) & \cdots & f_p(z) \\ c_{p-q+1} & c_{p-q+2} & \cdots & c_{p+1} \\ \vdots & \vdots & & \vdots \\ c_p & c_{p+1} & \cdots & c_{p+q} \end{vmatrix}}{\begin{vmatrix} z^q & z^{q-1} & \cdots & 1 \\ c_{p-q+1} & c_{p-q+2} & \cdots & c_{p+1} \\ \vdots & \vdots & & \vdots \\ c_p & c_{p+1} & \cdots & c_{p+q} \end{vmatrix}}.$$

Let us now assume that $f(0) = c_0 \neq 0$ and let g, the reciprocal series of f, be formally defined by

$$f(z)g(z) = 1.$$

Setting $g(z) = d_0 + d_1 z + d_2 z^2 + \cdots$ we have

$$c_0 d_0 = 1$$
$$c_0 d_i + c_1 d_{i-1} + \cdots + c_i d_0 = 0, \quad i \geq 1.$$

Then we have

PROPERTY 3.1. $\forall p, q, \; [p/q]_f(z)[q/p]_g(z) = 1$.

PROOF. Let us set $[p/q]_f(z) = N(z)/D(z)$. Then, by definition

$$N(z) - D(z)f(z) = O(z^{p+q+1}).$$

Multiplying both sides by $g(z)$ and using the definition of g, we obtain

$$g(z)N(z) - D(z) = O(z^{p+q+1})$$

since $d_0 \neq 0$, which shows that $D(z)/N(z) = [q/p]_g(z)$ by the uniqueness of Padé approximants and the result follows. □

This property is very useful since it relates the two halves of the Padé table. The other algebraic properties deal with transformations on the variable and on the series. They have been gathered in the two following properties.

PROPERTY 3.2.
   (i) Let $g(z) = f(az)$, $a \neq 0$. Then $[p/q]_g(z) = [p/q]_f(az)$.
   (ii) Let $g(z) = f(z^k)$, $k > 0$. Then, $\forall i, j$ such that $i + j \leq k - 1$, $[pk + i/qk + j]_g(z) = [p/q]_f(z^k)$.
   (iii) Let $T(z) = Az^k/R(z)$, $A \neq 0$ and R being a polynomial of degree $k > 0$ such that $R(0) \neq 0$. Let $g(z) = f(T(z))$. Then, $\forall i, j$ such that $i + j \leq k - 1$, $[pk + i/qk + j]_g(z) = [p/q]_f(T(z))$.

PROOF.
   (i) This is obvious.
   (ii) Let us set $[p/q]_f(z) = N(z)/D(z)$. Then

$$f(z^k)D(z^k) - N(z^k) = g(z)D(z^k) - N(z^k)$$
$$= O((z^k)^{p+q+1}) = O(z^{pk+qk+k}).$$

But $D(z^k)$ has the degree qk in z and $N(z^k)$ has the degree pk and the result follows from Theorem 2.1.
   (iii) This property is due to LUBINSKY [1980]. Its proof is quite tedious and it will not be given here. □

PROPERTY 3.3.
   (i) Let $g(z) = z^k f(z)$. Then $[p + k/q]_g(z) = z^k [p/q]_f(z)$.
   (ii) If $c_0 = \cdots = c_{k-1} = 0$ and $c_k \neq 0$ and if we set $g(z) = z^{-k} f(z)$ then $[p/q]_g(z) = z^{-k}[p + k/q]_f(z)$.
   (iii) Let R be a polynomial of degree k. If $p \geq q + k$ then $[p/q]_{f+R}(z) = [p/q]_f(z) + R(z)$.
   (iv) Let $g(z) = [A + Bf(z)]/[C + Df(z)]$ with $C + Dc_0 \neq 0$. Then

$$[p/p]_g(z) = \frac{A + B[p/p]_f(z)}{C + D[p/p]_f(z)}.$$

   (v) Let $g(z) = af(z)$, $a \neq 0$. Then $[p/q]_g(z) = a[p/q]_f(z)$.

PROOF.
(i) We set $[p/q]_z(z) = N(z)/D(z)$. Thus

$$z^k N(z) - z^k f(z)D(z) = O(z^{k+p+q+1})$$

which shows that $z^k N(z)/D(z)$ is the Padé approximant $[k + p/q]$ of the series g.

(ii) Since $f(z) = z^k g(z)$ the preceding property gives the result.

(iii) We set $[p/q]_f(z) = N(z)/D(z)$. Thus

$$\frac{N(z)}{D(z)} + R(z) = \frac{N(z) + R(z)D(z)}{D(z)} = f(z) + R(z) + O(z^{p+q+1}).$$

If $p \geq q + k$, then the degree of the numerator is less than or equal to p and the result follows from the uniqueness of Padé approximants.

(iv) We set $[p/p]_f(z) = N(z)/D(z)$. Then

$$\frac{A + B[p/p]_f(z)}{C + D[p/p]_f(z)} = \frac{AD(z) + BN(z)}{CD(z) + DN(z)}$$

$$= \frac{AD(z) + BD(z)[f(z) + O(z^{2p+1})]}{CD(z) + DD(z)[f(z) + O(z^{2p+1})]}$$

$$= \frac{A + Bf(z) + O(z^{2p+1})}{C + Df(z) + O(z^{2p+1})}$$

$$= \frac{A + Bf(z)}{C + Df(z)} + O(z^{2p+1})$$

if the constant term of the denominator, $C + Dc_0$, is different from zero and the result again follows from the uniqueness of the approximant.

(v) Obvious. □

An important property is that of consistency.

PROPERTY 3.4. *Let f be the power series expansion of a rational function with a numerator of degree p and a denominator of degree q. Then $\forall i, j \geq 0$, $[p + i/q + j]_f(z) \equiv f(z)$.*

PROOF. Let us write f as $f(z) = N(z)/D(z)$. Then $\forall i, j \geq 0$, we have

$$N(z)/D(z) = f(z) + O(z^{p+i+q+j+1})$$

which shows, by the uniqueness of the approximant, that

$$N(z)/D(z) = [p + i/q + j]_f(z). \qquad \square$$

A useful formula is the so-called Nuttall's compact formula, obtained by NUTTALL [1967]. A generalization of it is

PROPERTY 3.5. *Let $\{q_n\}$ be an arbitrary family of polynomials such that $\forall n$, q_n has the exact degree n. Let V be the $k \times k$ matrix with elements $v_{ij} = c((1 - xz)q_{i-1}(x)q_{j-1}(x))$ for $i, j = 1, \ldots, k$, let v' be the vector with components $v'_i = c(q_{i-1}(x)(1 - v_k(x)/v_k(z^{-1})))$ for $i = 1, \ldots, k$ and let u be the vector with components $u_i = c(q_{i-1}(x))$ for $i = 1, \ldots, k$. Then*

$$(k - 1/k)_f(z) = (u, V^{-1}v')$$

where v_k is the generating polynomial of $(k - 1/k)$. If $v_k \equiv P_k$ then

$$[k - 1/k]_f(z) = (u, V^{-1}v').$$

PROOF. From Theorem 2.3, we know that R_k is a polynomial of degree $k - 1$. Thus we have

$$\frac{1}{v_k(z^{-1})} \frac{v_k(z^{-1}) - v_k(x)}{1 - xz} = \beta_0 q_0(x) + \cdots + \beta_{k-1} q_{k-1}(x)$$

and it follows that

$$(k - 1/k)_f(z) = \beta_0 c(q_0) + \cdots + \beta_{k-1} c(q_{k-1}).$$

For $i = 0, \ldots, k - 1$ we have

$$c[q_i(x)(1 - v_k(x)/v_k(z^{-1}))] = c[q_i(x)(1 - xz)(\beta_0 q_0(x) + \cdots + \beta_{k-1} q_{k-1}(x))]$$

which is equivalent to the formulae of the property. □

If $q_n(x) = x^n$, then $v_{ij} = c_{i+j-2} - zc_{i+j-1}$, $u_i = c_{i-1}$ and the formula for $[k-1/k]$ exactly reduces to Nuttall's. Since $(k - 1/k)$ only depends on $c_0, \ldots, c_{k-1}$ then, in the preceding formula, $c_k, \ldots, c_{2k-1}$ can be arbitrarily chosen. In particular they can be set to zero. If $q_n(x) = P_n(x)$, the preceding extension of Nuttall's formula is closely related to the matrix interpretation of Padé approximants, see GRAGG [1972].

4. Formal orthogonal polynomials

As seen in Section 2, Padé approximants are based on formal orthogonal polynomials. Thus we shall now open a parenthesis to treat this subject. The other approximants of the table are related to other families of orthogonal polynomials, called adjacent families of orthogonal polynomials, which will be studied in Section 5.

Let c be the linear functional on the space of complex polynomials defined by its moments c_i

$$c(x^i) = c_i, \quad i \geqslant 0.$$

Let $\{P_k\}$ be a family of polynomials. $\{P_k\}$ is said to be the family of formal orthogonal polynomials with respect to c if, $\forall k \geq 0$,
  (i) P_k has the exact degree k,
  (ii) $c(x^i P_k(x)) = 0$ for $i = 0, \ldots, k-1$.
(ii) are the so-called orthogonality relations. They are equivalent to

$$c(p(x)P_k(x)) = 0$$

for any polynomial p of degree at most $k-1$ or to

$$c(P_n(x)P_k(x)) = 0 \quad \forall n \neq k.$$

The usual orthogonal polynomials (that is those orthogonal with respect to $c(\cdot) = \int_a^b \cdot \, d\alpha(x)$ with α bounded and nondecreasing in $[a,b]$) are known to satisfy a group of interesting properties such as a three-term recurrence relationship, the Christoffel–Darboux identity, properties of their zeros, ... We shall see that most of these properties still hold for formal orthogonal polynomials. However, in that case, the first question is that of existence. Let us write P_k as

$$P_k(x) = a_0 + a_1 x + \cdots + a_k x^k.$$

Then the orthogonality relations are equivalent to the system

$$a_0 c_i + a_1 c_{i+1} + \cdots + a_k c_{i+k} = 0, \quad i = 0, \ldots, k-1.$$

Since P_k must have the exact degree k, a_k must be different from zero or, in other words, the Hankel determinant

$$H_k^{(0)} = \begin{vmatrix} c_0 & \cdots & c_{k-1} \\ c_1 & \cdots & c_k \\ \vdots & & \vdots \\ c_{k-1} & \cdots & c_{2k-2} \end{vmatrix}$$

must not vanish. Thus, in the sequel, we shall assume that $\forall k > 0$, $H_k^{(0)} \neq 0$. In that case, we shall say that the functional c is definite, a property clearly related to the normality of the Padé table. The case when the functional c is nondefinite has been extensively studied by DRAUX [1983].

In the definite case, the polynomial P_k is uniquely determined apart from an arbitrary nonzero constant. Moreover we have the following determinantal formula

$$P_k(x) = D_k \begin{vmatrix} c_0 & c_1 & \cdots & c_k \\ c_1 & c_2 & \cdots & c_{k+1} \\ \vdots & \vdots & & \vdots \\ c_{k-1} & c_k & \cdots & c_{2k-1} \\ 1 & x & \cdots & x^k \end{vmatrix}$$

with $D_k \neq 0$ and $P_0(x) = D_0$. Let us set $P_k(x) = t_k x^k + s_k x^{k-1} + \cdots$. For a family of formal orthogonal polynomials we have

THEOREM 4.1. $\forall k \geq 0$

$$P_{k+1}(x) = (A_{k+1}x + B_{k+1})P_k(x) - C_{k+1}P_{k-1}(x)$$

with $P_{-1}(x) = 0, P_0(x) = t_0$,

$$A_{k+1} = t_{k+1}/t_k, \quad B_{k+1} = -\frac{\alpha_k t_{k+1}}{h_k t_k}, \quad C_{k+1} = \frac{t_{k-1}t_{k+1}}{t_k^2} \frac{h_k}{h_{k-1}}$$

$$\alpha_k = c(xP_k^2(x)), \quad h_k = c(P_k^2(x)).$$

Since P_k is determined apart from a multiplying factor, the t_k's in the preceding recurrence relationship can be arbitrarily chosen and thus this relation can be used to compute the P_k's recursively. In particular the choice $t_k = 1$ leads to monic orthogonal polynomials.

The reciprocal of this theorem was first proved by FAVARD [1935] for classical orthogonal polynomials. It was extended by SHOHAT [1938] (see also VAN ROSSUM [1953]) to the formal case.

THEOREM 4.2. *Let $\{P_k\}$ be a family of polynomials such that the relation of Theorem 4.1 holds with $t_0 \neq 0$ and $\forall k, A_k C_k \neq 0$. Then $\{P_k\}$ is a family of formal orthogonal polynomials with respect to a linear functional c whose moments c_i can be computed.*

A consequence of Theorem 4.1 is the so-called Christoffel–Darboux identity

THEOREM 4.3. $\forall k \geq 0$

$$\frac{t_k}{h_k t_{k+1}}[P_{k+1}(x)P_k(t) - P_{k+1}(t)P_k(x)] = (x-t)\sum_{i=0}^{k} h_i^{-1} P_i(x)P_i(t).$$

Usually this identity is proved using the three-term recurrence relationship. However, a direct proof of it was recently found by BREZINSKI [1990b] who also showed that if a family of polynomials satisfies a relation of the same form as the Christoffel–Darboux identity then it also satisfies a three-term recurrence relationship, which means, by the extension of Favard's theorem, that it is a family of formal orthogonal polynomials. Thus the Christoffel–Darboux identity and the three-term recurrence relationship are completely equivalent. They are both characterizations of orthogonal polynomials.

Let us now define the associated polynomials Q_k by

$$Q_k(z) = c\left(\frac{P_k(x) - P_k(z)}{x - z}\right)$$

where c acts on x and where z is a parameter. It is easy to see that Q_k is a polynomial of degree $k-1$ in z and that

$$Q_k(z) = D_k \begin{vmatrix} c_0 & c_1 & c_2 & \cdots & c_k \\ \vdots & \vdots & \vdots & & \vdots \\ c_{k-1} & c_k & c_{k+1} & \cdots & c_{2k-1} \\ 0 & c_0 & c_0 z + c_1 & \cdots & (c_0 z^{k-1} + c_1 z^{k-2} + \cdots + c_{k-1}) \end{vmatrix},$$

for $k > 1$, and $Q_0(z) = 0$.

THEOREM 4.4. *The family $\{Q_k\}$ satisfies the three-term recurrence relationship of Theorem 4.1 with $Q_{-1}(x) = -1, Q_0(x) = 0$ and $C_1 = A_1 c(P_0(x))$, and the Christoffel–Darboux identity. Moreover, $\forall k \geqslant 0$.*

$$P_k(x) Q_{k+1}(x) - Q_k(x) P_{k+1}(x) = A_{k+1} h_k.$$

Some other relations satisfied by the P_k's and the Q_k's are given in the definite case by BREZINSKI [1980, Chapter 2]. They are

THEOREM 4.5. $\forall k \geqslant 0$

$$1 + \frac{t_k}{h_k t_{k+1}} [P_{k+1}(x) Q_k(t) - Q_{k+1}(t) P_k(x)] = (x-t) \sum_{i=0}^{k} h_i^{-1} P_i(x) Q_i(t),$$

$$Q_k(x) P'_{k+1}(x) - Q_{k+1}(x) P'_k(x) = A_{k+1} h_k \sum_{i=0}^{k} h_i^{-1} P_i(x) Q_i(x),$$

$$P_k(x) Q'_{k+1}(x) - P_{k+1}(x) Q'_k(x) = A_{k+1} h_k \sum_{i=0}^{k} h_i^{-1} P_i(x) Q_i(x).$$

From these relations we have

$$A_1 \cdots A_k c(x^k P_k(x)) = h_k,$$
$$A_{k+1} h_k = C_1 \cdots C_{k+1},$$
$$c(x^{k+1} P_k(x)) = -[B_2 A_2^{-1} + \cdots + B_{k+1} A_{k+1}^{-1}] c(x^k P_k(x))$$

which can be useful in the implementation of the recurrence relationship.

The first relation of Theorem 4.5 generalizes that of Theorem 4.4 which is recovered for $x = t$. The last two relations imply

$$(Q_k(x) P_{k+1}(x))' = (P_k(x) Q_{k+1}(x))',$$

that is $Q_k(x) P_{k+1}(x) - P_k(x) Q_{k+1}(x)$ equals a constant which can be found to be equal to $-A_{k+1} h_k$, thus giving the relation of Theorem 4.4. It follows that

$$[k/k+1]_f(z) = [k-1/k]_f(z) + \frac{A_{k+1} h_k}{\tilde{P}_k(z) \tilde{P}_{k+1}(z)} z^{2k},$$

a relation known as the Euler–Minding identity and which follows directly from the theory of continued fractions (see Section 8).

These relations were extended to the nondefinite case by DRAUX [1983].

The zeros of the classical orthogonal polynomials are known to have certain properties. Not all of these properties extend to the formal case. In particular the zeros of formal orthogonal polynomials need not be simple or real. However, we have

THEOREM 4.6. *If c is definite, then $\forall k \geq 0$*
  (i) P_k *and* P_{k+1} *have no common zero,*
  (ii) Q_k *and* Q_{k+1} *have no common zero,*
  (iii) P_k *and* Q_k *have no common zero.*

PROOF. Let x be a common zero of P_k and P_{k+1}. Then, in the relation of Theorem 4.4, the left-hand side is zero while the right-hand side is different from zero. Thus P_k and P_{k+1} cannot have a common zero. The same result can be proved similarly for Q_k and Q_{k+1} and for P_k and Q_k. □

To end this section let us mention that a matrix formalism of orthogonality can be given via tridiagonal matrices. Orthogonal polynomials are known to play an important rôle in numerical analysis. In particular they are closely connected with projection methods used in the theory of linear operators, for example with the method of moments, Lanczos' method and the conjugate gradient method. All these connections were reviewed by BREZINSKI [1980, Section 2.7].

The notion of orthogonality studied in this section is a particular case of the more general notion of biorthogonality between a family of elements of a vector space and a family of elements of its dual. The notion of biorthogonality is extensively studied in BREZINSKI [1991a].

5. Adjacent families of orthogonal polynomials

Let us now define the linear functionals $c^{(n)}$ by

$$c^{(n)}(x^i) = c_{n+i}.$$

With the same convention as above, namely that $c_i = 0$ for $i < 0$, these linear functionals $c^{(n)}$ can be defined even for negative values of the upper index n. Let us denote by $\{P_k^{(n)}\}$ the family of formal orthogonal polynomials with respect to $c^{(n)}$. The family $\{P_k^{(n)}\}$ studied in Section 4 corresponds to $n = 0$. Such families are called adjacent families of orthogonal polynomials. For such families the same properties as above hold by replacing c by $c^{(n)}$ or, in other words, the sequence $c_0, c_1, \ldots$ by the sequence $c_n, c_{n+1}, \ldots$. In particular $\{P_k^{(n)}\}$ exists only if $\forall k, n$

$$H_k^{(n)} = \begin{vmatrix} c_n & \cdots & c_{n+k-1} \\ \vdots & & \vdots \\ c_{n+k-1} & \cdots & c_{n+2k-2} \end{vmatrix} \neq 0.$$

In that case we shall say that the linear functional c is completely definite. For the noncompletely definite case we again refer the interested reader to DRAUX [1983].

The polynomials $P_k^{(n)}$ are usually placed in a double-entry table similar to the Padé table

$$
\begin{array}{cccc}
P_{-1}^{(0)} & P_0^{(-1)} & P_1^{(-2)} & P_2^{(-3)} \cdots \\
P_{-1}^{(1)} & P_0^{(0)} & P_1^{(-1)} & P_2^{(-2)} \cdots \\
P_{-1}^{(2)} & P_0^{(1)} & P_1^{(0)} & P_2^{(-1)} \cdots \\
P_{-1}^{(3)} & P_0^{(2)} & P_1^{(1)} & P_2^{(0)} \cdots \\
\vdots & \vdots & \vdots & \vdots & \ddots
\end{array}
$$

Many relationships exist between adjacent polynomials of this table. First of all, each family of orthogonal polynomials satisfies a three-term recurrence relation similar to that of Theorem 4.1. Assuming all the polynomials to be monic we shall write this relation as

$$P_{-1}^{(n)}(x) = 0, \qquad P_0^{(n)}(x) = 1,$$

$$\begin{array}{c} \bullet \\ \bullet \\ * \end{array}$$

$$P_{k+1}^{(n)}(x) = (x - q_{k+1}^{(n)} - e_k^{(n)})P_k^{(n)}(x) - q_k^{(n)}e_k^{(n)}P_{k-1}^{(n)}(x).$$

The • indicates the position of the polynomials which are known in the table, while the ∗ indicates the position of the polynomial which is computed by the relation.

We also have

$$P_k^{(n+1)}(x) = P_k^{(n)}(x) - e_k^{(n)}P_{k-1}^{(n+1)}(x),$$

$$\begin{array}{cc} \bullet & \bullet \\ & * \end{array}$$

$$P_{k+1}^{(n)}(x) = xP_k^{(n+1)}(x) - q_{k+1}^{(n)}P_k^{(n)}(x).$$

$$\begin{array}{cc} & \bullet \\ \bullet & * \end{array}$$

Using these two relations alternately, allows us to compute recursively the two adjacent families $\{P_k^{(n)}\}$ and $\{P_k^{(n+1)}\}$. It can be proved (see, for example, BREZINSKI [1980, Section 2.8] where all these relations and the following ones are given) that the numbers $e_k^{(n)}$ and $q_k^{(n)}$ are related by

$$e_0^{(n)} = 0, \qquad q_1^{(n)} = c_{n+1}/c_n,$$
$$q_{k+1}^{(n)} + e_{k+1}^{(n)} = q_{k+1}^{(n+1)} + e_k^{(n+1)},$$
$$e_k^{(n)}q_{k+1}^{(n)} = e_k^{(n+1)}q_k^{(n+1)}$$

which is the so-called qd-algorithm. This algorithm can be used for their recursive computation. It is due to RUTISHAUSER [1954] (see also HENRICI [1974]) and was the basis for the development of the LR-algorithm for the computation of the eigenvalues of a matrix. Setting $x = 0$ in the preceding relations, it is easy to see that

$$q_k^{(n)} = H_k^{(n+1)} H_{k-1}^{(n)} / H_k^{(n)} H_{k-1}^{(n+1)},$$
$$e_k^{(n)} = H_{k-1}^{(n+1)} H_{k+1}^{(n)} / H_k^{(n)} H_k^{(n+1)}.$$

From these determinantal expressions and from the three preceding relations we can obtain the following ones

$$H_k^{(n+2)} H_k^{(n)} P_k^{(n)}(x) = [H_k^{(n+1)}]^2 P_k^{(n+1)}(x) + H_{k+1}^{(n)} H_{k-1}^{(n+2)} P_{k-1}^{(n+2)}(x), \qquad \substack{* \\ \bullet \ \bullet}$$

$$H_k^{(n+1)} H_{k+1}^{(n-1)} P_{k+1}^{(n-1)}(x) = x H_{k+1}^{(n-1)} H_k^{(n+1)} P_k^{(n+1)}(x) - H_{k+1}^{(n)} H_k^{(n)} P_k^{(n)}(x), \qquad \substack{\bullet \\ \bullet \\ *}$$

$$x H_k^{(n)} H_{k+1}^{(n-1)} H_k^{(n+1)} P_k^{(n+1)}(x)$$
$$= [x H_k^{(n+1)} H_{k+1}^{(n-1)} + H_{k+1}^{(n)} H_k^{(n)}] H_k^{(n)} P_k^{(n)}(x) \qquad \substack{\bullet \\ \bullet \\ *}$$
$$- H_{k+1}^{(n)} H_k^{(n+1)} H_k^{(n-1)} P_k^{(n-1)}(x),$$

$$H_k^{(n)} H_k^{(n+1)} H_{k+1}^{(n-1)} P_{k+1}^{(n-1)}(x)$$
$$= [x H_{k+1}^{(n-1)} H_k^{(n+1)} - H_k^{(n)} H_{k+1}^{(n)}] H_k^{(n)} P_k^{(n)}(x) \qquad \substack{\bullet \ \bullet \ *}$$
$$- x H_{k+1}^{(n-1)} H_{k+1}^{(n)} H_{k-1}^{(n+1)} P_{k-1}^{(n+1)}(x).$$

Combining these relations leads to many new ones. However, the preceding eight relations are sufficient to follow any path in the table of the adjacent families of orthogonal polynomials. Of course, similar relations hold among the associated polynomials

$$Q_k^{(n)}(z) = c^{(n)} \left(\frac{P_k^{(n)}(x) - P_k^{(n)}(z)}{x - z} \right).$$

Let us end this section by a result on the zeros of adjacent families of orthogonal polynomials. We have

THEOREM 5.1. $\forall k, n$, $P_k^{(n)}$ has no common zero with $P_k^{(n+1)}$, $P_{k-1}^{(n+1)}$, $P_k^{(n-1)}$ and $P_{k+1}^{(n-1)}$. Moreover $P_k^{(n)}(0) \neq 0$.

PROOF. From the above relations between adjacent orthogonal polynomials we see, for example, that if x is a common zero of $P_k^{(n)}$ and $P_k^{(n+1)}$ then it is also a zero of $P_{k+1}^{(n)}$, which is impossible by Theorem 4.6. Similar proofs can be given for the other pairs of polynomials. Moreover if 0 is a zero of $P_k^{(n)}$ then

$$P_{k+1}^{(n)}(0) = 0 \cdot P_k^{(n+1)}(0) - q_{k+1}^{(n)} P_k^{(n)}(0) = 0$$

which again is impossible by Theorem 4.6. □

6. Recursive computation of Padé approximants

Let us first relate all the approximants of the Padé table to the adjacent families of orthogonal polynomials defined in Section 5. Thus the recurrence relations given there will provide recursive methods for computing any sequence of Padé approximants.

In Section 2, we saw that

$$[k-1/k]_f(z) = \tilde{Q}_k^{(0)}(z)/\tilde{P}_k^{(0)}(z).$$

Making use of the convention that a sum with a negative upper index is equal to zero, it is easy to see that we have

THEOREM 6.1. $\forall k \geqslant 0, \forall n \geqslant -k$

$$[n+k/k]_f(z) = \sum_{i=0}^{n} c_i z^i + z^{n+1} \tilde{Q}_k^{(n+1)}(z)/\tilde{P}_k^{(n+1)}(z)$$

with $\tilde{P}_k^{(n+1)}(z) = z^k P_k^{(n+1)}(z^{-1})$ and $\tilde{Q}_k^{(n+1)}(z) = z^{k-1} Q_k^{(n+1)}(z^{-1})$.

PROOF. For $n \geqslant -1$, we set

$$f_n(z) = c_{n+1} + c_{n+2}z + \cdots.$$

We already know, from Section 2, that

$$\tilde{Q}_k^{(n+1)}(z)/\tilde{P}_k^{(n+1)}(z) = [k-1/k]_{f_n}(z) = f_n(z) + O(z^{2k}).$$

Thus

$$\sum_{i=0}^{n} c_i z^i + z^{n+1} \tilde{Q}_k^{(n+1)}(z)/\tilde{P}_k^{(n+1)}(z) = \sum_{i=0}^{n} c_i z^i + z^{n+1} f_n(z) + O(z^{n+2k+1})$$
$$= f(z) + O(z^{n+2k+1})$$

and the result follows from the uniqueness of Padé approximants since $n + 2k = (n+k) + k$.

With the convention that $c_i = 0$ if $i < 0$, the result also holds when $n < -1$. □

Let us set

$$[n+k/k]_f(z) = \tilde{N}_k^{(n+1)}(z)/\tilde{P}_k^{(n+1)}(z)$$

and

$$\tilde{P}_k^{(n)}(z) = \sum_{i=0}^{k} b_i^{(k,n)} z^i,$$

$$\tilde{N}_k^{(n)}(z) = \sum_{i=0}^{n+k-1} a_i^{(k,n)} z^i.$$

The relations of Section 5 give

$$\frac{\tilde{N}^{(n)}_{k+1}(z)}{\tilde{P}^{(n)}_{k+1}(z)} = \frac{a^{(k,n+1)}_{n+k}\tilde{N}^{(n+2)}_{k}(z) - za^{(k,n+2)}_{n+k+1}\tilde{N}^{(n+1)}_{k}(z)}{a^{(k,n+1)}_{n+k}\tilde{P}^{(n+2)}_{k}(z) - za^{(k,n+2)}_{n+k+1}\tilde{P}^{(n+1)}_{k}(z)},$$

• *
•

$$\frac{\tilde{N}^{(n)}_{k}(z)}{\tilde{P}^{(n)}_{k}(z)} = \frac{a^{(k-1,n+2)}_{n+k}\tilde{N}^{(n+1)}_{k}(z) - a^{(k,n+1)}_{n+k}\tilde{N}^{(n+2)}_{k-1}(z)}{a^{(k-1,n+2)}_{n+k}\tilde{P}^{(n+1)}_{k}(z) - a^{(k,n+1)}_{n+k}\tilde{P}^{(n+2)}_{k-1}(z)}.$$

*
• •

These two relations are identical with a method due to LONGMAN [1971] to compute recursively approximants located on an ascending staircase of the Padé table. They also cover an algorithm due to BAKER [1970].

We have

$$\frac{\tilde{N}^{(n+1)}_{k}(z)}{\tilde{P}^{(n+1)}_{k}(z)} = \frac{\tilde{N}^{(n)}_{k}(z) - e^{(n)}_{k}z\tilde{N}^{(n+1)}_{k-1}(z)}{\tilde{P}^{(n)}_{k}(z) - e^{(n)}_{k}z\tilde{P}^{(n+1)}_{k-1}(z)},$$

• •
*

$$\frac{\tilde{N}^{(n)}_{k+1}(z)}{\tilde{P}^{(n)}_{k+1}(z)} = \frac{\tilde{N}^{(n+1)}_{k}(z) - q^{(n)}_{k+1}z\tilde{N}^{(n)}_{k}(z)}{\tilde{P}^{(n+1)}_{k}(z) - q^{(n)}_{k+1}z\tilde{P}^{(n)}_{k}(z)},$$

•
• *

with $e^{(n)}_{k} = h^{(n)}_{k}/h^{(n+1)}_{k-1}$, $q^{(n)}_{k+1} = h^{(n+1)}_{k}/h^{(n)}_{k}$ and $h^{(n)}_{k} = c^{(n)}(P^{(n)^2}_{k}(x)) = \sum_{i=0}^{k} c_{n+k+i}b^{(k,n)}_{k-i}$. These two relations are identical to a method due to WATSON [1973] to compute recursively approximants located on a descending staircase of the Padé table.

We also have

$$\frac{\tilde{N}^{(n+2)}_{k}(z)}{\tilde{P}^{(n+2)}_{k}(z)} = \frac{b^{(k,n+1)}_{k}\tilde{N}^{(n)}_{k+1}(z) - zb^{(k+1,n)}_{k+1}\tilde{N}^{(n+1)}_{k}(z)}{b^{(k,n+1)}_{k}\tilde{P}^{(n)}_{k+1}(z) - zb^{(k+1,n)}_{k+1}\tilde{P}^{(n+1)}_{k}(z)},$$

• •
*

$$\frac{\tilde{N}^{(n+2)}_{k-1}(z)}{\tilde{P}^{(n+2)}_{k-1}(z)} = \frac{b^{(k,n+1)}_{k}\tilde{N}^{(n)}_{k}(z) - b^{(k,n)}_{k}\tilde{N}^{(n+1)}_{k}(z)}{b^{(k,n+1)}_{k}\tilde{P}^{(n)}_{k}(z) - b^{(k,n)}_{k}\tilde{P}^{(n+1)}_{k}(z)},$$

•
* •

$$\frac{\tilde{N}^{(n+1)}_{k-1}(z)}{\tilde{P}^{(n+1)}_{k-1}(z)} = \frac{\tilde{N}^{(n)}_{k}(z) - \tilde{N}^{(n+1)}_{k}(z)}{\tilde{P}^{(n)}_{k}(z) - \tilde{P}^{(n+1)}_{k}(z)},$$

* •
•

$$\frac{\tilde{N}^{(n)}_{k}(z)}{\tilde{P}^{(n)}_{k}(z)} = \frac{\tilde{N}^{(n+1)}_{k}(z) - \tilde{N}^{(n)}_{k+1}(z)}{\tilde{P}^{(n+1)}_{k}(z) - \tilde{P}^{(n)}_{k+1}(z)}.$$

*
• •

Combining these relations together allows us to obtain the relations

• • ∗   and   ∗ • •

•   ∗
    • and •
  ∗   •

•   ∗
• and   •
∗   •

Eight of these relations were used in a conversational program to compute recursively any sequence of Padé approximants in the normal case, see BREZINSKI [1980, Appendix].

All these recurrence relations were extended by DRAUX [1983] to the nonnormal case. A universal conversational program for computing any sequence of Padé approximants in the nonnormal case was given by DRAUX and VAN INGELANDT [1986]. In order to avoid numerical instability and also for the detection of the block structure of the Padé table, it was necessary to program these relations in exact arithmetic, that is in rational arithmetic coded on several words. All these programs are written in FORTRAN.

Setting for simplicity

$$[n+k/k-1] = W \quad \begin{matrix} [n+k-1/k] = N \\ [n+k/k] = C \\ [n+k+1/k] = S \end{matrix} \quad [n+k/k+1] = E$$

we obtain after elimination among the preceding identities, the so-called cross rule of WYNN [1966]

$$(N-C)^{-1} + (S-C)^{-1} = (W-C)^{-1} + (E-C)^{-1}.$$

When a square block occurs in the Padé table, this cross rule was extended by CORDELLIER [1979] who proved that

$$(N_i - C)^{-1} + (S_i - C)^{-1} = (W_i - C)^{-1} + (E_i - C)^{-1}$$

where we have

The initial values are

$$[-1/q]_f(z) = 0, \qquad [p/-1]_f(z) = \infty,$$

$$[p/0]_f(z) = \sum_{i=0}^{p} c_i z^i, \qquad [0/q]_f(z) = ([q/0]_g(z))^{-1} = \left(\sum_{i=0}^{q} d_i z^i\right)^{-1}$$

where the d_i's are the coefficients of the reciprocal series g of f.

Thus the theory of formal orthogonal polynomials provided a basis for rediscovering known recursive methods for the computation of sequences of Padé approximants which were found more or less heuristically by various authors. This theory also gave us the possibility of computing any sequence of approximants by new algorithms. It was possible to extend the theory to the nonnormal case, thus leading for the first time to all the possible recurrence relationships among the entries of a nonnormal Padé table and to write the only existing complete subroutine. As we shall see in Section 9 the theory of orthogonal polynomials will also provide us a natural basis for the extension of Kronrod's method for estimating the error in Padé approximation.

7. The ε-algorithm

We shall now deal with a subject which, a priori, has nothing to do with Padé approximation but which is, in fact, closely related to it: convergence acceleration.

Let (S_n) be a sequence converging to S. If the convergence is slow, one can try to accelerate its convergence. For that purpose we shall transform the sequence (S_n) into another sequence (T_n) such that, if possible, (T_n) converges to S faster than (S_n), that is

$$\lim_{n \to \infty} (T_n - S)/(S_n - S) = 0.$$

One of the most popular sequence transformations for that purpose is certainly Aitken's Δ^2 process which corresponds to

$$T_n = S_n - (\Delta S_n)^2 / \Delta^2 S_n, \quad n = 0, 1, \ldots.$$

If the sequence (S_n) is such that $\exists a \neq 1$, $\lim_{n \to \infty} (S_{n+1} - S)/(S_n - S) = a$ then (T_n) obtained by Aitken's process converges to S faster than (S_n).

In 1955, SHANKS [1955] gave a generalization of Aitken's process. He considered the various transformations $e_k : (S_n) \to (e_k(S_n))$ where

$$e_k(S_n) = \frac{\begin{vmatrix} S_n & \cdots & S_{n+k} \\ \vdots & & \vdots \\ S_{n+k} & \cdots & S_{n+2k} \\ \Delta^2 S_n & \cdots & \Delta^2 S_{n+k-1} \\ \vdots & & \vdots \\ \Delta^2 S_{n+k-1} & \cdots & \Delta^2 S_{n+2k-2} \end{vmatrix}}{}.$$

A recursive algorithm to compute the $e_k(S_n)$'s without computing the determinants involved in their definition was found one year later by WYNN [1956]. It is the so-called ε-algorithm whose rules are

$$\varepsilon_{-1}^{(n)} = 0, \qquad \varepsilon_0^{(n)} = S_n, \qquad n = 0, 1, \ldots,$$
$$\varepsilon_{k+1}^{(n)} = \varepsilon_{k-1}^{(n+1)} + [\varepsilon_k^{(n+1)} - \varepsilon_k^{(n)}]^{-1}, \quad n, k = 0, 1, \ldots.$$

It is related to Shanks's transformation by

$$\varepsilon_{2k}^{(n)} = e_k(S_n).$$

The $\varepsilon_{2k+1}^{(n)}$'s are only intermediate quantities. The ε-algorithm is a quite powerful acceleration process which has been widely studied. For its theory one can consult, for example, BREZINSKI [1977] and for subroutines and applications BREZINSKI [1978] and BREZINSKI and REDIVO ZAGLIA [1991]. The ε-algorithm is related to Padé approximants in the following way: if it is applied to the partial sums of the series f, that is if

$$S_n = \sum_{i=0}^{n} c_i z^i, \quad n = 0, 1, \ldots,$$

then

$$\varepsilon_{2k}^{(n)} = [n + k/k]_f(z).$$

Thus the ε-algorithm can be used to compute recursively the lower half of the Padé table. The upper half of the Padé table can be computed by applying the ε-algorithm to the partial sums of the reciprocal series g of f as stated in Property 3.1. Let us mention that the elimination of the ε's with an odd lower index leads to Wynn's cross rule mentioned in Section 6.

Since the ε-algorithm is related to Padé approximants, it is also connected with formal orthogonal polynomials. We have

$$\varepsilon_{2k}^{(n)} = S_n + Q_k^{(n+1)}(1)/P_k^{(n+1)}(1)$$

and thus the relations of Section 6 can be used for the recursive computation of these quantities. This topic was developed by BREZINSKI [1980, Section 3.3].

8. Continued fractions

Since orthogonal polynomials and continued fractions both satisfy a three-term recurrence relation, the connections between Padé approximants and continued fractions is not surprising. In fact, historically, Padé approximants were first obtained by several authors as the convergents of some continued fractions although these authors did not realize that the power series expansion of the convergent matches the original series as far as possible. An analysis of the process leading to Padé approximants, which is quite similar to the algorithm for finding the g.c.d. of two numbers, can be found in BREZINSKI [1985] and the whole history of the subject in BREZINSKI [1990c].

In this section we shall not develop this subject which has received much attention for several centuries but we shall only give the basic connections between the two topics. We shall refer the interested reader to the many books on continued fractions and, in particular, to the most recent ones by JONES AND THRON [1980], LORENTZEN and WAADELAND [1992] and PATRY [1991]. A chapter on this topic can also be found in BREZINSKI [1977].

Let us consider the monic orthogonal polynomials of Section 4 and their associated polynomials. As before, let us set

$$\tilde{P}_k(z) = z^k P_k(z^{-1}) \quad \text{and} \quad \tilde{Q}_k(z) = z^{k-1} Q_k(z^{-1}).$$

We have

$$\tilde{Q}_0(z) = 0, \quad \tilde{Q}_{-1}(z) = -1,$$
$$\tilde{P}_0(z) = 1, \quad \tilde{P}_{-1}(z) = 0,$$
$$\tilde{Q}_{k+1}(z) = (1 + B_{k+1}z)\tilde{Q}_k(z) - C_{k+1}z^2\tilde{Q}_{k-1}(z),$$
$$\tilde{P}_{k+1}(z) = (1 + B_{k+1}z)\tilde{P}_k(z) - C_{k+1}z^2\tilde{P}_{k-1}(z).$$

On the other hand let us consider the continued fraction

$$\tilde{C}(z) = \frac{C_1}{1 + B_1 z} - \frac{C_2 z^2}{1 + B_2 z} - \frac{C_3 z^2}{1 + B_3 z} - \cdots.$$

From the recurrence relations among the successive convergents of a continued fraction, we immediately see that the kth convergent $\tilde{C}_k(z)$ of this continued fraction is equal to $\tilde{Q}_k(z)/\tilde{P}_k(z)$ and thus

$$\tilde{C}_k(z) = [k-1/k]_f(z).$$

The continued fraction $\tilde{C}$ is called the continued fraction associated with the series f (or the associated continued fraction). Obviously this property can be extended to the other diagonals of the Padé table.

Let us now consider the continued fraction

$$\tilde{D}(z) = \frac{c_0}{1} - \frac{q_1^{(0)} z}{1} - \frac{e_1^{(0)} z}{1} - \frac{q_2^{(0)} z}{1} - \frac{e_2^{(0)} z}{1} - \cdots.$$

The convergents $\tilde{D}_k(z) = \tilde{V}_k(z)/\tilde{U}_k(z)$ of $\tilde{D}$ satisfy

$$\tilde{U}_{2k+1}(z) = \tilde{U}_{2k}(z) - e_k^{(0)} z^2 \tilde{U}_{2k-1}(z),$$
$$\tilde{U}_{2k+2}(z) = \tilde{U}_{2k+1}(z) - q_{k+1}^{(0)} z^2 \tilde{U}_{2k}(z)$$

with $\tilde{U}_0(z) = 1$ and $\tilde{U}_1(z) = 1$. Similar relations hold for $\tilde{V}_k$ with $\tilde{V}_0(z) = 0$ and $\tilde{V}_{-1}(z) = -1$. Thus, comparing with the relations given in Section 6, shows that

$$\tilde{D}_{2k}(z) = [k-1/k]_f(z),$$
$$\tilde{D}_{2k+1}(z) = [k/k]_f(z).$$

The continued fraction $\tilde{D}$ is called the continued fraction corresponding to the series f (or the corresponding continued fraction). The associated continued fraction can be obtained by a contraction of the corresponding continued fraction since

$$\tilde{C}_k(z) = \tilde{D}_{2k}(z).$$

The other descending staircases of the Padé table can be related to corresponding continued fractions in a similar way. For that purpose we have to consider the continued fractions

$$D^{(n)}(z) = c_0 + c_1 z + \cdots + c_n z^n + \frac{c_{n+1} z^n}{1} - \frac{q_1^{(n+1)} z}{1} - \frac{e_1^{(n+1)} z}{1} - \frac{q_2^{(n+1)} z}{1} - \cdots .$$

for $n \geq -1$. The successive convergents $D_k^{(n)}(z)$ of these continued fractions satisfy

$$D_{2k}^{(n)}(z) = [n+k/k]_f(z) = \varepsilon_{2k}^{(n)},$$
$$D_{2k+1}^{(n)}(z) = [n+k+1/k]_f(z) = \varepsilon_{2k}^{(n+1)}$$

if the ε-algorithm is applied to the partial sums of f.

Thus $D_{2k}^{(n+1)}(z)$ is identical to $D_{2k+1}^{(n)}(z)$, a connection leading to the qd-algorithm again and to the determinantal formulae for the $e_k^{(n)}$'s and $q_k^{(n)}$'s. Writing the classical relations between the convergents of a continued fraction and its elements gives

$$e_{k+1}^{(n+1)} z = \frac{\varepsilon_{2k}^{(n+1)} - \varepsilon_{2k}^{(n)}}{\varepsilon_{2k+2}^{(n)} - \varepsilon_{2k}^{(n)}} \frac{\varepsilon_{2k+2}^{(n+1)} - \varepsilon_{2k+2}^{(n)}}{\varepsilon_{2k+2}^{(n+1)} - \varepsilon_{2k}^{(n+1)}},$$

$$q_{k+1}^{(n+1)} z = \frac{\varepsilon_{2k}^{(n)} - \varepsilon_{2k-2}^{(n+1)}}{\varepsilon_{2k}^{(n+1)} - \varepsilon_{2k-2}^{(n+1)}} \frac{\varepsilon_{2k+2}^{(n)} - \varepsilon_{2k}^{(n+1)}}{\varepsilon_{2k+2}^{(n)} - \varepsilon_{2k}^{(n)}}.$$

Thus, ratios such as $q_i^{(j)}/e_k^{(n)}$ are independent of z for all i, j, k and n.

9. Error estimation

KRONROD's procedure [1965] is well known for estimating the error in Gaussian quadrature methods. Since Padé approximants can be looked at as formal Gaussian quadratures for the function $(1-xz)^{-1}$, as explained in Section 2, BREZINSKI

[1988b] proposed to use this procedure for the estimation of the error in Padé approximation.

Kronrod's method consists in building a new quadrature formula by using an interpolating polynomial on the k points of the Gaussian quadrature plus $k+1$ new points chosen in an optimal way, that is so that the new quadrature formula thus obtained be exact for polynomials of the highest possible degree. Then the difference between the two quadrature formulae gives an estimation of the error on that of the lowest precision, that is on the Gaussian one.

Thus let R_k be the Hermite interpolation polynomial of $(1-xz)^{-1}$ at the zeros of P_k, the polynomial of degree k of the family of orthogonal polynomials with respect to c. Then, as we saw above,

$$c(R_k(x)) = [k-1/k]_f(z).$$

To these k interpolation points let us add n new ones which can be considered as the zeros of the monic polynomial V_n. Then let us construct the interpolation polynomial R_{k+n} of $(1-xz)^{-1}$ at these $k+n$ points and compute $c(R_{k+n}(x))$. This procedure is identical to the construction of the Padé-type approximant $(n+k-1/n+k)$ with $v(x) = P_k(x)V_n(x)$ as a generating polynomial.

From the expression of the error given in Section 2, we have

$$f(z) - (n+k-1/n+k)_f(z) = \frac{z^{n+k}}{\tilde{P}_k(z)\tilde{V}_n(z)} c\left(\frac{P_k(x)V_n(x)}{1-xz}\right)$$

where $\tilde{V}_n(z) = z^n V_n(z^{-1})$. Moreover, if we set

$$W_n(z) = c\left(P_k(x)\frac{V_n(x)-V_n(z)}{x-z}\right),$$

$$w(z) = c\left(\frac{P_k(x)V_n(x)-P_k(z)V_n(z)}{x-z}\right)$$

we have

$$w(z) = W_n(z) + Q_k(z)V_n(z)$$

where Q_k is the polynomial associated with P_k.

Then it follows that

$$(n+k-1/n+k)_f(z) - [k-1/k]_f(z) = z^k \frac{\tilde{W}_n(z)}{\tilde{P}_k(z)\tilde{V}_n(z)}$$

where $\tilde{W}_n(z) = z^{n-1}W_n(z^{-1})$.

Let us now choose V_n in an optimal way, that is so that the precision be maximum. From the above expression of the error we have

$$f(z) - (n+k-1/n+k)_f(z)$$

$$= \frac{z^{n+k}}{\tilde{P}_k(z)\tilde{V}_n(z)} c\left[P_k(x)V_n(x)\left(1+xz+\ldots+x^{n-1}z^{n-1}+\frac{x^n z^n}{1-xz}\right)\right].$$

Thus V_n will be chosen so that

$$c(x^i P_k(x) V_n(x)) = 0 \quad \text{for } i = 0, \ldots, n-1.$$

In that case we shall have

$$f(z) - (n+k-1/n+k)_f(z) = O(z^{2n+k}).$$

$[V_n(x) - V_n(z)]/(x - z)$ is a polynomial of degree $n - 1$ in x. Thus, due to the orthogonality of P_k, W_n will be identically zero for $n \leqslant k$, and in that case $(n+k-1/n+k)$ will reduce to $[k-1/k]$. Thus we must take $n > k$ and the smallest possible value for n is $n = k+1$ which is exactly Kronrod's procedure. It is easy to see that such a V_{k+1} exists if and only if $H_k^{(0)} \neq 0$ and we have

THEOREM 9.1. *Let V_{k+1} be such that*

$$c(x^i P_k(x) V_{k+1}(x)) = 0 \quad \text{for } i = 0, \ldots, k.$$

Let $(2k/2k+1)$ be the Padé-type approximant of f with the generating polynomial $P_k(x) V_{k+1}(x)$. Then

$$f(z) - (2k/2k+1)_f(z) = \frac{z^{3k+2}}{\tilde{P}_k(z) \tilde{V}_{k+1}(z)} c \left(\frac{x^{k+1} P_k(x) V_{k+1}(x)}{1 - xz} \right),$$

$$(2k/2k+1)_f(z) - [k-1/k]_f(z) = \frac{z^{2k}}{\tilde{P}_k(z) \tilde{V}_{k+1}(z)} c(x^k P_k(x)),$$

$$\frac{f(z) - [k-1/k]_f(z)}{(2k/2k+1)_f(z) - [k-1/k]_f(z)}$$

$$= 1 + z^{k+2} c \left(\frac{x^{k+1} P_k(x) V_{k+1}(x)}{1 - xz} \right) \bigg/ c(x^k P_k(x)).$$

PROOF. From the preceding relations we have, for $n = k + 1$

$$f(z) - (2k/2k+1)_f(z)$$

$$= \frac{z^{2k+1}}{\tilde{P}_k(z) \tilde{V}_{k+1}(z)} c \left[P_k(x) V_{k+1}(x) \left(1 + xz + \cdots + x^k z^k + \frac{x^{k+1} z^{k+1}}{1 - xz} \right) \right]$$

and the first formula follows from the choice of V_{k+1}.

Obviously $W_{k+1}(x) = c(x^k P_k(x))$ since V_{k+1} is monic and P_k is orthogonal to any polynomial of degree strictly less than k. Thus $\tilde{W}_{k+1}(z) = z^k c(x^k P_k(x))$ and the second formula follows.

For proving the last relation, let e be the linear functional defined by

$$e(x^i) = e_i = c(x^i P_k(x)), \quad i = 0, 1, \ldots$$

and let $g(z) = e_0 + e_1 z + \cdots$. By definition of V_{k+1}, it is the orthogonal polynomial of degree $k+1$ with respect to e and W_{k+1} is its associated polynomial. Thus

$$\tilde{W}_{k+1}(z)/\tilde{V}_{k+1}(z) = [k/k+1]_g(z).$$

But, because P_k is orthogonal with respect to c, then $e_i = 0$ for $i = 0, \ldots, k-1$. Thus we set $g(z) = z^k g_k(z)$ and by Property 3.3(ii), we have

$$[k/k+1]_g(z) = z^k [0/k+1]_{g_k}(z).$$

Since $\tilde{W}_{k+1}(z) = e_k z^k$, it follows that

$$e_k/\tilde{V}_{k+1}(z) = [0/k+1]_{g_k}(z) = g_k(z) \frac{z^{k+2}}{\tilde{V}_{k+1}(z)} c \left(\frac{x^{k+1} P_k(x) V_{k+1}(x)}{1-xz} \right)$$

and we get, from the two preceding relations

$$(2k/2k+1)_g(z) - [k-1/k]_g(z) = \frac{e_k z^{2k}}{\tilde{P}_k(z) \tilde{V}_{k+1}(z)}.$$

From the error formula given in Section 2, we obtain

$$f(z) - [k-1/k]_f(z) = \frac{z^{2k}}{\tilde{P}_k(z)} c \left(\frac{x^k P_k(x)}{1-xz} \right) = \frac{z^{2k}}{\tilde{P}_k(z)} g_k(z)$$

and the result follows. □

This last relation shows that $(2k/2k+1)_f(z) - [k-1/k]_f(z)$ provides an approximation of the error $f(z) - [k-1/k]_f(z)$ and that this estimation of the error is very effective around the origin.

The polynomials V_{k+1} are called Stieltjes polynomials because they were introduced by Stieltjes in a letter to Hermite dated November 8, 1894, less than two months before his death. They have been studied by PRÉVOST [1988] in the formal case.

Contrarily to Kronrod's procedure for integrals, the knowledge of the zeros of V_{k+1} is not needed, nor do those zeros need to be real, distinct and in the interval of integration, which is a major simplification in the practical use of Kronrod's procedure for Padé approximants. The application of this procedure needs the knowledge of $c_0, \ldots, c_{3k+1}$.

Let us now give some numerical examples.

The first one deals with $f(z) = \exp(z)$. We obtain the results in Table 9.1.

As we see this procedure does not only give the order of magnitude of the error but a quite precise value of it.

We shall now take $f(z) = \exp(z)$ for complex values of z given by $z = x + iy$ with $x^2 + y^2 = r^2$. The results obtained are in Table 9.2 for $r = 1$, in Table 9.3 for $r = 0.5$, and in Table 9.4 for $r = 0.1$.

Table 9.1. $f(z) = \exp(z)$.

z	$(2/3)-[0/1]$	$\exp(z)-[0/1]$	$(4/5)-[1/2]$	$\exp(z)-[1/2]$
−3.0	−0.236842	−0.200213	0.512535×10^{-1}	0.497871×10^{-1}
−1.5	−0.184615	−0.176870	0.126534×10^{-1}	0.126038×10^{-1}
−1.0	−0.134328	−0.132121	0.424741×10^{-2}	0.424308×10^{-2}
−0.5	−0.060301	−0.060136	0.470093×10^{-3}	0.470053×10^{-3}
−0.3	−0.028431	−0.028412	0.774809×10^{-4}	0.774799×10^{-4}
−0.1	−0.004253	−0.004253	0.122459×10^{-5}	0.122459×10^{-5}
0.1	−0.005940	−0.005940	0.157761×10^{-5}	0.157761×10^{-5}
0.3	−0.078637	−0.078712	0.165559×10^{-3}	0.165556×10^{-3}
0.5	−0.349515	−0.351279	0.166270×10^{-2}	0.166245×10^{-2}
1.1	12.0531	13.0042	0.864646×10^{-1}	0.860166×10^{-1}

Table 9.2. $r = 1$.

x	$(2/3)-[0/1]$	$\exp(z)-[0/1]$
0.8	1.371070−i0.302249	1.336818−i0.243365
0.1	0.089950+i0.373320	0.101780+i0.374194
0.0	0.031757+i0.336627	0.040302+i0.341471
−0.6	−0.119060+i0.143426	−0.117639+i0.143693

Table 9.3. $r = 0.5$.

x	$(2/3)-[0/1]$	$\exp(z)-[0/1]$
0.3	0.167072−i0.090205	0.166379−i0.089725
0.1	0.117975+i0.053957	0.118039+i0.053453
0.0	0.077217+i0.079609	0.077583+i0.079426
−0.1	0.039494+i0.087744	0.039790+i0.087898
−0.3	0.020187+i0.072123	−0.020364+i0.072272

Instead of using Kronrod's method to estimate the error, one can use any other approximation of f needing the same coefficients $c_0, \ldots, c_{3k+1}$ of the initial series. In particular one can use the simplest one, namely the partial sum of the series up to the term of degree $3k + 1$, $f_{3k+1}(z)$.

TABLE 9.4. $r = 0.1$.

x	(2/3)–[0/1]	$\exp(z)$–[0/1]
+0.08	$-0.10154 \times 10^{-2} - i0.56300 \times 10^{-2}$	$-0.10152 \times 10^{-2} - i0.56300 \times 10^{-2}$
+0.00	$+0.49051 \times 10^{-2} + i0.82366 \times 10^{-3}$	$+0.49051 \times 10^{-2} + i0.82351 \times 10^{-2}$
−0.08	$-0.16215 \times 10^{-2} + i0.40717 \times 10^{-2}$	$-0.16216 \times 10^{-2} + i0.40717 \times 10^{-2}$

Let us consider the ratio

$$r(z) = \frac{\dfrac{(2k/2k+1)_f(z) - [k-1/k]_f(z)}{f(z) - [k-1/k]_f(z)} - 1}{\dfrac{f_{3k+1}(z) - [k-1/k]_f(z)}{f(z) - [k-1/k]_f(z)} - 1} = \frac{(2k/2k+1)_f(z) - f(z)}{f_{3k+1}(z) - f(z)}.$$

If $|r(z)| < 1$, $(2k/2k+1)_f(z) - [k-1/k]_f(z)$ is a better approximation of the error $f(z) - [k-1/k]_f(z)$ than $f_{3k+1}(z) - [k-1/k]_f(z)$. Otherwise it is the contrary.

Of course, in practice, $r(z)$ cannot be computed. However, if c_{3k+2} is known, then $r(0)$ can be obtained since

$$r(0) = c(x^{k+1} P_k(x) V_{k+1}(x))/(\tilde{P}_k(0)\tilde{V}_{k+1}(0) c_{3k+2}).$$

Thus, if $|r(0)| < 1$, Kronrod's procedure provides a better estimation of the error than $f_{3k+1}(z) - [k-1/k]_f(z)$, at least in a neighbourhood of the origin. Numerical examples can be found in BREZINSKI [1988b]. Due to the connection between Padé approximation and the ε-algorithm, a similar procedure can be applied for estimating the error in accelarating the convergence by this algorithm.

Kronrod's procedure provides good estimates of the error but is expensive since it needs the knowledge of $c_0, \ldots, c_{3k+1}$ which is not always available. We shall now describe other methods for the estimation of the error that use fewer coefficients of the initial series but that will, on the other hand, give less accurate estimates. The details can be found in BREZINSKI [1989].

In Section 2, we saw three different expressions for the error of Padé approximation

$$E_1: f(z) - [k-1/k]_f(z) = \frac{z^k}{\tilde{P}_k(z)} c\left(\frac{P_k(x)}{1-xz}\right),$$

$$E_2: f(z) - [k-1/k]_f(z) = \frac{z^{2k}}{\tilde{P}_k(z)} c\left(\frac{x^k P_k(x)}{1-xz}\right),$$

$$E_3: f(z) - [k-1/k]_f(z) = \frac{z^{2k}}{\tilde{P}_k^2(z)} c\left(\frac{P_k^2(x)}{1-xz}\right).$$

The basic idea of these new methods for estimating the error is to replace $(1 - xz)^{-1}$ in the right-hand side of these three expressions by its Hermite interpolation polynomial at the zeros of an arbitrary polynomial V_n.

We shall thus obtain three new procedures for estimating the error. Then the optimal choice of such a V_n will lead to three other procedures. We shall call R_n the interpolation polynomial of $(1-xz)^{-1}$ at the zeros of V_n, e_k the error and $e_k^{(n)}$ the estimation of the error obtained by replacing $(1-xz)^{-1}$ by R_n in the three expressions above. We have

THEOREM 9.2. *Replacing $(1-xz)^{-1}$ by R_n in E_1 leads to*

$$e_k^{(n)} = z^k \tilde{W}_n(z)/(\tilde{P}_k(z)\tilde{V}_n(z))$$

with $W_n(z) = c[P_k(x)(V_n(x) - V_n(z))/(x-z)]$ and $\tilde{W}_n(z) = z^{n-1}W_n(z^{-1})$. We have

$$\frac{e_k^{(n)}}{e_k} = 1 - \frac{z^{n-k}}{\tilde{V}_n(z)} \frac{c(P_k(x)V_n(x)/(1-xz))}{c(x^k P_k(x)/(1-xz))}.$$

If V_n is chosen so that

$$c(x^i P_k(x) V_n(x)) = 0 \quad \text{for } i = 0, \ldots, n-1 \quad (n > k)$$

then

$$\frac{e_k^{(n)}}{e_k} = 1 - \frac{z^{2n-k}}{\tilde{V}_n(z)} \frac{c(x^n P_k(x) V_n(x)/(1-xz))}{c(x^k P_k(x)/(1-xz))}.$$

PROOF. We have

$$e_k^{(n)} = \frac{z^k}{\tilde{P}_k(z)} c\left(P_k(x) R_n(x)\right)$$

and the first result immediately follows from the expression of R_n given in Theorem 2.3. From the expression of $e_k = f(z) - [k-1/k]_f(z)$, we have

$$\frac{e_k^{(n)}}{e_k} = \frac{\tilde{W}_n(z)}{\tilde{V}_n(z)} c\left(\frac{P_k(x)}{1-xz}\right).$$

But

$$\tilde{W}_n(z) = z^{n-1} c\left(P_k(x) \frac{V_n(x) - V_n(z^{-1})}{x - z^{-1}}\right)$$

$$= \tilde{V}_n(z) c\left(\frac{P_k(x)}{1-xz}\right) - z^n c\left(\frac{P_k(x) V_n(z)}{1-xz}\right).$$

Using the relation

$$c\left(\frac{P_k(x)}{1-xz}\right) = c\left(\frac{1 - x^k z^k + x^k z^k}{1 - xz} P_k(x)\right) = z^k c\left(\frac{x^k P_k(x)}{1-xz}\right)$$

we obtain the expression for $e_k^{(n)}/e_k$.

We have

$$c\left(\frac{P_k(x)V_n(x)}{1-xz}\right) = c\left(P_k(x)V_n(x)(1+xz+\cdots+x^{n-1}z^{n-1}+\frac{x^n z^n}{1-xz})\right)$$

and the last result immediately follows from the optimal choice of V_n. □

For $n = k+1$, this optimal choice of V_n reduces to Kronrod's procedure as explained above. The computation of $e_k^{(n)}$ requires $c_0, \ldots, c_{n+k-1}$ and $c_0, \ldots, c_{2n+k-1}$ in its optimal version.

Since the proofs of the two following theorems are quite similar to the preceding one, they will be omitted.

THEOREM 9.3. *Replacing $(1-xz)^{-1}$ by R_n in E_2 leads to*

$$e_k^{(n)} = z^{2k}\tilde{W}_n(z)/(\tilde{P}_k(z)\tilde{V}_n(z))$$

with $W_n(z) = c\left[x^k P_k(x)(V_n(x)-V_n(z))/(x-z)\right]$ *and* $\tilde{W}_n(z) = z^{n-1}W_n(z^{-1})$.

We have

$$e_k^{(n)}/e_k = 1 - \frac{z^n}{\tilde{V}_n(z)} \frac{c(P_k^2(x)V_n(x)/(1-xz))}{c(P_k^2(x)/(1-xz))}.$$

If V_n is chosen so that

$$c(x^i P_k^2(x)V_n(x)) = 0 \quad \text{for } i = 0, \ldots, n-1$$

then

$$e_k^{(n)}/e_k = 1 - \frac{z^{2n}}{\tilde{V}_n(z)} \frac{c(x^n P_k^2(x)V_n(x)/(1-xz))}{c(P_k^2(x)/(1-xz))}.$$

THEOREM 9.4. *Replacing $(1-xz)^{-1}$ by R_n in E_3 leads to*

$$e_k^{(n)} = z^{2k}\tilde{W}_n(z)/(\tilde{P}_k^2(z)\tilde{V}_n(z))$$

with $W_n(z) = c[P_k^2(x)(V_n(x)-V_n(z))/(x-z)]$ *and* $\tilde{W}_n(z) = z^{n-1}W_n(z^{-1})$.

We have

$$e_k^{(n)}/e_k = 1 - \frac{z^n}{\tilde{V}_n(z)} \frac{c(P_k^2(x)V_n(x)/(1-xz))}{c(P_k^2(x)/(1-xz))}.$$

If V_n is chosen so that

$$c(x^i P_k^2(x)V_n(x)) = 0 \quad \text{for } i = 0, \ldots, n-1$$

then

$$e_k^{(n)}/e_k = 1 - \frac{z^{2n}}{\tilde{V}_n(z)} \frac{c(x^n P_k^2(x) V_n(x)/(1-xz))}{c(P_k^2(x)/(1-xz))}.$$

In the last two cases, the computation of $e_k^{(n)}$ needs the knowledge of $c_0, \ldots, c_{2k+n-1}$ and $c_0, \ldots, c_{2k+2n-1}$ in the optimal version.

In their nonoptimal versions, these three procedures are not independent. In the first one if n is replaced by $n+k$ and if we take $V_{n+k}(z) = z^k V_n(z)$ where V_n is the polynomial of the second procedure, then both procedures are identical. If $V_{n+k}(z) = P_k(z) V_n(z)$ in the first procedure where V_n is the polynomial of the third one, then both procedures are the same.

For the details concerning the implementation of these procedures, their comparison and some numerical results we refer the interested reader to BREZINSKI [1989].

Of course all the procedures described in this section can be easily extended to the other approximants of the table.

10. Duality

In Section 2 we saw that the Padé-type approximant $(k-1/k)$ of f is defined by

$$(k-1/k)_f(z) = c(R_k(x))$$

where R_k is the Hermite interpolation polynomial of $(1-xz)^{-1}$ at the zeros of an arbitrary polynomial v_k of degree k and that when v_k is identical to P_k then $(k-1/k)$ is identical to $[k-1/k]$. We also saw that $f(z) = c((1-xz)^{-1})$.

We shall now look for the linear functional d (depending on v_k) such that $(k-1/k)$ can be expressed as

$$(k-1/k)_f(z) = d((1-xz)^{-1}).$$

For convenience we shall make use of the notation of duality $\langle L, g \rangle$ to denote the action of the linear functional L on the element g of a vector space E. Thus L belongs to E^*, the dual space of E. If T is a linear mapping on E, its dual mapping T^* is the mapping on E^* uniquely defined by

$$\langle T^*(L), g \rangle = \langle L, Tg \rangle.$$

Let E be the vector space of functions which are holomorphic in a neighbourhood of the origin and let v_k be an arbitrary polynomial of degree $k = k_1 + \cdots + k_n$ with distinct zeros $x_1, \ldots, x_n$ of respective multiplicities $k_1, \ldots, k_n$.

We shall denote by $I(v_k)$ the linear operator mapping $g \in E$ into its Hermite interpolation polynomial R_k at the zeros of v_k. Thus, as seen before,

$$I(v_k)(1-xz)^{-1} = (1-xz)^{-1}(1 - v_k(x)/v_k(z^{-1}))$$

and

$$\langle c, I(v_k)(1 - xz)^{-1}\rangle = (k - 1/k)_f(z).$$

Thus

$$\langle I^*(v_k)(c), (1 - xz)^{-1}\rangle = (k - 1/k)_f(z).$$

The aim of this section is to study some properties of the operator

$$d(v_k) = I^*(v_k)(c).$$

Let $\tilde{v}_k(x) = x^k v_k(x^{-1})$ and let $u_k(x) = u_0 + u_1 x + u_2 x^2 + \cdots$ be the reciprocal series of $\tilde{v}_k$ formally defined by

$$\tilde{v}_k(x) u_k(x) = 1.$$

Setting $v_k(x) = v_0 + v_1 x + \cdots + v_k x^k$, we have

$$u_0 v_k = 1,$$
$$u_0 v_{k-1} + u_1 v_k = 0,$$
$$\vdots$$
$$u_0 v_0 + u_1 v_1 + \cdots + u_k v_k = 0,$$
$$u_1 v_0 + u_2 v_1 + \cdots + u_{k+1} v_k = 0,$$
$$\vdots$$

That is, with the convention that $u_i = 0$ for $i < 0$

$$u_0 v_k = 1,$$
$$v_0 u_i + v_1 u_{i+1} + \cdots + v_k u_{i+k} = 0, \quad i \neq k.$$

If we set

$$r_i(x) = \sum_{j=0}^{i} u_j x^{i-j}, \quad i \geq 0,$$
$$r_i(x) = 0, \quad i < 0,$$

then $\forall i \geq 0$ we have

$$x^i - r_{i-k}(x) v_k(x) = -\sum_{j=0}^{k-1} a_j^{(i)} x^j$$

with $a_j^{(i)} = \sum_{m=0}^{j} v_m u_{i-k+m-j}$ and $I(v_k)x^i = x^i - r_{i-k}(x) v_k(x)$. From these two relations it is easy to obtain the expression of $R_k(x) = I(v_k)(1 - xz)^{-1}$.

Let us now set

$$d_i = \langle d(v_k), x^i \rangle = \langle c, I(v_k)x^i \rangle = \langle c, x^i r_{i-k}(x)v_k(x) \rangle.$$

Then

$$(k - 1/k)_f(z) = \langle d(v_k), (1 - xz)^{-1} \rangle = d_0 + d_1 z + d_2 z^2 + \cdots.$$

$I^*(v_k)$ is the mapping of E^* into itself which maps c into $d(v_k)$; it depends on c. Thus, if v_k does not depend on c, then $I^*(v_k)$ is a linear mapping (as is usually the case in Padé-type approximation if v_k is arbitrarily chosen). If $v_k \equiv P_k$ then v_k depends on c and, in general, $I^*(P_k)$ is not linear.

Let us now study some properties of $d(v_k)$. We have

$$\langle d(v_k), x^i \rangle = \langle c, x^i \rangle \quad \text{for } i = 0, \ldots, k - 1$$

and $\forall i \geq 0$, $\langle d(v_k), x^i v_k(x) \rangle = 0$ which generalizes a property given by BREZINSKI [1980, p. 23] when v_k has distinct simple zeros. A recursive formula for the d_i's then follows

$$d_{i+k} = -(v_0 d_i + \cdots + v_{k-1} d_{i+k-1})/v_k, \quad i = 0, 1, \ldots$$

with $d_i = c_i$ for $i = 0, \ldots, k - 1$.

In several physical applications, Padé-type and Padé approximants are used to obtain approximate values of the unknown coefficients of a series, an idea introduced by GILEWICZ [1973]. Thus, from the relations given above, we have

$$c_i - d_i = \langle c, r_{i-k}(x)v_k(x) \rangle = c_i + \sum_{j=0}^{k-1} a_j^{(i)} c_j$$

where the $a_j^{(i)}$ can be recursively computed by

$$a_0^{(i+1)} = u_{i-k+1} v_0,$$
$$a_j^{(i+1)} = a_{j-1}^{(i)} + u_{i-k+1} v_j \quad \text{for } j = 1, \ldots, k - 1,$$

with $a_j^{(k-1)} = 0$ for $j = 0, \ldots, k - 1$.

This formula cannot be used in practive to compute the error $c_i - d_i$ since its computation needs the knowledge of the unknown coefficient c_i. However, it can be useful in some cases. For example, if

$$c(x^i) = \int_a^b x^i \alpha(x) \, dx, \quad i \geq 0,$$

where α is positive in $[a, b]$, then $\exists t \in [a, b]$ such that

$$c_i - d_i = c_0 r_{i-k}(t) v_k(t)$$

and bounds for $c_i - d_i$ can be obtained.

Other applications of duality will be given in Section 23. For the proofs of the results given in this section see BREZINSKI [1990a].

The continuity of the operator mapping a formal power series into the table of its Padé approximants (which is obviously related to the operator d considered in this section) was studied by WERNER and WUYTACK [1983].

11. The method of moments

We shall now describe the method of moments of VOROBYEV [1965] and its connection with Padé approximants.

Let E be an indefinite inner product space with an inner product denoted by $(\cdot,\cdot)$. Let $x_0, x_1, \ldots, x_k$ be linearly independent elements of E and let $E_k = \text{span}\{x_0, \ldots, x_{k-1}\}$. The method of moments consists of constructing a linear operator A_k on E_k such that

$$x_1 = A_k x_0,$$
$$x_2 = A_k x_1,$$
$$\vdots$$
$$x_{k-1} = A_k x_{k-2},$$
$$H_k x_k = A_k x_{k-1}$$

where H_k denotes the projection operator on E_k. Of course

$$x_i = A_k^i x_0, \quad i = 0, \ldots, k-1$$

and A_k is completely defined by these equations since $\forall v \in E_k$, $v = a_0 x_0 + \cdots + a_{k-1} x_{k-1}$ and $A_k v_k = a_0 x_1 + \cdots + a_{k-2} x_{k-1} + a_{k-1} H_k x_k$.

Since $H_k x_k \in E_k$ it can be written as

$$H_k x_k = -\alpha_0 x_0 - \cdots - \alpha_{k-1} x_{k-1}.$$

But $x_k - H_k x_k$ is orthogonal to E_k, that is

$$(x_k - H_k x_k, x_i) = 0, \quad i = 0, \ldots, k-1$$

or

$$\alpha_0 (x_0, x_i) + \cdots + \alpha_{k-1}(x_{k-1}, x_i) + (x_k, x_i) = 0 \quad \text{for } i = 0, \ldots, k-1.$$

Since $x_0, \ldots, x_{k-1}$ are linearly independent, the determinant of this system is different from zero and $\alpha_0, \ldots, \alpha_{k-1}$ are uniquely determined. Let us set

$$P_k(t) = \alpha_0 + \alpha_1 t + \cdots + \alpha_{k-1} t^{k-1} + t^k.$$

Algebraic theory

We have

$$P_k(A_k)x_0 = \alpha_0 x_0 + \cdots + \alpha_{k-1} x_{k-1} + H_k x_k = 0$$

and

$$A_k^i P_k(A_k)x_0 = P_k(A_k) A_k^i x_0 = P_k(A_k) x_i = 0$$

for $i = 0, \ldots, k-1$.

Thus, by linear combinations, $\forall u \in E_k$ we have $P_k(A_k)u = 0$. In particular if u is an eigenvector of A_k then

$$P_k(A_k)u = P_k(\lambda I)u = 0$$

which shows that the zeros of P_k are eigenvalues of A_k.

Let us now consider the Fredholm equation

$$u = zAu + x_0$$

where z is a parameter and the approximate equation

$$u_k = zA_k u_k + x_0$$

where A_k is the operator obtained by the method of moments when applied to $x_i = A^i x_0$ for $i = 0, \ldots, k$.

We can formally write

$$(I - Az)^{-1} = I + Az + A^2 z^2 + \cdots,$$
$$(I - A_k z)^{-1} = I + A_k z + A_k^2 z^2 + \cdots,$$

and

$$u = (I - Az)^{-1} x_0 = x_0 + zAx_0 + z^2 A^2 x_0 + \cdots,$$
$$u_k = (I - A_k z)^{-1} x_0 = x_0 + zA_k x_0 + z^2 A_k^2 x_0 + \cdots.$$

Since E_k has dimension k, then $k+1$ elements of E_k are linearly dependent and there exist $e_0, \ldots, e_k$ not all zero such that

$$e_0 x_0 + e_1 A_k x_0 + \cdots + e_k A_k^k x_0 = 0.$$

Thus, $\forall n \geq 0$

$$e_0 A_k^n x_0 + e_1 A_k^{n+1} x_0 + \cdots + e_k A_k^{n+k} x_0 = 0.$$

Let y be an arbitrary element of E and let us set for $i \geq 0$

$$d_i = (y, A_k^i x_0).$$

Then, $\forall n \geq 0$

$$e_0 d_n + \cdots + e_k d_{n+k} = 0,$$

which shows that the series

$$(y, u_k) = (y, (I - A_k z)^{-1} x_0) = d_0 + d_1 z + d_2 z^2 + \cdots$$

is a rational function with a numerator of degree $k - 1$ and a denominator of degree k. Let P_k be the polynomial obtained from the method of moments. Then the denominator of the preceding rational function is $\tilde{P}_k(z) = z^k P_k(z^{-1})$ since if z is a zero of $\tilde{P}_k$ then $I - A_k z$ is singular, which shows that z^{-1} is an eigenvalue of A_k, that is a zero of P_k.

If we set

$$c_i = (y, A^i x_0)$$

then, by assumption, $c_i = d_i$ for $i = 0, \ldots, k$. Thus

$$(y, (I - A_k z)^{-1} x_0) = f(z) + O(z^{k+1})$$

where

$$f(z) = c_0 + c_1 z + c_2 z^2 + \cdots = (y, u),$$

which shows that $(y, (I - A_k z)^{-1} x_0)$ is the Padé-type approximant $(k - 1/k)$ of f constructed with the generating polynomial P_k (this is not the Padé-type approximant defined in Section 2 since it agrees with f up to the term of degree k instead of the term of degree $k-1$ only, but a so-called Padé-type approximant of higher order as defined in Section 19).

Of course, the Padé approximant $[k - 1/k]$ of $d_0 + d_1 z + \cdots$ is identical to the series $d_0 + d_1 z + \cdots$ by Property 3.4.

We have

$$P_k(A) x_0 = \alpha_0 x_0 + \cdots + \alpha_{k-1} x_{k-1} + x_k,$$
$$P_k(A_k) x_0 = \alpha_0 x_0 + \ldots + \alpha_{k-1} x_{k-1} + H_k x_k.$$

Thus

$$P_k(A) x_0 - P_k(A_k) x_0 = x_k - H_k x_k$$

and it follows that

$$(x_i, P_k(A) x_0 - P_k(A_k) x_0) = 0 \quad \text{for } i = 0, \ldots, k - 1.$$

But $P_k(A_k) x_0 = 0$ and then

$$(x_i, P_k(A) x_0) = 0 \quad \text{for } i = 0, \ldots, k - 1.$$

Thus if A is self-adjoint (that is, $A = A^*$) or if it is simple (that is, $\text{span}(u_0, Au_0, \ldots, A^{n-1}u_0) = \text{span}(u_0, A^*u_0, \ldots, A^{*n-1}u_0))$ (see HENDRIKSEN and VAN ROSSUM [1982]) and if $y = x_0$ then

$$\begin{aligned} c(x^i P_k(x)) &= (y, A^i P_k(A)x_0) \\ &= (A^i x_0, P_k(A)x_0) \\ &= (x_i, P_k(A)x_0) = 0 \end{aligned}$$

for $i = 0, \ldots, k-1$ where c is the linear functional defined by

$$c(x^i) = c_i = (x_0, A^i x_0).$$

Thus P_k is the polynomial of degree k belonging to the family of orthogonal polynomials with respect to c and we have

$$(y, (I - A_k z)^{-1} x_0) = (y, u_k) = [k - 1/k]_f(z).$$

If the above assumption on A is not satisfied, Padé approximants can still be recovered by using an oblique projection instead of an orthogonal one. These results will be useful later in the convergence theory of Padé approximants (see Section 13).

The method of moments (and thus Padé approximants) has important connections with Lanczos' biorthogonalization process and with the conjugate and bi-conjugate gradient methods for solving systems of linear equations. These connections were given by BREZINSKI [1980, pp. 79–91, 184–189]. They are also related to a generalization of the ε-algorithm, called the topological ε-algorithm, which deals with sequences of elements of a topological vector space. This algorithm is useful in defining new quadratically convergent derivative free methods for solving systems of nonlinear equations. Such projection methods have recently received much attention; see, for example, the works of SMITH, FORD and SIDI [1987], BREZINSKI and SADOK [1987], JBILOU and SADOK [1991], the thesis of SADOK [1988] and BREZINSKI, REDIVO ZAGLIA and SADOK [1992].

CHAPTER II

Convergence

12. Introduction to the convergence problem

The problem of convergence is central to the present chapter. It is a difficult problem which can be studied from various points of view. The first one is, a function being given, to study the sequences of Padé approximants which may converge to it and Theorem 12.1 is an example of such a study done by PADÉ [1984] for the exponential function.

On the other hand, it is possible to imagine convergence results for a whole class of functions, and this leads to the last part of the chapter: convergence in capacity. This is the most theoretical part, and between these two extreme points of view we will study different classes of functions for the classical uniform convergence on compact subsets of $\mathbb{C}$. Each time the problems are different if the sequences considered are column sequences, diagonal or paradiagonal sequences; close to these are, for example, sectorial sequences where m/n has lower and upper bounds as n goes to infinity. Other cases can also be considered.

We will first quote two results to show the most optimistic result that can be hoped for, and a counterexample to limit our ambitions.

THEOREM 12.1. *For any sequence (m_i, n_i), $i \geq 1$, where $m_i + n_i$ tends to infinity, the poles of the Padé approximants of e^z tend to infinity and*

$$\lim_{i \to \infty} [m_i/n_i](z) = e^z$$

uniformly on any compact set of $\mathbb{C}$.

The following result is due to WALLIN [1974].

THEOREM 12.2. *There exists an entire function f such that the sequence of diagonal Padé approximants $([n/n]_f)_n$ is unbounded at every point of the complex plane except zero, and so no convergence result can be expected on any open set of the plane.*

We will not give all the proofs, but only some of them to show how the assumptions are used, and in which cases it is hopeless to wait for an extension of the result. As often as possible, we shall give a first result, improvements of it, examples and counterexamples.

As we shall see below, the location of the poles of the approximants is of primary importance for studying convergence.

In Section 13 about meromorphic functions, the locations are supposed to be known, and so we deduce Montessus De Ballore's theorem.

In Sections 14, 15, 16 the locations are sought by means of the coefficients of the series. Section 15, about Stieltjes functions, extensively uses the link with orthogonal polynomials which are, in that case, defined by a positive definite functional, and so properties of the zeros are known. Section 17, about convergence to f in capacity, follows other considerations. In a sense it characterizes sets of functions fastly approximated by rational functions.

As a consequence, functions with branch points, for example, belong to these sets and convergence will be obtained on extremal subsets of $\mathbb{C}$ which localize the set of zeros and poles of the Padé approximants as a barrier to convergence.

Let us give a very simple example showing the difficulties associated with the convergence of Padé approximants (that is, the convergence of a sequence of approximants). We consider the series, taken from BENDER and ORSZAG [1978],

$$f(z) = \frac{10 + z}{1 - z^2} = \sum_{i=0}^{\infty} c_i z^i$$

with $c_{2i} = 10$ and $c_{2i+1} = 1$. It converges for $|z| < 1$. We have

$$[k/1]_f(z) = \sum_{i=0}^{k-1} c_i z^i + \frac{c_k z^k}{1 - c_{k+1} z / c_k}.$$

When k is odd, $[k/1]$ has a simple pole at $z = 1/10$ while f has no pole. Thus the sequence $([k/1])$ cannot converge to f in $|z| < 1$.

This example shows that the poles of the Padé approximants can prevent convergence and that a sequence of approximants can be nonconvergent in a domain where the series is. In order to prove the convergence of a sequence of Padé approximants in a domain D of the complex plane, it must be proved that the spurious poles of the approximants (that is, the poles which do not approximate poles of f) move out of D when the degree(s) of the approximants tend to infinity.

Another more paradoxical situation can arise: the zeros of the Padé approximants can also prevent convergence. Let us take the reciprocal series g of the series f of the preceding example:

$$g(z) = \frac{1 - z^2}{10 + z}.$$

It converges in $|z| < 10$. We have

$$[1/k]_g(z) = 1/[k/1]_f(z).$$

Since $[1/2k+1]_g(0.1) = 0$ and $g(0.1) \neq 0$ the sequence $([1/k]_g)$ cannot converge in $|z| < 10$ where the series g does.

These examples show that it is important for the study of the convergence of Padé approximants to have information about the location of their zeros and poles. Zero-free regions for sequences of polynomials generated by recurrence relations have been widely studied in the literature. It is not our aim, here, to give an extensive treatment of the subject. We shall only present a few results of this kind and refer the interested reader to the surveys by VARGA [1982] and DE BRUIN, GILEWICZ and RUNCKEL [1987].

The following result is due to SAFF and VARGA [1976a].

THEOREM 12.3. *Let $\{P_k\}_{k=0}^n$ be a finite sequence of polynomials of respective degrees k which satisfy the recurrence relation*

$$P_{-1}(z) = 0, \qquad P_0(z) \neq 0,$$

$$P_k(z) = (1 + z/b_k)P_{k-1}(z) - \frac{z}{c_k}P_{k-2}(z), \quad k = 1, \ldots, n,$$

where the b_k's and the c_k's are real positive numbers. Set

$$\alpha = \min_{1 \leqslant k \leqslant n} b_k(1 - b_{k-1}/c_k), \quad \text{where } b_0 = 0.$$

If $\alpha > 0$, then the parabolic region

$$P_\alpha = \{z = x + iy \in \mathbb{C}, \ y^2 \leqslant 4\alpha(x + \alpha), \ x > -\alpha\}$$

contains no zeros of $\{P_k\}_{k=1}^n$.

PROOF. Let z be any fixed point in P_α which is not a zero of P_k for $k = 1, \ldots, n$. We set

$$\mu_k = zP_{k-1}(z)/b_k P_k(z) \quad \text{for } k = 1, \ldots, n.$$

By the recurrence relationship of P_k, we have

$$\mu_k = \mu_k(z) = z/(z + b_k - b_k c_k^{-1} b_{k-1} \mu_{k-1}), \quad k = 2, \ldots, n.$$

We shall now prove, by induction, that

$$\operatorname{Re} \mu_k \leqslant 1 \quad \text{for } k = 1, \ldots, n.$$

Setting

$$\xi = T_k(w) = z/(z + b_k - b_k c_k^{-1} w).$$

We have

$$\mu_k = T_k(\mu_{k-1}).$$

For $k=1$, we have $\mu_1 = z/(z+b_1)$ and thus $\text{Re}\,\mu_1 \leq 1$ if and only if $\text{Re}\,z \geq b_1$. But, since $z \in P_\alpha$, $\text{Re}\,z > -\alpha \geq -b_1$ by the definition of α and thus $\text{Re}\,\mu_1 \leq 1$.

Let us now assume that $\text{Re}\,\mu_{k-1} \leq 1$. μ_k belongs to the image of the half-plane $\text{Re}\,w \leq 1$ by T_k. The pole $w_k = (z+b_k)c_k/b_k b_{k-1}$ of T_k satisfies $\text{Re}\,w_k > 1$, since $\text{Re}\,z > -\alpha$.

Thus, T_k maps the half-plane onto a closed disc D_k in the ξ-plane. Let r_k be the radius of D_k and ξ_k its center. By geometrical considerations, it can be proved that $r_k + \text{Re}\,\xi_k \leq 1$, that is $\text{Re}\,\mu_k \leq 1$, and the proof by induction is completed.

Now, from the recurrence relation, $P_0(0) = P_1(0) = \cdots = P_k(0) \neq 0$, and P_k and P_{k-1} have no common zeros. If there exists $z_0 \in P_\alpha$ such that $P_k(z_0) = 0$ then

$$c_k(z_0 + b_k)/b_k b_{k-1} = \mu_{k-1}(z_0).$$

By continuity considerations, $\text{Re}\,\mu_k \leq 1$ implies that $\text{Re}\,\mu_{k-1}(z_0) \leq 1$ and thus $\text{Re}\,z_0 \leq -\alpha$, which contradicts the assumption that $z_0 \in P_\alpha$. It follows that P_k has no zero in P_α for $k = 1, \ldots, n$. □

A recurrence relation of this form holds among the numerators of the sequence $([n+k/k])_n$ and among the denominators of the sequence $([n+k/k])_k$ (see Section 6) and we obtain the following results.

THEOREM 12.4. *Let f be a formal power series. If the Hankel determinants of the coefficients of f satisfy, for q fixed,*

$$H_q^{(p-q+1)} > 0, \quad H_{q+1}^{(p-q)} > 0 \quad \text{for } p = 0, \ldots, n,$$
$$H_{q+2}^{(p-q-1)} > 0 \quad \text{for } p = 0, \ldots, n-1$$

and if α is defined as

$$\alpha = \min_{p=1,\ldots,n} \frac{H_q^{(p-q+1)} H_{q+2}^{(p-q+2)}}{H_{q+1}^{(p-q-1)} H_{q+1}^{(p-q)}},$$

then the numerators of $[p/q]_f$ for $p = 1, \ldots, n$ have no zeros in P_α.

If, for p fixed,

$$H_q^{(p-q+1)} > 0, \quad H_q^{(p-q+2)} > 0 \quad \text{for } q = 1, \ldots, n,$$
$$H_q^{(p-q+3)} > 0 \quad \text{for } q = 1, \ldots, n-1$$

and if α is defined as

$$\alpha = \min_{q=1,\ldots,n} \frac{H_q^{(p-q+1)} H_{q-1}^{(p-q+4)}}{H_{q-1}^{(p-q+3)} H_q^{(p-q+2)}},$$

then the denominators of $[p/q]_f$ for $q = 1,\ldots,n$ have no zeros in

$$\bar{P}_\alpha = \{z = x + iy \in \mathbb{C},\ y^2 \leqslant 4\alpha(\alpha - x),\ x < \alpha\}.$$

PROOF. We shall only give a hint about it. From the relations given in Section 5 and from Theorem 6.1, the numerators of the approximants $[p/q]$ satisfy a recurrence relation of the form considered in Theorem 12.3.

Moreover the assumptions on the Hankel determinants imply that the coefficients in this relation are positive. Using the recurrence relation between Hankel determinants, it can be proved that the quantities α in Theorems 12.3 and 12.4 are the same and, thus, the first result follows from Theorem 12.3. A similar proof can be given for the second part of the theorem. □

Other results similar to those of Theorem 12.4 (but too complicated to be given here) can be found in the review paper of DE BRUIN, GILEWICZ and RUNCKEL [1987] already mentioned, where an extensive bibliography is given, or in GILEWICZ and LÉOPOLD [1985a,b] and LÉOPOLD [1985].

An interesting related question is to study how sharp are the results given in these theorems. This will not be done in the general case but we shall come back to this question in the case of the exponential function, see Section 28. General results can be found in GILEWICZ and LÉOPOLD [1985].

Let us now give another example, also taken from BENDER and ORSZAG [1978], which shows how to study the convergence of Padé approximants. We consider the series

$$f(z) = \frac{1}{4} - \frac{z}{10} + \frac{z^2}{32} - \frac{5z^3}{256} + \cdots = \frac{1}{4}\sum_{i=0}^{\infty} \frac{(-1)^i \Gamma(i+1/2)}{(i+1)!\Gamma(1/2)} z^i.$$

For $|z| < 1$, it converges to $f(z) = (\sqrt{1+z} - 1)/2z$. Let us consider the sequence $C_0(z) = [0/0]_f(z)$, $C_1(z) = [0/1]_f(z)$, $C_2(z) = [1/1]_f(z)$, $C_3(z) = [1/2]_f(z)$, ... We set $C_k(z) = A_k(z)/B_k(z)$.

Using the relations of Sections 5 and 6 among adjacent families of formal orthogonal polynomials, we have

$$B_0(z) = 1, \quad B_1(z) = 1 + z/4,$$

$$B_{k+1}(z) = B_k(z) + \frac{z}{4}B_{k-1}(z), \quad k = 1, 2, \ldots$$

and a similar relation for the A_k's with the initial conditions

$$A_0(z) = A_1(z) = 1/4.$$

In order to study the convergence of this sequence of Padé approximants, we have to study the asymptotic behaviours of the A_k's and B_k's which is, in this example, particularly easy since they satisfy a second-order difference equation with constant coefficients. This difference equation can be solved directly and we have

$$A_k(z) = \frac{1}{4\sqrt{1+z}} \left[\left(\frac{1+\sqrt{1+z}}{2} \right)^{k+1} + \left(\frac{1-\sqrt{1+z}}{2} \right)^{k+1} \right],$$

$$B_k(z) = \frac{1}{\sqrt{1+z}} \left[\left(\frac{1+\sqrt{1+z}}{2} \right)^{k+2} - \left(\frac{1-\sqrt{1+z}}{2} \right)^{k+2} \right]$$

and thus

$$C_k(z) = \frac{\sqrt{1+z}-1}{2z} \left[1 + O\left(\left(\frac{1-\sqrt{1+z}}{1+\sqrt{1+z}} \right)^{k+1} \right) \right].$$

When $|\arg(1+z)| < \pi$ then $|1 - \sqrt{1+z}| < |1 + \sqrt{1+z}|$ and

$$\lim_{k \to \infty} C_k(z) = f(z).$$

When $z < -1$ then $\arg(1+z) = \pi$, $|1 - \sqrt{1+z}| = |1 + \sqrt{1+z}|$ and the sequence $(C_k(z))$ oscillates and does not converge. Thus the sequence $(C_k(z))$ converges in the whole complex plane cut from -1 to $-\infty$.

Usually study of the convergence is not so easy because the difference equation to be solved has coefficients which depend on k and thus one has to perform an asymptotic analysis of the solutions of the difference equation since it cannot be solved exactly (worked examples of this situation can be found in BENDER and ORSZAG [1978]). Or, in other words and due to the connection with orthogonal polynomials described in the first chapter, one has to study the asymptotics of formal orthogonal polynomials, a difficult question which was mostly studied only for the classical orthogonal polynomials, as in VAN ASSCHE [1987].

Let us end this section by a quite general convergence theorem, given by JONES and THRON [1980], and which is a consequence of the Stieltjes–Vitali theorem

THEOREM 12.5. *Let (m_k) and (n_k) be two sequences of nonnegative integers such that*

$$\lim_{k \to \infty} \max(m_k, n_k) = \infty.$$

Let $R_k(z) = [m_k/n_k]_f(z)$ and let D be a domain of the complex plane containing the origin. Then
- *(R_k) converges uniformly on every compact subset of D if and only if $\{R_k(z)\}$ is uniformly bounded on every compact subset of D.*
- *If (R_k) converges uniformly on every compact subset of D, then $f(z) = \lim_{k \to \infty} R_k(z)$ is holomorphic in D and the series is the Taylor expansion of the function f about the origin.*

13. Meromorphic functions

Let us first consider the convergence of columns $([m/n])_m$ of the Padé table.

The most famous theorem is that of MONTESSUS DE BALLORE [1902]. It is concerned with meromorphic functions with a known fixed number of poles in the disc of radius R, centered at the origin.

An extension of this result has been given by SAFF [1972], for the case of interpolating rational functions instead of Padé approximants. Montessus's theorem is then a particular case of it when all the interpolation points are zero.

The proof, given below, is due to Saff, and is written here for the Padé case.

THEOREM 13.1. *Let f be analytic at $z = 0$, and meromorphic with exactly n poles $\alpha_1, \ldots, \alpha_n$, counted with their multiplicity, in the disc $D_R = \{z, |z| < R\}$. Let D be the domain $D_R - \{\alpha_i\}_{i=1,\ldots,n}$, and R_{mn} the Padé approximant $[m/n]$.*

The sequence $(R_{mn})_{m \geqslant 0}$ converges to f uniformly on every compact subset of D. The poles of R_{mn} approach the poles of f as m tends to infinity.

PROOF. Let $Q_0, \ldots, Q_n$ be the polynomials defined by

$$Q_0(z) = 1, \qquad Q_k(z) = \prod_1^k (z - \alpha_i), \quad 1 \leqslant k \leqslant n.$$

For any monic polynomial of degree less than n, we get

$$q_m(z) = \sum_{k=1}^n a_k^m Q_{k-1}(z) + Q_n(z).$$

The unique polynomial of degree $m + n$ which interpolates $q_m(z)Q_n(z)f(z)$ at zero, with the order $m + n$ is defined by the Hermite formula

$$\Pi_{m+n}(z) = \frac{1}{2i\pi} \int_{|t|=\rho} \left(1 - \frac{z^{m+n+1}}{t^{m+n+1}}\right) \frac{q_m(t)Q_n(t)f(t)}{t - z} \, dt,$$

where all the α_i's lie in D_ρ the disc of radius $\rho < R$. Suppose first that f has only simple poles in D_ρ. The a_k^m's, $k = 1, \ldots, n$, can be chosen such that Q_n

divides Π_{m+n}

$$\sum_{k=1}^{n} a_k^m c_{jk}^m = d_j^m, \quad j = 1, \ldots, n,$$

$$c_{jk}^m = \frac{1}{2i\pi} \int_{|t|=\rho} \left(1 - \frac{\alpha_j^{m+n+1}}{t^{m+n+1}}\right) \frac{Q_{k-1}(t)Q_n(t)f(t)}{t - \alpha_j} \, dt, \quad k = 1, \ldots, n,$$

$$d_j^m = -\frac{1}{2i\pi} \int_{|t|=\rho} \left(1 - \frac{\alpha_j^{m+n+1}}{t^{m+n+1}}\right) \frac{Q_n^2(t)f(t)}{t - \alpha_j} \, dt,$$

$$\lim_{m \to \infty} c_{jk}^m = c_{jk} = \frac{1}{2i\pi} \int_{|z|=\rho} \frac{Q_{k-1}(t)Q_n(t)f(t)}{t - \alpha_j} \, dt,$$

$$\lim_{m \to \infty} d_j^m = d_j = \frac{1}{2i\pi} \int_{|t|=\rho} \frac{Q_n^2(t)f(t)}{t - \alpha_j} \, dt.$$

By Cauchy's integral formula, we have

$c_{jk} = 0$, for $k > j$,
$c_{jk} \neq 0$, for $k = j$,
$d_j = 0$, for all j,
$\lim_{m \to \infty} \det(c_{jk}^m) = \det(c_{jk}) \neq 0$.

So, for m large enough, the system has a solution, and because the right-hand side tends to zero, the solution a_k^m tends to zero as m tends to infinity. Since the q_m's are polynomials, we finally get

$$\lim_{m \to \infty} q_m(z) = Q_n(z) \tag{13.1}$$

uniformly on compact subsets of the plane.

Suppose now that the α_i's are not simple poles of f, but of order m_i. So we get r distinct poles $\alpha_1, \ldots, \alpha_r$, each of order m_i for $i = 1, \ldots, r$.

The equations of the linear system with a_k^m as unknowns are obtained by setting the derivatives $\Pi_{m+n}^{(\mu)}(\alpha_j)$ equal to zero

$$\Pi_{m+n}^{(\mu)}(\alpha_j) = 0, \quad \mu = 0, \ldots, m_j - 1, \quad j = 1, \ldots, r.$$

Then the limits of the coefficients $c_{jk\mu}^m$ are

$$c_{jk\mu} = \frac{(\mu - 1)!}{2i\pi} \int_{|z|=\rho} \frac{Q_{k-1}(t)Q_n(t)f(t)}{(t - \alpha_j)^{\mu+1}} \, dt, \quad \mu = 0, \ldots, m_j - 1, \quad j = 1, \ldots, r.$$

The matrix is still triangular, with nonzero diagonal terms, and so the conclusion (13.1) holds.

Let K be a compact subset of D. Then there exist σ, ρ such that

$$\sigma < \rho < R,$$
$$K \subset D_\sigma \quad \text{and} \quad \alpha_i \in D_\rho,$$

$$q_m(z)Q_n(z)f(z) - \Pi_{m+n}(z) = \frac{1}{2i\pi} \int_{|t|=\rho} \frac{z^{m+n+1}}{t^{m+n+1}} \frac{q_m(t)Q_n(t)f(t)}{t-z} \, dt,$$

$$|q_m(z)Q_n(z)f(z) - \Pi_{m+n}(z)| \leq M \left|\frac{\sigma}{\rho}\right|^{m+n+1}.$$

By Eq. (13.1) and because K contains no zero of Q_n, $q_m(z)Q_n(z)$ is bounded from below on K, for m large enough. So we get

$$\limsup_{m \to \infty} \left| f(z) - \frac{\Pi_{m+n}(z)/Q_n(z)}{q_m(z)} \right|^{1/n} \leq \frac{\sigma}{\rho} < 1. \tag{13.2}$$

The last point is to prove that $\dfrac{\Pi_{m+n}/Q_n}{q_m}$ is the Padé approximant $[m/n]$ of f: it is a rational function of type (m,n), and

$$f(z) - \frac{\Pi_{m+n}/Q_n}{q_m}(z)$$
$$= \frac{z^{m+n+1}}{q_m(z)Q_n(z)} \frac{1}{2i\pi} \int_{|t|=\rho} \frac{q_m(t)Q_n(t)f(t)}{t^{m+n}(t-z)} \, dt = O(z^{m+n+1})$$

for z in the neighbourhood of 0 defined by $|z| < \inf_i |\alpha_i|/2$.

Since $\lim_{m \to \infty} \Pi_{m+n}/Q_n = Q_n f$ in K, no zero of Π_{m+n}/Q_n can be a zero of q_m, and finally R_{mn} has n actual poles. □

Montessus's theorem gives a result only if the exact number n of poles is known, and only for the column sequence $(R_{mn})_{m \geq 0}$. The poles of f serve as *attractors* for the poles of $[m/n]$. But if f has less than n poles, then only some of the poles of $[m/n]$ are attracted, and the other ones may go anywhere, destroying the convergence. If another column is considered, no result can be obtained as it can be seen from the following counterexamples. The first one, due to BENDER and ORSZAG [1978], has already been quoted in Section 12 of this chapter; it concerns the series $f(z) = (10+z)/(1-z^2)$ where the first column $(R_{m1})_{m \geq 0}$ cannot converge.

The second counterexample is due to PERRON [1957].

Let an arbitrary sequence $(z_n)_n$ of points of $\mathbb{C}$ be given, and let us define the following function

$$f(z) = \sum_{i=0}^{\infty} c_i z^i,$$

if $|z_n| \leq 1$, $c_{3n} = z_n/(3n+2)!$,
$$c_{3n+1} = c_{3n+2} = 1/(3n+2)!,$$
if $|z_n| > 1$, $c_{3n} = c_{3n+1} = 1/(3n+2)!$,
$$c_{3n+2} = z_n^{-1}/(3n+2)!.$$

We have $|c_i| < 1/i!$, $\forall i \geq 0$.

So f is an entire function, and either $[3n/1]$ or $[3n+1/1]$ has a pole in z_n.

The sequence (z_n) is a subsequence of the poles of $([m/1])_m$, and if $(z_n)_n$ is dense in $\mathbb{C}$, the sequence $([m/1])_m$ cannot converge in any open set of the complex plane.

So coming back to a meromorphic function with n poles, it is now obvious that it is impossible to obtain a convergence result for all the sequences $([m/k])_m$, k smaller or greater than n. It is a conjecture, made by BAKER and GRAVES-MORRIS [1977], that at least a subsequence of $([m/k])_{m \geq 0}$ converges for $k \geq n$.

Such a result has been proved by BEARDON [1968] for the column $([m/1])_{m \geq 0}$.

THEOREM 13.2. *Let f be analytic in $|z| < R$. Then, for $r < R$, there exists a subsequence of $([m/1])_{m \geq 0}$ converging uniformly to f in the disc $|z| \leq r$.*

PROOF.

$$f(z) = \sum_{i=0}^{\infty} c_i z^i.$$

If a subsequence of the c_i's are zero, then, for the corresponding indexes, $[i-1/1]$ is the Taylor polynomial of degree $(i-1)$ and this subsequence converges to f uniformly on $|z| \leq r$.

We now suppose that all the c_i's are different from zero for i large enough. There exists a subsequence (c_{i_k}) of (c_i) such that

$$\lim_{k \to \infty} \left| \frac{c_{i_k}}{c_{i_k+1}} \right| = R.$$

For these indexes $|1 - (c_{m+1}/c_m)z|$ is bounded from below for $|z| \leq r$ and m large enough. From the expression of the approximant $[m/1]$ it follows that

$$|f(z) - [m/1]| \leq \left| \sum_{m}^{\infty} c_i z^i \right| + M|c_m z^m|.$$

So $([m/1])_{m \in S}$ converges to f uniformly for $|z| \leq r$. □

The same result has been proved by BAKER and GRAVES-MORRIS [1977] for the second and third columns.

BUSLAEV, GONČAR and SUETIN [1984] establish the conjecture for entire functions; for $R < \infty$ they show that the conjecture is still true in a neighbourhood of zero, and they give a counterexample for the whole disc.

To end this section about the convergence of the columns of the Padé table for meromorphic functions, let us quote a result of divergence, due to WALLIN [1987], in the more general case of multipoint Padé approximants.

The important assumption is that f is a meromorphic function with a finite number of poles in D, and a pole on the boundary of D. Then divergence occurs outside $\mathbb{C} - D$. More precisely we get the following result, with the usual uniform norm on each compact set K

THEOREM 13.3. *Let f be analytic in D_σ, except at n poles $z_1, \ldots, z_n$ different from zero, and let it have a pole on ∂D_σ.*
Let $R_{mn} = [m/n]_f = N_{mn}/D_{mn}$; then, for any compact subset K of D_σ, we get the following results
  (i) $K \subset D_\sigma$: $\limsup_{m \to \infty} \|R_{mn}\|_K^{1/m} \leqslant r/\sigma$.
  (ii) $\forall K$: $\limsup_{m \to \infty} \|Q - D_{mn}\|_K^{1/m} \leqslant \sup_i |z_i|/\sigma$, where $Q(z) = \prod_{i=1}^{n}(z - z_i)$,
  (iii) *for any z of $\mathbb{C} - \bar{D}_\sigma$,*

$$\limsup_{m \to \infty} |N_{mn}(z)|^{1/m} > \frac{|z|}{\sigma}.$$

The convergence of $(D_{mn})_m$ on K (and so everywhere) and the divergence of $(N_{mn})_m$ outside $\bar{D}_\sigma$ produce the divergence of the $(R_{mn})_m$ outside $\bar{D}_\sigma$.

The preceding study is satisfactory if f is meromorphic with a finite number of poles, and the convergence is obtained in a disc. If f has an infinite number of poles, as $\tan z$, $\cotan z$, $\Gamma'(z)/\Gamma(z) \cdots$, there is divergence of the column $([m/n])_m$ outside the disc of radius equal to ρ, the modulus of the $(n+1)$th pole, and so it is natural to study the para-diagonal sequences $([m + p/m])_m$. From the result of Wallin (Theorem 12.2), there is no hope of a complete study for all meromorphic functions, but some results for certain classes of meromorphic functions have been obtained by FRANZEN [1972]. Let us consider functions of the following form

$$f(x) = c_0 + c_1 x + \cdots + c_{r-1} x^{r-1}$$
$$+ \sum_{i=1}^{\infty} A_i \left(\frac{1}{a_i - x} - \frac{1}{a_i} - \frac{x}{a_i^2} - \cdots - \frac{x^{r-1}}{a_i^r} \right)$$

satisfying the conditions
  (i) the c_i's, $i = 0, \ldots, r-1$ are arbitrary complex numbers,
  (ii) the A_i's are real,
  (iii) the a_i's lie on a line $L : a_i = d_i e^{i\theta}$, d_i real,
  (iv) $0 < |d_1| < |d_2| < \cdots$ with $\sum_{i=0}^{\infty} A_i/d_i^{r+1} < \infty$.
Then we get the following theorem

THEOREM 13.4. *Let f be as just described; if p is an integer such that $p \geqslant r-1$, and if $A_i/d_i^p > 0$ for all i, then the sequence $([m + p/m])_m$ converges to f, uniformly on any compact set bounded away from S_θ where S_θ is defined by*

$\forall i \quad d_i > 0, S_\theta = \{z, \arg(z) = \theta, |z| > |d_1|\}$,
$\exists i \quad d_i < 0, S_\theta = \{z, z \in L, |z| > |d_1|\}$.

If the c_n's are the coefficients of the power series expansion of f, then for $n > r$, we get

$$c_n = \sum_{i=1}^{\infty} \frac{A_i}{a_i^{n+1}},$$

and only these c_n $(n > r)$ are concerned in the denominators of the Padé approximants $[m+p/m]$. Then the proof consists in finding asymptotics for the determinants $H_m^{(p+1)}$ and $H_m^{(p+1)}(x)$ (numerator of the approximant) and then to study the convergence of the denominator $D_{m+p,m}$ to $\prod_{i=1}^{m}(1-x/a_i)$.

Using this method, it is obvious that conditions on f are only sufficient conditions for the convergence.

The same idea of finding asymptotics for the denominator will be used in the next section.

The method of moments (see Section 11) can also be used in Padé approximation. Such a link has been made by HENDRIKSEN and VAN ROSSUM [1982]. The two basic theorems are the following, where H is the space l_2 and $(e_n)_n$ the unit vector basis of H.

THEOREM 13.5. *Let $f(z) = \sum_{n=0}^{\infty} c_n z^n$ have radius of convergence R. Let $c_0 = 1$. Then*

(a) *There exists a bounded linear operator A such that $\langle A^n e_0, e_0 \rangle = c_n$ $(n \geq 0)$ if and only if $R > 0$,*

(b) *if $R = \infty$ then there is a linear compact operator A in H with $\langle A^n e_0, e_0 \rangle = c_n$ $(n \geq 0)$.*

Moreover for meromorphic functions, we get

THEOREM 13.6. *Let $\sum_{n=0}^{\infty} c_n z^n$ have a positive radius of convergence and let $c_0 = 1$. Then the following results are equivalent:*

(a) *There exists a compact linear operator A in H such that $\langle A^n e_0, e_0 \rangle = c_n$, $n \geq 0$.*

(b) *There is a meromorphic function f on $\mathbb{C}$ such that $f(z) = \sum_{n=0}^{\infty} c_n z^n$ in some neighbourhood of 0.*

Let us define the following notations

$$x = zAx + u_0, \quad A \text{ operator on } H, \ x, u_0 \in H, \ z \in \mathbb{C}$$
$$x_n = zA_n x_n + u_0, \quad \text{equation in } U_n = \text{span}(u_0, Au_0, \ldots, A^{n-1}u_0)$$

where, if E_n is the orthogonal projection of H onto U_n, A_n is defined from U_n on U_n, and satisfies

$$u_i = A^i u_0, \quad i \geq 0,$$
$$A_n^k u_0 = A^k u_0, \quad k = 0, \ldots, n-1,$$
$$A_n^n u_0 = E_n u_n.$$

So, setting $\langle A^n u_0, u_0 \rangle = c_n$, we have

$$\langle x, u_0 \rangle = \sum_n c_n z^n = f(z).$$

If the operator A is supposed to be simple (i.e. with $u_i = A^i u_0$ and $v_j = A^{*j} u_0$, then span $(u_0, \ldots, u_{n-1})$ = span $(u_0, v_1, \ldots, v_{n-1}))$, we get

$$\langle x_n, u_0 \rangle = [n - 1/n]_f(z).$$

Following VOROBYEV ([1965], pp. 25–29), the next theorem, concerning the convergence of the moment method, can be proved.

THEOREM 13.7. *If A is a compact operator in a Hilbert space H, then the sequence of operators $(A_n)_n$ converges in norm in H, A_n being considered as an operator on H, that is $\lim_{n \to \infty} \|A - A_n\| = 0$.*

If a solution x of the equation $x = zAx + f$ exists (that is, if z is a regular value of the equation), and if A is compact, then, for n large enough, the equation $x_n = zA_n x_n + f$ has a solution, and the sequence $(x_n)_n$ converges to x.

PROOF. Let us notice that E_n, the projection mapping H on U_n, satisfies: $E_n = E_n^*$, $\|E_n\| = 1$, $\|I - E_n\| = 1$, and $\forall h \in H$, $\lim_n E_n h = h$.

The first assertion is proved by contradiction. Suppose $\|A - A_n\|$ does not approach zero when n goes to infinity. Then, there exists $(f_n)_n$, $\|f_n\| = 1$, $\|(A - A_n)(f_n)\| > q$. Because A is compact, there exists a subsequence such that $(Af_n)_n$ and $(A(I - E_n)(f_n))_n$ converge; let $g = \lim_n Af_n$, $h = \lim_n A(I - E_n)f_n$,

$$A - A_n = (I - E_n)A + E_n A(I - E_n),$$
$$\|(I - E_n)Af_n\| \leq \|(I - E_n)(Af_n - g)\| + \|(I - E_n)g\|$$
$$\leq \|(Af_n - g)\| + \|g - E_n g\|$$
$$\to 0,$$
$$\|E_n A(I - E_n)f_n\| \leq \|A(I - E_n)f_n\|$$
$$\to \|h\|.$$

But, $\|h\|^2 = \lim_n (A(I - E_n)f_n, h) = \lim_n (f_n, (I - E_n)A^* h) = 0$, and it follows that $\lim_n \|(A - A_n)(f_n)\| = 0$. This contradicts the assumption and so $\lim_n \|(A - A_n)\| = 0$.

The proof of the second assertion is as follows: first of all, let us remark that the equation $x = zAx + f$ has, as its solution, the series $(I + zA + z^2 A^2 + \cdots)f$ if $|z| < \|A\|^{-1}$. Then $x_n = zA_n x_n + f$ can be written as

$$x_n - zAx_n + z(A - A_n)x_n = f,$$
$$x_n - z(I - zA)^{-1}(A_n - A)x_n = (I - zA)^{-1}f = x$$

and so it has a solution if $\|z(I - zA)^{-1}(A_n - A)\| < 1$. But this last assertion is satisfied, for n large enough, because $\lim_n \|(A - A_n)\| = 0$.

The last point to prove is the convergence of the sequence $(x_n)_n$, $x_n = (I - zA_n)^{-1}f$. It is sufficient to prove the convergence of $(I - zA_n)^{-1}$ to $(I - zA)^{-1}$.

$$(I - zA_n)^{-1} = (I - z(I - zA)^{-1}(A_n - A))^{-1}(I - zA)^{-1},$$

$$\|(I - zA_n)^{-1}\| \leq \|(I - zA)^{-1}\| \sum_{k=0}^{\infty} |z^k| \cdot \|(I - zA)^{-1}\|^k \|A_n - A\|^k$$

$$\leq \frac{\|(I - zA)^{-1}\|}{1 - |z| \cdot \|(I - zA)^{-1}\| \cdot \|A_n - A\|},$$

which proves that the sequence $(\|(I - zA_n)^{-1}\|)_n$ is uniformly bounded.

$$\|(I - zA_n)^{-1} - (I - zA)^{-1}\| \leq \|(I - zA)^{-1}\| \sum_{k=1}^{\infty} |z^k| \cdot \|(I - zA)^{-1}\|^k \|A_n - A\|^k$$

$$\leq \frac{|z| \cdot \|(I - zA)^{-1}\|^2}{1 - |z| \cdot \|(I - zA)^{-1}\| \cdot \|A_n - A\|}$$

and this ends the proof. □

This, with the results of Section 11, is used for the convergence of sequences of Padé approximants. We get the following theorems.

THEOREM 13.8. *Let A be simple and compact and let the sequence $(c_n)_n$ be normal (i.e. all the Hankel determinants $H_n^{(0)}$ are nonzero). Then the sequence $([n-1/n])_n$ of Padé approximants of $f(z) = \sum_n c_n z^n$ converges to f for all z satisfying $|z| < \|A\|^{-1}$.*

If A is compact, but not simple, it is possible to get a result concerning Padé-type approximants, $\langle x_n, u_0 \rangle$ being such an approximant

THEOREM 13.9. *Let A be compact and the sequence $(c_n)_n$ of its moments be normal. Then the sequence of $\langle x_n, u_0 \rangle$ is a sequence of Padé-type approximants $(n - 1/n)$ of $f(z) = \sum_n c_n z^n$ which converges to f for all z, $|z|$ smaller than $\|A\|^{-1}$.*

In these last two cases, the sequences have a geometric rate of convergence. If A is not simple, then, using an oblique projection, instead of an orthogonal one, again leads to Padé approximants.

14. Functions with smooth Taylor series coefficients. Entire functions

The counterexamples of the preceding section show that there is no hope for very general convergence results. The first method for investigating the problem is to consider special classes of functions; this has been done by LUBINSKY [1985, 1987, 1988], who considers functions with slow and smooth growth. He characterizes the *slow and smooth* growth by the following condition on the coefficients

$$\lim_{j \to \infty} \left| \frac{c_{j-1} c_{j+1}}{c_j^2} \right| = q.$$

The case where $c_{j-1}c_{j+1}/c_j^2 = q$ is of course of interest, because the c_i's can be completely described by

$$\frac{c_{j-1}c_{j+1}}{c_j^2} = q, \quad \frac{c_{j+1}}{c_j} = q\frac{c_j}{c_{j-1}} = \cdots = aq^j, \quad a = c_1/c_0.$$
$$c_n = \alpha a^n q^{n(n-1)/2}, \quad \alpha = c_1, \ a = c_0.$$

So with $q = \rho^2$ and a replaced by a/ρ, c_n has the form $c_n = \alpha a^n \rho^{n^2}$.

The same series can become *oscillating* if $c_n = \varepsilon_n \alpha a^n \rho^{n^2}$, $|\varepsilon_n| = 1$ and then we only have $\left|c_{j-1}c_{j+1}/c_j^2\right| = q$.

If we come back to the assumption

$$\lim_{j \to \infty} \left|\frac{c_{j-1}c_{j+1}}{c_j^2}\right| = q,$$

then two important sets of entire functions will satisfy it with $q = 1$:

$$f(z) = \sum_{j \geq 0} z^j (j!)^{1/\lambda},$$
$$f(z) = \sum_{j \geq 0} z^j / \Gamma(1 + j/\lambda) \quad \text{(Mittag–Leffler functions)}.$$

These two functions are both entire of order λ ($\lambda > 0$).

It must be noticed that if $|q| > 1$, f has a zero radius of convergence, while, if $|q| < 1$, f is an entire function of order zero. In the case $|q| = 1$, f may have a zero, a finite or an infinite radius of convergence, and be of any order.

The first results given here (LUBINSKY [1987]) are concerned with the convergence of the sequence $(R_{mn})_{m \geq 0}$, $R_{mn} = [m/n]$, that is with the convergence of the columns of the Padé table (having transposed the Padé table, Lubinsky speaks of convergence of the rows).

The idea of the proofs is to study the asymptotic behaviour of the denominator D_{mn} by using asymptotics of the Hankel determinants: q being given, define the polynomials $B_n(u) = B_n(u, q)$ (Rogers–Szegö polynomials) by

$$\begin{cases} B_0(u) = 1, \\ B_n(u) = B_{n-1}(u) - uq^{n-1}B_{n-1}(u/q). \end{cases}$$

It follows that $B_n(0) = 1$, so all the zeros of B_n are nonzero. Then the following theorem holds

THEOREM 14.1. *Let* $f(z) = \sum_{j=0}^{\infty} c_j z^j$, *with* $c_j \neq 0$ *for* j *large enough. It is supposed that*

$$\lim_{j \to \infty} \frac{c_{j-1}c_{j+1}}{c_j^2} = q.$$

Then

$$\lim_{m\to\infty} \frac{H_n^{(m-n+1)}}{c_m^n} = \prod_{j=1}^{n-1}(1-q^j)^{n-j}.$$

If $q^i \neq 1, i = 1, \ldots, n-1$, then, denoting by D_{mn} the denominator of R_{mn}, we have

$$\lim_{m\to\infty} D_{mn}(u\frac{c_m}{c_{m+1}}) = B_n(u) \tag{a}$$

uniformly on compact sets of $\mathbb{C}$.

If $q \neq 0$ and if $u_1, \ldots, u_n$ are the zeros of B_n, then with a suitable ordering for the zeros z_{ni} of D_{mn}

$$\lim_{m\to\infty} (z_{mi}\frac{c_m}{c_{m+1}}) = u_i, \quad i = 1, \ldots, n. \tag{b}$$

It must be noticed that $(u_i)_i$ does not depend on f but only on q.

In the case $q = 1$, the estimate for $H_n^{(m-n+1)}$ is of no use but the relations (a) and (b) of the theorem can still be proved in the case

$$q_j = \frac{c_{j-1}c_{j+1}}{c_j^2}.$$

The assumption $\lim_{j\to\infty} q_j = q$ can be transformed into $q_j = q(1+c/j+O(j^{-1}))$, $c \neq 0$, and an even more precise treatment can be done if $c = 0$ (LUBINSKY [1987]). And so the result about the convergence of the sequence $(R_{mn})_m$ follows

THEOREM 14.2. *Let n be fixed, and f a power series. We assume that $c_j \neq 0$ for j large enough,*

$$\frac{c_{j-1}c_{j+1}}{c_j^2} = q_j, \quad \lim_{j\to\infty} q_j = q,$$
$$q^\alpha \neq 1, \quad \alpha = 0, \ldots, n-1, \quad \text{or} \quad q_j = q(1+c/j+O(1/j)), \quad c \neq 0.$$

Let D_{mn} be the denominator of R_{mn}, normalized by $D_{mn}(0) = 1$. Then, on every compact subset of $\mathbb{C}$, we get

$$\lim_{m\to\infty} D_{mn}(u \cdot c_m/c_{m+1}) = B_n(u),$$
$$\lim_{m\to\infty} z_{mj}/(c_m/c_{m+1}) = u_j, \quad j = 1, \ldots, n, \ u_j \text{ zeros of } B_n.$$

Moreover, if $R = \liminf_{m\to\infty} |c_m/c_{m+1}|$ and $\sigma = \inf_j |u_j|$ then $\lim_{m\to\infty} R_{mn}(z) = f(z)$, $|z| < \sigma R$.

So for these classes of functions, the poles of R_{mn} go to infinity (with m), and all the columns converge, but if $R < \infty$, the convergence is not true for the whole disc where f is analytic.

If $\lim_{j\to\infty} c_{j-1}c_{j+1}/c_j^2 = q = 1$ (and not $|q| = 1$), it has been proved by LUBINSKY and SAFF [1988], that $\sigma = 1$. As an example of this case, they consider the partial theta function, for which

$$c_n = q^{n(n-1)/2}, \quad q = e^{i\theta},$$
$$q_j = q, \quad j \geq 1.$$

If θ is taken such that $\theta/2\pi$ is irrational, then q^j is always different from 1, and all the columns can be studied.

It is proved that there exists $\sigma_n < 1$ such that each R_{mn} ($m \geq n-1$) has a pole on $|z| = \sigma_n$, and so the domain of convergence of $(R_{mn})_n$ is strictly smaller than the unit disc.

For the diagonal sequence $(R_{nn})_n$ of this function, it is proved that some subsequences converge to f, locally uniformly on the unit disc, while some others do not.

To avoid such an oscillatory behaviour, we suppose, from now, that $|q| < 1$ in order to have a quickly decreasing sequence $|c_i|$.

Let us come now to other convergence results, not concerning the columns, but the diagonal or near diagonal sequences, as in the results of Padé for the exponential function, quoted at the beginning of this chapter (Theorem 12.1). We still assume the same condition of smoothness

$$\frac{c_{j-1}c_{j+1}}{c_j^2} = q \quad \text{or} \quad \lim_{j\to\infty} \frac{c_{j-1}c_{j+1}}{c_j^2} = q.$$

These results were obtained by LUBINSKY [1985, 1988]. The first method consists in transforming the Hankel determinant involved in D_{mn}, i.e. $H_n^{(m-n+1)}$, into the determinant of a diagonally dominant matrix which is possible only if

$$\left|\frac{c_{j-1}c_{j+1}}{c_j^2}\right| \leq \rho_0^2, \quad j \geq 1,$$

where $\rho_0 = 0.45\ldots$ is the positive zero of $\sum_1^\infty \rho^{j^2} = 1$. Of course this condition implies $\limsup_{j\to\infty} |c_j|^{1/j^2} \leq \rho_0$ and so only a limited class of entire functions with very quickly decreasing coefficients is concerned. The following result is obtained

THEOREM 14.3. *Let f be a power series with $c_j \neq 0$ for j large enough,*

$$\left|\frac{c_{j-1}c_{j+1}}{c_j^2}\right| \leq \rho_0^2$$

with ρ_0 as defined above. Then the Padé table is normal, and for any nonnegative integer sequence $(M_L)_L$

$$\lim_{L \to \infty} R_{LM_L}(z) = f(z),$$

uniformly on compact subsets of $\mathbb{C}$.

The second method deals with stronger asymptotics for Hankel determinants. Then with a condition linking m and n, such that n goes to infinity not too fast with respect to m, we get the following convergence result

THEOREM 14.4. *Let f be a power series with $c_j \neq 0$ for j large enough,*

$$\frac{c_{j-1}c_{j+1}}{c_j^2} = q_j, \quad \lim_{j \to \infty} q_j = q \quad \text{and} \quad |q| \leqslant 1,$$

then there exists a constant C such that for any sequence of pairs of integers (m_k, n_k) satisfying $\lim_{k \to \infty} m_k = \infty$ and

$$\lim_{k \to \infty} n_k \max_{j < C \ln n_k^{1/2}} \left| \frac{q_{m_k+j}}{q_{m_k}} - 1 \right| = 0,$$

we get, for $(m, n) = (m_k, n_k)$,

$$- \lim_{k \to \infty} H_n^{(m-n+1)} \left\{ c_m^n \prod_{j=1}^{n-1} (1 - q_m^j)^{m-j} \right\}^{-1} = 1,$$

- *for $\eta > 1$ and m large enough, the poles of R_{mn} lie in $\{z, |z| > \eta \left| \frac{c_m}{c_{m+1}} q_m^{1/2} \right| \}$,*
- $\lim_{k \to \infty} R_{mn}(z) = f(z)$ *on compact subsets of* $\mathbb{C}$.

If this result is applied to the series

$$c_n = \alpha a^n q^{n(n-1)/2}, \quad |q| < 1,$$

then not all the sequences (R_{mn}) converge, but in particular $(R_{nn})_n$ does.

Finally this part shows that the smooth character of $|c_n|$ and even of c_n is not sufficient to warrant convergence. It must be noticed that none of the above results imply the result concerning the exponential function, showing that general results are difficult to prove when only the coefficients are known.

15. Stieltjes series

The main references for this section are BAKER [1975] and BAKER and GRAVES-MORRIS [1981]. The complete proofs can be found in the last reference. A study of the subject can also be found in KARLSON and VON SYDOW [1976].

At the end of this section, we will deal with generalizations of Stieltjes functions to the meromorphic case, i.e. the convergence of sequences of Padé approximants associated with the power series expansion of f,

$$f(z) = f^*(z) + r(z),$$

where f^* is a Stieltjes function and r a rational function. These results are due to WYNN [1972], GONČAR [1975a,b], RACHMANOV [1977] and LOPEZ [1981].

A Stieltjes series is a power series of the form

$$S(z) = \sum_{i \geq 0} f_i(-z)^i, \quad f_i = \int_0^\infty x^i \, d\varphi(x), \tag{15.1}$$

where φ is a positive, bounded, nondecreasing measure. The Stieltjes function associated with the Stieltjes series is

$$f(z) = \int_0^\infty \frac{d\varphi(x)}{1 + xz}. \tag{15.2}$$

So the series $S(z)$ is formally the expansion of $f(z)$ into a power series, although this series may not converge except for $z = 0$ as for the Euler series, while the function is analytic in the cut plane $\mathbb{C}-]-\infty, 0[$

$$f(z) = \int_0^\infty \frac{e^{-t} \, dt}{1 + tz}, \quad S(z) = \sum_0^\infty n!(-z)^n.$$

Another problem is the *moment problem*, i.e. the existence and unicity of f corresponding to the moments $(f_i)_{i \geq 0}$. If φ takes only a finite number of values, it is a step function: φ is constant on $]u_i, u_{i+1}[$ for a finite number of u_i and so

$$f(z) = \sum_1^p \frac{\lambda_i}{1 + zu_i}.$$

To avoid this too simple case, φ is supposed in the sequel to take an infinite number of different values.

The characteristic of Stieltjes series is that the special form of the coefficients f_i allows us to study the corresponding Hankel determinants and so to locate the zeros of the orthogonal polynomials $P_n^{(m)}$ where

$$D_{mn}(z) = z^n P_n^{(m)}(1/z)$$

is the denominator of $[m+n-1/n]$.

So the most natural sequences to be considered are the paradiagonal sequences $([n + J/n])_n$, $J \geq -1$. From Chapter I, Theorem 4.1, we know that for each J the $P_n^{(n+J)}(= P_n)$ satisfy the three-term recurrence relation

$$P_{n+1} = (x - \beta_n^{n+J})P_n - \gamma_n^{n+J}P_{n-1},$$
$$\gamma_n^{n+J} = h_n/h_{n-1},$$
$$h_n = c^{(J-1)}(P_n^2) = c^{(J-1)}(x^n P_n) = H_{n+1}^{(J-1)}/H_n^{(J-1)}.$$

Let us set

$$\Delta(m, n) = \begin{vmatrix} f_m & \cdots & f_{m+n} \\ \vdots & & \vdots \\ f_{m+n} & \cdots & f_{m+2n} \end{vmatrix},$$

then as $f_m = (-1)^m c_m$, it is easy to prove that $\Delta(m, n) = (-1)^{(n+1)m} H_{n+1}^{(m)}$. We get the following result

THEOREM 15.1. *If f is a Stieltjes function, then all the determinants $\Delta(m, n)$, $m \geq 0$, $n \geq 0$, are strictly positive.*

PROOF. For m fixed, consider the quadratic form in $n + 1$ variables $x_0, \ldots, x_n$

$$\int_0^\infty u^m(x_0 + x_1 u + \cdots + x_n u^n)^2 \, d\varphi(u) = \sum_{p,q=0}^n f_{p+q+m} x_p x_q.$$

It is a real symmetric, positive quadratic form, so all the eigenvalues of the matrix $\Delta(m, n)$ are real and positive. The only case to avoid is $\lambda = 0$: if an eigenvalue is zero, then there exists a polynomial p such that $\int_0^\infty u^m p^2 \, d\varphi(u) = 0$, and this implies $d\varphi(u) = 0$ except at the zeros of p. This is impossible if φ takes an infinite range of values, and so all the eigenvalues are nonzero. As a product of these forms, the determinant $\Delta(m, n)$ is positive. □

A consequence of this theorem is that all the Padé approximants exist. So the Padé table is normal. Then in the recurrence relation of $P_n^{(m)}$, all the γ_n^m are positive. From the theory of orthogonal polynomials, it means that each diagonal sequence $(P_n^{(m)})_n$, m fixed, is orthogonal with respect to a positive definite functional. So $P_n^{(m)}$ has n real distinct zeros and the zeros of $P_n^{(m)}$ and $P_{n+1}^{(m)}$ interlace.

THEOREM 15.2. *All the zeros of $P_n^{(m)}$ are real, distinct and negative, for $m \geq n - 1 \geq 0$.*

PROOF.

$$P_1^{(m)} = \begin{vmatrix} c_m & c_{m+1} \\ 1 & x \end{vmatrix},$$
$$= c_m\left(x - \frac{c_{m+1}}{c_m}\right)$$
$$= c_m\left(x + \frac{f_{m+1}}{f_m}\right).$$

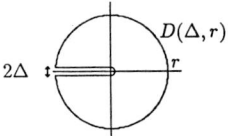

FIG. 15.1. $D(\Delta, r)$.

The zero of $P_1^{(m)}$ is negative, because all the f_i's are positive. From the interlacing property, each $P_n^{(m)}$ has at least one negative zero. Let $x_1, \ldots, x_k$ be the positive distinct zeros of $P_n^{(m)}$, and $V(x) = \prod_1^k (x - x_i)$.

$c(V(x) \cdot P_n^{(m)}(x)) = 0$, $k < n$, by the orthogonality property and $c(V(x) \cdot P_n^{(m)}(x))$ is positive because $V(x) P_n^{(m)}(x) > 0$ for $x > 0$ and c is a positive functional.

This is impossible and so all the zeros of $P_n^{(m)}$ are real, negative. □

Let us now consider the convergence of paradiagonal sequences. As $P_n^{(m)}$ has n simple negative zeros α_i, the denominator D_{mn} also has n simple negative zeros $1/\alpha_i$, so all the poles of the Padé approximants $([n+J/n])_n$ lie on the cut, and there is no impossibility to the convergence in the cut plane $\mathbb{C} -]-\infty, 0]$.

We get the following theorem

THEOREM 15.3. *Let $D(\Delta, r) = \{z \in \mathbb{C}, |z| \leqslant r,$ and $\forall x \leqslant 0, d(z, x) \geqslant \Delta\}$, then for each $J \geqslant -1$ the sequence $([n+J/n])_n$ converges uniformly on $D(\Delta, r)$ to a function f^J analytic in the cut plane $\mathbb{C} -]-\infty, 0]$.*

PROOF. Let us give a hint of the proof. First of all,

$$f(z) = \int_0^\infty \frac{d\varphi(x)}{1+xt}$$

$$= \sum_{i=0}^{J-1} (-1)^i f_i z^i + z^J \int_0^\infty \frac{x^J d\varphi(x)}{1+xt}$$

$$= \sum_{i=0}^{J-1} (-1)^i f_i z^i + z^J \varphi_J(z)$$

$$[n+J-1/n](z) = \sum_{i=0}^{J-1} (-1)^i f_i z^i + z^J [n-1/n]_{\varphi_J}(z).$$

Because φ_J is also a Stieltjes function for any J, it is sufficient to prove the convergence of the sequence $([n-1/n]_f)_n$.

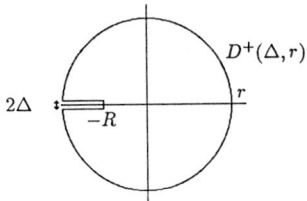

Fig. 15.2. $D^+(\Delta, r)$.

Then, $[n-1/n](z) = \sum_0^n a_i/(1+b_i z)$, with $a_i > 0$, and $b_i > 0$, and, because $\sum_0^n a_i = f_0$ and $\sum_0^n a_i b_i = f_1$, the sequence is shown to be equicontinuous and bounded on $D(\Delta, r)$. Then there exists a convergent subsequence.

The sequence is monotically increasing for z real, positive, so the whole sequence converges on $\mathbb{R}_+$. And finally, by Vitali's theorem, the whole sequence converges in $D(\Delta, r)$, uniformly. □

If the moment problem is determinate, then all the f^J are identical to f. The problem will be guaranteed to be determinate if the Stieltjes series has a nonzero radius of convergence R, or if $R = 0$ but the f_i's satisfying Carleman's condition: $\sum_{i \geq 1} (f_i)^{-1/2i}$ is diverging.

For the Euler series, the Carleman condition is satisfied since

$$\sum_{n \geq 1} \left(\frac{1}{n!}\right)^{1/2n} \text{ is equivalent to } \sum_{n \geq 1} \frac{1}{n},$$

which diverges and so the last theorem holds for the Euler function

$$f(z) = \int_0^\infty \frac{e^{-t}\, dt}{1+tz}.$$

For such sequences, Padé approximants can be useful for reconstructing the function from its power series expansion.

In the case of convergent Stieltjes series of radius R, the last theorem can be put into a more precise form due to MARKOV [1948]

THEOREM 15.4. $f(z) = \int_0^{1/R}(1+uz)^{-1}\, d\varphi(u)$ *is analytic in the cut plane* $\mathbb{C} -]-\infty, -R]$.

All the poles of $[n+J/n]$ *lie in* $]-\infty, -R]$.

The convergence of the sequence $([n+J/n])_n$ *is uniform in* $D^+(\Delta, r)$,

$$D^+(\Delta, r) = \{z,\ |z| \leq r,\ \forall x \in]-\infty, R],\ d(x, z) \geq \Delta\}.$$

A result of convergence has also been proved by PRÉVOST [1990b] concerning the product of two Stieltjes functions

THEOREM 15.5. *Let $f(z) = \int_0^a (1 - xz)^{-1} d\alpha(x)$ and $g(z) = \int_{-b}^0 (1 - xz)^{-1} d\beta(x)$, where a and b are finite and positive, α and β are positive, bounded, non decreasing measures. The integral $\int_{-b}^0 \int_0^a z/(z - x) d\alpha(x) d\beta(z)$ is assumed to exist.*
Then $f \cdot g(z) = \int_{-b}^a d\gamma(x)/(1 - xz)$ is a Stieltjes function, and so the sequence $([m_k + J, m_k]_{f \cdot g})_{m_k}$ ($J \geq -1$ and $\lim_{k \to \infty} m_k = +\infty$) of Padé approximants of $f \cdot g$ converges uniformly on every compact subset of $\mathbb{C} - (]-\infty, -b^{-1}] \cup [a^{-1}, +\infty[)$.

PROOF. The function f (resp. g) defines a linear form c (resp. d)

$$f(t) = \int_0^a \frac{d\alpha(x)}{1 - xt} = \left(c, \frac{1}{1 - xt}\right), \quad (c, P) = \int_0^a P(x) d\alpha(x),$$

$$f(t) = \sum_{n \geq 0} c_n t^n, \quad c_n = (c, t^n).$$

The tensorial product $c \otimes d$ and the product $c \cdot d$ are respectively defined by

$$(c \otimes d)_{nm} = (c \otimes d, x^n y^m) = c_n d_m,$$
$$(c \otimes d, p(x) \cdot q(y)) = (c, p(x)) \cdot (d, q(y)),$$
$$(c \cdot d)_n = \sum_{k=0}^n c_{n-k} d_k = (c \cdot d, z^n) = \left(c \otimes d, \frac{x^{n+1} - y^{n+1}}{x - y}\right),$$
$$(c \cdot d, p) = \left(c \otimes d, \frac{xp(x) - yp(y)}{x - y}\right).$$

So, $c \cdot d$ corresponds to the product of the two series f and g. Then, if $f(z^{-1}) \cdot d$ and $g(z^{-1}) \cdot c$ exist,

$$c \cdot d = f(z^{-1}) \cdot d + g(z^{-1}) \cdot c.$$

The proof is as follows, c acting on x,

$$f(z^{-1}) = \sum_{i \geq 0} c_i z^{-i} = c\left(\frac{z}{z - x}\right).$$

In the space of linear forms, $f(z^{-1}) \cdot d$ is defined (if it exists) by

$$(f(z^{-1}) \cdot d, p) = \langle d, f(z^{-1}) \cdot p(z) \rangle \quad \forall p \in \mathbb{C}[X],$$
$$(c \cdot d, p(z)) = \left(c_x \otimes d_y, \frac{xp(x) - yp(y)}{x - y}\right),$$

$$(f(z^{-1}) \cdot d_z + g(z^{-1}) \cdot c_z, p(z)) = (d_z, f(z^{-1})p(z)) + (c_z, g(z^{-1})p(z))$$
$$= \left(d_z, c_x\left(\frac{zp(z)}{z - x}\right)\right) + \left(c_z, d_y\left(\frac{zp(z)}{z - y}\right)\right)$$
$$= \left(c_x \otimes d_z, \frac{zp(z)}{z - x}\right) + \left(c_z \otimes d_y, \frac{zp(z)}{z - y}\right)$$
$$= \left(c_x \otimes d_y, \frac{yp(y) - xp(x)}{x - y}\right).$$

Now if c and d have an integral representation

$$(f(z^{-1}) \cdot d, p(z)) = \int_{-b}^{0} f(z^{-1}) p(z) \, d\beta(z) = \int_{-b}^{0} \int_{0}^{a} \frac{z}{z-x} p(z) \, d\alpha(x) \, d\beta(z),$$

the last equality being valid because $z(z-x)^{-1} \, d\alpha(x) \, d\beta(z)$ has been supposed to be integrable on the domain $[0, a] \times [-b, 0]$. Moreover it is a positive distribution. The same thing holds for $g(z^{-1}) \cdot c$, and so in terms of weight function, it follows that

$$f \cdot g(t) = \int_{-b}^{a} \frac{d\gamma(x)}{1 - xt},$$

$$d\gamma(x) = f(x^{-1}) \, d\beta(x) + g(x^{-1}) \, d\alpha(x).$$

So, because the functional $c \cdot d$ is positive, definite, the sequence of Padé approximants $([m + J/m])_m$ converges on every compact subset of $\mathbb{C} - (]-\infty, -b^{-1}] \cup [a^{-1}, +\infty[)$. □

In order to use high-order Padé approximants, without too much computation, an idea can be to follow ray sequences $[m/n]$ with $m = (\gamma + 1)n$, $\gamma \geq 0$. BAKER [1975], for the function $z^{-1} \ln(1 + z)$, proved the convergence of ray sequences in a domain and divergence in a larger one, and gave numerical experiments showing that convergence can occur in a region with a heart-shaped boundary.

GRAVES-MORRIS [1981] proved the same result of convergence for all Stieltjes series with a nonzero radius of convergence, in a domain which is very close to the biggest possible one.

Let f be the Stieltjes function $\int_0^1 (1 + uz)^{-1} \, d\varphi(u)$, whose series has a radius of convergence equal to one. For any J, the error term has the expression

$$E_J(z) = f(z) - [m + J/m](z)$$

$$= \frac{(-z)^{2m+J+1}}{(D_{m+J,m}(z))^2} \int_0^1 \frac{(P_m^{(m+J)}(u))^2 u^{J+1} \, d\varphi(u)}{1 + uz},$$

where $D_{m+J,m}$ is the denominator of $[m + J/m]$, associated with $P_m^{(m+J)}$, the polynomial of degree m of the family of orthogonal polynomials with respect to the functional $c^{(J+1)}$, with moments c_i

$$\sum_{J+1}^{\infty} c_i z^i = z^{J+1} \int_0^1 \frac{u^{J+1} \, d\varphi(u)}{1 + uz}.$$

If $d(z) = \inf\{d(x, z), x \in \,]-\infty, -1]\}$, then

$$|E_J(z)| \leq \frac{|z|^{2m+J+1}}{|D_{m+j,m}(z)|^2 \, d(z)} \int_0^1 (P_m^{(m+J)}(u))^2 u^J \, d\varphi(u),$$

$$\leq \frac{|z|^J}{d(z) \cdot |P_m^{(m+J)}(-z^{-1})|^2},$$

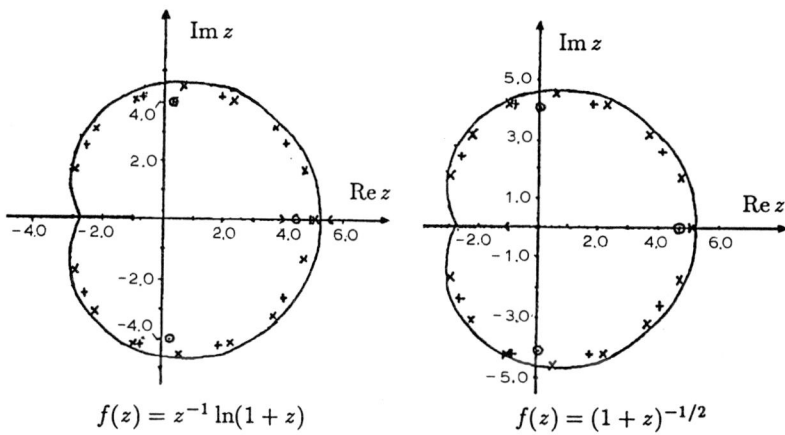

FIG. 15.3. The circled points denote a zero of [4/1], + a zero of [12/3], and × a zero of [20/5].

and so, for $J = \gamma m$, geometric convergence occurs in the domain

$$|z|^\gamma < \liminf_{m\to\infty} |P_m^{((\gamma+1)m)}(-z^{-1})|^{2/m}.$$

Then the problem is restricted to find asymptotics for $P_m^{((\gamma+1)m)}$. For the function $z^{-1}\ln(1+z)$, $P_m^{((\gamma+1)m)}(u) = k_m \bar{P}_m^{\gamma m,0}(1-2u)$ where the $\bar{P}_m^{\gamma m,0}$'s are the Jacobi polynomials.

Results concerning these ray sequences are extended to all Stieltjes series of radius 1. Complete proofs can be found in GRAVES-MORRIS [1981].

The boundary Γ of the convergence region represents a *wall* of zeros of the sequence $S_\gamma = ([m(1+\gamma)/m])_m$: for each approximant there are m poles and m zeros on the cut $]-\infty,-1]$, and the γm remaining zeros seem to accumulate on Γ. As $f(z)$ is not zero everywhere outside a (large enough) compact set, Γ is a natural boundary for the convergence of S_γ.

Let us now study the extension to the meromorphic case

$$f(z) = f^*(z) + r(z),$$
$$f^*(z) = \int \frac{d\varphi(z)}{1+xz},$$
$r(z)$ a rational function.

The cases are quite different, according to the support of the measure φ.
WYNN [1972] made the following assumptions

$$r(z) = \sum_{\gamma=1}^{n} \frac{M_\gamma}{1+b_\gamma z}, \quad b_1 > \cdots > b_n > b, \quad M_\gamma > 0, \quad \gamma = 1,\ldots,n,$$

and φ is a bounded nondecreasing measure with an infinite support included in $[a,b]$.

Let us define a progressive sequence of Padé approximants by $(R_{pq})_{pq}$: if $R_{p'q'}$ is the successor of R_{pq} then

$$p' \geq p, \quad q' \geq q, \quad p'+q' > p+q.$$

Then the result is

THEOREM 15.6. *Any progressive sequence* (R_{pq}), $p \geq n$ *and* $q \geq n$, *converges uniformly to* f *on any compact set of* $D = \{z, |z| < 1/b\} -]-1/b, -1/b_1]$.

That means that all the sequences between the column $(R_{mn})_m$ and the diagonal $(R_{nn})_n$, converge in D. The result is obtained by using Montessus De Ballore's and Markov's theorems. Moreover uniform boundedness of $(R_{n+r+h,n+r})_h$ in D' (part of D from which points lying in a neighbourhood of the negative real axis have been excluded), must be used.

Later GONČAR [1975a] proved the convergence of the diagonal sequence $(R_{nn})_n$ of the Padé table for some classes of meromorphic functions. For the sake of simplicity, Padé approximants are taken at infinity; α is a nonnegative measure of bounded variation whose support is infinite and contained in $\Delta = [-1, +1]$.

$$f(z) = f^*(z) + r(z),$$
$$f^*(z) = \int \frac{d\alpha(t)}{z-t},$$

α is said to satisfy the Szegö condition, i.e. $\alpha \in S$, if

$$\int_\Delta \frac{\ln(\alpha'(t))}{\sqrt{1-t^2}} \, dt > -\infty.$$

The Szegö condition is satisfied by

$$d\alpha(t) = (t-t_1)^{\gamma_1} \cdots (t-t_N)^{\gamma_N} w_0(t) \, dt,$$
$$t_i \in \Delta, \quad \gamma_i > -1,$$
w_0 any continous positive function on Δ.

Then the following theorem holds

THEOREM 15.7. *Let* $f = f^* + r$, $f^*(z) = \int_\Delta (z-t)^{-1} \, d\alpha(t)$ *and* $\alpha \in S$, r *a rational function with poles in* $D = \mathbb{C} - \Delta$, $f^*(\infty) = r(\infty) = 0$, *then*

(1) *For any open bounded set* $U \subset D$, *and for* n *large enough*, f *and* R_{nn} *have the same number of poles in* U, *counting their multiplicity*,

(2) *The sequence* $(R_{nn})_n$ *converges to* f *in* $D' = D - \{$poles of $f\}$. *For any compact set* K *of* D'

$$\varphi(z) = z + \sqrt{z^2-1} \quad (|z + \sqrt{z^2-1}| > 1, \, z \in D),$$
$$\rho(K) = \inf\{|\varphi(z)|, z \in K\},$$
$$\limsup_{n \to \infty} \|f - R_{nn}\|_K^{1/n} \leq \frac{1}{\rho(K)} < 1.$$

Statement (1) means that every pole of f in D attracts the same number of poles of R_{nn} counting their multiplicity; the remaining poles of R_{nn} superimpose on the interval Δ. Thus the poles of f can be found as the limit points of the set of poles of (R_{nn}) lying in D.

The proof can be based only on the following asymptotic formula, due to Szegö, for the unitary polynomials L_n, orthogonal with respect to α

$$\lim_{n\to\infty} \frac{L_{n+1}}{L_n}(z) = \tfrac{1}{2}\varphi(z), \quad z \in D.$$

And so the last theorem is proved for functions f such that the preceding relation is satisfied, (i.e. $\alpha \in S$).

The link between D_n, denominator of the Padé approximant R_{nn} of f, and L_n, denominator of the Padé approximant of f^*, is given by

$$f(z) = f^*(z) + r(z),$$
$$f^*(z) = \int_\Delta \frac{d\alpha(t)}{z-t}, \quad \alpha \in S,$$
$$r(z) = \sum_{j=1}^{l}\sum_{k=1}^{m_j} \frac{A_{jk}}{(k-1)!}\frac{1}{(z-a_j)^k}, \quad \sum_{j=1}^{l} m_j = m, \quad a_i \in D.$$

Then we get

$$\lim_{n\to\infty} \frac{D_n}{L_n}(z) = \frac{\prod_{j=1}^{l}(\varphi(z) - \varphi(a_j))^{2m_j}}{2^m \varphi^m(z) \cdot \prod_{j=1}^{l}(z-a_j)^{m_j}},$$

uniformly on compact subsets of D. And so it follows that $\lim_{n\to\infty} |D_n(z)|^{1/n} = \tfrac{1}{2}|\varphi(z)|$ uniformly on $D' = D - \{a_j, j = 1, \ldots, l\}$.

RACHMANOV [1977] also studied this type of function and generalized the condition on the measure $d\alpha$. He also proved that the result of the last theorem is not true in general for special measures $d\alpha$ and if r has complex coefficients. Then the denominator D_n of R_{nn} has more than m (number of poles of r) zeros outside Δ, and this does rule out uniform convergence on compact subsets of D, even if it does not rule out convergence in capacity.

LOPEZ [1981] studied the convergence problem for the diagonal Padé approximants for functions of the form $f = f^* + r$ where f^* is defined by a positive measure on $[0, +\infty[$, and r is a rational function with real coefficients. It is known that the diagonal sequence of Padé approximants of f^* converges in $D = \mathbb{C} - \Delta$ if the moment problem is assumed to be determinate, so if the coefficients c_i^* of the power series expansion of f^* satisfy the Carleman condition

$$\sum_{i=1}^{\infty}(c_i^*)^{-1/2i} = +\infty.$$

The generalization of this result to the meromorphic case is the following

THEOREM 15.8. *Let α be such that $\Delta = [0, \infty[$ and Carleman's condition is satisfied; let $f = f^* + r$ where r is a rational function with real coefficients, whose poles are in $D = \mathbb{C} - \Delta$ with $r(\infty) = 0$, and let $(R_{nn})_n$ be the diagonal sequence of Padé approximants of f. Then we get*

(1) For all n large enough, R_{nn} exists. The number of poles of R_{nn} in D equals the number of poles of r, and the poles of R_{nn} in D tend (as $n \to \infty$) to the poles of r.

(2) The sequence $(R_{nn})_n$ converges uniformly to f on compact sets in $D' = D - \{poles\ of\ r\}$.

The extension of the result to functions where r has complex coefficients is still open.

16. Pólya frequency series

The results about Pólya frequency series have been reviewed by BAKER and GRAVES-MORRIS [1981].

These series generalize the exponential function. For the exponential function (see Section 28), all the numerators and denominators of Padé approximants are explicitly known from their determinantal expression, using

$$H_m^{(l-m+1)} = (-1)^{m(m-1)/2} \prod_{k=1}^{m} \frac{1}{k(k+1)\cdots(k+l-1)}.$$

The class of Pólya frequency series, also called functions generated by a totally positive sequence of coefficients, are characterized by

$$(-1)^{m(m-1)/2} H_m^{(l-m+1)} > 0.$$

It has been proved by SCHOENBERG [1949] and EDREI [1953] that there is an equivalence between functions generated by a totally positive sequence and functions of class S

$$\begin{cases} f(z) = a_0 e^{\gamma z} \prod_{i \geq 0} \frac{1 + \alpha_i z}{1 - \beta_i z}, \\ a_0 > 0,\ \gamma \geq 0,\ \alpha_i \geq 0,\ \beta_i \geq 0,\ \sum_i \alpha_i + \beta_i < +\infty. \end{cases}$$

Let $g(z) = (1 + \alpha z)f(z)$, $\alpha \geq 0$; then the numerators and the denominators of the Padé approximants of f and g satisfy the following relations

$$[l/m]_g = \tilde{N}_{lg}^{(j)}/\tilde{P}_{mg}^{(j)}, \quad j = l - n,$$

$$\tilde{N}_{l,g}^{(j)}(z) = \tilde{N}_{lf}^{(j)}(z) + \alpha z \tilde{N}_{l-1,f}^{(j-1)}(z) \frac{\tilde{P}_{mf}^{(j)}(-1/\alpha)}{\tilde{P}_{mf}^{(j-1)}(-1/\alpha)},$$

$$\tilde{P}_{mg}^{(j)}(z) = \frac{\tilde{P}_{mf}^{(j-1)}(-1/\alpha)\tilde{P}_{mf}^{(j)}(z) + \alpha z \tilde{P}_{nf}^{(j-1)}(z) \cdot \tilde{P}_{mf}^{(j)}(-1/\alpha)}{\tilde{P}_{mf}^{(j-1)}(-1/\alpha)(1 + \alpha z)}.$$

For the exponential function, $\tilde{N}_l^{(j)}(z)$ and $\tilde{P}_m^{(j)}(z)$ have all their coefficients nonnegative, then it is also true for Pólya frequency series, because, from the preceding relations, each coefficient of $P_{lg}^{(j)}$ is greater than the corresponding coefficient of $P_{lf}^{(j)}$.

Other such relations can be found in the work of ARMS and EDREI [1970] where the most important result about convergence of Padé approximants is proved

THEOREM 16.1. *Let $\sum_{i \geq 0} c_i z^i$ be the expansion of a function of class S*

$$f(z) = a_0 e^{\gamma z} \prod_{i \geq 0} \left(\frac{1 + \alpha_i z}{1 - \beta_i z} \right),$$

$$a_0 > 0, \quad \gamma \geq 0, \quad \alpha_i \geq 0, \quad \beta_i \geq 0, \quad \sum_i \alpha_i + \beta_i < +\infty.$$

Then
  (1) *the Padé table is normal, and $(-1)^{m(m-1)/2} H_n^{(n-m+1)} > 0$.*
  (2) *Let (m_k, n_k) be a ray sequence*

$$\lim_{k \to \infty} m_k = \infty, \quad \lim_{k \to \infty} \frac{m_k}{n_k} = \omega, \quad 0 \leq \omega \leq +\infty.$$

and let $[m_k/n_k] = \tilde{N}_{m_k, n_k} / \tilde{P}_{m_k, n_k}$; then

$$\lim_{k \to \infty} \tilde{N}_{m_k, n_k}(z) = a_0 e^{\omega \gamma z / (1+\omega)} \prod_{i \geq 0} (1 + \alpha_i z),$$

$$\lim_{k \to \infty} \tilde{P}_{m_k, n_k}(z) = e^{-\gamma z / (1+\omega)} \prod_{i \geq 0} (1 - \beta_i z).$$

The convergence of both sequences is uniform on any compact subset of the complex plane.

The ability to separate numerators and denominators comes from the fact that, as for the exponential function, $1/f(-z)$ is also of class S.

The last result has been extended by EDREI [1974]: the convergence on compact sets is obtained for any sequence of Padé approximants $[m_k/n_k]$ only with the assumption $\lim_{k \to \infty} m_k = \lim_{k \to \infty} n_k = \infty$. Nevertheless the separate convergence of numerators and denominators is lost.

17. Convergence in capacity

As Wallin's counterexample has shown (Theorem 12.2), locally uniform convergence of Padé approximants requires specific structural properties of the function f, and cannot be summarized by analyticity.

However, it is possible to prove convergence results for analytic functions if we ask only for convergence in capacity, i.e. a type of convergence that allows non-convergence on exceptionnal sets of *small dimension*. Moreover convergence in capacity implies convergence with respect to the planar Lebesgue measure (i.e. almost everywhere).

Let us, first, recall the definition of convergence in capacity.

Let K be a compact set of $\mathbb{C}$ and Π_n the set of monic polynomials of degree n. The logarithmic capacity of K is defined by

$$\operatorname{cap} K = \left(\lim_{n \to \infty} \inf_{P_n \in \Pi_n} \max_{z \in K} |P_n(z)|^{1/n} \right). \tag{17.1}$$

If A is an arbitrary set, then

$$\operatorname{cap} A = \sup_{K \subset A} (\operatorname{cap} K). \tag{17.2}$$

The capacity of a denumerable set is zero, and the capacity of a disc of radius r is r. If a set contains a continuous arc, its capacity is positive. Now a sequence (f_n) is said to converge to f on A, in capacity, if and only if

$$\forall \varepsilon, \quad \lim_{n \to \infty} \operatorname{cap}(E_n) = 0,$$

where $E_n = \{z, z \in A$ and $\operatorname{cap}\{|f_n(z - f(z)| > \varepsilon\}$.

We will use the following result: if $(A_i)_{i=1,\ldots,N}$ are sets satisfying $\operatorname{cap} A_i < \alpha$, then $\operatorname{cap}(A_1 \cup \cdots \cup A_N) \leqslant \operatorname{diam}(A_1 \cup \cdots \cup A_N)^{1-1/N}$.

Let us define A^0 as the set of all functions f analytic on $\mathbb{C}$ except on a set E_f of capacity zero.

Of course all the meromorphic functions are in A^0; A^0 may contain functions with essential isolated singularities, but not with branch points. The following result has been proved by POMMERENKE [1973], after a first result concerning convergence almost everywhere by NUTTALL [1970].

The sequences of Padé approximants considered are sectorial sequences with indexes $(m_k, n_k)_k$ defined by $(m,n) \in S: (m,n) = (m_k, n_k)$, $1/c \leqslant n_k/m_k \leqslant c$ and $\lim_S (m+n) = \lim_{k \to \infty} m_k + n_k = \infty$.

For the sake of notational simplicity, Padé approximants are considered at infinity

$$q_{mn}(z)f(z) - p_{mn}(z) = O\left(\frac{1}{z^{m+n+1}}\right) \quad (z \to \infty).$$

q_{mn} and p_{mn} are polynomials in $1/z$ of degrees n and m respectively.

THEOREM 17.1. *Let f be a function in A^0, analytic on $\mathbb{C} - E$ where E is a compact set of capacity zero, and let D_r be the closed disc of radius r ($r > 1$). For $\varepsilon > 0$, $r > 1$, $c > 1$, there exists n_0 such that $n > n_0$ and $c^{-1} < m/n < c \Longrightarrow (p_{mn}/q_{mn} - f)(z) < \varepsilon^n$ for $z \in D_r - E_{mn}$, where $\operatorname{cap} E_{mn} < 3r\varepsilon^{1/3}$.*

PROOF. The proof is given, to show how, following the simple idea of representing the remainder term by Cauchy's formula, the notion of capacity occurs. The proof can be extended to the case where E is not compact.

From the definition of capacity, there exist an integer k and a polynomial h of Π_k such that

$$E \subset C \subset E_0,$$

$C = \{z, |h(z)| = \delta^k\}$ oriented such that the point at infinity is in the interior of C, $E_0 = \{z, |h(z)| \leq \varepsilon^k\}$, $\delta < \varepsilon$ and $r > 1$ be large enough so that $E_0 \subset D_r$, $q_{mn}^*(z) = z^n q_{mn}(z)$ is a polynomial of degree n in z, normalized by the condition $\sup_{|z|=r} |q_{mn}^*(z)| = 1$.

We consider an index n large enough such that $n - k > n/\alpha$, α fixed.

Let l be an integer satisfying $(n-k)/k < l \leq n/k$, so h^l is of degree kl, smaller than n.

Then

$$z^m h^l(z)(q_{mn}f - p_{mn})(z) = z^{m-n} h^l(z) q_{mn}^*(z) f(z) - h^l(z) z^m p_{mn}(z).$$

For $z \notin E_0$: $\int_C h^l(t) \cdot t^m p_{mn}(t)(t-z)^{-1} dt = 0$ and finally, by Cauchy's formula we get

$$z^m h^l(z)(q_{mn}f - p_{mn})(z) = \frac{1}{2i\pi} \int_C \frac{t^{m-n} h^l(t) q_{mn}^*(t)}{t - z} f(t) dt.$$

$C \subset D_r$, so, because of the normalizing condition, we get $|q_{mn}^*(t)| \leq 1$ for $t \in C$. Let us suppose, for the moment, that $n \leq m \leq cn$, $c > 1$, then

$$0 \leq m - n \leq (c-1) \cdot n.$$

For $|z| \leq r$ and $z \in E_0$

$$|z^m h^l(z)(q_{mn}f - p_{mn})(z)| \leq M r^{(c-1)n} \delta^{kl},$$

$$|(f - p_{mn}/q_{mn})(z)| \leq \frac{M r^{(c-1)n} \delta^{kl}}{|z^m h^l(z) q_{mn}(z)|} \leq \frac{M r^{(c-1)n} \delta^{kl}}{|z^{m-n} h^l(z) q_{mn}^*(z)|}$$

$$\leq M \frac{r^{(c-1)n} \delta^{n-k}}{\varepsilon^{(c+1)n}} \frac{1}{|q_{mn}^*(z)|} \leq M \left(\frac{r^{c-1} \delta^{1/\alpha}}{\varepsilon^{c+1}}\right)^n \frac{1}{|q_{mn}^*(z)|}.$$

We will prove in the next lemma that, with the actual assumptions, there exists a set Δ_{mn}, such that

$$|q_{mn}^*(z)| \geq \varepsilon^n, \quad z \in D_r - D_{mn}, \quad \text{cap } \Delta_{mn} \leq 3r\varepsilon,$$

and so, defining δ by

$$\frac{r^{c-1}}{\varepsilon^{c+1}} \delta^{1/\alpha} = \varepsilon, \quad \text{i.e. } \delta = \left(\frac{\varepsilon^{c+2}}{r^{c-1}}\right)^\alpha,$$

$|(f - p_{mn}/q_{mn})(z)| < \varepsilon^n$ for n large enough and $z \in D_r - E_{mn}$, where E_{mn} is

$$E_{mn} = \{z, \ |z| \leqslant \varepsilon\} \cup E_0 \cup \Delta_{mn}.$$

From the result, recalled at the beginning, about the capacities of a union of sets, we get

$$\text{cap } E_{mn} < 3r\varepsilon^{1/3}.$$

And this proves the assertion for $m \geqslant n$. If now $c^{-1}n \leqslant m \leqslant n$, we know that

$$R_{mn}(f) = \frac{1}{R_{mn}(1/f)}, \quad \text{if } f(0) \neq 0,$$
$$|R_{mn}(f) - f| = |1/R_{mn}(f^*) - 1/f^*| \quad (f^* = 1/f)$$
$$\leqslant \frac{|f^* - R_{mn}(f^*)|}{|f^*| \cdot (|f^*| - |f^* R_{mn}(f^*)|)}.$$

Let

$$E^* = E \cup \{\text{zeros of } f\}, \quad \text{cap } E^* = 0,$$
$$C^* = \mathbb{C} - E^*.$$

As f is nonzero on E^*, it will be bounded from below by a nonzero constant A for $z \in D_r - E_1^*$, and $\text{cap } E_1^* < \eta^*$.

Applying the preceding result to f^*, we get

$$|(R_{mn}(f) - f)(z)| \leqslant \frac{\varepsilon^{2n}}{A(A - \varepsilon^{2n})} < \varepsilon^n \quad \text{for } n \text{ large enough,}$$
$$z \in D_r - E_{mn}, \quad E_{mn} = E_{mn}^* \cup E_1^*$$

and, still from the relation between capacities, $\text{cap } E_{mn}$ can be made as small as necessary. □

It remains to prove that $\text{cap } D_{mn} < 3r\varepsilon$. This is implied by the following lemma

LEMMA 17.1. *Let $r > 0$ and q of degree n be such that*

$$\max_{|z|=r} |q(z)| \geqslant 1.$$

Let $0 < \varepsilon < 1/3$, $B = \{z, |z| \leqslant r \text{ and } |q(z)| < \varepsilon^n\}$. Then $\text{cap } B \leqslant 3r\varepsilon$.

PROOF.

$$q(z) = c \prod_1^k (z - z_i) \prod_{k+1}^n (z - z_i),$$

where for $i \leqslant k$, $|z_i| \leqslant 2r$.
From the maximum principle

$$1 \leqslant |c|(3r)^k \prod_{k+1}^{n}(|z_i| + r).$$

Let

$$h(z) = \prod_{1}^{k}(z - z_i),$$

$$z \in B: \quad |h(z)| \leqslant \frac{\varepsilon^n}{|c|\prod_{k+1}^{n}|z - z_i|}|c|(3r)^k \prod_{k+1}^{n}(|z_i| + r)$$

$$\leqslant \varepsilon^n (3r)^k z^{n-k} \leqslant \varepsilon^n 3^n r^k \quad (r > 1)$$

$$\leqslant 3^k \varepsilon^k r^k, \quad 3\varepsilon < 1.$$

$$\max_B |h(z)|^{1/k} \leqslant 3\varepsilon r.$$

For all h^l, we have the same upper bound with respect to a polynomial h^{kl} of degree kl, and so we get cap $B \leqslant 3\varepsilon r$. □

The lemma can be applied in the proof of the theorem with $q^* = q$, and if ε has been taken smaller than $1/3$ at the beginning.

It must be noticed that the theorem proves geometric convergence.

The class of functions to which the Nuttall–Pommerenke theorem has been extended is the set R_0 defined as follows:

$f \in R_0$: f analytic at zero, if $K = \{|z| < \delta\}$ for an arbitrary number δ depending on f and $\rho_n(f, K) = \inf \sup_{z \in K} |(f - r_n)(z)|$, (inf taken on all (n, n) rational functions) then $\liminf_{n \to \infty} (\rho_n(f, K))^{1/n} = 0$.

The link between fast approximability by rational functions and single-valuedness has been given by GONČAR [1972].

Obviously entire and meromorphic functions are in R_0. If f is a single-valued analytic function whose set of singularities has zero capacity, then f is in R_0. Other functions than these are in R_0.

The Nuttall-Pommerenke theorem has been extended to the set R_0 by GONČAR [1973].

If we consider the set R^* of functions locally analytic in $\mathbb{C} - E_f$ with cap $E_f = 0$, then such functions are multivalued. Functions with branch points and more particularly algebraic functions are in R^*, and obviously cannot satisfy fast approximability by rational functions.

Results about these sets of functions can be found in STAHL [1989]. It is possible to prove convergence in capacity to f of close-to-diagonal sequences (that is, n/m equivalent to 1) in a domain D, called extremal and linked to the branch points of f.

Other types of singularities have been studied. Let

$$f(z) = \int \frac{\mathrm{d}\mu(x)}{x - z}.$$

The convergence depends on the asymptotic behaviour of the orthogonal polynomials, here associated with complex-valued measures.

We will end with the following negative result from STAHL [1985]. Let I be the interval $[-1, +1]$, and $\mathcal{M}(I)$ the set of complex-valued Borel measures on I

THEOREM 17.2. *There exist measures* $\mu \in \mathcal{M}(I)$ *such that the sequence of Padé approximants* $(R_{nn})_n$ *to f converges neither pointwise nor in capacity on any open set in* $\mathbb{C} - I$.

18. Inverse problem

In the theory of Padé approximations, direct results on the convergence of the columns or diagonals have been given in the previous sections of this chapter. Recently much attention has been paid to inverse problems, in which a conclusion is to be drawn about the meromorphic continuation of f and about its singular points on the basis of the asymptotic behaviour of the poles of sequences of Padé approximants of f.

In what follows, each pole is counted with its multiplicity, and the sequence $(R_{nn})_n$ is considered only for the indices for which R_{nn} exists. So if R_{nn} exists for $n \in \Lambda$, $\lim_{n \to \infty} R_{nn}$ means $\lim_{n \to \infty, n \in \Lambda} R_{nn}$. Let us first consider the column sequence of Padé approximants of f, given by a power series expansion

$$f(z) = \sum_0^\infty c_k z^k.$$

$R_m(f)$ is the mth radius of meromorphy of f, i.e. it is the radius of the maximal open disc D_m centered at zero, in which f extends meromorphically and has at most m poles.

THEOREM 18.1. *Suppose that for all n (large enough) and m fixed, R_{nm}, approximant in the mth column of the Padé table of the series f, has exactly m poles $\tau_{n1}, \ldots, \tau_{nm}$, and that*

$$\lim_{n \to \infty} \tau_{np} = \lambda_p, \quad p = 1, \ldots, m.$$

Then

(1) $R_{m-1}(f) = \sup_{p=1,\ldots,m} |\lambda_p|$. *If* $|\lambda_p| < R_{m-1}(f)$, *then λ_p is a pole of f, and the only poles of f are the λ_p's satisfying such an inequality.*

(2) if $|\lambda_p| = R_{m-1}(f)$, then λ_p is a singular point of f.

These two results were conjectured by GONČAR [1982], the first being proved in the same paper, and the second by SUETIN [1985]. The case where only one λ_p has the maximum modulus $R_{m-1}(f)$ was first studied by VAVILOV, LOPEZ and PROKHOROV [1985]. The result is then a generalization of Fabry's theorem which states the following: for $m = 1$, $\lim_{n\to\infty} c_n/c_{n-1} = \lim_{n\to\infty} \tau_{n1} = \lambda_1$ is a singular point of f and f is holomorphic in the open disc $D(0, \lambda_1) = D_0$.

BUSLAEV [1988] gave this result in another form; the idea is to extend Poincaré's theorem, joined to Fabry's theorem.

Poincaré's theorem is the following: suppose that the terms of a sequence (f_n) satisfy the relations (infinitely many f_n being nonzero)

$$\begin{cases} f_{n+l} + \alpha_{n1} f_{n+l-1} + \cdots + \alpha_{nl} f_n = 0, \\ \lim_{n\to\infty} \alpha_{np} = \alpha_p, \quad p = 1, \ldots, l. \end{cases}$$

Suppose, moreover, that the roots of the polynomial $z^l + \alpha_1 z^{l-1} + \cdots + \alpha_l$ are distinct in modulus, then the limit of the ratio f_{n+1}/f_n exists and is equal to one of these roots. To recover the case of several points lying on $|z| = R_{m-1}(f)$, the assumptions are transformed into the following form:

from $f_{n+1} + \beta_n f_n = 0$, $\lim \beta_n = \beta$, $(z + \beta)$ divides $z^l + \alpha_1 z^{l-1} + \cdots + \alpha_l$,

it becomes

$f_{n+k} + \beta_{n1} f_{n+k-1} + \cdots + \beta_{nk} f_n = 0,$
$\lim_{n\to\infty} \beta_{ni} = \beta_i,$
$z^k + \beta_1 z^{k-1} + \cdots + \beta_k$ divides $z^l + \alpha_1 z^{l-1} + \cdots + \alpha_l$.

Moreover the conclusions remain true if the recurrence relation on (α_{ni}) is replaced by an infinite relation. Finally the following theorem supplements both Poincaré's theorem and the Fabry quotient theorem.

The following notations are used

$$f(z) = \sum_0^\infty c_n z^n,$$
$$R(f) = R_0(f) = (\limsup_{n\to\infty} |c_n|^{1/n})^{-1},$$
$U_\delta(f) = \{z, R(f)e^{-\delta} < |z| < R(f)e^\delta\},$
$U_{\delta,m}(f) = \{z, R(f)e^{-\delta} < |z| < R_{m-1}(f)e^\delta\},$
$H(U) = \{\text{functions holomorphic in } U\},$
$[f \cdot g]_n =$ partial sum, truncated at the power n, of the product of the two series.

THEOREM 18.2. *Let f be a power series with a finite radius of convergence R ($R \neq 0$). Suppose that there exists $\delta > 0$, and for $n \geqslant 0$, functions $\alpha_n(z)$ of $H(U_\delta(f))$ with $\lim_{n\to\infty} \alpha_n(z) = \alpha(z)$ for $z \in U_\delta(f)$, such that*

$$[f(z) \cdot \alpha_n(z)]_n = O(R^{-n}e^{-n\delta}) \quad (n \to \infty).$$

Then α has at least one zero on the circle $|z| = R$, and the c_n's satisfy

$$c_{n+k} + \beta_{n1}c_{n+k-1} + \cdots + \beta_{nk}c_n = 0,$$

where

$$\lim_{n \to \infty} \beta_{ni} = \beta_i, \quad i = 1, \ldots, k.$$

The polynomial $z^k + \beta_1 z^{k-1} + \cdots + \beta_k$ divides α, all its roots are equal in modulus to R, and at least one of them is a singular point of f.

Theorem 18.1 can be put into the same form, with the assumptions written as recurrence relations satisfied by the c_n

THEOREM 18.3. *Suppose that f is a nonrational function, having at most $m - 1$ poles, and the coefficient c_k satisfying a system of m linear relations,*

$$[f(z)\alpha_n(z)]_{n+\gamma} = 0, \quad \gamma = 1, \ldots, m, \ n \geq 1,$$

where the α_n's are polynomials of degree m and $\lim_{n \to \infty} \alpha_n(z) = \prod_{p=1}^{m}(z - \lambda_p)$. Then the conclusion of Theorem 18.1 holds: if $|\lambda_p| < R_{m-1}(f)$, λ_p is a pole of f and the only poles of f are these λ_p's; if $|\lambda_p| = R_{m-1}(f)$, λ_p is a singular point of f.

In the same paper Buslaev gave an extension of these results, whose main application is the proof of similar results for the mth row of multipoint Padé approximants.

Let us consider now the inverse problem concerning diagonal sequences of Padé approximants associated to a given power series. The results are taken from a paper of GONČAR and LUNGU [1981]. The Padé approximants are considered at infinity.

In these results, the asymptotic behaviour of the sequence $(R_{nn})_n$ leads to the conclusion that one can define an analytic continuation of the series f in a corresponding domain. The conclusion of holomorphic extension follows from the regular distribution of the poles of R_{nn} or from the fact that the poles of this sequence have accumulation points.

The notations are as follows
- $R_{nn} = P_n/Q_n$,
- L: set of limit points of the table $(\zeta_{nj})_{,j=1...n}$, $n \geq 0$ of the poles of $(R_{nn})_{n \geq 0}$,
  - $f \in \mathcal{M}(D)$: f has a meromorphic extension in D,
  - $f \in \mathcal{M}_k(D)$: f has a meromorphic extension in D with k poles,
  - $K_n(U)$ = number of poles of R_{nn} in U,

– A set is said to be compact if it is compact in $\bar{\mathbb{C}}$.

THEOREM 18.4. *Let f be a formal series, D a regular region in $\bar{\mathbb{C}}$, containing the point $z = \infty$, and $E = \bar{\mathbb{C}} - D$.*
Assume the following conditions
  (1) $\limsup_{n \to \infty} K_n(U) = K(U) < +\infty$ *for any compact U of D,*
  (2) $\lim_{n \to \infty} \|Q_n\|_E^{1/n} = \operatorname{cap} E$.
Then $f \in \mathcal{M}(D)$. If in addition $K(U) \leqslant k$ for any compact set U of D then $f \in \mathcal{M}_k(D)$. If $E = L$, then f has a holomorphic extension in D.

For any a of $\mathbb{C}$, we set

$$U_\varepsilon(a) = \{z, \ |z - a| < \varepsilon\},$$
$$\lambda(a) = \lim_{\varepsilon \to 0} \liminf_{n \to \infty} \frac{1}{n} K_n(U_\varepsilon(a)).$$

THEOREM 18.5. *Let f be a formal power series, D an arbitrary region containing the point $z = \infty$, and $E = \bar{\mathbb{C}} - D$. Assume the following conditions*
  (1) $\limsup_{n \to \infty} K_n(U) = K(U) < +\infty$ *for any compact set $U \subset D$,*
  (2) *there exists $a \in E$: $\lambda(a) > 0$.*
Then $f \in \mathcal{M}(D)$. If, moreover, $K(U) \leqslant k$ for any compact set $U \subset D$, then $f \in \mathcal{M}_k(D)$.

Some particular consequences must be noticed: if the assumptions of Theorem 18.4 or Theorem 18.5 are fulfilled, the sequence $(R_{nn})_n$ defines a single-valued function.

If, moreover, $\liminf_{n \to \infty} K_n(U) = p$ for any neighbourhood of a, then a is a pole of order p of f.

The assumptions of Theorem 18.4 or Theorem 18.5 are fulfilled by the meromorphic extension of the Stieltjes case: $f = f^* + r$,

$$f^*(z) = \int_\Delta \frac{d\mu(t)}{z - t}$$

where μ a finite positive measure whose support is infinite and lies in a segment Δ of $\mathbb{R}$ and r a rational fraction with poles in $\mathbb{C} - \Delta$.

With the same methods, it is possible to prove the following theorem

THEOREM 18.6. *Let f be a formal power series and D_R the disc of radius R. If $\limsup_{n \to \infty} K_n(D_R) \leqslant k$, then $f \in \mathcal{M}_k(D_{cR})$ where $c > 0$ is an absolute constant (independent of f). The constant c satisfies*

$$c \leqslant c_0, \quad c_0 = 2 + \sqrt{5}.$$

CHAPTER III

Generalizations

19. Padé-type approximants

Padé-type approximants are a generalization of Padé approximants. They were earlier introduced in Section 2 and we shall now study them in more detail. The advantage (which can also be a drawback) of Padé-type approximants is that their denominator is arbitrarily chosen and then the numerator is calculated so that their power series expansion agrees with that of the series f as far as possible. A *good* choice of the denominator (that is, of the poles of the rational approximant) can lead to interesting approximation and convergence properties while a *bad* choice can destroy them.

Let us recall the construction of the Padé-type approximant with a numerator of degree $k-1$ and a denominator of degree k as explained in Section 2.

Let v_k be an arbitrary polynomial of degree k. It is assumed to have $x_1, \ldots, x_n$ as distinct zeros with the respective multiplicities $k_1, \ldots, k_n$ and $k = k_1 + \cdots + k_n$. Thus

$$v_k(x) = (x - x_1)^{k_1} \cdots (x - x_n)^{k_n}.$$

Let R_k be the Hermite interpolation polynomial of the function $x \to (1-xz)^{-1}$ at $x_1, \ldots, x_n$. R_k is given by Theorem 2.3.

$c(R_k(x))$ is a rational function with a numerator of degree $k-1$ and a denominator of degree k in z, which is denoted $(k-1/k)_f(z)$, and is such that

$$(k-1/k)_f(z) = f(z) + O(z^k).$$

More precisely

$$(k-1/k)_f(z) = f(z) - \frac{z^k}{\tilde{v}_k(z)} c(v_k(z)(1-xz)^{-1})$$

with $\tilde{v}_k(z) = z^k v_k(z^{-1})$.

If we set

$$w_{k-1}(z) = c\left(\frac{v_k(z) - v_k(x)}{z - x}\right)$$

and

$$\tilde{w}_{k-1}(z) = z^{k-1}w_{k-1}(z^{-1})$$

then it is easy to see that

$$(k-1/k)_f(z) = \tilde{w}_{k-1}(z)/\tilde{v}_k(z).$$

$(k-1/k)$ is a so-called Padé-type approximant of f and v_k is called its generating polynomial.

Let us now show how to construct Padé-type approximants with arbitrary degrees in the numerator and in the denominator.

Let v_q be an arbitrary polynomial of degree q. We set

$$w_p(z) = c\left(\frac{x^{p-q+1}v_q(x) - z^{p-q+1}v_q(z)}{x-z}\right)$$

where c acts on x (with the convention that $c(x^i) = 0$ if $i < 0$) and z is a parameter.

It is easy to see that w_p is a polynomial of degree p. Indeed if we write

$$v_q(x) = a_0 + a_1 x + \cdots + a_q x^q$$

then

$$[x^{p-q+1}v_q(x) - z^{p-q+1}v_q(z)](x-z)^{-1}$$
$$= a_0(x^{p-q} + x^{p-q-1}z + \cdots + xz^{p-q-1} + z^{p-q})$$
$$+ \cdots + a_q(x^p + x^{p-1}z + \cdots + xz^{p-1} + z^p).$$

Let us now consider the rational fraction

$$\tilde{w}_p(z)/\tilde{v}_q(z)$$

with $\tilde{v}_q(z) = z^q v_q(z^{-1})$ and $\tilde{w}_p(z) = z^p w_p(z^{-1})$. Then we have

$$\tilde{w}_p(z) = c\left(\frac{z^q v_q(z^{-1}) - z^{p+1}x^{p-q+1}v_q(x)}{1-xz}\right)$$
$$= \tilde{v}_q(z)c((1-xz)^{-1}) - z^{p+1}c(x^{p-q+1}v_q(x)(1-xz)^{-1})$$

and thus

$$\tilde{w}_p(z)/\tilde{v}_q(z) = f(z) + O(z^{p+1})$$

which shows that it is a rational fraction with a numerator of degree p and a denominator of degree q whose series expansion coincides with that of f up to the degree p. Such a rational function is called a Padé-type approximant

Section 19 — Generalizations

of f. If $p = k - 1$ and $q = k$ all the results of Section 2 are recovered. Let us recall that the Padé approximant with the same degrees matches f up to the degree $p + q$. It must be noticed that the computation of (p/q) needs the knowledge of $c_0, \ldots, c_p$ while that of $[p/q]$ needs $c_0, \ldots, c_{p+q}$. It is also possible to construct approximants with an order of approximation between p and $p + q$. Such approximants, called Padé-type approximants of higher order, are obtained by choosing a part of the denominator (that is, some of the poles of the approximant) and calculating the other part (that is, the other poles) and the numerator such that the order of approximation be maximum. For that let us write

$$v_q(x) = r_m(x)s_{q-m}(x)$$

where s_{q-m} is arbitrarily chosen (the index indicates the degree). From the above expression of the error we have

$$\tilde{w}_p(z) = \tilde{v}_q(z)f(z) - z^{p+1}c(x^{p-q+1}r_m(x)s_{q-m}(x)$$
$$\times (1 + xz + \cdots + x^{m-1}z^{m-1} + x^m z^m(1 - xz)^{-1})).$$

Now if r_m is calculated so that

$$c(x^{p-q+1+i}r_m(x)s_{q-m}(x)) = 0 \quad \text{for } i = 0, \ldots, m - 1$$

then we shall have

$$\tilde{w}_p(z)/\tilde{v}_q(z) = f(z) + O(z^{p+m+1}).$$

The computation of this approximant, called a Padé-type approximant of order $p + m$, needs the knowledge of $c_0, \ldots, c_{p+m}$. Of course, if $m = q$ we recover the ordinary Padé approximant $[p/q]$ where no arbitrary choice is left, while, when $m = 0$, the preceding Padé-type approximant (p/q) with s_q as a generating polynomial is again obtained. In Section 20 we shall study a further generalization of this idea where a part of the numerator and a part of the denominator are arbitrarily chosen.

Let us now come back to the ordinary Padé-type approximants, as defined at the beginning of this section, and study their algebraic properties. As we shall see below, Padé-type approximants can exhibit the same properties as Padé approximants if some further conditions are imposed on their generating polynomials. Since the proofs of these results are quite similar to those of Properties 3.1, 3.2 and 3.3, they will be omitted.

The first property concerns the approximants of the reciprocal series g (that is, the series formally defined by $f(z)g(z) = 1$). While, in the Padé case, this property occurred for all the approximants of the table, it now holds only when $p = q = k$.

Let v_k be the generating polynomial of $(k/k)_f$ and let V_k be the generating polynomial of $(k/k)_g$ where

$$V_k(x) = c_0 v_k(x) + w(x)$$

with

$$w(z) = c\left(x\frac{v_k(x) - v_k(z)}{x - z}\right).$$

Then we have

PROPERTY 19.1.

$$(k/k)_f(z)(k/k)_g(z) = 1$$

if the generating polynomials v_k and V_k satisfy the above relations.

The other algebraic properties are gathered in

PROPERTY 19.2. *If the generating polynomials of the approximants are the same then the following relations hold*
  (i) *Let a be a constant and R a polynomial of degree $k \leqslant p - q$. Then*

$$(p/q)_{af+R}(z) = a(p/q)_f(z) + R(z).$$

  (ii) *If $c_0 = 0$ and if g is defined by $zg(z) = f(z)$ then $z(k - 1/k)_g(z) = (k/k)_f(z)$.*
  (iii) *Let $h(z) = (p/q)_f(z) + (p/q)_g(z)$. Then $(p/q)_{f+g}(z) = (p/q)_h(z)$.*

For Padé-type approximants a property of homographic covariance also holds (see Property 3.3, (iv)). We have

PROPERTY 19.3. *Let $W(z)/V(z) = (k/k)_f(z)$ and*

$$g(z) = \frac{A + Bf(az/(1 + bz))}{C + Df(az/(1 + bz))}$$

with $a \neq 0$ and $C + Dc_0 \neq 0$. If the generating polynomial of $(k/k)_g$ is chosen such that its denominator is

$$(1 + bz)^k[CV(az/(1 + bz)) + DW(az/(1 + bz))]$$

then

$$(k/k)_g(z) = \frac{A + B(k/k)_f(az/(1 + bz))}{C + D(k/k)_f(az/(1 + bz))}.$$

The last algebraic property is the following

PROPERTY 19.4. *Let $(p/q)_f(z) = P_1(z)/Q(z) = f(z) + Az^{p+1} + O(z^{p+2})$ and $(p + 1/q)_f(z) = P_2(z)/Q(z)$. Then $P_2(z) = P_1(z) - AQ(0)z^{p+1}$.*

PROOF. We have

$$P_1(z) = f(z)Q(z) + AQ(z)z^{p+1} + O(z^{p+2})$$

and

$$P_2(z) = f(z)Q(z) + O(z^{p+2}).$$

Subtracting we obtain

$$P_2(z) - P_1(z) = -AQ(z)z^{p+1} + O(z^{p+2})$$

and the result follows since $P_2 - P_1$ is a polynomial of degree $p + 1$. □

As we saw before a Nuttall's type compact formula for Padé-type approximants holds (see Property 3.5).

Padé-type approximants were introduced by BREZINSKI [1979]. The proofs of the preceding results can be found in BREZINSKI [1980].

Let us now illustrate the power (and also the weakness) of Padé-type approximants by a numerical example. If the generating polynomials are chosen properly then the approximants can present much better approximation properties than the classical Padé approximants. But, on the other hand, the difficulty lies in the proper choice of the generating polynomials.

We consider the series

$$f(z) = z^{-1}\ln(1+z) = 1 - \frac{z}{2} + \frac{z^2}{3} - \frac{z^3}{4} + \cdots$$

which has a cut in the complex plane from -1 to $-\infty$. Let us compare the relative errors obtained with [1/2] and with (3/4) with $v_4(z) = (z+1)(z+\frac{1}{2})(z+\frac{1}{3})(z+\frac{1}{4})$. We have

TABLE 19.1.

z	[1/2]	(3/4)
-0.8	-0.27×10^{-1}	0.29×10^{-1}
-0.5	-0.12×10^{-2}	0.73×10^{-3}
0.1	-0.46×10^{-6}	0.92×10^{-7}
0.5	-0.15×10^{-3}	0.56×10^{-5}
1.0	-0.12×10^{-2}	-0.13×10^{-3}
1.5	-0.35×10^{-2}	-0.77×10^{-3}
2.0	-0.70×10^{-2}	-0.21×10^{-2}
4.0	-0.27×10^{-1}	-0.14×10^{-1}

Both approximations require the knowledge of $c_0, \ldots, c_3$ and we have

$$[1/2]_f(z) = \frac{6 + 3z}{6 + 6z + z^2},$$

$$(3/4)_f(z) = \frac{24 + 38z + 18z^2 + 19z^3/6}{24 + 50z + 35z^2 + 10z^3 + z^4}.$$

General theoretical results concerning the choice of the generating polynomials were obtained by EIERMANN [1984]. Since the approximants $(n + k/k)$ of f can be constructed from the approximants $(k - 1/k)$ of the series $f_{n+1}(z) = c_{n+1} + c_{n+2}z + \cdots$ and since the singularities of f and f_{n+1} are the same, it is sufficient to consider the case $n = -1$ only. The following results were proved by EIERMANN [1984] from an extension of Okada's theorem.

THEOREM 19.1. *Let f be analytic in a domain D of the complex plane. If the generating polynomials of the Padé-type approximants $(k - 1/k)$ satisfy*

$$\lim_{k \to \infty} v_k(x)/v_k(z^{-1}) = 0$$

uniformly with respect to x and z on any compact subset of an open set $A \subset \mathbb{C}^2$ containing $\{(x,0) \mid x \in \mathbb{C}\}$, then

$$\lim_{k \to \infty} (k - 1/k)_f(z) = f(z).$$

The convergence is uniform on any compact subset of

$$\{z \in \mathbb{C} \mid \lim_{k \to \infty} v_k(t^{-1})/v_k(z^{-1}) = 0, \ \forall t \in \bar{\mathbb{C}} \setminus D\}.$$

Before trying to apply this general result (which also gives a convergence result for Padé approximants if $v_k \equiv P_k$ satisfies the above conditions), let us give a result which is easier to use in practical situations.

THEOREM 19.2. *Assume that*

$$\sigma(x, z) = \limsup_{k \to \infty} \left[v_{k+1}(x)/v_{k+1}(z^{-1}) \right]^{1/k}$$

is continuous in an open set $\wedge \subseteq \mathbb{C}^2$ containing $\{(x,0) \mid x \in \mathbb{C}\}$. Then the sequence $((k - 1/k)_f(z))$ converges to $f(z)$ on

$$\{z \in \mathbb{C} \mid \sigma(t^{-1}, z) < 1, \forall t \in \bar{\mathbb{C}} \setminus D\}$$

uniformly and geometrically on each compact subset of this set. More precisely

$$\limsup_{k \to \infty} |f(z) - (k - 1/k)_f(z)|^{1/(k-1)} \leqslant r < 1$$

for all z contained in

$$\{z \in \mathbb{C} \mid \sigma(t^{-1}, z) \leqslant r, \ \forall t \in \bar{\mathbb{C}} \setminus D\}.$$

These two theorems can be applied to some particular choices of the generating polynomials and the following results are obtained.

Let us first consider the case where the generating polynomials are given by

$$v_k(x) = (x - a)^k$$

where $a \in \mathbb{C}$. If $a = 0$ then $(k - 1/k)$ are the partial sums of f, while the generalized Euler transformation is recovered if $a = 1$. In that case $\sigma(x, z) = |x - a|/|z^{-1} - a|$ which is continuous for all $(x, z) \in \mathbb{C}^2 \setminus \{(x, z), \ z^{-1} = a\}$ and thus we have

THEOREM 19.3. *Let f be analytic in a domain D of the complex plane containing the origin and let the generating polynomials be chosen as above. Then the sequence $((k - 1/k)_f(z))$ converges to $f(z)$ uniformly on any compact subset of $\{z \in \mathbb{C} \mid |z^{-1} - a| > \sup_{t \in \bar{\mathbb{C}} \setminus D} |t^{-1} - a|\}$ and we have*

$$\lim_{k \to \infty} |f(z) - (k - 1/k)_f(z)|^{1/(k-1)} = \frac{1}{|z^{-1} - a|} \sup_{t \in \bar{\mathbb{C}} \setminus D} |t^{-1} - a|.$$

THEOREM 19.4. *Let f be analytic in the half-plane $D_a = \{z \in \mathbb{C} \mid \mathrm{Re}(za) < 1/2, \ a \in \mathbb{C}, \ a \neq 0\}$. Then $\forall z \in D_a$, $\lim_{k \to \infty} (k - 1/k)_f(z) = f(z)$, the convergence being uniform on any compact subset of D_a if the generating polynomials are chosen as above. More precisely*

$$\limsup_{k \to \infty} |f(z) - (k - 1/k)_f(z)|^{1/(k-1)} \leqslant r < 1$$

$\forall z$ *contained in the closed disk of center $-r^2 a^{-1}/(1 - r^2)$ and radius $r|a|^{-1}/(1 - r^2)$.*

PROOF. Since $\{\xi^{-1}, \xi \in \bar{\mathbb{C}} \setminus D_a\}$ is the closed disc of center a and radius $|a|$, then, from the preceding theorem, the sequence $((k - 1/k)_f)$ converges to f uniformly on every compact subset of $\{z \in \mathbb{C} \mid |z^{-1} - a| > |a|\}$. But $|z^{-1} - a| > |a|$ is equivalent to $\mathrm{Re}(az) < 1/2$ and the first assertion follows. From the preceding theorem, the asymptotic rate of convergence is at most r if $|a|/|z^{-1} - a| \leqslant r$ holds. Using a result about the reflection of circles (see HENRICI [1974], Lemma 5.4.a), the closed disc $\{z, |a|/|z^{-1} - a| \leqslant r\}$ is the same as that of the theorem. □

We shall now take the generating polynomials as

$$v_k(z) = \sum_{i=1}^{k} (z - a_i), \quad a_i \in \mathbb{C}$$

with $\lim_{i\to\infty} a_i = a$. For that choice we have

THEOREM 19.5. *If f is an entire function and if the generating polynomials are chosen as above, then*

(i) *if $a = 0$, $\lim_{k\to\infty}(k-1/k)_f(z) = f(z)$ uniformly on any compact subset of $\mathbb{C}$. Moreover, $\forall z \in \mathbb{C}$*

$$\limsup_{k\to\infty} |f(z) - (k-1/k)_f(z)|^{1/(k-1)} = 0.$$

(ii) *if $a \neq 0$, $\lim_{k\to\infty}(k-1/k)_f(z) = f(z)$ uniformly on any compact subset of the half-plane $\{z \in \mathbb{C} \,|\, \mathrm{Re}\,(za) < 1/2\}$ and*

$$\limsup_{k\to\infty} |f(z) - (k-1/k)_f(z)|^{1/(k-1)} \leqslant r < 1$$

$\forall z$ *contained in the closed disk of center $-r^2 a^{-1}/(1-r^2)$ and radius $r|a|^{-1}/(1-r^2)$.*

PROOF. It can be proved that

$$\sigma(x,z) = \lim_{k\to\infty} \left| \prod_{i=0}^{k} \frac{x - a_i}{z^{-1} - a_i} \right|^{1/k} = \left| \frac{x - a}{z^{-1} - a} \right|.$$

Since the mapping σ is the same as in Theorem 19.3 and since the assumption of Theorem 19.2 only involves σ, then the sequences of Padé-type approximants have the same convergence properties as those of Theorem 19.3. Moreover since f is an entire function $\{\xi^{-1}, \xi \in \bar{\mathbb{C}} \setminus D\} = \{0\}$. By Theorems 19.1 and 19.2, $\lim_{k\to\infty}(k-1/k)_f(z) = f(z)$ if $|z^{-1} - a| > |a|$. The rate of convergence follows from the previous results. □

The results of this theorem are still valid if

$$v_k(z) = (z - a_k)^k, \quad a_k \in \mathbb{C}$$

with $\lim_{i\to\infty} a_i = a$. An application of this result will be given in Section 29.

We shall now assume that $v_k(z) = \prod_{i=1}^{k}(z - a_i)$ where the a_i's have m cyclic limit points, that is

$$\lim_{n\to\infty} a_{nm+j} = \gamma_j, \quad j = 0, \ldots, m-1$$

where $\gamma_0, \ldots, \gamma_{m-1}$ are nonnecessarily distinct points in the complex plane. Let L_ρ be the interior of the lemniscate with foci at $\gamma_0, \ldots, \gamma_{m-1}$ and radius ρ, that is

$$L_\rho = \{z \in \mathbb{C} \,|\, \prod_{i=0}^{m-1} |z - \gamma_i| < \rho\}$$

and let $\bar{L}_\rho$ be its closure. We have

THEOREM 19.6. *Let f be analytic in a domain D of the complex plane containing the origin and let the generating polynomials satisfy the preceding conditions. Let $\rho_0 = \sup_{t \in \bar{\mathbb{C}} \setminus D} \prod_{i=0}^{m-1} |t^{-1} - \gamma_i|$. Then $\lim_{k \to \infty} (k - 1/k)_f(z) = f(z)$ uniformly and geometrically on every compact subset of $\{z \in \mathbb{C} \mid z^{-1} \notin \bar{L}_{\rho_0}\}$. More precisely, $\forall z^{-1} \in L_{\rho_0/\rho^m}$*

$$\limsup_{k \to \infty} |f(z) - (k - 1/k)_f(z)|^{1/(k-1)} \leq \rho.$$

PROOF. Let us set $q_k(x) = \prod_{i=0}^{k-1}(x - \gamma_i)$. It can be proved that $\sigma(x, z) = |q_k(x)/q_k(z^{-1})|^{1/k}$ which is continuous for all $(x, z) \in \mathbb{C}^2 \setminus \bigcup_{i=0}^{k-1}\{(x, z), z^{-1} = \gamma_i\}$. Then the result follows from Theorem 19.2. □

The last choice consists in $v_k(x) = T_k(x) = \cos(k \arccos x)$. We have

THEOREM 19.7. *Let f be analytic in a domain D of the complex plane containing the origin and let the generating polynomials be chosen as above. Then the sequence $((k - 1/k)_f(z))$ converges to $f(z)$ uniformly and geometrically on any compact subset of*

$$\{z \in \mathbb{C} \mid |z^{-1} - 1| + |z^{-1} + 1| > \sup_{t \in \bar{\mathbb{C}} \setminus D} (|t^{-1} - 1| + |t^{-1} + 1|)\}.$$

In particular if D is the cut plane $\mathbb{C} -]-\infty, -1] \cup [1, +\infty[$ the previous set is D and $\forall z \in D$

$$\limsup_{k \to \infty} |f(z) - (k - 1/k)_f(z)|^{1/(k-1)} = |(1 - \sqrt{1 - z^2})/z|.$$

This theorem is again an application of Theorem 19.2.

This is not the only case where v_k can be chosen as an orthogonal polynomial. The following result was obtained by PRÉVOST [1983].

THEOREM 19.8. *Let $f(z) = \int_a^b d\alpha(x)/(1 - xz), z^{-1} \in \mathbb{C} \setminus [a, b]$, α bounded and nondecreasing. Let*

$$\tau(x) = \frac{x - (a+b)/2}{(b-a)/2}$$

and let R_k be the polynomial of degree k belonging to the family of orthogonal polynomials with respect to a distribution $d\mu$ with support in $[-1, +1]$ and $\mu'(x) > 0$ for almost all $x \in [-1, 1]$ (this last condition can be replaced by $\limsup_{k \to \infty} [R_k(x)]^{1/k} \leq 1$, $\forall x \in [-1, +1]$).
Let us choose $v_k(x) = R_k(\tau(x))$. Then, $\forall z^{-1} \in \mathbb{C} \setminus [a, b]$

$$\limsup_{k \to \infty} |f(z) - (k - 1/k)_f(z)|^{1/k} \leq |B| < 1$$

with $B = A - \sqrt{A^2 - 1}$ and $A = \tau(z^{-1})$.

Let us mention that Padé approximants satisfy the conditions of the preceding Theorem and that, in the last inequality, $|B|$ can be replaced by $|B|^2$.

Instead of replacing, as in the Padé-type case, the function $x \to (1 - xz)^{-1}$ by its Hermite interpolation polynomial, it is possible to replace it by its best approximation polynomial, or by its truncated expansion in a series of Chebyshev polynomials of the first or second kind, or by its L^1 or L^2 approximation. All these extensions were treated by PRÉVOST [1983].

The convergence of sequences of Padé-type approximants of higher order was studied by MAGNUS [1981] who extended the Montessus De Ballore Theorem and proved geometric convergence for meromorphic functions.

The case of Stieltjes series was investigated by KARLBERG and WALLIN [1990, 1991]. They considered the Stieltjes function

$$f(z) = \int_{-1}^{1} \frac{d\alpha(z)}{1 - xz}$$

where α is a finite positive measure whose support is an infinite subset of $[-1, +1]$ and the Padé-type approximants $(k - 1/k)$ of order $2k - 2$ with only one preassigned pole at the point 1, and they proved

THEOREM 19.9. *Let* $f(z) = \int_{-1}^{1} d\alpha(x)/(1 - xz)$ *and let* $(k - 1/k)$ *be the Padé-type approximant of order* $2k - 2$ *of* f *with one preassigned pole at the point 1, then*

$$\limsup_{k \to \infty} \max_{z \in K} |f(z) - (k - 1/k)_f(z)|^{1/k} < 1$$

on every compact set K of $\mathbb{C} -]-\infty, -1] \cup [1, +\infty[$.

When several poles are preassigned, the following result holds

THEOREM 19.10. *Let* $f(z) = \int_{-1}^{1} d\alpha(x)/(1 - xz)$ *and let* $(k - 1/k)$ *be the Padé-type approximant of order* $2k - n - 1$ *of* f *with n preassigned poles which are* -1 *and* $+1$ *with arbitrary multiplicities and points in* $]-\infty, -1] \cup [1, +\infty[$ *with even multiplicities. Then the $k - n$ other poles of $(k - 1/k)$ are simple and in* $]-\infty, -1] \cup [1, +\infty[$.

Moreover, if $n = n(k)$ and $\lim_{k \to \infty} n(k)/k = 0$, *then*

$$\limsup_{k \to \infty} \max_{z \in K} |f(z) - (k - 1/k)_f(z)|^{1/k} < 1$$

on every compact set K of $\mathbb{C} -]-\infty, -1] \cup [1, +\infty[$.

20. Partial Padé approximants

In Section 19 we saw that one of the interests of Padé-type approximants was that the denominator (that is, the poles) can be arbitrarily chosen. We also

Generalizations

saw that, in Padé-type approximants of higher order, a part of the denominator (that is, some of the poles) can be arbitrarily chosen and the remaining part of denominator and the numerator are then obtained by imposing the highest possible degree of approximation to the approximant. So, if some of the poles of the function are known, this information can be included in the approximant, thus leading to better approximation properties. We shall now do the same thing with the zeros. We shall choose arbitrarily a part of the numerator (that is, some of the zeros) and a part of the denominator (that is, some of the poles) and determine the remaining parts of the numerator and the denominator in order to obtain the highest possible order of approximation. Such rational approximants, called *partial Padé approximants*, were introduced by BREZINSKI [1988a].

Let v_k and w_r be given polynomials of the respective degrees k and r. We shall determine the polynomials p_m and q_n of the respective degrees m and n, such that

$$\tilde{P}(z) - f(z)\tilde{Q}(z) = O(z^{m+n+1})$$

where

$$\tilde{P}(z) = \tilde{p}_m(z)\tilde{v}_k(z), \quad \tilde{v}_k(z) = z^k v_k(z^{-1}), \quad \tilde{p}_m(z) = z^m p_m(z^{-1}),$$

and

$$\tilde{Q}(z) = \tilde{q}_n(z)\tilde{w}_r(z), \quad \tilde{w}_r(z) = z^r w_r(z^{-1}), \quad \tilde{q}_n(z) = z^n q_n(z^{-1}).$$

The rational function $\tilde{P}(z)/\tilde{Q}(z)$ is called a partial Padé approximant of f and it is denoted by

$$\{m, v_k/n, w_r\}_f(z).$$

They generalize Padé and Padé-type approximants since if $v_k(z) = z^k$ and $w_r(z) = z^r$ (or if $k = r = 0$) then

$$\{m, v_k/n, w_r\}_f \equiv [m/n]_f.$$

If $v_k(z) = z^k$ (or if $k = 0$) and $n > 0$ then $\{m, v_k/n, w_r\}_f$ is the Padé-type approximant $(m/n + r)_f$ of higher order $m + n$.

The first problem is the effective construction of the polynomials p_m and q_n. We have

$$\tilde{p}_m(z)\tilde{v}_k(z) - \tilde{q}_n(z)\tilde{w}_r(z)f(z) = O(z^{m+n+1})$$

or

$$\tilde{p}_m(z) - \tilde{q}_n(z)\tilde{w}_r(z)f(z)/\tilde{v}_k(z) = O(z^{m+n+1})$$

since v_k has the exact degree k and thus $\tilde{v}_k(0) \neq 0$. This relation shows that $\tilde{p}_m(z)/\tilde{q}_n(z)$ is the Padé approximant $[m/n]$ of the series $f\tilde{w}_r/\tilde{v}_k$ or, equivalently, that $\tilde{p}_m(z)/\tilde{q}_n(z)\tilde{w}_r(z)$ is the Padé-type approximant $(m/n+r)$ of higher order $m+n$ of the series $f/\tilde{v}_k$. Both approaches will, of course, lead to the same partial Padé approximants. Anyway the first step is to compute the coefficients of the series $f/\tilde{v}_k$. We set

$$\tilde{v}_k(z) = v_0 + \cdots + v_k z^k,$$
$$g(z) = f(z)/\tilde{v}_k(z) = g_0 + g_1 z + g_2 z^2 + \cdots.$$

We have

$$c_0 = v_0 g_0,$$
$$c_1 = v_0 g_1 + v_1 g_0,$$
$$\vdots$$
$$c_k = v_0 g_k + v_1 g_{k-1} + \cdots + v_k g_0,$$
$$c_{k+1} = v_0 g_{k+1} + v_1 g_k + \cdots + v_k g_1,$$
$$c_{k+2} = v_0 g_{k+2} + v_1 g_{k+1} + \cdots + v_k g_2,$$
$$\vdots$$

Since $\tilde{v}_k(0) = v_0 \neq 0$, these relations give the g_i's. Let us now construct the Padé-type approximant $(m/n+r)$ of order $m+n$ of g. For that purpose we define the linear functionals $g^{(j)}$ by

$$g^{(j)}(x^i) = g_{i+j}, \quad i \geq 0$$

with the convention that $g_s = 0$ if $s < 0$.

From the theory of Padé-type approximation of higher order (see Section 19) we know that q_n must satisfy the relations

$$g^{(m-n-r+1)}(x^i q_n(x) w_r(x)) = 0 \quad \text{for } i = 0, \ldots, n-1$$

and that

$$(m/n+r)_g(z) = \sum_{i=0}^{m-n-r} g_i z^i + z^{m-n-r+1} \tilde{u}(z)/\tilde{q}_n(z)\tilde{w}_r(z)$$

with the convention that the sum is identically zero if $m - n - r < 0$ and with

$$\tilde{u}(z) = z^{n+r-1} u(z^{-1})$$

and

$$u(z) = g^{(m-n-r+1)}\left(\frac{q_n(x)w_r(x) - q_n(z)w_r(z)}{x - z}\right).$$

Thus

$$\tilde{p}_m(z) = \tilde{q}_n(z)\tilde{w}_r(z) \sum_{i=0}^{m-n-r} g_i z^i + z^{m-n-r+1}\tilde{u}(z)$$

that is,

$$p_m(z) = q_n(z)w_r(z) \sum_{i=0}^{m-n-r} g_i z^{m-n-r-i} + u(z).$$

For the following it will be useful to use the second approach to partial Padé approximants as Padé approximants of the series $f\tilde{w}_r/\tilde{v}_k$. We have first to compute the coefficients of this series. We set

$$\tilde{w}_r(z) = w_0 + \cdots + w_r z^r,$$
$$h(z) = g(z)\tilde{w}_r(z) = h_0 + h_1 z + h_2 z^2 + \cdots.$$

We have

$$h_0 = w_0 g_0,$$
$$h_1 = w_0 g_1 + w_1 g_0,$$
$$\vdots$$
$$h_r = w_0 g_r + w_1 g_{r-1} + \cdots + w_r g_0,$$
$$h_{r+1} = w_0 g_{r+1} + w_1 g_r + \cdots + w_r g_1,$$
$$h_{r+2} = w_0 g_{r+2} + w_1 g_{r+1} + \cdots + w_r g_2,$$
$$\vdots$$

which directly gives the h_i's. Let us now construct the Padé approximant $[m/n]$ of the series h. For that purpose we define the linear functionals $h^{(j)}$ by

$$h^{(j)}(x^i) = h_{i+j}, \quad i \geq 0$$

with the convention that $h_s = 0$ if $s < 0$. Since $\tilde{p}_m(z)/\tilde{q}_n(z) = [m/n]_h(z)$ it is well known (see Section 2) that q_n must satisfy the orthogonality relations

$$h^{(m-n+1)}(x^i q_n(x)) = 0 \quad \text{for } i = 0, \ldots, n-1$$

and that we have

$$[m/n]_h(z) = \sum_{i=0}^{m-n} h_i z^i + z^{m-n+1}\tilde{v}(z)/\tilde{q}_n(z)$$

with the convention that the sum is identically zero if $m - n < 0$ and with

$$\tilde{v}(z) = z^{n-1}v(z^{-1})$$

and

$$v(z) = h^{(m-n+1)} \left(\frac{q_n(x) - q_n(z)}{x - z} \right).$$

Thus

$$\tilde{p}_m(z) = \tilde{q}_n(z) \sum_{i=0}^{m-n} h_i z^i + z^{m-n+1} \tilde{v}(z)$$

that is,

$$p_m(z) = q_n(z) \sum_{i=0}^{m-n} h_i z^{m-n-i} + v(z).$$

From the theory of Padé approximation we know that such a unique polynomial q_n exists if the Hankel determinant

$$\begin{vmatrix} h_{m-n+1} & h_{m-n+2} & \cdots & h_m \\ \vdots & & & \vdots \\ h_m & h_{m+1} & \cdots & h_{m+n-1} \end{vmatrix}$$

is different from zero. We shall assume in the sequel that this condition is satisfied for all n, which ensures the existence and uniqueness of $\{m, v_k/n, w_r\}$.

A few lines of calculation show that both approaches lead to the same partial Padé approximant. This is due to the relation

$$h^{(r+s)}(x^i) = g^{(s)}(x^i w_r(x))$$

which will be useful later.

The usual determinantal formula of Section 3 gives

$$\tilde{p}_m(z) = \begin{vmatrix} \sum_{i=0}^{m-n} h_i z^{n+i} & \cdots & \sum_{i=0}^{m} h_i z^i \\ h_{m-n+1} & \cdots & h_{m+1} \\ \vdots & & \vdots \\ h_m & \cdots & h_{m+n} \end{vmatrix},$$

$$\tilde{q}_n(z) = \begin{vmatrix} z^n & \cdots & 1 \\ h_{m-n+1} & \cdots & h_{m+1} \\ \vdots & & \vdots \\ h_m & \cdots & h_{m+n} \end{vmatrix}.$$

Thus we get a first determinantal formula for the partial Padé approximants. It shows that the construction of $\{m, v_k/n, w_r\}$ needs the knowledge of $c_0, \ldots, c_{m+n}$. Another determinantal formula was obtained by PRÉVOST [1990a]. We set

$$\tilde{v}_k(z) = \prod_{i=1}^{k}(z - \alpha_i),$$

$$\tilde{w}_r(z) = \prod_{i=k+1}^{k+r}(z - \alpha_i)$$

if the α_i's are distinct. Let $N_m(z)/D_n(z)$ be the $[m/n]$ Padé approximant of f. Then $\{m, v_k/n, w_r\}$ is the ratio of two determinants of dimension $k + r + 1$. The numerator is

$$\begin{vmatrix} N_m(z)z^p & \alpha_1^p N_m(\alpha_1) & \cdots & \alpha_k^p N_m(\alpha_k) & \alpha_{k+1}^p D_n(\alpha_{k+1}) & \cdots & \alpha_p^p D_n(\alpha_{k+r}) \\ \vdots & \vdots & & \vdots & \vdots & & \vdots \\ N_{m+p}(z) & N_{m+p}(\alpha_1) & \cdots & N_{m+p}(\alpha_k) & D_{n+p}(\alpha_{k+1}) & \cdots & D_{n+p}(\alpha_{k+r}) \end{vmatrix}$$

with $p = k + r$. The denominator is the same after replacing the first column by $D_n(z)z^p, \ldots, D_{n+p}(z)$. The E-algorithm can be used for the computation of this partial Padé approximant.

From the error formulae for Padé and Padé-type approximants we have

$$f(z) - \{m, v_k/n, w_r\}_f(z) = \frac{z^{m+n+1}\tilde{v}_k(z)}{\tilde{q}_n(z)\tilde{w}_r(z)} g^{(m-n-r+1)}\left(\frac{x^n w_r(x) q_n(x)}{1 - xz}\right)$$

$$= \frac{z^{m+n+1}\tilde{v}_k(z)}{\tilde{q}_n(z)\tilde{w}_r(z)} g^{(m-r+1)}\left(\frac{w_r(x) q_n(x)}{1 - xz}\right)$$

$$= \frac{z^{m+n+1}\tilde{v}_k(z)}{[\tilde{q}_n(z)]^2 \tilde{w}_r(z)} g^{(m-n-r+1)}\left(\frac{w_r(x) q_n^2(x)}{1 - xz}\right).$$

Partial Padé approximants also share some algebraic properties with Padé approximants.

Let e be the reciprocal series of f which exists if $c_0 \neq 0$ and is formally defined by

$$f(z)e(z) = 1.$$

Then

$$\{m, v_k/n, w_r\}_f(z)\{n, w_r/m, v_k\}_e(z) = 1.$$

If we set $F(z) = z^s f(z)$ then

$$\{m + s, v_k/n, w_r\}_F(z) = z^s \{m, v_k/n, w_r\}_f(z).$$

Obviously, if a is a constant

$$\{m, v_k/n, w_r\}_{af}(z) = a\{m, v_k/n, w_r\}_f(z).$$

If we set $F(z) = f(az)$, $a \neq 0$, $\tilde{V}_k(z) = \tilde{v}_k(az)$ and $\tilde{W}_r(z) = \tilde{w}_r(az)$ then

$$\{m, V_k/n, W_r\}_F(z) = \{m, v_k/n, w_r\}_f(az).$$

If we set $F(z) = f(z^s)$, $s > 0$, $\tilde{V}_k(z) = \tilde{v}_k(z^s)$ and $\tilde{W}_r(z) = \tilde{w}_r(z^s)$ then, $\forall i, j$ such that $i + j \leq s - 1$ we have

$$\{ms + i, V_k/ns + j, W_r\}_F(z) = \{m, v_k/n, w_r\}_f(z^s).$$

If we set $F(z) = f(az(1+bz)^{-1})$, $\tilde{V}_k(z) = (1+bz)^k \tilde{v}_k(az(1+bz)^{-1})$ and $\tilde{W}_r(z) = (1+bz)^r \tilde{w}_r(az(1+bz)^{-1})$ with $a \neq 0$ then, if $m + k = n + r$, we have

$$\{m, V_k/n, W_r\}_F(z) = \{m, v_k/n, w_r\}_f(az(1+bz)^{-1}).$$

As is the case for Padé and Padé-type approximants, let us now relate partial Padé approximants to interpolation. We previously saw that the functionals $h^{(r+s)}$ and $g^{(s)}$ were related. Let us first connect the functionals $c^{(k+s)}$ and $g^{(s)}$. It is easy to see, from the relations between the c_i's and the g_i's that

$$c^{(k+s)}(x^i) = g^{(s)}(x^i v_k(x)).$$

Let now $u_k(x) = x^{-k}(u_0 + u_1 x^{-1} + u_2 x^{-2} + \cdots)$ be formally defined by

$$v_k(x) u_k(x) = 1.$$

After some calculations, one can prove that

$$\{m, v_k/n, w_r\}_f(z) = c(S(x)) = c(R(x))$$

where

$$S(x) = \frac{1}{1-xz}\left(1 - \frac{z^{m+n+1}\tilde{v}_k(z)}{\tilde{q}_n(z)\tilde{w}_r(z)} x^{m+k-r+1} w_r(x) q_n(x) u_k(x)\right)$$

and

$$R(x) = \frac{1}{1-xz}\left(1 - \frac{z^{m+1}\tilde{v}_k(z)}{\tilde{q}_n(z)\tilde{w}_r(z)} x^{m+k-r-n+1} w_r(x) q_n(x) u_k(x)\right).$$

If $m + k = n + r - 1$ then

$$R(x) = \frac{1}{1-xz}\left(1 - \frac{z^{m+1}\tilde{v}_k(z)}{\tilde{q}_n(z)\tilde{w}_r(z)} w_r(x) q_n(x) u_k(x)\right)$$

TABLE 20.1.

z	$f(z)$	$\{1,v_1/1,w_1\}_f(z)$	$[1/1]_f(z)$
−0.9	3.3025850	4.6039730	2.6363636
−0.5	1.6931471	1.7097808	1.6666666
−0.3	1.3566749	1.3584556	1.3529411
−0.1	1.1053605	1.1053971	1.1052631
0.1	0.9046898	0.9046680	0.9047619
0.3	0.7376357	0.7372726	0.7391304
0.8	0.4122133	0.4100425	0.4285714
1.5	0.0837092	0.0821464	0.1428570
1.7	0.0067482	0.0065906	0.0810810
2.5	−0.2527629	−0.2416952	−0.1111111
4.0	−0.6094379	−0.5587768	−0.3333333

which shows that R interpolates $(1-xz)^{-1}$ in the Hermite sense at the zeros of $q_n(x)w_r(x)$. Thus we obtain, in that case, a connection similar to the connection for Padé and Padé-type approximants.

Let us now give a numerical example showing the interest of partial Padé approximants. We consider the series

$$f(z) = 1 - \ln(1+z) = 1 - z + \frac{z^2}{2} - \frac{z^3}{3} + \cdots$$

which has a zero at $e - 1$ and a logarithmic branch point at -1. Choosing $\tilde{w}_1(z) = z+1$ and $\tilde{v}_1(z) = z+1-e$ we obtain the numbers as shown in Table 20.1.

Both approximants use c_0, c_1 and c_2 only.

If no information on the zeros and poles of f is known, one can choose

$$\tilde{v}_k(z)/\tilde{w}_r(z) = [k/r]_f(z).$$

In that case

$$h(z) = 1 + \frac{z^{k+r+1}}{\tilde{v}_k(z)} c^{(k+1)} \left(\frac{w_r(x)}{1-xz} \right)$$

and, due to the block structure of the Padé table,

$$[m/n]_h(z) = 1 \quad \text{for } m, n = 0, \ldots, k+r.$$

Thus $\{m, v_k/n, w_r\}_f$ reduces to $[k/r]_f$ for $m, n = 0, \ldots, k+r$. If $m > k+r$ or $n > k+r$, we have

$$\{m, v_k/n, w_r\}_f(z) = [k/r]_f(z)[m/n]_h(z).$$

TABLE 20.2.

z	$\{2,v_0/1,w_1\}$	$\{3,v_1/1,w_1\}$	$\{1,v_1/3,w_1\}$
-0.9	4.2142857	2.9275619	2.9637199
-0.5	1.7000000	1.5898148	1.6901408
-0.3	1.3571428	1.3565224	1.3565319
-0.1	1.1053639	1.1053601	1.1053601
0.1	0.9046920	0.9046900	0.9046901
0.3	0.7377622	0.7376843	0.7376871
0.8	0.4152046	0.4155102	0.4158964
1.5	0.1000000	0.1198979	0.1230769
1.7	0.0287628	0.0631373	0.0663888
2.5	-0.2012987	-0.0468106	-0.0703812
4.0	-0.4857142	0.2592592	-0.1200000

Taking again $f(z) = 1 - \ln(1+z)$, we obtain for this choice the numbers shown in Table 20.2.

Another possible choice for $\tilde{v}_k$ and $\tilde{w}_r$ is

$$\tilde{v}_k(z)/\tilde{w}_r(z) = (k/r)_f(z).$$

In that case

$$h(z) = 1 + \frac{z^{k+1}}{\tilde{v}_k(z)} c^{(k-r+1)}\left(\frac{w_r(x)}{1-xz}\right)$$

and, due to the block structure of the Padé table,

$$[m/n]_h(z) = 1 \quad \text{for } m, n = 0, \ldots, k.$$

Thus $\{m, v_k/n, w_r\}_f$ reduces to $(k/r)_f$ for $m, n = 0, \ldots, k$. If $m > k$ or $n > k$, we have

$$\{m, v_k/n, w_r\}_f(z) = (k/r)_f(z)[m/n]_h(z).$$

With the same example and $\tilde{w}_2(z) = 6 + 7z + 2z^2$, we obtain for this choice the numbers presented in Table 20.3.

In both cases (which only need the knowledge of $c_0, \ldots, c_{m+n}$) the computation of the h_i's simplifies since the g_i's are no longer needed. We directly have

$$h_0 = 1, \quad h_1 = \cdots = h_k = 0,$$

$$v_0 h_{k+1} = c^{(k-r+1)}(w_r(x)),$$

$$v_0 h_{k+2} + v_1 h_{k+1} = c^{(k-r+1)}(xw_r(x)),$$

$$\vdots$$

$$v_0 h_{2k+1} + v_1 h_{2k} + \cdots + v_k h_{k+1} = c^{(k-r+1)}(x^k w_r(x)),$$

$$v_0 h_{2k+2} + v_1 h_{2k+1} + \cdots + v_k h_{k+2} = c^{(k-r+1)}(x^{k+1} w_r(x)),$$

$$\vdots$$

TABLE 20.3.

z	$\{2,v_1/1,w_2\}$
−0.9	2.8932346
−0.5	1.6866666
−0.3	1.3561692
−0.1	1.1053563
0.1	0.9046868
0.3	0.7374581
0.8	0.4072759
1.5	0.0510204
1.7	−0.0397779
2.5	−0.3852339
4.0	−1.0606060

with

$$c^{(k-r+1)}(x^i w_r(x)) = w_0 c_{k+i+1} + w_1 c_{k+i} + \cdots + w_r c_{k-r+i+1}.$$

If $\tilde{v}_k(z)/\tilde{w}_r(z) = [k/r]_f(z)$ then, due to the orthogonality of w_r, we have $c^{(k-r+1)}(x^i w_r(x)) = 0$ for $i = 0, \ldots, r-1$ and thus $h_{r+1} = \cdots = h_{r+k} = 0$. These two particular cases deserve further studies.

If we take $r = m = 0$ in partial Padé approximants then only the zeros of the approximant are arbitrarily chosen contrarily to the case of Padé-type approximants where only the poles of the approximant are chosen. Such approximants have been called inverse Padé-type approximants since

$$\{0, v_k/n, w_0\}_f(z) = 1/(n/k)_e(z)$$

where e is the reciprocal series of f and where $(n/k)_e$ is constructed from the generating polynomial v_k.

The concept of partial Padé approximation was extended by DE BRUIN [1988] to the simultaneous approximation of several power series by rational functions with a common denominator. We consider d power series

$$f_j(z) = \sum_{i=0}^{\infty} c_{j,i} z^i, \quad j = 1, \ldots, d.$$

Let v_j ($j = 1, \ldots, d$) and w_r be given polynomials of the respective degrees k_j ($j = 1, \ldots, d$) and r. We shall determine the polynomials P_j ($j = 1, \ldots, d$) of degree m_j and q_n of degree n such that

$$\tilde{P}_j(z) - f_j(z)\tilde{Q}(z) = O(z^{m_j+[n/d]+r_j+1}), \quad j = 1, \ldots, d$$

where

$$\tilde{P}_j(z) = \tilde{p}_j(z)\tilde{v}_j(z), \qquad \tilde{Q}(z) = \tilde{q}_n(z)\tilde{w}_r(z).$$

(the notation $\tilde{r}$ on a polynomial r of degree k designates $\tilde{r}(z) = z^k r(z^{-1})$), and

$$r_j = 1, \quad j = 1, \ldots, n - d[n/d],$$
$$r_j = 0, \quad j = n - d[n/d] + 1, \ldots, d,$$

$[x]$ being the integer part of the real number x.

The unique solution of this problem with $\tilde{Q}(0) = 1$, which is assumed to exist, is called a simultaneous partial Padé approximant. The choice $v_j(z) = z^{k_j}, w_r(z) = z^r$ (or $k_j = r = 0$) leads to the ordinary simultaneous Padé approximants while the simultaneous Padé-type approximants are recovered for $v_j(z) = z^{k_j}$ (or $k = n = 0$).

As in the case of partial Padé approximation, these simultaneous approximants can be obtained by two approaches which are proved to be equivalent. The first one consists in writing

$$\tilde{P}_j(z)\tilde{v}_j(z) - f_j(z)\tilde{q}_n(z)\tilde{w}_r(z) = O(z^{m_j+[n/d]+r_j+1}), \quad j = 1, \ldots, d$$

and thus $\tilde{P}_j(z)/\tilde{q}_n(z)$ is a simultaneous Padé approximant of the series $f_j\tilde{w}_r/\tilde{v}_j$. The second approach consists in writing

$$\tilde{P}_j(z) - \tilde{q}_n(z)\tilde{w}_r(z)f_j(z)/\tilde{v}_j(z) = O(z^{m_j+[n/d]+r_j+1}), \quad j = 1, \ldots, d$$

which shows that $\tilde{P}_j(z)/\tilde{q}_n(z)\tilde{w}_r(z)$ is a simultaneous Padé-type approximant of the series $f_j/\tilde{v}_j$.

A very interesting example showing the advantages of simultaneous partial Padé approximants over the ordinary simultaneous Padé approximants was given by DE BRUIN [1988]. We consider the two series

$$f_1(z) = e^z/(1-z), \quad f_2(z) = \cos z/(1+z).$$

The presence of the poles is imitated by taking

$$v_1(z) = z + 1, \quad v_2(z) = z - 1, \quad w_2(z) = z^2 - 1.$$

With $m_1 = m_2 = 1$ and $n = 2$, we obtain the approximation problem

$$\tilde{p}_1(z) - \tilde{q}_2(z)e^z = O(z^3),$$
$$\tilde{p}_2(z) - \tilde{q}_2(z)\cos z = O(z^3),$$

whose solution is $\tilde{q}_2(z) = 1 - z + z^2/2$, $\tilde{p}_1(z) = -(1+z)$ and $\tilde{p}_2(z) = -(1-z)^2$.

Thus it is possible to find simultaneous partial Padé approximants which, although they have the same denominator before cancellation of the common factors between the denominator and the numerators, mimic the behaviour of both functions near the poles because of this cancellation. In ordinary simultaneous Padé approximation one can never be sure that such a cancellation would occur, thus leading to good behaviour near the poles. Other examples are also given in the same paper by DE BRUIN [1988].

21. Multipoint Padé approximants

Interpolation by polynomials has a long history, and it has been extended to interpolation by rational functions. An extensive review has been given by WALSH [1969], and this has opened the way to many new developments. Two extreme cases have been considered first: when all the interpolation points coincide and when they are all distinct. The first of these two cases is the Padé case.

The problem is to define a rational function R_{nm} of type (n, m) interpolating a given function f in $(n + m + 1)$ points β_i. If going from R_{nm} to $R_{n+1,m}$, $R_{n,m+1}$, the same first β_i are used, then the β_i can be considered as a sequence $(\beta_i)_{i \geq 1}$, and f is a formal Newton series. This is the point of view of GALLUCI and JONES [1976] who defined Newton–Padé approximants.

A more general case is the following: R_{nm} interpolates f in $n + m + 1$ points $(\beta_1^{n+m+1}, \ldots, \beta_{n+m+1}^{n+m+1})$. Problems of convergence and divergence have been studied in that case for column or diagonal sequences by WALLIN [1982, 1987].

At the other extreme, special attention has been paid to the case where there are only two distinct points β_i which can be considered as 0 and ∞ (JONES and THRON [1977]). Orthogonality for Laurent polynomials can be defined. The case of a finite number of interpolation points $(\beta_1, \ldots, \beta_p)$ was studied by NJÅSTAD [1989]. A review and new developments have been given by BULTHEEL [1987], and because no task is ever finished, Laurent–Hermite interpolation problems are now arising (BULTHEEL [1987]).

Let us first consider the problem of interpolation with a sequence of points (β_i). The following results are taken from GALLUCI and JONES [1976]. A formal Newton series $(f.n.s.)$ is defined from two sequences $(a_n)_{n \geq 0}$ $(\beta_n)_{n \geq 1}$ as follows

$$\begin{cases} f(z) = \sum_n a_n \omega_n(z), \\ \omega_0(z) = 1, \quad \omega_n(z) = \omega_{n-1}(z).(z - \beta_n). \end{cases}$$

As $z \cdot f(z) = a_0 \beta_1 \omega_0(z) + \sum_{k \geq 1} (a_{k-1} + a_k \beta_{k+1}) \omega_k(z)$, the product of an $(f.n.s.)$ and a polynomial is also an $(f.n.s.)$ based on the same points β_i. Then we get the following theorem (GALLUCI and JONES [1976])

THEOREM 21.1. *Let* $u(z) = c_0 + c_1 z + \cdots + c_n z^n$, $v(z) = d_0 + d_1 z + \cdots + d_m z^m$. *Then a necessary and sufficient condition that the $(f.n.s.)$ $vf - u$ be of the form*

$$v(z)f(z) - u(z) = b_{n+m+1} \omega_{n+m+1}(z) + \cdots$$

is that the c_i and d_i satisfy the system of equations

$$\begin{aligned} d_0 A_{00} &+ \cdots + d_m A_{0m} &= c_0, \\ &\vdots &\vdots \\ d_0 A_{n0} &+ \cdots + d_m A_{n,m} &= c_n, \\ d_0 A_{n+1,0} &+ \cdots + d_m A_{n+1,0} &= 0, \\ &\vdots &\vdots \\ d_0 A_{n+m,0} &+ \cdots + d_m A_{n+m,m} &= 0 \end{aligned}$$

where the A_{ij} are defined by $z^p.f(z) = \sum_{k \geq 0} A_{kp}\omega_k(z)$.

The system defines a unique rational function u/v. R_{nm} is defined by u/v of the preceding theorem; it exists and is unique if the determinant of the system is not zero. If all these determinants are not zero, the table $(R_{nm})_{n,m}$ is said to be normal. There is no equivalence with the interpolatory point of view, since we only have

$$v(\beta_i) \neq 0 \Rightarrow f(\beta_i) = u(\beta_i)/v(\beta_i).$$

Let us turn now to convergence problems (WALLIN [1982, 1987]). The first paper deals with convergence of columns of the table, i.e. sequences of approximants with a fixed number of poles. In the case of Padé approximants, this is exactly Montessus De Ballore's theorem (proved in Section 13), generalized by SAFF [1972] to the case of multipoint Padé approximants. The assumptions are made to guarantee that the (β_i) are not in too large a set. The β_i are no longer a sequence, but a set of interpolation points as follows

THEOREM 21.2. *Let E be a closed bounded point set whose complement K (with respect to the extended plane) is connected and regular in the sense that K possesses a Green's function $G(z)$ with a pole at infinity. Let Γ_σ ($\sigma > 1$) denote generically the locus $G(z) = \ln \sigma$, and let E_σ be the interior of Γ_σ. Let the points*

$$\begin{aligned} &\beta_1^{(1)}, \\ &\beta_1^{(2)}, \beta_2^{(2)}, \\ &\quad \vdots \\ &\beta_1^{(n)}, \beta_2^{(n)}, \ldots, \beta_n^{(n)}, \\ &\quad \vdots \end{aligned} \tag{21.1}$$

(which may not all be distinct) have no limit point exterior to E and satisfy the relation

$$\lim_{n \to \infty} \left| \prod_{i=1}^n (z - \beta_i^{(n)}) \right|^{1/n} = \Delta \exp G(z), \tag{21.2}$$

uniformly in z on each closed bounded subset of K, where Δ is the transfinite diameter of E.

Suppose that the function $f(z)$ is analytic on E and meromorphic with precisely v poles in E_ρ ($\rho > 1$). Let D_ρ denote the region obtained from E_ρ by deleting the v poles of $f(z)$. Then, for all n sufficiently large, there exists a unique rational function $R_{nv}(z)$ of type (n, v), which interpolates $f(z)$ at the points $\beta_1^{(n+v+1)}, \beta_2^{(n+v+1)}, \ldots, \beta_{n+v+1}^{(n+v+1)}$. Each $R_{nv}(z)$ has precisely v finite poles and, as $n \to \infty$, these poles approach, respectively, the v poles of $f(z)$ in E_ρ. The sequence $(R_{nv}(z))$ converges to $f(z)$ throughout D_ρ, uniformly on any compact subset of D_ρ.

These results are the extension to rational approximation of the results for the Taylor series of f, which is the interpolation polynomial with all $\beta_i = 0$.

In the case of the Taylor series, results about divergence are also obtained. If the smallest singularity (in modulus) is of modulus R, the Taylor series is divergent outside D_R. This result has been extended to polynomial interpolation by KAKEHASHI [1955, 1956], and following the same ideas, to rational interpolation by WALLIN [1987]. The first result by Kakehashi is the following

THEOREM 21.3. *Let the sequence of points*

$$\begin{array}{l} \beta_1^{(1)} \\ \beta_1^{(2)}, \beta_2^{(2)}, \\ \phantom{\beta_1^{(2)},} \vdots \\ \beta_1^{(n)}, \beta_2^{(n)}, \beta_3^{(n)}, \ldots, \beta_n^{(n)} \\ \phantom{\beta_1^{(n)},} \vdots \end{array} \tag{P}$$

which do not lie outside the unit circle $C: |z| = 1$, *satisfy the condition that the sequence*

$$\frac{W_n(z)}{z^n} = \frac{(z - \beta_1^{(n)})(z - \beta_2^{(n)}) \cdots (z - \beta_n^{(n)})}{z^n}$$

converges to a function $\lambda(z)$, *single-valued, analytic and nonvanishing for* z *outside* C, *and converges uniformly on any bounded closed point set exterior to* C, *that is*

$$\lim_{n \to \infty} \frac{W_n(z)}{z^n} = \lambda(z) \quad \text{for } |z| > 1.$$

Let the function $f(z)$ *be single-valued and analytic throughout the interior of the circle* $C_\rho : |z| = \rho > 1$ *but not analytic regular on* C_ρ. *Then the sequence of polynomials* $P_n(z; f)$ *of respective degrees* n *found by interpolation of* $f(z)$ *at all the zeros of* $W_{n+1}(z)$ *diverges at every point outside* C_ρ. *Moreover we have*

$$\lim_{n \to \infty} |P_n(z; f)|^{1/n} = \frac{|z|}{\rho} \quad \text{for } |z| > \rho.$$

The result can be transformed to a set of points (β_i^j) lying in a bounded set D. Mapping the complement K of D onto the exterior of the unit disc permits more general results.

THEOREM 21.4. *Let* D *be a closed limited point set whose complement* K *with respect to the extended plane is connected and regular in the sense that* K *possesses a Green's function with a pole at infinity. Let* $W = \varphi(z)$ *map* K *onto the region* $|w| > 1$ *so that the points at infinity correspond to each other.*

Let the function $f(z)$ *be single-valued and analytic throughout the interior of the level curve* $\Gamma_\rho : |w| = |\varphi(z)| = \rho > 1$ *but not analytic regular on* Γ_ρ, *and* (P) *be a sequence of points which satisfies the condition*

$$\lim_{n \to \infty} \frac{\prod_{j=1}^n (z - \beta_j^n)}{(\Delta \varphi(z))^n} = \lambda(w)$$

where $w = \varphi(z)$, λ is a function single-valued analytic and nonvanishing for $|w| > 1$, and Δ is the capacity of D, the limit being uniform in w on bounded closed sets exterior to the unit circle.

Then the sequence of polynomials $P_n(z;f)$ of respective degrees n found by interpolation of $f(z)$ at all the zeros of $W_{n+1}(z)$ converges to $f(z)$ at every point interior to Γ_ρ, uniformly on any closed set interior to Γ_ρ, and diverges at every point outside Γ_ρ. Moreover, we have

$$\limsup_{n\to\infty} |R_n(z;f)|^{1/n} = \frac{|w|}{\rho} \quad \text{for } 1 < |w| = |\varphi(z)| < \rho,$$

and

$$\limsup_{n\to\infty} |P_n(z;f)|^{1/n} = \frac{|w|}{\rho} \quad \text{for } |w| = |\varphi(z)| > \rho > 1.$$

The results are extended to the rational case for the convergence problem. The result of divergence is obtained in particular cases and no counterexample is known so far.

The notations are as follows:

(a) β_i^j are points of a compact set E, with positive logarithmic capacity (cap $E > 0$). The complement $\mathbb{C} - E$ is connected and regular (i.e. $\mathbb{C} - E$ has a classical Green's function G, with a pole at infinity, and $G = 0$ on E).

$$E_\sigma = \{z \in \mathbb{C}, G(z) < \ln\sigma\}, \quad \sigma > 1,$$
$$\Gamma_\sigma = \partial E_\sigma = \{z, G(z) = \ln\sigma\}, \quad \sigma > 1.$$

(b) The sequence of multipoint Padé approximants considered is a column sequence (m fixed), the β_i^j are in E , and

$$\lim_{n\to\infty} \left| \prod_1^{n+m+1} (z - \beta_i^{n+m+1}) \right|^{1/n} = \text{cap } E \cdot \exp(G(z)).$$

The limit is uniform on compact subsets of $\mathbb{C} - E$.

(c) f is analytic on E_σ for some $\sigma > 1$, except at m poles $z_1, \ldots, z_m$ of E_σ ($z_j \neq \beta_i$) counted with their multiplicities.

Let σ' be the supremum of such σ ($\sigma' = \infty$ if and only if f is meromorphic with m poles).

THEOREM 21.5. *Assume that the conditions (a), (b) and (c) hold and that $R_{nm} = P_{nm}/Q_{nm}$ is the multipoint Padé approximant of f of type (n,m), at the points $(\beta_1^{n+m+1}, \ldots, \beta_{n+m+1}^{n+m+1})$. Then taking the uniform norm on each compact K*

$$K \subset \bar{E}_\sigma - \{z_j\}, \quad \sigma < \sigma', \quad \lim_{n\to\infty} \|f - R_{nm}\|_K^{1/n} \geqslant \sigma/\sigma'.$$

R_{nm} has m poles in $\mathbb{C}$ for n large enough, which converge to $(z_j)_{j=1,\ldots,m}$ as n tends to infinity. If $Q_m(z) = \prod_1^m(z-z_j)$, and if Q_{nm} is monic, define σ_j as

$$G(z_j) = \ln \sigma_j, \quad 1 \geqslant j \geqslant m;$$

assume that $\sigma_1 = \sup \sigma_j$, then for all compact K of $\mathbb{C}$

$$\limsup_{n\to\infty} \|Q_{nm} - Q_m\|_K^{1/n} \geqslant \sigma_1/\sigma' < 1.$$

The problem of divergence is divergence outside $\bar{E}_{\sigma'}$, so f has a singularity on $\partial E_{\sigma'}$. It is proved in the three following cases, with the same notations as above:

(1) For $\sigma > \sigma'$, f has a simple pole α on $\partial E_{\sigma'}$ and finitely many poles $\alpha_1, \ldots, \alpha_k$ in $E_\sigma - \bar{E}_\sigma$, then $(R_{nm}(z))_n$ diverges for $z \in E_{\sigma'} - (\bar{E}_\sigma, \cup \{\alpha_1, \ldots, \alpha_k\})$.

(2) The points β_i^j are independent of n, i.e. they form a sequence (β_i) as described for the $(f.n.s.)$, then $(R_{nm}(z))_n$ diverges on $\mathbb{C} - \bar{E}_{\sigma'}$.

(3) It is the generalization of Kakehaski's theorem (Theorem 21.3): let H be the conjugate of G in $\mathbb{C} - E$ and

$$w = \varphi(z) = \exp(G(z) + iH(z)).$$

Then E_σ becomes $E_\sigma = \{z : |w| = |\varphi(z)| < \sigma\}$ and ∂E_σ corresponds to the circle of radius σ in the w-plane and

$$w_n(z) = \prod_{j=1}^n (z - \beta_j^n).$$

Let the (β_i^j) satisfy the following condition, where $w = \varphi(z)$:

$$\lambda(w) = \lim_{n\to\infty} \left(\frac{w_{n+m+1}(z)}{\operatorname{cap} E \cdot (\varphi(z))^n} \right)$$

exists for $|w| > 1$, nonzero, the limit being uniform on compact subsets of $\{|w| > 1\}$.

Then with the assumptions of Theorem 21.5, the sequence $(R_{nm}(z))_m$ diverges pointwise on $\mathbb{C} - \bar{E}_\sigma, = \{z, |\varphi(z)| > \sigma'\}$.

Furthermore

$$\lim_{n\to\infty} |P_{nm}(z)|^{1/n} = |\varphi(z)|/\sigma' > 1, \quad z \in \mathbb{C} - \bar{E}_\sigma.$$

The geometric degree of divergence of $(P_{mn})_n$ is to be compared first with the divergence of a power series, and also to the geometric degree of convergence of the sequence $(Q_{mn})_n$.

For diagonal sequences, as for Padé approximants, it can be seen that the poles of R_{nn} may cluster everywhere in $\mathbb{C}$, even for entire functions. We may, in general, expect convergence of $(R_{nn})_n$ to f outside a certain exceptional set only. The results are generalizations of those obtained in the Padé case. The interested reader is referred to WALLIN [1982], KARLSON and SAFF [1981], KARLSON and VON SYDOW [1976], LOPEZ [1979]. The convergence to functions of Stieltjes type has been studied in these last two papers.

The link between multipoint Padé approximants and continued fractions has been studied through several papers of NJÅSTAD [1989] (see other references there).

Let us define the continued fraction $K_{n=1}^{\infty} a_n(z)/b_n(z)$, as follows. Let a sequence (a_i) be given, and three sequences $(A_n)_n$, $(B_n)_n$, (C_n), B_n and C_n nonzero for all n. We set

$$a_1(z) = \frac{c_1}{z - z_1}, \qquad b_1(z) = \frac{A_1}{z - a_1} + B_1,$$

$$a_2(z) = \frac{c_2}{z - z_2}, \qquad b_2(z) = \frac{A_2(z - a_1)}{z - a_2} + \frac{B_2}{z - a_2},$$

$$a_n(z) = \frac{c_n(z - a_{n-2})}{z - a_n}, \qquad b_n(z) = \frac{A_n(z - a_{n-1}) + B_n(z - a_{n-2})}{z - a_n}, \qquad n \geq 3.$$

In the case studied, (a_i) is a periodic sequence of period p: if $n = pq + r$ then $a_n = a_r$. Then the continued fraction $K_{n=1}^{\infty} a_n(z)/b_n(z)$ is called a multipoint Padé continued fraction (MP-fraction).

The nth convergent is denoted by P_n/Q_n. The P_n's and the Q_n's satisfy the recurrence relations of the convergents of continued fractions,

$$Q_n(z) = a_n(z)Q_{n-1}(z) + b_n(z)Q_{n-2}(z), \quad n \geq 1$$
with $Q_{-1} = 0$, $Q_0 = 1$

and a similar relation for P_n with $P_{-1} = 1, P_0 = 0$.

So P_n and Q_n are rational functions with the same denominator: if $n = pq + r$, we get

$$N_n(z) = \prod_{i=1}^{r}(z - a_i)^{q+1} \cdot \prod_{i=r+1}^{p}(z - a_i)^q.$$

P_n/Q_n is equal to U_n/V_n with degree $(U_n) = n - 1$ and degree $(V_n) = n$ if Q_n is of *exact degree* (i.e. the terms $\beta/(z - a_n)^{q+1}$ is nonzero in the decomposition of Q_n).

Every MP-fraction whose denominators are of exact degree defines a system of p formal power series $L_0 = c_0/z$, $L_i = -\sum_{j=1}^{\infty} c_j^i (z - a_i)^{j-1}$, $i = 1, \ldots, p$ such that the convergents of the MP-fraction are multipoint Padé approximants of type $(n - 1, n)$ of these series.

Orthogonality and a Favard Theorem can be proved for R-functions (meromorphic with p fixed poles) (HENDRIKSEN and NJÅSTAD [1989]).

The studies concerning the approximation of a function known by its Taylor developments around p fixed points $a_1, \ldots, a_p$ are generalizations of the case $p = 2$ which has been developed in recent years.

By homography, these two points can be considered as 0 and ∞. So f is represented by two power series

$$\sum_{i \geq 0} c_i z^i \quad \text{and} \quad \sum_{i \geq 1} c_i z^{-i}$$

or by one Laurent series $\sum_{-\infty}^{+\infty} c_i z^i$.

The first paper on the subject was that of JONES and THRON [1977]. It deals with T-fractions defined by

$$1 + d_0 z + \frac{z}{1 + d_1 z} + \frac{z}{1 + d_2 z} \cdots, \quad d_n \in \mathbb{C}.$$

Under conditions of regularity, the nth convergent A_n/B_n is of degree $(n+1, n)$ and corresponds to two series

$$L = 1 + c_1 z + \cdots,$$
$$L^* = c_{-1}^* z + c_0^* + \frac{c_1^*}{z} + \frac{c_2^*}{z^2} + \cdots, \quad c_{-1}^* \neq 0,$$

in the sense that

$$\frac{A_n(z)}{B_n(z)} - L = O(z^{n+1}), \quad z \text{ in a neighbourhood of zero,}$$

$$\frac{A_n(z)}{B_n(z)} - L^* = O(1/z^n), \quad z \text{ in a neighbourhood of } \infty.$$

Conversely, L and L^* being given, the $(d_n)_n$ can be computed. Orthogonal Laurent polynomials have been defined. A complete study of the orthogonality and of the tables of two-point Padé approximants can be found in DRAUX [1983] in the normal and nonnormal cases.

22. Cauchy-type approximants

We shall now study a new type of approximants, called Cauchy-type approximants, which generalize Padé-type approximants. Again we want to construct approximations of the series

$$f(z) = \sum_{i=0}^{\infty} c_i z^i.$$

We assume that $\exists c \neq 0$ such that $\lim_{n \to \infty} c_{n+1}/c_n = c$. Thus the series f has a radius of convergence $1/|c|$.

We are given a second series

$$g(z) = \sum_{i=0}^{\infty} b_i z^i$$

whose radius of convergence R is strictly greater than $1/|c|$, and we consider the series h which is the Cauchy product of f and g

$$h(z) = \sum_{i=0}^{\infty} a_i z^i = f(z)g(z).$$

It is well known that the a_i's are given by

$$a_i = c_0 b_i + c_1 b_{i-1} + \cdots + c_{i-1} b_1 + c_i b_0, \quad i = 0, 1, 2, \ldots,$$

that h converges in $|z| < 1/|c|$, and that $z = 1/c$ is a singular point of f. We shall denote by f_n, g_n and h_n the partial sums of the series f, g and h respectively up to the terms of degree n inclusively and we shall set

$$S_n(z) = h_n(z)/g(z).$$

S_n will be called a *Cauchy-type approximant* of f.

The idea of such approximants, first introduced by BREZINSKI [1991c], emerged when reading an old result, initially proved by SZÁSZ [1921] (see also PÓLYA and SZEGÖ [1972], Vol. 1, pp. 39 and 218), and rediscovered and improved by VAN DEN BERG [1987] by means of nonstandard analysis. This theorem is as follows

THEOREM 22.1. *Under the preceding assumptions on f and g, then*
  (i) $\lim_{n\to\infty} a_n/c_n = g(1/c)$,
  (ii) *if* $g(1/c) \neq 0$ *then* $\lim_{n\to\infty} a_{n+1}/a_n = c$,
  (iii) *if* $c_{n+1}/c_n = c + o(n^{-1/2})$ *then* $a_n/c_n = g(1/c) + o(n^{-1/2})$. *Moreover if* $g(1/c) \neq 0$ *then* $a_{n+1}/a_n = c + o(n^{-1/2})$.

We have, $\forall |z| < 1/|c|$ such that $g(z) \neq 0$,

$$\frac{S_{n+1}(z) - S_n(z)}{f_{n+1}(z) - f_n(z)} = \frac{a_{n+1}}{c_{n+1}g(z)}$$

which tends to $g(1/c)/g(z)$ when n tends to infinity by the preceding theorem. Thus if $g(1/c) = 0$, the sequence $(S_{n+1}(z) - S_n(z))$ converges faster than the sequence $(f_{n+1}(z) - f_n(z))$ for all z in the open disc of radius $1/|c|$ such that $g(z) \neq 0$. Of course, with the preceding restrictions on z, $S_n(z)$ tends to $f(z)$ and we have

THEOREM 22.2. *Let* $|z| < 1/|c|$ *and be such that* $g(z) \neq 0$. *If* $\lim_{n\to\infty} c_{n+1}/c_n = c \neq 0$, *if* $g(1/c) = 0$ *and if one of the following conditions is satisfied*
  (i) $\exists a, |c| \leq |a|$ *such that* $\lim_{n\to\infty} a_{n+1}/a_n = a$,

(ii) $\exists \rho \in [0, 1[, \exists \lambda \in [0, 1/2], \exists N, \forall n \geq N, |(a_{n+1}/a_n)z| \leq \rho, |(c_{n+1}/c_n)z| \leq \lambda$,
(iii) $f_n(z)$ is monotone,
then $\lim_{n \to \infty} (S_n(z) - f(z))/(f_n(z) - f(z)) = 0$.

Of course the choice $g(z) = 1 - cz$ forces itself and we have

$$h(z) = f(z) - czf(z),$$
$$h_n(z) = f_n(z) - czf_{n-1}(z),$$
$$S_n(z) = f_n(z) + cc_n z^{n+1}/(1 - cz).$$

We have also

$$(f(z) - f_{n-1}(z))/c_n z^n = 1 + \frac{c_{n+1}}{c_n} z + \frac{c_{n+2}}{c_n} z^2 + \cdots$$

which shows that this ratio tends to $(1 - cz)^{-1}$ when n goes to infinity and thus we obtain

THEOREM 22.3. *If* $\lim_{n \to \infty} c_{n+1}/c_n = c \neq 0$ *and if* $g(z) = 1 - cz$ *then* $\forall z$ *such that* $|z| < 1/|c|$, $(S_n(z))$ *converges to* $f(z)$ *faster than* $(f_n(z))$, *that is*

$$\lim_{n \to \infty} (S_n(z) - f(z))/(f_n(z) - f(z)) = 0.$$

An extension of this result to the case where $c_n = 0$ if $n \neq pk + q$ and $\lim_{n \to \infty} c_{(n+1)k+q}/c_{nk+q} = c \neq 0$ is given in BREZINSKI [1991c].

The choice $g(z) = 1 - cz$ leads to a rational approximation $S_n(z)$. In fact we have the more general result

THEOREM 22.4. *If* g *is a polynomial of degree* k *with* $g(0) \neq 0$ *then* S_n *is the Padé-type approximant* (n/k) *of* f *whose generating polynomial is* $z^k g(z^{-1})$.

PROOF. We have

$$f_n(z)g(z) = h_n(z) + O(z^{n+1}),$$

that is, since $g(0) \neq 0$,

$$h_n(z)/g(z) = f_n(z) + O(z^{n+1}) = f(z) + O(z^{n+1})$$

which is the definition of the Padé-type approximant $(n/k)_f$. □

Thus Cauchy-type approximants generalize Padé and Padé-type approximants.

Instead of considering S_n as given above, one can consider the following rational approximants

$$V_{n/k}(z) = h_n(z)/g_k(z).$$

We have

$$f_n(z)g_k(z) = h_k(z) + O(z^{k+1}) \quad \text{if} \quad k \leq n,$$
$$= h_n(z) + O(z^{n+1}) \quad \text{if} \quad n \leq k,$$

and thus there folllows

THEOREM 22.5. *If $g(0) \neq 0$ then, for $n \leq k$, $V_{n/k}$ is the Padé-type approximant (n/k) of f whose generating polynomial is $z^k g_k(z^{-1})$.*

We have

$$\frac{V_{n+1/k}(z) - V_{n/k}(z)}{f_{n+1}(z) - f_n(z)} = \frac{a_{n+1}}{c_{n+1}g_k(z)}$$

which tends to $g(1/c)/g_k(z)$ when n goes to infinity. Thus, for a fixed value of k, the results of Theorem 22.2 are still valid by replacing the condition $g(z) \neq 0$ by $g_k(z) \neq 0$, which again shows the importance of the knowledge of the zeros of sections of power series studied by EDREI, SAFF and VARGA [1983].

Let us give a numerical example. We consider the series

$$f(z) = \ln(1 + z) = z - z^2/2 + z^3/3 - \cdots.$$

Since $\lim_{n \to \infty} c_{n+1}/c_n = -1$ we shall take $g(z) = 1 + z$ and thus

$$h(z) = z - z \sum_{n=1}^{\infty} (-1)^n z^n / n(n+1),$$

which shows, for example, that the computation of $\ln 2$ with a precision of 10^{-k} will need 10^k terms of f and only $10^{k/2}$ terms with S_n.

In Theorem 22.2, it was assumed that $g(1/c) = 0$. If this condition is not satisfied we shall consider the approximants defined by

$$\theta_n(z) = f_n(z) - \frac{S_n(z) - f_n(z)}{\Delta S_n(z) - \Delta f_n(z)} \Delta f_n(z).$$

It can be proved that the following result holds

THEOREM 22.6. *Let $|z| < 1/|c|$ and be such that $g(z) \neq 0$ and $g(z) \neq g(1/c)$. If $\lim_{n \to \infty} c_{n+1}/c_n = c \neq 0$ and if $g(1/c) \neq 0$ then $(\theta_n(z))$ converges to $f(z)$ faster than $(f_n(z))$.*

PROOF. We have

$$\frac{\theta_n(z) - f(z)}{f_n(z) - f(z)} = 1 - \frac{(S_n(z) - f(z))/(f_n(z) - f(z)) - 1}{\Delta S_n(z)/\Delta f_n(z) - 1}.$$

Under the assumptions of the theorem, there exists $a \neq 1$ such that

$$\lim_{n\to\infty} \frac{S_n(z) - f(z)}{f_n(z) - f(z)} = \lim_{n\to\infty} \frac{\Delta S_n(z)}{\Delta f_n(z)} = a$$

and the result immediately follows. □

All the results presented in this section are only preliminary work on a subject which deserves further research, see MATOS [1991a,b].

23. Series of functions

Let us now assume that f is a series of functions

$$f(z) = \sum_{i=0}^{\infty} c_i g_i(z)$$

and try to extend Padé-type and Padé approximants. Such cases have already been studied when the g_i are orthogonal polynomials. All the authors were looking for approximations of the form

$$r(z) = \sum_{i=0}^{p} a_i g_i(z) \bigg/ \sum_{i=0}^{q} b_i g_i(z)$$

and the a_i's and the b_i's were obtained by multiplying by the denominator and identifying the coefficients of the successive g_i's in

$$\sum_{i=0}^{p} a_i g_i(z) - f(z) \sum_{i=0}^{q} b_i g_i(z) = O(g_{p+q+1}(z))$$

where the notation $O(g_j(z))$ means a series of functions beginning with $g_j(z)$. Of course, such an identification requires the use of the multiplication law of the family $\{g_i\}$

$$g_i(z) g_j(z) = \sum_k d_k^{(i,j)} g_k(z),$$

thus leading to tedious computations since this law is, in general, much more complicated than the multiplication law for polynomials, $z^i z^j = z^{i+j}$, which ensures the simplicity of Padé approximants.

We shall follow and generalize a different approach due to HORNECKER [1959a,b] and simplified by PASZKOWSKI [1963, 1975] in the case where the g_i's are the Chebyshev polynomials. It consists in constructing a rational function of the variable z such that its power series expansion agrees with f as far as possible.

Let G be the generating function of the family $\{g_i\}$ defined by

$$G(x, z) = \sum_{i=0}^{\infty} x^i g_i(z)$$

and let c be the linear functional on the space of polynomials defined as above by

$$c(x^i) = c_i, \quad i = 0, 1, \ldots$$

with the convention that $c_i = 0$ for $i < 0$.

Obviously, we formally have

$$f(z) = c(G(x, z))$$

where c acts on x and z is a parameter.

As in the case of Padé-type approximants, we obtain an approximation of f by replacing $G(\cdot, z)$ by its interpolation polynomial R_k and then computing $c(R_k(x))$. In the case of a power series this was easy because the Hermite interpolation polynomial of the generating function $G(x, z) = (1 - xz)^{-1}$ had a very simple expression (see Theorem 2.3). In general, this is not the case and we have to use Lagrange interpolation. In that case we know that if $x_1, \ldots, x_k$ are distinct points in the complex plane then the interpolation polynomial of $G(x, z)$ at $x_1, \ldots, x_k$ is given by

$$R_k(x) = \sum_{i=1}^{k} L_i(x) G(x_i, z)$$

where

$$L_i(x) = \frac{v_k(x)}{(x - x_i) v_k'(x_i)} \quad \text{and} \quad v_k(x) = (x - x_1) \cdots (x - x_k).$$

Thus we obtain

$$c(R_k(x)) = \sum_{i=1}^{k} A_i G(x_i, z)$$

where the A_i's, which depend on k, are given by

$$A_i = c(L_i(x)) = w_{k-1}(x_i) / v_k'(x_i)$$

with

$$w_{k-1}(z) = c\left(\frac{v_k(x) - v_k(z)}{x - z}\right).$$

Generalizations

By analogy with Section 19 we shall denote $c(R_k(x))$ by $(k-1/k)_f(z)$ although it is not always a rational function. We have the following results

THEOREM 23.1. $(k-1/k)_f(z) = \sum_{i=0}^{\infty} d_i g_i(z)$ *with* $d_i = \sum_{j=1}^{k} A_j x_j^i$ *and* $d_i = c_i$ *for* $i = 0, \ldots, k-1$. *Thus*

$$f(z) - (k-1/k)_f(z) = \sum_{i=k}^{\infty}(c_i - d_i)g_i(z) = O(g_k(z)).$$

If the interpolation points $x_1, \ldots, x_k$ *are the zeros (assumed to be distinct) of* P_k, *the polynomial of degree k belonging to the family of orthogonal polynomials with respect to c, then* $d_i = c_i$ *for* $i = 0, \ldots, 2k-1$ *and*

$$f(z) - (k-1/k)_f(z) = O(g_{2k-1}(z)).$$

PROOF. From Lagrange's polynomial interpolation formula, we have

$$x^i = \sum_{j=1}^{k} L_j(x) x_j^i \quad \text{for } i = 0, \ldots, k-1.$$

Thus

$$c_i = c(x^i) = \sum_{j=1}^{k} A_j x_j^i, \quad i = 0, \ldots, k-1.$$

But

$$(k-1/k)_f(z) = \sum_{j=1}^{k} A_j G(x_j, z) = \sum_{j=1}^{k} A_j \sum_{i=0}^{\infty} x_j^i g_i(z)$$

$$= \sum_{i=0}^{\infty} \left(\sum_{j=1}^{k} A_j x_j^i \right) g_i(z)$$

and the results follow. □

In the last case the approximant will be denoted by $[k-1/k]$ and called a Padé approximant of the series of functions.

Thus, this Theorem shows that the characteristic property of Padé-type and Padé approximants for power series has been extended to series of functions.

In the construction of such approximants for series of functions there is a fundamental point which must be clearly understood. The preceding series f can also be written as

$$f(z) = \sum_{i=0}^{\infty} e_i h_i(z)$$

with $e_i = 1$ and $h_i(z) = c_i g_i(z)$. The approximant $(k - 1/k)$ obtained by replacing $G(x, z)$ by its interpolation polynomial at $x_1, \ldots, x_k$ and then applying the functional c will, in general, be different from the approximant $(k - 1/k)$ obtained by replacing $H(x, z) = \sum_{i=0}^{\infty} x^i h_i(z)$ by its interpolation polynomial at the same points and then applying the functional e defined by $e(x^i) = e_i = 1$.

Now let L be a linear functional transformation. We shall use the following notations which, though not strictly correct, are more appropriate since both variables clearly appear. We shall set

$$h_i(p) = L g_i(z)$$

and

$$F(p) = L f(z) = \sum_{i=0}^{\infty} c_i h_i(p).$$

Of course this notation comes from the Laplace transform in which

$$F(p) = \int_0^{\infty} e^{-pz} f(z) \, dz.$$

We shall now relate the Padé-type and Padé approximants of the series f and F as explained by BREZINSKI and VAN ISEGHEM [1984].

Let H be the generating function of the family $\{h_i\}$

$$H(x, p) = \sum_{i=0}^{\infty} x^i h_i(p).$$

Obviously, we have

$$H(x, p) = L G(x, z).$$

The interpolation polynomial of $G(\cdot, z)$ depends on z and we shall now denote it by $R_k(\cdot, z)$. We set

$$S_k(x, p) = L R_k(x, z).$$

Since L acts on z then S_k is a polynomial of degree at most $k - 1$ in x and it is easy to see that $S_k(\cdot, p)$ is the interpolation polynomial of $H(\cdot, p)$ at the same points and we have

$$c(S_k(x, p)) = c(L R_k(x, z)) = L c(R_k(x, z))$$

since L acts on z and c on x. Thus

$$(k - 1/k)_F(p) = L(k - 1/k)_f(z).$$

SECTION 23 — Generalizations

As pointed out above, this result is only valid if the coefficients c_i are the same for both series. For example, if

$$F(p) = Lf(z) = f'(p) = \sum_{i=0}^{\infty} i c_i p^{i-1},$$

$(k-1/k)_{f'}(p) = (d/dz)(k-1/k)_f(z)$ if the approximant of f' is constructed with the same c_i and with $h_i(p) = Lz^i = ip^{i-1}$.

If the interpolation points are the zeros of P_k, then the preceding property holds since the interpolation points are the same because they are the zeros of P_k which only depends on the c_i's which are the same for both series.

Thus we have proved

THEOREM 23.2. *Let $F(p) = Lf(z)$. Then $(k-1/k)_F(p) = L(k-1/k)_f(z)$ if both approximants are constructed from the same interpolation points and the same linear functional c. This is, in particular, the case when the interpolation points are the zeros of P_k.*

If $g_i(z) = z^i$, we recover the definition of Padé approximants for series of functions used by VAN ROSSUM [1980] and also our previous approach.

From the approximant $(k-1/k)$ it is possible to construct the whole set of approximants (p/q) for arbitrary values of p and q.

We can write

$$f(z) = \sum_{i=0}^{n} c_i g_i(z) + c^{(n+1)}(G_n(x,z))$$

where $c^{(n+1)}$ is defined by $c^{(n+1)}(x^i) = c_{n+i+1}$ and where G_n is the generating function of the family $\{g_{n+i+1}\}$,

$$G_n(x,z) = \sum_{i=0}^{\infty} x^i g_{n+i+1}(z).$$

Replacing, in this expression, G_n by its interpolation polynomial R_k leads to approximants denoted by $(n+k/k)_f(z)$. Similarly we can write

$$f(z) = c^{(-n+1)}(G_{-n}(x,z))$$

where $c^{(-n+1)}$ is defined by $c^{(-n+1)}(x^i) = c_{i-n+1}$ with the convention that $c_j = 0$ if $j < 0$ and where $G_{-n}(x,z) = x^{n-1}G(x,z)$. Replacing, in this expression, G_{-n} by its interpolation polynomial R_{n+k} leads to approximants denoted by $(k/n+k)_f(z)$. In both cases we have

THEOREM 23.3.

$$(p/q)_f(z) = f(z) + O(g_{p+1}(z)).$$

Moreover if the interpolation points $x_1,\ldots,x_q$ are the zeros (assumed to be distinct) of the polynomial $P_q^{(p-q+1)}$ of degree q belonging to the family of orthogonal polynomials with respect to $c^{(p-q+1)}$ then

$$(p/q)_f(z) = f(z) + O(g_{p+q+1}(z)).$$

PROOF. Coming back to the notations of Theorem 23.1 and using the same arguments, we have $d_i = c_i$ for $i = 0,\ldots,p+q$. □

In the last case the approximant (called a Padé approximant of the series of functions) will be denoted by $[p/q]$.

Let us now turn to an interesting particular case. We saw that the construction of Padé approximants for series of functions needs the knowledge of the zeros $x_1,\ldots,x_q$ of the polynomial $P_q^{(p-q+1)}$ contrarily to the case of Padé approximants for power series. This was the procedure followed by HORNECKER [1959a]. However in the particular case where the g_i are the Chebyshev polynomials of the first kind, this knowledge is not needed, as demonstrated by PASZKOWSKI [1963, 1975].

Thus

$$g_i(z) = T_i(z) = \cos(i \arccos z), \quad i = 0, 1, \ldots$$

and let us write f as

$$f(z) = c_0/2 + \sum_{i=1}^{\infty} c_i T_i(z).$$

The generating function is given by

$$G(x,z) = 1/2 + \sum_{i=1}^{\infty} x^i T_i(z) = \frac{1-x^2}{2(1-2xz+x^2)}.$$

Let $P_k^{(n+1)}$ be the polynomial of degree k belonging to the family of orthogonal polynomials with respect to $c^{(n+1)}$. We set

$$P_k^{(n+1)}(x) = a_0 + a_1 x + \cdots + a_k x^k$$

and

$$(n+k/k)_f(z) = R(z)/S(z).$$

We have

$$S(z) = P_k^{(n+1)}(z)P_k^{(n+1)}(z^{-1})/2 = \frac{1}{2}\prod_{i=1}^{k}(1-2x_i z + x_i^2)$$

and

THEOREM 23.4.

$$S(z) = e_0/2 + e_1 T_1(z) + \cdots + e_k T_k(z),$$
$$R(z) = h_0/2 + h_1 T_1(z) + \cdots + h_{n+k} T_{n+k}(z)$$

with

$$e_i = \sum_{j=0}^{k-i} a_j a_{j+i}, \quad i = 0, \ldots, k,$$

$$h_0 = c_0 e_0/2 + \sum_{i=1}^{k} c_i e_i,$$

$$h_i = (c_i e_0 + \sum_{j=1}^{k} (c_{|i-j|} + c_{i+j}) e_j)/2, \quad i = 1, \ldots, n+k.$$

The proof of this result is based on the multiplication law of Chebyshev polynomials,

$$T_i(z) T_j(z) = (T_{|i-j|}(z) + T_{i+j}(z))/2.$$

More recent and advanced results on Padé–Chebyshev approximation and an extensive bibliography can be found in TREFETHEN and GUTKNECHT [1987].

SABLONNIÈRE [1984] has extended the results of this Section to multivariate series of functions using the generalization of Padé-type approximants to multivariate power series given in SABLONNIÈRE [1983] and the Hakopian interpolation polynomial (see Section 27).

24. Padé–Hermite approximants

The Padé approximation problem consists in finding two polynomials P_1 and P_2 of the respective degrees n_1 and n_2 at most such that

$$P_1(z) f_1(z) + P_2(z) f_2(z) = \mathrm{O}(z^{n_1+n_2+1})$$

where f_1 and f_2 are given power series. With this notation $P_1(z)/P_2(z)$ is the Padé approximant $[n_1/n_2]$ of the series $f(z) = -f_2(z)/f_1(z)$.

This problem was extended to more than two series by HERMITE [1893] and PADÉ [1894] and it is now called the Padé–Hermite approximation problem. Let $f_1, \ldots, f_k$ be k formal power series. The Padé–Hermite approximation problem consists in finding the polynomials $P_1, \ldots, P_k$ of the respective degrees $n_1, \ldots, n_k$ at most such that

$$P_1(z) f_1(z) + \cdots + P_k(z) f_k(z) = \mathrm{O}(z^{n_1+\cdots+n_k+k-1}).$$

These past few years an abundant literature on the subject has arisen. It is not our purpose here to give a review of the known results about Padé–Hermite approximants but only to guide the interested reader through the literature and to give some examples showing the interest of such approximants.

The first problem to be studied is that of the existence and the practical computation of the Padé–Hermite approximants, that is the k-uple of polynomials $(P_1, \ldots, P_k)$. This problem was studied by DELLA DORA and DI CRESCENZO [1984a,b]. These authors gave some recursive algorithms generalizing those for the classical Padé approximants. Other algorithms are due to PASZKOWSKI [1987]. Some results about the block structure of the Padé–Hermite table of approximants are reviewed by PASZKOWSKI [1990]. More recently a theory of vector orthogonal polynomials related to Padé–Hermite approximants has been built up by DRAUX and MAANAOUI [1990]. These orthogonal polynomials can be put into the framework of biorthogonality as explained by BREZINSKI [1991a]. The block structure of the table was studied by DELLA DORA [1981].

After having constructed the approximants and studied their algebraic aspects, the next problem to deal with is that of convergence. A conjecture about the asymptotic behaviour of the polynomials P_i was given by NUTTALL [1984]. It asserts, in the case where $\forall i, n_i = n$, that the asymptotic form of P_i when n tends to infinity is given by the solution of a boundary value problem on an appropriate Riemann surface. Some examples and partial results for supporting this conjecture are given. The convergence problem was mainly studied by STAHL [1988] who gave results about nth root asymptotics of the polynomials P_n. He also studied the convergence of two important classes of Padé–Hermite approximants, namely the algebraic approximants which correspond to $f_i = f^i$ and generalize the case treated by SHAFER [1974] where $k = 3$, and the integral approximants which correspond to $f_i = f^{(i-1)}$ and generalize the D-log approximants of BAKER [1961] for which $k = 2$ (see also BAKER [1988]). The asymptotic behaviour of the zeros of the polynomials was considered in these two cases and the domains of convergence were characterized by certain logarithmic potentials. The interested reader will find more references in the works just quoted.

Let us now give examples to illustrate the interest of Padé–Hermite approximation. We take $k = 3$ and $f_1 = 1$, $f_2 = f$ and $f_3 = f^2$. Such approximants were introduced by SHAFER [1974] and are called quadratic approximants, see also LOI and McINNES [1984].

Let us consider the function $f(z) = \arctan z$. The ordinary Padé approximants do not have the correct behaviour when z approaches infinity. In order to obtain a finite value for the approximants when z tends to infinity we have to construct the approximants of $F(t) = f^2(z)$ with $t = z^2$ and then take their square root as explained by GAMMEL [1973].

By this trick we obtain an approximant tending to a constant as $O(z^{-2})$ when $z \to \infty$ which is wrong since $\tan z$ tends to a constant as $O(z^{-1})$. If we use the quadratic approximants with $n_1 = 2$, $n_2 = 1$ and $n_3 = 2$, we obtain by solving the quadratic equation, an approximation of the form

$$\frac{8z}{3 + \sqrt{25 + 80z^2/3}}$$

which has the correct behaviour at infinity and is much more accurate than the corresponding Padé approximant. In fact the maximum error is 1.5 %.

Let us now consider

$$f(z) = (1 - 3z)^{-1} + (1 - z/2)^{-1/2}.$$

We have $f(1) = 0.91422356237\ldots$. With $n_1 = n_2 = n_3 = 3$, the quadratic approximants provide a value of $0.914213562\ldots$, while $[5/5] = 0.91421\ldots$. Both approximants use the same number of coefficients of the series f.

Sometimes the Padé approximants give better results than the quadratic approximants. For example if $f(z) = \frac{1}{2}\ln(1 + z)$ we obtain $f(2) = 0.549306144\ldots$, $[5/5] = 0.549306\ldots$, while with $n_1 = n_2 = n_3 = 3$ the quadratic approximants give $0.54930\ldots$.

Usually the quadratic approximants provide better results for functions with branch points.

25. Vector Padé approximants

The term vector approximants is used for rational functions with a common denominator approximating simultaneously several functions $f_1, \ldots, f_d$. The name of Padé is joined to the name of these approximants because the main ideas of scalar approximation are kept (VAN ISEGHEM [1985, 1987b]): first, giving m and n as the degrees of the numerator and the denominator is sufficient (in the normal case) to determine completely the approximant; secondly the Padé approximant is best in a sense to be explained. For vector Padé approximants, to give m and n as the common degree m of all the numerators, and n as the degree of the common denominator defines completely the vector Padé approximants, and secondly the vector Padé approximant $\mathbb{R}(t) = (P^\alpha/Q)_{\alpha=1,\ldots,d}$ is the best in the following sense: it is impossible to improve simultaneously the order of approximation of all the components.

The first point is what makes the difference from the simultaneous approximants defined by DE BRUIN [1984] which need auxilliary choices for the degrees of the P^α. For the second point, if $d = 1$ then the usual Padé approximation for one function is recovered. Let us define first the vector Padé-type approximants.

Let $\mathbb{F} = (f_1, \ldots, f_d)$. $\mathbb{F}$ is supposed to be expanded into a power series with coefficients in $\mathbb{C}^d$

$$\mathbb{F}(t) = \sum_{i \geq 0} \Gamma_i t^i, \quad \Gamma_i \in \mathbb{C}^d, \ t \in \mathbb{C}.$$

If, for each $\alpha = 1, \ldots, d$,

$$f_\alpha(t) = \sum_{i \geq 0} c_i^\alpha t^i, \quad \text{then } \Gamma_i = (c_i^1, \ldots, c_i^d)^T.$$

Then let us define a linear functional $\Gamma: \mathbb{C}[[x]] \to \mathbb{C}^d$ by $\Gamma(x^i) = \Gamma_i$. Taking as components of the vector approximant, the Padé-type approximants of the f_α's, we get the following theorem

THEOREM 25.1. *Let P be the Hermite interpolation polynomial of $1/(1-xt)$ at $x_1, \ldots, x_n$, let*

$$v(t) = \prod_{i=1}^{n}(t - x_i), \quad \tilde{v}(t) = t^n v(t^{-1}),$$

and

$$\mathbb{W}(t) = \Gamma(\frac{v(t) - v(x)}{t - x}) \quad (\Gamma \text{ acting on } x),$$

then

$$\Gamma(P(t)) = \tilde{\mathbb{W}}(t)/\tilde{v}(t),$$

$$\mathbb{F}(t) - \Gamma(P(t)) = \frac{t^n}{\tilde{v}(t)} \Gamma(\frac{v(x)}{1-xt}),$$

$$= \frac{t^n}{\tilde{v}(t)} \sum_{i \geq 0} D_i t^i, \quad D_i = \Gamma(x^i \cdot v(x)).$$

$\tilde{\mathbb{W}}(t)/\tilde{v}(t)$ is called the *Padé-type approximant* $(n-1/n)$ of $\mathbb{F}$.

The proof is similar to the scalar case (cf. Section 19), because each component $(\tilde{\mathbb{W}}(t)/\tilde{v}(t))_\alpha$ is the Padé-type approximant of f_α, for $\alpha = 1, \ldots, d$.

In order to improve the order of approximation on all the components, we have to choose the polynomial v such that a maximum number of D_i are zero. D_i is a vector of $\mathbb{C}^d$ so $D_i = 0$ represents d scalar equations with respect to the coefficients of v as unknowns. And so if n is the degree of the denominator, the best order of approximation by rational functions of type $(n-1, n)$, is $n + [n/d]$ where $[n/d]$ is the integer part of n/d.

Padé-type approximants for all degrees (s/r) can be defined as in Section 19 for the scalar case. For any integer h, positive or not, we get

$$\mathbb{F}(t) = \sum_{i=0}^{h-1} \Gamma_i t^i + t^h \mathbb{F}_h(t), \quad \Gamma_i = 0 \quad \text{if} \quad i < 0,$$

$$(r+h-1/r)_\mathbb{F}(t) = \sum_{i=0}^{h-1} \Gamma_i t^i + t^h (r-1/r)_{\mathbb{F}_h}(t).$$

The order of approximation is $r+h-1$; it can be improved up to $r+h-1+[r/d]$.

We can now choose the generating polynomials v of the vector Padé-type approximants to improve the order of approximation. Let r be an arbitrary integer, written in the form $r = nd + k$, $0 \leqslant k < d$; let us denote by P_{nd+k} the polynomial defined by the following equations

$$\begin{aligned} \Gamma(x^i \cdot P_{nd+k}(x)) &= 0, \quad i = 0, \ldots, n-1, \\ c^\alpha(x^n \cdot P_{nd+k}(x)) &= 0, \quad \alpha = 1, \ldots, k. \end{aligned} \tag{R}$$

The Padé-type approximant $(r - 1/r)$ generated by P_{nd+k} will be of maximal order of approximation: the order of approximation is $r + n - 1$ at least, $r + n$ for the first k components. It will be called the *vector Padé approximant* $[r - 1/r]_\mathbb{F}$.

Writing the conditions (R) as a linear system, we get an expression of P_r as a ratio of two determinants

$$P_r(x) = \frac{\begin{vmatrix} \Gamma_0 & \cdots & \Gamma_r \\ \vdots & & \vdots \\ \Gamma_{n-1} & \cdots & \Gamma_{n+r-1} \\ \Gamma_n^{(k)} & \cdots & \Gamma_{n+r}^{(k)} \\ 1 & \cdots & x^r \end{vmatrix}}{\begin{vmatrix} \Gamma_0 & \cdots & \Gamma_{r-1} \\ \vdots & & \vdots \\ \Gamma_{n-1} & \cdots & \Gamma_{n+r-2} \\ \Gamma_n^{(k)} & \cdots & \Gamma_{n+r-1}^{(k)} \end{vmatrix}}$$

where each row $(\Gamma_i \cdots \Gamma_{r+i})$ represents d scalar rows formed by the components. The last row $(\Gamma_n^{(k)} \cdots \Gamma_{n+r}^{(k)})$ represents the k first components of $(\Gamma_n \cdots \Gamma_{n+r})$. Similarly to the scalar case, the polynomials $(P_r^{(s)})_{r \geqslant 0}$ are the generating polynomials of $[s + r - 1/r]$ and, for each s, they satisfy a recurrence formula, which, here, is of order $d + 1$ (i.e. with $d + 2$ terms)

$$P_{r+1}^{(s)}(x) = (x - \beta_r^s) P_r^{(s)}(x) - \sum_{\mu=1}^{d} \gamma_\mu^s P_{r-\mu}^{(s)}. \tag{D}$$

If all the $P_r^{(s)}$'s exist, then the last term γ_d^s is not zero. Then a theory analogous to the theory of orthogonal polynomials can be developed, and thus these polynomials have been called *vector orthogonal polynomials* (or of dimension d) (VAN ISEGHEM [1985, 1987b, 1989]). A Shohat–Favard theorem is proved: given a family $(P_r)_{r \geqslant 0}$ satisfying a relation of type (D), there exist d functionals $c^1, \ldots, c^d$ such that the P_r's satisfy the relation (R) with respect to $\Gamma = (c^1, \ldots, c^d)$. The space of all the possible Γ is a vector space of dimension $(d!)$. And so there is, as in the scalar case, an equivalence between the vector-orthogonality, defined by the relations of orthogonality (R), and the family of polynomials defined by the recurrence relations (D). The $1/d$-orthogonality was defined by MARONI [1981]. It is easy to see that a family of polynomials defined by the recurrence relation (D) is $1/d$-orthogonal with respect to c^1.

The vector Padé approximants can now be studied.

The determinantal expression for $P_r^{(s)}$ gives rise to a determinantal expression for the vector Padé approximants.

$$\mathbb{F}(t) = \sum_{i=0}^{h-1} \Gamma_i t^i + t^h \mathbb{F}_h(t) = \Sigma_h + t^h \mathbb{F}_h(t),$$

$$t^h[r+h-1/r]_\mathbb{F}(t) = \Sigma_h + t^h[r-1/r]_{\mathbb{F}_h}(t),$$

$$[r-1/r]_\mathbb{F}(t) = \tilde{\mathbb{W}}(t)/\tilde{P}_r(t)$$

and finally we get (with $r = nd + k$)

$$[r+h-1/r]_\mathbb{F}(t) = \frac{\begin{vmatrix} \Gamma_h & \cdots & \Gamma_{r+h} \\ \vdots & & \vdots \\ \Gamma_{h+n-1} & \cdots & \Gamma_{h+n+r-1} \\ \Gamma_{h+n}^{(k)} & \cdots & \Gamma_{h+n+r}^{(k)} \\ t^r \Sigma_{h-1} & \cdots & \Sigma_{r+h-1} \end{vmatrix}}{\begin{vmatrix} \Gamma_h & \cdots & \Gamma_{r+h} \\ \vdots & & \vdots \\ \Gamma_{h+n}^{(k)} & \cdots & \Gamma_{h+n+r}^{(k)} \\ t^r & \cdots & 1 \end{vmatrix}}$$

where only the last row of the numerator is a vector, all the other rows being put for d scalar rows.

This expression can be transformed in terms of $\Delta^i \Sigma_h$; the first row being the vector row, we get for any p, q and $h = p - q$

$$[p/q] = \frac{\begin{vmatrix} \Sigma_h & \Delta \Sigma_h & \cdots & \Delta \Sigma_{p-1} \\ \Delta \Sigma_h & \Delta^2 \Sigma_h & \cdots & \Delta^2 \Sigma_{p-1} \\ \vdots & \vdots & & \vdots \\ \Delta^{n+1} \Sigma_h^{(k)} & \Delta^{n+2} \Sigma_h^{(k)} & \cdots & \Delta^{n+2} \Sigma_{p-1}^{(k)} \end{vmatrix}}{\begin{vmatrix} \Delta^2 \Sigma_h & \cdots & \Delta^2 \Sigma_{p-1} \\ \vdots & & \vdots \\ \Delta^{n+2} \Sigma_h^{(k)} & \cdots & \Delta^{n+2} \Sigma_{p-1}^{(k)} \end{vmatrix}}.$$

And so the approximants can be computed by algorithms like the recursive projection algorithm (R.P.A.) or the compact recursive projection algorithm (C.R.P.A.) of BREZINSKI [1983c].

It is also possible to generalize the cross rule of Wynn given in Section 6 (VAN ISEGHEM [1986]).

In the scalar case, the cross rule involves five approximants in the array

$$\begin{matrix} & N & \\ W & C & E \\ & S & \end{matrix}$$

and can be written in two forms

$$(E-N)(C-W)(S-C) = (C-N)(E-C)(S-W),$$
$$\frac{1}{C-N} + \frac{1}{C-S} = \frac{1}{C-E} + \frac{1}{C-W}.$$

The proof can be extended to the vector case. The approximants involved are the following, W_i and N_i lying on diagonals

$$\begin{matrix} W_d & N_d & & & \\ & \ddots & \ddots & & \\ & & \ddots & N_1 & N \\ & & & W_1 & C & E \\ & & & & S & \end{matrix}$$

The result, given in the implicit form, is the following: the determinants are $d \times d$ determinants, the indicated vectors are the columns of the determinants

$$(E-N) \cdot |C - W_1, W_d - W_{d-1}, \ldots, W_2 - W_1|$$
$$\times |S - C, N_{d-1} - N_{d-2}, \ldots, N_1 - C|$$
$$= (C-N) \cdot |S - W_1, W_d - W_{d-1}, \ldots, W_2 - W_1|$$
$$\times |E_C, N_{d-1} - N_{d-2}, \ldots, N_1 - C|.$$

The explicit form is given for all the components $(E-C)^\alpha$, $\alpha = 1, \ldots, d$,

$$D_1 = |C - W_1, W_d - W_{d-1}, \cdots, W_2 - W_1|,$$
$$D_2 = |S - C, N_{d-1} - N_{d-2}, \ldots, N_1 - C|,$$
$$D_3 = |S - W_1, W_d - W_{d-1}, \ldots, W_2 - W_1|,$$
$$D_4 = |C - N, N_{d-1} - N_{d-2}, \ldots, N_1 - C|,$$
$$\frac{1}{(E-C)^\alpha} + \frac{1}{(C-N)^\alpha} = \frac{1}{(C-N)^\alpha} \frac{D_3 D_4}{D_1 D_2}, \quad \alpha = 1, \ldots, d.$$

As in the scalar case, symbolic negative columns are defined, so that the algorithm can be used with the center term C in column zero, and so it computes E from the first column. All the approximants $[p/q]$ with $p \geq q - 1$ can be computed by this algorithm.

The natural link between two consecutive diagonals of the table of $P_r^{(s)}$ is a vector qd-algorithm, i.e. a generalization of the classical qd-algorithm of RUTISHAUSER [1954] (see Section 5),

$$P_r^{(s+1)}(x) = xP_r^{(s+1)}(x) - q_{r+1}^s P_r^{(s)}(x), \quad r \geq 0,$$
$$P_r^{(s+1)}(x) = P_r^{(s)}(x) - \sum_{i=r-d}^{r-1} e_{r,i}^s P_i^{(s+1)}(x), \quad r \geq d.$$

As for the recurrence relation between the $P_r^{(s)}$, s fixed, the last term $e_{r,r-d}^s$ is nonzero if the functional is nondegenerate, i.e. if all the polynomials $P_r^{(s)}$ exist. The q_{r+1}^s and the $(e_{ri}^s)_{i=r-1,\ldots,r-d}$ satisfy a pseudo-rhombus algorithm

$$\begin{cases} q_{r+1}^{r+1} + e_{r,r-1}^{s+1} = q_{r+1}^s + e_{r+1,r}^s, \\ e_{ri}^{s+1} q_{i+1}^{s+1} + e_{r,i-1}^{s+1} = e_{r,i}^s q_{r+1}^s + e_{r+1,i}^s, \quad i = r-d+1, \ldots, r-1 \\ e_{r,r-d}^{s+1} \cdot q_{r-d+1}^{s+1} = e_{r,r-d}^s \cdot q_{r+1}^s. \end{cases}$$

The q_{r+1}^s can be written in terms of generalized Hankel determinants

$$q_{r+1}^s = \frac{H_{r+1}^{s+1} H_r^s}{H_{r+1}^s H_r^{s+1}},$$

where H_r^s is the denominator of the monic polynomial $P_r^{(s)}$.

In the case where all the $(f_\alpha)_{\alpha=1,\ldots,d}$ are meromorphic functions in a disc, asymptotics for H_r^s can be found, and so we get

$$\lim_{s \to \infty} q_r^s = u_r, \quad u_r^{-1} \in \bigcup_\alpha \{\text{poles of } f_\alpha\}.$$

It is, more or less, possible to find for which f_α, u_r^{-1} is a pole (VAN ISEGHEM [1987b, 1989]).

From the relation defining q_{r+1}^s,

$$P_{r+1}^{(s+1)}(x) = x P_r^{(s+1)}(x) - q_{r+1}^s P_r^{(s)}(x),$$

or from an asymptotic of the numerator $H_r^s(x)$ of $P_r^{(s)}$, it is easy to see that $\lim_{s \to \infty} (q_{r+1}^s)^{-1}$ in a zero of the limit of the denominators of the Padé approximants. This gives rise to a Montessus de Ballore type Theorem for vector Padé approximants.

Such a Theorem has also been proved for simultaneous approximants by GRAVES-MORRIS and SAFF [1984]. In both cases, the key assumption for the $(f_\alpha)_{\alpha=1,\ldots,d}$ is to be polewise independent with respect to integers ρ_i. Let us just recall this definition.

Let $f_1, \ldots, f_d$ be meromorphic in the disc D, and let nonnegative integers ρ_i be given, for which $\sum_{i=1}^d \rho_i > 0$.

The functions are said to be polewise independent with respect to the numbers ρ_i if there do not exist polynomials $\Pi_1, \ldots, \Pi_d$, at least one of which is non null (with degree $(\Pi_i) \leq \rho_i - 1$ if $\rho_i \geq 1$ and $\Pi_i \equiv 0$ if $\rho_i = 0$), and such that $\psi(z) = \sum_i \Pi_i(z) \cdot f_i(z)$ is analytic through D.

Let us now study the application of the vector Padé approximants to the acceleration of vector sequences.

If $\mathbb{F}$ is a power series $\sum_{i \geq 0} \Gamma_i t^i$, a vector sequence (S_n) is canonically associated with $\mathbb{F}$ by $\Gamma_i = \Delta S_i$, so S_n is the partial sum of $\mathbb{F}(1)$ and the vector Padé approximants are associated with a transformation of sequences. From combinations of the rows of the determinantal expression of the vector approximant of $\mathbb{F}$, it follows that

$$[r+h/r]_{\mathbb{F}}(1) = \psi_r(S_h) = \frac{\begin{vmatrix} S_h & \cdots & S_{h+r} \\ \Delta S_h & \cdots & \Delta S_{h+r} \\ \vdots & & \vdots \\ \Delta S_{h+n-1} & \cdots & \Delta S_{h+r+n-1} \\ \Delta S_{h+n}^{(k)} & \cdots & \Delta S_{h+r+n}^{(k)} \end{vmatrix}}{\begin{vmatrix} 1 & \cdots & 1 \\ \Delta S_h & \cdots & \Delta S_{h+r} \\ \vdots & & \vdots \\ \Delta S_{h+n-1} & \cdots & \Delta S_{h+r+n-1} \\ \Delta S_{h+n}^{(k)} & \cdots & \Delta S_{h+r+n}^{(k)} \end{vmatrix}}.$$

The first row is formed of vectors, the following rows are put for the d rows of their components, except as usual the last ones which contain only the first k components.

The basic result is the following.

A necessary and sufficient condition to have $\psi_r(S_h) = S$ for all h large enough, is that the sequence (S_n) satisfies a linear recurrence relation

$$\sum_{i=0}^{r} a_i (S_{h+i} - S) = 0,$$

$$\sum_{i=0}^{r} a_i \neq 0, \quad a_i \in \mathbb{C}.$$

In the scalar case, if $r = 2$, we recover the Δ^2-process, if $r \geq 2$ we recover the Padé table, the Shanks transformation or the ε-algorithm. If d is not equal to one, if $r < d$ we recover the MPE algorithm (minimal polynomial extrapolation) studied by SMITH, FORD and SIDI [1987], if $r = d$ we recover Henrici's transformation, if $r > d$ the transform seems not to have been studied yet independently from vector Padé approximants (VAN ISEGHEM's thesis [1987b]).

The condition for $\psi_r(S_h)$ to be equal to S is necessary and sufficient, and not only sufficient as is the case for the vector ε-algorithm or the topological ε-algorithm. So the general results are extensions of those obtained in the scalar case by BREZINSKI [1980]. Let us just quote two kinds of results.

For linear systems $X = AX + B$, with A a $d \times d$ matrix, the recurrence relation for the sequence (X_n) given by $X_{n+1} = AX_n + B$ is of order $r \leq d$, and so we recover Henrici's transformation.

$$X = \begin{pmatrix} 0.2 & 11 & 3 \\ 0 & 0.1 & 5 \\ 0 & 0 & 0.5 \end{pmatrix} X \quad (d=3, \text{ rank}(X)=3), \quad \text{see Table 25.1,}$$

TABLE 25.1.

0.100D+01			
0.100D+01			
0.100D+01			
0.142D+02	−0.427D+01		
0.510D+01	−0.638D+00		
0.500D+00	0.120D+01		
0.604D+02	0.494D+02	0.388D+02	
0.301D+01	0.351D+01	0.269D+01	
0.250D+00	0.310D+00	0.485D+00	
0.459D+02	0.104D+03	0.356D+01	−0.295D−16
0.155D+01	0.739D+01	0.247D+00	−0.152D−17
0.125D+00	0.625D+00	0.444D−01	−0.156D−18
0.266D+02	−0.903D+01	0.212D+00	
0.780D+00	−0.643D+00	0.147D−01	
0.625D−01	−0.528D+01	0.264D−02	
0.141D+02	−0.119D+01		
0.391D+00	−0.846D−01		
0.313D−01	−0.686D−02		
0.721D+01			
0.195D+00			
0.156D−01			

$$X = \begin{pmatrix} 1 & 2 & 3 \\ 3 & 2 & 1 \\ 0 & 1 & 2 \end{pmatrix} X \quad (d=3, \text{rank}(X) = 2), \quad \text{see Table 25.2.}$$

The second kind of example is a system of nonlinear equations

$$\begin{cases} x = \dfrac{y^2}{2} + x - 1/2, \\ y = \sin x + \sin(y-1) + 1. \end{cases}$$

The solution is $(0, 1)$ and the Jacobian matrix at the solution $\begin{pmatrix} 1 & 1 \\ 1 & 1 \end{pmatrix}$ is singular.

The computations have been performed, in double precision, with the extended cross rule. With $x_0 = 0.5$ and $y_0 = 1$ we get the numbers as shown in Tables 25.3 and 25.4.

26. The noncommutative case

Padé approximants for series whose coefficients are square matrices have been used by physicists for a long time because they have many applications in theoretical physics, in the partial realization problem in system theory, in statistics

TABLE 25.2.

0.100D+01			
0.100D+01			
0.100D+01			
0.600D+01	−0.562D+00		
0.600D+01	−0.562D+00		
0.300D+01	0.375D+00		
0.270D+02	0.556D+00	0.909D−01	
0.330D+02	−0.100D+01	−0.818D+00	
0.120D+02	0.667D+00	0.545D+00	
0.129D+03	0.116D+00	0.714D−16	0.598D−16
0.159D+03	−0.209D+00	0.795D−16	0.250D−16
0.570D+02	0.140D+00	0.732D−16	0.350D−17
0.618D+03	0.243D−01	0.425D−17	
0.762D+03	−0.437D−01	0.235D−15	
0.273D+03	0.291D−01	−0.906D−16	
0.296D+04	0.507D−02		
0.365D+04	−0.912D−02		
0.131D+04	0.608D−02		
0.142D+05			
0.175D+05			
0.627D+04			

TABLE 25.3. Vector ε-algorithm.

n	x_n	y_n
1	0.28	1.22
2	0.15	0.907
3	0.11×10^{-1}	0.9928
4	0.51×10^{-4}	0.999957
5	0.19×10^{-8}	0.9999999983
6	0.52×10^{-17}	1

and so on. However, as in the scalar case, Padé approximants for such series can be more easily understood as a special case of Padé-type approximants corresponding to a particular choice of the generating polynomials. We shall follow this presentation, due to DRAUX [1984], since it also leads, in a very natural way, to recursive methods for their computation.

Let $\mathcal{A}$ be a noncommutative algebra on a commutative field K of characteristic 0 and with a unit element I. Let f be a formal power series with coefficients c_i

TABLE 25.4. Vector Padé approximants.

n	x_n	y_n
1	0.21	0.984
2	0.14×10^{-1}	1
3	0.18×10^{-2}	1
4	0.10×10^{-4}	1
5	0.48×10^{-9}	1
6	0.11×10^{-17}	1

in $\mathcal{A}$

$$f(z) = \sum_{i=0}^{\infty} c_i z^i, \quad z \in K,$$

and let us define two linear functionals $^R c$ and $^L c$ on the space of polynomials with coefficients in $\mathcal{A}$ by

$$^L c(ax^i) = c_i a, \qquad {}^R c(ax^i) = a c_i,$$

where $a \in \mathcal{A}$.

Let v_k be an arbitrary polynomial of degree k with coefficients in $\mathcal{A}$ and such that the coefficient of z^k be invertible (such a polynomial is called quasi-monic) and let us set

$$\begin{aligned}
{}^L w_{k-1}(z) &= {}^L c((v_k(x) - v_k(z))(x-z)^{-1}), \\
{}^R w_{k-1}(z) &= {}^R c((v_k(x) - v_k(z))(x-z)^{-1}), \\
\tilde{v}_k(z) &= z^k v_k(z^{-1}), \\
{}^L \tilde{w}_{k-1}(z) &= z^{k-1} \, {}^L w_{k-1}(z^{-1}), \\
{}^R \tilde{w}_{k-1}(z) &= z^{k-1} \, {}^R w_{k-1}(z^{-1}).
\end{aligned}$$

We shall set

$$\begin{aligned}
{}^L (k-1/k)_f(z) &= {}^L \tilde{w}_{k-1}(z)(\tilde{v}_k(z))^{-1}, \\
{}^R (k-1/k)_f(z) &= (\tilde{v}_k(z))^{-1} \, {}^R \tilde{w}_{k-1}(z),
\end{aligned}$$

and call them respectively left and right Padé-type approximants. Generally these two approximants are not identical but we have

THEOREM 26.1.

$$\begin{aligned}
{}^L (k-1/k)_f(z) - f(z) &= \mathrm{O}(z^k), \\
{}^R (k-1/k)_f(z) - f(z) &= \mathrm{O}(z^k).
\end{aligned}$$

PROOF. Let us give only the proof for the left approximants since the other case is similar. We set

$$v_k(z) = b_0 + \cdots + b_k z^k.$$

Thus

$$^L\tilde{w}_{k-1}(z) - f(z)\tilde{v}_k(z) = \sum_{i=0}^{k-1} z^{k-i-1} \sum_{j=0}^{k-i-1} c_i b_{i+j+1} - \left(\sum_{i=0}^{\infty} c_i z^i\right)\left(\sum_{j=0}^{k} b_j z^{k-j}\right)$$

$$= \sum_{i=k}^{\infty} z^i \sum_{j=0}^{k} c_{i+j-k} b_j = O(z^k). \qquad \square$$

v_k is called the generating polynomial of the approximant. Following a procedure similar to that used in the scalar case, left and right Padé-type approximants with arbitrary degrees in the numerator and in the denominator can be constructed from the preceding ones. They can be proved to satisfy algebraic properties similar to those of the scalar case. An expression for the error can also be obtained

THEOREM 26.2.

$$f(z) - {}^L(k-1/k)_f(z) = z^k {}^L c(v_k(x)(1-xz)^{-1})(\tilde{v}_k(z))^{-1},$$
$$f(z) - {}^R(k-1/k)_f(z) = z^k (\tilde{v}_k(z))^{-1} {}^R c(v_k(x)(1-xz)^{-1}).$$

PROOF. Similarly, let us give only the proof for the left approximants. We have

$$^L\tilde{w}_{k-1}(z) = z^k {}^L c((v_k(z^{-1}) - v_k(x))(1-xz)^{-1})$$
$$= z^k {}^L c(I(1-xz)^{-1})v_k(z^{-1}) - z^k {}^L c(v_k(x)(1-xz)^{-1})$$
$$= f(z)\tilde{v}_k(z) - z^k {}^L c(v_k(x)(1-xz)^{-1}). \qquad \square$$

Thus we shall now try to improve the order of approximation and we shall choose v_k such that

$$^L c(x^i v_k(x)) = 0, \quad i = 0, \ldots, k-1.$$

Such a family of polynomials is called orthogonal with respect to ${}^L c$ and the corresponding Padé-type approximant (called a Padé approximant) will be denoted by ${}^L[k - 1/k]$. Similarly we can construct right Padé approximants and we have

THEOREM 26.3.

$$f(z) - {}^L[k-1/k]_f(z) = O(z^{2k}),$$
$$f(z) - {}^R[k-1/k]_f(z) = O(z^{2k}).$$

Moreover

$$^L[k-1/k] \equiv {}^R[k-1/k].$$

PROOF. The first result immediately follows from Theorem 26.2 and the orthogonality conditions on the polynomial v_k.

Subtracting the second relation from the first one gives

$$^L[k-1/k]_f(z) = {}^R[k-1/k]_f(z) + \mathrm{O}(z^{2k}).$$

Multiplying on the left by $^R\tilde{v}_k$ and on the right by $^L\tilde{v}_k$ gives

$$^R\tilde{v}_k(z)\,^L\tilde{w}_{k-1}(z) - {}^R\tilde{w}_{k-1}(z)\,^L\tilde{v}_k(z) = \mathrm{O}(z^{2k}).$$

This is identically zero since there are no terms of degree $2k$ in the left-hand side and thus

$$^R\tilde{v}_k(z)\,^L\tilde{w}_{k-1}(z) = {}^R\tilde{w}_{k-1}(z)\,^L\tilde{v}_k(z),$$

that is

$$^L\tilde{w}_{k-1}(z)(^L\tilde{v}_k(z))^{-1} = (^R\tilde{v}_k(z))^{-1}(^R\tilde{w}_{k-1}(z)). \qquad \square$$

These Padé approximants, which are thus uniquely defined, satisfy the same algebraic properties as the scalar Padé approximants. The block structure of the Padé table (which is no longer made up of square blocks) has been studied and recursive algorithms for the computation of any sequence of Padé approximants have been obtained via the connection with orthogonal polynomials. A cross rule, similar to that of Wynn, also holds and an ε-algorithm as well. We refer the interested reader to DRAUX [1984].

27. Multivariate approximants

Many attempts have been made to define Padé-type approximants and Padé approximants in several variables. The case of two variables is only considered here, the generalization to more variables being straightforward. With no hope of being complete, we will summarize the main ideas of these definitions.

One possibility is to generalize the determinantal expression, in the aim of generalizing the fundamental identity of Padé approximants

$$\text{degree}(P) = m, \quad \text{degree}(Q) = n,$$
$$Q(z) \cdot f(z) - P(z) = \mathrm{O}(z^p),$$

$p = m+1$ for Padé-type approximants, and $p = m+n+1$ for Padé approximants.

The first problem is to find a link with a generating function and the interpolation point of view

$$f(z) = c(1/(1 - xz)),$$
$$P/Q(z) = c(\Pi)(z), \quad \Pi \text{ interpolation polynomial of } (1-xz)^{-1}.$$

The second step would be to go from Padé-type approximants to Padé approximants by a suitable choice of the denominator Q, i.e. by defining orthogonal polynomials. In the case of two variables, it has not yet been possible to connect all these points of view.

LEVIN [1976] gave a definition of general-order Padé-type approximants in terms of a ratio for two determinants. The numerators and denominators are similar in form to those of the scalar Padé table and satisfy an approximation property of the same type. Let

$$f(x,y) = \sum_{i,j \geq 0} c_{ij} x^i y^j,$$
$$c_{ij} = 0, \quad \text{if } i < 0 \text{ or } j < 0.$$

Let Ω (resp. Ω^+) denote the set of all pairs of (resp. positive) integers. If M is a subset of Ω, then

$$M^+ = M \cap \Omega^+,$$
$$M_{ij} = \{(k,m), (k+i, m+j) \in M\}, \quad \text{the } (i,j) \text{ translation of } M.$$

M is also called the rank of the polynomial

$$P(x,y) = \sum_{i,j \in M} p_{ij} x^i y^j.$$

We choose three sets of indices A, S and M:
S has s elements (s finite) in Ω^+,
$A \subset M$ and $R = M - A$ has $(s-1)$ elements in Ω^+.
By this choice, the number of conditions imposed on $[A/S]$ is equal to the number of free coefficients in it.
Let $(i_1, j_1), (i_2, j_2), \ldots, (i_s, j_s)$ be the elements of S, and $(m_2, k_2), (m_3, k_3), \cdots, (m_s, k_s)$ the elements of R^+.
The approximant $[A/S]_M$ is formally defined by $P_{ASM}(x,y)/Q_{ASM}(x,y)$

$$P_{A,S,M}(x,y) = \begin{vmatrix} x^{i_1} y^{j_1} A_{i_1 j_1}(x,y) & x^{i_2} y^{j_2} A_{i_2 j_2}(x,y) & \cdots & x^{i_s} y^{j_s} A_{i_s j_s}(x,y) \\ c_{m_2-i_1, k_2-j_1} & c_{m_2-i_2, k_2-j_2} & \cdots & c_{m_2-i_s, k_2-j_s} \\ c_{m_3-i_1, k_3-j_1} & c_{m_3-i_2, k_3-j_2} & \cdots & c_{m_3-i_s, k_3-j_s} \\ \vdots & \vdots & & \vdots \\ c_{m_s-i_1, k_s-j_1} & c_{m_s-i_2, k_s-j_2} & \cdots & c_{m_s-i_s, k_s-j_s} \end{vmatrix}$$

where $A_{ij}(x,y)$ is the partial sum of rank A_{ij} of the series representing f

$$A_{ij}(x,y) = \sum_{(m,k) \in A_{ij}^+} c_{mk} x^m y^k.$$

A_{ij} is the (i, j) translation of A, and

$$Q_{A,S,M}(x,y) = \begin{vmatrix} x^{i_1}y^{j_1} & x^{i_2}y^{j_2} & \cdots & x^{i_s}y^{j_s} \\ c_{m_2-i_1,k_2-j_1} & c_{m_2-i_2,k_2-j_2} & \cdots & c_{m_2-i_s,k_2-j_s} \\ c_{m_3-i_1,k_3-j_1} & c_{m_3-i_2,k_3-j_2} & \cdots & c_{m_3-i_s,k_3-j_s} \\ \vdots & \vdots & & \vdots \\ c_{m_s-i_1,k_s-j_1} & c_{m_s-i_2,k_s-j_2} & \cdots & c_{m_s-i_s,k_s-j_s} \end{vmatrix}.$$

Choices of A, S and M must be made to avoid P_{ASM} or Q_{ASM} being identically zero. These cases must be examined separately.

The main result is the following

$$\begin{cases} f(x,y) \cdot Q_{ASM}(x,y) - P_{ASM}(x,y) = \sum_{i,j \in \bar{M}^+} d_{mk} x^m y^k, \\ f(x,y) - [A/S]_M(x,y) = O(x^i y^j) \quad (i,j) \in \bar{M}^+. \end{cases}$$

If

$A = \{(i,j),\ i,j \leq 1\} = \{(0,0),(1,0),(0,1),(1,1)\}$,
$S = \{(i,j),\ i+j \leq 1\} = \{(0,0),(1,0),(0,1)\}$,
$M = \{(i,j),\ i+j \leq 2\} = \{(0,0),(1,0),(0,1),(2,0),(1,1),(0,2)\}$,
$R = M - A = \{(2,0),(0,2)\}$,
$f(x,y) - [A/S]_M = O(x^i y^{3-i}),\quad i \geq 0$.

If $A = \{(i,j),\ i,j \leq m\}$, $S = \{(i,j),\ i,j \leq n\}$, $M = \{(i,j),\ i+j \leq m+n\} \cup \{(i,j),\ i,j \leq \max(m,n)\}$, it is possible to recover the Chisholm approximants (CHISHOLM [1973]) but supplementary conditions must be added. In the case $m = n$, these conditions are

$$d_{i,2m-i} + d_{2m-i,i} = 0, \quad i = 0, \ldots, m,$$

and they imply the symmetry property

$$[A/A]_M(x,y) = [A/A]_M(y,x).$$

Other types of conditions can be added to the definition as a ratio of determinants, to define uniquely the approximants, but obviously these are extra conditions, not linked to the optimal character of the accuracy principle which is the basic idea of Padé approximation.

In the same way, CUYT [1986] describes approximants determined by the accuracy-through-order principle. The sets A, S and M satisfy the following assumptions
  (a) $A \subset M$,
  (b) $M - A$ has $s - 1$ elements and S has s elements (s finite),
  (c) M satisfies the inclusion property meaning that, when a point belongs to the index set M, then the rectangular subset of points emanating from the origin, with the given point as its furthermost corner, also lies in M.

Then the approximants exist.

What is gained is the existence of a recursive algorithm, similar to the ε-algorithm, but a special case of the more general E-algorithm. So the univariate equivalence of the techniques for Padé approximants is also established for the multivariate case: algebraic relations and recurrence relations.

Starting from the generating function, with a generating polynomial for the approximant, leads to completely different approximants

$$f(t) = c(1/(1-xt)),$$
$$P(t) = \frac{1}{1-tx}\left(1 - \frac{V(x)}{V(t^{-1})}\right), \text{ interpolation polynomial at the zeros of } V,$$
$$(k-1/k)_f(t) = c(P) = \frac{\tilde{W}(t)}{\tilde{V}(t)}.$$

An error formula is then automatically obtained

$$f(t) - (k-1/k)_f(t) = \frac{t^k}{\tilde{V}(t)} c\left(\frac{V(x)}{1-xt}\right).$$

Different generalizations exist, starting from this point of view. They differ mainly in the generating function they use, or in the functional c.

BREZINSKI [1980, 1986] defined Padé-type approximants from the standpoint of the rectangular form

$$f(t,s) = \sum_{i=0}^{\infty} \sum_{j=0}^{\infty} c_{ij} t^i s^j,$$
$$= c((1-xt)^{-1} \cdot (1-ys)^{-1}),$$

c being the linear functional, acting on x and y, defined by $c(x^i y^j) = c_{ij}$. Let V be an arbitrary polynomial, the concerned powers lying in a rectangle,

$$V(x,y) = \sum_{i=0}^{k_1} \sum_{j=0}^{k_2} b_{ij} x^i y^j,$$

and let W be

$$W(t,s) = c\left(\frac{V(x,y) + V(t,s) - V(t,y) - V(x,s)}{(x-t)(y-s)}\right).$$

We set

$$\tilde{V}(t,s) = t^{k_1} s^{k_2} V(t^{-1}, s^{-1}),$$
$$\tilde{W}(t,s) = t^{k_1-1} s^{k_2-1} W(t^{-1}, s^{-1}).$$

Then the series $\tilde{W}(t,s) - \tilde{V}(t,s).f(t,s)$ has no terms in $t^i s^j$ for $i = 0, \ldots, k_1 - 1$ and $j = 0, \ldots, k_2 - 1$.

$\tilde{W}(t,s)/\tilde{V}(t,s)$ is the ratio of a polynomial of degree $(k_1 - 1, k_2 - 1)$ to a polynomial of degree (k_1, k_2) in (t, s). This fundamental result can be written in the form

$$(k_1 - 1, k_2 - 1/k_1, k_2)(t, s) = \tilde{W}(t,s)/\tilde{V}(t,s),$$
$$(k_1 - 1, k_2 - 1/k_1, k_2)(t, s) = f(t, s) + O(t^i s^{k_2}) + O(t^{k_1} s^i), \quad i \geqslant 0.$$

Padé-type approximants for all degrees in both variables can be defined with the same ideas as in the one dimensional case. We get

$$(p_1, p_2/q_1, q_2)(t, s) - f(t, s) = O(t^i s^{p_2}) + O(t^{p_1} s^i), \quad i \geqslant 0.$$

The form of the generating function $(1 - xt)^{-1} \cdot (1 - ys)^{-1}$ invites us to consider generating polynomials of the form $V(x, y) = u(x) \cdot v(y)$. Then Padé-type approximants are related to polynomial interpolation

THEOREM 27.1. *Let u and v be arbitrary polynomials of respective degrees k_1 and k_2. The Padé-type approximant $(k_1 - 1, k_2 - 1/k_1, k_2)$ whose generating polynomial is $V(x, y) = u(x) \cdot v(y)$ is such that*

$$(k_1 - 1, k_2 - 1/k_1, k_2) = c(P(x, y)),$$

where P is the Hermite interpolation polynomial of $(1 - xs)^{-1}(1 - ys)^{-1}$ at the nodes (x_i, y_j) where the x_i's are the zeros of u, and the y_j's the zeros of v.

PROOF. Let us set $g(x) = (1 - xt)^{-1}$ and $h(y) = (1 - ys)^{-1}$ and let P_1 and P_2 be the Hermite interpolation polynomials of g and h at the zeros of u and v respectively. Then P, the interpolation polynomial of $g(x)h(y)$ is given by

$$P(x, y) = P_1(x) P_2(y).$$

But, from Theorem 2.3 it follows that

$$\frac{\partial^{n+m}}{\partial x^n \partial y^m} P(x_i, y_j) = \frac{\partial^{n+m}}{\partial x^n \partial y^m} [(1 - x_i t)^{-1} (1 - y_j s)^{-1}]$$

for $i = 1, \ldots, p$, $j = 1, \ldots, q$, $n = 0, \ldots, n_i - 1$ and $m = 0, \ldots, m_j - 1$ if

$$u(x) = (x - x_1)^{n_1} \cdots (x - x_p)^{n_p}, \quad n_1 + \cdots + n_p = k_1$$
$$v(y) = (y - y_1)^{m_1} \cdots (y - y_q)^{m_q}, \quad m_1 + \cdots + m_q = k_2.$$

Thus P is the Hermite interpolation polynomial of $g(x)h(y)$ at the nodes (x_i, y_i) for $i = 1, \ldots, p$ and $j = 1, \ldots, q$. □

Unfortunately it can be shown (BREZINSKI [1986]) that all the terms $t^i s^{p_2}$, $i = 0, \ldots, p_1 - 1$, $t^{p_1} s^j$, $j = 0, \ldots, p_2 - 1$, and $t^{p_1} s^{p_2}$, cannot be automatically cancelled by a suitable choice of the generating polynomial, if it has the form $u(x).v(y)$. And so there is no canonical continuation to Padé approximants by this method.

Similar ideas were followed by ARIOKA [1987], but with a triangular form

$$f(t,s) = \sum_{p=0}^{\infty} \sum_{q=0}^{p} c_{pq} t^{p-q} s^q,$$
$$= c((1 - (xt + ys))^{-1}).$$

So the linear functional c, operating on the polynomials in two variables, is defined by

$$c(x^{p-q} y^q) = c_{pq} / \binom{p}{q}, \quad q = 0, \ldots, p, \ p \geq 0.$$

Consider an arbitrary polynomial $V(x,y)$ of (total) degree k, and define $W(t,s)$,

$$V(x,y) = \sum_{i=0}^{k} \sum_{j=0}^{i} b_{ij} t^{i-j} s^j \quad (b_{k,0} \neq 0),$$
$$W(t,s) = c\left(\frac{V(t,s) - V(x+ys,s)}{t - (x+ys)}\right).$$

Then $W(t,s)$, where the roles of t and s can be exchanged, is a polynomial of degree $k - 1$. The Padé-type approximant is defined by

$$\tilde{V}(t,s) = t^k V(t^{-1}, t^{-1}s),$$
$$\tilde{W}(t,s) = t^{k-1} W(t^{-1}, t^{-1}s),$$
$$(k - 1/k)(t,s) = \tilde{W}(t,s) / \tilde{V}(t,s),$$

and the result for accuracy-through-order follows

$$((k - 1/k) - f)(t,s) = O\left(\left(\sqrt{t^2 + s^2}\right)^k\right) \quad \text{as } (t,s) \to (0,0).$$

Such Padé-type approximants can be defined for all degrees (l,m); similarly we get

$$(l/m)(t,s) - f(t,s) = O\left(\left(\sqrt{t^2 + s^2}\right)^{l+1}\right).$$

As for the Padé-type approximants defined by Brezinski, fundamental algebraic properties are proved.

The connection with interpolation is obtained through the Kergin interpolation polynomial

$$h(u) = \frac{1}{1-u}, \quad u \in \mathbb{R},$$

$$\frac{1}{1-(tx+sy)} = \frac{1}{1-T \cdot X}.$$

$T = (t,s)$, $X = (x,y)$ and $T \cdot X$ is the scalar product in $\mathbb{R}^2$.

Then, $X_1, \ldots, X_k$ being given, the Kergin interpolation polynomial of $g(x) = 1/(1-TX)$ is defined through the divided difference of the real function $1/(1-u)$ at the points $u_i = TX_i$, $i = 1, \ldots, k$

$$P(X,T) = \frac{1}{1-TX_1} + \frac{T(X-X_1)}{(1-TX_1)(1-TX_2)} + \cdots$$
$$+ \frac{T(X-X_1)\cdots T(X-X_{k-1})}{(1-TX_1)\cdots(1-TX_k)}$$

with

$$\begin{cases} \tilde{V}(T) = \prod_i (1 - X_i T), \\ c(P(X,T)) = \dfrac{\tilde{W}(T)}{\tilde{V}(T)} = (k - 1/k)_f. \end{cases}$$

Very similar to these approximants, are those of SABLONNIÈRE [1983] starting from the Hakopian interpolation polynomial at $\binom{r+1}{k}$ points x_i for $g(X,T) = (1 - X \cdot T)^{-k}$. The functional, denoted here by $\bar{c}$, and the generating function are different from the Arioka case. He defines the Padé-type approximant of f as

$$f(T) = \bar{c}(g(X,T)),$$
$$(r - k + 1/r + 1)_f(T) = \bar{c}(P(X,T)).$$

The denominator is the same

$$\tilde{V}(T) = \prod_{i=1}^{k} (1 - X_i T).$$

$$g(x,T) = \frac{1}{(1-XT)^k} = \sum_{p=0}^{\infty} \sum_{|i|=p} \binom{p}{i} x^i g_i(t),$$

where $i = (i_1, i_2)$, $|i| = i_1 + i_2$, and

$$\binom{p}{i} = \frac{p!}{i_1! i_2!}.$$

Recently KIDA [1990a,b] defined Padé-type and Padé approximants following the same way, i.e. generating functions and polynomial interpolation. The idea is to define

$$f(T) = c\left(\frac{1}{1-X}\right),$$
$$= \sum_{i \geq 0} c_i, \quad c(X^i) = c_i$$

where the c_i are homogeneous polynomials in $T = (t_1, t_2)$, of degree i, and so c is a functional with values in the set of homogeneous polynomials in T: $\mathbb{C}[t_1, t_2]$. Let V be a homogeneous polynomial of degree $m+q$ in t_1, t_2, X,

$$V(X) = b_m X^q + b_{m+1} X^{q-1} + \cdots + b_{m+q-1} X + b_{m+q}, \quad b_m \neq 0,$$

where the b_{m+i}'s are homogeneous polynomials of degree $m+i$ in $t_1 t_2$. Such polynomials are called g-polynomials. For such a V, let W^n be

$$W^n(T) = c\left(\frac{V(1) - X^n V(X)}{1-X}\right).$$

Notice that $V(1) = b_m + \cdots + b_{m+q}$ is a polynomial in T. $W^n(T)$ is a polynomial in $T = (t_1, t_2)$, of degree $m+q+n-1$. Its order (smallest power of T) is m. Let, as usual, the functional $c^{(n)}$ be defined by

$$c^{(n)}(X^i) = c_{n+i},$$

where c takes its values not in $\mathbb{C}$, but in the space of homogeneous polynomials in T. Then

$$f(t) \cdot V(T) - W^n(T) = c^{(n)}\left(\frac{V(X)}{1-X}\right) = O(T^{m+q+n}).$$

For any p and q, the Padé-type approximant of f is then defined

$$W(T) = W^{p-q+1}(T),$$
$$\text{degree}(W(T)) = m+p, \quad \text{degree}(V(1)) = m+q,$$
$$(p/q)_f^m(T) = \frac{W(T)}{V(1)}.$$

The g-polynomial $V(X)$ is the generating polynomial of the approximant and we have

$$f(T)V(1) - W(T) = O(T^{m+p+1}).$$

The algebraic properties can be proved as for the univariate case. More interesting is the fact that the choice of $V(X)$ can be made to improve the accuracy.

If $V(X) = b_m X^q + \cdots + b_{m+q}$, $b_m \neq 0$, then

$$f(T) \cdot V(1) - W(T) = O(T^{m+p+r+1}),$$

if and only if

$$c^{(p-q+1)}(X^i V(X)) = 0, \quad i = 0, \ldots, r-1.$$

Let $V_q(X)$

$$V_q(X) = \begin{vmatrix} c_{p-q+1} & \cdots & c_{p+1} \\ \vdots & & \vdots \\ c_p & \cdots & c_{p+q} \\ 1 & \cdots & X^q \end{vmatrix}.$$

Then V_q satisfies the *orthogonality relations* for $r = q$, and it is a g-polynomial of degree $pq+q$ and of order pq. So the Padé-type approximant, with generating polynomial $V_q(X)$, is called a Padé approximant and satisfies

$$f(T) \cdot V_q(1) - W_p(T) = [p/q]_f^{pq}(T)$$

$$= c^{(p-q+1)}\left(\frac{X^q V_q(X)}{1-X}\right)$$

$$= O(T^{pq+p+q+1})$$

$$= \frac{\begin{vmatrix} c_{p-q+1} & \cdots & c_{p+1} \\ \vdots & & \vdots \\ c_p & \cdots & c_{p+q} \\ \sum_0^{p-q} c_i & \cdots & \sum_0^p c_i \end{vmatrix}}{\begin{vmatrix} c_{p-q+1} & \cdots & c_{p+1} \\ \vdots & & \vdots \\ c_p & \cdots & c_{p+q} \\ 1 & \cdots & 1 \end{vmatrix}}.$$

Because the c_i's are homogeneous polynomials in (t_1, t_2), such approximants have been called homogeneous Padé approximants. We have

$$\sum_{m=0}^{\infty} \sum_{i+j=m} \bar{c}_{ij} t_1^i t_2^j \quad \text{(Cuyt's notations)},$$

$$= \sum_{m=0}^{\infty} c_m \quad \text{(Kida's notations)}.$$

And in that case it is well known that a theory of orthogonal polynomials very similar to the univariate case can be developed (CHAFFY [1984], CUYT [1982]).

Kida's view of the problem brings a logical framework, very useful to derive recurrence relations, and to develop all the tools of the univariate case.

Completely different is the point of view of CHAFFY [1988a]. The very simple basic idea is to take successively the Padé approximant $R(x,y)$ of $f(x,y)$ with respect to x, and then the Padé approximant of $R(x,y)$ with respect to y. From a practical point of view, this is only possible with formal computation of the successive approximants. If $R(x,y)$, of degree (m,n), is denoted Padé(f,x,m,n), then the *(Padé) ○ (Padé) approximants* are

$$\text{Padé}(\text{Padé}(f,x,m,n),y,p,q) = [p/q]_y \circ [m/n]_x(f).$$

The variable is put as an index to remind us that the approximant is taken with respect to this variable. They are obviously rational functions with respect to x and y. If f is a rational function, then it is exactly recovered. If f is the product $h(x) \cdot g(y)$ then

$$[p/q]_y \circ [m/n]_x(f) = [p/q]_y(g) \cdot [m/n]_x(h).$$

Such an approximant is constructed from the rectangular point of view. There is no problem in generalizing to more variables, especially from the computational point of view.

Finally there exist only two different kinds of multivariable Padé approximants (those of Cuyt and Chaffy already quoted); except in the particular case of homogeneous approximants, none of them leads to *orthogonal polynomials*.

CUYT [1990] and CHAFFY [1988b] proved in each case a Montessus De Ballore Theorem for meromorphic functions of the type $g(x,y)/Q(x,y)$, where g is holomorphic in a polydisc, and Q is a polynomial in x and y. Let us first consider the (Padé) ○ (Padé) approximants of CHAFFY [1988a],

$$f(x,y) = \frac{g(x,y)}{Q(x,y)},$$

where Q is a polynomial in x and y, of degree n in x, irreducible in $\mathbb{C}[X,Y]$:

$$\begin{cases} Q(x,y) = q_0(y) + q_1(y)x + \cdots + q_{n-1}(y)x^{n-1} + x^n, \\ \text{degree}(q_k) \leqslant p, \\ Q(0,0) \neq 0, \quad \text{i.e. } q_0(0) \neq 0. \end{cases}$$

For the sake of simplicity, it is assumed that the n zeros of $Q(x,0)$ are simple. Let β be defined by $\beta = \{\inf_i |y_i|, q_0(y_i) = 0\}$. The polynomial in x, $Q(x,y)$ has no multiple zeros except for a finite number of values of y, $(r \leqslant |y| \leqslant \beta)$. So, if $|y| < R$, $Q(x,y) = 0$ defines n holomorphic functions

$$\begin{cases} x_i = \alpha_i(y), \quad i = 1,\ldots,n, \\ Q(x_i,y) = 0. \end{cases}$$

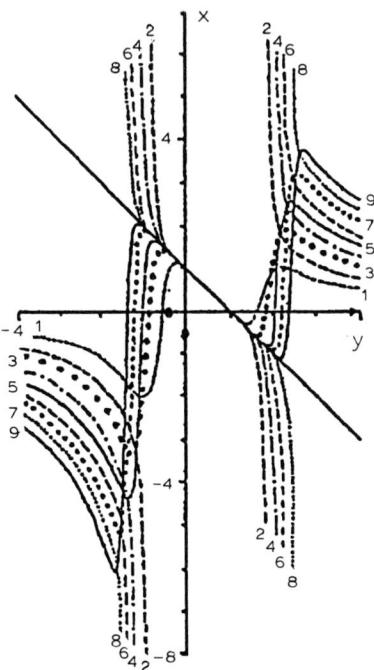

FIG. 27.1. Poles of $[l/1]_x$.

The holomorphic function g can be assumed to be holomorphic and non zero in $\mathbb{C} \times \{|y| < R\}$. Finally, for $|y| < R_2 < R$, the function $x \to f(x, y)$ has exactly n poles $\alpha_i(y)$, $i = 1, \ldots, n$ which lie in $\{|x| < R_1\}$, with

$$R_1 = \sup_i(|\alpha_i(y)|, |y| < R_2).$$

So, from the Montessus theorem in one variable, the column $(m/n)_x$ is to be used, as intermediate approximants, as shown by the following example where $f(x, y) = e^{x \cdot y}/(1 - x - y)$.

An intermediate result follows.

If Q_{mn} is the denominator of the fraction, in x, $[m/n]_x(f)$, the sequence $(Q_{mn})_m$ converges uniformly on compact subsets of $D_{R_1} \times D_{R_2} - \{Q(x, y) = 0\}$ to f when m tends to infinity.

For x_0 in the disc $D(0, R_1)$, $Q(x_0, y)$ has q simple zeros $y_1, \ldots, y_q$. And, finally, there exists r and (r_k), $k = 1, \ldots, q$ such that

$$\mathcal{K} = D_r \times D_{R_2} - \{\bigcup_{k=1,\ldots,q} D(y_k, r_k)\},$$

$$\lim_{m \to \infty} (\lim_{p \to \infty} [p/q]_y \circ [m/n]_x(f)) = f,$$

locally uniformly on $\mathcal{H}$.

Let us now quote A. Cuyt's *Montessus-type* theorem (CUYT [1990]); here $M \times N$ denotes the set $\{(i+k, j+l), (i,j) \in M, (k,l) \in N\}$:

THEOREM 27.2. *Let $f(x,y)$ be a function which is meromorphic in the polydisc $B(0; R_1, R_2) = \{(x,y): |x| < R_1, |y| < R_2\}$, meaning that there exists a polynomial*

$$R_M(x,y) = \sum_{(d,e) \in M \subseteq N^2} r_{de} x^d y^e = \sum_{i=0}^{m} r_{d_i e_i} x^{d_i} y^{e_i},$$

such that $(fR_M)(x,y)$ is analytic in the polydisc above. Furthermore, let there be no zero of R_M, in other words let $(0,0) \in M$. Let the coefficients $r_{d_i e_i}$ ($i = 1, \ldots, m$) be completely determined up to a constant factor by m zeros $(x_h, y_h) \in B(0; R_1, R_2)$ of $(R_M(x,y)$ with

$$(fR_M)(x_h, y_h) \neq 0, \quad h = 1, \ldots, m,$$

$$\begin{vmatrix} x_1^{d_1} y_1^{e_1} & \cdots & x_1^{d_m} y_1^{e_m} \\ \vdots & & \vdots \\ x_m^{d_1} y_m^{e_1} & \cdots & x_m^{d_m} y_m^{e_m} \end{vmatrix} \neq 0.$$

Then the $[N/M]_E = (p/q)(x,y)$ Padé approximant with M fixed as given above and N and E growing, converges to $f(x,y)$ uniformly on compact subsets of

$$\{(x,y): |x| < R_1, |y| < R_2, R_M(x,y) \neq 0\},$$

and its denominator

$$q(x,y) = \sum_{i=0}^{m} b_{d_i e_i} x^{d_i} y^{e_i}$$

converges to $R_M(x,y)$ under the following conditions for N and E: the range of the largest inscribed triangle in E and the range of the smallest triangle circumscribing $N \times M$ should both tend to infinity as the sets N and E grow along a column in the multivariate Padé table.

CHAPTER IV

Applications

28. The exponential function

The exponential function is sufficiently interesting in itself and has sufficiently many applications (see Section 29, for example) to have a section devoted to the study of its Padé approximants.
 They are given in closed form, as obtained by Padé in his thesis in 1892, see PADÉ [1984]. We have, for $f(z) = e^z$,

$$[p/q]_f(z) = N_{p,q}(z)/D_{p,q}(z)$$

with

$$N_{p,q}(z) = \sum_{i=0}^{p} \frac{(p+q-i)!p!}{(p+q)!i!(p-i)!} z^i,$$

$$D_{p,q}(z) = \sum_{i=0}^{q} \frac{(p+q-i)!q!}{(p+q)!i!(q-i)!} (-z)^i.$$

The Padé table of e^z is normal and, since $e^z = 1/e^{-z}$, $D_{p,q}(z) = N_{q,p}(-z)$. The location of the zeros and poles was studied, in a series of papers, by SAFF and VARGA [1975, 1976b,c, 1977, 1978]. Due to the above-mentioned property relating the numerators and the denominators of the approximants of e^z and e^{-z}, it is sufficient to study the location of the zeros of the Padé approximants to e^z as done by VARGA [1982]. We have the following results which are obtained as consequences of Theorem 12.4.

THEOREM 28.1. $\forall q$, the numerators of $[p/q]_e$ for $p = 1, 2, \ldots$ have no zeros in

$$P_{q+1} = \{z = x + iy \in \mathbb{C}, \ y^2 \leq 4(q+1)(x+q+1), \ x > -(q+1)\}.$$

PROOF. For the exponential function, it is known that, for $k \geq 1$,

$$H_k^{(n)} = \left[\prod_{i=1}^{k} i(i+1) \cdots (i+n+k-2) \right]^{-1}.$$

Thus the result follows directly from Theorem 12.4. □

We saw, in Section 12, that the question arises to know how sharp such a result is. This can be obtained by considering the normalized numerators $N_{p,q}((q+1)z)$ and we have

THEOREM 28.2. $\forall p, q$, the normalized Padé numerator $N_{p,q}((q+1)z)$ for e^z has no zeros in $P_1 = \{z = x + iy \in \mathbb{C}, \ y^2 \leqslant 4(x+1), \ x > -1\}$. Moreover each point on the boundary of P_1 is a limit point of the zeros of $\{N_{p,q}((q+1)z)\}_{p,q}$.

We shall not give the proof of this result since it is very technical and involves asymptotics for Whittaker's differential equation.

For other results of this type we refer the interested reader to the literature mentioned above where figures showing the remarkable behaviour of the zeros and poles of the Padé approximants to e^z can be found.

Let us define the remainders by

$$R_{p,q}(z) = D_{p,q}(z)e^z - N_{p,q}(z).$$

We set

$$R_{p,q}(z) = (-1)^q \frac{z^{p+q+1}}{(p+q+1)!} \varphi_{p,q}(z).$$

When z is real, the function $\varphi_{p,q}$ was studied by VAN ROSSUM [1987] who proved, using previous results by GAUTSCHI [1982] and BREZINSKI [1983b] on the successive remainders of the exponential series, the following

THEOREM 28.3. $\forall z > 0, \forall q$ fixed, the sequence $(\varphi_{p,q}(z))_p$ is totally monotonic. $\forall z < 0, \forall q$ fixed, the sequence $(\varphi_{q,p}(z))_p$ is totally monotonic.

We recall that a sequence (u_n) is said to be totally monotonic if $\forall k, n$, $(-1)^k \Delta^k u_n \geqslant 0$ or, in other words, if there exists α bounded and non-decreasing such that $u_n = \int_0^1 x^n \, d\alpha(x)$.

We have, for all $z \in \mathbb{C}$

$$e^z - [m/n]_e(z) = (-1)^n \frac{m!n!}{(m+n)!(m+n+1)!} z^{m+n+1} e^{\alpha z} (1 + o(1))$$

where $\alpha = 2n/(n+m)$, when $n + m$ tends to infinity.

If we restrict ourselves to the interval $[-1, +1]$, then it was proved by BRAESS [1986] that the preceding error term is divided by 2^{m+n}.

Let us now come to the convergence of the Padé approximants to e^z. Of course, the exponential function is a Pólya frequency series corresponding to $a_0 = \gamma = 1$ and $\alpha_j = \beta_j = 0$ for all j (see Section 16). Thus, Theorem 16.1 applies and we have

THEOREM 28.4. Let $([m_k/n_k]_e(z) = P_k(z)/Q_k(z))$ be a sequence of Padé approximants to e^z such that

$$\lim_{k \to \infty} m_k/n_k = w > 0.$$

Then

$$\lim_{k \to \infty} P_k(z) = \exp(wz/(w+1)),$$
$$\lim_{k \to \infty} Q_k(z) = \exp(-z/(w+1))$$

uniformly on every compact subset of the complex plane.

When z is on the negative real axis, the following results were proved by SAFF, VARGA and NI [1976]

THEOREM 28.5. *Let* $([m_k/n_k])$ *be a sequence of Padé approximants to* e^z *such that* $\exists \omega \in [0,1]$

$$\lim_{k \to \infty} m_k/n_k = \omega.$$

Then

$$\lim_{k \to \infty} \sup_{-\infty \leqslant x \leqslant 0} |e^x - [m_k/n_k]_e(x)|^{1/n_k} = \omega^\omega \left(\frac{1-\omega}{2}\right)^{1-\omega} = g(\omega).$$

The minimum of g is achieved for $\omega = 1/3$ and $g(1/3) = 1/3$. Thus the best rate of convergence is obtained for the ray sequence $([m/3m])$ for which we have

$$\sup_{-\infty \leqslant x \leqslant 0} |e^x - [m/3m]_e(x)| \sim (1/3)^{3m}.$$

Let us also recall the original convergence result given by PADÉ [1894], see Theorem 12.1.

29. A-acceptable approximations to the exponential function

Let us consider the differential equation

$$y'(x) = -\lambda y(x)$$

where λ is a complex number whose real part is strictly positive. Thus the solution will satisfy

$$\lim_{x \to \infty} y(x) = 0.$$

This differential equation (with the initial condition $y(0) = y_0$) is integrated by a numerical method which computes approximations y_n of the exact solution $y(nh)$, where h is the step size. This numerical method will be said to be *A-stable* if $\forall h\lambda$ such that $\text{Re}(h\lambda) > 0$, $\lim_{n \to \infty} y_n = 0$, which means that both the exact and the approximate solutions tend to zero at infinity.

Of course, since the exact solution is $y(x) = y_0 e^{-\lambda x}$, we have

$$y(x_{n+1}) = e^{-h\lambda} y(x_n)$$

with $x_n = nh$. When using either a one-step or a multistep method, it can be proved that the approximate solution satisfies

$$y_{n+1} = r(h\lambda) y_n$$

where r is a rational function. Thus, if the numerical method has order p, we have

$$r(z) = e^{-z} + O(z^{p+1}).$$

Moreover if the method is A-stable we must have $\forall z$ such that $\operatorname{Re}(z) > 0$

$$|r(z)| < 1$$

since $y_n = [r(h\lambda)]^n y_0$.

Such a rational approximation to the exponential function is called A-acceptable and, of course, Padé, Padé-type, and partial Padé approximants are candidates for such an r.

Using the maximum modulus principle it can be shown that r is A-acceptable if and only if $\forall t \in \mathbb{R}$, $|r(it)| \leqslant 1$, $\lim_{|z| \to \infty} |r(z)| \leqslant 1$ and r is analytic in the right-hand part of the complex plane (see ALT [1972]).

The A-acceptability of Padé approximants to the exponential function was studied by EHLE [1973] who proved

THEOREM 29.1. *The Padé approximants $[n/n]$, $[n-1/n]$ and $[n-2/n]$ of e^{-z} are A-acceptable for all n.*

Let us now turn to Padé-type approximants. We have

THEOREM 29.2. *Let r be a Padé-type approximant of e^{-z} with real coefficients, whose numerator has degree k and whose denominator has degree $n+k$ ($n \geqslant 0$). Let*

$$|r(it)|^2 = \frac{1 + \beta_1 t^2 + \cdots + \beta_k t^{2k}}{1 + \alpha_1 t^2 + \cdots + \alpha_{n+k} t^{2(n+k)}}.$$

If the zeros of the denominator of r have negative real parts, if $\beta_i \leqslant \alpha_i$ for $i = [k/2] + 1, \ldots, k$ and if $0 \leqslant \alpha_i$ for $i = k+1, \ldots, k+n$, then r is A-acceptable. ($[x]$ denotes the integer part of the real number x.)

PROOF. r is analytic in the right-hand part of the complex plane, since all the zeros of its denominator have negative real parts. Moreover, if $n \geqslant 1$,

$$\lim_{|t| \to \infty} |r(t)| = 0.$$

It remains to prove the first condition for A-acceptability. By definition of Padé-type approximants, we have

$$r(t) = e^{-t} + O(t^{k+1})$$

and thus

$$|r(it)|^2 = 1 + O(t^{k+1}).$$

This condition implies that $\alpha_i = \beta_i$ for $i = 1, \ldots, p = [k/2]$. Moreover, we have

$$|r(it)|^2 = 1 + \frac{(\beta_{p+1} - \alpha_{p+1})t^{2(p+1)} + \cdots + (\beta_{n+k} - \alpha_{n+k})t^{2(n+k)}}{1 + \alpha_1 t^2 + \cdots + \alpha_{n+k} t^{2(n+k)}}$$

with the convention that $\beta_i = 0$ for $i \geq k+1$. Thus, if $\beta_i \leq \alpha_i$ for $i = p+1, \ldots, n+k$ then $|r(it)|^2 \leq 1$.

If $n = 0$, then $\beta_k = a_0^2$ and $\alpha_k = b_0^2$, where a_0 and b_0 are the constant terms of the denominator and of the numerator respectively, which implies that $\lim_{|t| \to \infty} |r(t)| \leq 1$. □

The proof of this result is an adaptation of that of CROUZEIX and RUAMPS [1977] for rational approximants to the exponential function.

When solving a parabolic partial differential equation of the second order, one obtains after discretization of the space variable a differential system of the form

$$Cu'(t) = -Au(t) + v(t), \quad u(0) = u_0,$$

where C and A are real square matrices whose elements are independent of the time t. Using a one-step method for integrating this differential equation leads to

$$Q_k(Bh)u_{n+1} = P_m(Bh)u_n + T_n,$$

where $B = C^{-1}A$, where T_n is a matrix depending on k and m, where u_n is an approximation of the exact solution $u(t_n)$ at the point t_n, and where Q_k and P_m are matrix polynomials of the respective degrees k and m. As before, $[Q_k(Bh)]^{-1}P_m(Bh)$ must be an approximation of e^{-Bh} and the order of the method is determined by that of the approximation. This approximation must be A-acceptable if an A-stable one-step method is needed. The computation of u_{n+1} from u_n requires the computation of the inverse of the matrix $Q_k(Bh)$. This computation is greatly simplified if

$$Q_k(z) = (1 + \alpha_k z)^k.$$

Indeed, in that case, the computation of u_{n+1} reduces to the solution of k systems of linear equations with the same matrix

$$(I + \alpha_k Bh)v_{p+1} = v_p, \quad \text{for } p = 0, \ldots, k-1,$$

with $v_0 = P_m(Bh)u_n + T_n$ and we obtain

$$v_k = u_{n+1}.$$

Of course this simplification is not possible with Padé approximations to the exponential function but it becomes possible with Padé-type approximants. For convergence reasons, since $\lim_{k\to\infty}(1 + z/k)^k = e^z$ we shall make the choice $\alpha_k = 1/k$ which corresponds to the generating polynomials $v_k(x) = (x + 1/k)^k$. The following result can be proved

THEOREM 29.3. *The Padé-type approximants $(k-1/k)$ of e^{-z} constructed with the generating polynomials $v_k(x) = (x + 1/k)^k$ are A-acceptable for $k = 1, 2, 3$. The Padé-type approximants (k/k) constructed with the same generating polynomials are A-acceptable for $k = 1, \ldots, 4$. $(6/6)$ is not A-acceptable.*

The study of the convergence of these approximants is due to VAN ISEGHEM [1984] who proved the following results

THEOREM 29.4. *The sequences $((k-1/k))$ and $((k/k))$ of Padé-type approximants to $\exp(-z)$ constructed with the generating polynomials $v_k(x) = (x + 1/k)^k$ converge to $\exp(-z)$ uniformly on every compact subset of the complex plane. Moreover, $\forall K$, $\exists$ an integer k_0 (depending on K) such that the convergence of the two sequences of Padé-type approximants is geometric on K for $k = k_0+1, k_0+2, \ldots$.*

The approximants and the error as well can be expressed with the help of Laguerre's polynomials. We have

$$(k-1/k) = \sum_{i=0}^{k-1} z^i D^{k-i} R_k(0) / \sum_{i=0}^{k} z^i D^{k-i} R_k(1),$$

$$(k/k) = \sum_{i=0}^{k} z^i D^{k-i} R_k(0) / \sum_{i=0}^{k} z^i D^{k-i} R_k(1),$$

where $R_k(z) = k^{-k} L_k(k(1-z))$ and D^j designates the jth derivative.

Complementary results on the A-acceptability of Padé-type approximants with a single pole were given by GONZÁLEZ CONCEPCIÓN [1987].

See WANNER [1987] for a review on the A-acceptability of Padé approximants of the exponential function.

30. Borel transform

In many branches of applied mathematics one has often to deal with diverging perturbation series. In order to obtain a meaningful finite answer from such series two techniques have been used: Padé approximation and the Borel transform. However, each of these techniques presents some drawbacks. Padé approximants can either not converge at all or they can tend to a wrong limit. Borel transform provides, in principle, a correct answer even in most cases where Padé approximants fail, but its practical implementation is quite difficult since it is based on conformal mapping in the complex plane.

The drawbacks of both methods were avoided in the past by combining them in the so-called Borel–Padé method. Very good results were thus obtained in practice but the physicists were then faced with another problem: the proof of the convergence of the method. Quite recently MARZIANI [1987] took up the method and replaced the Padé approximants involved in the Borel–Padé method by Padé-type approximants. He thus obtained the Borel–Padé-type method and was able to prove its convergence for a suitable choice of the generating polynomials of the Padé-type approximants. We shall now present his method and begin by recalling a result about the Borel transform, namely the Watson–Nevanlinna theorem.

THEOREM 30.1. *Let $\alpha > 0$, $R > 0$ and $A > 0$ be given. We set*

$$D_{\alpha,R} = \{z \in \mathbb{C}, \ 0 < |z| < R, \ |\arg z| \leqslant \alpha + \pi/2\},$$
$$T_{\alpha,A} = \{z \in \mathbb{C}, \ |z| < 1/A\} \cup \{z \in \mathbb{C}, \ |\arg z| < \alpha\}.$$

Let f be analytic in $D_{\alpha,R}$, continuous on $\bar{D}_{\alpha,R}$ and have there the asymptotic expansion

$$f(z) = \sum_{n=0}^{\infty} c_n z^n \quad (z \to 0).$$

We assume that there exists $C > 0$ such that $\forall z \in D_{\alpha,R}$ and $\forall N$

$$\left| f(z) - \sum_{n=0}^{N} c_n z^n \right| \leqslant C(N+1)! A^{N+1} |z|^{N+1}.$$

Then
  (i) *the Borel transform series*

$$B(z) = \sum_{n=0}^{\infty} \frac{c_n}{n!} z^n$$

converges in $\{z \in \mathbb{C}, \ |z| < 1/A\}$,
  (ii) $B(z)$ *has an analytic continuation $g(z)$ in $T_{\alpha,A}$,*
  (iii) *the integral*

$$F(z) = \frac{1}{z} \int_0^{\infty} e^{-t/z} g(t) \, dt$$

is absolutely convergent $\forall z \in \{z \in \mathbb{C}, \ |z| < R, \ |\arg z| < \alpha\}$ and

$$F(z) = f(z).$$

Thus the integral $F(z)$ provides a formal sum for the asymptotic series $f(z)$ and the Taylor expansion of F around the origin coincides with the series f.

The main drawback of this method is that usually g is not known since, in practice, only a finite set of numerically computed coefficients c_n is available. The series B cannot be used either since it converges only for $|z| < 1/A$. Thus, the idea was to replace $g(t)$ in the definition of F by $[n+k/k]_B(t)$ with $n \geqslant -1$, giving rise to the Borel–Padé approximants

$$F_B^{[n+k/k]}(z) = \frac{1}{z} \int_0^\infty e^{-t/z} [n+k/k]_B(t)\,dt.$$

For proving that these Borel–Padé approximants tend to $f(z)$ when k tends to infinity, one has first to prove that $[n + k/k]_B$ tends to B uniformly when $k \to \infty$. Usually this is not possible and that was the reason why MARZIANI [1987] replaced the Padé approximant $[n+k/k]_B$ by the Padé-type approximant $(n+k/k)$ thus obtaining the so-called Borel–Padé-type approximant denoted by $F_B^{(n+k/k)}$.

Using the convergence results of EIERMANN [1984] (see Section 19) he was able to prove

THEOREM 30.2. *Let f be an analytic function satisfying the assumptions of Theorem 30.1 with α arbitrarily close to π. If the generating polynomials v_k are the Chebyshev polynomials of the first kind $v_k(x) = T_k(2x/A+1)$, then $\forall n \geqslant -1$*

$$f(z) = \lim_{k \to \infty} F_B^{(n+k/k)}(z)$$

for every z in the half plane $\{z, \mathrm{Re}(z) > 0\}$.

The numerical results given by MARZIANI [1987] show that the Borel–Padé-type approximants converge at almost the same rate as the Borel–Padé approximants. The major advantage is that one has complete control of the poles with Padé-type approximants and thus a proof of the convergence of the method can be obtained.

31. z-transform

The z-transform is a functional transformation of sequences which can be considered as equivalent to the Laplace transform for functions. While the Laplace transform is useful in solving differential equations, the z-transform plays a central rôle in the solution of difference equations. By changing z into z^{-1} it is identical to the method of generating functions introduced by the French mathematician François Nicole (1683–1758) and developed by Joseph Louis Lagrange (1736–1813). It has many applications in digital filtering and in signal processing as exemplified by VICH [1987]. By signal processing is understood the transformation of a function of time $f(t)$, called the input signal, into an output signal

$h(t)$. This transformation is realized via a system G called a digital filter. f can be known for all values of t, in which case we speak of a continuous signal and a continuous filter, or it can only be known at equally spaced values of t, $t_n = nT$ for $n = 0, 1, \ldots$ where T is the period and in that case we speak of a discrete signal and a discrete filter. The z-transform of a discrete signal is given by

$$F(z) = \sum_{n=0}^{\infty} f_n z^{-n}$$

where $f_n = f(nT)$. Corresponding to the input sequence (f_n) is the output sequence $(h_n = h(nT))$. If we set

$$H(z) = \sum_{n=0}^{\infty} h_n z^{-n}$$

then the system G can be represented by its so-called transfer function $G(z)$ such that

$$H(z) = G(z)F(z).$$

In other words, if we write $G(z) = \sum_{n=0}^{\infty} g_n z^{-n}$ then

$$h_n = \sum_{k=0}^{n} f_k g_{n-k}, \quad n = 0, 1, \ldots .$$

Thus if (f_n) and (h_n) are known, then (g_n) can be computed. An important problem in the analysis of digital filters is the identification of the transfer function when (f_n) and (h_n) are known (that is, when (g_n) is known). If the filter is linear then G is a rational function of z, if not its transfer function can be approximated by a rational function $R(z) = P(z)/Q(z)$.

If we set

$$P(z) = a_0 z^s + a_1 z^{s-1} + \cdots + a_s,$$
$$Q(z) = z^s + b_1 z^{s-1} + \cdots + b_s$$

it was shown by VICH [1987, p. 183] that the b_i's are solution of the system

$$\begin{pmatrix} g_s & g_{s-1} & \cdots & g_1 \\ \vdots & \vdots & & \vdots \\ g_{2s-1} & g_{2s-2} & \cdots & g_s \end{pmatrix} \begin{pmatrix} b_1 \\ \vdots \\ b_s \end{pmatrix} = - \begin{pmatrix} g_{s+1} \\ \vdots \\ g_{2s} \end{pmatrix}$$

and the a_i's are then given by

$$a_0 = g_0,$$
$$a_1 = g_1 + b_1 g_0,$$
$$\vdots$$
$$a_s = g_s + b_1 g_{s-1} + \cdots + b_s g_0.$$

Thus, comparing with the relations given in Section 2, we have

$$R(z) = [s/s]_G(z)$$

which shows the equivalence between the z-transform method and Padé approximation.

As proved by WEISS and MC DONOUGH [1963] it is also equivalent to a method for interpolation by a sum of exponential functions due to Gaspard De Prony (1755–1839) which is as follows. The problem is to find the A_j's and the a_j's ($j = 1, \ldots, s$) such that

$$\sum_{j=1}^{s} A_j e^{a_j t_i} = g_i, \quad i = 1, \ldots, 2s,$$

where the g_i's are given numbers and $t_i = iT$. Thus, setting

$$z_j = e^{a_j T}$$

the preceding system can be written as

$$\sum_{j=1}^{s} A_j z_j^i = g_i, \quad i = 1, \ldots, 2s.$$

We set

$$Q(z) = b_s + b_{s-1}z + \cdots + b_1 z^{s-1} + z^s = \prod_{j=1}^{s}(z - z_j)$$

and we shall first calculate the b_i's. Setting $b_0 = 1$, we multiply the first equation by b_s, the second one by b_{s-1} and so on up to the $(s+1)$th equation which is multiplied by b_0. Then these equations are summed. We begin again the same process by multiplying the second equation by b_s, the third one by $b_{s-1}, \ldots$, the $(s+2)$th by b_0 and then summing these. And so on. We thus obtain

$$\sum_{i=0}^{s} b_{s-i} \sum_{j=1}^{s} A_j z_j^{i+k} = \sum_{i=0}^{s} b_{s-i} g_{i+k}, \quad k = 1, \ldots, s,$$

which can also be written as

$$\sum_{i=0}^{s} b_{s-i} g_{i+k} = \sum_{j=1}^{s} A_j z_j^k \sum_{i=0}^{s} b_{s-i} z_j^i = \sum_{j=1}^{s} A_j z_j^k Q(z_j) = 0.$$

Thus the b_i's are solution of the system

$$\sum_{i=0}^{s-1} b_{s-i} g_{i+k} = -g_{s+k}, \quad k = 1, \ldots, s,$$

which is exactly the system solved above to find the denominator of the Padé approximant $R(z) = [s/s]_G(z)$. Once the b_i's have been obtained, the z_i's are the zeros of $Q(z)$ and $a_i = T^{-1} \ln z_i$ for $i = 1, \ldots, s$. Then the A_i's can be uniquely determined from the z_i's by solving a non-singular sub-system extracted from the initial one or with the help of Padé approximants.

As we know from Theorem 6.1

$$[s/s]_G(z) = g_0 + z[s - 1/s]_{G_1}(z)$$

where $G_1(z) = g_1 + g_2 z + g_3 z^2 + \cdots$.

Thus the partial fraction decomposition of $[s - 1/s]_{G_1}$ also gives the A_i's since

$$[s - 1/s]_{G_1}(z) = \sum_{i=1}^{s} A_i (z - z_i)^{-1}$$

if the z_i's are distinct. If it is not the case it means that at least two a_i's are identical and thus s has to be replaced by a lower value. This shows the complete equivalence between Prony's method and Padé approximation in the z-transform domain.

A survey of the applications of Padé approximation and continued fractions to model reduction problems and an extensive bibliography are given by BULTHEEL and VAN BAREL [1986].

32. Laplace transform inversion

The Laplace transform of a function f is defined by

$$\bar{f}(p) = \int_0^\infty e^{-pt} f(t) \, dt.$$

It is used in several cases: if f satisfies a functional equation, $\bar{f}$ satisfies a simpler one that can be solved more easily. For example, an ordinary differential equation is replaced by an algebraic equation, a partial differential equation is replaced by an ordinary differential equation, and so forth. For example, the following partial differential equation is transformed, with respect to x

$$\left[\frac{\partial^2}{\partial r^2} - 2 \frac{\partial^2}{\partial r \partial x} + \frac{1}{r} \left(\frac{\partial}{\partial r} - \frac{\partial}{\partial x} \right) - \frac{m^2}{r^2} \right] R(x, r) = 0$$

into

$$\left[\frac{\partial}{\partial r^2} + \left(\frac{1}{r} - 2p \right) \frac{\partial}{\partial r} - \left(\frac{p}{r} + \frac{m^2}{r^2} \right) \right] \bar{R}(p, x) = 0.$$

Then the problem is to find $f(t)$ from $\bar{f}(p)$. This necessitates the construction of approximate methods for computing inverse Laplace transforms that permit us to find the original function in a broad class of cases.

It must be noticed at once that the problem is always instable: if $\bar{f}(p) = 1/(p - \alpha)$, then $f(t) = e^{\alpha t}$. So if there is an error on α, say ε, then there is an amplification of the error: $f_\varepsilon = e^{\varepsilon t} f$. Conversely, if f is modified on a small interval, then $\bar{f}$ will have a very smooth change.

An extensive literature exists on the subject and on the different methods for inverting the Laplace transform. A review can be found for example in LUKE [1969]. We will only deal with the problem of inversion by use of rational approximants.

In many applications, one knows $\bar{f}(p)$ explicitly and wants to find $f(t)$ numerically. One way of obtaining approximations to the inverse $f(t)$ of $\bar{f}(p)$ is by approximating $\bar{f}(p)$ by a sequence of rational functions $\bar{f}_n(p)$, $n \geq 1$, and then inverting the $\bar{f}_n(p)$ exactly to obtain the sequence $f_n(t)$, $n \geq 1$. The hope is that if the sequence $(\bar{f}(p))_n$ converge to $\bar{f}(p)$ quickly, then the sequence $(f_n(t))_n$ will converge to $f(t)$ also, more or less quickly. There are several ways of obtaining rational approximations to a given function, one of them being by expanding this function into a Taylor series, and then forming the Padé table associated with the Taylor series. Detailed discussions and references to various applications can be found in the paper by LONGMAN [1973].

The link with Prony's method (see Section 31) is obvious and has been generalized by SIDI [1981].

If $\bar{f}_n(p)$ has n distinct poles then we get

$$\bar{f}_n(p) = \sum_{i=1}^{n} \frac{A_i}{p - \alpha_i} \Leftrightarrow f_n(t) = \sum_{i=1}^{n} A_i e^{\alpha_i t}.$$

If the poles are not distinct but of order n_i, with $\sum_1^m n_i \leq n$,

$$\bar{f}_n(p) = \sum_{i=1}^{m} \sum_{j=1}^{n_i} \frac{A_{ij}}{(p - \alpha_i)^j} \Leftrightarrow f_n(t) = \sum_{i=1}^{m} \sum_{j=1}^{n_i} A_{ij} t^{j-1} e^{\alpha_i t}.$$

So the problem is the approximation of $f(t)$ by functions of the same type as $f_n(t)$.

The result proved by SIDI [1981], which generalizes the link between Prony's method and Padé approximation, is the following

THEOREM 32.1. *Define the set G_n as follows*

$$G_n = \{g(t) = \sum_{i=1}^{m} \sum_{j=1}^{n_i} B_{i,j} t^{j-1} e^{\alpha_i t}, \ \alpha_i \neq \alpha_j, \ \sum_{1}^{m} n_i \leq n, B_{ij} \in \mathbb{C}\}.$$

Now let $g_n(t)$ be the function, if it exists, belonging to G_n, which approximates $f(t)$ in $[0, \infty[$ in the following weak sense

$$\int_0^\infty t^N e^{-wt} (f(t) - g_n(t)) t^i \, dt = 0, \quad i = 0 \cdots 2n - 1,$$

then $\bar{g}_n(p)$, the Laplace transform of $g_n(t)$, is the Padé approximant $[n-1/n]$ of $\bar{f}(p-w)$; furthermore, $g_n(t)$ is a real function of t if $\bar{f}(p)$ is real for real p.

PROOF. If the function $g_n(t)$ exists, it has the form

$$g_n(t) = \sum_{j=1}^{s}\sum_{k=1}^{\mu_j} \frac{A_{jk}}{(k-1)!} t^{k-1} e^{\alpha_j t}, \quad \sum_{1}^{s} \mu_j = n' \leqslant n.$$

Because

$$\int_0^\infty t^l e^{-pt} f(t)\,dt = (-1)^l \bar{f}^{(l)}(p) \quad \text{and} \quad \int_0^\infty t^\nu e^{-pt}\,dt = \frac{\nu!}{p^{\nu+1}} \quad (\nu > -1),$$

we get, by substituting

$$(-1)^{N+i}\bar{f}^{(N+i)}(w) = \sum_{j=1}^{s}\sum_{k=1}^{\mu_j}\frac{(N+i+k-1)!}{(k-1)!}\frac{A_{jk}}{(w-\alpha_j)^{N+i+k}},$$
$$i = 0,\ldots,2n-1,$$
$$\frac{\bar{f}^{(N+i)}(w)}{(N+i)!} = \sum_{j=1}^{s}\sum_{k=1}^{\mu_j}(-1)^k \binom{N+i+k-1}{N+i}\frac{A_{jk}}{(w-\alpha_j)^{N+i+k}},$$
$$i = 0,\ldots,2n-1,$$

which is the coefficient of the Taylor expansion of $F(z) = \bar{f}(p-w)$ in $p = 0$. If, as usual, $F(z) = R_{N-1}(z) + z^N F_N(z)$, ($R_{N-1}$ polynomial of degree $N-1$), then, by identification, it is possible to prove that

$$[n-1/n]_{F_N}(z) = \sum_{j=1}^{s}\sum_{k=1}^{\mu_j}\frac{A_{jk}}{(z-\alpha_j+w)^k}, \quad p = z+w,$$

and so

$$[n-1/n]_{F_N}(p-w) = \bar{g}_n(p).$$

Since $\bar{f}(p)$ is real for real p, the Padé approximants are real, and equivalently $\bar{g}_n(p)$ are real for real p, therefore $g_n(t)$ is a real function of t too. □

Then an oscillation theorem for the error $(f - g_n)(t)$ is proved

THEOREM 32.2. Let $f(t)$ be continuous in $[0,\infty[$, and $\bar{f}(p)$, its Laplace transform, be analytic for $\mathrm{Re}(p) > \gamma$, let $w > \gamma$ and $F(z) = \bar{f}(p-w)$ $(z = p-w)$. Let $\bar{g}_n(p)$ be the $[n-1/n]$ Padé approximant of $F(z)$, and assume that $\bar{g}_n(p)$ has no poles for $\mathrm{Re}(p) \geqslant w$, then $D(t) = f(t) - g_n(t)$ changes its sign $2n$ times in $[0,\infty[$, or is zero if $f \in G_n$.

As seen before, Padé-type approximants can give better numerical results than Padé approximants, if there is some information to choose good poles. Different investigations have been made in the last ten years in that direction.

SIDI and LUBINSKY [1983] proved general results in the case where $\bar{f}(p)$ is a Stieltjes function. The proofs used the Bromwich inversion formula

$$\bar{f}(p) = \int_0^\infty e^{-pt} f(t)\,dt, \qquad f(t) = \frac{1}{2i\pi} \int_{\Delta-i\infty}^{\Delta+i\infty} e^{pt} \bar{f}(p)\,dp.$$

Let $\bar{f}(p)$ be a Stieltjes function; let $\beta(x)$ be a real valued function, right continuous and of bounded variation in $[0, \infty[$. If

$$\bar{f}(p) = \int_0^\infty \frac{d\beta(x)}{1+px}, \qquad p \in \mathbb{C} - \,]-\infty, 0],$$

then $f(t) = \int_0^\infty x^{-1} e^{-t/x}\,d\beta(x)$, $\mathrm{Re}(t) > 0$, and f is analytic in the half plane $\mathrm{Re}(t) > 0$.

Similarly for a Padé-type approximant of $\bar{f}$, $\bar{f}_n(p) = (n-1/n)_{\bar{f}}(p)$ is a Stieltjes function for the step function β_n with discontinuity at each x_{n_k} such that $-1/x_{n_k}$ is a pole of $\bar{f}_n(p)$

$$\bar{f}_n(p) = \int_0^\infty \frac{d\beta_n(x)}{1+px},$$

$$f_n(t) = \int_0^\infty x^{-1} e^{-t/x}\,d\beta_n(x).$$

The uniform convergence of the sequence $(f_n)_n$ in infinite sectors of the right half plane $S(\varepsilon, \theta_0) = \{t = re^{i\theta}, r > \varepsilon, \theta \leqslant \theta_0 < \pi/2\}$ is obtained in several cases
– first the Padé case: $\bar{f}_n(p) = [n-1/n]_{\bar{f}}(p)$,
– secondly Padé-type approximants: let us suppose $\bar{f}(p) = \int_0^\infty d\alpha(x)/(1+px)$ and $\bar{f}(p) = \int_0^\infty d\beta(x)/(1+px)$ where β is as follows: β is a real valued function, right continuous in $[0, \infty[$ and of bounded variation. $\beta(x)$ is absolutely continuous with respect to $\alpha(x)$ i.e. there is a real valued function $(d\beta/d\alpha)(x)$ defined on $[0, \infty[$, such that $\beta(x) = \int_0^x d\beta/d\alpha(y)\,d\alpha(y)$ exists in $[0, \infty[$ except possibly at a discontinuity of α and $\int_0^\infty [d\beta/d\alpha(x)]^2\,d\alpha(x) < +\infty$. The β_n's are then defined as follows. We set

$$I(g) = \int_0^\infty g(x)\,d\beta(x),$$

$$I_n(g) = \sum_1^n \lambda_{n_j} g(x_{n_j}).$$

I_n is a quadrature formula, where the λ_{n_j}'s are such that $I_n(g) = I(g)$ for polynomials of degree less than n, and β_n is the weight function of I_n,

$$\beta_n(x) = \sum_{x_{n_j} \leqslant x} \lambda_{n_j}, \quad x \in [0, \infty[.$$

If more is assumed about the support of $d\alpha$, one obtains the rate of convergence: if $\mathrm{supp}(d\alpha) \subset [a, b]$ $(0 < a < b < +\infty)$ then $f(t)$ is entire and the convergence has a geometric character, that is

$$\limsup_{n \to \infty} |f_n(t) - f(t)|^{1/n} \leqslant \rho < 1.$$

Similar results are proved for Padé and Padé-type approximants at infinity.

Another line of research has been followed by VAN ISEGHEM [1987a] through orthogonal polynomials. The basic remark is the following, made by Tricomi (in SNEDDON [1972]), about the Laguerre polynomials of zero order

$$f(t) = e^{\lambda t} L_k(2\lambda t) \Leftrightarrow \bar{f}(p) = \frac{(p - \lambda)^k}{(p + \lambda)^{k+1}}.$$

So the Laplace transform formally achieves a correspondence between a series in powers of $(p - \lambda)/(p + \lambda)$ and an expansion into Laguerre polynomials. Convergence in the least squares sense is to be expected for $(f_n)_n$, but better results are obtained. We have

$$\bar{f}(p) = \frac{1}{p + \lambda} \sum_{k \geqslant 0} a_k \left(\frac{p - \lambda}{p + \lambda}\right)^k.$$

The partial sum $f_n(p)$ of this series is the $(n/n + 1)$ Padé-type approximant of $F(z)$ with denominator $(p + \lambda)^{n+1}$. If $\bar{f}(p) = \sum_{i \geqslant 0} c_i (z - \lambda)^i$, then the a_k's are easily computed

$$a_k = \sum_{i=0}^{k} \binom{k}{i} c_i (2\lambda)^i.$$

The following results are obtained

THEOREM 32.3. $\bar{f}$ is supposed to be analytic in the half plane $\mathrm{Re}(p) > 0$. $f(t)$ exists and $\int_0^\infty f^2(t)\, dt < \infty$. Then the sequence $(\bar{f}(p))_n$ converges to $\bar{f}$, uniformly on every compact set of the half plane $\mathrm{Re}(z) > 0$.

The sequence $(f_n(t))_n$ converges to f in the least squares sense. Furthermore if $(p + \lambda)\bar{f}(p)$ is analytic at infinity and if $\bar{f}(p)$ is analytic on $\mathrm{Re}(z) \geqslant 0$, then the sequence $(f_n(t))_n$ converges to $f(t)$ uniformly on compact sets of $\mathbb{R}^+$.

PROOF. Let $u = (p - \lambda)/(p + \lambda)$ and $\varphi(u) = \bar{f}(p)$. When p is in the half plane $\operatorname{Re} p > 0$, u lies in the unit disk. So $\varphi(u)$ and $\varphi(u)/(1-u)$ are analytic functions and may be expanded into power series with radius 1, which converge uniformly on every compact set of the unit disk. We have

$$\frac{\varphi(u)}{1-u} = \frac{1}{2\lambda}\sum_{n \geq 0} a_n u^n \iff \bar{f}(p) = \frac{1}{p+\lambda}\sum_{n \geq 0} a_n \left(\frac{p-\lambda}{p+\lambda}\right)^n.$$

The last series converges on every compact set of the half-plane, by a change of variables.

Let us now prove the convergence to f.

Because $\int_0^\infty f^2 < +\infty$, f admits an expansion in $\left(\sqrt{2\lambda}e^{-\lambda t}L_n(2\lambda t)\right)_n$ which forms an orthonormal family, and this expansion converges in the least squares sense. We have

$$f(t) = e^{-\lambda t}\sum_{n \geq 0} b_n \sqrt{2\lambda} L_n(2\lambda t),$$

$$b_n = \sqrt{2\lambda}\int_0^\infty e^{-\lambda t}L_n(2\lambda t)f(t)\,dt.$$

It remains to prove that $b_n\sqrt{2\lambda} = a_n$, $n \geq 0$.

$$\bar{f}(p) - \sum_0^N b_n \sqrt{2\lambda}\left(\frac{p-\lambda}{p+\lambda}\right)^n$$

$$= \int_0^\infty e^{-pt}f(t)\left(1 - \sum_0^N \frac{(z-\lambda)^n}{(z+\lambda)^{n+1}}2\lambda \cdot L_n(2\lambda t)\right)dt,$$

$$\left|\bar{f}(p) - \sum_0^N b_n\sqrt{2\lambda}\left(\frac{p-\lambda}{p+\lambda}\right)^n\right|^2$$

$$\leq \int_0^\infty f^2(t)\,dt \cdot \int_0^\infty \left|e^{-pt} - 2\lambda e^{-\lambda t}\sum_0^N \frac{(p-\lambda)^n}{(p+\lambda)^{n+1}}L_n(2\lambda t)\right|^2 dt.$$

For $p \geq 0$, e^{-pt} may be expanded into a series of $(\sqrt{2\lambda}e^{-\lambda t}L_n(2\lambda t))$, whose coefficients are

$$\sqrt{2\lambda}\int_0^\infty e^{-\lambda t}L_n(2\lambda t)e^{-pt}\,dt = \frac{(p-\lambda)^n}{(p+\lambda)^{n+1}}.$$

This proves that the second integral tends to zero as N tends to infinity, and finally, for convergence in the least squares sense

$$f(t) = \lim_N \sum_0^N e^{-\lambda t}a_n L_n(2\lambda t), \quad \text{with } \bar{f}(p) = \sum_0^\infty a_n \frac{(p-\lambda)^n}{(p+\lambda)^{n+1}}.$$

Furthermore, under the last assumption, the convergence is uniform in compact sets of $\mathbb{R}^+$.

First the radius of convergence of $(\sum_n a_n u^n)$ is strictly greater than one: the singularities of $\bar{f}$ are transformed (by homography) into points exterior to the unit disc because they lie in $\{\operatorname{Re} z < 0\}$. The point at infinity is transformed into 1, and is a regular point for $(p+\lambda)\bar{f}(p)$, so 1 is not a singularity of $(\sum_n a_n u^n)$, and the radius R is strictly greater than 1. Let $1 < \rho < R$. By Cauchy's formula we get $|a_n| < A(\rho)/\rho^n$,

$$\left| \sum_{n \geq 0} e^{-\lambda t} a_n L_n(2\lambda t) \right| \leq A(\rho) e^{-\lambda t} \sum_{n \geq 0} \frac{1}{\rho^n} \sum_{r=0}^{n} \binom{n}{r} \frac{(2\lambda t)^r}{r!} \quad (t \geq 0)$$

$$\leq A(\rho) e^{-\lambda t} \sum_{r \geq 0} \frac{(2\lambda t)^r}{r!} \sum_{n \geq r} \binom{n}{r} \frac{1}{\rho^n}$$

$$\leq A(\rho) e^{-\lambda t} \sum_{r \geq 0} \frac{(2\lambda t)^r}{r!} \frac{1/\rho^r}{(1-1/\rho)^{r+1}} \quad (1/\rho < 1)$$

$$\leq \frac{\rho A(\rho) e^{-\lambda t}}{\rho - 1} e^{-2\lambda t/(\rho-1)}.$$

The series converges absolutely for any $t \in \mathbb{R}^+$, and uniformly on compact subsets of $\mathbb{R}^+$. The sum of this series is $f(t)$, which can be proved by taking the Laplace transform of it. □

This theorem can be improved in two directions
(i) $\bar{f}$ analytic in $\operatorname{Re}(p) > w$ (instead of $w = 0$),
(ii) $(p+\lambda)\bar{f}^{(k)}(p)$ is analytic at infinity (instead of $k = 0$).
With the first assumption, we get the following sequence $(h_n(t))$

$$h_n(t) = \frac{1}{t^k} e^{(w-\lambda)t} \sum_{0}^{n} a_i L_i(2\lambda t),$$

$$\lim_{n \to \infty} \int_0^\infty t^{2k} e^{-2wt} (f(t) - h_n(t))^2 \, dt = 0.$$

With the second one, the same sequence converges uniformly to f on compact sets of $\mathbb{R}^+$.

The idea is to obtain a quickly decreasing sequence $(a_i(\lambda))$, and the computations are very sensitive to that choice, even if the theoretical results are not. The choice of λ must be made to speed up the convergence of the power series $\sum_{i \geq 0} a_i u^i$ (i.e. the convergence of $\bar{f}_n(p)$ to $\bar{f}(p)$). Let

$$\varphi(u) = \Sigma a_i u^i, \quad (p+\lambda)\bar{f}(p) = \varphi(u), \quad u = \frac{p-\lambda}{p+\lambda}.$$

The singularities of φ are $(\alpha - \lambda)/(\alpha + \lambda)$ with α a singularity of $\bar{f}$.

So R_λ, the radius of convergence of φ, is

$$R_\lambda = \frac{1}{\max_i |LA_i|},$$

L being the point 1, and A_i the point $2\lambda/(\lambda - \alpha_i)$.

And so the best λ is obtained by minimizing $\max_i |LA_i|$.

Computations have been made, and compared with those of LONGMAN [1973] with Padé approximants. For the examples studied (with poles, branch points or isolated essential singularities) they give better results.

We now sum up three examples, the last line of each array containing the exact results when they are known.

TABLE 32.1. $f(z) = 1/(z + 1)(z + 2)$; $F(t) = e^{-t} - e^{-2t}$; Approximant $F_7(t)$.

λ	$t=4$	$t=3$	$t=2$	$t=1$	$t=0.5$
1	0.01797	0.04739	0.11695	0.23263	0.23866
1.2	0.01797971	0.04730743	0.11702114	0.23254302	0.23865336
1.4	0.01798023	0.04730826	0.11701970	0.23254407	0.23865132
	0.01798018	0.04730832	0.11701964	0.23254416	0.23865122

The case $\lambda = 1$ has been obtained by Ward (in SNEDDON [1972]). For the second example, the results are obtained with the weight function, depending on k, $t^{2k}e^{-2kt}$,

TABLE 32.2. $f(z) = (1/z)\ln(1 + z)$.

k	$t=4$	$t=3$	$t=2$	$t=1$	$t=0.5$
0	0.00610753	0.02783664	0.03565157	0.18681021	0.61903884
1	0.00367911	0.01317950	0.04913335	0.21905461	0.55836858
2	0.00381005	0.01302425	0.04893459	0.21946490	0.55968527
3	0.00378606	0.01304452	0.04889932	0.21937999	0.55983595
4	0.00377835	0.01304889	0.04889975	0.21938201	0.55975173
5	0.00377870	0.01304862	0.04890096	0.21938555	0.55978776
6	0.00477197	0.01305021	0.04890073	0.21938696	0.55979929
7	0.00373412	0.01305411	0.04889717	0.21938630	0.55966299
			0.04890051	0.21938393	0.55977359

Nevertheless, it is obvious that for such unstable problems, no single method gives optimal results for all purposes and all occasions.

TABLE 32.3. $f(z) = (1/z)\exp(-z/\sqrt{1+\sigma z})$.

t	$\sigma=0.2$	$\sigma=0.4$	$\sigma=0.6$	$\sigma=0.8$	$\sigma=1$
0.5	0.1022010	0.2200330	0.2983019	0.3548312	0.3983875
1	0.5673705	0.5956933	0.6173415	0.6352666	0.6506315
1.5	0.8684599	0.8179220	0.7988473	0.7909833	0.7882222
2	0.9691488	0.9239090	0.8964390	0.8797707	0.869366
2.5	0.9948563	0.9697096	0.9474830	0.9308438	0.9187462
3	0.9989072	0.9883548	0.9736810	0.9602775	0.9492417
3.5	0.9998211	0.9956401	0.9869363	0.9772277	0.9682182
4	0.9999725	0.9984017	0.9935675	0.9869720	0.9800756

As the Borel transform is also a Laplace transform, there are also some applications of Padé and Padé-type approximants for the inversion of that transform, as has been seen by MARZIANI [1987] (see Section 30 concerning the Borel transform).

Laplace transform inversion can also be performed by using interpolation rational functions, see BREZINSKI [1978].

References

ALT, R. (1972), Deux théorèmes sur la A-stabilité des schémas de Runge–Kutta simplement implicites, *RAIRO* **R3**, 99–104.

ARIOKA, S. (1987), Padé-type approximants in multivariables, *Appl. Numer. Math.* **3**, 497–511.

ARMS, R.J. and A. EDREI (1970), The Padé tables and continued fractions generated by totally positive sequences, in: *Mathematical Essays* (Ohio University Press, Athens, OH) 1–21.

BAKER, G.A. JR. (1961), Application of the Padé approximation method to the investigation of some magnetic properties of the Ising model, *Phys. Rev.* **124**, 768–774.

BAKER, G.A. JR. (1970), The Padé approximant method and some related generalizations, in: G.A. BAKER JR. and J.L. GAMMEL, eds., *The Padé Approximant in Theoretical Physics* (Academic Press, New York).

BAKER, G.A. JR. (1975), *Essentials of Padé Approximants* (Academic Press, New York).

BAKER, G.A. JR. (1988), Integral approximants for functions of higher monodromic dimension, in: A. CUYT, ed., *Nonlinear Numerical Methods and Rational Approximation* (Reidel, Dordrecht) 3–22.

BAKER, G.A. JR. and P.R. GRAVES-MORRIS (1977), Convergence of rows of the Padé table, *J. Math. Anal. Appl.* **57**, 323–329.

BAKER, G.A. JR. and P.R. GRAVES-MORRIS (1981), *Padé Approximants* (Addison-Wesley, Reading, MA).

BEARDON, A.F. (1968), The convergence of Padé approximants, *J. Math. Anal. Appl.* **21**, 344–346.

BENDER, C.M. and S.A. ORSZAG (1978), *Advanced Mathematical Methods for Scientists and Engineers* (McGraw-Hill, Kogakusha).

BRAESS, D. (1986), *Nonlinear Approximation Theory* (Springer, Berlin).

BREZINSKI, C. (1977), *Accélération de la Convergence en Analyse Numérique*, Lecture Notes in Math. **584** (Springer, Berlin).

BREZINSKI, C. (1978), *Algorithmes d'Accélération de la Convergence. Etude Numérique* (Technip, Paris).

BREZINSKI, C. (1979), Rational approximation to formal power series, *J. Approx. Theory* **25**, 295–317.

BREZINSKI, C. (1980), *Padé-Type Approximation and General Orthogonal Polynomials*, Intern. Ser. Numer. Math. **50** (Birkhäuser, Basel).

BREZINSKI, C. (1983a), Outlines of Padé approximation, in: H. WERNER et al., eds., *Computational Aspects of Complex Analysis* (Reidel, Dordrecht) 1–50.

BREZINSKI, C. (1983b), On the successive remainders of the exponential series, *Elem. Math.* **38**, 86–89.

BREZINSKI, C. (1983c), Recursive interpolation, extrapolation and projection, *J. Comput. Appl. Math.* **9**, 369–376.

BREZINSKI, C. (1985), The birth and early developments of Padé approximants, in: G.M. RASSIAS and T.M. RASSIAS, eds., *Differential Geometry, Calculus of Variations, and their Applications* (Dekker, New York) 105–121.

BREZINSKI, C. (1986), On interpolatory multivariate Padé-type approximants, *BIT* **26**, 234–288.

BREZINSKI, C. (1988a), Partial Padé approximation, *J. Approx. Theory* **54**, 210–233.

BREZINSKI, C. (1988b), Error estimate in Padé approximation, in: M. ALFARO et al., eds., *Orthogonal Polynomials and their Applications*, Lecture Notes in Math. **1329** (Springer, Berlin) 1–19.
BREZINSKI, C. (1989), Procedures for estimating the error in Padé approximation, *Math. Comp.* **54**, 565–574.
BREZINSKI, C. (1990a), Duality in Padé-type approximation, *J. Comput. Appl. Math.* **30**, 351–357.
BREZINSKI, C. (1990b), A direct proof of the Christoffel–Darboux identity and its equivalence to the recurrence relationship, *J. Comput. Appl. Math.* **32**, 17–25.
BREZINSKI, C. (1990c), *History of Continued Fractions and Padé Approximants* (Springer, Berlin).
BREZINSKI, C. (1991a), *Biorthogonality and its Applications to Numerical Analysis* (Dekker, New York).
BREZINSKI, C. (1991b), *A Bibliography on Continued Fractions, Padé Approximation, Extrapolation and Related Subjects* (Prensas Universitarias de Zaragoza, Zaragoza).
BREZINSKI, C. (1991c), The asymptotic behaviour of sequences and new series transformations based on the Cauchy product, *Rocky Mountain J. Math.* **21**, 71–84.
BREZINSKI, C. and M. REDIVO ZAGLIA (1991), *Extrapolation Methods. Theory and Practice* (North-Holland, Amsterdam).
BREZINSKI, C., M. REDIVO ZAGLIA and H. SADOK (1992), A breakdown-free Lanczos type algorithm for solving linear systems, *Numer. Math.* **63**, 29–38.
BREZINSKI, C. and H. SADOK (1987), Vector sequence transformations and fixed point methods, in: C. TAYLOR et al., eds., *Numerical Methods in Laminar and Turbulent Flows, Vol. 1* (Pineridge Press, Swansea) 3–11.
BREZINSKI, C. and J. VAN ISEGHEM (1984), Padé-type approximants and linear functional transformations, in: P.R. GRAVES-MORRIS et al., eds., *Rational Approximation and Interpolation*, Lecture Notes in Math. **1105** (Springer, Berlin) 100-108.
BULTHEEL, A. (1982), On a special Laurent–Hermite interpolation problem, in: L. COLLATZ et al., eds., *Proc. Conf. Numerische Methoden der Approximations Theorie* (Birkhäuser, Basel).
BULTHEEL, A. (1987), *Laurent Series and their Padé Approximation* (Birkhäuser, Basel).
BULTHEEL, A. and M. VAN BAREL (1986), Padé techniques for model reduction in linear system theory: a survey, *J. Comput. Appl. Math.* **14**, 401–438.
BUSLAEV, V.I. (1988), Relations for the coefficients and singular points of a function, *Math. USSR-Sb.* **59**, 349–377.
BUSLAEV, V.I., A.A. GONČAR and S.P. SUETIN (1984), On the convergence of subsequences of the mth row of the Padé table, *Math. USSR-Sb.* **48**, 535–540.
CHAFFY, C. (1984), A homogeneous process for Padé approximants in two variables, *Numer. Math.* **45**, 149–164.
CHAFFY, C. (1988a), (Padé)$_y$ of (Padé)$_x$ approximants of $F(x, y)$, in: A. CUYT, ed., *Nonlinear Numerical Methods and Rational Approximation* (Reidel, Dordrecht) 155–166.
CHAFFY, C. (1988b), Uniform convergence of a new kind of multivariate Padé approximants, *C. R. Acad. Sci. Paris, Sér. I Math.* **306**, 387–392.
CHISHOLM, J.S.R. (1973), Rational approximants defined from double power series, *Math. Comp.* **27**, 841–848.
CORDELLIER, F. (1979), Démonstration algébrique de l'extension de l'identité de Wynn aux tables de Padé non normales, in: L. WUYTACK, ed., *Padé Approximation and its Applications*, Lecture Notes in Math. **765** (Springer, Berlin) 36–60.
CROUZEIX, M. and F. RUAMPS (1977), On rational approximations to the exponential, *RAIRO Anal. Numer.* **R11**, 241–243.
CUYT, A. (1982), *Abstract Padé Approximants for Operators: Theory and Applications*, Thesis, Universiteit Antwerpen.
CUYT, A. (1986), Multivariate Padé approximants revisited, *BIT* **26**, 71–79.
CUYT, A. (1990), A multivariate convergence theorem of the "de Montessus De Ballore" type, *J. Comput. Appl. Math.* **32**, 47-57.
DE BRUIN, M.G. (1984), Simultaneous Padé Approximation and orthogonality, in: C. BREZINSKI et al., eds., *Polynômes Orthogonaux et Applications*, Lecture Notes in Math. **1171** (Springer, Berlin) 74–83.

DE BRUIN, M.G. (1988), Simultaneous partial Padé approximants, *J. Comput. Appl. Math.* **21**, 343–355.
DE BRUIN, M.G., J. GILEWICZ and H.J. RUNCKEL (1987), A survey of bounds for the zeros of analytic functions obtained by continued fraction methods, in: J. GILEWICZ et al., eds., *Rational Approximation and its Applications in Mathematics and Physics*, Lecture Notes in Math. **1237** (Springer, Berlin) 1–23.
DE BRUIN, M.G. and H. VAN ROSSUM (1975), Formal Padé approximation, *Nieuw Arch. Wisk. (23)* **3**, 115–130.
DELLA DORA, J. (1981), Quelques résultats sur la structure des tables de Padé–Hermite, in: M.G. DE BRUIN and H. VAN ROSSUM, eds., *Padé Approximation and its Applications. Amsterdam 1980* (Springer, Berlin) 173–184.
DELLA DORA, J. and C. DI CRESCENZO (1984a), Approximants de Padé–Hermite. Première partie: théorie, *Numer. Math.* **43**, 23–39.
DELLA DORA, J. and C. DI CRESCENZO (1984b), Approximants de Padé–Hermite. Deuxième partie: programmation, *Numer. Math.* **43**, 41–57.
DRAUX, A. (1983), *Polynômes Orthogonaux Formels. Applications*, Lecture Notes in Math. **974** (Springer, Berlin).
DRAUX, A. (1984), The Padé approximants in a non-commutative algebra and their applications, in: H. WERNER and H.J. BÜNGER, eds., *Padé Approximation and its Applications. Bad Honnef 1983*, Lecture Notes in Math. **1071** (Springer, Berlin) 117–131.
DRAUX, A. and A. MAANAOUI (1990), Vector orthogonal polynomials, *J. Comput. Appl. Math.* **32**, 59–68.
DRAUX, A. and P. VAN INGELANDT (1986), *Polynômes Orthogonaux et Approximants de Padé. Logiciels* (Technip, Paris).
EDREI, A. (1953), On the generating functions of totally positive sequences, II, *J. Anal. Math.* **2**, 104–109.
EDREI, A. (1974), The Padé table of meromorphic functions of small order with negative zeros and positive poles, *Rocky Mountain J. Math.* **4**, 175–180.
EDREI, A., E.B. SAFF and R.S. VARGA (1983), *Zeros of Sections of Power Series*, Lecture Notes in Math. **1002** (Springer, Berlin).
EHLE, B.L. (1973), A-stable methods and Padé approximation to the exponential, *SIAM J. Math. Anal.* **4**, 671–680.
EIERMANN, M. (1984), On the convergence of Padé-type approximants to analytic functions, *J. Comput. Appl. Math.* **10**, 219–227.
FAVARD, J. (1935), Sur les polynômes de Tchebicheff, *C. R. Acad. Sci. Paris* **200**, 2052–2053.
FRANZEN, N.R. (1972), Convergence of Padé approximants for a certain class of meromorphic functions, *J. Approx. Theory* **6**, 264–271.
GALLUCI, M.A. and W.B. JONES (1976), Rational approximations corresponding to Newton Series (Newton Padé Approximants), *J. Approx. Theory* **17**, 366–392.
GAMMEL, J.L. (1973), Review of two recent generalizations of the Padé approximants, in: P.R. GRAVES-MORRIS, ed., *Padé Approximants and their Applications* (Academic Press, New York) 3–9.
GAUTSCHI, W. (1982), A note on the successive remainders of the exponential series, *Elem. Math.* **37**, 46–49.
GILEWICZ, J. (1973), Numerical detection of the best Padé approximant and determination of the Fourier coefficients of the insufficiently sampled functions, in: P.R. GRAVES-MORRIS, ed., *Padé Approximants and their Applications* (Academic Press, New York) 99–103.
GILEWICZ, J. (1978), *Approximants de Padé*, Lecture Notes in Math. **667**, (Springer, Berlin).
GILEWICZ, J. and E. LÉOPOLD (1985a), On the sharpness of results in the theory of location of zeros of polynomials defined by three term recurrence relations, in: C. BREZINSKI et al., eds., *Polynômes Orthogonaux et Applications*, Lecture Notes in Math. **1171** (Springer, Berlin) 259–266.
GILEWICZ, J. and E. LÉOPOLD (1985b), Location of the zeros of polynomials satisfying three-term recurrence relations. I. General case with complex coefficients, *J. Approx. Theory* **43**, 1–14.
GONČAR, A.A. (1972), A local condition for the single-valuedness of analytic functions, *Math. USSR-Sb.* **18**, 151–157.

GONČAR, A.A. (1973), On the convergence of Padé approximants, *Math. USSR-Sb.* **21**, 155–166.
GONČAR, A.A. (1975a), On convergence of Padé approximants for some classes of meromorphic functions, *Math. USSR-Sb.* **26**, 555–575.
GONČAR, A.A. (1975b), On the convergence of generalized Padé approximants of meromorphic functions, *Math. USSR-Sb.* **27**, 503–514.
GONČAR, A.A. (1982), Poles of rows of the Padé table and meromorphic continuation of functions, *Math. USSR-Sb.* **43**, 527–546.
GONČAR, A.A. and N.K. LUNGU (1981), Poles of diagonal Padé approximants and the analytic continuation of functions, *Math. USSR-Sb.* **39**, 255–266.
GONZÁLEZ CONCEPCIÓN, C. (1987), On the A-acceptability of Padé-type approximants to the exponential with a single pole, *J. Comput. Appl. Math.* **19**, 133–140.
GRAGG, W.B. (1972), The Padé table and its relation to certain algorithms of numerical analysis, *SIAM Rev.* **14**, 1–62.
GRAVES-MORRIS, P.R. (1981), The convergence of ray sequences of Padé Approximants of Stieltjes functions, *J. Comput. Appl. Math.* **7**, 191–201.
GRAVES-MORRIS, P.R. and E.B. SAFF (1984), A Montessus De Ballore theorem for vector valued rational interpolants, in: P.R. GRAVES-MORRIS et al., eds., *Rational Approximation and Interpolation.*, Lecture Notes in Math. **1105** (Springer, Berlin) 227–242.
GUTTMANN, A.J. (1989), Asymptotic analysis of power-series expansions, in: C. DOMB and J.L. LEBOWITZ, eds., *Phase Transitions and Critical Phenomena* (Academic Press, New York) 1–234.
HENDRIKSEN, E. and O. NJÅSTAD (1989), A Favard theorem for rational functions, *J. Math. Appl.* **142**, 508–520.
HENDRIKSEN, E. and H. VAN ROSSUM (1982), Moment methods in Padé approximation, *J. Approx. Theory* **35**, 250–263.
HENRICI, P. (1974), *Applied and Computational Complex Analysis, Vol. 1* (Wiley, New York).
HERMITE, C. (1893), Sur la généralisation des fractions continues algébriques, *Ann. Mat. Pura Appl., Ser. II* **21**, 289–308.
HORNECKER, G. (1959a), Approximations rationnelles voisines de la meilleur approximation au sens de Tchebyscheff, *C. R. Acad. Sci. Paris* **249**, 939–941.
HORNECKER, G. (1959b), Détermination des meilleures approximations rationnelles (au sens de Tchebycheff), des fonctions réelles d'une variable sur un segment fini et des bornes d'erreur correspondantes, *C. R. Acad. Sci. Paris* **249**, 2265–2267.
JBILOU, K. and H. SADOK (1991), Some results about vector extrapolation methods and related fixed point iterations, *J. Comput. Appl. Math.* **36**, 385–398.
JONES, W.B. and W.J. THRON (1977), Two-point Padé tables and T-fractions, *Bull. Amer. Math. Soc.* **43**, 388–390.
JONES, W.B. and W.J. THRON (1980), *Continued Fractions. Analytic Theory and Applications* (Addison-Wesley, Reading, MA).
JONES, W.B. and W.J. THRON (1988), Continued fractions in numerical analysis, *Appl. Numer. Math.* **4**, 143–230.
KAKEHASHI, T. (1955), The decomposition of coefficients of power series and the divergence of interpolation polynomials, *Proc. Japan Acad.* **31**, 517.
KAKEHASHI, T. (1956), On interpolation of analytic functions, I and II, *Proc. Japan Acad.* **32**, 707–713.
KARLBERG, L. and H. WALLIN (1990), Padé-type approximants and orthogonal polynomials for Markov–Stieltjes functions, *J. Comput. Appl. Math.* **32**, 153–157.
KARLBERG, L. and H. WALLIN (1991), Padé-type approximants for functions for Markov–Stieltjes type, *Rocky Mount. J. Math.* **21**, 437–449.
KARLSON, J. and E.B. SAFF (1981), Singularities of functions determined by the poles of Padé approximants, in: M.G. DE BRUIN, and H. VAN ROSSUM, eds., *Padé Approximation and its Applications. Amsterdam 1980*, Lecture Notes in Math. **888** (Springer, Berlin) 239–254.
KARLSON, J. and B. VON SYDOW (1976), The convergence of Padé approximants to series of Stieltjes, *Ark. Math.* **14**, 44–53.
KIDA, S. (1990a), Padé-type and Padé-approximations in several variables, *Appl. Numer. Math.* **5**, 371–391.

KIDA, S. (1990b), Relation between Padé-type approximation, and polynomial interpolation in several variables, *Appl. Numer. Math.* **5**, 393–404.
KRONROD, A.S. (1965), *Nodes and Weight of Quadrature Formulas* (Consultants Bureau, New York).
LÉOPOLD, E. (1985), Location of the zeros of polynomials satisfying three-term recurrence relations. III. Positive coefficients case, *J. Approx. Theory* **43**, 15–24.
LEVIN, D. (1976), General order Padé-type approximants defined from double power series, *J. Inst. Math. Applics.* **18**, 1–8.
LOI, S.L. and A.W. MCINNES (1984), An algorithm for the quadratic approximation, *J. Comput. Appl. Math.* **11**, 161–174.
LONGMAN, I. (1971), Computation of the Padé table, *Internat. J. Comput. Math.* **3B**, 53–64.
LONGMAN, I. (1973), On the generation of rational function approximations for Laplace transform inversion with an application to viscoelasticity, *SIAM J. Appl. Math.* **24**, 429–440.
LOPEZ, G. (1979), Conditions for convergence of multipoint Padé approximants for functions of Stieltjes type, *Math. USSR-Sb.* **14**, 43–53.
LOPEZ, G. (1981), On the convergence of the Padé approximants for meromorphic functions of Stieltjes type, *Math. USSR-Sb.* **39**, 281–288.
LORENTZEN, L. and H. WAADELAND (1992), *Continued Fractions with Applications* (North-Holland, Amsterdam).
LUBINSKY, D.S. (1980), *Exceptional Sets of Padé Approximants*, Ph.D. Thesis, University of Witwatersrand, Johannesburg.
LUBINSKY, D.S. (1985), Padé tables of entire functions of very slow and smooth growth, *Constr. Approx.* **1**, 349–358.
LUBINSKY, D.S. (1987), Uniform convergence of rows of the Padé table, *Constr. Approx.* **3**, 307–330.
LUBINSKY, D.S. (1988), Padé tables of entire functions of very slow and smooth growth, II, *Constr. Approx.* **4**, 321–339.
LUKE, Y. (1969), *The Special Functions and their Approximation, Vol. III* (Academic Press, New York).
MAGNUS, A.P. (1981), Rate of convergence of sequences of Padé-type approximants and pole detection in the complex plane, in: M.G. DE BRUIN and H. VAN ROSSUM, eds., *Padé Approximation and its Applications. Amsterdam 1980*, Lecture Notes in Math. **888** (Springer, Berlin) 300–308.
MAGNUS, A.P. (1988), *Approximations Complexes Quantitatives*, Cours de questions spéciales en Mathématiques (Facultés Universitaires Notre Dame de la Paix, Namur).
MARKOV, A.A. (1948), in: N.I. ACHYESER, ed., *Selected Papers on Continued Fractions and the Theory of Functions Deviating Least from Zero* (Ogiz, Moscow) (in Russian).
MARONI, P. (1981), Une généralisation du théorème de Shohat–Favard sur les polynômes orthogonaux, *C. R. Acad. Sci. Paris* **293**, I, 19–22.
MARZIANI, M.F. (1987), Convergence of a class of Borel–Padé type approximants, *Nuovo Cimento* **99B**, 145–154.
MATOS, A.C. (1991a), Construction of new transformations for lacunary power series based on the Cauchy-type approximants, *Appl. Numer. Math.* **7**, 493–507.
MATOS, A.C. (1991b), Some new acceleration methods for periodico-linearly convergent power series, *BIT* **31**, 686–696.
MONTESSUS DE BALLORE, R. DE (1902), Sur les fractions continues algébriques, *Bull. Soc. Math. France* **30**, 28–36.
NJÅSTAD, O. (1989), Multipoint Padé approximants and related continued fractions, in: L. JACOBSEN, ed., *Analytic Theory of Continued Fractions III*, Lecture Notes in Math. **1406** (Springer, Berlin) 76–87.
NUTTALL, J. (1967), Convergence of Padé approximants for the Bethe–Salpeter amplitude, *Phys. Rev.* **157**, 1312–1316.
NUTTALL, J. (1970), The convergence of Padé approximants of meromorphic functions, *J. Math. Anal. Appl.* **31**, 147–153.
NUTTALL, J. (1984), Asymptotics of diagonal Hermite–Padé polynomials, *J. Approx. Theory* **42**, 299–386.
PADÉ, H. (1894), Sur la généralisation des fractions continues algébriques, *J. Math. Pures Appl.* **IV**, Sér. 10, 291–329.

PADÉ, H. (1984), *Oeuvres*, C. BREZINSKI, ed. (Libraire Scientifique et Technique Albert Blanchard, Paris).
PASZKOWSKI, S. (1963), Approximation uniforme des fonctions continues par les fonctions rationnelles, *Zastos. Mat.* **6**, 441–458.
PASZKOWSKI, S. (1975), *Zastosowania Numeryczne Wielomianów i Szeregów Czebyszewa* (Państwowe Wydawnictwo Naukowe, Warsaw).
PASZKOWSKI, S. (1987), Recurrence relations in Padé–Hermite approximation, *J. Comput. Appl. Math.* **19**, 99–107.
PASZKOWSKI, S. (1990), Padé–Hermite appproximation (basic notions and theorem), *J. Comput. Appl. Math.* **32**, 229–236.
PATRY, J. (1991), *Les Fractions Continues. Théorie et Applications* (Technip, Paris).
PERRON, O. (1957), *Die Lehre von den Kettenbrüchen* (Teubner, Stuttgart).
PÓLYA, G. and G. SZEGÖ (1972), *Problems and Theorems in Analysis* (Springer, Berlin).
POMMERENKE, J. (1973), Padé approximants and convergence in capacity, *J. Math. Anal. Appl.* **41**, 775–780.
PRÉVOST, M. (1983), Padé-type approximants with orthogonal generating polynomials, *J. Comput. Appl. Math.* **9**, 333–346.
PRÉVOST, M. (1988), Stieltjes- and Geronimus-type polynomials, *J. Comput. Appl. Math.* **21**, 133–144.
PRÉVOST, M. (1990a), Determinantal expression for partial Padé approximants, *Appl. Numer. Math.* **3**, 221–224.
PRÉVOST, M. (1990b), Cauchy product of distributions with applications to Padé approximants, Publication ANO 229, Université des Sciences et Technologies de Lille, May 1990.
RACHMANOV, E.A. (1977), Convergence of diagonal Padé approximants, *Math. USSR-Sb.* **33**, 243–260.
RUTISHAUSER, H. (1954), Der Quotienten-Differenzen-Algorithms, *Z. Angew. Math. Phys.* **5**, 233–251.
SABLONNIÈRE, P. (1983), A new family of Padé-type approximants, in $\mathbb{R}^n$, *J. Comput. Appl. Math.* **9**, 347–359.
SABLONNIÈRE, P. (1984), Padé-type approximants for multivariate series of functions, in: H. WERNER and H.J. BÜNGER, eds., *Padé Approximation and its Applications - Bad Honnef 1983*, Lecture Notes in Math. **1071** (Springer, Berlin) 238–251.
SADOK, H. (1988), *Accélération de la Convergence de Suites Vectorielles et Méthodes de Point Fixe*, Thesis, University of Lille I.
SAFF, E.B. (1972), An extension of Montessus De Ballore's theorem on the convergence of interpolating rational functions, *J. Approx. Theory* **6**, 63–67.
SAFF, E.B. and R.S. VARGA (1975), On the zeros and poles of Padé approximants to e^z, *Numer. Math.* **25**, 1–14.
SAFF, E.B. and R.S. VARGA (1976a), Zero-free parabolic regions for sequences of polynomials, *SIAM J. Math. Anal.* **7**, 344–357.
SAFF, E.B. and R.S. VARGA (1976b), On the sharpness of theorems concerning zero-free regions for certain sequences of polynomials, *Numer. Math.* **26**, 345–354.
SAFF, E.B. and R.S. VARGA (1976c), The behavior of the Padé table for the exponential, in: G.G. LORENTZ et al., eds., *Approximation Theory II* (Academic Press, New York) 519–531.
SAFF, E.B. and R.S. VARGA (1977), On the zeros and poles of Padé approximpants to e^z, II, in: E.B. SAFF and R.S. VARGA, eds., *Padé and Rational Approximation: Theory and Applications* (Academic Press, New York) 195–213.
SAFF, E.B. and R.S. VARGA (1978), On the zeros and poles of Padé approximants to e^z, III, *Numer. Math.* **30**, 241–266.
SAFF, E.B., R.S. VARGA and W.C. NI (1976), Geometric convergence of rational approximations to e^{-z} in infinite sectors, *Numer. Math.* **26**, 211–225.
SCHOENBERG, I.J. (1949), Sur la positivité des déterminants de translation des fonctions de fréquence de Pólya, *C. R. Acad. Sci. Paris* **228A**, 1996–1998.
SHAFER, R.E. (1974), On quadratic approximation, *SIAM J. Numer. Anal.* **11**, 447–460.
SHANKS, D. (1955), Nonlinear transformations of divergent and slowly convergent sequences, *J. Math. Phys.* **34**, 1–42 .

SHOHAT, J. (1938), Sur les polynômes orthogonaux généralisés, *C. R. Acad. Sci. Paris* **207**, 556–558.
SIDI, A. (1981), The Padé table and its connection with some weak exponential function approximations to Laplace transform inversion, in: M.G. DE BRUIN and H. VAN ROSSUM, eds., *Padé Approximation and its Applications. Amsterdam 1980*, Lecture Notes in Math. **888** (Springer, Berlin).
SIDI, A. and D.S. LUBINSKY (1983), Convergence of exponential interpolation for completely bounded functions, *J. Approx. Theory* **39**, 185–201.
SMITH, D.A., W.F. FORD and A. SIDI (1987), Extrapolation methods for vector sequences, *SIAM Rev.* **29**,199–233, correction, *SIAM Rev.* **30**, 623–624.
SNEDDON, I.N. (1972), *The Use of Integral Transforms* (Tata-McGraw-Hill, New York).
STAHL, H. (1985), Divergence of diagonal Padé approximants and the asymptotic behavior of orthogonal polynomials associated with non positive measures, *Constr. Approx.* **1**, 249–270.
STAHL, H. (1988), Asymptotics of Hermite–Padé polynomials and related convergence results, in: A. CUYT, ed., *Nonlinear Numerical Methods and Rational Approximation* (Reidel, Dordrecht) 23–65.
STAHL, H. (1989), On the convergence of generalized Padé approximants, *Constr. Approx.* **5**, 221–240.
SUETIN, S.P. (1985), On an inverse problem for the mth row of the Padé table, *Math. USSR-Sb.* **52**, 231–244.
SZÁSZ, O. (1921), Ein Grenzwertsatz über Potenzreihen, *Sitzungesber. Berlin Math. Gesel.* **21**, 25–29.
TREFETHEN, L.N. and M.H. GUTKNECHT (1987), Padé, stable Padé and Chebyshev–Padé approximation, in: J.C. MASON and M.G. COX, eds., *Algorithms for Approximation* (Clarendon Press, Oxford) 227–264.
VAN ASSCHE, W. (1987), *Asymptotics for Orthogonal Polynomials*, Lecture Notes in Math. **1265** (Springer, Berlin).
VAN DEN BERG, I. (1987), *Nonstandard Asymptotic Analysis*, Lecture Notes in Math. **1249** (Springer, Berlin).
VAN ISEGHEM, J. (1984), Padé-type approximants of $\exp(-z)$ whose denominators are $(1 + z/n)^n$, *Numer. Math.* **43**, 282–292.
VAN ISEGHEM, J. (1985), Vector Padé approximants, in: R. VICHNEVETSKY and J. VIGNES, eds., *Numerical Mathematics and Applications*, (North-Holland, Amsterdam) 73–77.
VAN ISEGHEM, J. (1986), An extended cross rule for vector Padé approximants, *Appl. Numer. Math.* **2**, 143–155.
VAN ISEGHEM, J. (1987a), Laplace transform inversion and Padé-type approximants, *Appl. Numer. Math.* **3** , 529–538.
VAN ISEGHEM, J. (1987b), *Approximants de Padé Vectoriels*, Thesis, University of Lille I.
VAN ISEGHEM, J. (1989), Convergence of the vector qd algorithm. Zeros of vector orthogonal polynomials, *J. Comput. Appl. Math.* **25**, 33–46.
VAN ROSSUM, H. (1953), *A Theory of Orthogonal Polynomials Based on the Padé Table*, Thesis, University of Utrecht (Van Gorcum, Assen).
VAN ROSSUM, H. (1980), Generalized Padé approximants, in: E.W. CHENEY, ed., *Approximation Theory III* (Academic Press, New York).
VAN ROSSUM, H. (1987), On the successive Padé remainders of $\exp(x)$, *J. Approx. Theory* **50**, 294–296.
VARGA, R.S. (1982), *Topics in Polynomial and Rational Interpolation and Approximation* (Les Presses de l'Université de Montréal, Montréal).
VAVILOV, V.V., G. LOPEZ, and V.A. PROKHOROV (1985), The poles of the mth row of the Padé table and the singular points of a function, *Math. USSR-Sb.* **50**, 457–463.
VICH, R. (1987), *z-Transform. Theory and Applications* (Reidel, Dordrecht).
VOROBYEV, Yu V. (1965), *Method of Moments in Applied Mathematics* (Gordon and Breach, New York).
WALL, H.S. (1948), *Analytic Theory of Continued Fractions* (Van Nostrand, New York).
WALLIN, H. (1974), The convergence of Padé approximants and the size of the power series coefficients, *Appl. Anal.* **4**, 235–251.

WALLIN, H. (1982), *Interpolation by Rational Functions with Free Poles in the Complex Plane*, Univ. of Umeå, **8**, Sweden.
WALLIN, H. (1987), The divergence problem for multipoint Padé approximants of meromorphic functions, *J. Comput. Appl. Math.* **19**, 61–68.
WALSH, J.L. (1969), *Interpolation and Approximation by Rational Functions in the Complex Domain*, Coll. Publ. XX (Amer. Math. Soc., Providence, RI).
WANNER, G. (1987), Order stars and stability, in: A. ISERLES and M.J.D. POWELL, eds., *The State of the Art in Numerical Analysis* (Clarendon Press, Oxford) 451–471.
WATSON, P.J.S. (1973), Algorithms for differentiation and integration, in: P.R. GRAVES-MORRIS, ed., *Padé Approximants and their Applications* (Academic Press, New York) 93–97.
WEISS, L. and R.N. McDONOUGH (1963), Prony's method, z-transforms, and Padé approximation, *SIAM Rev.* **5**, 145–149.
WERNER, H. and L. WUYTACK (1983), On the continuity of the Padé operator, *SIAM J. Numer. Anal.* **20**, 1273–1280.
WYNN, P. (1956), On a device for computing the $e_m(S_n)$ transformation, *MTAC* **10**, 91–96.
WYNN, P. (1966), Upon systems of recursions which obtain among the quotients of the Padé table, *Numer. Math.* **8**, 264–269.
WYNN, P. (1972), Upon a convergence result in the theory of the Padé table, *Trans. Amer. Math. Soc.* **165**, 239–249.

Subject Index

A-acceptability, 195
A-stability, 195
Adjacent families, 68
Aitken Δ^2 process, 74
Algebraic approximants, 168
Algebraic properties, 61
Associated continued fraction, 76
Associated polynomials, 66, 70

Biorthogonality, 68
Block structure, 57, 73
Borel transform, 200
Borel–Padé method, 200
Borel–Padé-type method, 200
Bromwich inversion formula, 206

Capacity, 122
Carleman condition, 114
Cauchy-type approximants, 157
Chebyshev polynomials, 161
Chisholm approximants, 182
Christoffel–Darboux identity, 66
Class S, 120
Compact operator, 104
Compact recursive projection algorithm, 172
Conjugate gradient method, 68, 91
Consistency property, 63
Continued fractions, 75, 156
Convergence in capacity, 121
Convergents, 76
Cordellier identity, 73
Corresponding continued fraction, 77
Cross rule, 73, 172
Cyclic limit points, 138

D-log approximants, 168
$1/d$-orthogonality, 171
Definite functional, 65
δ^2-process, 74

Determinantal formula, 61, 144, 145, 172, 182, 188
Diagonal sequence, 93, 109, 112, 128
Differential equations, 195
Digital filter, 200
Duality, 85

Entire function, 93, 102, 106
ε-algorithm, 74, 91
Error estimation, 77
Error formula, 60, 145
Euler series, 114
Euler–Minding identity, 68
Exponential function, 93, 193

Fabry theorem, 127
Favard theorem, 66
Formal Newton series, 151
Formal orthogonal polynomials, 60, 64
Fredholm equation, 89

g-polynomials, 187
Gaussian quadrature formula, 58
Generating function, 162
Generating polynomial, 132

Hakopian interpolation polynomial, 167, 186
Hankel determinant, 65, 68
Henrici transformation, 175
Homogeneous Padé approximants, 188
Homographic covariance, 63, 134

Integral approximants, 168
Interpolation polynomial, 58, 184, 186
Inverse Padé-type approximants, 149
Inverse problem, 126

Kergin interpolation polynomial, 186

Kronrod method, 78, 79

Laguerre polynomials, 198, 207
Lanczos method, 68, 91
Laplace transform, 203
Laplace transform inversion, 203
Linear functional, 57, 65, 67
Linear functional transformation, 164
Logarithmic capacity, 122
LR-algorithm, 70

Matrix formalism, 68
Meromorphic functions, 99, 117
Method of moments, 68, 88, 104
Minimal polynomial extrapolation, 175
Mittag–Leffler function, 107
Model reduction problem, 203
Moment problem, 111
Moments, 64, 88, 111
Monic orthogonal polynomials, 66
Montessus de Ballore, 99, 174, 190
Multiplication law, 161
Multipoint Padé approximant, 151
Multipoint Padé fraction, 156
Multivariate approximants, 180

Newton–Padé approximant, 152
Non-commutative case, 176
Non-definite functional, 65
Non-normal Padé table, 57, 73
Normal Padé table, 57
Nuttall formula, 63

Okada theorem, 136
Orthogonal projection, 91
Orthogonality relations, 60, 65

Padé approximants, 56
Padé table, 57
Padé-type approximants, 60, 131
    higher order, 133
Padé–Hermite approximants, 167
Padé ∘ Padé approximants, 189
Paradiagonal sequence, 93, 112
Partial Padé approximants, 140
Partial theta function, 109
Poincaré theorem, 127
Poles, 94
Pólya frequency series, 120, 194

Progressive sequence, 118
Projection method, 68, 91
Prony method, 202, 203

qd-algorithm, 69, 77, 173
Quadratic approximants, 168
Quadrature formula, 58
Quasi-monic polynomials, 178

R-function, 156
Radius of meromorphy, 126
Ray sequence, 116
Reciprocal series, 61
Recurrence relation, 66, 171
Recursive computation, 71
Recursive projection algorithm, 172
Rogers–Szegö polynomials, 107

Schrödinger equation, 53, 55
Sectorial sequence, 93, 122
Series of functions, 161
Shanks transformation, 74
Signal processing, 200
Simple operator, 104
Simultaneous approximation, 149, 169
Simultaneous partial Padé approximants, 150
Slow and smooth growth, 106
Stieltjes polynomials, 80
Stieltjes series, 110, 129, 142, 150
Stieltjes–Vitali theorem, 114
Subroutines, 74

Totally monotonic sequence, 194
Transfer function, 203

Unknown coefficients, 87

Vector ε-algorithm, 175
Vector orthogonal polynomials, 171
Vector Padé approximants, 169
Vector Padé-type approximants, 170
Vector qd-algorithm, 173

Wall of zeros, 117
Watson–Nevanlinna theorem, 199

z-transform, 200
Zero-free regions, 95, 194
Zeros of orthogonal polynomials, 68, 70, 112

Approximation and Interpolation Theory

Blagovest Sendov and Andrei Andreev

Institute of Mathematics
Bulgarian Academy of Sciences
Acad. G. Bonchev bl. 8
1113 Sofia, Bulgaria

Contents

PREFACE	227
CHAPTER I. Interpolation	229
1. Interpolation of functions	229
2. Lagrange's interpolation polynomial	232
3. Divided differences and Newton interpolation polynomial	234
4. Aitken's scheme	238
5. Finite differences	239
6. Interpolation polynomials with finite differences	241
7. Frazer's diagram (Lozenge diagram)	245
8. Utilization of the interpolation formulas	246
9. Inverse interpolation	247
10. The Hermite–Birkhoff interpolation problem (H–B problem)	248
11. The Abel–Gontcharov interpolation problem (A–G problem)	252
12. The Hermite interpolation problem (H problem)	254
13. The divided differences with repeating knots and Hermite interpolation	257
14. Interpolation by means of trigonometric polynomials	262
15. Interpolation of complex functions	266
16. Chakalov's approach for divided differences	270
17. Interpolation of functions of several variables	274
18. Multivariate Hermite interpolation	281
19. Convergence of the interpolation processes	284
20. The Lagrange interpolation process	284
21. Discrete Fourier transforms	289
22. Fast Fourier transforms (FFTs)	290
23. Applications of FFTs	295
CHAPTER II. Uniform Approximation	301
24. Uniform distance and best approximation	301
25. Characterization of the element of the best approximation	304
26. Uniqueness of the polynomial of the best uniform approximation	309
27. The uniform rational approximation	311
28. The Vallee-Poussin and Chebyshev theorems for rational functions	313
29. The possibility for approximation of continuous functions	316
30. Moduli of functions	317
30.1. Moduli of smoothness	318
30.2. Integral moduli	319
30.3. Averaged moduli	320
31. Approximation of functions by means of linear operators	323
32. Whitney's theorem	325
33. On the order of the uniform approximation by polynomials	333
34. Newman's results and approximation by means of rational functions	339

35. Chebyshev polynomials	342
36. Approximation of functions on a discrete point set	347
37. The discrete Remez algorithm	354
38. The second Remez algorithm	357
39. Remez algorithm—Multidimensional case	360
40. A second Remez algorithm for rational functions	365
41. The differential correction algorithm	367
42. Algorithms for rational approximation	372
43. Stability of numerical methods	374

CHAPTER III. Numerical Integration 381

44. Quadrature formulas	381
45. Optimal knots	386
46. An estimate of the error of quadrature formulas	392
47. Estimates for classical quadrature formulas	395
48. Quadrature formulas with restrictions	397
49. The Runge principle. Romberg's quadrature formulas	399
50. Integration of periodic functions	401
51. Obreshkov–Chakalov quadrature formulas	403
52. A concept for the best quadrature formulas	404
53. Monte Carlo methods	406
53.1. Convergence and error of the MC method	407
54. Ordinary and geometric MC methods for integrals	408
54.1. Ordinary MC method	408
54.2. Geometric MC method	409
55. Effective MC methods	410
55.1. Separation of the principal part	411
55.2. Symmetrization of the integrand	411
55.3. Important sampling method	412
56. MC methods with increased rate of convergence	412
57. Random interpolation quadrature formulas	414
58. Quasi-MC methods	416
59. MC methods for continual integrals, weight functions, splitting method	418
59.1. Continual integrals	418
59.2. Weight functions	420
59.3. Splitting method	421

CHAPTER IV. Hausdorff Approximation 423

60. Segment functions and Hausdorff distance	423
61. The metric space $\mathbb{F}_\Omega$ and H-distance in $\mathbb{A}_\Omega$	425
62. Relationships between the uniform distance and the Hausdorff distance	427
63. Convergence of sequences of positive operators	429
64. Approximation of periodic functions by positive integral operators	431
65. Approximation by partial sums of Fourier series	434
66. The best Hausdorff approximation	438
67. Universal estimates	442
68. Numerical methods for calculating the polynomial of best Hausdorff approximation	443
69. Multidimensional Hausdorff approximation	447

REFERENCES 451

SUBJECT INDEX 461

Preface

An important field of modern mathematics is approximation theory. The necessary of representing complicated mathematical objects by more simple ones arises in purely theoretical problems of mathematics, as well as in concrete methods of computation. Approximation theory is especially valuable not only as the base of numerical analysis, but also in control theory, mathematical programming and in other fields of mathematics and its application.

The goal of this article is to present together classical and recent results in interpolation and approximation of functions. Because the commonly used tools for approximation such as spline functions are subject of other articles in the project the main attention goes to polynomials and rational functions. Approximation by means of polynomials is the basis of almost all modern numerical methods, and in spite of the long history and big amount of theoretical results accumulated during the last 200 years significant theorems and algorithms were obtained in the last three decades. Here it is worthwhile mentioning the approximate properties of rational functions, see NEWMAN [1964] and POPOV [1977]. Briefly, rational functions are much more powerful for approximation of non-smooth functions, e.g. the function $|x|$ or functions with bounded variation.

The article consists of four chapters which are connected.

The first chapter considers the basic facts of interpolation in the one-dimensional case. Even in this "simple" case BIRKHOFF's [1906] general statement of a question is still open. In connection with the application of different interpolation polynomials in numerical methods a detailed representation is given of the main theorems and algorithms. The multidimensional case of interpolation by means of polynomials is also an open problem and there are no satisfactory theoretical results from a numerical point of view for the existence of an interpolation polynomial.

The fast Fourier transform (FFT) of COOLEY and TUKEY [1965] is a special case of interpolation with wide applications in techniques and a series of the best known algorithms (with respect to the number of arithmetic operations) follows after an appropriate use of FFT.

Uniform approximation of functions has several important points in its history:

– CHEBYSHEV [1857] proved his famous theorem for alternation and so he gave a full constructive characterization of the polynomial of the best uniform approximation;

– JACKSON [1911] obtained the rate of convergence for approximation of continuous functions by means of polynomials in uniform metric;

– REMEZ [1934] using Chebyshev's result proposed an efficient algorithm for iterative numerical determination of the polynomial of the best uniform approximation.

Together with such "pure" mathematical problems for existence, uniqueness and characterizations of the polynomials of the best approximation the rapid computer progress stimulates the investigations for obtaining robust and convenient numerical algorithms for their determination. The commonly used algorithms can be found in Chapter 2.

Parallel with classical modules of functions a new one is described—so-called averaged modules of smoothness. It seems that this modulus is deeply connected with a series of numerical methods and it is a natural tool for representation of the remainder terms of quadrature formulas, interpolation, methods for numerical integration of differential equations, etc.

Chapter 3 is divided into two parts:

– Newton–Cotes and Gauss quadrature formulas and their interesting generalization by CHAKALOV [1938]. A new approach for representation of the remainder term by means of the averaged modules of smoothness of the integrand;

– Monte-Carlo methods as a useful tool for multivariate numerical integration.

Hausdorff approximation of functions has a relatively short history starting with the basic paper of SENDOV [1962]. This distance does not generate normed space in the set of bounded functions and it requires special techniques and ideas. For example, the polynomial of the best Hausdorff approximation is not always unique and this fact shows that big difficulties arise in numerical methods for approximate determination of the best elements by means of polynomials or rational functions.

In any case, for bounded functions with points of discontinuities the Hausdorff metric gives natural criteria for proximity between the functions. The proposed numerical methods for determination of polynomial and rational functions of the best Hausdorff approximation are illustrated by a series of examples.

We are thankful to our colleagues, I. Dimov, P. Marinov and R. Georgiev, for their help and also to the Ministry of Education and Science in Bulgaria for the financial support—contract MM-27/91.

CHAPTER I

Interpolation

In this chapter the basic facts are considered in the field of interpolation theory of functions by means of polynomials. In spite of the fact that spline interpolation is widely used as an instrument for approximation of functions and numerical computations polynomials preserve their basic significant role in numerical methods. Side by side with classical results for interpolation polynomials the recent investigations are given.

Some new approaches for representation of the well-known divided differences (Section 16) and Newton interpolation polynomial (Section 6) are used and the problems connected with the convergence of the interpolation processes are discussed and illustrated by numerical examples in real (also multivariate) and complex case.

The Hermite–Birkhoff interpolation problem is a general case in the interpolation theory of functions. All kinds of interpolations by means of algebraic polynomials can be considered as special cases and therefore the theorems and ideas in Section 10 play an important role.

Fast Fourier transform (FFT) is the basis of many fast, efficient and optimal algorithms. The last three sections of this chapter offer an opportunity for a detailed acquaintance with the nature of FFT and its applications.

The formulas and the theorems, together with the numerical examples, can be used for practical goals and are a fast theoretical reference source as well.

1. Interpolation of functions

Let F be a set of functions and $l_0, l_1, \ldots, l_n$ be linear functionals, which are defined for every $f \in F$. Denote by F_n ($F_n \subset F$) an $n+1$ dimensional subset of F and let F_n be generated by the functions $\{\varphi_i\}_{i=0}^{N}$, i.e. $F_n = \{\varphi \in F: \varphi = a_0\varphi_0 + a_1\varphi_1 + \cdots + a_n\varphi_n\}$, where $a_0, a_1, \ldots, a_n$ are numbers.

The general interpolation problem can be formulated in the following way. For a given function $f \in F$ a function $\varphi \in F_n$ has to be found such that

$$l_i(\varphi) = l_i(f), \quad i = 0, 1, \ldots, n. \tag{1.1}$$

Since $\varphi = \sum_{i=0}^{n} a_i \varphi_i$ and because of the linearity of l_i the conditions (1.1) can be written as

$$l_i(\varphi) = l_i\left(\sum_{j=0}^{n} a_j \varphi_j\right) = \sum_{j=0}^{n} a_j l_i(\varphi_j) = l_i(f), \quad i = 0, 1, \ldots, n.$$

So, the general interpolation problem (1.1) has a solution if there exist $n+1$ numbers $\{a_i\}_{i=0}^{n}$ that satisfy the linear system of equations

$$\sum_{j=0}^{n} a_j l_i(\varphi_j) = l_i(f), \quad i = 0, 1, \ldots, n.$$

THEOREM 1.1. *The general interpolation problem* (1.1) *has a unique solution if the following condition is fulfilled:*

$$D = \begin{vmatrix} l_0(\varphi_0) & l_0(\varphi_1) & \cdots & l_0(\varphi_n) \\ l_1(\varphi_0) & l_1(\varphi_1) & \cdots & l_1(\varphi_n) \\ \vdots & \vdots & & \vdots \\ l_n(\varphi_0) & l_n(\varphi_1) & \cdots & l_n(\varphi_n) \end{vmatrix} \neq 0. \tag{1.2}$$

If the condition (1.2) holds then the solution can be found via Cramer's formulas in the form $\varphi = \sum_{i=0}^{n} \Delta_i \varphi_i / D$, where Δ_i is the determinant obtained from the determinant D by changing the ith column by the vector $(l_0(f), l_1(f), \ldots, l_n(f))$. The unique function $\varphi = \sum_{i=0}^{n} \Delta_i \varphi_i / D$ derived under the conditions (1.2) is called the generalized interpolation polynomial of the function f over the system $\{\varphi_i\}_{i=0}^{n}$.

Expanding the matrix Δ_i in the elements of the ith column

$$\Delta_i = \sum_{j=0}^{n} l_j(f) \Delta_{ji},$$

where Δ_{ji} are the cofactors of the elements of the ith column of D, it follows that

$$\varphi = \sum_{j=0}^{n} l_j(f) \Phi_j, \tag{1.3}$$

where the functions $\Phi_j = \sum_{i=0}^{n} \Delta_{ji} \varphi_i / D$ belong to F_n and do not depend on the function f. The formula (1.3) is usually called the Lagrange interpolation formula and Φ_j the basic Lagrange polynomials. They satisfy

$$l_i(\Phi_j) = \delta_{ij} = \begin{cases} 0, & i \neq j, \\ 1, & i = j. \end{cases}$$

Depending on the choice of the functions $\{\varphi_i\}_{i=0}^{n}$ and on the sequences of the functionals $\{l_i\}_{i=0}^{n}$ different interpolation problems can be defined.

REMARK 1.1. The above considerations relate to the case of linear interpolation. The more general approach is: for a given function f the approximate function φ has to be found in the form $\varphi(x; a_0, a_1, \ldots, a_n)$. Let the parameters $a_0, a_1, \ldots, a_n$ be determined by the conditions $f(x_i) = \varphi(x_i; a_0, a_1, \ldots, a_n)$, where $\{x_i\}_{i=0}^{n}$ are the points at which interpolation is carried out. Such a method for the approximation of f is called interpolation.

REMARK 1.2. The system of functions $\{\varphi_i\}_{i=0}^n$ is called Chebyshev's system on the set Δ if every function $\varphi = \sum_{i=0}^n a_i \varphi_i$ has at most n zeros in Δ, where a_i are arbitrary real numbers for which $\sum_{i=0}^n |a_i| > 0$. Usually φ is called a generalized polynomial over the functions $\{\varphi_i\}_{i=0}^n$. In the case when the linear functionals l_i in (1.1) are given by $l_i(f) = f(x_i)$, $i = 0, 1, \ldots, n$, the Theorem 1.1 takes the form

THEOREM 1.2. *A necessary and sufficient condition for the interpolation problem $\varphi(x_i) = f(x_i)$, $i = 0, 1, \ldots, n$, $\varphi = \sum_{i=0}^n a_i \varphi_i$ to have a unique solution for every function f defined on the set Δ and for every choice of the points $\{x_i\}_{i=0}^n$ ($x_i \in \Delta$, $x_i \neq x_j$ for $i \neq j$) is for the system $\{\varphi_i\}_{i=0}^n$ to be a Chebyshev system.*

PROOF. *Necessity.* Let the system of functions $\{\varphi_i\}_{i=0}^n$ not be a Chebyshev system on the set Δ. Then there exists a polynomial $P = \sum_{i=0}^n a_i \varphi_i$ that has $n + 1$ zeros $\{x_i\}_{i=0}^n$ in Δ, where a_i are real numbers such that $\sum_{i=0}^n |a_i| > 0$; i.e.

$$P(x_i) = \sum_{i=0}^n a_i \varphi_i(x_i) = 0, \quad i = 0, 1, \ldots, n. \tag{1.4}$$

It follows from (1.4) that

$$D = \begin{vmatrix} \varphi_0(x_0) & \varphi_1(x_0) & \cdots & \varphi_n(x_0) \\ \varphi_0(x_1) & \varphi_1(x_1) & \cdots & \varphi_n(x_1) \\ \vdots & \vdots & & \vdots \\ \varphi_0(x_n) & \varphi_1(x_n) & \cdots & \varphi_n(x_n) \end{vmatrix} = 0. \tag{1.5}$$

Hence there exists a function f and a selection of points $\{x_i\}_{i=0}^n$ for which the interpolation problem has no solution.

Sufficiency. Let the system of functions $\{\varphi_i\}_{i=0}^n$ be Chebyshev system on the set Δ. If for every choice of $n + 1$ different points the determinant D from (1.5) does not vanish, the theorem follows from Theorem 1.1.

Let us assume that there exist $n + 1$ different points $\{x_i\}_{i=0}^n$ in Δ for which $D = 0$. From $D = 0$ a linear dependence between the columns of D follows,

$$\sum_{j=0}^n b_j \varphi_j(x_i) = 0, \quad \sum_{j=0}^n |b_j| > 0, \quad i = 0, 1, \ldots, n.$$

Therefore the polynomial $\sum_{j=0}^n b_j \varphi_j$ has $n + 1$ zeros and this contradicts the assumption that $\{\varphi_i\}_{i=0}^n$ is a Chebyshev system. □

Some simple examples for the Chebyshev systems follow.

(a) The functions $1, x, x^2, \ldots, x^n$ form a Chebyshev system on every interval $[a, b]$. The same is true for the system $1, \exp(\alpha_1 x), \ldots, \exp(\alpha_n x)$ if $\alpha_i \neq \alpha_j$ for $i \neq j$;

(b) The functions $1, \sin x, \cos x, \sin 2x, \cos 2x, \ldots, \sin nx, \cos nx$ form a Chebyshev system on every interval $(a, a + 2\pi]$ or $[a, a + 2\pi)$;

(c) If $\{\varphi_i\}_{i=0}^n$ is a Chebyshev system then $\{p\varphi_i\}_{i=0}^n$ is also such a system for every positive function p.

For Chebyshev systems see KARLIN and STUDDEN [1966].

2. Lagrange's interpolation polynomial

The algebraic polynomial of nth degree

$$L_n(f; x) = \sum_{i=0}^{n} f(x_i) \frac{(x - x_0) \cdots (x - x_{i-1})(x - x_{i+1}) \cdots (x - x_n)}{(x_i - x_1) \cdots (x_i - x_{i-1})(x_i - x_{i+1}) \cdots (x_i - x_n)} \quad (2.1)$$

satisfies the conditions $L_n(f; x_i) = f(x_i)$, $i = 0, 1, \ldots, n$. This polynomial exists for every function f when the points of interpolation satisfy $x_i \neq x_j$ for $i \neq j$— LAGRANGE ([1795], p. 286). The formula (2.1) can be represented as

$$L_n(f; x) = \sum_{i=0}^{n} f(x_i) \frac{\omega(x)}{(x - x_i)\omega'(x_i)}, \quad \omega(x) = \prod_{i=0}^{n} (x - x_i). \quad (2.2)$$

The polynomials of nth degree

$$L_{n,i}(x) = \frac{\omega(x)}{(x - x_i)\omega'(x_i)}$$

are called the basic Lagrange polynomials constructed on the points $\{x_i\}_{i=0}^{n}$ and they satisfy

$$L_{n,i}(x_j) = \delta_{ij} = \begin{cases} 0, & i \neq j, \\ 1, & i = j. \end{cases}$$

The polynomial L_n can be used as an approximation of the function f, i.e. $f(x) = L_n(f; x) + R_n(f; x)$, where $R_n(f; x)$ is the remainder term. For a given function $f \in C^{n+1}$ and points $\{x_i\}_{i=0}^{n}$, CAUCHY ([1840], p. 409), R_n is represented in the form

$$R_n(f; x) = f^{(n+1)}(\xi) \frac{\omega(x)}{(n + 1)!}, \quad (2.3)$$

where $\min\{\min_{0 \leq i \leq n} x_i, x\} \leq \xi \leq \max\{\max_{0 \leq i \leq n} x_i, x\}$.

Because of the fact that the derivative $f^{(n+1)}$ is, as a rule, an unknown function, one approach for the minimization of R_n in (2.3) is the minimization of ω. Supposing that the knots $\{x_i\}_{i=0}^{n}$ lie in the interval $[a, b]$ then the problem consists of the minimization of

$$\max_{a \leq x \leq b} \left| \prod_{i=0}^{n} (x - x_i) \right| = \max_{a \leq x \leq b} \left| x^{n+1} + \sum_{k=0}^{n} a_k x^k \right|;$$

i.e. a polynomial $C_{n+1}(x) = x^{n+1} + \sum_{k=0}^{n} a_k x^k$ of $(n + 1)$th degree that deviates from zero in the interval $[a, b]$ at least has to be found.

THEOREM 2.1. *Let the knots*

$$x_i = \frac{1}{2}\left((b - a)\cos\frac{2i + 1}{2n + 2}\pi + a + b\right), \quad i = 0, 1, \ldots, n,$$

be the zeros of the $(n + 1)$th Chebyshev polynomial in the interval $[a, b]$. Then

$$\min_{a \leq t_i \leq b} \max_{a \leq x \leq b} \left| \prod_{i=0}^{n} (x - t_i) \right| = \max_{a \leq x \leq b} \left| \prod_{i=0}^{n} (x - x_i) \right| = \frac{(b - a)^{n+1}}{2^{2n+1}} = r_n. \quad (2.4)$$

PROOF. The proof of this theorem follows immediately from the results in Section 35. □

Let us compare the error of the commonly used type of interpolation over equidistant points with the estimation (2.4) for the interval $[-1, 1]$. Here

$$r'_n = \max_{-1 \leq x \leq 1} \left| \prod_{i=0}^{n} \left(x - \frac{2i-n}{n} \right) \right| \geq \left| \prod_{i=0}^{n} \left(1 - \frac{1}{n} - \frac{2i-n}{n} \right) \right|$$

$$= \left(2 - \frac{1}{n} \right) \left(2 - \frac{3}{n} \right) \left(2 - \frac{5}{n} \right) \cdots \frac{3}{n} \frac{1}{n} \frac{1}{n} = \frac{(2n)!}{n! n^{n+1} 2^n},$$

and using Stirling's formula $n! = n^n e^{-n} \sqrt{2\pi n} \exp(\vartheta_n / 12n)$, $0 < \vartheta_n < 1$, then

$$r'_n \geq \frac{(2n)^{2n} e^{-2n} \sqrt{4\pi n}}{n^n e^{-n+1} \sqrt{2\pi n} n^{n+1} 2^n} \geq \frac{3}{n} \left(\frac{2}{e} \right)^n.$$

Compare r_n from (2.4) for the interval $[-1, 1]$ and the lower estimate for r'_n. Then

$$r'_n \geq \frac{3}{n} \left(\frac{4}{e} \right)^n r_n.$$

The fact that

$$\lim_{n \to \infty} \frac{3}{n} \left(\frac{4}{e} \right)^n = \infty$$

shows the advantage of the selection of the interpolation knots as the roots of the Chebyshev polynomials. For instance $r'_{20} \geq 3700$.

REMARK 2.1. The representation (2.2) is a particular case of (1.3) when

$$l_i(f) = f(x_i), \quad \Phi_i(x) = \frac{\omega(x)}{(x - x_i)\omega'(x_i)}, \quad \varphi_i(x) = x^i, \quad i = 0, 1, \ldots, n.$$

REMARK 2.2. In the case of equidistant knots when $x_i = x_0 + ih$, $h > 0$, the formula (2.2) takes the form

$$L_n(f; x) = L_n(f; x_0 + th) = \frac{t(t-1)\cdots(t-n)}{n!} \sum_{i=0}^{n} (-1)^{n+i} \binom{n}{i} \frac{f(x_i)}{t-i}. \quad (2.5)$$

The coefficients in front of $f(x_i)$ in (2.5) do not depend on the step h or on the function f. These coefficients are tabulated in so-called Lagrange coefficient tables.

Using equidistant knots, the quantity

$$\omega(x) = \omega(x_0 + th) = h^{n+1} t(t-1) \cdots (t-n),$$

involved in the remainder term (2.3) and its behavior play an important role.

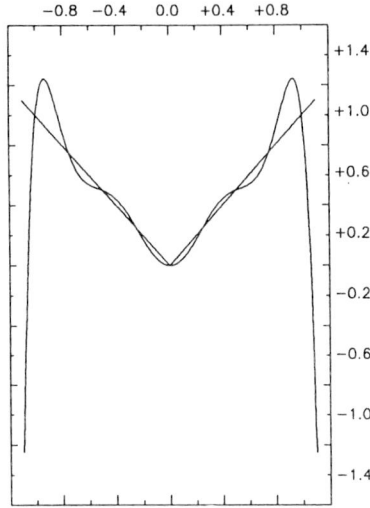

Fig. 2.1. The graphs of the function $|x|$ and its interpolation polynomial L_8.

The function $\varphi(t) = t(t-1)\cdots(t-n)$ is an even (odd) function in respect to the point $n/2$ depending on n. This follows from $\varphi(t) = (-1)^{n+1}\varphi(n-t)$. The equality $\varphi(t+1) = (t+1)/(t-n)\varphi(t)$ shows that the values of the function φ in the interval $[i, i+1]$ are the values of φ in the previous interval $[i-1, i]$ multiplied by $(t+1)/(t-n)$. Because of $|(t+1)/(t-n)| < 1$ for $0 \le t < (n-1)/2$ the extremal values of $|\varphi|$ decrease from 0 to $n/2$. Outside of the interval $[0, n]$ the function $|\varphi|$ increases quickly. The conclusions that can be derived are the following.

(a) $|R_n(f;x)|$ is smaller if x lies in the middle of the interpolation interval.

(b) For so-called extrapolation, when $x \notin [x_0, x_n]$ the absolute value of the remainder term $R_n(f;x)$ can be too large. In Fig. 2.1 the graphs of the function $|x|$ and its interpolation polynomial L_8 are given in the interval $[-1.1, 1.1]$. The polynomial L_8 coincides with $|x|$ at the points $x_i = -1 + i/4$, $i = 0, 1, \ldots, 8$, and it is evident that L_8 does not approximate $|x|$ outside of the interval $[-1, 1]$.

3. Divided differences and Newton interpolation polynomial

If the function f is defined at the points $\{x_i\}_{i=0}^{\infty}$, the ratio

$$f(x_i; x_{i+1}; \ldots; x_{i+k+1}) = \frac{f(x_{i+1}; \ldots; x_{i+k+1}) - f(x_i; \ldots; x_{i+k})}{x_{i+k+1} - x_i}$$

is the divided difference of $(k+1)$th degree defined recursively by the divided differences of the kth degree. The table of divided differences of f is

Interpolation

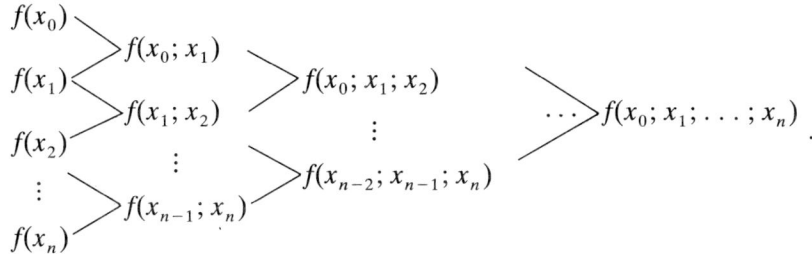

The main properties of the divided differences are as follows.

(a) $f(x_i; \ldots ; x_{i+k}) = \sum_{j=i}^{i+k} f(x_j)/\omega'_{i,k}(x_j)$, $\omega_{i,k}(x) = \prod_{j=i}^{i+k} (x - x_j)$;

the proof follows immediately by induction on k.

(b) If $f(x) = \alpha g(x) + \beta \varphi(x)$, α and β are real numbers, then

$$f(x_i; \ldots ; x_{i+k}) = \alpha g(x_i; \ldots ; x_{i+k}) + \beta \varphi(x_i; \ldots ; x_{i+k}).$$

(c) The divided difference is a symmetric function of the arguments, e.g.

$$f(x_i; x_{i+1}; \ldots ; x_{i+k}) = f(x_{i+1}; x_i; \ldots ; x_{i+k}) = \cdots$$
$$= f(x_i; \ldots ; x_{i+k-1}; x_{i+k}).$$

This property follows from (a).

(d) If $f(x) = x^n$ then

$$f(x_i; \ldots ; x_{i+k}) = \begin{cases} 0, & k > n, \\ 1, & k = n, \\ \sum_{\alpha_0 + \cdots + \alpha_k = n-k} x_i^{\alpha_0} x_{i+1}^{\alpha_1} \cdots x_{i+k}^{\alpha_k}, & k < n. \end{cases}$$

PROOF OF (d). By induction. For the differences of first order (d) is true because

$$f(x_i; x_{i+1}) = \frac{x_{i+1}^n - x_i^n}{x_{i+1} - x_i} = x_{i+1}^{n-1} + x_{i+1}^{n-2} x_i + \cdots + x_i^{n-1}.$$

Let us assume that

$$f(x_i; \ldots ; x_{i+k}) = \sum_{\alpha_0 + \cdots + \alpha_k = n-k} x_i^{\alpha_0} x_{i+1}^{\alpha_1} \cdots x_{i+k}^{\alpha_k}.$$

Then

$$f(x_i; x_{i+1}; \ldots ; x_{i+k+1}) = \frac{f(x_{i+1}; \ldots ; x_{i+k+1}) - f(x_i; \ldots ; x_{i+k})}{x_{i+k+1} - x_i}$$

$$= \frac{\sum_{\alpha_0 + \cdots + \alpha_k = n-k} x_{i+1}^{\alpha_0} x_{i+2}^{\alpha_1} \cdots x_{i+k+1}^{\alpha_k} - \sum_{\alpha_0 + \cdots + \alpha_k = n-k} x_i^{\alpha_0} x_{i+1}^{\alpha_1} \cdots x_{i+k}^{\alpha_k}}{x_{i+k+1} - x_i}$$

$$= \frac{\sum_{\alpha_0+\cdots+\alpha_k=n-k} x_{i+k+1}^{\alpha_0} x_{i+1}^{\alpha_1} \cdots x_{i+k+1}^{\alpha_k} - \sum_{\alpha_0+\cdots+\alpha_k=n-k} x_i^{\alpha_0} x_{i+1}^{\alpha_1} \cdots x_{i+k}^{\alpha_k}}{x_{i+k+1} - x_i}$$

$$= \sum_{\alpha_0+\cdots+\alpha_k=n-k} x_{i+1}^{\alpha_1} \cdots x_{i+k}^{\alpha_k} \frac{x_{i+k+1}^{\alpha_0} - x_i^{\alpha_0}}{x_{i+k+1} - x_i}$$

$$= \sum_{\beta_0+\cdots+\beta_{k+1}=n-k-1} x_i^{\beta_0} x_{i+1}^{\beta_1} \cdots x_{i+k+1}^{\beta_{k+1}}. \qquad \square$$

(e) If $f \in C^k$ then

$$f(x_i; x_{i+1}; \ldots; x_{i+k})$$

$$= \int_0^1 \left\{ \int_0^{t_1} \left[\cdots \int_0^{t_{k-1}} f^{(k)}\left(x_i + \sum_{j=i+1}^{i+k} t_{j-1}(x_j - x_{j-1}) \right) dt_k \cdots \right] dt_2 \right\} dt_1.$$

PROOF OF (e). By induction. When $k = 1$, $\int_0^1 f'(x_i + t_1(x_{i+1} - x_i)) dt_1 = f(x_i; x_{i+1})$. Assuming that the assertion holds for k, then

$$\int_0^1 \left\{ \int_0^{t_1} \left[\cdots \int_0^{t_k} f^{(k+1)}\left(x_i + \sum_{j=i+1}^{i+k+1} t_{j-1}(x_j - x_{j-1}) \right) dt_{k+1} \cdots \right] dt_2 \right\} dt_1$$

$$= \frac{1}{x_{i+k+1} - x_{i+k}} \int_0^1 \left\{ \int_0^{t_1} \left[\cdots \int_0^{t_{k-1}} f^{(k)}(x_i + t_1(x_{i+1} - x_i) \right.\right.$$

$$+ \cdots + t_k(x_{i+k} - x_{i+k-1}) + t_k(x_{i+k+1} - x_{i+k})) - f^{(k)}(x_i + t_1(x_{i+1} - x_i)$$

$$\left.\left. + \cdots + t_k(x_{i+k} - x_{i+k-1})) dt_k \cdots \right] dt_2 \right\} dt_1$$

$$= \frac{1}{x_{i+k+1} - x_{i+k}} [f(x_i; x_{i+1}; \ldots; x_{i+k-1}; x_{i+k+1}) - f(x_i; \ldots; x_{i+k})]$$

$$= \frac{1}{x_{i+k+1} - x_{i+k}} [f(x_{i+k+1}; x_i; x_{i+1}; \ldots; x_{i+k-1}) - f(x_i; \ldots; x_{i+k})]$$

$$= f(x_i; x_{i+1}; \ldots; x_{i+k+1}). \qquad \square$$

(f) If $f \in C^k$ then

$$f(x_i; x_{i+1}; \ldots; x_{i+k}) = f^{(k)}(\xi)/k!,$$

where $\min_{i \leq j \leq i+k} x_j \leq \xi \leq \max_{i \leq j \leq i+k} x_j$. The proof follows immediately from the representations (2.3) and (3.2) of the remainder term of the interpolation polynomial.

(g) $f(x_i; x_{i+1}; \ldots; x_{i+k}) = \dfrac{\begin{vmatrix} 1 & x_i & \cdots & x_i^{k-1} & f(x_i) \\ 1 & x_{i+1} & \cdots & x_{i+1}^{k-1} & f(x_{i+1}) \\ \vdots & \vdots & & \vdots & \vdots \\ 1 & x_{i+k} & \cdots & x_{i+k}^{k-1} & f(x_{i+k}) \end{vmatrix}}{\begin{vmatrix} 1 & x_i & \cdots & x_i^{k-1} & x_i^k \\ 1 & x_{i+1} & \cdots & x_{i+1}^{k-1} & x_{i+1}^k \\ \vdots & \vdots & & \vdots & \vdots \\ 1 & x_{i+k} & \cdots & x_{i+k}^{k-1} & x_{i+k}^k \end{vmatrix}}.$

PROOF OF (g). Without loss of generality the proof will be given for the points $x_0, x_1, \ldots, x_n$. If the polynomial L_n from (3.1) is written in the form $L_n(f; x) = \sum_{s=0}^{n} a_s x^s$, then from the interpolation conditions we have that $L_n(f; x_i) = f(x_i)$, $i = 0, 1, \ldots, n$. The coefficient a_n is the factor of x^n. It means that $a_n = f(x_0; x_1; \ldots; x_n)$. The property (g) follows by the determination of a_n via Cramer's formulas from the linear system

$$\sum_{s=0}^{n} a_s x_i^s = f(x_i), \quad i = 0, 1, \ldots, n. \qquad \square$$

THEOREM 3.1. *The interpolation polynomial* (2.1) *can be written as*

$$L_n(f; x) = f(x_0) + (x - x_0)f(x_0; x_1) + (x - x_0)(x - x_1)f(x_0; x_1; x_2)$$
$$+ \cdots + (x - x_0)(x - x_1)\cdots(x - x_{n-1})f(x_0; x_1; \ldots; x_n), \quad (3.1)$$

and the remainder term in (2.3) R_n *takes the form*

$$R_n(f; x) = (x - x_0)(x - x_1)\cdots(x - x_n)f(x; x_0; x_1; \ldots; x_n). \quad (3.2)$$

PROOF. If L_k is Lagrange interpolation polynomial for the function f on the points $x_0, x_1, \ldots, x_k$, then $L_n = L_0 + (L_1 - L_0) + \cdots + (L_n - L_{n-1})$. The difference $L_k - L_{k-1}$ is an algebraic polynomial of degree k that vanishes at the points $x_0, x_1, \ldots, x_{k-1}$. Therefore

$$L_k(f; x) - L_{k-1}(f; x) = A_k(x - x_0)(x - x_1)\cdots(x - x_{k-1})$$

and

$$f(x_k) - L_{k-1}(f; x_k) = A_k(x_k - x_0)(x_k - x_1)\cdots(x_k - x_{k-1}).$$

Finally

$$A_k = \dfrac{f(x_k)}{(x_k - x_0)\cdots(x_k - x_{k-1})} - \dfrac{1}{(x_k - x_0)\cdots(x_k - x_{k-1})}$$
$$\times \sum_{i=0}^{k-1} f(x_i) \dfrac{\omega(x_k)}{(x_k - x_i)\omega'(x_i)}$$
$$= \sum_{i=0}^{k} f(x_i)/\omega_k'(x_i) = f(x_0; x_1; \ldots; x_k), \quad \text{where } \omega_k(x) = \prod_{i=0}^{k}(x - x_i).$$

The representation (3.1) is proved. For the error $f(x) - L_n(f; x)$ let us consider

$$f(x; x_0; x_1; \ldots; x_n) = \frac{f(x)}{(x - x_0)(x - x_1) \cdots (x - x_n)}$$

$$+ \frac{f(x_0)}{(x_0 - x)(x_0 - x_1) \cdots (x_0 - x_n)}$$

$$+ \cdots + \frac{f(x_n)}{(x_n - x)(x_n - x_0) \cdots (x_n - x_{n-1})}.$$

From here

$$f(x) = \sum_{i=0}^{n} f(x_i) \frac{(x - x_0) \cdots (x - x_{i-1})(x - x_{i+1}) \cdots (x - x_n)}{(x_i - x_1) \cdots (x_i - x_{i-1})(x_i - x_{i+1}) \cdots (x_i - x_n)}$$

$$+ (x - x_0)(x - x_1) \cdots (x - x_n) f(x; x_0; x_1; \ldots; x_n)$$

$$= L_n(f; x) + R_n(f; x). \qquad \square$$

The representation (3.1) is called the Newton interpolation polynomial and the advantage of (3.1) for (2.1) is that by adding additional points it is not necessary to compute all the terms again.

4. Aitken's scheme

Let $L_{(k,l)}(f)$ be an algebraic polynomial of degree $l - k$ that satisfies $L_{(k,l)}(f; x_i) = f(x_i)$, $i = k, k+1, \ldots, l$. Then

$$L_{(k,l+1)}(f; x) = \frac{L_{(k+1,l+1)}(f; x)(x - x_k) - L_{(k,l)}(f; x)(x - x_{l+1})}{x_{l+1} - x_k}.$$

Aitken's scheme which was devised by AITKEN [1932] and NEVILLE [1934] for the computation of $L_{(0,n)}(f; x)$ at the point x makes use of the above identity to fill Table 4.1.

TABLE 4.1.

$L_{(0,0)}(f; x)$				
	$L_{(0,1)}(f; x)$			
$L_{(1,1)}(f; x)$		$L_{(0,2)}(f; x)$		
	$L_{(1,2)}(f; x)$			
$L_{(2,2)}(f; x)$		$\vdots$	$\cdots$	$L_{(0,n)}(f; x)$
	$\vdots$	$L_{(n-2,n)}(f; x)$		
$\vdots$	$L_{(n-1,n)}(f; x)$			
$L_{(n,n)}(f; x)$				

A practical application of Aitken's scheme is given in BACHVALOV, JIDKOV and KOBELKOV ([1987], p. 46). Let x be a fixed point and the points $\{x_i\}_{i=0}^n$ be renumbered in increasing order of $|x - x_i|$. From

$$f(x) - L_{(0,m)}(f; x) = f(x; x_0; \ldots ; x_m) \prod_{i=0}^{m} (x - x_i)$$

and

$$L_{(0,m+1)}(f; x) - L_{(0,m)}(f; x) = f(x_0; \ldots ; x_m) \prod_{i=0}^{m} (x - x_i),$$

under the assumption that $|x - x_i|$ is a small number, it follows that

$$f(x; x_0; \ldots ; x_m) \approx \frac{f^{(m+1)}(x)}{(m+1)!} \approx f(x_0; \ldots ; x_{m+1}).$$

From here

$$f(x) - L_{(0,m)}(f; x) \approx L_{(0,m+1)}(f; x) - L_{(0,m)}(f; x).$$

So $\varepsilon_m = |L_{(0,m+1)}(f; x) - L_{(0,m)}(f; x)|$ can be taken as a measure of the proximity between f and $L_{(0,m)}(f; x)$. Computing successively $L_{(0,0)}(f; x)$, ε_0, $L_{(0,1)}(f; x)$, ε_1, ..., ε_{m_0} has to be found such that $\varepsilon_{m_0} = \min_m \varepsilon_m$ and $f(x) \approx L_{(0,m_0)}(f; x)$.

5. Finite differences

Let the function f be defined at the points $\{x_i\}_{i=0}^n$ that form an equidistant set of points with a step size of h, e.g. $x_i = x_0 + ih$, $i = 0, 1, \ldots, n$, and let f_i denote $f_i = f(x_0 + ih)$. The numbers $\Delta f_i = f_{i+1} - f_i$, $i = 0, 1, \ldots, n-1$, are called forward finite differences of the first order. Inductively, forward finite differences of order $k+1$ are determined by

$$\Delta^{k+1} f_i = \Delta^k f_{i+1} - \Delta^k f_i, \quad k = 0, 1, \ldots. \tag{5.1}$$

Another notation is also used for finite differences:

$$\Delta f_i = \nabla f_{i+1} = \delta f_{i+1/2} = f^1_{i+1/2} = f_{i+1} - f_i,$$

$$\nabla^{k+1} f_i = \nabla^k f_i - \nabla^k f_{i-1},$$

$$\delta^{k+1} f_i = \delta^k f_{i+1/2} - \delta^k f_{i-1/2},$$

$$f_i^{k+1} = f^k_{i+1/2} - f^k_{i-1/2},$$

where $\nabla^k f_i$ is the backward finite difference, and $\delta^k f_i$ or f_i^k is the central finite difference.

For a function f that is defined at the points $\{x_i\}_{i=0}^n$ its finite differences can be arranged in the so-called finite-difference table (Table 5.1).

TABLE 5.1. The finite-difference table.

Table of forward finite differences	Table of backward finite differences

$f_0, f_1, f_2, \ldots, f_n$ with forward differences $\Delta f_0, \Delta f_1, \ldots, \Delta f_{n-1}$; $\Delta^2 f_0, \ldots, \Delta^2 f_{n-2}$; $\ldots$; $\Delta^n f_0$.

$f_0, f_1, f_2, \ldots, f_n$ with backward differences $\nabla f_1, \nabla f_2, \ldots, \nabla f_n$; $\nabla^2 f_2, \ldots, \nabla^2 f_n$; $\ldots$; $\nabla^n f_n$.

$f_0, f_1, f_2, \ldots, f_n$ with $f^1_{1/2}, f^1_{3/2}, \ldots, f^1_{n-1/2}$; $f^2_1, \ldots, f^2_{n-1}$; $\ldots$; $f^n_{n/2}$.

The main properties of the finite differences are as follows.

(a) $\Delta^k f_i = \sum_{j=0}^{k} (-1)^{k+j} \binom{k}{j} f_{i+j}$.

The proof is trivial by induction using the identity

$$\binom{l}{k+1} + \binom{l}{k} = \binom{l+1}{k+1}.$$

(b) $\nabla^k f_i = \Delta^k f_{i-k}$, $f^k_i = \Delta^k f_{i-k/2}$, $\Delta^k f_i = f^k_{i+k/2}$.

(c) $\Delta^k f_i = h^k k! f(x_i; x_{i+1}; \ldots; x_{i+k})$.

PROOF OF (c). By induction. For $k = 0$ the assumption is true. Let us assume that it is true for k. Then

$$f(x_i; x_{i+1}; \ldots; x_{i+k+1}) = \frac{f(x_{i+1}; \ldots; x_{i+k+1}) - f(x_i; \ldots; x_{i+k})}{x_{i+k+1} - x_i}$$

$$= \frac{1}{(k+1)h} \left(\frac{\Delta^k f_{i+1}}{k! h^k} + \frac{\Delta^k f_i}{k! h^k} \right) = \frac{\Delta^{k+1} f_i}{(k+1)! h^{k+1}}. \qquad \square$$

(d) If $f(x) = \alpha g(x) + \beta \varphi(x)$, α and β are real numbers, then

$$\Delta^k f_i = \alpha \Delta^k g_i + \beta \Delta^k \varphi_i;$$

(e) $\Delta^k f_i = \int_0^h \cdots \int_0^h f^{(k)}(x_1 + t_1 + \cdots + t_k) \, dt_1 \cdots dt_k$. The proof is by simple induction on k.

(f) If $f \in C^k$ then $\Delta^k f_i = h^k f^{(k)}(\xi)$, where $\xi \in [x_i, x_i + kh]$. This property is a consequence of (e).

6. Interpolation polynomials with finite differences

The sequence of points $\{x_i\}_{i=0}^{\infty}$ is called regular with a step size of h if
$$\max_{0 \leq i \leq k} x_i - \min_{0 \leq i \leq k} x_i = kh, \quad k = 1, 2, \ldots.$$

THEOREM 6.1. *Let $\{x_i\}_{i=0}^{\infty}$ be a regular sequence of points with a step size of h and*
$$m_k = (x_0 - \min_{0 \leq i \leq k} x_i)/h, \quad k = 0, 1, \ldots.$$

The interpolation polynomial (2.1) of the function f at the points $\{x_i\}_{i=0}^n$ can be written as
$$L_n(f; x) = \sum_{k=0}^{n} \binom{t + m_{k-1}}{k} \Delta^k f_{-m_k}, \tag{6.1}$$

where $t = (x - x_0)/h$ and $\Delta^k f_{-m_k} = \Delta^k f(x_0 - m_k h)$.

PROOF. Since $\{x_i\}_{i=0}^{\infty}$ is a regular sequence of points then the points $x_0, x_1, \ldots, x_{k-1}$, up to reordering are the points $x_0 - m_{k-1}h$, $x_0 - (m_{k-1} - 1)h, \ldots, x_0 - (m_{k-1} - k + 1)h$. The theorem follows from (3.1),
$$(x - x_0)(x - x_1) \cdots (x - x_k)$$
$$= (x - x_0 + m_{k-1}h)[x - x_0 + (m_{k-1} - 1)h] \cdots [x - x_0 + (m_{k-1} - k + 1)h]$$
$$= h^k(t + m_{k-1})(t + m_{k-1} - 1)(t + m_{k-1} - k + 1) = k!h^k \binom{t + m_{k-1}}{k}$$

and
$$f(x_0; x_1; \ldots; x_k) = f(x_0 - m_k h; x_0 - (m_k - 1)h; \ldots; x_0 - (m_k - k + 1)h)$$
$$= \Delta^k f_{-m_k}/k!h^k. \quad \square$$

As a consequence of Theorem 6.1 a series of interpolation formulas can be obtained.

(1) The *Newton forward* interpolation formula. This formula corresponds to the regular sequence $\{x_i\}_{i=0}^n$, $x_k = x_0 + kh$, $k = 1, 2, \ldots, n$. For this sequence $m_k = 0$ and (6.1) takes the form
$$L_n(f; x) = \sum_{k=0}^{n} \binom{t}{k} \Delta^k f_0.$$

(2) The *Newton backward* interpolation formula. Here the regular sequence of points is $\{x_i\}_{i=0}^n$, $x_k = x_0 - kh$, $k = 1, 2, \ldots, n$, and $m_k = k$. The formula (6.1) turns into

$$L_n(f; x) = \sum_{k=0}^n \binom{t+k-1}{k} \Delta^k f_{-k}.$$

(3) The *Gauss forward* interpolation formula corresponds to the regular sequence

$$\{x_i\}_{i=0}^n, \quad x_i = x_0 + (-1)^{i+1}\left(\left[\frac{i-1}{2}\right] + 1\right)h,$$

i.e.

$$x_0, \ x_0 + h, \ x_0 - h, \ x_0 + 2h, \ x_0 - 2h, \ldots,$$
$$x_0 + (-1)^{n+1}([n-1)/2] + 1)h. \tag{6.2}$$

In view of the fact that for this sequence $m_k = [k/2]$ the polynomial from (6.1) is

$$L_n(f; x) = \sum_{k=0}^n \binom{t + [(k-1)/2]}{k} \Delta^k f_{-[k/2]}$$

$$= f_0 + \binom{t}{1} \Delta f_0 + \binom{t}{2} \Delta^2 f_{-1} + \binom{t+1}{3} \Delta^3 f_{-1}$$

$$+ \cdots + \binom{t + [(n-1)/2]}{n} \Delta^n f_{-[n/2]}. \tag{6.3}$$

(4) The *Gauss backward* interpolation polynomial utilizes the regular sequence

$$\{x_i\}_{i=0}^n, \quad x_i = x_0 + (-1)^i\left(\left[\frac{i-1}{2}\right] + 1\right)h,$$
$$x_0, \ x_0 - h, \ x_0 + h, \ x_0 - 2h, \ x_0 + 2h, \ldots,$$
$$x_0 + (-1)^n([(n-1)/2] + 1)h,$$

and taking into account that for this sequence $m_k = [(k+1)/2]$ the polynomial from (6.1) is

$$L_n(f; x) = \sum_{k=0}^n \binom{t + [k/2]}{k} \Delta^k f_{-[(k+1)/2]}$$

$$= f_0 + \binom{t}{1} \Delta f_{-1} + \binom{t+1}{2} \Delta^2 f_{-1} + \binom{t+1}{3} \Delta^3 f_{-2}$$

$$+ \cdots + \binom{t + [n/2]}{n} \Delta^n f_{-[(n+1)/2]}. \tag{6.4}$$

(5) The *Stirling* interpolation polynomial for the function f is a halfsum of the polynomials given by (6.3) and (6.4),

$$L_n(f;x) = f_0 + \frac{1}{2}\binom{t}{1}(\Delta f_{-1} + \Delta f_0) + \frac{1}{2}\left\{\binom{t}{2} + \binom{t+1}{2}\right\}\Delta^2 f_{-1}$$

$$+ \frac{1}{2}\binom{t+1}{3}(\Delta^3 f_{-2} + \Delta^3 f_{-1}) + \cdots$$

$$+ \frac{1}{2}\left\{\left[\begin{array}{c}t + [(n-1)/2]\\n\end{array}\right]\Delta^n f_{-[n/2]}\right.$$

$$\left. + \binom{t + [n/2]}{n}\Delta^n f_{-[(n+1)/2]}\right\},$$

and passing on to central finite differences with the notation

$$\tilde{f}_0^{2n-1} = \tfrac{1}{2}\{f_{-1/2}^{2n-1} + f_{1/2}^{2n-1}\}.$$

Stirling's formula takes the form:

(a) for $n = 2m - 1$,

$$L_n(f;x) = f_0 + t\tilde{f}_0^1 + \frac{t^2}{2!}f_0^2 + \cdots + \frac{t(t^2-1)\cdots[t^2-(m-1)^2]}{(2m-1)!}\tilde{f}_0^{2m-1},$$

(b) for $n = 2m$,

$$L_n(f;x) = f_0 + t\tilde{f}_0^1 + \frac{t^2}{2!}f_0^2 + \cdots + \frac{t^2(t^2-1)\cdots[t^2-(m-1)^2]}{(2m)!}f_0^{2m}.$$

(6) The *Bessel* interpolation polynomial. The Gauss backward interpolation polynomial (6.4) with initial point $x_0 + h$ instead of x_0 and $t' = (x - x_0 - h)/h$ over the points (6.2) when $n = 2m + 1$ is of the form

$$L_n(f;x) = \sum_{k=0}^{n}\binom{t' + [k/2]}{k}\Delta^k f_{-[(k+1)/2]+1}$$

$$= f_1 + \binom{t-1}{1}\Delta f_0 + \binom{t}{2}\Delta^2 f_0 + \binom{t}{3}\Delta^3 f_{-1} + \cdots$$

$$+ \binom{t-1+m}{2m+1}\Delta^{2m+1} f_{-m}.$$

The Bessel interpolation formula is a half sum of the Gauss forward polynomial (6.3) and the above polynomial

$$L_{2m+1}(f;x) = \frac{1}{2}(f_0 + f_1) + (t - 1/2)\Delta f_0 + \frac{1}{2}\binom{t}{2}\{\Delta^2 f_0 + \Delta^2 f_{-1}\}$$

$$+ \frac{t(t-1)(t-1/2)}{6}\Delta^3 f_{-1} + \cdots$$

$$+ \frac{1}{2}\binom{t-1+m}{2m}\{\Delta^{2m}f_{-m} + \Delta^{2m}f_{-m+1}\}$$

$$+ \frac{t(t^2-1)\cdots[t^2-(n-1)^2](t-n)(t-1/2)}{(2n+1)!}\Delta^{2m+1}f_{-m},$$

and with the notation

$$\tilde{f}_{1/2}^{2s} = \tfrac{1}{2}(f_0^{2s} + f_1^{2s}) = \tfrac{1}{2}\{\Delta^{2s}f_{-s} + \Delta^{2s}f_{-s+1}\},$$

$$L_{2m+1}(f;x) = \tilde{f}_{1/2} + (t-1/2)f_{1/2}^1 + \tfrac{1}{2}t(t-1)\tilde{f}_{1/2}^2$$

$$+ \frac{t(t-1)(t-1/2)}{6} f_{1/2}^3 + \cdots$$

$$+ \frac{t(t^2-1)\cdots[t^2-(n-1)^2](t-n)}{(2n)!} \tilde{f}_{1/2}^{2m}$$

$$+ \frac{t(t^2-1)\cdots[t^2-(n-1)^2](t-n)(t-1/2)}{(2n+1)!} f_{1/2}^{2m+1}.$$

(7) The *first* Everett interpolation polynomial. Starting with the formula (6.3) terminated with an odd difference, e.g., $n = 2m + 1$,

$$L_{2m+1}(f;x) = \sum_{k=0}^{2m+1} \binom{t+[(k-1)/2]}{k} \Delta^k f_{-[k/2]}$$

$$= \sum_{k=0}^{m} \left\{ \binom{t+k-1}{2k} \Delta^{2k} f_{-k} + \binom{t+k}{2k+1} \Delta^{2k+1} f_{-k} \right\},$$

and using the relation $\Delta^{2k+1}f_{-k} = \Delta^{2k}f_{-k+1} - \Delta^{2k}f_{-k}$ it follows that

$$L_{2m+1}(f;x) = \sum_{k=0}^{m} \left\{ \left[\binom{t+k-1}{2k} - \binom{t+k}{2k+1} \right] \Delta^{2k} f_{-k} \right.$$

$$\left. + \binom{t+k}{2k+1} \Delta^{2k} f_{-k+1} \right\}$$

$$= \sum_{k=0}^{m} \left\{ \left[\binom{\xi+k}{2k+1} \right] \Delta^{2k} f_{-k} + \binom{t+k}{2k+1} \Delta^{2k} f_{-k+1} \right\},$$

where $\xi = 1 - t$.

(8) The *second* Everett (*Steffensen*) interpolation polynomial. Similarly to the first Everett polynomial in the Gauss forward formula (6.3) terminated with an even difference, e.g., $n = 2m$, the even finite differences can be substituted by $\Delta^{2k}f_{-k} = \Delta^{2k-1}f_{-k+1} + \Delta^{2k-1}f_{-k}$. So the formula (6.3) takes the form

$$L_{2m}(f;x) = \sum_{k=0}^{2m} \binom{t+[(k-1)/2]}{k} \Delta^k f_{-[k/2]}$$

$$= \sum_{k=0}^{m} \left\{ \binom{t+k-1}{2k} \Delta^{2k} f_{-k} + \sum_{k=1}^{m} \binom{t+k-1}{2k-1} \Delta^{2k-1} f_{-k+1} \right\}$$

$$= f_0 + \sum_{k=1}^{m} \left\{ \binom{t+k-1}{2k} \left[\Delta^{2k-1} f_{-k+1} - \Delta^{2k-1} f_{-k} \right] \right.$$

$$\left. + \binom{t+k-1}{2k-1} \Delta^{2k-1} f_{-k+1} \right\}$$

$$= f_0 + \sum_{k=1}^{m} \left\{ \binom{t+k-1}{2k-1} \frac{t+k}{2k} \Delta^{2k-1} f_{-k+1} \right.$$
$$\left. - \binom{t+k-1}{2k} \Delta^{2k-1} f_{-k} \right\}.$$

7. Frazer's diagram (Lozenge diagram)

The common way to obtain different interpolation formulas for a given function f defined on the equidistant set of points $\{x_i\}_{i=-\infty}^{\infty}$ (f can be defined on a part of these points) is the so-called Frazer diagram (see Table 7.1). Linking the corresponding finite differences and setting in every rhombus the binomial coefficient $\binom{t}{k}$, keeping the rule that in the rhombuses of the first column the numbers $\binom{t-i}{1}$ are set, in the rhombuses of the second column $\binom{t-i}{2}$ and so on, the arbitrary interpolation polynomial can be derived in the following way.

(a) Starting from f_i in the first column (functional values) set $t = (x - x_i)/h$ and choose one of the two paths to a first-order difference in the second column, from this difference choose one of the three outgoing paths and so on. The path finishes in some finite difference.

(b) The formula can be built as follows:

(b1) write the functional values from which the path starts;

(b2) for every cut-off from left to right add the term that consists of the finite difference in which this cut-off finishes multiplied by the binomial

TABLE 7.1.

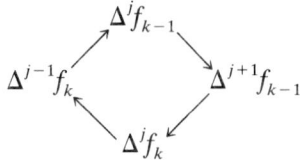

Fig. 7.1. Closed path in Frazer's diagram.

coefficient lying under (above) it when the inclination is positive (negative);

(b3) for every cut-off from right to left subtract the term that consists of the finite difference from which this cut-off comes multiplied by the binomial coefficient lying under (above) it when the inclination is positive (negative).

REMARK 7.1. The formula obtained from Frazer's diagram according to the rules (a) and (b) above that finishes at the finite difference $\Delta^s f_k$ coincides with the Lagrange polynomial constructed over the equidistant set of points $\{x_n\}_{n=k}^{k+s}$ with a step size of h. The proof of this proposition is based on the fact that every closed path of the kind given in Fig. 7.1 does not add anything in the interpolation formula or the path

$$\Delta^{j-1} f_k \Rightarrow \Delta^j f_{k-1} \Rightarrow \Delta^{j+1} f_{k-1}$$

has the same contribution as the path

$$\Delta^{j-1} f_k \Rightarrow \Delta^j f_k \Rightarrow \Delta^{j+1} f_{k-1} \, .$$

8. Utilization of the interpolation formulas

All the interpolation formulas derived in Section 6 represent Lagrange interpolation polynomials written in different forms. The general advantage of the formulas using finite differences is that by adding one additional knot, only one more term has to be computed.

Usually working with the interpolation polynomials with finite differences the highest order finite difference that takes part in the formula must be "small" (if that is possible). It is recommended that the various polynomials are used in the following situations.

(a) If x is situated near the beginning (end) of the interval where the function is tabulated, then use the Newton forward (backward) interpolation polynomial.

(b) The Gauss, Bessel and Stirling interpolation polynomials are recommended if x is in the middle of the interval where the function is tabulated. Bessel's formula is most appropriate when either $t = (x - x_0)/h \approx \frac{1}{2}$ and the last finite difference is of even order or $t = (x - x_0)/h \approx 0$ and the last finite difference is of odd order.

(c) Everett's formula is used for subtabulations when from a table of a given function with step h it is necessary to obtain additional tables with steps $h/2$, $h/4, \ldots$.

9. Inverse interpolation

Let the function f be tabulated at the points $\{x_i\}_{i=0}^n$. Then using the values $\{f(x_i)\}_{i=0}^n$ for a given number y a point z has to be found such that $f(z) = y$. If $y = 0$ the equation $f(x) = 0$ must be solved. One approach for solving this problem is the inverse interpolation.

Suppose that the points $\{x_i\}_{i=0}^n$ are in increasing order and $f'(x) \neq 0$ for $x_0 \leq x \leq x_n$; i.e. the inverse function g of the function f exists in the interval $[x_0, x_n]$. Build the interpolation polynomial P of nth degree for the function g which takes values $\{x_i\}_{i=0}^n$ at the points $\{f(x_i)\}_{i=0}^n$. Then $P(y)$ can be considered as an approximation of z.

In the case when the function f is not strict monotone (the values $\{f(x_i)\}_{i=0}^n$ are not strict monotone) the above procedure cannot always be applied. The error in the inverse interpolation expressed by the function g is [see (2.3)]

$$z = g(y) = P(y) + \omega_n(y)g^{(n+1)}(\xi)/(n+1)!.$$

From the equalities

$$g'(y) = 1/f'(z), \quad g''(y) = -f''(z)/f'^3(z), \ldots;$$

i.e. the degrees of $f'(z)$ take part in the denominators of the derivatives of the function g from which it follows that if f' vanishes near the point x then $g^{(n+1)}(\xi)$ can be too large and a satisfactory approximation of the inverse function g is not certain. To avoid this difficulty another two alternatives exist.

(a) Build the interpolation polynomial L of nth degree for f which takes values $\{f(x_i)\}_{i=0}^n$ at the points $\{x_i\}_{i=0}^n$. The solution of the equation $L(x) = y$ is an approximation of z. Note that the solution is not unique.

(b) Perform the following iterative procedure:

(b1) find two abscissas x_a and x_b between $\{x_i\}_{i=0}^n$ such that $f(x_a) \leq y \leq f(x_b)$ (if possible);

(b2) apply inverse interpolation using only the points x_a and x_b. Let the obtained point be x_c;

(b3) compute $f(x_c)$ approximately using the interpolation polynomial for f over the points $\{x_i\}_{i=0}^n$ (some of these can also be used);

(b4) if $f(x_c) < y$ then set $x_a = x_c$ and substitute $f(x_a)$ by $f(x_c)$, otherwise set $x_b = x_c$ and substitute $f(x_b)$ by $f(x_c)$;

(b5) go to (b1).

This iterative procedure produces a sequence of points and if it converges the cycle of operations has to be repeated as often as necessary.

10. The Hermite–Birkhoff interpolation problem (H–B problem)

In BIRKHOFF [1906] the most general interpolation problem involving algebraic polynomials was formulated. The exact definition of the H–B problem uses the concept of incidence matrix. Let E be a matrix with $m+1$ rows and $n+1$ columns. The elements of E are e_{ij}:

$$E = \begin{Vmatrix} e_{00} & e_{01} & \cdots & e_{0n} \\ e_{10} & e_{11} & \cdots & e_{1n} \\ \vdots & \vdots & & \vdots \\ e_{m0} & e_{m1} & \cdots & e_{mn} \end{Vmatrix}.$$

This matrix is called an incidence matrix if its elements are 0 or 1 and the number of unit elements in the matrix is $|E| = n+1$.

Let e be the set of couples (i, j) for which $e_{ij} = 1$ and $X = \{x_i\}_{i=0}^m$, $x_0 < x_1 < \cdots < x_m$, are knots on the real axes.

The interpolation H–B problem is characterized by the couples (E, X). For a given couple (E, X) and function f a function $\varphi \in F_n$ (F_n is an $n+1$ dimensional set of functions) must be found such that $\varphi^{(j)}(x_i) = f^{(j)}(x_i)$ for $(i, j) \in e$. According to Section 1 the H–B problem is characterized by the linear functionals $l_{ij}(f) = f^{(j)}(x_i)$ for $(i, j) \in e$.

In the case when $F_n = H_n$ (algebraic polynomials of degree at most n) the H–B problem reduces to the determination of a polynomial P_n of nth degree that satisfies

$$P_n^{(j)}(x_i) = f^{(j)}(x_i) \quad \text{for } (i, j) \in e. \tag{10.1}$$

This is a generalization of a series of interpolation problems.

(a) The Taylor formula $P_n(x) = \sum_{k=0}^n f^{(k)}(x_0)(x-x_0)^k/k!$ corresponds to a matrix $E = \|1\ 1\ 1\ \cdots\ 1\|$.

(b) Lagrange's interpolation polynomial—see Section 2. For this problem E is a square matrix and only the first column consists of $n+1$ units

$$E = \begin{Vmatrix} 1 & 0 & 0 & \cdots & 0 \\ 1 & 0 & 0 & \cdots & 0 \\ \vdots & \vdots & \vdots & & \vdots \\ 1 & 0 & 0 & \cdots & 0 \end{Vmatrix}.$$

(c) The A–G (Abel–Gontcharoff) interpolation problem—see Section 11. For this problem E is a square matrix and only the main diagonal consists of $n+1$ units

$$E = \begin{Vmatrix} 1 & 0 & 0 & \cdots & 0 \\ 0 & 1 & 0 & \cdots & 0 \\ \vdots & \vdots & \vdots & & \vdots \\ 0 & 0 & 0 & \cdots & 1 \end{Vmatrix}.$$

(d) Hermite interpolation—see Section 12. The matrix of incidence for the Hermite problem is characterized by the property that every row begins with units followed by zeros. For example,

$$E = \begin{Vmatrix} 1 & 0 & 0 & 0 & 0 & 0 & 0 & 0 & 0 \\ 1 & 1 & 1 & 0 & 0 & 0 & 0 & 0 & 0 \\ 1 & 0 & 0 & 0 & 0 & 0 & 0 & 0 & 0 \\ 1 & 1 & 1 & 1 & 0 & 0 & 0 & 0 & 0 \end{Vmatrix}.$$

The H–B problem does not always have a solution, or it can have more than one solution. For the incidence matrix

$$E = \begin{Vmatrix} 0 & 1 \\ 0 & 1 \end{Vmatrix}$$

the number of unit elements is two and the linear functionals $l_{01}(f) = f'(x_0)$, $l_{11}(f) = f'(x_1)$ describe the problem; i.e. a polynomial of first degree $P(x) = ax + b$ must be found such that $P'(x_0) = f'(x_0)$ and $P'(x_1) = f'(x_1)$. As $P'(x) = a$, if $f'(x_0) = f'(x_1)$ the problem has infinitely many solutions, otherwise it has no solution.

The question for the characterization of the incidence matrices for which the H–B problem has a unique solution is still open.

The couple (E, X) is called regular if the system (10.1) has a unique solution for every smooth function f. This means that the determinant $D(E, X)$ of the linear system (10.1) according to the coefficients of the polynomial P does not vanish.

The incidence matrix E is called poised if the couple (E, X) is regular for every set X.

THEOREM 10.1 (LORENTZ, JETTER and RIEMANSCNEIDER [1983]). *If*

$$M_j := \sum_{k=0}^{j} \sum_{i=0}^{m} e_{ik} \geq j + 1 \quad \text{for } j = 0, 1, \ldots, n, \tag{10.2}$$

then the determinant $D(E, X)$ of the linear system (10.1) is a polynomial of $x_0, x_1, \ldots, x_n$ of total degree $\frac{1}{2}n(n+1) - \Sigma_{e_{ik}=1} k$. If $M_j \leq j$ for some j, $0 \leq j \leq n$, then $D(E, X) \equiv 0$.

The necessary condition (10.2) is known as the Polya condition and was found by SCHOENBERG [1966]. The proof for the necessity of (10.2) is simple. Indeed, note that the row in $D(E, X)$ that corresponds to $e_{ik} = 1$, $k > 0$, begins with k zeros. If $M_j \leq j$ for some j, $0 \leq j \leq n$, then all rows in $D(E, X)$ except at most j begin with $j + 1$ zeros. Therefore the first $j + 1$ columns of $D(E, X)$ are not linearly independent; i.e. $D(E, X) = 0$.

On the contrary the condition (10.2) is not sufficient for a matrix of incidence to be poised. To prove this let us consider the matrix

$$E = \begin{Vmatrix} 1 & 0 & 1 \\ 0 & 1 & 0 \\ 1 & 0 & 0 \end{Vmatrix}$$

that satisfies Polya's condition (10.2). The H–B problem (10.1) for this matrix is $P_2^{(j)}(x_i) = f^{(j)}(x_i)$ for $(i, j) \in e$; i.e. $P_2(x_0) = f(x_0)$, $P_2(x_2) = f(x_2)$, $P_2'(x_1) =$

$f'(x_1)$. For simplicity let $f \equiv 0$. Then $P_2(x) = a_0(x - x_0)(x - x_2)$ and $P_2'(x) = 2a_0[x - (x_0 - x_2)/2]$. The last equality shows that if $x_1 = (x_0 + x_2)/2$ then the H–B problem has infinitely many solutions, otherwise $P_2 \equiv 0$ is a unique solution.

In the case that E consists of two rows (10.2) is also a sufficient condition— POLYA [1931] and WHITTAKER [1935]. Every sequence from units in one row of E

$$e_{ik} = e_{i,k+1} = \cdots = e_{i,k+l-1} = 1 \tag{10.3}$$

is called a block if one of the following conditions is fulfilled:
 (a) it is bounded by zeros from both sides;
 (b) it is bounded by zeros from one side and begins (ends) at the beginning (end) of the row;
 (c) it fills the row.
The block (10.3) is called:
 (a) odd (even) if l is odd (even);
 (b) Hermitian if $k = 0$ (non-Hermitian if $k \neq 0$);
 (c) supported if there exist indexes i_1, i_2, k_1, k_2, such that $i_1 < i$, $k_1 < k$, $e_{i_1 k_1} = 1$, $i_2 > i$, $k_2 > k$, $e_{i_2 k_2} = 1$.

It is proved by FERGUSON [1969] that if the incidence matrix E satisfies Polya's condition (10.2) and has only non-Hermitian even blocks, then E is a poised matrix.

The most general sufficient condition is given in ATKINSON and SHARMA [1969].

THEOREM 10.2. *If the incidence matrix E satisfies Polya's condition* (10.2) *and does not have odd supported blocks, then E is a poised matrix.*

PROOF. It is sufficient to prove that the unique polynomial $P_n \in H_n$ that satisfies the conditions $P_n^{(k)}(x_i) = 0$ for $e_{ik} \in e$ is $P_n \equiv 0$. For this aim let us denote by $\tilde{m}_j$, $j = 0, 1, \ldots, n$, the number of the zeros of $P_n^{(j)}$ taking into account their multiplicities and omitting those zeros of $P_n^{(j)}$ that are already included in the numbers $\tilde{m}_0, \tilde{m}_1, \ldots, \tilde{m}_{j-1}$. Let $\tilde{M}_k = \Sigma_{j=0}^k \tilde{m}_j$, $k = 0, 1, \ldots, n$. It follows from the definition that $M_k \leq \tilde{M}_k$ for $k = 0, 1, \ldots, n$. Let us prove that for each k, $0 \leq k \leq n$, the polynomial $P_n^{(k)}$ has at least $\tilde{M}_k - k$ different zeros taking into account their multiplicities. For $k = 0$ the assertion is true because $\tilde{m}_0 = \tilde{M}_0 - 0$. Let us assume that $P_n^{(k-1)}$ has at least $\tilde{M}_{k-1} - (k-1)$ zeros. By Rolle's theorem $P_n^{(k)}$ has $\tilde{M}_{k-1} - (k-1) - 1$ zeros, which are either zeros of $P_n^{(k-1)}$ or zeros with an odd multiplicity. Since $P_n^{(k)}(x_i) = 0$ for $e_{ik} = 1$ it follows that the incidence matrix E assigns to $P_n^{(k)}$ $\tilde{m}_k$ zeros that are not zeros of $P_n^{(k-1)}$. On the other hand, these $\tilde{m}_k$ zeros are either of even multiplicity or they cannot coincide with the zero obtained by Rolle's theorem. Therefore the zeros of $P_n^{(k)}$ are at least $\tilde{M}_{k-1} - k + \tilde{m}_k = \tilde{M}_k - k$; i.e. $P_n^{(k)}$ has at least $\tilde{M}_k - k$ zeros for $k = 0, 1, \ldots, n$. By Polya's condition $M_k \geq k + 1$ and

$M_k \leq \tilde{M}_k$ it follows that for every $k = 0, 1, \ldots, n$, the polynomial $P_n^{(k)}$ has at least one zero; i.e. $P_n^{(k)} \equiv 0$. □

The Atkinson and Sharma condition is not necessary. For instance, the matrices

$$E = \begin{Vmatrix} 1 & 1 & 0 & 0 & 0 & 0 \\ 0 & 1 & 0 & 0 & 1 & 0 \\ 1 & 1 & 0 & 0 & 0 & 0 \end{Vmatrix}, \quad E = \begin{Vmatrix} 1 & 0 & 0 & 0 & 0 & 0 \\ 0 & 0 & 1 & 0 & 1 & 0 \\ 1 & 1 & 1 & 0 & 0 & 0 \end{Vmatrix},$$

$$E = \begin{Vmatrix} 1 & 1 & 1 & 0 & 0 & 0 & 0 & 0 \\ 0 & 1 & 0 & 0 & 0 & 0 & 1 & 0 \\ 1 & 1 & 1 & 0 & 0 & 0 & 0 & 0 \end{Vmatrix}$$

are poised and do not satisfy the Atkinson and Sharma condition.

Some authors tried to characterize the so-called quasi-Hermite incidence matrices. Denote by $E(p, q; k_1, k_2)$ the incidence matrix with three rows, the first and third containing only one Hermite block with lengths p and q respectively and the second having two unit elements—$e_{2k_1} = e_{2k_2} = 1$, $k_1 < k_2$. The results of LORENTZ [1975], LORENTZ, STANGLER and ZELLER [1976], DE VORE, MEIR and SHARMA [1973] can be summarized in the following theorem.

THEOREM 10.3. *Let $k_1 + k_2 = p + q + 1$, $k_2 > q$. Then $E(p, q; k_1, k_2)$ is a poised matrix if $p = q$ and it is not poised otherwise.*

In the case

$$p \leq k_1, \quad k_2 < q + 1,$$

$$\rho(k_1, k_2) = (q + 2)(k_1 + k_2 - 1)^2 - 4(q - 1)k_1 k_2,$$

it follows that $E(1, q; k_1, k_2)$ is a poised matrix if $\rho(k_1, k_2) < 0$ and it is not a poised one if $\rho(k_1, k_2) \geq 0$.

DIMITROV [1991] presents an algorithm for the representation of the determinant $D(E, X)$ in the form

$$D(E, X) = \sum_{|\alpha| = n(n+1)/2 - \Sigma_{e_{ik}=1} k} (-1)^{s(\alpha)} g(\alpha) \prod_{j<i} (x_i - x_j)^{\alpha_{ij}},$$

where $\alpha = \{\alpha_{ij}\}_{1 \leq j < i \leq m}$, $\alpha_{ij} \geq 0$, $|\alpha| = \Sigma_{1 \leq j < i \leq m} \alpha_{ij}$, $s(\alpha)$ and $g(\alpha)$ are natural numbers that depend on α and E, $s(\alpha) \in \{0, 1\}$. For an arbitrary incidence matrix E the algorithm gives an array of numbers g and s. It allows the determination of an explicit representation of the interpolation polynomial

$$P_n(f; x) = \sum_{e_{ik}=1} f^{(k)}(x_i) p_{ik}(x),$$

where the basic interpolation polynomials p_{ik} satisfy

$$p_{ik}^{(j)}(x_\nu) = \delta_{i\nu} \delta_{kj} \quad \text{for } e_{ik} = 1, \; \delta_{ij} = \begin{cases} 1, & i = j, \\ 0, & i \neq j. \end{cases}$$

For example,
(1) let

$$E = \begin{Vmatrix} 1 & 1 & 0 & 0 & 0 & 0 & 0 \\ 0 & 1 & 0 & 1 & 0 & 0 & 0 \\ 1 & 1 & 1 & 0 & 0 & 0 & 0 \end{Vmatrix},$$

then

$$D(E, X) = 24\{(x_1 - x_0)(x_2 - x_0)^6(x_2 - x_1)^6$$
$$- 6(x_1 - x_0)^2(x_2 - x_0)^6(x_2 - x_1)^5$$
$$+ 9(x_1 - x_0)^3(x_2 - x_0)^6(x_2 - x_1)^4$$
$$- 4(x_1 - x_0)^4(x_2 - x_0)^6(x_2 - x_1)^3\},$$

from which it is easy to derive that the couple (E, X) is singular if and only if $x_1 = (x_0 + x_2)/2$;
(2) let $x_0 = 0$, $x_1 = 1$ and

$$E = \begin{Vmatrix} 1 & 0 & 1 & 1 & 0 & 0 \\ 0 & 1 & 1 & 0 & 1 & 0 \end{Vmatrix},$$

then $D(E, X) = 11\,520$ and the basic polynomials that correspond to the elements $e_{ij} = 1$ have the following forms:

$$p_{00}(x) = 1, \qquad p_{02}(x) = (x^5 - 5x^4 + 20x^2 - 25x)/40,$$
$$p_{03}(x) = (3x^5 - 15x^4 + 20x^3 - 15x)/120,$$
$$p_{11}(x) = x, \qquad p_{12}(x) = (-x^5 + 5x^4 - 15x)/40,$$
$$p_{14}(x) = (6x^5 - 10x^4 + 10x)/480.$$

BALAZS and TURAN [1957, 1958] consider the couples (E, X) with fixed X (e.g., the zeros of the Legendre polynomial) and FREUD [1958] obtained some convergent results for the Birkhoff interpolation.

11. The Abel–Gontcharov interpolation problem (A–G problem)

Following GONTCHAROV [1930, 1954] an algebraic polynomial of nth degree P_n must be built such that

$$P_n^{(i)}(x_i) = f^{(i)}(x_i), \quad i = 0, 1, \ldots, n. \tag{11.1}$$

The determinant of the linear system (11.1)

$$D = \begin{vmatrix} 1 & x_0 & x_0^2 & \cdots & x_0^n \\ 0 & 1! & 2x_1 & \cdots & nx_1^{n-1} \\ 0 & 0 & 2! & \cdots & n(n-1)x_2^{n-2} \\ \vdots & \vdots & \ddots & \ddots & \vdots \\ 0 & 0 & \cdots & 0 & n! \end{vmatrix} = 1 \cdot 1! \cdot 2! \cdots n!$$

is always different from zero and the problem (11.1) has a unique solution.

An explicit form of the polynomial P_n can be obtained using the polynomials

$$A_0(x) = 1, \quad A_1(x) = x - x_0, \ldots, \quad A_k(x) = \int_{x_0}^{x} dt_1 \int_{x_1}^{t_1} dt_2 \cdots \int_{x_{k-1}}^{t_{k-1}} dt_k, \ldots,$$

$k = 1, 2, \ldots, n$.

The polynomial A_k is of the kth degree and satisfies $A_k^{(s)}(x_s) = 0$, $A_k^{(k)}(x) = 1$, $s = 0, 1, \ldots, k-1$. The final equalities allow the so-called Abel–Gontcharov interpolation polynomial P_n to be written in the form

$$P_n(x) = \sum_{k=0}^{n} f^{(k)}(x_k) A_k(x) = \sum_{k=0}^{n} f^{(k)}(x_k) \int_{x_0}^{x} dt_1 \int_{x_1}^{t_1} dt_2 \cdots \int_{x_{k-1}}^{t_{k-1}} dt_k. \quad (11.2)$$

The following are special cases of the polynomial (11.2).

(a) When all the knots coincide $(x_0 = x_1 = \cdots = x_n)$ then the problem (11.1) is called a Taylor interpolation problem and P_n takes the form

$$P_n(x) = \sum_{k=0}^{n} f^{(k)}(x_0)(x - x_0)^k / k! \, .$$

(b) Let the points $\{x_i\}_{i=0}^{n}$ form an arithmetic progression $x_i = x_0 + ih$, $i = 0, 1, \ldots, n$, $n > 0$. In this particular case the solution was given by Abel and is

$$P_n(x) = \sum_{k=0}^{n} f^{(k)}(x_0)(x - x_0)(x - x_0 - kh)^{k-1} / k! \, . \quad (11.3)$$

The remainder term $R_n(f; x) = f(x) - P_n(x)$, where P_n is the polynomial from (11.1), can be represented in the form

$$R_n(f; x) = \int_{x_0}^{x} dt_1 \int_{x_1}^{t_1} dt_2 \cdots \int_{x_n}^{t_n} f^{(n+1)}(t_{n+1}) \, dt_{n+1} \, .$$

This follows from the properties $R_n^{(k)}(f; x_k) = f^{(k)}(x_k) - P_n^{(k)}(x_k) = 0$, $k = 0, 1, \ldots, n$, and $R_n^{(n+1)}(f; x) = f^{(n+1)}(x)$. If the knots $x, x_0, x_1, \ldots, x_n$ lie in the interval $[a, b]$ in order to minimize the remainder term R_n the knots $\{x_i\}_{i=0}^{n}$ must be chosen in such way that

$$r = \max_{a \le x \le b} \left| \int_{x_0}^{x} dt_1 \int_{x_1}^{t_1} dt_2 \cdots \int_{x_n}^{t_n} t_{n+1} \, dt_{n+1} \right| \quad (11.4)$$

is minimal. This problem leads to the Chebyshev polynomials. Indeed,

$$\varphi(x) = \int_{x_0}^{x} dt_1 \int_{x_1}^{t_1} dt_2 \cdots \int_{x_n}^{t_n} t_{n+1} \, dt_{n+1}$$

is an algebraic polynomial of degree $n + 1$ with leading coefficient $1/(n + 1)!$.

Therefore, the number r will be the smallest one if $\varphi(x) = C_{n+1}(x)/2^n(n+1)!$ (see Section 35). The optimal choice of the knots is when x_i is a zero of $C_{n+1}^{(i)}$, $i = 0, 1, \ldots, n$. According to this choice of the knots

$$r' = \inf_{x_0,\ldots,x_n \in [a,b]} \max_{a \leq x \leq b} \left| \int_{x_0}^{x} dt_1 \int_{x_1}^{t_1} dt_2 \cdots \int_{x_n}^{t_n} t_{n+1}\, dt_{n+1} \right|$$

$$= (b-a)^{(n+1)} 2^{-2n-1}/(n+1)! \,.$$

Another case is when $x_i = a + i(b-a)/n$, $i = 0, 1, \ldots, n$ (see 11.3). Here

$$\int_{x_0}^{x} dt_1 \int_{x_1}^{t_1} dt_2 \cdots \int_{x_n}^{t_n} t_{n+1}\, dt_{n+1} = (x-a)[x - b - (b-a)/n]^n/(n+1)!$$

and if

$$r'' = \max_{a \leq x \leq b} \left| \int_{x_0}^{x} dt_1 \int_{x_1}^{t_1} dt_2 \cdots \int_{x_n}^{t_n} t_{n+1}\, dt_{n+1} \right|,$$

then

$$r'' = (b-a)^{n+1}/(n+1)!n \,.$$

Comparison between r' and r'' shows the importance of the choice of knots.

12. The Hermite interpolation problem (H problem)

According to Section 1 the H problem for a smooth enough function f is characterized by the sequence of linear functionals $l_{i,p_i}(f) = f^{(p_i)}(x_i)$, $p_i = 0, 1, \ldots, \alpha_i$, $i = 0, 1, \ldots, m$, where $\{x_i\}_{i=0}^{m}$ are different points. The number of the functionals is $n = \alpha_0 + \alpha_1 + \cdots + \alpha_m + m + 1$ and n must be the dimension of the subset F_n.

When the interpolation is by means of algebraic polynomials the basic theorem is the following one.

THEOREM 12.1. *Let f be a sufficiently smooth function in the interval $[a, b]$ and $\{x_i\}_{i=0}^{m}$ be different points from this interval. For arbitrary non-negative integer numbers $\{\alpha_i\}_{i=0}^{m}$ there exists a unique algebraic polynomial $P_n \in H_n$, $n = \alpha_0 + \alpha_1 + \cdots + \alpha_m + m$, which satisfies the conditions*

$$P_n^{(s_i)}(x_i) = f^{(s_i)}(x_i), \quad s_i = 0, 1, \ldots, \alpha_i, \quad i = 0, 1, \ldots, m \,. \tag{12.1}$$

PROOF. Let us show that the polynomial

$$P_n(x) = \sum_{k=0}^{m} \sum_{s_k=0}^{\alpha_k} f^{(s_k)}(x_k) L_{k,s_k}(x) \,,$$

satisfies the conditions (12.1), where

$$L_{k,s_k}(x) = \frac{Q(x)}{s_k!(x-x_k)^{\alpha_k+1-s_k}} S_{\alpha_k-s_k}\left(\frac{(x-x_k)^{\alpha_k+1}}{Q(x)};x\right)_{(x_k)},$$

$$Q(x) = (x-x_0)^{\alpha_0+1}(x-x_1)^{\alpha_1+1}\cdots(x-x_m)^{\alpha_m+1},$$

$$S_r(\varphi;x)_{(a)} = \sum_{k=0}^{r}\frac{\varphi^{(k)}(a)}{k!}(x-a)^k.$$

For this aim it is sufficient to prove that the polynomials L_{k,s_k} are of degree at most n and that they satisfy

$$L_{k,s_k}^{(j)}(x_k) = \begin{cases} 0, & j \neq s_k, \\ 1, & j = s_k, \end{cases} \quad j=0,1,\ldots,\alpha_k. \tag{12.2}$$

Since the polynomial $\varphi(x) = Q(x)/(x-x_k)^{\alpha_k+1-s_k}$ has a degree of $n - \alpha_k + s_k$ and $S_{\alpha_k-s_k}(\varphi;x)_{(x_k)}$ is of degree $\alpha_k - s_k$ it is clear that the degree of L_{k,s_k} is at most n. For $j = 0, 1, \ldots, \alpha_k$,

$$\left\{\varphi(x)S_p\left(\frac{(x-a)^{s_k}}{\varphi(x)};x\right)_{(a)}\right\}^{(j)}_{x=a} = \left\{\varphi(x)\frac{(x-a)^{s_k}}{\varphi(x)}\right\}^{(j)}_{x=a} = \{(x-a)^{s_k}\}^{(j)}_{x=a},$$

and therefore

$$L_{k,s_k}^{(j)}(x_k) = \{(x-x_k)^{s_k}\}^{(j)}_{x=x_k}/s_k!.$$

The equality (12.2) is proved and the polynomial P_n of nth degree satisfies (12.1).

Let us assume that there is another polynomial $\bar{P}_n$ of nth degree that satisfies (12.1). Then $\bar{P}_n^{(s_k)}(x_k) - P_n^{(s_k)}(x_k) = 0$ for $s_k = 0, 1, \ldots, \alpha_k$, $k = 0, 1, \ldots, m$; i.e. $\bar{P}_n \equiv P_n$. □

Particular cases of the H problem are:
(a) if $\alpha_i = 0$, for $i = 0, 1, \ldots, m$, then the H problem coincides with Lagrange's interpolation problem considered in Section 1;
(b) if $m = 0$ then the algebraic polynomial P_n from Theorem 12.1 represents the Taylor formula

$$P_n(x) = \sum_{i=0}^{n}(x-x_0)^i f^{(i)}(x_0)/i!;$$

(c) if $m = 2$ then the algebraic polynomial P_n from Theorem 12.1 is the Obreshkov–Chakalov (Section 51) interpolation polynomial,

$$P_n(x) = \sum_{s=0}^{\alpha_0} f^{(s)}(x_0) \frac{(x-x_1)^{\alpha_1+1}(x-x_0)^s}{s!(x_0-x_1)^{\alpha_1+1}} \sum_{i=0}^{\alpha_0-s}\binom{\alpha_1+i}{i}\frac{(x-x_0)^i}{(x_1-x_0)^i}$$

$$+ \sum_{s=0}^{\alpha_1} f^{(s)}(x_1) \frac{(x-x_0)^{\alpha_0+1}(x-x_1)^s}{s!(x_1-x_0)^{\alpha_0+1}}$$

$$\times \sum_{i=0}^{\alpha_1-s}\binom{\alpha_0+i}{i}(x-x_1)^i/(x_1-x_0)^i;$$

(d) if $\alpha_i = 1$, $i = 0, 1, \ldots, m$, the polynomial P_n from Theorem 12.1 takes the form

$$P_{2m+1}(x) = \sum_{k=0}^{m} f(x_k)\left(1 - \frac{\omega''(x_k)}{\omega'(x_k)}(x - x_k)\right) \frac{\omega^2(x)}{(x - x_k)^2 \omega'^2(x_k)}$$

$$+ \sum_{k=0}^{m} f'(x_k) \frac{\omega^2(x)}{(x - x_k)\omega'^2(x_k)}, \quad \text{where } \omega(x) = \prod_{k=0}^{m}(x - x_k).$$

Let the function $f \in C_{[a,b]}^{n+1}$ and the algebraic polynomial $P_n \in H_n$ satisfy

$$P_n^{(p_i)}(x_i) = f^{(p_i)}(x_i), \quad p_i = 0, 1, \ldots, \alpha_i, \ i = 0, 1, \ldots, m,$$

where $\{x_i\}_{i=0}^m$ are different points in $[a, b]$ and $n = \alpha_0 + \alpha_1 + \cdots + \alpha_m + m$. Let us estimate the quantity $\max_{a \leq x \leq b} |P_n(x) - f(x)|$. Evidently

$$P_n(x) - f(x) = \lambda(x) \prod_{i=0}^{m}(x - x_i)^{\alpha_i + 1}$$

and to determine the function λ let us consider the function

$$\varphi(t) = f(t) - P_n(t) - [f(x) - P_n(x)] \prod_{i=0}^{m}(t - x_i)^{\alpha_i + 1} \bigg/ \prod_{i=0}^{m}(x - x_i)^{\alpha_i + 1}.$$

For a fixed point $x \in [a, b]$ the function φ has at the point x_k zero of multiplicity $\alpha_k + 1$, $k = 0, 1, \ldots, m$, and including the point x the function φ has $n + 2$ zeros in the interval $[a, b]$. It follows from Rolle's theorem that there exists a point $\xi \in (a, b)$ for which

$$\varphi^{(n+1)}(\xi) = f^{(n+1)}(\xi) - (n+1)![f(x) - P_n(x)] \bigg/ \prod_{i=0}^{m}(x - x_i)^{\alpha_i + 1} = 0$$

and the last equality is valid for every $x \in [a, b]$. Therefore

$$R_n(f, x) = f(x) - P_n(x) = f^{(n+1)}(\xi) \prod_{i=0}^{m}(x - x_i)^{\alpha_i + 1}/(n+1)!. \tag{12.3}$$

From the error representation (12.3) there follows:
(a) the estimation (2.3) for Lagrange's interpolation polynomial when $\alpha_i = 0$, $i = 0, 1, \ldots, m$;
(b) the remainder term for the Taylor interpolation formula

$$f(x) - P_n(x) = f(x) - \sum_{i=0}^{n}(x - x_0)^i f^{(i)}(x_0)/i!$$

$$= f^{(n+1)}(\xi)(x - x_i)^{n+1}/(n+1)!,$$

when $m = 0$ and $\alpha_0 = n$.

REMARK 12.1. FEJER [1916] considered the special case when the knots are the roots of the $(n+1)$th Chebyshev polynomial C_{n+1} in the interval $[-1, 1]$; i.e. $x_k = \cos[(2k+1)\pi/2n+1]$, $k = 0, 1, \ldots, n$, and let $\Phi_{2n+1} \in H_{2n+1}$ be an algebraic polynomial that satisfies $\Phi_{2n+1}(x_k) = f(x_k)$, $\Phi'_{2n+1}(x_k) = 0$, $k = 0, 1, \ldots, n$, for a given function f. Explicitly (see the particular case (d) in this section)

$$\Phi_{2n+1}(x_k) = \sum_{k=0}^{n} f(x_k)\left(1 - \frac{\omega''(x_k)}{\omega'(x_k)}(x - x_k)\right)\left(\frac{\omega(x)}{(x - x_k)\omega'(x_k)}\right)^2,$$

where $\omega(x) = C_{n+1}(x) = 2^{-n} \cos[(n+1)\cos^{-1}x]$. Calculating $\omega'(x_k)$ and $\omega''(x_k)$ the polynomial Φ_{2n+1} takes the form

$$\Phi_{2n+1}(x_k) = \sum_{k=0}^{n} f(x_k)(1 - x_k x)\left(\frac{C_{n+1}(x)}{(n+1)(x - x_k)}\right)^2.$$

The basic result of Fejer is that if $f \in C_{[-1,1]}$ then $\lim_{n\to\infty} \|f - \Phi_{2n+1}\| = 0$ and he observed that this uniform convergence remains valid for arbitrary knots for which

$$\min_{-1 \leq x \leq 1} \left(1 - \frac{\omega''(x_k)}{\omega'(x_k)}(x - x_k)\right) \geq 0, \quad k = 0, 1, \ldots, n, \ n = 1, 2, \ldots.$$

The last condition leads to the fact that if the function f is non-negative then Φ_{2n+1} is also non-negative. For details see Section 31.

13. The divided differences with repeating knots and Hermite interpolation

Let us define

$$f(\underbrace{x_0; x_0; \ldots; x_0}_{\leftarrow k_0 \text{ times} \rightarrow}; \underbrace{x_1; x_1; \ldots; x_1}_{\leftarrow k_1 \text{ times} \rightarrow}; \ldots; \underbrace{x_n; x_n; \ldots; x_n}_{\leftarrow k_n \text{ times} \rightarrow})$$

$$= \lim_{x_i^{(j)} \to x_i} f(x_0; x_0^{(1)}; \ldots; x_0^{(k_0-1)}; x_1; x_1^{(1)}; \ldots; x_1^{(k_1-1)};$$

$$\ldots; x_n; x_n^{(1)}; \ldots; x_n^{(k_n-1)}), \tag{13.1}$$

where all the points that take part in the last divided difference are different. For the existence of the limit it is necessary for the function f to be smooth enough. For example,

$$f(x; x) = \lim_{y \to x} f(x; y) = \lim_{y \to x} \frac{f(y) - f(x)}{y - x} = f'(x).$$

For the proof of the correctness of the definition (13.1) let us follow BEREZIN and JIDKOV [1966], p. 120). Using property (g) in Section 3 it follows that

$$f(x_0; x_1; \ldots; x_n) = \begin{vmatrix} 1 & x_0 & \cdots & x_0^{n-1} & f(x_0) \\ 1 & x_1 & \cdots & x_1^{n-1} & f(x_1) \\ \vdots & \vdots & & \vdots & \vdots \\ 1 & x_n & \cdots & x_n^{n-1} & f(x_n) \end{vmatrix} : \begin{vmatrix} 1 & x_0 & \cdots & x_0^{n-1} & x_0^n \\ 1 & x_1 & \cdots & x_1^{n-1} & x_1^n \\ \vdots & \vdots & & \vdots & \vdots \\ 1 & x_n & \cdots & x_n^{n-1} & x_n^n \end{vmatrix}$$

and let us denote by $D(x_0; x_1; \ldots; x_n)$ the determinant in the denominator and by $D(x_0; x_1; \ldots; x_n; f)$ the determinant in the numerator. The definition (13.1) can be rewritten as

$$f(\underbrace{x_0; x_0; \ldots; x_0}_{\leftarrow k_0 \text{ times} \rightarrow}; \underbrace{x_1; x_1; \ldots; x_1}_{\leftarrow k_1 \text{ times} \rightarrow}; \ldots; \underbrace{x_n; x_n; \ldots; x_n}_{\leftarrow k_n \text{ times} \rightarrow})$$

$$= \lim_{x_i^{(j)} \to x_i} \{ D(x_0; x_0^{(1)}; \ldots; x_0^{(k_0-1)}; x_1; x_1^{(1)}; \ldots; x_1^{(k_1-1)}; \ldots;$$

$$x_n; x_n^{(1)}; \ldots; x_n^{(k_n-1)}; f) / D(x_0; x_0^{(1)}; \ldots; x_0^{(k_0-1)}; x_1;$$

$$x_1^{(1)}; \ldots; x_1^{(k_1-1)}; \ldots; x_n; x_n^{(1)}; \ldots; x_n^{(k_n-1)}) \}.$$

Direct substitution of x_0 instead of $x_0^{(1)}$ leads to an expression in the form $0/0$. Using l'Hopital's rule let us first differentiate the numerator and denominator and then substitute $x_0^{(1)}$ by x_0. The second row in the numerator becomes

$$0 \quad 1 \quad 2x_0 \quad \cdots \quad (p-1)x_0^{p-2} \quad f'(x_0)$$

and the second row in the denominator takes the form

$$0 \quad 1 \quad 2x_0 \quad \cdots \quad (p-1)x_0^{p-2} \quad px_0^{p-1},$$

where $p = k_0 + k_1 + \cdots + k_n - 1$. After double differentiation on $x_0^{(2)}$ of the numerator and denominator and substitution of $x_0^{(2)}$ by x_0 the third rows will be, respectively,

$$0 \quad 0 \quad 2 \quad 2.3x_0 \quad \cdots \quad (p-2)(p-1)x_0^{p-3} \quad f''(x_0)$$

and

$$0 \quad 0 \quad 2 \quad 2.3x_0 \quad \cdots \quad (p-2)(p-1)x_0^{p-3} \quad (p-1)px_0^{p-2}.$$

Continuing this process further the first k_0 rows in the numerator take the form

$$\begin{matrix} 1 & x_0 & x_0^2 & \cdots & x_0^{p-1} & f(x_0) \\ 0 & 1 & 2x_0 & \cdots & (p-1)x_0^{p-2} & f'(x_0) \\ 0 & 0 & 2 & \cdots & (p-1)(p-2)x_0^{p-3} & f''(x_0) \\ \vdots & \vdots & \vdots & & \vdots & \vdots \\ 0 & 0 & 0 & \cdots & (p-1)(p-2)\cdots(p-k_0+1)x_0^{p-k_0} & f^{(k_0-1)}(x_0) \end{matrix}$$

The denominator is similar with only this difference that instead of the function f the function x^p has to be taken.

The same operation must be carried out with $x_1^{(1)}, x_1^{(2)}, \ldots, x_n^{(k_n-1)}$, and then the form of the final determinants in the numerator and in the denominator is clear.

For the application of l'Hopital's rule it is necessary that all the denominators be different from zero. Let us prove this. It is known for the Wandermond's determinant that

$$D(x_0; x_0^{(1)}; \ldots; x_0^{(k_0-1)}; x_1; x_1^{(1)}; \ldots; x_1^{(k_1-1)}; \ldots; x_n; x_n^{(1)}; \ldots; x_n^{(k_n-1)})$$

$$= \prod (x_i^{(j)} - x_k^{(s)})$$

Section 13   Interpolation

for $i > k$ or $i = k$, $j > s$, and distinguishing the factors that contain $x_0^{(1)}$

$$D(x_0; x_0^{(1)}; \ldots; x_n^{(k_n-1)})$$
$$= (x_0^{(1)} - x_0)(x_0^{(2)} - x_0^{(1)}) \cdots (x_n^{(k_n-1)} - x_0^{(1)}) D(x_0; x_0^{(2)}; \ldots; x_n^{(k_n-1)}).$$

So the derivative of the denominator on $x_0^{(1)}$ is, on setting $x_0^{(1)} = x_0$,

$$(x_0^{(2)} - x_0)(x_0^{(3)} - x_0) \cdots (x_n^{(k_n-1)} - x_0) D(x_0; x_0^{(2)}; \ldots; x_n^{(k_n-1)}).$$

Distinguishing further the factors that contain $x_0^{(2)}$

$$(x_0^{(2)} - x_0)^2 (x_0^{(3)} - x_0^{(2)}) \cdots (x_n^{(k_n-1)} - x_0^{(2)})(x_0^{(3)} - x_0)(x_0^{(4)} - x_0)$$
$$\cdots (x_n^{(k_n-1)} - x_0) D(x_0; x_0^{(3)}; \ldots; x_n^{(k_n-1)}),$$

and differentiating two times on $x_0^{(2)}$ and setting $x_0^{(2)} = x_0$ the result is

$$2!(x_0^{(3)} - x_0)^2 (x_0^{(4)} - x_0)^2 \cdots (x_n^{(k_n-1)} - x_0)^2 D(x_0; x_0^{(3)}; \ldots; x_n^{(k_n-1)}).$$

Similarly the third derivative of the above expression on $x_0^{(3)}$ is, on setting $x_0^{(3)} = x_0$, equal to

$$2!3!(x_0^{(4)} - x_0)^3 \cdots (x_n^{(k_n-1)} - x_0)^3 D(x_0; x_0^{(4)}; \ldots; x_n^{(k_n-1)}).$$

Continue this process with $x_0^{(j)}$, $j = 4, 5, \ldots, k_0 - 1$, the result is

$$2!3! \cdots (k_0 - 1)!(x_1 - x_0)^{k_0-1}(x_1^{(1)} - x_0)^{k_0-1}$$
$$\cdots (x_n^{(k_n-1)} - x_0)^{k_0-1} D(x_0; x_1; \ldots; x_n^{(k_n-1)}).$$

Distinguishing now $x_1^{(1)}$ from the last expression

$$2!3! \cdots (k_0 - 1)!(x_1 - x_0)^{k_0-1}(x_1^{(1)} - x_0)^{k_0}(x_1^{(2)} - x_0)^{k_0-1} \cdots (x_n^{(k_n-1)} - x_0)^{k_0-1}$$
$$\times (x_1^{(1)} - x_1)(x_1^{(2)} - x_1^{(1)}) \cdots (x_n^{(k_n-1)} - x_1^{(1)}) D(x_0; x_1; x_1^{(2)}; \ldots; x_n^{(k_n-1)})$$

and differentiating on $x_1^{(1)}$, setting x_1 instead of $x_1^{(1)}$ it follows that

$$2!3! \cdots (k_0 - 1)!(x_1 - x_0)^{2k_0-1}(x_1^{(2)} - x_0)^{k_0-1} \cdots (x_n^{(k_n-1)} - x_0)^{k_0-1}$$
$$\times (x_1^{(2)} - x_1) \cdots (x_n^{(k_n-1)} - x_1) D(x_0; x_1; x_1^{(2)}; \ldots; x_n^{(k_n-1)}).$$

Continuing, let us distinguish from the last factor of the above expression the differences $x_1^{(2)} - x_i^{(j)}$, then differentiate two times on $x_1^{(2)}$ and set $x_1^{(2)} = x_1$. This gives

$$2!3! \cdots (k_0 - 1)!2!(x_1 - x_0)^{3k_0-1}(x_1^{(3)} - x_0)^{k_0-1} \cdots (x_n^{(k_n-1)} - x_0)^{k_0-1}$$
$$\times (x_1^{(3)} - x_1)^2 \cdots (x_n^{(k_n-1)} - x_1)^2 D(x_0; x_1; x_1^{(3)}; \ldots; x_n^{(k_n-1)}).$$

After exhaustion of this process according to the next $x_1^{(i)}$, $i = 3, 4, \ldots, k_1 - 1$, the result is

$$2!3! \cdots (k_0 - 1)! 2! 3! \cdots (k_1 - 1)! (x_1 - x_0)^{k_1 k_0 - 1} (x_2 - x_0)^{k_0 - 1}$$
$$\cdots (x_n^{(k_n-1)} - x_0)^{k_0 - 1} (x_2 - x_1)^{k_1 - 1} \cdots (x_n^{(k_n-1)} - x_1)^{k_1 - 1}$$
$$\times D(x_0; x_1; x_2; x_2^{(1)}; \ldots; x_n^{(k_n-1)}) .$$

It is clear that on completing this process with $x_n^{(k_n-1)}$ the initial determinant

$$D(x_0; x_0^{(1)}; \ldots; x_0^{(k_0-1)}; x_1; x_1^{(1)}; \ldots; x_1^{(k_1-1)}; \ldots; x_n^{(k_n-1)})$$

turns into

$$2!3! \cdots (k_0 - 1)! \cdots 2!3! \cdots (k_n - 1)! \prod_{i>j} (x_i - x_j)^{k_i k_j - 1} D(x_0; x_1; \ldots; x_n)$$

and on evaluating $D(x_0; x_1; \ldots; x_n)$ the final result is

$$\left(\prod_{i=0}^{n} \prod_{j=2}^{k_i-1} j! \right) \prod_{i>j} (x_i - x_j)^{k_i k_j} .$$

Under the assumption that all the points in the initial determinant are different it follows that all the obtained determinants do not vanish. So the correctness of the definition (13.1) is proved. □

The definition (13.1) gives the rule for the computation of the divided differences with repeated knots:
(a) if at least two knots are different, e.g., $x_0 \neq x_n$,

$$f(\underbrace{x_0; x_0; \ldots; x_0}_{k_0 \text{ times}}; \underbrace{x_1; x_1; \ldots; x_1}_{k_1 \text{ times}}; \ldots; \underbrace{x_n; x_n; \ldots; x_n}_{k_n \text{ times}})$$

$$= \frac{1}{x_n - x_0} \{ f(\underbrace{x_0; x_0; \ldots; x_0}_{k_0 - 1 \text{ times}}; \underbrace{x_1; x_1; \ldots; x_1}_{k_1 \text{ times}}; \ldots; \underbrace{x_n; x_n; \ldots; x_n}_{k_n \text{ times}})$$

$$- f(\underbrace{x_0; x_0; \ldots; x_0}_{k_0 \text{ times}}; \underbrace{x_1; x_1; \ldots; x_1}_{k_1 \text{ times}}; \ldots; \underbrace{x_n; x_n; \ldots; x_n}_{k_n - 1 \text{ times}}) \} ;$$

(b) if all the knots coincide, e.g.,

$$f(\underbrace{x_0; x_0; \ldots; x_0}_{k_0 \text{ times}})$$

$$= \frac{\begin{vmatrix} 1 & x_0 & x_0^2 & \cdots & x_0^{k-2} & f(x_0) \\ 0 & 1 & 2x_0 & \cdots & (k-2)x_0^{k-3} & f'(x_0) \\ \vdots & \vdots & \vdots & & \vdots & \vdots \\ 0 & 0 & 0 & \cdots & (k-2)! & f^{(k-2)}(x_0) \\ 0 & 0 & 0 & \cdots & 0 & f^{(k-1)}(x_0) \end{vmatrix}}{\begin{vmatrix} 1 & x_0 & x_0^2 & \cdots & x_0^{k-2} & x_0^{k-1} \\ 0 & 1 & 2x_0 & \cdots & (k-2)x_0^{k-3} & (k-1)x_0^{k-2} \\ \vdots & \vdots & \vdots & & \vdots & \vdots \\ 0 & 0 & 0 & \cdots & (k-2)! & (k-1)!x_0 \\ 0 & 0 & 0 & \cdots & 0 & (k-1)! \end{vmatrix}} = \frac{f^{(k-1)}(x_0)}{(k-1)!} .$$

According to (3.1) the polynomial

$$\hat{H}_m(x) = f(x_0) + (x - x_0)f(x_0; x_0^{(1)}) + (x - x_0)(x - x_0^{(1)})f(x_0; x_0^{(1)}; x_0^{(2)}) + \cdots$$
$$+ (x - x_0)(x - x_0^{(1)}) \cdots (x - x_0^{(k_0 - 1)})f(x_0; x_0^{(1)}; \ldots; x_0^{(k_0 - 1)}; x_1)$$
$$+ \cdots + (x - x_0)(x - x_0^{(1)}) \cdots (x - x_0^{(k_0 - 1)})(x - x_1)$$
$$\times f(x_0; x_0^{(1)}; \ldots; x_0^{(k_0 - 1)}; x_1; x_1^{(1)}) + \cdots$$
$$+ (x - x_0)(x - x_0^{(1)}) \cdots (x - x_n^{(k_n - 2)})f(x_0; x_0^{(1)}; \ldots; x_n^{(k_n - 1)})$$

is of degree $m = k_0 + k_1 + \cdots + k_n - 1$ and satisfies

$$\hat{H}_m(x_s^{(j_s)}) = f(x_s^{(j_s)}) \quad \text{for } s = 0, 1, \ldots, n, \; j_s = 0, 1, \ldots, k_s - 1$$
$$(x_s^{(0)} = x_s).$$

If the function f has the necessary derivatives on passing on to $x_s^{(j_s)} \to x_s$ the polynomial $\hat{H}_m$ turns into H_m,

$$H_m(x) = f(x_0) + (x - x_0)f(x_0; x_0) + (x - x_0)^2 f(x_0; x_0; x_0) + \cdots$$
$$+ (x - x_0)^{k_0 - 1} f(\underbrace{x_0; x_0; \ldots; x_0}_{\leftarrow k_0 \text{ times} \rightarrow}) + (x - x_0)^{k_0} f(\underbrace{x_0; x_0; \ldots; x_0}_{\leftarrow k_0 \text{ times} \rightarrow}; x_1)$$
$$+ (x - x_0)^{k_0}(x - x_1) f(\underbrace{x_0; x_0; \ldots; x_0}_{\leftarrow k_0 \text{ times} \rightarrow}; x_1; x_1) + \cdots$$
$$+ (x - x_0)^{k_0}(x - x_1)^{k_1} \cdots (x - x_n)^{k_n - 1}$$
$$\times f(\underbrace{x_0; x_0; \ldots; x_0}_{\leftarrow k_0 \text{ times} \rightarrow}; \underbrace{x_1; x_1; \ldots; x_1}_{\leftarrow k_1 \text{ times} \rightarrow}; \ldots; \underbrace{x_n; x_n; \ldots; x_n}_{\leftarrow k_n \text{ times} \rightarrow}).$$
(13.2)

The polynomial H_m satisfies $H_m^{(j)}(x_0) = f^{(j)}(x_0)$ for $j = 0, 1, \ldots, k_0 - 1$. Because of the fact that the divided differences are symmetric functions of their arguments [see Section 3, (c)] before the limit passage $x_s^{(j_s)} \to x_s$ in $\hat{H}_m$ the polynomial obtained will be the same as H_m from (13.2) but in the form

$$H_m(x) = f(x_i) + (x - x_i)f(x_i; x_i) + (x - x_i)^2 f(x_i; x_i; x_i) + \cdots$$
$$+ (x - x_i)^{k_i - 1} f(\underbrace{x_i; x_i; \ldots; x_i}_{\leftarrow k_i \text{ times} \rightarrow}) + (x - x_i)^{k_i} f(\underbrace{x_i; x_i; \ldots; x_i}_{\leftarrow k_i \text{ times} \rightarrow}; x_j) + \cdots.$$

Evidently $H_m^{(j_i)}(x_i) = f^{(j_i)}(x_i)$ for $j_i = 0, 1, \ldots, k_i - 1, \; i = 0, 1, \ldots, n$.

According to Section 12 H_m is a Hermite polynomial for the function f and on combining the expression for $\hat{H}_m$ with the remainder term for $\hat{H}_m$ from (3.2) it follows that

$$f(x) = H_m(x) + R_m(f; x)$$
$$= H_m(x) + (x - x_0)^{k_0}(x - x_1)^{k_1} \cdots (x - x_n)^{k_n}$$
$$\times f(x; \underbrace{x_0; x_0; \ldots; x_0}_{\leftarrow k_0 \text{ times} \rightarrow}; \underbrace{x_1; x_1; \ldots; x_1}_{\leftarrow k_1 \text{ times} \rightarrow}; \ldots; \underbrace{x_n; x_n; \ldots; x_n}_{\leftarrow k_n \text{ times} \rightarrow}). \quad (13.3)$$

REMARK 13.1. Comparing the representations of the remainder terms from (12.1) and (13.3) the following expression results for the divided differences with repeated knots

$$f(x; \underbrace{x_0; x_0; \ldots; x_0}_{\leftarrow k_0 \text{ times} \rightarrow}; \underbrace{x_1; x_1; \ldots; x_1}_{\leftarrow k_1 \text{ times} \rightarrow}; \ldots; \underbrace{x_n; x_n; \ldots; x_n}_{\leftarrow k_n \text{ times} \rightarrow}) = \frac{f^{(m+1)}(\xi)}{(m+1)!},$$

where $m = k_0 + k_1 + \cdots + k_n - 1$.

14. Interpolation by means of trigonometric polynomials

Let f be a function defined in the interval $[0, 2\pi)$ and $\{x_i\}_{i=0}^{2m}$ be different points in this interval. There exists a unique trigonometric polynomial

$$\tau_m(x) = a_0 + \sum_{i=1}^{m} (a_i \cos ix + b_i \sin ix)$$

that satisfies $\tau_m(x_i) = f(x_i)$, $i = 0, 1, \ldots, 2m$. This polynomial can be written in the form

$$\tau_m(x) = \sum_{i=0}^{2m} f(x_i) \left(\prod_{s=0, s \neq i}^{2m} \sin \frac{x - x_s}{2} \bigg/ \prod_{s=0, s \neq i}^{2m} \sin \frac{x_i - x_s}{2} \right). \tag{14.1}$$

Really $\tau_m \in T_m$ because of the relations:

$\sin(x - \alpha)/2 \sin(x - \beta)/2$
$\quad = [\cos(\alpha - \beta)/2 - \cos(\alpha + \beta)/2 \cos x - \sin(\alpha + \beta)/2 \sin x]/2,$

$\sin kx \sin lx = [\cos(k - l)x - \cos(k + l)x]/2,$

$\sin kx \cos lx = [\sin(k - l)x + \sin(k + l)x]/2,$

$\cos kx \cos lx = [\cos(k - l)x + \cos(k + l)x]/2.$

The trigonometric polynomials

$$t_{m,i}(x) = \prod_{s=0, s \neq i}^{2m} \sin \frac{x - x_s}{2} \bigg/ \prod_{s=0, s \neq i}^{2m} \sin \frac{x_i - x_s}{2}, \quad i = 0, 1, \ldots, 2m,$$

satisfy $t_{m,i}(x_k) = \delta_{i,k}$ for $i, k = 0, 1, \ldots, 2m$ (see the basic Lagrange polynomials in Section 1) and $\tau_m(x) = \sum_{i=0}^{2m} f(x_i) t_{m,i}(x)$. The uniqueness of τ_m follows from the fact that the linear system

$$a_0 + \sum_{i=1}^{m} (a_i \cos ix_j + b_i \sin ix_j) = f(x_j), \quad j = 0, 1, \ldots, 2m,$$

has the determinant

$$D = \begin{vmatrix} 1 & \cos x_0 & \sin x_0 & \cos 2x_0 & \sin 2x_0 & \cdots & \sin 2mx_0 \\ 1 & \cos x_1 & \sin x_1 & \cos 2x_1 & \sin 2x_1 & \cdots & \sin 2mx_1 \\ 1 & \cos x_2 & \sin x_2 & \cos 2x_2 & \sin 2x_2 & \cdots & \sin 2mx_2 \\ \vdots & \vdots & \vdots & \vdots & \vdots & & \vdots \\ 1 & \cos x_{2m} & \sin x_{2m} & \cos 2x_{2m} & \sin 2x_{2m} & \cdots & \sin 2mx_{2m} \end{vmatrix}$$

$$= 2^{2m^2} \prod_{p>q} \sin \frac{x_p - x_q}{2} \neq 0, \quad \text{for } x_i \neq x_j, \ i \neq j \text{ and } x_i \in [a, a+2\pi),$$

$$i = 0, 1, \ldots, 2m, \tag{14.2}$$

and a is an arbitrary real number [compare with (1.2)]. To prove (14.2) let us multiply the third, fifth, ..., $(2m+1)$th columns by $2i$ and add them to the second, fourth, ..., $2m$th columns, then multiply the third, fifth, ..., $(2m+1)$th columns by $-2i$, with $i^2 = -1$, and add to them the second, fourth, ..., $2m$th columns. The kth row of the obtained matrix D_1 is

$$|1 \quad \exp(ix_k) \quad \exp(-ix_k) \quad \exp(2ix_k) \quad \exp(-2ix_k) \quad \cdots$$
$$\exp(mix_k) \quad \exp(-mix_k)|$$

and $(-2i)^m D = D_1$. Changing the columns of D_1 so that the kth row of the new obtained matrix D_2 is

$$|\exp(-mix_k) \quad \exp[-(m-1)ix_k] \quad \cdots \quad \exp(-ix_k) \quad 1$$
$$\exp(ix_k) \quad \cdots \quad \exp(mix_k)|$$

and then multiplying the kth row of D_2 by $\exp(mix_k)$, $k = 0, 1, \ldots, 2m$, the obtained matrix D_3 has a kth row

$$|1 \quad \exp(ix_k) \quad \exp(2ix_k) \quad \exp(3ix_k) \quad \cdots \quad \exp[(2m-1)ix_k] \quad \exp(2mix_k)|$$

and

$$(-1)^{m(m+1)}(-2i)^m \exp\left(mi \sum_{s=0}^{2m} x_s\right) D = D_3.$$

Setting $\exp(ix_k) = t_k$ the matrix D_3 turns into the Wandermond matrix. Hence

$$D_3 = \prod_{p>q}(t_p - t_q) = \prod_{p>q}[\exp(ix_p) - \exp(ix_q)]$$

$$= \prod_{p>q}(\cos x_p + i \sin x_p - \cos x_q - i \sin x_q)$$

$$= 2(i)^{m(2m+1)} \exp\left(mi \sum_{s=0}^{2m} x_s\right) \prod_{p>q} \sin \frac{x_p - x_q}{2}.$$

From the connection between D and D_3 and from the last equality taking into account that $i^{2m^2} = 1$ if m is an even number and $i^{2m^2} = -1$ if m is an odd number the assertion follows. □

REMARK 14.1. In the case of equidistant knots, $x_i = 2\pi i/(2m+1)$, $i = 0, 1, \ldots, 2m$, the interpolation polynomial (14.1) has an explicit form

$$T_m(x) = a_0 + \sum_{i=1}^{m}(a_i \cos ix + b_i \sin ix),$$

where

$$a_0 = \frac{1}{2m} \sum_{i=0}^{2m} f(x_i), \quad a_k = \frac{2}{(2m+1)} \sum_{i=0}^{2m} f(x_i) \cos kx_i,$$

$$b_k = \frac{2}{(2m+1)} \sum_{i=0}^{2m} f(x_i) \sin kx_i, \quad k = 1, 2, \ldots, m.$$

REMARK 14.2. If the function f is defined in the interval $[a, b]$ and $f(a) = f(b)$, the function $g(t) = f[a + t(b-a)/2\pi]$ is defined in $[0, 2\pi]$ and it is possible to consider g as a 2π-periodic function.

REMARK 14.3. If f is a 2π-periodic and even function it is natural to interpolate it using the basic functions $1, \cos x, \cos 2x, \cos 3x, \ldots$. In this case if $\{x_i\}_{i=0}^n$ are different points in the interval $[0, \pi)$, then the even trigonometric polynomial

$$\tau_n(x) = \sum_{i=0}^{n} f(x_i) \left(\prod_{s=0, s\neq i}^{n} (\cos x - \cos x_s) \right) \bigg/ \prod_{s=0, s\neq i}^{n} (\cos x_i - \cos x_s) \quad (14.3)$$

is the unique one that satisfies: $\tau_n \in T_n$ and $\tau_n(x_i) = f(x_i)$, $i = 0, 1, \ldots, n$.

Similarly if f is a 2π-periodic and odd function and $\{x_i\}_{i=1}^n$ are different points in the interval $[0, \pi)$, then the odd trigonometric polynomial of nth degree

$$\tau_n(x) = \sum_{i=1}^{n} f(x_i) \left(\sin x \prod_{s=1, s\neq i}^{n} (\cos x - \cos x_s) \right) \bigg/ \sin x_i \prod_{s=1, s\neq i}^{n} (\cos x_i - \cos x_s) \quad (14.4)$$

is the unique one that satisfies $\tau_n(x_i) = f(x_i)$, $i = 1, 2, \ldots, n$.

The uniqueness of the polynomials (14.3) and (14.4) follows from

$$D_{\cos}(x_0; x_1; \ldots; x_n) = \begin{vmatrix} 1 & \cos x_0 & \cos 2x_0 & \cdots & \cos nx_0 \\ 1 & \cos x_1 & \cos 2x_1 & \cdots & \cos nx_1 \\ 1 & \cos x_2 & \cos 2x_2 & \cdots & \cos nx_2 \\ \vdots & \vdots & \vdots & & \vdots \\ 1 & \cos x_n & \cos 2x_n & \cdots & \cos nx_n \end{vmatrix} \neq 0,$$

$$D_{\sin}(x_1; x_2; \ldots; x_n) = \begin{vmatrix} \sin x_1 & \sin 2x_1 & \cdots & \sin nx_1 \\ \sin x_2 & \sin 2x_2 & \cdots & \sin nx_2 \\ \sin x_3 & \sin 2x_3 & \cdots & \sin nx_3 \\ \vdots & \vdots & & \vdots \\ \sin x_n & \sin 2x_n & \cdots & \sin nx_n \end{vmatrix} \neq 0,$$

similarly to the uniqueness of the polynomial (14.1) using inequality (14.2). More exactly

$$D_{\cos} = 2^{n(n-1)/2} \prod_{p>q} (\cos x_p - \cos x_q), \quad (14.5)$$

$$D_{\sin} = 2^{n(n-1)/2} \prod_{s=1}^{n} \sin x_s \prod_{p>q} (\cos x_p - \cos x_q). \quad (14.6)$$

To prove (14.5) let us use the fact that $D_{\cos}(x_0; x_1; \ldots; x_{n-1}; x)$ is an even trigonometric polynomial of x of nth degree with zeros $\pm x_0, \pm x_1, \ldots, \pm x_{n-1}$.

This means that

$$D_{\cos}(x_0; x_1; \ldots; x_{n-1}; x) = C \prod_{q=0}^{n-1} (\cos x - \cos x_q). \tag{14.7}$$

Since $\cos nx = 2^{n-1} \cos^n x + \cdots$ the coefficient C can be determined by comparison of the factors of $\cos^n x$ on both sides of (14.7); so

$$C = 2^{n-1} D_{\cos}(x_0; x_1; \ldots; x_{n-1}),$$

$$D_{\cos}(x_0; x_1; \ldots; x_{n-1}; x)$$

$$= 2^{n-1} D_{\cos}(x_0; x_1; \ldots; x_{n-1}) \prod_{q=0}^{n-1} (\cos x - \cos x_q).$$

The identity (14.5) follows by applying the above relation recursively, substituting x by x_n. The proof of (14.6) is similar using

$$D_{\sin}(x_1; x_2; \ldots; x_{n-1}; x)/\sin x = S \prod_{q=0}^{n-1} (\cos x - \cos x_q)$$

$$\sin nx / \sin x = 2 \cos(n-1)x + \cdots.$$

REMARK 14.4. The Taylor interpolation problem by means of trigonometric polynomials consists of the determination of the polynomial $\tau_m \in T_m$ that satisfies for a given function f the conditions

$$\tau_m^{(k)}(x_0) = f^{(k)}(x_0), \quad k = 0, 1, \ldots, 2m. \tag{14.8}$$

The conditions (14.8) lead to a system of linear equations. For instance let $x_0 = 0$. Then to determine the coefficients of the polynomial

$$\tau_m(x) = a_0 + \sum_{k=1}^{m} (a_k \cos kx + b_k \sin kx)$$

it is necessary for the following two systems to be solved:

$$\begin{aligned}
a_0 + a_1 + a_2 + a_3 + \cdots + a_m &= f(0), \\
a_1 + 2^2 a_2 + 3^2 a_3 + \cdots + m^2 a_m &= -f''(0), \\
a_1 + 2^4 a_2 + 3^4 a_3 + \cdots + m^4 a_m &= f^{(4)}(0), \\
\vdots \quad \vdots \quad \vdots \quad \vdots \quad \vdots & \\
a_1 + 2^{2m} a_2 + 3^{2m} a_3 + \cdots + m^{2m} a_m &= (-1)^m f^{(2m)}(0),
\end{aligned}$$

and

$$\begin{aligned}
b_1 + 2b_2 + 3b_3 + \cdots + mb_m &= f'(0), \\
b_1 + 2^3 b_2 + 3^3 b_3 + \cdots + m^3 b_m &= -f'''(0), \\
b_1 + 2^5 b_2 + 3^5 b_3 + \cdots + m^5 b_m &= f^{(5)}(0), \\
\vdots \quad \vdots \quad \vdots \quad \vdots \quad \vdots & \\
b_1 + 2^{2m-1} b_2 + 3^{2m-1} b_3 + \cdots + m^{2m-1} b_m &= (-1)^{m-1} f^{(2m-1)}(0).
\end{aligned}$$

For $m = 1$ and $m = 2$ the corresponding polynomials are

$$T_1(x) = f(0) + f''(0) - f''(0)\cos x + f'(0)\sin x\,;$$

$$T_2(x) = f(0) + \tfrac{15}{12}f''(0) + \tfrac{1}{4}f^{(4)}(0) - \tfrac{1}{3}[4f''(0) + f^{(4)}(0)]\cos x$$
$$+ \tfrac{1}{3}[4f'(0) + f'''(0)]\sin x + \tfrac{1}{12}[f''(0) + f^{(4)}(0)]\cos 2x$$
$$- \tfrac{1}{6}[f'(0) + f'''(0)]\sin 2x\,.$$

15. Interpolation of complex functions

The Lagrange interpolation formula (2.2) is suitable for complex functions. Indeed, let the function f be an analytic function in the domain G of the complex plane and let L be a closed Jordan rectifiable curve that belongs to G together with its interior D. Suppose that the knots $\{z_i\}_{i=0}^n$ belong to D and let us consider the integral

$$P_n(f;z) = \frac{1}{2\pi i}\int_L \frac{\omega(\zeta) - \omega(z)}{\omega(\zeta)(\zeta - z)} f(\zeta)\,d\zeta\,, \tag{15.1}$$

where $\omega(z) = (z - z_0)(z - z_1)\cdots(z - z_n)$. Using the residual theorem and the equality $\lim_{\alpha \to z_k}(\zeta - z_k)/\omega(\zeta) = 1/\omega'(z_k)$ it follows that

$$P_n(f;z) = \sum_{k=0}^n \lim_{\zeta \to z_k} \frac{\omega(\zeta) - \omega(z)}{\omega(\zeta)(\zeta - z)} f(\zeta)(\zeta - z_k)$$

$$= \sum_{k=0}^n f(z_k) \frac{\omega(z)}{\omega'(z_k)(z - z_k)}\,;$$

i.e. P_n is Lagrange's interpolation polynomial. By virtue of the Cauchy formula

$$f(z) = \frac{1}{2\pi i}\int_L \frac{f(\zeta)}{\zeta - z}\,d\zeta$$

and (15.1) it follows that $f(z) = P_n(f;z) + R_n(f;z)$, where the remainder R_n has the form

$$R_n(f;z) = \frac{\omega(z)}{2\pi i}\int_L \frac{f(\zeta)}{\omega(\zeta)(\zeta - z)}\,d\zeta\,.$$

Let us mention that similarly to the interpolation of a real function the smoothness of the functions plays an important role for the accuracy. For instance, let us consider the functions $f_1(z) = |z|$ and $f_2(z) = e^z$ and their interpolation polynomials $p_8(f_s)$, of eighth degree such that

$$p_8(f_s; z_{kl}) = f_s(z_{kl})\,, \quad s = 1, 2\,,$$

$$z_{kl} = -1 + k + i(-1 + l)\,, \quad k, l = 0, 1, 2,\ i^2 = -1\,.$$

In Figs. 15.1 and 15.2 the graphs of $|f_s(z) - p_8(f_s; z)|$, $s = 1, 2$, are given in

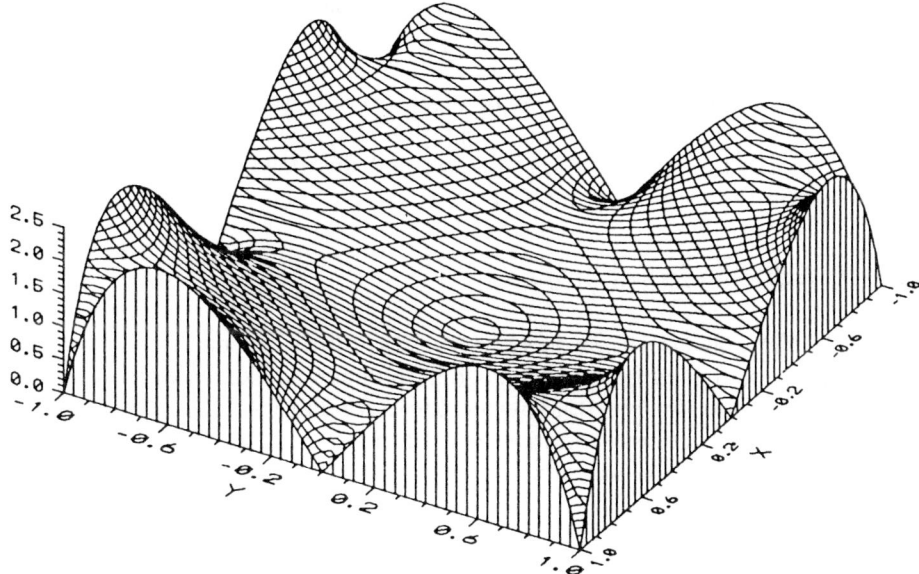

Fig. 15.1. The graph of $||z| - p_8(\cdot; z)|$.

the unit square $D = \{z = x + \mathrm{i}y: -1 \leq x \leq 1, -1 \leq y \leq 1\}$. For the deviation the results are:

$$\max_{z \in D} |f_1(z) - p_8(f_1; z)| \leq 2.2964 \ldots,$$

$$\max_{z \in D} |f_2(z) - p_8(f_2; z)| \leq 0.0000298 \ldots.$$

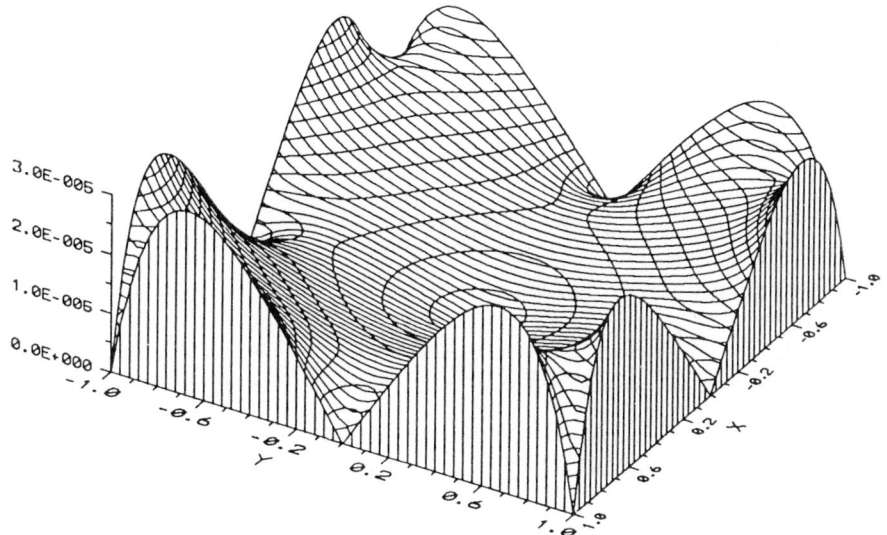

Fig. 15.2. The graph of $|e^z - p_8(\cdot; z)|$.

The Hermite interpolation problem from Section 12 can also be considered for complex functions. Let the function f be smooth enough in the domain G and $\{z_i\}_{i=0}^m$ be different points from G. For arbitrary non-negative integer numbers $\{\alpha_i\}_{i=0}^m$ there exists a unique algebraic polynomial P_n of nth degree, $n = \alpha_0 + \alpha_1 + \cdots + \alpha_m + m$, which satisfies the conditions $P_n^{(s_i)}(f; z_i) = f^{(s_i)}(z_i)$, $s_i = 0, 1, \ldots, \alpha_i$, $i = 0, 1, \ldots, m$, and this polynomial evidently can be written in the form

$$P_n(f; z) = \sum_{k=0}^{m} \sum_{i=0}^{\alpha_k} L_{ki}(z) f^{(i)}(z_k),$$

where L_{ki} are polynomials of degree at most n, which depend on the knots z_k and on their multiplicities α_k. It is possible to obtain an explicit expression for L_{ki}. Let us follow KRILOV, BOBKOV and MONASTIRNII ([1972], p. 380).

For this aim let us consider the Hermite interpolation polynomial $P_n(1/(w-z); z)$ for the function $1/(w-z)$. The remainder term

$$R_n\left(\frac{1}{w-z}; z\right) = \frac{1}{w-z} - P_n\left(\frac{1}{w-z}; z\right)$$

$$= \frac{1}{w-z} - \sum_{k=0}^{m} \sum_{i=0}^{\alpha_k} L_{ki}(z) \frac{i!}{(w-z_k)^{i+1}}$$

is a rational fraction on w and

$$R_n\left(\frac{1}{w-z}; z\right) = \frac{B(w, z)}{(w-z)A(w)}.$$

For $|w| > |z|$,

$$\frac{1}{w-z} = \sum_{\nu=0}^{\infty} \frac{z^\nu}{w^{\nu+1}}, \qquad R_n\left(\frac{1}{w-z}; z\right) = \sum_{\nu=0}^{\infty} w^{-\nu-1} R_n(z^\nu; z).$$

Because of $R_n(z^\nu; z) = 0$ for $\nu = 0, 1, \ldots, n$ it follows that

$$R_n\left(\frac{1}{w-z}; z\right) = \sum_{\nu=n+1}^{\infty} w^{-\nu-1} R_n(z^\nu; z).$$

The last equality shows that when $w \to \infty$,

$$R_n\left(\frac{1}{w-z}; z\right) = \frac{B(w, z)}{(w-z)A(w)} \to 0$$

not slower than w^{-n-2}. As $A(w) = w^{n+1} + \cdots$, it comes out that $B(w, z)$ does not depend on w. Leaving $z \to w$ in

$$\frac{1}{w-z} - \sum_{k=0}^{m} \sum_{i=0}^{\alpha_k} L_{ki}(z) \frac{i!}{(w-z_k)^{i+1}} = \frac{B(z)}{(w-z)A(w)}$$

Interpolation

it follows that $B(z) = A(z)$ and

$$R_n\left(\frac{1}{w-z}; z\right) = \frac{A(z)}{(w-z)A(w)}.$$

From the last equality using the Cauchy formula and the residual theorem the following expression for the remainder term results:

$$R_n(f; z) = \frac{1}{2\pi i} \int_L R_n\left(\frac{1}{w-z}; z\right) f(w) \, dw = \frac{A(z)}{2\pi i} \int_L \frac{f(w)}{(w-z)A(w)} \, dw$$

$$= A(z)\left(\text{Res}\, \frac{f(w)}{(w-z)A(w)}\bigg|_{w=z} + \sum_{k=0}^{m} \text{Res}\, \frac{f(w)}{(w-z)A(w)}\bigg|_{w=z_k}\right)$$

$$= f(z) + A(z) \sum_{k=0}^{m} \text{Res}\, \frac{f(w)}{(w-z)A(w)}\bigg|_{w=z_k}.$$

When w is near to z_k let us consider the series

$$f(w) = \sum_{i=0}^{\infty} \frac{1}{i!} f^{(i)}(z_k)(w - z_k)^i,$$

$$\frac{1}{w-z} = \frac{1}{(w-z_k) - (z-z_k)} = -\sum_{i=0}^{\infty} \frac{(w-z_k)^i}{(z-z_k)^{i+1}},$$

$$\frac{(w-z_k)^{\alpha_k+1}}{A(w)} = \sum_{i=0}^{\infty} c_i^{(k)} (w-z_k)^i.$$

Multiplying the above three series together,

$$\text{Res}\, \frac{f(w)}{(w-z)A(w)}\bigg|_{w=z_k}$$

is the coefficient of $(w - z_k)^{-1}$ in the Loran series of the function

$$\frac{1}{(w-z_k)^{\alpha_k+1}} \frac{f(w)(w-z_k)^{\alpha_k+1}}{(w-z)A(w)} = \sum_{i=-\infty}^{\infty} d_i^{(k)} (w-z_k)^i.$$

The evaluation shows that

$$d_{-1}^{(k)} = -\sum_{i=0}^{\alpha_k} \frac{1}{i!} f^{(i)}(z_k) \sum_{s=0}^{\alpha_k-i} c_s^{(k)} (x - z_k)^{-\alpha_k+s+i-1}$$

and finally the Hermite polynomial takes the form

$$P_n(f; z) = \sum_{k=0}^{m} \sum_{i=0}^{\alpha_k} \frac{1}{i!} f^{(i)}(z_k) \frac{A(z)}{(z-z_k)^{\alpha_k+1}} \sum_{s=0}^{\alpha_k-i} c_s^{(k)} (x - z_k)^{s+i}, \qquad (15.2)$$

where $A(z) = \Pi_{k=0}^{m} (z - z_k)^{\alpha_k+1}$. Only the values $f^{(i)}(z_k)$, $i = 0, 1, \ldots, \alpha_k$, $k = 0, 1, \ldots, m$, in the representation (15.2) take part. This means that the representation (15.2) is valid not only for analytic functions but for all functions for which the values $f^{(i)}(z_k)$ are determined.

16. Chakalov's approach for divided differences

By Section 3, properties (a) and (b), the divided difference is a linear functional of the type $D[f] = \sum_{k=0}^{n} A_k f(x_k)$, which satisfies the condition (d). These conditions entirely determine the coefficients A_k because they must satisfy the linear system

$$A_0 x_0^n + A_1 x_1^n + \cdots + A_n x_n^n = 1,$$
$$A_0 x_0^m + A_1 x_1^m + \cdots + A_n x_n^m = 0, \quad m = 0, 1, \ldots, n-1,$$

with the Wandermond determinant.

CHAKALOV [1957] gives an equivalent definition of the divided difference with multiple knots. Let us denote by

$$D\left[f \left| \begin{matrix} x_0, x_1, \ldots, x_n \\ \nu_0, \nu_1, \ldots, \nu_n \end{matrix} \right. \right]$$

the divided difference of the function f at the points $x_0, x_1, \ldots, x_n$ with multiplicities $\nu_0, \nu_1, \ldots, \nu_n$. Such a divided difference is an expression of the type

$$D[f] = \sum_{k=0}^{n} \sum_{\lambda=0}^{\nu_k - 1} A_{k\lambda} f^{(\lambda)}(x_k),$$

with coefficients $A_{k\lambda}$ that do not depend on f and satisfy the conditions:
(1) $D[f] = 0$ for $f \in H_{N-1}$;
(2) $D[f] = 1$ for $f = x^N$, $N = \nu_0 + \nu_1 + \cdots \nu_n - 1$.
The next two theorems are due to CHAKALOV [1957].

THEOREM 16.1. *Let* $P(z) = (z - x_0)^{\nu_0}(z - x_1)^{\nu_1} \cdots (z - x_n)^{\nu_n}$. *If*

$$\frac{1}{P(z)} = \sum_{k=0}^{n} \sum_{\lambda=0}^{\nu_k - 1} A_{k\lambda} \frac{\lambda!}{(z - x_k)^{\lambda+1}},$$

then the linear functional

$$D[f] = \sum_{k=0}^{n} \sum_{\lambda=0}^{\nu_k - 1} A_{k\lambda} f^{(\lambda)}(x_k) \tag{16.1}$$

satisfies the conditions (1) *and* (2) *and is a unique expression of this type.*

PROOF. Let $D[f]$ satisfy (1) and (2). For the function

$$f(x) = P(z)/(z - x)$$

the relation

$$D[f] = D[P(z)/(z - x)] = P(z) \sum_{k=0}^{n} \sum_{\lambda=0}^{\nu_k - 1} A_{k\lambda} \frac{\lambda!}{(z - x_k)^{\lambda+1}}, \tag{16.2}$$

SECTION 16   *Interpolation*   271

is fulfilled because $[1/(z-x)]^{(\lambda)}_{x=x_k} = \lambda!/(z-x_k)^{\lambda+1}$. On the other hand, $f = f_1 + f_2$, where

$$f_1(x) = [P(z) - P(x)]/(z-x), \qquad f_2(x) = P(x)/(z-x).$$

The function f_1 is a polynomial of degree N with respect to x with a leading coefficient of one and therefore $D[f_1] = 1$, $D[f_2] = 0$; i.e. $D[f] = 1$. This equality and (16.2) give

$$\frac{1}{P(z)} = \sum_{k=0}^{n} \sum_{\lambda=0}^{\nu_k - 1} A_{k\lambda} \frac{\lambda!}{(z-x_k)^{\lambda+1}}.$$

It is proved that if there is an expression of the type (16.1) that satisfies the conditions (1), (2) then its coefficients must be determined by the expansion of $1/P(z)$ and therefore this expression is unique.

Conversely, let us prove that if

$$\frac{1}{P(z)} = \sum_{k=0}^{n} \sum_{\lambda=0}^{\nu_k - 1} B_{k\lambda} \frac{\lambda!}{(z-x_k)^{\lambda+1}}$$

then the expression (16.1) with coefficients $A_{k\lambda} = B_{k\lambda}/\lambda!$ satisfies the conditions (1) and (2). Let $A_{k\lambda} = B_{k\lambda}/\lambda!$. From

$$D[P(z)/(z-x)] = P(z) \sum_{k=0}^{n} \sum_{\lambda=0}^{\nu_k - 1} B_{k\lambda}/(z-x_k)^{\lambda+1} = 1,$$

which is true for every z and $P(z)/(z-x) = f_1(x) + f_2(x)$, it follows that

$$D[f_1] = D[f_1] + D[f_2] = 1.$$

Since

$$f_1(x) = z^N + \varphi_1(x) z^{N-1} + \cdots + \varphi_N(x),$$

where

$$\varphi_k(x) = x^k + c_{k1} x^{k-1} + \cdots + c_{kk}, \qquad k = 1, 2, \ldots, N,$$

it follows that for every z it is fulfilled that

$$1 = D[f_1] = D[1] z^N + D[\varphi_1] z^{N-1} + \cdots + D[\varphi_N].$$

The last equality implies $D[1] = D[\varphi_1] = \cdots = D[\varphi_{N-1}] = 0$ and $D[\varphi_N] = 1$. As the polynomials $1, \varphi_1, \ldots, \varphi_{N-1}$ are linearly independent the condition (1) follows. The condition (2) follows from $D[\varphi_N] = 1$. □

THEOREM 16.2. *If the function f has a partially continuous Nth derivative in $[x_0, x_n]$, $x_0 < x_1 < \cdots < x_n$, $\nu_0 + \nu_1 + \cdots + \nu_n - 1 = N$, then*

$$D\left[f \left| \begin{matrix} x_0, x_1, \ldots, x_n \\ \nu_0, \nu_1, \ldots, \nu_n \end{matrix} \right. \right] = \int_{x_0}^{x_n} U(t) f^{(N)}(t) \, dt,$$

where

$$U(t) = \frac{D_x[(x-t)_+^{N-1}]}{(N-1)!} = \sum_{k=0}^{n} \sum_{\lambda=0}^{\nu_k-1} \frac{A_{k\lambda}(x_k-t)_+^{N-\lambda-1}}{(N-\lambda-1)!},$$

$$U(t) \begin{cases} >0 & \text{for } t \in (x_0, x_n), \\ =0 & \text{for } t \notin (x_0, x_n). \end{cases}$$

(16.3)

PROOF. By property (1) $D[f]=0$ for polynomials f of degree $N-1$ and by Theorem 44.1 the integral representation follows. Let us prove by induction that U is positive. Assume that the theorem is true for an arbitrary choice of the knots with multiplicities whose sum is less or equal to N. Let us build the divided difference

$$D\left[f \middle| \begin{array}{c} x_0, x_1, \ldots, x_n \\ \nu_0, \nu_1, \ldots, \nu_n \end{array}\right],$$

such that $\nu_0 + \nu_1 + \cdots + \nu_n = N+1$ and U is defined by (16.3). The expression

$$\sum_{\lambda=0}^{\nu_k-1} \frac{A_{k\lambda}(x_k-t)_+^{N-\lambda-1}}{(N-\lambda-1)!}$$

is the residual r_k of the function

$$\frac{(z-x)^{N-1}}{(N-1)!P(z)},$$

which corresponds to the pole $z = x_k$. Indeed, if C_k is a closed curve around x_k then

$$r_k = \frac{1}{2\pi i} \int_{C_k} \frac{(z-x)^{N-1}}{(N-1)!P(z)} dz = \frac{1}{2\pi i} \int_{C_k} \sum_{j=0}^{n} \sum_{\lambda=0}^{\nu_j-1} \frac{\lambda! A_{j\lambda}(z-x)^{N-1}}{(N-1)!(z-x_j)^{\lambda+1}} dz$$

$$= \sum_{\lambda=0}^{\nu_k-1} \frac{A_{k\lambda}}{(N-1)!} \frac{\lambda!}{2\pi i} \int_{C_k} \frac{(z-x)^{N-1}}{(z-x_k)^{\lambda+1}} dz.$$

The equality

$$r_k = \sum_{\lambda=0}^{\nu_k-1} \frac{A_{k\lambda}}{(N-1)!} [(z-x)^{N-1}]_{x=x_k}^{(\lambda)} = \sum_{\lambda=0}^{\nu_k-1} \frac{A_{k\lambda}}{(N-\lambda-1)!}(x_k-x)^{N-\lambda-1}$$

gives

$$U(x) = \frac{1}{2\pi i} \int_{C_s} \frac{(z-x)^{N-1}}{(N-1)!} \frac{1}{P(z)} dz$$

for $x \in [x_{s-1}, x_s]$, where C_s is a closed curve such that the points $x_0, x_1, \ldots, x_{s-1}$ lie outside of C_s and $x_s, x_{s+1}, \ldots, x_n$ are in C_s.

For every $x \in (x_{s-1}, x_s)$

$$\frac{d}{dx}\left[\frac{U(x)}{(x_n - x)^{N-1}}\right] = \frac{1}{(x_n - x)^N} \frac{1}{2\pi i} \int_{C_s} \frac{(z-x)^{N-1}}{(N-1)!} \frac{1}{P_1(z)} dz,$$

where $P_1(z) = P(z)/(z - x_n)$. Since the function

$$U_1(x) = \frac{1}{2\pi i} \int_{C_s} \frac{(z-x)^{N-1}}{(N-1)!} \frac{1}{P_1(z)} dz$$

corresponds to the divided difference

$$D\left[f \left| \begin{array}{c} x_0, x_1, \ldots, x_{n-1} \\ \nu_0, \nu_1, \ldots, \nu_{n-1} \end{array} \right.\right] \quad \text{for } \nu_n = 1$$

or

$$D\left[f \left| \begin{array}{c} x_0, x_1, \ldots, x_n \\ \nu_0, \nu_1, \ldots, \nu_n \end{array} \right.\right] \quad \text{for } \nu_n > 1$$

the recurrence relation

$$\frac{d}{dx}\left[\frac{U(x)}{(x_n - x)^{N-1}}\right] = \frac{U_1(x)}{(x_n - x)^N} \tag{16.4}$$

is true. By assumption $U_1(x) > 0$ for $x \in (x_0, x_n)$ (or for $x \in (x_0, x_{n-1})$ if $\nu_n = 1$). From (16.4) it follows that $U(x)/(x_n - x)^{N-1}$ and also $U(x)$ must be positive if $U(x_0) \geq 0$. It is clear that $U(x) = 0$ for $x \notin (x_0, x_n)$ because of

$$(x_k - x)_+ = \begin{cases} x_k - x & \text{for } x < x_0, \\ 0 & \text{for } x > 0, \end{cases} \quad k = 0, 1, \ldots, n,$$

which gives $U(x) = D[(z-x)^{N-1}] = 0$ in the first case and $U(x) = D[0] = 0$ in the second case. Since U is a continuous function for $\nu_0 < N$ it follows that

$$U(x_0) = \lim_{x \to x_0} U(x) = 0.$$

Similarly $U(x_n) = 0$. The case $\nu_0 = N$ is possible only for $n = 1$, $\nu_1 = 1$ and

$$U(x) = \frac{1}{2\pi i} \int_{C_1} \frac{(z-x)^{N-1}}{(N-1)!(z-x_0)^N(z-x_1)} dz$$

$$= \frac{1}{(N-1)!} \operatorname*{res}_{z=x_1} \frac{(z-x)^{N-1}}{(z-x_0)^N(z-x_1)}$$

$$= \frac{1}{(N-1)!} \frac{(x_1 - x)^{N-1}}{(x_1 - x_0)^N} > 0 \quad \text{for } x \in [x_0, x_1].$$

So for arbitrary N the theorem is true for $\nu_0 = N$, $\nu_1 = 1$ and $U(x_0) \geq 0$. All this together with the recursive relation (16.4) completes the proof by induction. □

Remark 13.1 is a direct consequence of Theorem 16.2. Indeed, for $\varphi(x) = x^N$ it follows that

$$1 = D[\varphi] = N! \int_{x_0}^{x_n} U(t)\,dt$$

and by the mean value theorem

$$D[f] = \int_{x_0}^{x_n} U(t)f^{(N)}(t)\,dt = f^{(N)}(\xi)\int_{x_0}^{x_n} U(t)\,dt = \frac{f^{(N)}(\xi)}{N!}.$$

17. Interpolation of functions of several variables

Let the function f be defined at the points $\{(x_i, y_i)\}_{i=0}^{n}$, which belong to the set G in the plane. The algebraic polynomial of two variables of mth degree is an expression of the kind $P_m(x, y) = \sum_{i+j \le m} a_{ij} x^i y^j$, where a_{ij} are constants. The interpolation problem consists of the determination of a polynomial P_m such that

$$P_m(x_i, y_i) = f(x_i, y_i), \quad i = 0, 1, \ldots, n. \tag{17.1}$$

The interest in multivariate interpolation, a particular case of which is (17.1), increased with the development of the finite-element method—see NICOLAIDES [1972]. A simple example given by ZLAMAL [1968, 1969] in this connection is that for any triangle $\triangle$ in the plane with the vertices A_i, $i = 1, 2, 3$, there is a unique polynomial $P_2(x, y) = \sum_{i+j \le 2} a_{ij} x^i y^j$ such that

$$P_2(A_i) = \varphi(A_i), \quad P_2(B_i) = \varphi(B_i), \quad i = 1, 2, 3,$$

where B_i are the midpoints of the sides of $\triangle$ and φ is an arbitrary function defined on $\triangle$. For the error he derived the relations

$$\sup_{P \in \triangle} |P_2(P) - \varphi(P)| \le c M_3 h^3,$$

$$\sup_{P \in \triangle} \left| \frac{\partial}{\partial x_i} [P_2(P) - \varphi(P)] \right| \le \frac{c_1 M_3 h^2}{\sin \theta},$$

where h is the greatest length of the sides of $\triangle$, θ is the smallest angle of $\triangle$,

$$M_3 = \sup_{P \in \triangle} \left| \frac{\partial^3 \varphi(P)}{\partial x_i \partial x_j \partial x_k} \right|, \quad 1 \le i, j, k \le 2,$$

and c, c_1 are constants.

CIARLET and WAGSCHAL [1970] generalized this result for an arbitrary n-simplex $\triangle$ in $\mathbb{R}^n$, with the vertices A_i, $i = 1, 2, \ldots, n+1$. Using a multipoint Taylor formula they proved that there exists a unique polynomial

$$P_2(x_1, x_2, \ldots, x_n) = \sum_{i_1 + \cdots + i_n \le 2} a_{i_1 i_2 \cdots i_n} x_1^{i_1} x_2^{i_2} \cdots x_n^{i_n},$$

such that

$$P_2(A_i) = \varphi(A_i), \qquad P_2(A_{ij}) = \varphi(A_{ij}),$$

where A_{ij} is the midpoint of the segment A_iA_j. Note that the number of interpolation conditions is $(n+1)(n+2)/2$ and there are so many coefficients in P_2.

Further important generalizations of Lagrange interpolation in $\mathbb{R}^n$ are given in CIARLET and RAVIART [1972]. They derived an explicit form of the interpolation polynomial for a special point set in $\mathbb{R}^n$ (e.g., the vertices and the midpoints of the edges of a non-degenerate n-simplex in $\mathbb{R}^n$) as well as the estimation of the remainder term.

Two difficulties arise in solving the linear system (17.1).

(1) The number of the basic functions

$$1, x, y, x^2, xy, y^2, \ldots, x^m, x^{m-1}y, \ldots, y^m$$

taking part in P_m is $(m+1)(m+2)/2$ and this means that the number of the interpolation knots (x_i, y_i) must be $(m+1)(m+2)/2$.

(2) If the knots $(x_i, y_i) \in G$ are arbitrarily distributed there is no guarantee that the system (17.1) has a unique solution. For example, let $m=1$, $n=2$ and the points (x_0, y_0), (x_1, y_1), (x_2, y_2) be collinear; i.e.

$$\begin{vmatrix} 1 & x_0 & y_0 \\ 1 & x_1 & y_1 \\ 1 & x_2 & y_2 \end{vmatrix} = 0.$$

This example shows that the algebraic polynomial P_1 for which $P_1(x_i, y_i) = f(x_i, y_i)$, $i = 0, 1, 2$, either does not exist or there exist many polynomials of first degree satisfying these conditions.

THEOREM 17.1. *Let* $Q_i = (x_i, y_i)$, $i = 0, 1, \ldots, (m+1)(m+2)/2 - 1$, *be different points in the plane that do not lie on the algebraic curve of mth degree* $(\Sigma_{i+j \leq m} a_{ij} x^i y^j = 0)$. *Then for every function f defined at the points* Q_i *there exist a unique algebraic polynomial* P_m *of mth degree that satisfies* $P_m(x_i, y_i) = f(x_i, y_i)$, $i = 0, 1, \ldots, (m+1)(m+2)/2 - 1$.

The proof of the theorem follows directly from Theorem 1.1 regarding $l_i(f) = f(x_i, y_i)$.

The explicit form of the interpolation polynomial of two variables can be obtained in the case of the $(m+1)(m+2)/2$ knots

$$\begin{aligned} &(x_0, y_0), \ (x_0, y_1), \ldots, (x_0, y_2), \ (x_0, y_m), \\ &(x_1, y_0), \ (x_1, y_1), \ldots, (x_1, y_{m-1}), \\ &\quad \vdots \qquad \vdots \qquad \ddots \\ &(x_{m-1}, y_0), (x_{m-1}, y_1), \\ &(x_m, y_0), \end{aligned} \qquad (17.2)$$

where $x_i \neq x_j$ and $y_i \neq y_j$ for $i \neq j$. They do not lie on an algebraic curve of mth degree. Indeed, assume that the points (17.2) lie on the algebraic curve ϕ_m of mth degree. Because the $m+1$ points from the first row (x_0, y_i), $i = 0, 1, \ldots, m$ lie together on ϕ_m and on the straight line $\lambda_0: x = x_0$ the curve ϕ_m must decompose to an algebraic curve ϕ_{m-1} of degree $m-1$ and a straight line λ_0. It follows that $\phi_m = \lambda_0 \phi_{m-1}$. Similarly using the points (x_1, y_i), $i = 0, 1, \ldots, m-1$, from the second row of (17.2), which lie on the straight line $\lambda_1: x = x_1$ and on the algebraic curve ϕ_{m-1} it follows that $\phi_{m-1} = \lambda_1 \phi_{m-2}$, where ϕ_{m-2} is an algebraic curve of degree $m-2$. Continuing in this way it turns out that the points (x_{m-1}, y_0), (x_{m-1}, y_1), (x_m, y_0) lie on a straight line. This is impossible.

The points (17.2) are ordered regularly in the right-angled triangle with vertices (x_0, y_0), (x_0, y_m), (x_m, y_m). For an arbitrary triangle in the plane let $(m+1)(m+2)/2$ points $P_{ij} = (x_i, y_j)$ be situated as is shown in Fig. 17.1, where the segments $[P_{m0}, P_{0m}]$, $[P_{m0}, P_{00}]$, $[P_{00}, P_{0m}]$ are divided into m equal segments and the other points are intersection points of the straight lines that are parallel to the sides of the triangle with vertexes P_{00}, P_{m0}, and P_{0m}. The proof that the points P_{ij} obtained do not lie on a curve of mth degree is similar to the proof for the points (17.2).

CHUNG and YAO [1977] gave a geometric characterization GC of the distribution of the points in $\mathbb{R}^n$ which ensures the existence and uniqueness of the Lagrange-type interpolant.

Let a node mean a point in $\mathbb{R}^n$, a lattice mean a set of nodes, and a polynomial always mean a polynomial in n variables. If the degree of the polynomial is k then it has $N = \binom{n+k}{k}$ terms. If $X = \{P_1, P_2, \ldots, P_m\}$ is a lattice, then X admits interpolations of degree, less than or equal to k if and only if for any $f: X \to \mathbb{C}$ ($\mathbb{C}$ is the complex plane) there exists a unique complex polynomial P of degree less than or equal to k such that $P(P_i) = f(P_i)$, $i = 1, 2, \ldots, m$.

Following COATMELEC [1966] and similar to Theorem 17.1, X admits a unique

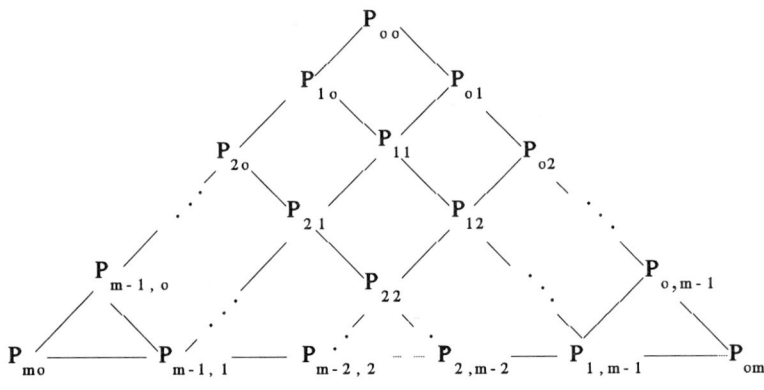

FIG. 17.1.

interpolation of degree less than or equal to k if and only if $m = N$ and X is not a subset of any algebraic surface of degree less than or equal to k. Also if $m = N$ and X admits an interpolation of degree less than or equal to k then X admits a unique interpolation of degree less than or equal to k and the polynomial has the form

$$P(\mathrm{P}) = \sum_{i=1}^{N} p_i(\mathrm{P})f(\mathrm{P}_i),$$

where the polynomials p_i satisfy: p_i is a real polynomial of degree exactly k; p_i does not have a factor u^2, where u is a real polynomial of degree greater than or equal to 1; p_i depends only on X and $p_i(\mathrm{P}_j) = \delta_{ij}$.

A lattice $X = \{\mathrm{P}_1, \mathrm{P}_2, \ldots, \mathrm{P}_N\}$ of N nodes in $\mathbb{R}^n$ satisfies the GC condition if to each node P_i there exist k distinct hyperplanes $G_{i1}, G_{i2}, \ldots, G_{ik}$ such that $\mathrm{P}_i \not\in G_{is}$, $s = 1, 2, \ldots, k$, and all the other nodes of X lie on at least one of these hyperplanes.

Let k be any positive integer. Suppose that there exist $M = k + n$ distinct hyperplanes $H_1, \ldots, H_M$ in $\mathbb{R}^n$ such that the intersection of any n distinct hyperplanes chosen from $H_1, \ldots, H_M$ is a point and different choices give different points, then the set of all the above points is called the kth-order natural lattice in $\mathbb{R}^n$ generated by $H_1, \ldots, H_M$.

The next three theorems are due to CHUNG and YAO [1977].

THEOREM 17.2. *Let $X = \{\mathrm{P}_1, \mathrm{P}_2, \ldots, \mathrm{P}_N\}$ be a lattice of N nodes in $\mathbb{R}^n$. If X satisfies the condition GC, then X admits a unique interpolation $P(\mathrm{P}) = \Sigma_{i=1}^{N} p_i(\mathrm{P})f(\mathrm{P}_i)$ of degree less than or equal to k. Furthermore, for each $i = 1, \ldots, N$, the real polynomial p_i is in the form $p_i = u_{i1}u_{i2} \cdots u_{ik}$, where $u_{ij}(t) = 0$ is the equation of the hyperplane G_{ij} given in condition GC.*

The converse is also true: if X admits a unique interpolation of degree less than or equal to k and for each $i = 1, \ldots, N$, the real polynomial p_i in $P(\mathrm{P}) = \Sigma_{i=1}^{N} p_i(\mathrm{P})f(\mathrm{P}_i)$ is a product of real polynomials of first degree, then the lattice X satisfies condition GC.

THEOREM 17.3. *For each n and each k, there always exist a set of $n + k$ hyperplanes in $\mathbb{R}^n$ generating a kth-order natural lattice.*

THEOREM 17.4. *Every kth-order natural lattice satisfies the condition GC.*

NICOLAIDES [1972] gave the conditions for a lattice of an n-simplex Δ to admit a unique interpolation and express the interpolation polynomial via barycentric coordinates of the nodes. CHUNG and YAO [1977] tried to characterize the set of all lattices of N nodes in $\mathbb{R}^n$ admitting a unique interpolation and they give some examples of lattices on the plane that satisfy the GC condition—see Fig. 17.2.

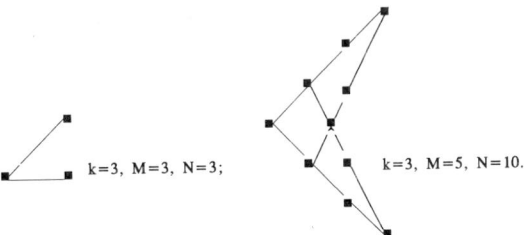

k=3, M=3, N=3;   k=3, M=5, N=10.

FIG. 17.2. Lattices that satisfy the GC condition.

Let us determine inductively

$$f(x_i; \ldots; x_{i+k+1}; y_j; \ldots; y_{j+s}) = [f(x_{i+1}; \ldots; x_{i+k+1}; y_j; \ldots; y_{j+s})$$
$$- f(x_i; \ldots; x_{i+k}; y_j; \ldots; y_{j+s})]/(x_{i+k+1} - x_i),$$
$$f(x_i; \ldots; x_{i+k}; y_j; \ldots; y_{j+s+1}) = [f(x_i; \ldots; x_i; y_{j+1}; \ldots; y_{j+s+1})$$
$$- f(x_i; \ldots; x_{i+k}; y_j; \ldots; y_{j+s})]/(y_{j+s+1} - y_j)$$

the divided differences of kth and sth degrees, respectively, of the function f according to the variables x and y. For the divided differences of a function of one variable and for details see Sections 3 and 16.

Let the unique polynomial P_m of mth degree that interpolates a given function f at the knots (17.2) have the form

$$P_m(x, y) = \sum_{i+j \leq m} a_{ij}(x - x_0)\cdots(x - x_{i-1})(y - y_0)\cdots(y - y_{j-1}).$$

All the coefficients a_{ij} can be expressed by the divided differences of the function f. Indeed the polynomial

$$P_m(x, y_0) = a_{00} + a_{10}(x - x_0) + a_{20}(x - x_0)(x - x_1) + \cdots$$
$$+ a_{m0}(x - x_0)\cdots(x - x_{m-1})$$

interpolates the function $f(x, y_0)$ as a function of one variable at the points x_i, $i = 0, 1, \ldots, m$. From (3.1) it follows that

$$a_{i0} = f(x_0; x_1; \ldots; x_i, y_0).$$

Let us now consider the polynomial

$$P_m(x, y_1) = [a_{00} + a_{01}(y_1 - y_0)] + [a_{10} + a_{11}(y_1 - y_0)](x - x_0) + \cdots$$
$$+ [a_{m-1,0} + a_{m-1,1}(y_1 - y_0)](x - x_0)\cdots(x - x_{m-2})$$
$$+ a_{m0}(x - x_0)\cdots(x - x_{m-1})$$

that interpolates the function $f(x, y_1)$ at the points x_i, $i = 0, 1, \ldots, m$. Applying (3.1) again it follows that $a_{i0} + a_{i1}(y_1 - y_0) = f(x_0; x_1; \ldots; x_i, y)$. Hence

$$a_{i1} = [f(x_0; x_1; \ldots; x_i, y_1) - f(x_0; x_1; \ldots; x_i, y_1)]/(y_1 - y_0)$$
$$= f(x_0; x_1; \ldots; x_i, y_0; y_1).$$

Section 17 — Interpolation

Continuing this process the polynomial P_m takes the form

$$P_m(x, y) = \sum_{k=0}^{m} \sum_{i+j=k} (x - x_0) \cdots (x - x_{i-1})(y - y_0) \cdots (y - y_{j-1})$$
$$\times f(x_0; x_1; \ldots; x_i, y_0; y_1; \ldots; y_j). \quad (17.3)$$

The last formula is called the Newton interpolation formula for interpolation of the functions of two variables.

In the case of equidistant knots $x_i - x_{i-1} = h$, $y_i - y_{i-1} = k$, $i = 1, 2, \ldots, m$, it is convenient to introduce finite differences for the function of two or more variables as follows:

$$f(x_{i+1}, y_j) - f(x_i, y_j) = \Delta_x f(x_i, y_j), \quad f(x_i, y_{j+1}) - f(x_i, y_j) = \Delta_y f(x_i, y_j),$$

$$\Delta_x f(x_{i+1}, y_j) - \Delta_x f(x_i, y_j) = \Delta_{x^2}^2 f(x_i, y_j),$$

$$\Delta_y f(x_i, y_{j+1}) - \Delta_y f(x_i, y_j) = \Delta_{y^2}^2 f(x_i, y_j),$$

$$\Delta_x f(x_i, y_{j+1}) - \Delta_x f(x_i, y_j) = \Delta_{xy}^2 f(x_i, y_j),$$

and so on. Using the property (c) of Section 5 the relation between finite and divided differences can be derived in the form

$$f(x_0; x_1; \ldots; x_i, y_0; y_1; \ldots; y_j) = \frac{1}{i! j! h^i k^j} \Delta_{x^i y^j}^{i+j} f(x_0, y_0). \quad (17.4)$$

Combining (17.3) and (17.4) the Newton interpolation polynomial (17.3) takes the form

$$P_m(x_0 + ht, y_0 + kt) = \sum_{k=0}^{m} \sum_{i+j=k} \binom{t}{i}\binom{u}{j} \Delta_{x^i y^j}^{i+j} f(x_0, y_0)$$

$$= f(x_0, y_0) + t\Delta_x f(x_0, y_0) + u\Delta_y f(x_0, y_0)$$

$$+ \binom{t}{2}\Delta_{x^2}^2 f(x_0, y_0) + \binom{t}{1}\binom{u}{1}\Delta_{xy}^2 f(x_0, y_0) + \binom{u}{2}\Delta_{y^2}^2 f(x_0, y_0) + \cdots$$

$$+ \binom{t}{m}\Delta_{x^m}^m f(x_0, y_0) + \cdots + \binom{u}{m}\Delta_{y^m}^m f(x_0, y_0),$$

where $t = (x - x_0)/h$, $u = (y - y_0)/k$.

Let the condition for uniqueness of the interpolation polynomial be not necessary, the interpolation knots be

$$(x_0, y_0), (x_1, y_0), \ldots, (x_n, y_0),$$
$$(x_0, y_1), (x_1, y_1), \ldots, (x_n, y_1), \quad (17.5)$$
$$\vdots \quad \vdots \quad \vdots$$
$$(x_0, y_m), (x_1, y_m), \ldots, (x_n, y_m),$$

and the values of the function f be given at these knots. The next method for building the interpolation polynomial P_{nm} of degree nm for the function f can now be proposed.

Since (3.1) and (3.2) the function f has the representation

$$f(x, y) = f(x, y_0) + (y - y_0)f(x, y_0; y_1) + \cdots$$
$$+ (y - y_0)(y - y_1) \cdots (y - y_{m-1})f(x, y_0; y_1; \ldots; y_m)$$
$$+ (y - y_0)(y - y_1) \cdots (y - y_m)f(x, y_0; y_1; \ldots; y_m; y). \quad (17.6)$$

Similarly the function $f(x, y_0; y_1; \ldots; y_k)$ can be represented by its interpolation polynomial as

$$f(x, y_0; y_1; \ldots; y_k) = f(x_0, y_0; y_1; \ldots; y_k)$$
$$+ (x - x_0)f(x_0; x_1, y_0; y_1; \ldots; y_m) + \cdots$$
$$+ (x - x_0)(x - x_1) \cdots (x - x_{n-1})f(x_0; x_1; \ldots; x_n, y_0; y_1; \ldots; y_m)$$
$$+ (x - x_0)(x - x_1) \cdots (x - x_n)f(x_0; x_1; \ldots; x_n, y_0; y_1; \ldots; y_m).$$

Substituting the last expression for $f(x, y_0; y_1; \ldots; y_k)$ in (17.6) the result is

$$f(x, y)$$
$$= \sum_{i=0}^{n} \sum_{j=0}^{m} (x - x_0)(x - x_1) \cdots (x - x_{i-1})(y - y_0)(y - y_1) \cdots (y - y_{j-1})$$
$$\times f(x_0; x_1; \ldots; x_i, y_0; y_1; \ldots; y_j)$$
$$+ (x - x_0)(x - x_1) \cdots (x - x_n) \sum_{j=0}^{m} (y - y_0)(y - y_1) \cdots (y - y_{j-1})$$
$$\times f(x; x_0; x_1; \ldots; x_n, y_0; y_1; \ldots; y_j)$$
$$+ (y - y_0)(y - y_1) \cdots (y - y_m)f(x, y; y_0; y_1; \ldots; y_m), \quad (17.7)$$

setting in above formula $(x - x_{-1}) = (y - y_{-1}) = 1$. Taking into account the fact that

$$f(x; x_0; x_1; \ldots; x_n, y)$$
$$= \sum_{j=0}^{m} (y - y_0)(y - y_1) \cdots (y - y_{j-1})f(x; x_0; x_1; \ldots; x_n, y_0; y_1; \ldots; y_j)$$
$$+ (y - y_0)(y - y_1) \cdots (y - y_m)f(x; x_0; x_1; \ldots; x_n, y_0; y_1; \ldots; y_m; y),$$

the formula (17.7) turns into

$$f(x, y) = \sum_{i=0}^{n} \sum_{j=0}^{m} (x - x_0)(x - x_1) \cdots (x - x_{i-1})(y - y_0)(y - y_1) \cdots (y - y_{j-1})$$
$$\times f(x_0; x_1; \ldots; x_i, y_0; y_1; \ldots; y_j)$$
$$+ (x - x_0)(x - x_1) \cdots (x - x_n)f(x; x_0; x_1; \ldots; x_n, y)$$
$$+ (y - y_0)(y - y_1) \cdots (y - y_m)f(x, y; y_0; y_1; \ldots; y_m)$$
$$- (x - x_0)(x - x_1) \cdots (x - x_n)(y - y_0)(y - y_1) \cdots (y - y_m)$$
$$\times f(x; x_0; x_1; \ldots; x_n, y; y_0; y_1; \ldots; y_m). \quad (17.8)$$

In the expression (17.8) under the double sum

$$P_{nm}(x, y) = \sum_{i=0}^{n} \sum_{j=0}^{m} (x - x_0)(x - x_1) \cdots (x - x_{i-1})(y - y_0)(y - y_1)$$
$$\cdots (y - y_{j-1}) f(x_0; x_1; \ldots ; x_i, y_0; y_1; \ldots ; y_j)$$

is the polynomial of nmth degree that interpolates the function f at the knots (17.5) and let us write (17.8) in the form

$$f(x, y) = P_{nm}(x, y) + R_{nm}(f; x, y). \tag{17.9}$$

The remainder term $R_{nm}(x, y)$ in (17.9) can be expressed by the derivatives of the function f using the following property of the divided differences:

$$f(x_0; x_1; \ldots ; x_n, y_0; y_1; \ldots ; y_m) = \frac{1}{n!m!} \frac{\partial^{m+n}}{\partial x^n \partial y^m} f(\xi, \eta),$$

where

$$\min\{x_0, x_1, \ldots, x_n\} < \xi < \max\{x_0, x_1, \ldots, x_n\},$$
$$\min\{y_0, y_1, \ldots, y_m\} < \eta < \max\{y_0, y_1, \ldots, y_m\}.$$

This property is a direct consequence from Section 3 and $R_{nm}(f)$ takes the form

$$R_{nm}(f; x, y) = (x - x_0)(x - x_1) \cdots (x - x_n) \frac{1}{(n+1)!} \frac{\partial^{n+1}}{\partial x^{n+1}} f(\xi, y)$$
$$+ (y - y_0)(y - y_1) \cdots (y - y_m) \frac{1}{(m+1)!} \frac{\partial^{m+1}}{\partial y^{m+1}} f(x, \eta)$$
$$- (x - x_0)(x - x_1) \cdots (x - x_n)(y - y_0)(y - y_1)$$
$$\cdots (y - y_m) \frac{1}{(n+1)!(m+1)!} \frac{\partial^{m+n+2}}{\partial x^{n+1} \partial y^{m+1}} f(\xi_1, \eta_1).$$

WERNER [1980] considers the case when not all the points (17.5) are interpolation nodes. Let $n \geq n_0 \geq n_1 \geq \cdots \geq n_m$ and the interpolation problem consists of the determination of the polynomial P that satisfies

$$P(x_i, y_k) = f(x_i, y_k), \quad i = 0, 1, \ldots, n_k, \quad j = 0, 1, \ldots, m.$$

The number of nodes is $N = \sum_{j=0}^{m} (1 + n_j)$ and evidently the nodes (17.2) are a particular case when $n_k = n - k$ and the points (17.5) are the case when $n_k = n$.

18. Multivariate Hermite interpolation

The Hermite interpolation problem is understood to be a set of points $\{P_i\}_{i=1}^{s}$, $P_i \in \mathbb{R}^m$, an n-dimensional linear space of functions V_n and a set of values $\{\alpha_{ij}\}_{i=1}^{s}$, $j = 0, 1, \ldots, n_i$, $s + n_1 + \cdots + n_s = n$. The solution is a function in V_n such that it and some of its derivatives take given values at the given points.

On the real line, there are choices for V_n (e.g., the algebraic polynomials of degree at most n) such that the Hermite interpolation problem has a unique solution for any choice of knots and any choice of values (see Section 12). In this case one says that the Hermite interpolation problem is regular. In the plane the situation becomes more complicated because the problem is not always regular (see, e.g., Section 17 for Lagrange interpolation).

As is noted in LORENTZ [1984] there are several ways to get around this problem.

(a) Particular choices of sets of points, for which the problem has a solution. This is done in the theory of finite element, CIARLET and RAVIART [1972], and for the natural lattices of CHUNG and YAO [1977].

(b) Instead of point evaluation functionals one could take special values, which lead to the regular problem—KERGIN [1980], HAKOPIAN [1982].

(c) The Newton-type methods of WERNER [1980], GASCA and MAETZU [1982], JETTER [1983], where for the chosen set of lines on the plane that induces the point set Z, associate with them an interpolating space $V_n(Z)$ such that the interpolation problem is always solvable. Of course $V_n(Z)$ depends on Z.

(d) The approach given in LORENTZ [1984], LORENTZ and LORENTZ [1991] on the plane is to fix the set of functions V_n (as a rule bivariate polynomials) and then to investigate for which values of the function and its derivatives for some set of points the interpolation problem has a solution. Note that because the interpolating space is a space of polynomials the problem will be solvable for almost all choices of points.

One of the main reasons for the considerable interest in the use of approximation theory in several variables for the Hermite interpolation is its application to the finite-element methods—see CIARLET [1978]. CIARLET and RAVIART [1972] consider the following situation: given a finite set $\Sigma \subset \mathbb{R}^n$ and given a function f, the interpolation problem consists in finding a polynomial P of degree less than or equal to k, in such a way that the values of f and P and some of their corresponding derivatives are equal at some specified points of Σ. Under the condition that this problem has a unique solution they proved the error estimate

$$\sup_{x \in K} \|D^m f(x) - D^m P(x)\| \leq CM_{k+1} h^{k+1}/\rho^m \quad \text{for } 0 \leq m \leq k,$$

where K is a closed convex hull of Σ, $M_{k+1} = \sup_{x \in K} \|D^{k+1} f(x)\|$, h is the diameter of K, ρ is the supremum of diameters of the inscribed spheres of K, C is a constant independent on Σ and $\|D^m f(x)\|$ satisfy

$$\left|\frac{\partial f(x)}{\partial x_i}\right| \leq \|Df(x)\| \leq c_1(n) \max_{1 \leq i \leq n} \left|\frac{\partial f(x)}{\partial x_i}\right|,$$

$$\left|\frac{\partial^2 f(x)}{\partial x_i \partial x_j}\right| \leq \|D^2 f(x)\| \leq c_2(n) \max_{1 \leq i, j \leq n} \left|\frac{\partial^2 f(x)}{\partial x_i \partial x_j}\right|, \text{ etc.}$$

Let

$$\Pi_n(\mathbb{R}^2) = \left\{P: P(x, y) = \sum_{i+j \leq n} a_{ij} x^i y^j\right\}, \quad T_n = \{(\alpha_1, \alpha_2): \alpha_1 + \alpha_2 \leq n\},$$

$$\Omega = \left\{ Q: Q = \{n_1, n_2, \ldots, n_k; n\}, \sum_{\nu=1}^{k} \bar{n}_\nu = \overline{n+1}, \bar{m} = 1 + 2 + \cdots + m \right\},$$

$$U = \{u_\nu = (x_\nu, y_\nu)\}_{\nu=1}^{k} \in \mathbb{R}^{2k}, \quad u_i \neq u_j \text{ for } i \neq j. \tag{18.1}$$

The Hermite interpolation problem (Q, U) is defined as follows: for arbitrary numbers

$$\Lambda = \{\lambda_{\alpha,\nu} \in \mathbb{R}^1 : \alpha \in T_{n_\nu - 1}, \nu = 1, 2, \ldots, k\} \tag{18.2}$$

find a unique polynomial $P \in \Pi_n(\mathbb{R}^2)$ such that

$$\left. \frac{\partial^{\alpha_1 + \alpha_2} P(x, y)}{\partial x^{\alpha_1} \partial y^{\alpha_2}} \right|_{(x_\nu, y_\nu)} = \lambda_{\alpha,\nu}, \quad \alpha = (\alpha_1, \alpha_2) \in T_{n_\nu - 1}. \tag{18.3}$$

Writing (18.3) in the form $D^Q P|_U = \Lambda$, the determination of the polynomial P that satisfies (18.1) consists in the solution of the linear system of $\sum_{\nu=1}^{k} \bar{n}_\nu$ equations with $\overline{n+1}$ unknowns with the determinant $d_Q(U)$ of order $\overline{n+1}$. By

{the problem (Q, U) is solvable} $\Leftrightarrow$ {$d_Q(U) \neq 0$}

$\Leftrightarrow$ {there is no $P \in \Pi_n(\mathbb{R}^2)$, $D^Q P|_U = 0$, $P \neq 0$}

it follows that two cases are possible:

(1) (Q, U) is solvable for some $U \in \mathbb{R}^{2k}$; i.e. for almost all $U \in \mathbb{R}^{2k}$. Let $R\Omega$ be the set of all such (Q, U);

(2) (Q, U) is not solvable for each $U \in \mathbb{R}^{2k}$. Then call Q singular and let $S\Omega$ be the set of all such (Q, U).

The case when (Q, U) is solvable for all U is possible only for $k = 1$—see LORENTZ and LORENTZ [1991]. RADON [1948], and CHUNG and YAO [1977] proved that if $n_1 = n_2 = \cdots = n_k = 1$ (Lagrange interpolation) then $Q \in R\Omega$. LORENTZ [1984], and LORENTZ and LORENTZ [1984, 1991], obtained sufficient conditions for the solvability or non-solvability of a given $Q \in \Omega$.

HAKOPIAN, GEVORGIAN and SAAKIAN ([1990], p. 137) develop the above mentioned investigations on two-dimensional Hermite interpolation. They characterize the sets $R\Omega$ and $S\Omega$ and consider the Polya condition in the two-dimensional Birkhoff interpolation (see Section 10), proving the next result: let

$$Q = \{n_1, n_2, \ldots, n_k; n\}, \quad 1 \leq n_\nu \leq n + 1, \quad \nu = 1, \ldots, k,$$

$$\sum_{\nu=1}^{k} n_\nu = \overline{n+1}, \tag{18.4}$$

$$L_n = \{(\alpha_1, \alpha_2) : \alpha_1 + \alpha_2 = n\}, \quad n = 0, 1, \ldots.$$

For the set U from (18.1) let us consider the Birkhoff interpolation problem $(Q, U)_0$, which is defined similarly to (Q, U) with $L_{n_\nu - 1}$ instead of $T_{n_\nu - 1}$ in (18.2) and (18.3). Then if Q satisfies (18.4) a necessary and sufficient condition for the problem $(Q, U)_0$ to be solvable for almost all $U \in \mathbb{R}^{2k}$ is the Polya condition $\sum_{\nu: n_\nu \leq j} n_\nu \geq \bar{j}$.

19. Convergence of the interpolation processes

Let us consider the infinite triangle matrix of functionals

$$
\begin{aligned}
&l_{0,0} \\
&l_{1,0}, l_{1,1} \\
&l_{2,0}, l_{2,1}, l_{2,2} \\
&\vdots \qquad\qquad\qquad \ddots \\
&l_{n,0}, l_{n,1}, l_{n,2}, \ldots, l_{n,n} \\
&\vdots
\end{aligned}
\tag{19.1}
$$

defined on a set of functions F. If $F_n \subset F$ is an $(n+1)$-dimensional subset of F, $n = 0, 1, 2, \ldots$, then the functionals $l_{n,0}, l_{n,1}, l_{n,2}, \ldots, l_{n,n}$ from the nth row of the matrix (19.1) and the set F_n define an interpolation problem—see Section 1. Let us suppose that this problem has a unique solution. This means that for a given function $f \in F$ there exists one function $f_n \in F_n$ such that $l_{n,k}(f_n) = l_{n,k}(f)$, $k = 0, 1, \ldots, n$. So for every function $f \in F$ the matrix (19.1) and the sets $\{F_n\}_{n=0}^{\infty}$ generate an *interpolation process* or a sequence of functions $\{f_n\}_{n=0}^{\infty}$ that satisfy $l_{n,k}(f_n) = l_{n,k}(f)$, $k = 0, 1, \ldots, n$, $n = 0, 1, 2, \ldots$. This interpolation process converges to the function f according to the functional l if

$$\lim_{n\to\infty} l(f_n) = l(f).$$

Usually the functional l has the form $l(f) = f(x')$, where x' is a point. In this case if $\lim_{n\to\infty} f_n(x') = f(x')$ then the interpolation process converges for the function f at the point x'. If

$$\lim_{n\to\infty} \max_{x\in[a,b]} |f_n(x) - f(x)| = 0,$$

then the interpolation process converges uniformly in the interval $[a, b]$ for the function f.

20. The Lagrange interpolation process

The Lagrange interpolation process is characterized by the functionals (19.1) when $l_{n,k}(f) = f(x_{n,k})$; i.e. the interpolation process is given by the infinite triangle matrix X of knots

$$
X = \left\| \begin{array}{llllll}
x_{0,0} & & & & & \\
x_{1,0} & x_{1,1} & & & & \\
x_{2,0} & x_{2,1} & x_{2,2} & & & \\
\vdots & & & \ddots & & \\
x_{n,0} & x_{n,1} & x_{n,2} & \cdots & x_{n,n} & \\
\vdots & & & & &
\end{array} \right\|,
\tag{20.1}
$$

where all the knots belong to the interval $[a, b]$.

Let the function f be defined on $[a, b]$ and

$$L_n(f; x) = \sum_{i=0}^{n} f(x_{n,i}) L_{n,i}(x)$$

$$= \sum_{i=0}^{n} f(x_{n,i}) \frac{(x - x_{n,0}) \cdots (x - x_{n,i-1})(x - x_{n,i+1}) \cdots (x - x_{n,n})}{(x_{n,i} - x_{n,1}) \cdots (x_{n,i} - x_{n,i-1})(x_{n,i} - x_{n,i+1}) \cdots (x_{n,i} - x_{n,n})}$$

be the Lagrange interpolation polynomial of nth degree for the function f that satisfies $L_n(f; x_{n,i}) = f(x_{n,i})$, $i = 0, 1, \ldots, n$; i.e. the polynomial $L_n(f)$ interpolates the function f at the knots of the nth row of the matrix (20.1).

The matrix X and the function f generate the sequence of polynomials $\{L_n(f)\}_{n=0}^{\infty}$. The problem is whether

$$\lim_{n \to \infty} \max_{x \in [a,b]} |L_n(f; x) - f(x)| = 0.$$

BERNSTEIN [1916] proved the following negative result: if the knots in (20.1) are $x_{n,k} = (2k - n)/n$, $k = 0, 1, \ldots, n$, $n = 0, 1, \ldots$, and $f(x) = |x|$, then the sequence $L_n(f; x)$ diverges for every point $x \in [-1, 1]$ different from $-1, 0, 1$. The points -1 and 1 are interpolation knots for every polynomial $L_n(f)$ and therefore $L_n(f; -1) = L_n(f; 1) = 1$. For the point zero it is proved in NATANSON ([1949] p. 523) that

$$\lim_{n \to \infty} L_n(f; 0) = 0.$$

This result is due to D.L. Berman in 1939 and S.M. Lozinskii showed more exactly that $|L_{2n}(f; 0)| < A/n$. The last estimate follows from

$$L_{2n}(f; 0) = \left(\frac{(2n - 3)!!}{2^{n-1}(n - 1)!} \right)^2.$$

For details see the book of Natanson cited above. DAVYDOV [1986] proved that the Lagrange interpolation polynomial does not converge over equidistant nodes in measure to the function $|x|$ on $[-1, 1]$.

To MARCINKIEWIEZ [1937a] is due the following theorem.

THEOREM 20.1. *For every function $f \in C_{[a,b]}$ there exists a matrix* (19.1) *such that*

$$\lim_{n \to \infty} \max_{x \in [a,b]} |L_n(f; x) - f(x)| = 0.$$

PROOF. Let the polynomial $P_n(f)$ of nth degree is the polynomial of the best uniform approximation for the function f on the interval $[a, b]$. By Theorem 25.3 there exist $n + 1$ points $\{x_{n,k}\}_{k=0}^{n}$ in $[a, b]$ such that $P_n(f; x_{n,k}) = f(x_{n,k})$, $k = 0, 1, \ldots, n$. If the points $\{x_{n,k}\}_{k=0}^{n}$ build the nth row of the matrix (20.1), then according to Theorem 29.1 the sequence of the interpolation polynomials $\{P_n(f)\}_{n=0}^{\infty}$ satisfy

$$\lim_{n \to \infty} \max_{x \in [a,b]} |P_n(f; x) - f(x)| = 0. \qquad \square$$

The following theorem proved by FABER [1914] solves the problem of the existence or non-existence of the universal matrix (20.1) such that for every function $f \in C_{[a,b]}$ the corresponding interpolation process converges.

THEOREM 20.2. *For every matrix* (20.1) *there exists a function* $f \in C_{[a,b]}$ *for which the corresponding interpolation polynomials* $\{L_n(f)\}_{n=0}^{\infty}$ *determined by the matrix* (20.1) *do not converge uniformly to the function* f.

PROOF. Let us suppose the contrary: there exists a universal matrix (20.1) such that for every function $f \in C_{[a,b]}$ the sequence $\{L_n(f)\}_{n=0}^{\infty}$ satisfies

$$\lim_{n \to \infty} \max_{x \in [a,b]} |L_n(f; x) - f(x)| = 0.$$

Introducing the uniform norm $\| \ \|_{C_{[a,b]}}$ (or, in shorthand notation, $\| \ \|_C$) in $C_{[a,b]}$ the set $C_{[a,b]}$ turns into a complete normed linear space; i.e. a Banach space.

The linear operators $\{L_n\}_{n=0}^{\infty}$ map the Banach space $C_{[a,b]}$ into itself. By the Banach–Steinhaus theorem the necessary condition for the convergence of the sequence of linear operators $\{L_n\}_{n=0}^{\infty}$ for every element $f \in C_{[a,b]}$ is the boundedness of the norms of the operators. So the condition $\|L_n\| \leq M < \infty$ must be valid for all n. Let us denote

$$\max_{x \in [a,b]} \sum_{i=0}^{n} |L_{n,i}(x)| = \sum_{i=0}^{n} |L_{n,i}(\xi)| = \lambda_n, \quad \xi \in [a, b], \tag{20.2}$$

and define the function φ as

$$\varphi(x) = \begin{cases} \operatorname{sgn} L_{n,i}(\xi) & \text{for } x = x_{n,i}, \\ \text{linear between the knots } x_{n,i}, \\ \text{constant in the intervals } [a, x_{n,0}], [x_{n,n}, b]. \end{cases}$$

Hence $\|\varphi\|_C = 1$ and

$$L_n(\varphi; \xi) = \sum_{i=0}^{n} \varphi(x_{n,i}) L_{n,i}(\xi) = \sum_{i=0}^{n} \operatorname{sgn} L_{n,i}(\xi) L_{n,i}(\xi) = \sum_{i=0}^{n} |L_{n,i}(\xi)| = \lambda_n,$$

$$\lambda_n = \sum_{i=0}^{n} \varphi(x_{n,i}) L_{n,i}(\xi) \leq \sup_{\|f\|_C = 1} \max_{x \in [a,b]} \left| \sum_{i=0}^{n} f(x_{n,i}) L_{n,i}(x) \right| = \|L_n\|.$$

From the last inequality it follows that $\lambda_n \leq \|L_n\|$. By Theorem 20.3 $\lambda_n \geq \ln n/8\sqrt{\pi}$ and the condition $\|L_n\| \leq M < \infty$ cannot be satisfied. □

ERDÖS and VERTESI [1980] sharpened the Theorem 20.2. They proved that if the knots of the matrix (20.1) lie in the interval $[-1, 1]$, then there is a continuous function $f \in C_{[-1,1]}$, so that

$$\overline{\lim_{n \to \infty}} |L_n(f; x)| = \infty$$

for almost all $x \in [-1, 1]$.

An analogous assertion is true in the complex and trigonometric case of interpolation. Following VERTESI [1982] (see also ALPER [1956], GERMAN [1980]) let the nodes in matrix (20.1) be the arbitrary numbers $x_{n,k} = \exp(iv_{n,k})$, $k = 0, 1, \ldots, n$, $n = 0, 1, \ldots$, $i^2 = -1$, where

$$0 \leq v_{n,0} < v_{n,1} < \cdots < v_{n,n} < 2\pi ;$$

i.e. X is an arbitrary triangular matrix on the unit circle $G = \{x: x = \exp(iv), 0 \leq v < 2\pi\}$. Then there is a function f that is analytic on $U = \{x: |x| < 1\}$ and continuous on the closure $[U] = \{x: |x| \leq 1\}$ such that the corresponding Lagrange interpolation polynomial

$$L_n(f; x) = \sum_{i=0}^{n} f(x_{n,i}) L_{n,i}(x), \quad L_{n,i}(x) = \prod_{j \neq i} (x - x_{n,j}) / (x_{n,i} - x_{n,j}),$$

satisfies $\overline{\lim}_{n \to \infty} |L_n(f; x)| = \infty$ for almost all $x \in G$.

For every matrix (20.1) the numbers λ_n, defined by (20.2), play an important role for the convergence of the interpolation processes generated by this matrix. The behavior of the numbers λ_n was investigated by FABER [1914] and BERNSTEIN [1916]. Their result is the following theorem.

THEOREM 20.3. *For an arbitrary matrix* (20.1) *the inequalities* $\lambda_n \geq (\ln n)/8\sqrt{\pi}$ *hold true.*

BERNSTEIN [1916] proved that in the special case when the knots of the matrix (20.1) are the roots of the Chebyshev polynomials

$$x_{n,k} = \cos[\pi(2k+1)/2(n+1)], \quad k = 0, 1, \ldots, n, \; n = 0, 1, \ldots, \quad (20.3)$$

then $\ln n/8\sqrt{\pi} < \lambda_n \leq 8 + 4\pi^{-1} \ln n$. This estimate together with Theorem 20.3 show that the knots (20.3) are "the best". As an illustration of this fact see the graphs of the functions $|x|$ and L_{15}, where L_{15} is the interpolation polynomial of the function $|x|$ in $[-1, 1]$ when the interpolation knots are:
 (1) $x_{15,k} = -1 + 2k/15$, $k = 0, 1, \ldots, 15$, Fig. 20.1;
 (2) $x_{15,k} = \cos[\pi(2k+1)/32]$, $k = 0, 1, \ldots, 15$, Fig. 20.2.

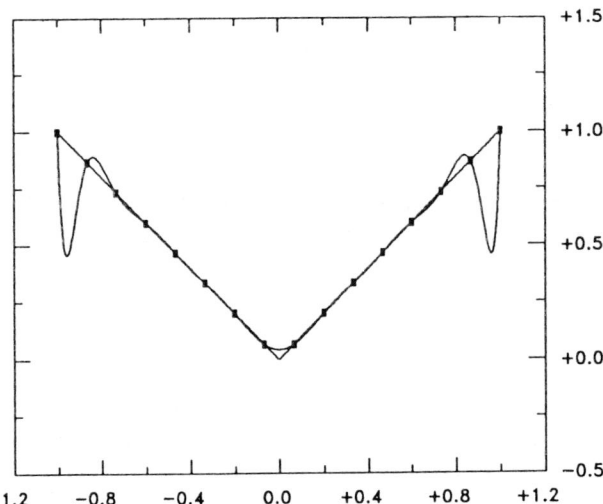

FIG. 20.1. Graphs of the functions $|x|$ and L_{15} with uniform interpolation knots.

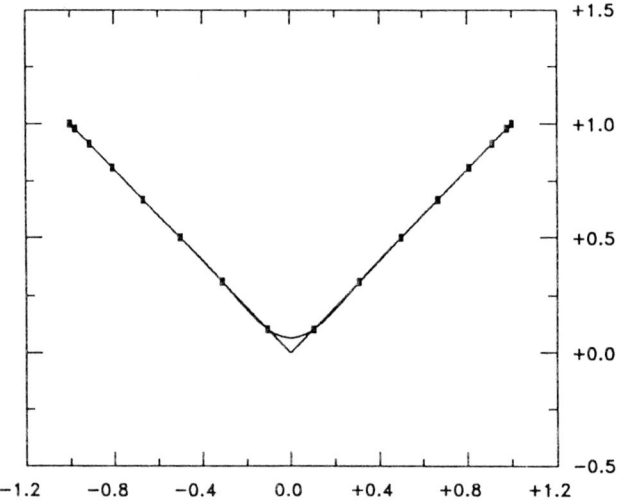

FIG. 20.2. Graphs of the functions $|x|$ and L_{15} with Chebyshev knots.

For the matrix (20.1) with knots (20.3) MARCINKIEWIEZ [1937b] and GRÜNWALD [1936] built continuous functions for which the interpolation process diverges at every point.

It is clear that the requirement for continuity of the interpolated function f cannot ensure convergence of the Lagrange interpolation polynomials. Increasing the demands on the smoothness of the interpolated function the convergence of the interpolation process can be obtained. This fact is connected with the following theorem.

THEOREM 20.4. *Consider the matrix* (20.1) *and the function* $f \in C_{[a,b]}$. *Let* $E_n(f)$ *be its best uniform approximation by algebraic polynomials of nth degree in the interval* $[a, b]$. *If* $\lim_{n\to\infty} E_{n-1}(f)\lambda_n = 0$, *then*

$$\lim_{n\to\infty} \max_{x\in[a,b]} |L_n(f; x) - f(x)| = 0.$$

PROOF. Let $P_n(f)$ be the polynomial of nth degree of the best uniform approximation for the function f in the interval $[a, b]$. Then

$$|L_n(f; x) - f(x)| \leq |L_n(f; x) - P_{n-1}(f; x)| + |P_{n-1}(f; x) - f(x)|$$
$$= |L_n(f; x) - L_n(P_{n-1}(f); x)| + E_{n-1}(f)$$
$$= |L_n(f - P_n(f); x)| + E_{n-1}(f)$$
$$\leq \|L_n\| \|f - P_n(f)\|_{C_{[a,b]}} + E_{n-1}(f)$$
$$= (\|L_n\| + 1)E_{n-1}(f) = (\lambda_n + 1)E_{n-1}(f). \qquad \square$$

Detailed information about the convergence of interpolation processes including analytic functions can be found in KRILOV, BOBKOV and MONASTIRNII ([1972], Chapter 3). WALSH [1960a,b] gives basic results in the interpolation of complex functions—see also the supplement to the Russian translation of this book.

21. Discrete Fourier transforms

Let us consider the interpolation problem described in Section 1 for a function f defined in the interval $[0, 1]$, $f(0) = f(1)$, and the linear functionals $l_k(f) = f(x_k)$, $x_k = k/N$, $k = 0, 1, \ldots, N-1$. Let the function $\varphi_k(x) = e^{2\pi i k x}$, $i^2 = -1$.

The problem is to find a function $\varphi = \sum_{k=0}^{N-1} a_k \varphi_k$, which interpolates f at the points x_k; i.e. $f(x_k) = \varphi(x_k)$, $k = 0, 1, \ldots, N-1$.

The functions $\{\varphi_k\}_{k=0}^{N-1}$ form an orthonormal system on the set $\{x_k\}_{k=0}^{N-1}$ according to the scalar product

$$(f, g) = \frac{1}{N} \sum_{k=0}^{N-1} f(x_k)\overline{g(x_k)} = \frac{1}{N} \sum_{k=0}^{N-1} f_k \bar{g}_k,$$

where $\bar{g}_k$ is a complex conjugate value of g_k. Indeed,

$$(\varphi_s, \varphi_j) = \frac{1}{N} \sum_{k=0}^{N-1} e^{2\pi i(s-j)k/N} = \begin{cases} \dfrac{1}{N} \dfrac{e^{2\pi i(s-j)} - 1}{e^{2\pi i(s-j)/N} - 1} = 0, & s \neq j, \\ 1, & s = j. \end{cases}$$

If the function $\varphi = \sum_{k=0}^{N-1} a_k \varphi_k$ interpolates f at the points $\{x_k\}_{k=0}^{N-1}$ then $f \equiv \varphi$ on the set $\{x_k\}_{k=0}^{N-1}$ and

$$(\varphi, \varphi_j) = (f, \varphi_j) = \sum_{k=0}^{N-1} a_k (\varphi_k, \varphi_j) = a_j$$

or

$$a_j = \frac{1}{N} \sum_{k=0}^{N-1} f_k e^{-2\pi i k j/N}, \quad j = 0, 1, \ldots, N-1. \tag{21.1}$$

Evidently, if $\varphi = \sum_{k=0}^{N-1} a_k \varphi_k$ interpolates the function f at the points $\{x_k\}_{k=0}^{N-1}$ then

$$f_j = \sum_{k=0}^{N-1} a_k e^{2\pi i k j/N}, \quad j = 0, 1, \ldots, N-1. \tag{21.2}$$

The formulas (21.1) and (21.2) are called the direct and inverse discrete Fourier transforms (DFTs)

$$(f_0, f_1, \ldots, f_{N-1}) \Leftrightarrow (a_0, a_1, \ldots, a_{N-1}). \tag{21.3}$$

REMARK 21.1. The transformations (21.1), (21.2) are discrete analogs of the Fourier transform. Indeed let the 1-periodic function f be defined on the interval $[0, 1]$; its Fourier-series expansion is

$$f(x) = \sum_{k=-\infty}^{\infty} b_k e^{2\pi i k x}, \quad \text{where} \quad \sum_{k=-\infty}^{\infty} |b_k| < \infty. \tag{21.4}$$

If the function f is considered on the discrete set of points $\{x_k = k/N\}_{k=0}^{N-1}$ the representation (21.4) turns into a finite sum. Really, for every $k_2 - k_1 = sN$, where s is an integer number, $k_2 x_m - k_1 x_m = sm$ and

$$\exp(2\pi i k_1 x_m) = \exp(2\pi i k_2 x_m), \quad m = 0, 1, \ldots, N-1.$$

Then at the points x_m, $m = 0, 1, \ldots, N-1$,

$$f(x_m) = f_m = \sum_{k=-\infty}^{\infty} b_k e^{2\pi i k m/N} = \sum_{k=0}^{N-1} \left(\sum_{s=-\infty}^{\infty} b_{k+sN} \right) e^{2\pi i k m/N}$$

$$= \sum_{k=0}^{N-1} a_k e^{2\pi i k m/N}.$$

22. Fast Fourier transforms (FFTs)

The transformations (21.3)

$$(f_0, f_1, \ldots, f_{N-1}) \leftrightarrow (a_0, a_1, \ldots, a_{N-1})$$

via formulas (21.1), (21.2) need $O(N^2)$ arithmetic operations (addition and multiplication) in both directions. Because of the wide utilization of (21.3) as a part of the solution of different problems the question of decreasing the number of operations will be considered. This idea is based on the fact that the formulas (21.1) and (21.2) contain groups of expressions that take part in the computations of different coefficients a_k or function values f_k, $k = 0, 1, \ldots, N-1$, when N is not a prime.

The numbers $e^{2\pi i m/N}$, $m = 0, 1, \ldots, N-1$, are the Nth roots of unity in the field of the complex numbers $\mathbb{C}$. The discrete Fourier transform (21.3) can be considered without complications in rings or fields.

Let $\mathbb{F}$ be a commutative ring with unity and let n be a positive integer. $\mathbb{F}$ is called to support the discrete Fourier transform (DFT) with length n, if:

(a) n has an inverse element in $\mathbb{F}$;

(b) there exists an element $\omega \in \mathbb{F}$, called the primitive nth root of unity for which $\omega^n = 1$ and $\omega^k \neq 1$ for $0 < k \leq n-1$;

(c) $\sum_{i=0}^{n-1} \omega^{ij} = 0$ for every $j = 1, 2, \ldots, n-1$.

For example, the field of the complex numbers $\mathbb{C}$ supports a DFT with arbitrary length, and the field of the real numbers $\mathbb{R}$ supports DFTs with lengths of only one and two.

If ω is a primitive nth root of unity in $\mathbb{F}$, then evidently $\omega^{-1} = \omega^{n-1}$ is also such a root.

If $\mathbb{F}$ supports DFT with length $n = rs$ (r and s are natural numbers), and ω is a primitive nth root of the unity in $\mathbb{F}$, then:

(a) ω^r and ω^s are primitive rth and sth roots of unity, respectively;

SECTION 22 Interpolation

(b) $\mathbb{F}$ supports the DFTs with lengths r and s.

Let $\mathbb{F}$ support the DFT with length n and let ω_n be a primitive nth root of the unity in $\mathbb{F}$. The direct and inverse DFT (21.3) in $\mathbb{F}$ can be written as

$$b_i = \sum_{j=0}^{n-1} a_j \omega^{ij}, \quad i = 0, 1, \ldots, n-1, \tag{22.1}$$

$$a_j = \frac{1}{n} \sum_{i=0}^{n-1} b_i \omega^{-ij}, \quad j = 0, 1, \ldots, n-1. \tag{22.2}$$

In matrix notation (22.1) and (22.2) look like:

$$b = W_n a, \quad a = W_n^{-1} b,$$

where

$$a = (a_0, a_1, \ldots, a_{n-1})^t, \quad b = (b_0, b_1, \ldots, b_{n-1})^t,$$

and the $n \times n$ matrices W_n and W_n^{-1} have elements

$$W_n = \{\omega^{ij}\}_{i,j=0}^{n-1}, \quad W_n^{-1} = \frac{1}{n} \{\omega^{-ij}\}_{i,j=0}^{n-1}.$$

The inverse DFT is similar to the direct one and can be performed using the same algorithms.

Direct computation via formulas (22.1), (22.2) needs n^2 multiplications and $n^2 - n$ additions in $\mathbb{F}$ (assuming that the constants ω^{ij}, ω^{-ij} are computed in advance). In fact the number of multiplications is $n^2 - 2n + 1$, taking into account the fact that $\omega^0 = 1$.

A more effective way to realize the formulas (22.1), (22.2), which is called the fast Fourier transform (FFT), was given by COOLEY and TUKEY [1965].

Let $n = rs$, where r and s are natural numbers that are larger than one. The integer numbers i and j, $0 \leq i, j \leq n-1$, have unique representations:

$$i = i_0 + i_1 s, \quad \text{where } 0 \leq i_0 \leq s-1, \; 0 \leq i_1 \leq r-1, \tag{22.3}$$

$$j = j_0 r + j_1, \quad \text{where } 0 \leq j_0 \leq s-1, \; 0 \leq j_1 \leq r-1. \tag{22.4}$$

The formula (22.3) maps one-to-one the elements a_i of the vector a into the elements a_{i_0, i_1} of an $(r \times s)$ matrix A. The formulas (22.4) maps the elements b_j of the vector b one-to-one into the elements b_{j_0, j_1} of an $(s \times r)$ matrix B.

The correspondence of the elements of the vectors a and b and the matrices A and B in the Cooley–Tukey algorithm in the case $n = 15$, $r = 3$, $s = 5$ are given in the Table 22.1.

For every i, j, $0 \leq i, j \leq n-1$, the following result is fulfilled:

$$ij = (i_0 + i_1 s)(j_0 r + j_1) = i_0 j_1 + i_1 j_1 s + i_0 j_0 r + i_1 j_0 n$$

and therefore

$$\omega_n^{ij} = \omega_n^{i_0 j_1} \omega_r^{i_1 j_1} \omega_s^{i_0 j_0}, \tag{22.5}$$

where $\omega_r = \omega_n^s$ and $\omega_s = \omega_n^r$ are primitive rth and sth roots of the unity in $\mathbb{F}$. By

TABLE 22.1. Vectors and matrices in the Cooley-Tukey algorithm in the case $n = 15$, $r = 3$, $s = 5$.

Matrix A

$i_1 \backslash i_0$	0	1	2	3	4
0	a_0	a_1	a_2	a_3	a_4
1	a_5	a_6	a_7	a_8	a_9
2	a_{10}	a_{11}	a_{12}	a_{13}	a_{14}

Matrix B

$j_1 \backslash j_0$	0	1	2	3	4
0	b_0	b_3	b_6	b_9	b_{12}
1	b_1	b_4	b_7	b_{10}	b_{13}
2	b_2	b_5	b_8	b_{11}	b_{14}

(22.3), (22.4) and (22.5) it follows that

$$b_j = b_{j_0, j_1} = \sum_{i_0=0}^{s-1} \left(\sum_{i_1=0}^{r-1} (a_{i_0,i_1} \omega_r^{i_1 j_1}) \omega_n^{i_0 j_1} \right) \omega_s^{i_0 j_0}.$$

Hence, the transformation (22.1) can be performed in the following way:

$$a_{i_0, i_1} = a_{i_0 + i_1 s}, \quad i_0 = 0, 1, \ldots, s-1, \quad i_1 = 0, 1, \ldots, r-1 \quad (22.6)$$

(the vector a maps into the matrix A);

$$c_{i_0, j_1} = \sum_{i_1=0}^{r-1} a_{i_0, i_1} \omega_r^{i_1 j_1}, \quad j_1 = 0, 1, \ldots, s-1 \quad (22.7)$$

(an FFT with length r of every column of A);

$$d_{i_0, j_1} = c_{i_0, j_1} \omega_n^{i_0 j_1}, \quad i_0 = 0, 1, \ldots, r-1, \quad j_1 = 0, 1, \ldots, s-1, \quad (22.8)$$

$$b_{j_0, j_1} = \sum_{i_0=0}^{r-1} d_{i_0, i_1} \omega_s^{i_0 j_0}, \quad j_0 = 0, 1, \ldots, r-1, \quad (22.9)$$

(an FFT with length s of every row);

$$b_{j_0 r + j_1} = b_{j_0, j_1}, \quad j_0 = 0, 1, \ldots, s-1, \quad j_1 = 0, 1, \ldots, r-1, \quad (22.10)$$

(the vector b is read in the matrix B by columns).

In the formulas (22.6) and (22.10) no arithmetic operations are used, the formulas (22.7) are s DFTs with length r and the formulas (22.9) represent r DFTs with length s. For their execution it is sufficient to perform:

$$s(r^2 - 2r + 1) + r(s^2 - 2s + 1) = n(r + s) - 4n + r + s \quad \text{multiplications}$$

and

$$s(r^2 - r) + r(s^2 - s) = n(r + s) - 2n \quad \text{additions}.$$

The multiplication by so-called "rotation factors" $\omega_n^{i_0 j_1}$ in (22.8) needs $n - r - s + 1$ multiplications in $\mathbb{F}$ (without $\omega^0 = 1$) and usually it is combined with (22.7) or with (22.9). Hence, the number of multiplications and additions taking part in the formulas (22.6)–(22.10) is approximately $n(r + s)$, which is significantly less than $n^2 = n(rs)$ for the direct execution of (22.1).

In matrix notation the Cooley–Tukey algorithm is a factorization of the DFT matrix W_n as a product of diagonal, block-diagonal and "permutation" matrices:

$$W_n = P_1 \begin{pmatrix} W_s & & 0 \\ & \ddots & \\ 0 & & W_s \end{pmatrix} P_2 D P_3 \begin{pmatrix} W_r & & 0 \\ & \ddots & \\ 0 & & W_r \end{pmatrix} P_4, \qquad (22.11)$$

where the diagonal matrix D consists of rotation factors and P_1, P_2, P_3 and P_4 are suitable "permutation" matrices.

If r or s are in turn composite numbers the above approach can be applied recursively and in the case $n = r_1 r_2 \cdots r_k$ the number of operations will be approximately $n(r_1 + r_2 + \cdots + r_k)$. Particularly if $n = r^k$ then the number of operations is $O(rn \log_r n)$.

The stability of the FFT has been the subject of investigation by many authors—see, e.g., RAMOS [1971], and WELCH [1969]. Roughly speaking, the conclusion is that the number of arithmetic operations in DFT and FFT is approximately linearly proportional to the round-off error in them: fewer arithmetic operations in FFT [compared with the direct execution of (21.1)–(21.2)] lead to a smaller round-off error. FFT is especially stable when $n = 2^k$ and $n = 4^k$.

Another algorithm for fast computation of (22.1) was proposed by GOOD [1958]:

Let r and s be relatively prime integer numbers and u and v be integer numbers such that:

$$ur \equiv 1 \ (\text{mod } s), \quad vs \equiv 1 \ (\text{mod } r), \qquad 0 \leq u \leq s - 1, \ 0 \leq v \leq r - 1.$$

Evidently

$$ur^2 \equiv r \ (\text{mod } n) \quad \text{and} \quad vs^2 \equiv s \ (\text{mod } n). \qquad (22.12)$$

Then another correspondence can be established between the vectors a and b and the matrices A and B, respectively.

$$i_0 = (ui) \bmod s, \qquad i_1 = (vi) \bmod r, \qquad (22.13)$$

$$j_0 = j \bmod s, \qquad j_1 = j \bmod r. \qquad (22.14)$$

By the Chinese remainder theorem (see BORODIN and MUNRO [1975], Chapter IV) the correspondences (22.13), (22.14) are one-to-one reversible

$$i = (i_0 r + i_1 s) \bmod n, \qquad j = (j_0 ur + j_1 vs) \bmod n.$$

The correspondence between the vectors a and b with the matrices A and B in Good's algorithm in the case $n = 15$, $r = 3$, $s = 5$, $u = 2$, $v = 2$ is given in Table 22.2.

TABLE 22.2. Vectors and matrices in Good's algorithm in the case $n = 15$, $r = 3$, $s = 5$.

Matrix A

i_1 \ i_0	0	1	2	3	4
0	a_0	a_3	a_6	a_9	a_{12}
1	a_5	a_8	a_{11}	a_{14}	a_2
2	a_{10}	a_{13}	a_1	a_4	a_7

Matrix B

j_1 \ j_0	0	1	2	3	4
0	b_0	b_6	b_{12}	b_3	b_9
1	b_{10}	b_1	b_7	b_{13}	b_4
2	b_5	b_{11}	b_2	b_8	b_{14}

For every i, j, $0 \leq i, j \leq n - 1$, the following result is fulfilled

$$ij = (i_0 r + i_1 s)(j_0 ur + j_1 vs) \pmod{n}$$

and from (22.12) it follows that

$$ij = i_0 j_0 r + i_1 j_1 s \pmod{n}.$$

Hence

$$\omega_n^{ij} = \omega_r^{i_1 j_1} \omega_s^{i_0 j_0}$$

or

$$b_j = b_{j_0, j_1} = \sum_{i_0=0}^{s-1} \left(\sum_{i_1=0}^{r-1} a_{i_0, i_1} \omega_r^{i_1 j_1} \right) \omega_s^{i_0 j_0}.$$

So the following algorithm is obtained for the transformation (22.1):

$$a_{i_0, i_1} = a_{(i_0 r + i_1 s) \bmod n}, \quad i_0 = 0, \ldots, s-1, \quad i_1 = 0, \ldots, r-1$$

(the vector a is written down as a matrix A—see Table 22.2);

$$c_{i_0, j_1} = \sum_{i_1=0}^{r-1} a_{i_0, i_1} \omega_r^{i_1 j_1}, \quad j_1 = 0, 1, \ldots, s-1$$

(an FFT with length r of every column of the matrix A)

$$b_{j_0, j_1} = \sum_{i_0=0}^{r-1} c_{i_0, i_1} \omega_s^{i_0 j_0}, \quad j_0 = 0, 1, \ldots, r-1$$

(an FFT with length s of every row);

$$b_{j_0 r + j_1} = b_{j_0, j_1}, \quad j_0 = 0, 1, \ldots, s-1, \quad j_1 = 0, 1, \ldots, r-1$$

(the vector b is read by the matrix B—see Table 22.2).

Similarly to (22.11), in matrix notation, the Good algorithm is a factorization of the matrix W_n:

$$W_n = P'_1 \begin{pmatrix} W_s & & 0 \\ & \ddots & \\ 0 & & W_s \end{pmatrix} P'_2 \begin{pmatrix} W_r & & 0 \\ & \ddots & \\ 0 & & W_r \end{pmatrix} P'_3,$$

where P'_1, P'_2 and P'_3 are suitable permutation matrices.

The advantage of the Good algorithm for the Cooley–Tukey algorithm is the lack of rotation factors, but a serious deficiency is the condition that r and s be relatively prime.

WINOGRAD [1978] gives another approach. The correspondences between a with A and b with B are the same as in the Good algorithm (the condition that r and s be relatively prime numbers remains valid) but using special algorithms for short DFTs Winograd was successful in decreasing the number of multiplications. The advantage of the Winograd algorithm lies in the case when the length of the DFT is at most several thousand points. This algorithm is asymptotically slower than the algorithms of Good and Cooley–Tukey.

The Cooley–Tukey algorithm is often used in the cases $n = 2^k$ and $n = 4^k$. These two cases can be easily implemented on binary arithmetic computers. They have a high stability according to round-off errors, and the restriction on the number n (to be an exact power of two) is not a difficult obstacle for the applications.

REMARK 22.1. The transformation

$$b_{i_1,\ldots,i_k} = \sum_{j_1=0}^{n-1} \cdots \sum_{j_k=0}^{n-1} a_{j_1,\ldots,j_k} \omega_{n_1}^{i_1 j_1} \cdots \omega_{n_k}^{i_k j_k},$$

$$a_{j_1,\ldots,j_k} = \sum_{i_1=0}^{n-1} \cdots \sum_{i_k=0}^{n-1} b_{i_1,\ldots,i_k} \omega_{n_1}^{i_1 j_1} \cdots \omega_{n_k}^{i_k j_k},$$
(22.15)

is called a k-dimensional DFT with length n according to k variables—respectively $n_1, n_2, \ldots, n_k$. Since the different sums in (22.15) do not depend on each other they can be performed in an arbitrary order. At every fixed set of values of $l, i_1, i_2, \ldots, i_{l-1}, i_{l+1}, \ldots, i_k$ $(0 \leq i_s < n_s, \; s \neq l, \; 1 \leq s \leq k)$ the transformation (22.15) is a one-dimensional DFT with length n_l.

All one-dimensional DFTs taking part in the multidimensional DFT can be performed by FFT algorithms. Vice versa, the Cooley–Tukey and Good algorithms can be regarded as a reduction of a one-dimensional DFT (with length $n = rs$) to a multidimensional DFT (with lengths r and s) plus, eventually, some multiplications by rotation factors.

23. Applications of FFTs

The cyclic convolution of the vectors a and $b \in \mathbb{F}^n$ is the vector $c \in \mathbb{F}^n$ for which

$$c_i = \sum_{j=0}^{n-1} a_j b_{(i-j) \bmod n}, \quad i = 0, 1, \ldots, n-1. \tag{23.1}$$

One important property of the DFT is the so-called "convolution property": if the vectors $\hat{c}$, $\hat{a}$ and $\hat{b}$ result after DFT with length n from vectors c, a and b, respectively, then

$$\hat{c}_i = \hat{a}_i \hat{b}_i, \quad i = 0, 1, \ldots, n-1.$$

Therefore, if $\mathbb{F}$ supports a DFT with length n, then a cyclic convolution with length n can be performed using two direct and one inverse FFT with length n and n additional multiplications. If n is an exact power of two for these operations $\frac{3}{2}n \log n$ multiplications and $3n \log n$ additions and subtractions are sufficient. The direct execution of (23.1) requires n^2 multiplications and $n^2 - n$ additions.

If $N \geq 2n$, the cyclic convolution (23.1) with length n can be performed as a part of the cyclic convolution with length N: let

$$\alpha_i = \begin{cases} a_i, & 0 \leq i \leq n-1, \\ 0, & n \leq i \leq N-1, \end{cases}$$

$$\beta_i = b_{i \bmod n}, \quad 0 \leq i \leq N-1$$

and

$$\gamma_i = \sum_{j=0}^{N-1} \alpha_j \beta_{(i-j) \bmod N}, \quad 0 \leq i \leq N-1.$$

Then $c_i = \gamma_{n+i}$, $0 \leq i \leq n-1$.

Hence, if n is not a power of two but $\mathbb{F}$ supports DFT with length $N \geq 2n$, N being a power of two, then the execution of the cyclic convolution (23.1) with length n can be reduced to one with length N for which $\frac{3}{2}N \log N$ multiplications and $3N \log N$ additions are sufficient. If N is chosen to be the power of two, for which $2n \leq N < 4n$ (i.e. $N = 2^{\lceil \log(2n) \rceil}$) then the number of arithmetic operations is $O(n \log n)$.

RADER [1968] proved that if n is a prime number then FFT with length n can be performed by $2n - 1$ additions and one cyclic convolution with length $n - 1$.

This result implies an interesting corollary: there exists a constant c, such that any complex DFT with length n can be performed by no more than $cn \log n$ arithmetic operations. More generally, if $\mathbb{F}$ supports a DFT with length $N = 2^v$ then there exists a constant c such that any DFT with length $n \leq N/2$ can be performed by no more than $cn \log n$ arithmetic operations.

Indeed, let $n = p_1 p_2 \cdots p_k$, where p_j are primes. Using the Cooley–Tukey algorithm, a DFT with length n can be reduced to n/p_1 DFTs with length p_1, n/p_2 DFTs with length p_2, ..., n/p_k DFTs with length p_k and $n(k-1) = O(n \log n)$ multiplications by rotation factors. Each DFT with length p_j can be reduced to $2p_j - 1$ additions and a cyclic convolution with length $p_j - 1$, which can be performed by $O(p_j \log p_j)$ operations, because $\mathbb{F}$ supports DFT with length $N \geq 2p_j$.

Let

$$P(x) = \sum_{i=0}^{n} p_i x^i \quad \text{and} \quad Q(x) = \sum_{i=0}^{m} q_i x^i$$

be two polynomials over the field $\mathbb{F}$. The multiplication of P and Q is a polynomial R and the problem consists of a fast determination of the coefficients r_i, $0 \leq i \leq n + m$, of R. Evidently

$$r_i = \sum_{j=0}^{n} p_j q_{i-j}, \quad i = 0, 1, \ldots, n + m, \tag{23.2}$$

where $q_i = 0$ if $i < 0$.

The direct execution of (23.2) needs nm additions and $nm + n + m + 1$ multiplications. Using FFT the polynomials P and Q can be multiplied faster.

The DFT (22.1) with length n can be treated as a transformation from the coefficient representation of the polynomial $P(x) = \sum_{i=0}^{n-1} a_i x^i$ of degree $n - 1$ to the representation of this polynomial by its values $P(\omega^i)$ at the special set of n points ω^i, $i = 0, 1, \ldots, n - 1$.

From this point of view the FFT is a method for making transformations between these two representations of the polynomial.

The polynomial multiplication (23.2) can be done as follows: let $N \geq m + n + 1$ be an exact power of two. Using two FFTs with length N it is possible to determine the values of P and Q at the points ω_N^j, $j = 0, 1, \ldots, N - 1$. Then using N multiplications for

$$R(\omega_N^j) = P(\omega_N^j) Q(\omega_N^j), \quad j = 0, 1, \ldots, N - 1,$$

with one inverse FFT with length N; from these values the coefficients of the polynomial R can be computed. For the described algorithm

$$\tfrac{3}{2} N \log N < 3(n + m + 1) \log(n + m + 1)$$

multiplications and

$$3 N \log N < 6(n + m + 1) \log(n + m + 1)$$

additions are sufficient.

MOENCK and BORODIN [1972] considered the division of polynomials via FFT. Let $\mathbb{F}$ support an FFT with length N that is an exact power of two and $N \geq n$. If the polynomials

$$P(x) = \sum_{i=0}^{2n} p_i x^i, \quad Q(x) = \sum_{i=0}^{n} q_i x^i,$$

are given by their coefficients then using $O(n \log n)$ arithmetic operations the coefficients of the polynomials D and R can be computed, where

$$P(x) \equiv Q(x) D(x) + R(x), \quad \deg R < \deg Q.$$

Let us consider the next problem. Let $P(x) = \sum_{i=0}^{n-1} p_i x^i$ be a polynomial of degree $n - 1$. The computation of $P(y)$, where y is a given point, using the classical Horner scheme needs $n - 1$ multiplications and $n - 1$ additions, and OSTROWSKI [1954] and PAN [1966] proved that this problem cannot be solved with fewer arithmetic operations. If n points are given

$$y_0, y_1, \ldots, y_{n-1},$$

then the values

$$P(y_0), P(y_1), \ldots, P(y_{n-1})$$

can be computed using Horner's scheme with $O(n^2)$ multiplications and additions. For this problem Horner's scheme is not optimal. The FFT allows this problem to be solved with $O(n \log^2 n)$ operations.

For simplicity let n be an exact power of two, let $\mathbb{F}$ support a DFT with length n and let

$$P = (x - y_0)(x - y_1) \cdots (x - y_{n/2-1})Q_1 + R_1, \quad \deg R_1 < n/2,$$
$$P = (x - y_{n/2})(x - y_{n/2+1}) \cdots (x - y_n)Q_2 + R_2, \quad \deg R_2 < n/2.$$

The following conditions are also fulfilled:

$$P(y_i) = \begin{cases} R_1(y_i), & \text{if } 0 \leq i < n/2, \\ R_2(y_i), & \text{if } n/2 \leq i < n. \end{cases}$$

If the coefficients of the polynomials

$$(x - y_0) \cdots (x - y_{n/2-1}), \quad (x - y_{n/2}) \cdots (x - y_n)$$

are computed in advance, then it is possible to determine the coefficients of the polynomials R_1 and R_2 by two divisions with a remainder. In this way the problem reduces to two problems of the same kind each with a dimension a half of the original one. Continuing this process recursively finally n problems for the computation of the value of a polynomial of degree zero have to be solved. The number of operations is subjected to the recursive equation

$$T(n) = 2T(n/2) + Cn \log n, \quad T(1) = 0, \tag{23.3}$$

where C is a constant. Hence $T(n) = O(n \log^2 n)$ if the coefficients of the following polynomials are known in advance:

$$\begin{aligned} &(x - y_0), \ldots, (x - y_{n-1}), \\ &(x - y_0)(x - y_1), \ldots, (x - y_{n-2})(x - y_{n-1}), \\ &\vdots \\ &(x - y_0) \cdots (x - y_{n/2-1}), \ldots, (x - y_{n/2}) \cdots (x - y_{n-1}). \end{aligned} \tag{23.4}$$

These coefficients can be computed by $O(n \log^2 n)$ operations, according to the graphs given in Figs. 23.1 and 23.2.

Thus the evaluation of an $n - 1$ degree polynomial at n points can be done in a time of $O(n \log^2 n)$.

Let us consider the problem for the determination of the coefficients of the Lagrange interpolation polynomial (23.5) when the numbers x_i, $f(x_i)$, $i = 0, \ldots, n - 1$, are given

$$L_{n-1}(f; x) = \sum_{i=0}^{n-1} f(x_i) \frac{\omega(x)}{(x - x_i)\omega'(x_i)}, \quad \omega(x) = \prod_{i=0}^{n-1} (x - x_i). \tag{23.5}$$

Remember that $L_{n-1}(f; x_i) = f(x_i)$, $i = 0, 1, \ldots, n - 1$.

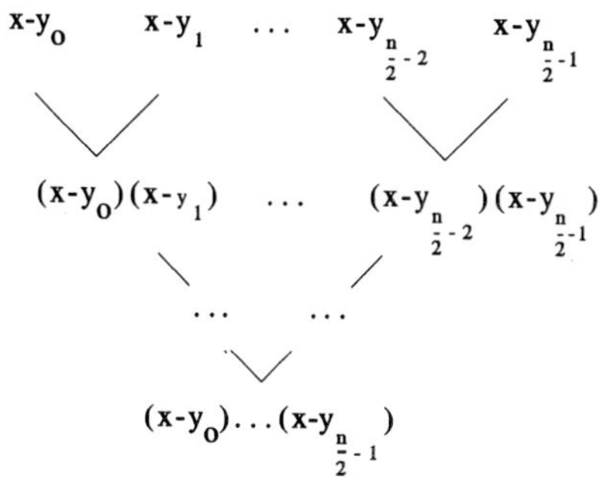

Interpolation

```
    x-y₀      x-y₁    ...    x-y_{n/2-2}    x-y_{n/2-1}
       \    /                    \    /
      (x-y₀)(x-y₁)      ...    (x-y_{n/2-2})(x-y_{n/2-1})
            \                           /
              ...                     ...
                         \    /
                    (x-y₀)...(x-y_{n/2-1})
```

FIG. 23.1.

HOROWITZ [1972] proved that an FFT allows the number of arithmetic operations for the solution of that problem to be decreased from $O(n^2)$ to $O(n \log^2 n)$.

Indeed, with $O(n \log^2 n)$ arithmetic operations the coefficients of the polynomials (23.4) can be computed. By multiplication of the final two of them the coefficients of ω are obtained. After that the computation of the coefficients of ω' need $O(n)$ operations and the computation of the values, $\omega'(x_i)$ and $a_i = f(x_i)/\omega'(x_i)$, $0 \le i < n$, needs an additional $O(n \log^2 n)$ arithmetic operations.

Finally by the help of the equality

$$\sum_{i=0}^{n-1} a_i \prod_{\substack{j=0 \\ j \ne i}}^{n-1} (x-x_j) = \left(\sum_{i=0}^{n/2-1} a_i \prod_{\substack{j=0 \\ j \ne i}}^{n/2-1} (x-x_j) \right) \prod_{j=n/2}^{n-1} (x-x_j)$$

$$+ \left(\sum_{i=n/2}^{n-1} a_i \prod_{\substack{j=n/2 \\ j \ne i}}^{n-1} (x-x_j) \right) \prod_{j=0}^{n/2-1} (x-x_j),$$

the problem reduces to two problems of the same kind with a dimension that is a half of the original one. The recursive continuation of this process shows that

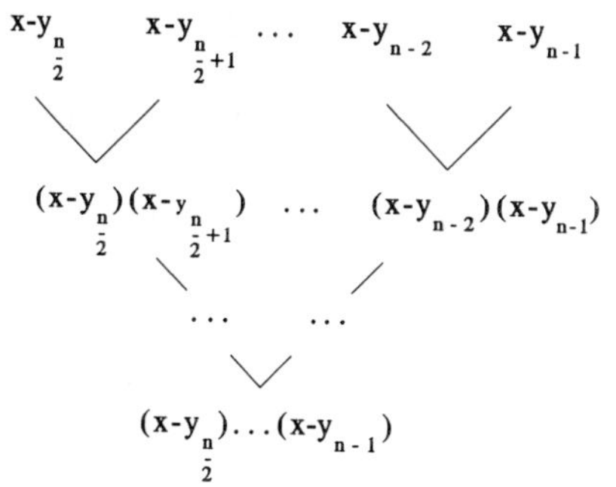

```
    x-y_{n/2}    x-y_{n/2+1}  ...  x-y_{n-2}    x-y_{n-1}
         \    /                        \    /
       (x-y_{n/2})(x-y_{n/2+1})  ... (x-y_{n-2})(x-y_{n-1})
              \                              /
                ...                        ...
                          \    /
                    (x-y_{n/2})...(x-y_{n-1})
```

FIG. 23.2.

the number of arithmetic operations is still given by Eq. (23.3). So the total number of arithmetic operations for Lagrange interpolation is $O(n \log^2 n)$.

The generalization of this result for Hermite interpolation (see Section 12) is given by GEORGIEV [1990]: let $\nu_1 + \nu_2 + \cdots + \nu_k = n$ and $\mathbb{F}$ support an FFT with length N that is an exact power of two, $N \geqslant 2n$. By a given x_m and $y_{\nu,m}$, $\nu = 0, 1, \ldots, \nu_k - 1$, $m = 1, 2, \ldots, k$ from $\mathbb{F}$ the coefficients of the polynomial H of degree $n - 1$,

$$H^{(\nu)}(x_m) = y_{\nu,m}, \quad \nu = 0, 1, \ldots, \nu_k - 1, \ m = 1, 2, \ldots, k,$$

with $\log(k+1)O(n \log n)$ arithmetic operations can be found.

The same number of operations is necessary for the inverse problem—using a given Hermite polynomial H to compute the values $H^{(\nu)}(x_m)$, $\nu = 0, 1, \ldots, \nu_k - 1$, $m = 1, 2, \ldots, k$.

Constructing an algorithm based on FFT and Schur sequences, NEFF [1990] proved an interesting theoretical result: the problem of approximating all the roots of a complex polynomial with a specified precision can be solved in a polylogarithmic parallel time using a polynomial number of processors. In particular, given the coefficients of an arbitrary nth degree polynomial $p(z)$ with integer coefficients, whose absolute values are bounded above by 2^m, and a specified integer μ, all the roots of p can be approximated with an error of less than $2^{-\mu}$ in at most $c_1 \log^3(n + m + \mu)$ parallel steps with at most $c_2(n + m + \mu)^c$ processors, where c_1, c_2, and c are constants.

CHAPTER II

Uniform Approximation

Uniform approximation of functions by means of polynomials and rational functions is a useful part of a series of methods for numerical computation of elementary functions, for convenient representation of functions given by complicated analytical expressions or by discrete data.

In recent time the theoretical investigations proved the excellent approximation properties of rational functions. Polynomials as a classical tool for approximation cannot enter into competition with rational functions especially for functions that are not smooth enough. The results of NEWMAN [1964] and POPOV [1977] motivated and proved this advantage.

At the same time polynomials do not lose their significance for approximation theory in many cases concerning smooth and analytical functions. As a rule the numerical determination of a polynomial or rational function of best uniform approximation is a difficult problem even in the one-dimensional case. In this chapter systematical presentation is given for numerical methods for approximate finding of the elements of best uniform approximation. Numerical examples (tables and figures) illustrate the behavior of the error and it can be compared with theoretical estimations.

Some theoretical problems are considered for approximation by positive linear operators, the possibility of approximation in a uniform metric, and properties of the important applications of Chebyshev polynomials.

Refinement of the Whitney constant allows us to obtain satisfactory theoretical estimates (improving the existed ones) for well-known and popular numerical methods, where the estimates are given by appropriate moduli of smoothness of the considered functions.

24. Uniform distance and best approximation

Let X be a compact set. The uniform distance between the continuous functions f and g defined on X is the number

$$\rho(f, g) = \max_{x \in X} |f(x) - g(x)|.$$

The number $\rho(f, g)$ has the following properties:
(a) $\rho(f, g) \geq 0$ and $\rho(f, g) = 0$ iff $f \equiv g$;

(b) $\rho(f, g) = \rho(g, f)$;
(c) $\rho(f, g) \leq \rho(f, \varphi) + \rho(\varphi, g)$.

Introducing the norm in the set $C(X)$ of continuous functions defined on X by

$$\|f\|_{C(X)} = \max_{x \in X} |f(x)| = \rho(f, 0),$$

the set $C(X)$ becomes a linear normed space and the number $\|f\|_{C(X)}$ satisfies the conditions (a)–(d) given below.

More generally, any real function $\|*\|$ defined on the set X which satisfies the conditions (a)–(c) is called a norm in X:

(a) $\|f\| \geq 0$ and $\|f\| = 0$ if and only if $f \equiv 0$;
(b) $\|\alpha f\| = |\alpha| \|f\|$;
(c) $\|f + g\| \leq \|f\| + \|g\|$;
(d) $\|f - g\| = \rho(f - g, 0) = \rho(f, g)$.

Let $\{\varphi_i\}_{i=0}^n$ be linear independent elements from $C(X)$ and the subset $L \subset X$ is generated by $\{\varphi_i\}_{i=0}^n$; i.e.

$$L = \left\{ \varphi \in C(X) \colon \varphi = \sum_{i=0}^n a_i \varphi_i, \ a_i \text{ are real numbers} \right\}.$$

For every element $f \in C(X)$ the best uniform approximation of f by means of the elements of L is defined as

$$E_L(f) = \inf_{\varphi \in L} \|\varphi - f\|.$$

Several questions arise:

(a) for every element $f \in C(X)$ does there exist an element $\varphi \in L$ of the best approximation that satisfies

$$E_L(f) = \|\varphi - f\| ? \tag{24.1}$$

(b) how many elements satisfy the condition (24.1)?
(c) how large is the quantity $E_L(f)$?
(d) given an element $f \in C(X)$ how can an element $\varphi \in L$ be constructed that satisfies (24.1)?

The answer to the first question gives the following theorem.

THEOREM 24.1. *Let L be the linear subspace of the normed space Y and $L \subset Y$ be generated by the linear independent elements $\{\varphi_i\}_{i=0}^n$. For every $f \in Y$ there exists an element $\varphi \in L$ of the best approximation such that*

$$E_L(f) = \|\varphi - f\|.$$

PROOF. The function $F(a_0, a_1, \ldots, a_n) = \|\sum_{i=0}^n a_i \varphi_i\|$ is a continuous one because of

$$\left| \left\|\sum_{i=0}^n a_i \varphi_i\right\| - \left\|\sum_{i=0}^n b_i \varphi_i\right\| \right| \leq \left\|\sum_{i=0}^n (a_i - b_i)\varphi_i\right\| \leq \sum_{i=0}^n |a_i - b_i| \|\varphi_i\|.$$

Therefore, on the unit ball $\sum_{i=0}^{n} a_i^2 = 1$ the function F achieves its minimum

$$\mu = \min\left\{\left\|\sum_{i=0}^{n} a_i \varphi_i\right\|: \sum_{i=0}^{n} a_i^2 = 1\right\}$$

and from the linear independence of $\{\varphi_i\}_{i=0}^{n}$ it follows that $\mu > 0$.

The function $\|f - \sum_{i=0}^{n} a_i \varphi_i\|$ is also a continuous one and on the ball $\sum_{i=0}^{n} a_i^2 = r^2$ the following relations are fulfilled

$$\left\|f - \sum_{i=0}^{n} a_i \varphi_i\right\| \geq \left\|\sum_{i=0}^{n} a_i \varphi_i\right\| - \|f\| = r\left\|\sum_{i=0}^{n} \frac{|a_i|}{r} \varphi_i\right\| - \|f\| \geq r\mu - \|f\|.$$

If $r > 2\|f\|/\mu = r_0$, then

$$\left\|f - \sum_{i=0}^{n} a_i \varphi_i\right\| \geq r\mu - \|f\| > \|f\| \geq E_L(f).$$

The last inequality shows that

$$E_L(f) = \inf_{\varphi \in L} \|\varphi - f\| = \inf\left\{\left\|f - \sum_{i=0}^{n} a_i \varphi_i\right\|: \sum_{i=0}^{n} a_i^2 \leq r_0^2\right\}.$$

The set

$$\left\{\{a_i\}_{i=0}^{n}: \sum_{i=0}^{n} a_i^2 \leq r_0^2\right\}$$

is a compact one and the continuous function

$$\left\|f - \sum_{i=0}^{n} a_i \varphi_i\right\|$$

achieves its minimum on this set; i.e. there exists a $\varphi \in L$ such that $E_L(f) = \|\varphi - f\|$. □

To answer the question (b) let us denote by $P(f)$ the set $P(f) = \{\varphi: E_L(f) = \|\varphi - f\|\}$. The last theorem shows that $P(f)$ is not an empty set.

THEOREM 24.2. *$P(f)$ is a convex and closed set.*

PROOF. If $\varphi \in P(f)$ and $\psi \in P(f)$ the convexity of $P(f)$ follows from

$$E_L(f) \leq \|f - [\alpha\varphi + (1-\alpha)\psi]\| \leq \alpha\|f - \varphi\| + (1-\alpha)\|f - \psi\| = E_L(f)$$

for $0 \leq \alpha \leq 1$; i.e. $\alpha\varphi + (1-\alpha)\psi \in P(f)$.

If $\{\psi_i\}_{i=0}^{\infty} \in P(f)$ and $\lim_{i \to \infty} \|\psi_i - \psi\| = 0$ the closure of $P(f)$ follows from

$$\|f - \psi\| \leq \|f - \psi_i\| + \|\psi_i - \psi\|$$
$$= E_L(f) + \|\psi_i - \psi\| \xrightarrow[i \to \infty]{} E_L(f). \quad \square$$

In the general case the element of the best approximation is not unique.

The normed linear space Y is called strongly normed if the equality

$$\|x+y\| = \|x\| + \|y\|, \quad y \neq 0,$$

implies the existence of a number α such that $x = \alpha y$.

THEOREM 24.3. *If the space Y is strongly normed space then for every element $f \in Y$ the set $P(f)$ consists of one element.*

PROOF. Suppose that for $f \in Y$ there exist two elements $\varphi \in L$, $\psi \in L$ such that

$$E_L(f) = \|\varphi - f\| = \|\psi - f\|.$$

By Theorem 24.2

$$E_L(f) = \|f - \tfrac{1}{2}(\varphi + \psi)\| \leq \tfrac{1}{2}\|\varphi - f\| + \tfrac{1}{2}\|\psi - f\| = E_L(f);$$

i.e.

$$\|f - \tfrac{1}{2}(\varphi + \psi)\| \leq \tfrac{1}{2}\|\varphi - f\| + \tfrac{1}{2}\|\psi - f\| \quad \text{or} \quad \varphi - f = \alpha(\psi - f),$$

where α is a number. If $\alpha \neq 1$ then $f \in L$ and $f = \varphi = \psi$. If $\alpha = 1$ then $\varphi = \psi$. □

Theorem 24.3 does not cover all the cases because there exist normed spaces that are not strongly normed for which the element of the best approximation is unique. For instance, the space $C(K)$ of the continuous functions on the compact K is not strongly normed. Let $K = [0, 1]$ and $f_1 = 1$, $f_2 = x$. According to the uniform norm

$$\|f_1\|_{C(K)} = 1, \quad \|f_2\|_{C(K)} = 1, \quad \|f_1 + f_2\|_{C(K)} = 2,$$

$$\|f_1\|_{C(K)} + \|f_2\|_{C(K)} = \|f_1 + f_2\|_{C(K)}.$$

At the same time the functions f_1 and f_2 do not satisfy $f_1 = \alpha f_2$. Nevertheless, even the space $C(K)$ is not strongly normed, under some conditions for the set $L \subset C(K)$ the element of the best approximation is unique—see Theorem 26.1.

25. Characterization of the element of the best approximation

Let f be a continuous function of complex variable $z = x + iy$, $i^2 = -1$, in the closed domain D. Given the positive continuous function q defined in D let us denote by

$$E_n(f) = \inf_{\varphi \in V_n} \max_{z \in D} q(z)|f(z) - \varphi(z)|$$

the best approximation of the function f by means of elements of $V_n = \{\varphi: \varphi = \sum_{i=0}^{n} b_i \varphi_i\}$, where the functions $\{\varphi_i\}_{i=0}^{n}$ are continuous and linearly independent. The generalized polynomial $\varphi \in V_n$ that satisfies

$$E_n(f) = \max_{z \in D} q(z)|f(z) - \varphi(z)|$$

is called the polynomial of the best uniform approximation for f. The weight function q can be omitted taking into account the fact that q is attributed to f and to φ_i.

KOLMOGOROV [1948] proved the following theorem (see also TONELLI [1908]).

THEOREM 25.1. *Let $E \subset D$ be the closed domain where*

$$\max_{z \in D} |f(z) - \varphi(z)| = \{|f(z) - \varphi(z)|: z \in E\}.$$

A necessary and sufficient condition from the generalized polynomial $\varphi \in V_n$ to satisfy $E_n(f) = \max_{z \in D} |f(z) - \varphi(z)|$ is for every $\psi \in V_n$ it is fulfilled that

$$\min_{z \in E} \operatorname{Re}\{\psi(z)\overline{[\varphi(z) - f(z)]}\} \leq 0.$$

PROOF. *Necessity.* Let us suppose that there exists a $\psi \in V_n$ and an $\varepsilon > 0$ such that

$$\min_{z \in E} \operatorname{Re}\{\psi(z)\overline{[\varphi(z) - f(z)]}\} > \varepsilon > 0. \tag{25.1}$$

By (25.1) the existence of the domain E_1 follows and the number $\delta > 0$ with the properties: $E \subset E_1 \subset D$, $\operatorname{dist}(E, E_1) < \delta$, $G = D \setminus E_1$ is a closed domain and

$$\min_{z \in E_1} \operatorname{Re}\{\psi(z)\overline{[\varphi(z) - f(z)]}\} > \varepsilon.$$

Let

$$L' = \max_{z \in G} |f(z) - \varphi(z)|, \qquad L = \max_{z \in D} |f(z) - \varphi(z)|,$$

$$H = \max_{z \in D} |\psi(z)|, \qquad h = L - L' > 0,$$

and $\lambda \leq \min[\varepsilon/H^2, h/2H]$. The polynomial $q = \varphi - \lambda\psi$ satisfies for $z \in E_1$ the following equalities:

$$|q(z) - f(z)|^2 = [q(z) - f(z)]\overline{[q(z) - f(z)]}$$
$$= [\varphi(z) - f(z) - \lambda\psi(z)][\overline{\varphi(z) - f(z)} - \lambda\overline{\psi(z)}]$$
$$= |\varphi(z) - f(z)|^2 - 2\lambda \operatorname{Re}\{\psi(z)\overline{[\varphi(z) - f(z)]}\} + \lambda^2|\psi(z)|^2$$
$$\leq L^2 - 2\lambda\varepsilon + \lambda^2 H^2 \leq L^2 - 2\lambda\varepsilon + \lambda\varepsilon = L^2 - \lambda\varepsilon < L^2.$$

If $z \in G$ then

$$|q(z) - f(z)| = |\varphi(z) - f(z) - \lambda\psi(z)|$$
$$\leq |\varphi(z) - f(z)| + \lambda|\psi(z)| \leq (L - h) + h/2 < L.$$

So $\max_{z \in D} |f(z) - q(z)| < L$ and φ is not the polynomial of the best approximation.

Sufficiency. Let the conditions of the theorem be fulfilled and q be an arbitrary polynomial that is different from φ. For some $z_0 \in E$ from

$$\operatorname{Re}\{[\varphi(z_0) - q(z_0)]\overline{[\varphi(z_0) - f(z_0)]}\} \leq 0$$

it follows that

$$\begin{aligned}|q(z_0) - f(z_0)|^2 &= |\varphi(z_0) - f(z_0) - \varphi(z_0) + q(z_0)|^2 \\ &= |\varphi(z_0) - f(z_0)|^2 - 2\operatorname{Re}\{[\varphi(z_0) - q(z_0)]\overline{[\varphi(z_0) - f(z_0)]}\} \\ &\quad + |\varphi(z_0) - q(z_0)|^2 \\ &\geq |\varphi(z_0) - f(z_0)|^2 + |\varphi(z_0) - q(z_0)|^2 \geq L^2 \,;\end{aligned}$$

i.e. the polynomial q cannot approximate f better than φ. □

Let

$$E_n(f) = \max_{z \in D} |f(z) - \varphi(z)| = \{|f(z) - \varphi(z)|: z \in E_0 \subseteq D\} \,,$$

where the finite set E_0 is such that for every set $E^* \subseteq E_0$, with $E_0 \setminus E^* \neq \emptyset$, the following inequality is fulfilled:

$$\inf_{\psi \in V_n} \max_{z \in E^*} |f(z) - \psi(z)| < E_n(f) \,.$$

The set E_0 is called the characteristic set of order n according to V_n. VALLEE-POUSSIN [1910] proved (see also SMIRNOV and LEBEDEV [1964], Chapters 3, 5, DZJADIK [1977], Chapter 1) that if D consists of at least $n + 2$ points, then:
 (a) there exist characteristic sets;
 (b) every characteristic set E_0 has m points, where $n + 2 \leq m \leq 2n + 3$ if V_n is a Chebyshev system on D and $1 \leq m \leq 2n + 3$ otherwise.

Theorem 25.1 is called Kolmogorov's criteria for the characterization of the element of the best uniform approximation and in the real case keeping the notation from Section 24, Theorem 25.1 takes the following form.

THEOREM 25.2. *Let $E \subset K$ be the set where*

$$\max_{x \in K} |f(x) - \varphi(x)| = \{|f(x) - \varphi(x)|: x \in E\} \,.$$

A necessary and sufficient condition for the polynomial $\varphi \in V_n$ to satisfy

$$E_n(f) = \max_{x \in K} |f(x) - \varphi(x)|$$

is: for every polynomial $\psi \in V_n$ the inequality $\min_{x \in E} \psi(x)[\varphi(x) - f(x)] \leq 0$ is fulfilled.

More convenient conditions from the practical point of view for the characterization of the element of the best approximation when the dimension of the compact K is one and $L = \{\psi: \psi = \sum_{i=0}^{n} b_i x^i\}$ are given by CHEBYSHEV [1857–1859]. Therefore the next theorem is called the Chebyshev theorem.

THEOREM 25.3. *Let the compact K belong to the interval $[a, b]$ and have at least $n + 2$ points. A necessary and sufficient condition for the polynomial $\varphi \in V_n$ ($V_n \subset C(K)$, and V_n is generated by a Chebyshev system $\{\varphi_i\}_{i=0}^{n}$) to be a* polynomial of the best approximation for the function $f \in C(K)$ is the existence of $n+2$ points $x_0 < x_1 < \cdots < x_{n+1}$, $x_i \in K$, such that

$$f(x_i) - \varphi(x_i) = \varepsilon(-1)^i \|f - \varphi\|_{C(K)} = \varepsilon(-1)^i \max_{x \in K} |f(x) - \varphi(x)|,$$

$i = 0, \ldots, n+1$, $\varepsilon = \pm 1$.

PROOF. The points $\{x_i\}_{i=0}^{n+1}$ are called points of Chebyshev alternation.

Necessity. Let there exist at most $q + 1 < n + 2$ points of alternation and let $x_0 < x_1 < \cdots < x_q$ be one collection of such points. Let us choose the points $y_0 < y_1 < y_2 < \cdots < y_q$, which satisfies:
  (a) $a = y_0 \leq x_0 < y_1 < x_1 < y_2 < x_2 < \cdots < y_q < x_q \leq b$, $s = 1, 2, \ldots, q$:
  (b) if a point $y_s \in K$ then $|f(y_s) - \varphi(y_s)| < \|f - \varphi\|_{C(K)}$;
  (c) in every interval $[y_s, y_{s+1}]$, $s = 0, 1, \ldots, q - 1$, the function $f - \varphi$ attains only one of the values $\|f - \varphi\|_{C(K)}$ or $-\|f - \varphi\|_{C(K)}$.

Let us choose the point $y \in (y_q, x_q)$, such that on the set $K \cap [y_q, y]$ the function $f - \varphi$ does not attain $\pm \|f - \varphi\|_{C(K)}$. Let the points $y_i \in (y_q, y)$, $i = q + 1, \ldots, q + 2m$, where m is the greatest number for which $q + 2m \leq n$. If $q + 2m = n - 1$ then let $y_n = b$. The polynomial $\psi \in V_n$,

$$\psi(x) = \begin{vmatrix} \varphi_0(x) & \varphi_1(x) & \cdots & \varphi_n(x) \\ \varphi_0(y_1) & \varphi_1(y_1) & \cdots & \varphi_n(y_1) \\ \varphi_0(y_2) & \varphi_1(y_2) & \cdots & \varphi_n(y_2) \\ \vdots & \vdots & & \vdots \\ \varphi_0(y_n) & \varphi_1(y_n) & \cdots & \varphi_n(y_n) \end{vmatrix},$$

has the properties:
  (a) $\psi(y_i) = 0$, $i = 1, 2, \ldots, n$, and ψ has no other zeros in $[a, b]$;
  (b) $\operatorname{sgn} \psi(y_s - \delta) = -\operatorname{sgn} \psi(y_s + \delta)$ for all sufficiently small $\delta > 0$.
The assertion (a) is evident and (b) follows from Theorem 25.5.

Without loss of generality let

$$\operatorname{sgn} \psi(x) = \operatorname{sgn}[f(x_0) - \varphi(x_0)]$$

for $x \in [a, y_1)$. Otherwise the polynomial $-\psi$ must be taken. This means that $\operatorname{sgn} \psi(x) = \operatorname{sgn}[f(x_s) - \varphi(x_s)]$ for $x \in (y_s, y_{s+1})$, $s = 1, 2, \ldots, q - 1$. On the interval (y_q, y_{q+2m}) the polynomial ψ changes $\operatorname{sgn} 2m$ times and therefore $\operatorname{sgn} \psi(x) = \operatorname{sgn}[f(x_q) - \varphi(x_q)]$ for $x \in (y_{q+2m}, b)$.

So if $q + 2m = n$ for $x \in E \subset K$, $E = \{x \in K : |f(x) - \varphi(x)| = \|f - \varphi\|_{C(K)}\}$, the inequality $\psi(x)[f(x) - \varphi(x)] > 0$ is fulfilled and by Theorem 25.2 φ is not the polynomial of the best uniform approximation for f. This conclusion remains valid in the case $q + 2m = n - 1$ and $|f(b) - \varphi(b)| \neq \|f - \varphi\|_{C(K)}$.

If $q + 2m = n - 1$ and $|f(b) - \varphi(b)| = \|f - \varphi\|_{C(K)}$ then the inequality $\psi(x)[f(x) - \varphi(x)] > 0$ holds for all $x \in E \setminus b$. Let $\phi \in V_n$ satisfy $\operatorname{sgn} \phi(b) = \operatorname{sgn}[f(b) - \varphi(b)]$. Then for sufficiently small $\lambda > 0$ the polynomial $\Psi = \psi + \lambda \phi$ satisfies $\Psi(x)[f(x) - \varphi(x)] > 0$ for $x \in E$.

Sufficiency. Let the conditions of the theorem be fulfilled but $\psi \in V_n$ is the polynomial of the best approximation for f. Then the polynomial $\psi - \varphi =$

$[f - \varphi] - [f - \psi]$ has different signs at the points $\{x_i\}_{i=0}^{n+1}$; i.e. the polynomial $\psi - \varphi$ has $n + 1$ zeros, which leads to $\varphi \equiv \psi$. □

Using the results of REMEZ [1953, 1957] and IVANOV [1951, 1952], VIDENSKII [1956, 1960] gives a necessary and sufficient condition that is more convenient for applications than Kolmogorov's criteria.

THEOREM 25.4. *Let f be continuous on the set D on the plane and let $\varphi \in V_n$. A necessary and sufficient condition for $E_n(f) = \|f - \varphi\|_{C(D)}$ is the existence of the points $\{z_k\}_{k=0}^m \subseteq D$ and positive numbers $\{\delta_k\}_{k=0}^m$, $1 \leq m \leq 2n + 3$, such that $E_n(f) = |f(z_k) - \varphi(z_k)|$ and for every $\psi \in V_n$ to be fulfilled $\sum_{k=1}^m \delta_k [f(z_k) - \psi(z_k)]\varphi(z_k) = 0$.*

THEOREM 25.5. *Let $a < x_1 < x_2 < \cdots < x_n < b$ and $\{\varphi_i\}_{i=0}^n$ be continuous functions that form a Chebyshev system on $[a, b]$. Then the function*

$$D(x) = (x, x_1, x_2, \ldots, x_n) = \begin{vmatrix} \varphi_0(x) & \varphi_1(x) & \cdots & \varphi_n(x) \\ \varphi_0(x_1) & \varphi_1(x_1) & \cdots & \varphi_n(x_1) \\ \varphi_0(x_2) & \varphi_1(x_2) & \cdots & \varphi_n(x_2) \\ \vdots & \vdots & & \vdots \\ \varphi_0(x_n) & \varphi_1(x_n) & \cdots & \varphi_n(x_n) \end{vmatrix},$$

preserves the sign on every interval $(a, x_1), (x_1, x_2), \ldots, (x_n, b)$ and the signs of D are different in adjacent intervals.

PROOF. The function D vanishes in the interval $[a, b]$ only at the points $x_1, x_2, \ldots, x_n$, because D has the form $D = \sum_{i=0}^n b_i \varphi_i$, and $\{\varphi_i\}_{i=0}^n$ are Chebyshev system on $[a, b]$. Having observed that the sign of $D(x)$ does not change moving the points $x, x_1, x_2, \ldots, x_n$ continuously in $[a, b]$ keeping their mutual disposition then for the points

$$x_1 < x_2 < \cdots < x_k < \xi < x_{k+1} < \eta < x_{k+2} < \cdots < x_n$$

it is fulfilled that

$$\operatorname{sgn} D(\xi) = \operatorname{sgn} D(\xi, x_1, x_2, \ldots, x_k, x_{k+1}, \ldots, x_n)$$
$$= \operatorname{sgn} D(x_{k+1}, x_1, \ldots, x_k, \eta, x_{k+2}, \ldots, x_n).$$

The determinant $D(x_{k+1}, x_1, \ldots, x_k, \eta, x_{k+2}, \ldots, x_n)$ can be obtained from $D(\eta, x_1, \ldots, x_k, x_{k+1}, x_{k+2}, \ldots, x_n)$ by permutation of two rows; i.e. $\operatorname{sgn} D(\xi) = -\operatorname{sgn} D(\eta)$. □

THEOREM 25.6. *Let $\{\varphi_i\}_{i=0}^n$ be a Chebyshev system on the compact K, $f \in C(K)$ and*

$$\varphi = \sum_{i=0}^n a_i \varphi_i, \quad \varphi \in L, \quad L = \left\{ \psi : \psi = \sum_{i=0}^n b_i \varphi_i, \varphi_i \in C(K) \right\}.$$

If the equation

$$|f(x) - \varphi(x)| = \|f - \varphi\|_{C(K)}$$

has less than $n + 2$ zeros in K then the polynomial φ cannot be a polynomial of the best approximation for f.

PROOF. Assuming that the equation $|f(x) - \varphi(x)| = \|f - \varphi\|_{C(K)}$ has $m + 1$ zeros $x_i \in K$, $i = 0, 1, \ldots, m$, $m \leq n$, then by Theorem 1.1 there exists a polynomial $\psi \in L$ that satisfies $\psi(x_i) = f(x_i) - \varphi(x_i)$, $i = 0, 1, \ldots, m$. Hence

$$\psi(x_i)\{f(x_i) - \varphi(x_i)\} = \|f - \varphi\|_{C(K)}^2 > 0, \quad i = 0, 1, \ldots, m.$$

By Theorem 25.2 φ cannot be the polynomial of the best approximation for f. □

Let us mention that Theorem 25.6 was proved in the complex case by TONELLI [1908].

26. Uniqueness of the polynomial of the best uniform approximation

The Theorem 24.3 can be used for the establishment of the uniqueness of the element of the best approximation. Unfortunately it does not work for a uniform distance. In this case the main result is the Theorem 26.1 due to HAAR [1918] given below.

Retaining the notation from Section 24 let the system of functions $\{\varphi_i\}_{i=0}^n$ be given, $\varphi_i \in C(K)$, where $C(K)$ is the space of all continuous functions on the compact K.

THEOREM 26.1. *Let the compact K contain at least $n + 2$ points. A necessary and sufficient condition for every function $f \in C(K)$ its element of the best uniform approximation $\varphi \in L$, $L \subset C(K)$,*

$$L = \left\{\psi \colon \psi = \sum_{i=0}^{n} b_i \varphi_i, \; \varphi_i \in C(K)\right\}$$

to be unique is for the system of functions $\{\varphi_i\}_{i=0}^n$ to build a Chebyshev system on K.

PROOF. *Necessity.* Let us assume that there exists a polynomial

$$\psi = \sum_{i=0}^{n} a_i \varphi_i, \quad \sum_{i=0}^{n} a_i^2 > 0,$$

and $n + 1$ points x_i, $x_i \in K$, $i = 0, 1, \ldots, n$, $x_i \neq x_j$, $i \neq j$, for which

$$\psi(x_j) = \sum_{i=0}^{n} a_i \varphi_i(x_j) = 0, \quad j = 0, 1, \ldots, n.$$

Because of $\sum_{i=0}^{n} a_i^2 > 0$ it is fulfilled that

$$\begin{vmatrix} \varphi_0(x_0) & \varphi_1(x_0) & \cdots & \varphi_n(x_0) \\ \varphi_0(x_1) & \varphi_1(x_1) & \cdots & \varphi_n(x_1) \\ \vdots & \vdots & & \vdots \\ \varphi_0(x_n) & \varphi_1(x_n) & \cdots & \varphi_n(x_n) \end{vmatrix} = 0.$$

Therefore the rows of this determinant are linearly dependent; i.e. there exist numbers b_i, $i = 0, 1, \ldots, n$, $\sum_{i=0}^{n} b_i^2 > 0$, such that

$$\sum_{j=0}^{n} b_j \varphi_i(x_j) = 0, \quad i = 0, 1, \ldots, n.$$

Hence for every generalized polynomial $g = \sum_{i=0}^{n} c_i \varphi_i$ the following equality is fulfilled

$$\sum_{j=0}^{n} b_j g(x_j) = 0. \tag{26.1}$$

Since $\sum_{j=0}^{n} b_j c_i \varphi_i(x_j) = 0$,

$$\sum_{i=0}^{n} c_i \sum_{j=0}^{n} b_j \varphi_i(x_j) = \sum_{j=0}^{n} b_j \sum_{i=0}^{n} c_i \varphi_i(x_j) = \sum_{j=0}^{n} b_j g(x_j) = 0.$$

There exists a function $h \in C(K)$ for which $\|h\| = 1$, $h(x_i) = 1$ if $b_i > 0$ and $h(x_i) = -1$ if $b_i < 0$ (in the case when K is an interval the existence of such a function is evident).

Let $\lambda > 0$ be such that $\lambda \|\psi\| \leq 1$. Then the function $g = h(1 - \lambda|\psi|)$ has the same properties as the function h. As

$$E_L(g) = \inf_{\varphi \in L} \|\varphi - g\| \leq \|0 - g\| = \|g\| = 1,$$

let us prove that $E_L(g) = 1$. Assuming the existence of the polynomial $q \in L$ for which $E_L(g) = \|q - g\| = \delta < 1$. This means that $|q(x_i) - g(x_i)| < 1$, $i = 0, 1, \ldots, n$, and therefore $q(x_i) > 0$ if $b_i > 0$ and $q(x_i) < 0$ if $b_i < 0$. Therefore, $\sum_{j=0}^{n} b_j q(x_j) > 0$, which contradicts (26.1).

For every $|\alpha| \leq 1$ the generalized polynomial $\alpha \lambda \psi \in L$ satisfies

$$|g(x) - \alpha\lambda\psi(x)| \leq |h(x)| |1 - \lambda| |\psi(x)| + |\alpha| |\lambda| |\psi(x)|$$
$$\leq 1 - \lambda|\psi(x)| + |\alpha| |\lambda| |\psi(x)| \leq 1;$$

i.e. the function g has more than one generalized polynomial of the best uniform approximation.

Sufficiency. Assume that for the function f there exist two elements

$$\varphi = \sum_{i=0}^{n} a_i \varphi_i, \quad \psi = \sum_{i=0}^{n} b_i \varphi$$

of the best approximation. By Theorem 24.2 the polynomial $g = (\varphi + \psi)/2$ is also the polynomial of the best approximation for f. By Theorem 25.6 there exist $n + 1$ points $x_i \in K$, such that

$$|f(x_i) - g(x_i)| = E_L(f), \quad i = 0, 1, \ldots, n.$$

From this equality and from

$$|f(x_i) - \varphi(x_i)| \leq E_L(f), \quad |f(x_i) - \psi(x_i)| \leq E_L(f),$$

it follows that

$$f(x_i) - \varphi(x_i) = f(x_i) - \psi(x_i), \quad i = 0, 1, \ldots, n. \tag{26.2}$$

The equalities (26.2) show that the polynomial $\varphi - \psi$ has $n + 1$ zeros, which contradicts the assumption that the functions $\{\varphi_i\}_{i=0}^n$ build a Chebyshev system on K. □

27. The uniform rational approximation

Let K be a compact set containing at least $n + m + 2$ points, $C(K)$ be the space of all real continuous functions on K and $\{\varphi_i\}_{i=0}^m$, $\{\psi_i\}_{i=0}^n$, $\varphi_i \in C(K)$, $\psi_i \in C(K)$, be Chebyshev systems on K; i.e. every polynomial $\sum_{i=0}^m a_i \varphi_i$ or $\sum_{i=0}^n b_i \psi_i$ has at most m, respectively, n zeros in K. Let us denote by L_{mn}

$$L_{mn} = \left\{ \varphi : \varphi = w \sum_{i=0}^m a_i \varphi_i \bigg/ \sum_{i=0}^n b_i \psi_i, \, w(x) > 0 \text{ for } x \in K, \, a_i, b_i \text{ real numbers} \right\},$$

and for the function $f \in C(K)$ let $E_{mn}(f)$ denote the best uniform approximation of f by elements of L_{mn}

$$E_{mn}(f) = \inf_{\varphi \in L_{mn}} \max_{x \in K} |f(x) - \varphi(x)| = \inf_{\varphi \in L_{mn}} \|f - \varphi\|.$$

The function $\psi \in L_{mn}$ is called the element of the best approximation for f if $E_{mn}(f) = \|f - \psi\|$.

If $\varphi_i = \psi_i = x^i$, $w \equiv 1$ and $K \in [a, b]$, L_{mn} is the space of ordinary rational functions.

For a given function $f \in C(K)$ the existence of its element of the best approximation from L_{mn} does not follow from Theorem 24.1 because L_{mn} is not a linear space, e.g., if $\varphi \in L_{mn}$ and $\psi \in L_{mn}$ it is not certain that $\varphi + \psi \in L_{mn}$.

THEOREM 27.1. *For every function $f \in C(K)$ there exists a function $\varphi \in L_{mn}$ such that $E_{mn}(f) = \|f - \varphi\|$.*

PROOF. By the definition of $E_{mn}(f)$ for $s = 1, 2, \ldots,$ there exist functions $r_s \in L_{mn}$ for which

$$E_{mn}(f) \leq \|f - r_s\| < E_{mn}(f) + 1/s.$$

Let the denominators of the functions

$$r_s = w \sum_{i=0}^m a_{is} \varphi_i \bigg/ \sum_{i=0}^n b_{is} \psi_i$$

be normed as follows, $\sum_{i=0}^{n} b_{is}^2 = 1$. The coefficients a_{is}, $i = 0, 1, \ldots, m$, $s = 0, 1, \ldots$, are also bounded. Indeed, from

$$\|r_s\| < E_{mn}(f) + 1/s + \|f\|$$

it follows for every $x \in K$ that

$$\left|\sum_{i=0}^{m} a_{is}\varphi_i(x)\right| \leq \left|\sum_{i=0}^{n} b_{is}\psi_i(x)\right| \frac{[E_{mn}(f) + \|f\|]}{w(x)} \leq C[E_{mn}(f) + \|f\|],$$

where

$$C = \max_{0 \leq i \leq n} \|\psi_i\| \sum_{i=0}^{n} |b_{is}| / \inf_{x \in K} w(x) \leq \sqrt{n+1} \max_{0 \leq i \leq n} \|\psi_i\| / \inf_{x \in K} w(x).$$

Because the polynomial $\sum_{i=0}^{m} a_{is}\varphi_i$ is bounded in K (it is sufficient for $\sum_{i=0}^{m} a_{is}\varphi_i$ to be bounded at $n+1$ different points in K) all the coefficients a_{is} are bounded.

Let us choose convergent sequences from the bounded numbers a_{is}, b_{js}, $i = 0, 1, \ldots, m$, $j = 0, 1, \ldots, n$, $s = 0, 1, 2, \ldots$,

$$\lim_{s_k \to \infty} a_{is_k} = a_i, \qquad \lim_{s_k \to \infty} b_{js_k} = b_j.$$

Denoting by $\varphi = w \sum_{i=0}^{m} a_i \varphi_i / \sum_{i=0}^{n} b_i \psi_i$ let $K_1 \subset K$ be the set

$$K_1 = \left\{ x \in K : \sum_{i=0}^{n} b_i \psi_i(x) = 0 \right\}.$$

For every point $\xi \notin K_1$ it is evident that

$$\varphi(\xi) = \lim_{s_k \to \infty} \varphi_{s_k}(\xi)$$

and

$$|\varphi(\xi)| \leq |f(\xi)| + |f(\xi) - \varphi_{s_k}(\xi)| + |\varphi(\xi) - \varphi_{s_k}(\xi)|$$
$$\leq \|f\| + E_{mn}(f) + 1/s_k + |\varphi(\xi) - \varphi_{s_k}(\xi)| \xrightarrow[s_k \to \infty]{} \|f\| + E_{mn}(f).$$

This last consideration shows that the function φ is bounded on $K \backslash K_1$. The set K_1 consists of at most m points and therefore φ is bounded on K. Hence, for every $\xi \in K$ it is fulfilled that $\varphi(\xi) = \lim_{s_k \to \infty} \varphi_{s_k}(\xi)$ and

$$\max_{x \in K} |f(x) - \varphi(x)| \leq \max_{x \in K} |f(x) - \varphi_{s_k}(x)| + \max_{x \in K} |\varphi_{s_k}(x) - \varphi(x)|$$
$$\leq E_{mn}(f) + 1/s_k + \|\varphi - \varphi_{s_k}\|,$$

for any integer s_k. The last inequality gives $\|f - \varphi\| \leq E_{mn}(f)$. □

In the case when $K = [a, b]$, $n = 0$, $w \equiv 1$, $\varphi_i(x) = x^i$, $i = 0, 1, \ldots, m$, the Theorem 27.1 is proved by BOREL [1905].

Without the requirement that the compact K contains at least $n + m + 2$ points the Theorem 27.1 is not true. Indeed, let $K = \{0, 1\}$, the function f is defined as $f(0) = 1$, $f(1) = 0$, $n = 1$, $m = 0$, $w \equiv 1$, $\psi_i(x) = x^i$, $i = 0, 1$. Then $E_{01}(f) = 0$ because the function $\varphi_a(x) = 1/(1 + ax)$ approximates f with arbitrary accuracy at the points 0 and 1 when $a \to \infty$.

The theorems for the existence of the rational function of the best approximation in the complex case for a given continuous function or when the domain is not bounded or the weight function w vanishes at some points can be found in WALSH [1960a,b], AHIEZER [1965], and SMIRNOV and LEBEDEV [1964].

28. The Vallee-Poussin and Chebyshev theorems for rational functions

The following theorem proved by VALLEE-POUSSIN [1910, 1919] in the polynomial case gives the estimation from below for the best uniform approximation of the continuous function by means of rational functions. Following RALSTON ([1965a], Chapter 7.8), or AHIEZER ([1965], Chapter 2), let us denote

$$L_{mn} = \left\{\varphi \colon \varphi(x) = w(x) \sum_{i=0}^{m} a_i x^i \Big/ \sum_{i=0}^{n} b_i x^i, \; w(x) > 0 \text{ for } x \in [a, b]\right\}.$$

If $[a, b] = (-\infty, \infty)$ it is posible that $w(\infty) = w(-\infty) = 0$, but for simplicity let $w \equiv 1$. The considerations are the same with and without the weight function w.

THEOREM 28.1. *Let $\varphi \in L_{mn}$ have the form*

$$\varphi(x) = w(x) \sum_{i=0}^{m-\mu} a_i x^i \Big/ \sum_{i=0}^{n-\nu} b_i x^i,$$

$0 \leq \mu \leq m$, $0 \leq \nu \leq n$, $d = \min\{\mu, \nu\}$, $b_0 \neq 0$.

Let the polynomials $\sum_{i=0}^{m-\mu} a_i x^i$ and $\sum_{i=0}^{n-\nu} b_i x^i$ be irreducible and for the continuous function f in $[a, b]$ the difference $f - \varphi$ is bounded in $[a, b]$. If at the points $a \leq x_1 < x_2 < \cdots < x_N \leq b$, $N = m + n - d + 2$, the following result is fulfilled

$$f(x_i) - \varphi(x_i) = \varepsilon(-1)^i \lambda_i, \quad \lambda_i > 0, \; i = 0, 1, \ldots, N, \; \varepsilon = \pm 1,$$

then for every function $\psi \in L_{mn}$

$$\max_{a \leq x \leq b} |f(x) - \psi(x)| = \|f - \psi\| \geq \min\{\lambda_1, \lambda_2, \ldots, \lambda_N\}.$$

This inequality holds if $\varphi \equiv 0$ and $N = m + 2$.

PROOF. Let for the function $\psi \in L_{mn}$ the following inequality be fulfilled

$$\|f - \psi\| < \min\{\lambda_1, \lambda_2, \ldots, \lambda_N\}.$$

Then the numbers

$$\psi(x_1) - \varphi(x_1) = [f(x_1) - \varphi(x_1)] - [f(x_1) - \psi(x_1)],$$
$$\psi(x_2) - \varphi(x_2), \ldots, \psi(x_N) - \varphi(x_N),$$

are different from zero and

$$-\mathrm{sgn}[\psi(x_i) - \varphi(x_i)] = \mathrm{sgn}[\psi(x_{i+1}) - \varphi(x_{i+1})], \quad i = 1, 2, \ldots, N.$$

This means that $\psi - \varphi$ has at least $N - 1 = m + n + 1 - d$ zeros in (a, b), which is impossible because the numerator of the rational function $\psi - \varphi$ is a polynomial of degree at most $N - 2$. □

The Chebyshev Theorem 25.3 remains valid for the approximation by rational functions. The importance of the next theorem is the full characterization of the rational function of the best uniform approximation for a given continuous function and therefore the possibility for numerical calculation.

THEOREM 28.2. *Let $\varphi \in L_{mn}$ have the form*

$$\varphi(x) = w(x) \sum_{i=0}^{m-\mu} a_i x^i \bigg/ \sum_{i=0}^{n-\nu} b_i x^i,$$

$$0 \leq \mu \leq m, \; 0 \leq \nu \leq n, \; d = \min\{\mu, \nu\}, \; b_0 \neq 0$$

and the polynomials $A(x) = \sum_{i=0}^{m-\mu} a_i x^i$, $B(x) = \sum_{i=0}^{n-\nu} b_i x^i$ be irreducible. A necessary and sufficient condition for the continuous function f in the interval $[a, b]$ and the rational function φ to satisfy

$$E_{mn}(f) = \inf_{\psi \in L_{mn}} \max_{a \leq x \leq b} |f(x) - \psi(x)| = \inf_{\psi \in L_{mn}} \|f - \psi\| = \|f - \varphi\|$$

is the existence of points $a \leq x_1 < x_2 < \cdots < x_N \leq b$, $N = m + n - d + 2$, such that

$$f(x_i) - \varphi(x_i) = \varepsilon(-1)^i \|f - \varphi\|, \quad i = 1, 2, \ldots, N, \; \varepsilon = \pm 1.$$

If $\varphi \equiv 0$ then $N \geq m + 2$.

PROOF. The *sufficiency* follows from Theorem 28.1.

Necessity. Let us assume that the rational function $\varphi \in L_{mn}$ satisfies $E_{mn}(f) = \|f - \varphi\|$ but the maximal number of points of alternation is $N' < m + n - d + 2$ (if $\varphi \equiv 0$ then $d = n$).

Then there exist N' subintervals

$$[a, \xi_1], [\xi_1, \xi_2], \ldots, [\xi_{N'-1}, b]$$

and a number $\alpha > 0$, such that: either

$$-\|f - \varphi\| \leq f(x) - \varphi(x) < \|f - \varphi\| - \alpha$$

or

$$-\|f - \varphi\| + \alpha < f(x) - \varphi(x) \leq \|f - \varphi\|$$

for $x \in [\xi_i, \xi_{i+1}]$. Let $\Phi(x) = (x - \xi_1)(x - \xi_2) \cdots (x - \xi_{N'-1})$. Since the polynomials A and B are irreducible there exist polynomials φ_{1n} and ψ_{1m} of degree n and m, respectively, for which $\Phi = B\psi_{1m} - A\varphi_{1n}$. Let the function $\psi \in L_{mn}$ be defined as $\psi = w(A\Omega - \omega\psi_{1m})/(B\Omega - \omega\varphi_{1n})$, where Ω is a polynomial of degree at most d (positive on $[a, b]$, $\Omega(x) = 1$) and ω is a real number. Then $f - \psi = f - \varphi + \omega w\Phi/(B^2\Omega - \omega B\varphi_{1n})$. The function $\omega w\Phi$ changes its sign at the points $\{\xi_i\}_{i=1}^{N'-1}$ and the polynomial $B^2\Omega - \omega B\varphi_{1n}$ is positive on $[a, b]$ for small enough $|\omega|$. So the number ω can be chosen in such a way that the function $\omega w\Phi/(B^2\Omega - \omega B\varphi_{1n})$ has the opposite sign to the function $f - \varphi$ in every subinterval

$$[a, \xi_1], [\xi_1, \xi_2], \ldots, [\xi_{N'-1}, b].$$

Hence, $\|f - \psi\| < \|f - \varphi\|$, which contradicts $E_{mn}(f) = \|f - \varphi\|$. □

If the interval $[a, b]$ is infinite, e.g., $a = -\infty$ or/and $b = \infty$ then Theorem 28.2 holds under some natural restrictions on the degrees of the numerator and denominator and on the weight function. For details see AHIEZER ([1965], Chapter 2). For example, in $(-\infty, \infty)$, if

$$\lim_{x \to -\infty} f(x) = \lim_{x \to \infty} f(x)$$

then

$$n - m = k \geq 0, \quad \nu \geq \mu, \quad \lim_{x \to -\infty} \omega(x)x^k = \lim_{x \to \infty} \omega(x)x^k.$$

The above theorem allows us to prove the uniqueness of the rational function of the best uniform approximation. Let us suppose the contrary that for the continuous function f there exist two functions $\varphi \in L_{mn}$ and $\psi \in L_{mn}$ of the best uniform approximation; i.e. $E_{mn}(f) = \|f - \varphi\| = \|f - \psi\|$. Let the numbers N', μ', ν', d' have the same meaning according to the function ψ as the numbers N, μ, ν, d for the function φ in Theorem 28.5. Let $N' \geq N$, where $N' \geq m + n + 2 - d'$, $N \geq m + n + 2 - d$. Let the points of alternation for the function ψ be $\beta_1, \beta_2, \ldots, \beta_{N'}$. From

$$\varphi(\beta_i) - \psi(\beta_i) = \varphi(\beta_i) - f(\beta_i) + f(\beta_i) - \psi(\beta_i),$$

it follows that

$$\mathrm{sgn}[f(\beta_i) - \psi(\beta_i)] = \mathrm{sgn}[\varphi(\beta_i) - \psi(\beta_i)].$$

Let, for example,

$$\varphi(\beta_{i-1}) - \psi(\beta_{i-1}) \neq 0, \quad \varphi(\beta_i) - \psi(\beta_i) = \cdots = \varphi(\beta_{i+k}) - \psi(\beta_{i+k}) = 0,$$
$$\varphi(\beta_{i+k+1}) - \psi(\beta_{i+k+1}) \neq 0,$$

then the numbers

$$(-1)^{i-1}[f(\beta_{i-1}) - \psi(\beta_{i-1})], \quad (-1)^{i+k+1}[f(\beta_{i+k+1}) - \psi(\beta_{i+k+1})]$$

have the same sign and this is also true for the numbers

$$\varphi(\beta_{i-1}) - \psi(\beta_{i-1}), \quad (-1)^k(\varphi(\beta_{i+k+1}) - \psi(\beta_{i+k+1})).$$

So the function $\varphi - \psi$ has at least $k + 2$ zeros in $[\beta_{i-1}, \beta_{i+k+1}]$.

The above considerations show that the function $\varphi - \psi$ has at least $N' - 1$ zeros in (a, b). This is impossible because the degree k of the numerator of the rational function $\varphi - \psi$ is less than $N' - 2$. Indeed,

$$k = \begin{cases} \max\{m + n - \mu' - \nu, m + n - \mu - \nu'\} \leq N' - 2, & \text{if } \varphi \neq 0, \psi \neq 0, \\ m - \mu' \leq N' - 2, & \text{if } \varphi \equiv 0, \\ m - \mu \leq N - 2 \leq N' - 2, & \text{if } \psi \equiv 0. \end{cases}$$

29. The possibility for approximation of continuous functions

Let $C(K)$ be the set of all continuous functions on the compact K and let A be a set of functions defined on K.

From a numerical point of view it is important that the set A be such as to ensure for every function $f \in C(K)$ and any positive number $\varepsilon > 0$ the existence of a function $g \in A$ for which $\sup_{x \in K} |f(x) - g(x)| < \varepsilon$; i.e. the function f can be approximated arbitrarily "well" in a uniform metric by elements of A.

In the case $K = [a, b]$ and

$$A = \left\{ f: f(x) = \sum_{k=0}^{n} a_k x^k, n = 0, 1, \ldots, a_k \text{ real numbers} \right\}$$

WEIERSTRASS [1885] proved the following theorem.

THEOREM 29.1. *For every continuous function f on $[a, b]$ and for any $\varepsilon > 0$ there exists an algebraic polynomial P such that*

$$\max_{x \in [a,b]} |f(x) - P(x)| < \varepsilon.$$

Of course the degree of the polynomial P depends on the function f, on the interval $[a, b]$ and on the number ε.

There exist many proofs of Theorem 29.1—see PICARD [1891], VOLTERRA [1897], LERCH [1903], RUNGE [1885a,b], LEBESQUE [1898], MITTAG-LEFFLER [1900], and BERNSTEIN [1912].

One proof of Theorem 29.1 is the inequality (31.5).

MÜNTZ [1914] generalized Theorem 29.1 as follows.

THEOREM 29.2. *For every continuous function f on the interval $[a, b]$ and for any $\varepsilon > 0$ there exists a function $g \in M$,*

$$M = \left\{ \varphi: \varphi(x) = \sum_{i=0}^{\infty} a_i x^{\lambda_i}, 0 = \lambda_0 < \lambda_1 < \cdots < \lambda_n < \cdots, \sum_{i=0}^{\infty} \frac{1}{\lambda_i} = \infty \right\},$$

such that $\max_{x \in [a,b]} |f(x) - g(x)| < \varepsilon$.

MERGELIAN [1951] completed the complex case by the next theorem.

THEOREM 29.3. *Let E be a closed bounded set on the plane and E does not divide the plane. If the function f is continuous on E and analytic in the interior of E, then for any $\varepsilon > 0$ there exists a polynomial P such that $\max_{z \in E} |f(z) - P(z)| < \varepsilon$.*

A very important generalization of the Weierstrass theorem was given by STOUN [1937, 1948].

Following DZJADIK ([1977], p. 105), the set of functions A is called a *Stoun algebra* on the point set S if:
  (a) if $\varphi \in A$ then $c\varphi \in A$ for any complex number c;
  (b) if $\varphi \in A$ and $\phi \in A$, then $\varphi + \phi \in A$, $\varphi\phi \in A$;
  (c) for every point $x_1 \in S$, $x_2 \in S$ there exists a function $\varphi \in A$ such that $\varphi(x_1) \neq \varphi(x_2)$;
  (d) for every point $x \in S$ there exists a function $\varphi \in A$ for which $\varphi(x) \neq 0$.

THEOREM 29.4. *Let A be a Stoun algebra on the compact K. Then for every continuous function f defined on K and any positive number $\varepsilon > 0$ there exists a function $\varphi \in A$ such that*

$$\sup_{x \in K} |f(x) - \varphi(x)| < \varepsilon \, .$$

The following are examples of Stoun algebras:

(1) $\quad A = \left\{ \varphi \colon \varphi(x) = a_0 + \sum_{i=1}^{\infty} (a_i \cos ix + b_i \sin ix) \right\}$

and $S = [a, b)$, where $b - a \leq 2\pi$. If $b - a > 2\pi$ then the condition (c) is not fulfilled;

(2) $\quad A = \left\{ \varphi \colon \varphi(x_1, x_2, \ldots, x_n) = \sum_{k_1 + k_2 + \cdots + k_n \leq \infty} a_{k_1 k_2 \cdots k_n} x_1^{k_1} x_2^{k_2} \cdots x_n^{k_n} \right\}$

and S is a bounded subspace of the n-dimensional Euclidean space;

(3) $\quad A = \left\{ \varphi \colon \varphi(x) = \sum_{i=0}^{n} a_i x^i \Big/ \sum_{i=0}^{m} b_i x^i \right\}$

and $S = [a, b]$.

The proof of the Stoun theorem and some other related topics can be found in LAURENT ([1972], Chapter 3.1), TIMAN ([1960], Chapter 1), and DZJADIK ([1977], Chapter 2).

30. Moduli of functions

To estimate the error of numerical methods sometimes it is convenient to use so-called moduli of considered functions which are characteristics closely connected with the properties of the functions.

30.1. Moduli of smoothness

Let the function f be defined in the interval $[a, b]$. Then the modulus of smoothness of order k is the following function of $\delta \in [0, (b-a)/k]$

$$\omega_k(f; \delta) = \sup\{|\Delta_h^k f(x)|: |h| \leq \delta, x, x + kh \in [a, b]\}, \tag{30.1}$$

where

$$\Delta_h^k f(x) = \sum_{i=0}^{k} (-1)^{k+i} \binom{k}{i} f(x + ih).$$

The basic properties of $\omega_k(f; \delta)$ are the following.
 (a) $\omega_k(f; \delta') \leq \omega_k(f; \delta'')$ for $\delta' \leq \delta''$.
 (b) $\omega_k(f + g; \delta) \leq \omega_k(f; \delta) + \omega_k(g; \delta)$.
 (c) $\omega_k(f; \delta) \leq 2\omega_{k-1}(f; \delta)$.
This property follows from $\Delta_h^k f(x) = \Delta_h^{k-1} f(x+h) - \Delta_h^{k-1} f(x)$.
 (d) $\omega_k(f; \delta) \leq \delta \omega_{k-1}(f'; \delta)$.
This property holds for absolutely continuous functions with bounded first derivatives. Indeed for $|h| \leq \delta$ the following relations are fulfilled:

$$|\Delta_h^k f(x)| = |\Delta_h^{k-1}[f(x+h) - f(x)]| = \left|\Delta_h^{k-1} \int_0^h f'(x+t)\,dt\right|$$

$$= \left|\int_0^h \Delta_h^{k-1} f'(x+t)\,dt\right| \leq \int_{\min(0,h)}^{\max(0,h)} |\Delta_h^{k-1} f'(x+t)|\,dt$$

$$\leq \int_{\min(0,h)}^{\max(0,h)} \omega_{k-1}(f'; \delta)\,dt \leq \delta \omega_{k-1}(f'; \delta)$$

and therefore

$$\omega_k(f; \delta) = \sup\{|\Delta_h^k f(x)|: |h| \leq \delta, x, x + kh \in [a, b]\} \leq \delta \omega_{k-1}(f'; \delta).$$

 (e) $\omega_k(f; n\delta) \leq n^k \omega_k(f; \delta)$, n is a natural number.
The proof follows from the identity

$$\Delta_{nh}^k f(x) = \sum_{i_1=0}^{n-1} \sum_{i_2=0}^{n-1} \cdots \sum_{i_k=0}^{n-1} \Delta_h^k f(x + i_1 h + i_2 h + \cdots + i_k h), \tag{30.2}$$

which can be proved by induction on k. Really, for $k = 1$,

$$\Delta_{nh} f(x) = f(x + nh) - f(x) = \sum_{i=0}^{n-1} \Delta_h f(x + ih).$$

Let (30.2) be true for some k. Then

$$\Delta_{nh}^{k+1} f(x) = \Delta_{nh}^k [f(x + nh) - f(x)] = \Delta_{nh}^k [\Delta_{nh} f(x)]$$

$$= \sum_{i_1=0}^{n-1} \sum_{i_2=0}^{n-1} \cdots \sum_{i_k=0}^{n-1} \Delta_h^k [\Delta_{nh} f(x + i_1 h + i_2 h + \cdots + i_k h)]$$

$$= \sum_{i_1=0}^{n-1} \sum_{i_2=0}^{n-1} \cdots \sum_{i_k=0}^{n-1} \Delta_h^k \left[\sum_{i_{k+1}=0}^{n-1} \Delta_h f(x + i_1 h + i_2 h + \cdots + i_k h + i_{k+1} h) \right]$$

$$= \sum_{i_1=0}^{n-1} \sum_{i_2=0}^{n-1} \cdots \sum_{i_{k+1}=0}^{n-1} \Delta_h^{k+1} f(x + i_1 h + i_2 h + \cdots + i_{k+1} h)$$

and for $|h| \leq \delta$ it follows that

$$|\Delta_{nh}^k f(x)| = \sum_{i_1=0}^{n-1} \sum_{i_2=0}^{n-1} \cdots \sum_{i_k=0}^{n-1} |\Delta_h^k f(x + i_1 h + i_2 h + \cdots + i_k h)| \leq n^k \omega_k(f; \delta).$$

(f) $\omega_k(f; \lambda \delta) \leq (\lambda + 1)^k \omega_k(f; \delta)$, $\lambda > 0$.
The proof follows from $\omega_k(f; \lambda \delta) \leq \omega_k(f; [\lambda + 1]\delta) \leq (\lambda + 1)^k \omega_k(f; \delta)$.
(g) $\omega(f; \delta) = \omega_1(f; \delta) \leq \delta \|f'\|_{C_{[a,b]}}$.
Indeed, for $f' \in C_{[a,b]}$ the proof follows from

$$|f(x + h) - f(x)| = \left| \int_x^{x+h} f'(t) \, dt \right| \leq |h| \, \|f'\|_{C_{[a,b]}};$$

(h) $\omega_k(f; \delta) \leq \delta^k \|f^{(k)}\|_{C_{[a,b]}}$.

30.2. Integral moduli

Let $f \in L_p[a, b]$, $1 \leq p \leq \infty$. The integral modulus of order k of the function f is the following function of $\delta \in [0, (b-a)/k]$

$$\omega_k(f; \delta)_{L_p} = \sup_{0 \leq h \leq \delta} \left(\int_a^{b-kh} |\Delta_h^k f(x)|^p \, dx \right)^{1/p}.$$

All the properties (a)–(h) of the moduli of smoothness from this section are also valid for the integral moduli substituting $\|f\|_C$ by $\|f\|_{L_p}$ everywhere. An important additional property is

$$\omega_1(f; \delta)_{L_1} = \omega(f; \delta)_L \leq \delta \bigvee_a^b f.$$

Indeed,

$$\int_a^{b-h} |f(x+h) - f(x)| \, dx \leq \int_a^{b-h} \bigvee_x^{x+h} f \, dx = \int_a^{b-h} \left(\bigvee_a^{x+h} f - \bigvee_a^x f \right) dx$$

$$= \int_{a+h}^b \bigvee_a^x f \, dx - \int_a^{b-h} \bigvee_a^x f \, dx \leq \int_{b-h}^b \bigvee_a^x f \, dx \leq h \bigvee_a^b f.$$

30.3. Averaged moduli

The local modulus of smoothness of the function f of order k at a point $x \in [a, b]$ is the following function of $\delta \in [0, (b-a)/k]$:

$$\omega_k(f, x; \delta) = \sup\{|\Delta_h^k f(t)|: t, t + kh \in [x - k\delta/2, x + k\delta/2] \cap [a, b]\}. \tag{30.3}$$

Obviously $\omega_k(f; \delta) = \|\omega_k(f, \cdot; \delta)\|_C$.

The averaged modulus of smoothness of order k (or τ-modulus) of the function $f \in M_{[a,b]}$ ($|f| \le M$) is the following function of $\delta \in [0, (b-a)/k]$:

$$\tau_k(f; \delta)_{L_p} = \|\omega_k(f, \cdot; \delta)\|_{L_p} = \left(\int_a^b (\omega_k(f, x; \delta))^p \, dx\right)^{1/p}, \quad 1 \le p \le \infty.$$

The τ modulus can be defined for $k = 1$ as (see also DOLZENKO and SEVASTJANOV [1976])

$$\tau_1(f; \delta)_{L_p} = \tau(f; \delta)_{L_p} = \|S(f, \delta; \cdot) - I(f, \delta; \cdot)\|_{L_p},$$

where

$$S(f, \delta; x) = \sup\{f(t): t \in [x - \delta/2, x + \delta/2] \cap [a, b]\},$$
$$I(f, \delta; x) = \inf\{f(t): t \in [x - \delta/2, x + \delta/2] \cap [a, b]\}.$$

For the first time moduli of such a type in a function space with arbitrary metric r were defined by SENDOV [1967] and KOROVKIN [1969] in the following way:

$$\tau(f; \delta)_r = r(S(f, \delta), I(f, \delta)).$$

The main properties of the averaged moduli of smoothness are (see SENDOV and POPOV [1988], p. 7) the following.
(a) $\tau_k(f; \delta')_{L_p} \le \tau_k(f; \delta'')_{L_p}$ for $\delta' \le \delta''$.
(b) $\tau_k(f + g; \delta)_{L_p} \le \tau_k(f; \delta)_{L_p} + \tau_k(g; \delta)_{L_p}$.
(c) $\tau_k(f; \delta)_{L_p} \le 2\tau_{k-1}\left(f; \dfrac{k}{k-1}\delta\right)_{L_p}$.
(d) $\tau_k(f; \delta)_{L_p} \le \delta\tau_{k-1}\left(f'; \dfrac{k}{k-1}\delta\right)_{L_p}$.

PROOF. From

$$|\Delta_h^k f(t)| = \left|\Delta_h^{k-1} \int_0^h f'(t+u) \, du\right|$$

it follows that
$$\sup\{|\Delta_h^k f(t)|: t, t+kh \in [x - k\delta/2, x + k\delta/2] \cap [a, b]\}$$
$$\leq \sup\left\{\left|\Delta_h^{k-1}\int_0^h f'(t+u)\,du\right|: t, t+kh \in [x - k\delta/2, x + k\delta/2] \cap [a, b]\right\}.$$

If $t, t + kh \in [x - k\delta/2, x + k\delta/2] \cap [a, b]$ and $h > 0$, then
$$t + u, t + u + (k-1)h \in [x - k\delta/2, x + k\delta/2] \cap [a, b],$$
and therefore
$$|\Delta_h^{k-1} f'(t+u)| \leq \omega_{k-1}\left(f', x; \frac{k}{k-1}\delta\right).$$

The last equality leads to
$$\omega_k(f, x; \delta) \leq \delta \omega_{k-1}\left(f', x; \frac{k}{k-1}\delta\right)$$
and taking the L_p norm of both sides the property is proved. $\square$

(e) $\tau_k(f; n\delta)_{L_p} \leq (2n)^{k+1} \tau_k(f; \delta)_{L_p}$, where n is a natural number.

PROOF. From (30.2) it follows that
$$\Delta_{nh}^k f(x) = \sum_{i=0}^{(n-1)k} A_i^{n,k} \Delta_h^k f(t+ih), \qquad (30.4)$$

where $A_i^{n,k} > 0$ are defined by
$$(1 + t + \cdots + t^{n-1})^k = \sum_{i=0}^{(n-1)k} A_i^{n,k} t^i.$$

This gives
$$\sum_{i=0}^{(n-1)k} A_i^{n,k} = n^k \qquad (30.5)$$

and using (30.3), (30.4) it follows that
$$|\Delta_{2nh}^k f(t)| \leq \sum_{i=0}^{(2n-1)k} A_i^{2n,k} |\Delta_h^k f(t+ih)|.$$

If $t, t + 2nkh \in [x - kn\delta/2, x + kn\delta/2] \cap [a, b]$, then
$$t + ih, t + ih + kh \in [x - kn\delta/2 + (j-1)k\delta/2, x - kn\delta/2 + (j+1)k\delta/2]$$
for some $j = 1, 2, \ldots, 2n - 1$. Therefore,
$$|\Delta_{2nh}^k f(t)| \leq \sum_{i=0}^{(2n-1)k} A_i^{2n,k} \sum_{j=1}^{2n-1}{}' \omega_k(f, x - (n-j)k\delta/2; \delta)$$

or

$$\omega_k(f, x; n\delta) \leq \sum_{i=0}^{(2n-1)k} A_i^{2n,k} \sideset{}{'}\sum_{j=1}^{2n-1} \omega_k(f, x - (n-j)k\delta/2; \delta),$$

where the second sum Σ' contains only the terms for which

$$x - (n-j)k\delta/2 \in [a, b].$$

Taking the L_p-norm of both sides of the last equality and using (30.5) it follows that

$$\tau_k(f; n\delta)_{L_p} \leq (2n)^k (2n-1) \tau_k(f; \delta)_{L_p}. \qquad \square$$

(f) $\tau_k(f; \lambda\delta)_{L_p} \leq [2(\lambda + 1)]^{k+1} \tau_k(f; \delta)_{L_p}$, $\lambda > 0$.
(g) $\tau(f; \delta)_{L_p} = \tau_1(f; \delta)_{L_p} \leq \delta \|f'\|_{L_p}$.

PROOF. Extending f outside the interval $[a, b]$, setting

$$f(x) = f(a) \quad \text{for } x < a \quad \text{and} \quad f(x) = f(b) \quad \text{for } x > b,$$

it follows that

$$\omega(f, x; \delta) = \sup\{|f(t') - f(t'')| : t', t'' \in [x - \delta/2, x + \delta/2]\}$$

$$\leq \sup\left\{ \left| \int_{t'}^{t''} f'(t)\,dt \right| : t', t'' \in [x - \delta/2, x + \delta/2] \right\}$$

$$\leq \int_{x-\delta/2}^{x+\delta/2} |f'(t)|\,dt = \int_{-\delta/2}^{\delta/2} |f'(x+t)|\,dt.$$

The property follows taking the L_p-norm; i.e.

$$\tau(f; \delta)_{L_p} = \|\omega(f, \cdot; \delta)\|_{L_p}$$

$$\leq \int_{\delta/2}^{\delta/2} \|f'(\cdot + t)\|_{L_p}\,dt = \delta\|f'\|_{L_p}. \qquad \square$$

(h) $\tau_k(f; \delta)_{L_p} \leq c(k)\delta^k \|f^{(k)}\|_{L_p}$.
(i) $\tau_1(f; \delta)_{L_1} = \tau(f; \delta)_L \leq \delta \overset{b}{\underset{a}{V}} f$.

PROOF. Let $f(x) = f(a)$ for $x < a$ and $f(x) = f(b)$ for $x > b$. Then

$$\omega(f, x; \delta) \leq \overset{x+\delta/2}{\underset{x-\delta/2}{V}} f$$

and therefore

$$\tau(f;\delta)_L \leq \int_a^b \bigvee_{x-\delta/2}^{x+\delta/2} f \, dx = \int_a^b \bigvee_{a-\delta/2}^{x+\delta/2} f \, dx - \int_a^b \bigvee_{a-\delta/2}^{x-\delta/2} f \, dx$$

$$= \int_{a+\delta/2}^{b+\delta/2} \bigvee_{a-\delta/2}^{t} f \, dt - \int_{a-\delta/2}^{b-\delta/2} \bigvee_{a-\delta/2}^{t} f \, dt$$

$$= \int_{a-\delta/2}^{b+\delta/2} \bigvee_{a-\delta/2}^{t} f \, dt - \int_{a-\delta/2}^{a+\delta/2} \bigvee_{a-\delta/2}^{t} f \, dt$$

$$\leq \int_{b-\delta/2}^{b+\delta/2} \bigvee_a^b f \, dt = \delta \bigvee_a^b f. \qquad \square$$

(j) A necessary and sufficient condition for the function f to be Riemann integrable is $\lim_{\delta \to +0} \tau(f;\delta)_L = 0$. The proof follows from

$$\tau(f;\delta)_L = \|S(f,\delta;\cdot) - I(f,\delta;\cdot)\|_L.$$

(k) $\omega_k(f;\delta)_{L_p} \leq \tau_k(f;\delta)_{L_p} \leq \omega_k(f;\delta)(b-a)^{1/p}$.

(l) If the function f is an absolutely continuous function on the interval $[a,b]$, then $\tau_k(f;\delta)_{L_p} \leq c(k)\delta\omega_{k-1}(f';\delta)_{L_p}$, $k \geq 2$.

This property is the Theorem 1.5 in SENDOV and POPOV [1988].

31. Approximation of functions by means of linear operators

Let A and B be two sets of functions. A mapping L is called an operator defined in A with values in B if $L(f) \in B$ for every $f \in A$.

The operator L is linear if $L(\alpha f + \beta g) = \alpha L(f) + \beta L(g)$, where $f, g \in A$ and α, β are numbers.

If the sets A and B are sets of functions defined, respectively, in $D(A)$ and $D(B)$, then the operator L is positive if for every $y \in D(B)$ and $x \in D(A)$ from $f(x) \geq 0$ it follows that $L(f;y) \geq 0$.

For example, let A, B be sets of bounded functions in the interval $[0,1]$; i.e. $D(A) = D(B) = [0,1]$. The Bernstein polynomial

$$B_n(f;x) = \sum_{i=0}^n \binom{n}{i} f\left(\frac{i}{n}\right) x^i (1-x)^{n-i} \qquad (31.1)$$

is a linear positive operator.

The linear operators play an important role as an explicit instrument for the approximation of the functions in different functional spaces and metrics.

The next theorem is due to KOROVKIN [1959] and MAMEDOV [1959].

THEOREM 31.1. *Let L be linear positive operator in the space $C_{[a,b]}$; i.e. $L: C_{[a,b]} \to C_{[a,b]}$, and*

$$L(1; x) = 1, \quad L(t; x) = t + \alpha(x), \quad L(t^2; x) = t^2 + \beta(x). \tag{31.2}$$

Then for every function $f \in C_{[a,b]}$ it is fulfilled that

$$\|L(f; \cdot) - f\|_{C_{[a,b]}} \leq 2\omega(f; \sqrt{d}), \tag{31.3}$$

where $d = \|\beta(x) - 2x\alpha(x)\|_{C_{[a,b]}}$.

PROOF. Let $x \in [a, b]$ be a fixed point and $t \in [a, b]$. For $\delta > 0$, using the properties of $\omega(f; \delta)$ and the inequality $2a \leq a^2 + 1$ it follows that

$$|f(t) - f(x)| \leq \omega(f; |t - x|) = \omega(f; \delta(|t - x|/\delta)) \leq (|t - x|/\delta + 1)\omega(f; \delta)$$
$$\leq [\{[(t - x)/\delta]^2 + 1\}/2 + 1]\omega(f; \delta)$$
$$= [\{[(t - x)/\delta]^2 + 3\}/2]\omega(f; \delta),$$

i.e.

$$-\{[(t - x)^2/\delta^2 + 3]/2\}\omega(f; \delta) \leq f(t) - f(x) \leq \{[(t - x)^2/\delta^2 + 3]/2\}\omega(f; \delta).$$

Applying the operator L to the last inequality according to the variable t the result is

$$-\tfrac{1}{2}\omega(f; \delta)(L((t - x)^2; x)/\delta^2 + 3) \leq L(f; x) - f(x)$$
$$\leq \tfrac{1}{2}\omega(f; \delta)(L((t - x)^2; x)/\delta^2 + 3). \tag{31.4}$$

By (31.2) it follows that

$$L((t - x)^2; x) = \beta(x) - 2x\alpha(x) \geq 0,$$

and setting $\delta = [\beta(x) - 2x\alpha(x)]^{1/2}$, the inequalities (31.4) give

$$|L(f; x) - f(x)| \leq 2\omega(f; \sqrt{\beta(x) - 2x\alpha(x)}). \quad \square$$

In the 2π-periodic case the estimation of the type (31.3) in terms of the numbers

$$\|L_n(f_i) - f_i\|_{C[0, 2\pi)}, \quad i = 1, 2, 3,$$
$$f_1(x) = 1, \quad f_2(x) = \sin x, \quad f_3(x) = \cos x,$$

is given by SHISHA and MOND [1968].

The Bernstein polynomial (31.1) satisfies

$$B_n(1; x) = 1, \quad B_n(t; x) = x, \quad B_n(t^2; x) = x^2 + x(1 - x)/n$$

and direct application of the Theorem 31.1, taking into account the fact that $x(1 - x) \leq \tfrac{1}{4}$, gives for every function $f \in C_{[0,1]}$ the result of POPOVICIU [1934]:

$$\|B_n(f; \cdot) - f\|_{C_{[0,1]}} \leq 2\omega(f; 1/2\sqrt{n}). \tag{31.5}$$

Let $K \subseteq \mathbb{R}^m$ be a compact subset of the m-dimensional Euclidean space $\mathbb{R}^m$ and $C(K)$ be the space of all continuous functions on K. VOLKOV [1957] has shown that the following $m+2$ functions are test functions for $C(K)$ (compare with the functions 1, x and x^2 in the one-dimensional case):

$$f_{0m}(x_1, x_2, \ldots, x_m) = 1;$$
$$f_{jm}(x_1, x_2, \ldots, x_m) = x_j, \quad j = 1, 2, \ldots, m;$$
$$f_{m+1,m}(x_1, x_2, \ldots, x_m) = x_1^2 + x_2^2 + \cdots + x_m^2.$$

In the periodic case when $f(x_1, x_2, \ldots, x_m)$ is 2π-periodic in each variable MOROZOV [1958] shows that the test functions are

$$f_{0m}(x_1, x_2, \ldots, x_m) = 1;$$
$$f_{jm}(x_1, x_2, \ldots, x_m) = \sin x_j, \quad j = 1, 2, \ldots, m;$$
$$f_{m+j,m}(x_1, x_2, \ldots, x_m) = \cos x_j, \quad j = 1, 2, \ldots, m.$$

If $\{L_i\}_{i=1}^{\infty}$ are linear positive operators defined on $C(K)$ and $L_n(1) = 1$, $n = 1, 2, \ldots$, then for every $f \in C(K)$ the following inequality is fulfilled

$$\|L_n(f) - f\|_{C(K)} \leq 2\omega(f; \mu_n),$$

where

$$\mu_n = \left\| L_n\left(\sum_{i=1}^{m} (\xi_i - x_i)^2; (x_1, x_2, \ldots, x_m) \right) \right\|_{C(K)}^{1/2},$$

$$\omega(f; \delta) = \max_{x, y \in K, \, d(x,y) \leq \delta} |f(x) - f(y)|, \quad d(x, y) = \left(\sum_{i=1}^{m} (x_i - y_i)^2 \right)^{1/2}.$$

32. Whitney's theorem

WHITNEY [1957] proved the following basic theorem in the approximation theory and numerical analysis.

THEOREM 32.1. *For each integer $n \geq 1$, there is a number W_n with the following property: for any interval $\Delta = [a, b]$ and for any continuous function f on Δ there exists a polynomial P of degree at most $n - 1$ such that*

$$|f(x) - P(x)| \leq W_n \omega_n(f; b - a) \quad \text{for } x \in \Delta. \tag{32.1}$$

The problem for the size of the constant W_n, which is called Whitney's constant, plays an important role for obtaining a more accurate estimation in different numerical methods. For a finite interval the constant W_n does not depend on its length and, furthermore, $\Delta = [0, 1]$. Whitney proved (32.1) using the Lagrange interpolation polynomial P that satisfies

$$P\left(\frac{i}{n-1}\right) = f\left(\frac{i}{n-1}\right), \quad i = 0, 1, \ldots, n-1.$$

The polynomial P satisfies (32.1) with some other constants. Let us denote them by W'_n. For the polynomial that interpolates at the points $i/(n+1)$, $i = 1, 2, \ldots, n$, let the constants be W''_n. Of course,

$$W_n \leq W'_n, \quad W_n \leq W''_n, \quad n = 1, 2, \ldots.$$

WHITNEY [1959] has shown that Theorem 32.1 is also valid for bounded functions and IVANOV [1980] proved this for Lebesque-integrable functions defined at each point.

WHITNEY [1957] and later, on the basis of linear programming, SENDOV [1982] estimated some constants of low order:

$$W_1 = W_2 = \tfrac{1}{2}, \quad W'_1 = W'_2 = 1,$$

$$\tfrac{8}{15} \leq W_3 \leq \tfrac{7}{10}, \quad \tfrac{1}{2} \leq W_4 \leq 3.2425, \quad \tfrac{1}{2} \leq W_5 \leq 10.4,$$

$$\tfrac{16}{15} \leq W'_3 \leq \tfrac{14}{9}, \quad 1 \leq W'_4 \leq 3.29525, \quad 1 \leq W'_5 \leq 10.4,$$

$$W_4 \leq 1.26, \quad W_5 \leq 1.31, \quad W_6 \leq 1.67,$$

$$W'_4 \leq 2.85, \quad W'_5 \leq 3.46, \quad W'_6 \leq 5.36.$$

Nevertheless, despite the pessimistic first estimation of W_n (BRUDNII [1970], SENDOV [1982]) that

$$W'_n \leq (n+1)n^n,$$

SENDOV [1982] conjectured that for all n:

$$W_n \leq 1, \quad W'_n \leq 2.$$

IVANOV and TAKEV [1985] showed that $W_n \leq O(n \ln n)$, and BINEV [1985] gave $W_n \leq O(n)$.

THEOREM 32.2 (SENDOV [1987]). *For any function f integrable on $[0, 1]$ and for each integer $n \geq 1$ there is a polynomial P of degree $n - 1$ such that*

$$|f(x) - P(x)| \leq 6\omega_n\left(f; \frac{1}{n+1}\right) \quad \text{for } x \in [0, 1].$$

The polynomial P can be the polynomial that interpolates f at the points $i/(n+1)$, $i = 1, 2, \ldots, n$; i.e. $W_n \leq W''_n \leq 6$, $n = 1, 2, \ldots$.

The proof of the Theorem 32.2 will be divided into five theorems.

THEOREM 32.2a. *If f is defined for every $x \in [0, 1]$ and is integrable on $[0, 1]$, then for each integer $n \geq 1$ the following relation is fulfilled*

$$f(x) = P_{n-1}(x) + \varphi_n(f; x) + \sum_{j=0}^{n} \frac{1}{h} \int_0^t \varphi_n(f; jh + v) L'_{n,j}\left(\frac{x-v}{h}\right) dv,$$

where $h = 1/(n+1)$, $x = vh + t$, $0 \leq t < h$,

$$\varphi_n(f; x) = \varphi_n(f; \nu h + t) = \frac{(-1)^{(n-\nu)}}{h\binom{n}{\nu}} \int_0^h \Delta_y^n f(x - \nu y) \, dy ,$$

and

$$L_{n,\nu}(x) = \prod_{j=0, j \neq \nu}^{n} \frac{x - j}{\nu - j}$$

are the basic Lagrange polynomials for interpolation at $0, 1, \ldots, n$.

PROOF. If $x \in [\nu h, (\nu - 1)h]$ then

$$\varphi_n(f; x) = f(x) + \frac{(-1)^{(n-\nu)}}{h\binom{n}{\nu}} \int_0^h \sum_{j=0, j \neq \nu}^{n} (-1)^{n-j} \binom{n}{j} f[x + (j - \nu)v] \, dv$$

$$= f(x) + \frac{(-1)^{\nu}}{h\binom{n}{\nu}} \sum_{j=0, j \neq \nu}^{n} \frac{(-1)^j}{j - \nu} \binom{n}{j} \int_{\nu h + t}^{jh + t} f(v) \, dv . \quad (32.2)$$

Let us define the functions

$$y_j(t) = \int_0^{jh + t} f(v) \, dv, \quad 0 \leq t \leq h, \; j = 0, 1, \ldots, n .$$

Then (32.2) may be written as a system of linear non-homogeneous differential equations

$$y'_\nu(t) = \frac{(-1)^{\nu - 1}}{h\binom{n}{\nu}} \sum_{j=0, j \neq \nu}^{n} \frac{(-1)^j}{j - \nu} \binom{n}{j} (y_j(t) - y_\nu(t)) + \varphi_n(f; \nu h + t) ,$$

$$\nu = 0, 1, \ldots, n .$$

The general solution of the homogeneous part of the above system is

$$y_\nu(t) = \sum_{s=0}^{n} C_s (\nu h + t)^s, \quad \nu = 0, 1, \ldots, n ,$$

where C_s are arbitrary constants. Indeed, for every s the function $(\nu h + t)^s$ satisfies

$$\frac{(-1)^{\nu - 1}}{h\binom{n}{\nu}} \sum_{j=0, j \neq \nu}^{n} \frac{(-1)^j}{j - \nu} \binom{n}{j} ((jh + t)^s - (\nu h + t)^s)$$

$$= \frac{(-1)^{\nu - 1}}{h\binom{n}{\nu}} \sum_{j=0, j \neq \nu}^{n} \frac{(-1)^j}{j - \nu} \binom{n}{j} (j - \nu) h \sum_{i=0}^{s-1} (jh + t)^i (\nu h + t)^{s-i-1}$$

$$= \frac{(-1)^{\nu-1}}{\binom{n}{\nu}} \sum_{i=0}^{s-1} (\nu h + t)^{s-i-1} \sum_{j=0,\, j\neq\nu}^{n} (-1)^j \binom{n}{j} (jh+t)^i$$

$$= \frac{(-1)^{\nu-1}}{\binom{n}{\nu}} \sum_{i=0}^{s-1} (\nu h + t)^{s-i-1} (-1)^{\nu-1} \binom{n}{\nu} (\nu h + t)^i$$

$$= s(\nu h + t)^{s-1} = [(\nu h + t)^s]'.$$

To find a general solution of the non-homogeneous system the method of variation of the parameters will be applied. Looking for a solution in the form

$$\eta_\nu(t) = \sum_{s=0}^{n} C_s(t)(\nu h + t)^s, \quad \nu = 0, 1, \ldots, n, \qquad (32.3)$$

the functions $C_s(t)$, $s = 0, 1, \ldots, n$, must satisfy the system

$$\sum_{s=0}^{n} C'_s(t)(\nu h + t)^s = \varphi_n(f; \nu h + t), \quad \nu = 0, 1, \ldots, n. \qquad (32.4)$$

Let $D(t)$ be the determinant

$$D(t) = \|a_{\nu,s}\|, \quad a_{\nu,s} = (\nu h + t)^s, \; s, \nu = 0, 1, \ldots, n,$$

and $D_{\nu,s}(t)$ be the conjugate value of $a_{\nu,s}$; i.e.

$$\sum_{\nu=0}^{n} a_{\nu,s} D_{\nu,s}(t) = D(t), \quad s = 0, 1, \ldots, n. \qquad (32.5)$$

From (32.4), (32.5) it follows that

$$C'_s(t) = \frac{1}{D(t)} \sum_{j=0}^{n} D_{j,s}(t) \varphi_n(f; jh + t)$$

or

$$C_s(t) = \int_0^t \frac{1}{D(v)} \sum_{j=0}^{n} D_{j,s}(v) \varphi_n(f; jh + v)\, dv, \quad s = 0, 1, \ldots, n. \qquad (32.6)$$

The equalities (32.3) and (32.6) give

$$\eta_\nu(t) = \sum_{s=0}^{n} (\nu h + t)^s \int_0^t \frac{1}{D(v)} \sum_{j=0}^{n} D_{j,s}(v) \varphi_n(f; jh + v)\, dv$$

$$= \int_0^t \sum_{j=0}^{n} \varphi_n(f; jh + v) \frac{1}{D(v)} \sum_{s=0}^{n} (\nu h + t)^s D_{j,s}(v)\, dv. \qquad (32.7)$$

As

$$\frac{1}{D(v)} \sum_{s=0}^{n} (\nu h + t)^s D_{j,s}(v) = L_{n,j}\left(\frac{\nu h + t - v}{h}\right) = L_{n,j}\left(\frac{x - v}{h}\right)$$

from (32.7) it follows that

$$\eta_\nu(t) = \int_0^t \sum_{j=0}^n \varphi_n(f; jh+v) L_{n,j}\left(\frac{vh+t-v}{h}\right) dv.$$

Hence the general solution of the non-homogeneous system is

$$y_\nu(t) = \int_0^{vh+t} f(v)\, dv = \sum_{s=0}^n (vh+t)^s L_{n,j}\left(\frac{vh+t-v}{h}\right) dv,$$

after one differentiation of the last identity the theorem follows. Indeed

$$f(x) = f(vh+t)$$

$$= \sum_{s=1}^n sC_s(vh+t)^{s-1} + \varphi_n(f;x)$$

$$+ \sum_{j=0}^n \frac{1}{h} \int_0^t \varphi_n(f; jh+v) L'_{n,j}\left(\frac{x-v}{h}\right) dv. \qquad \square$$

THEOREM 32.2b. *Let the polynomial $Q(f)$ of degree $n-1$ interpolate f at the points $h, 2h, \ldots, nh$; i.e.*

$$Q(f;x) = \sum_{j=1}^n f(jh) L_{n-1,j-1}(x/h - 1),$$

then

$$f(x) - Q(x) = \Delta_h^n f(0) L_{n,0}\left(\frac{x}{h}\right) + \varphi_n(f;x) - \sum_{j=0}^n \varphi_n(f; jh) L_{n,j}\left(\frac{x}{h}\right)$$

$$+ \sum_{j=0}^n \frac{1}{h} \int_0^t \varphi_n(f; jh+v) L'_{n,j}\left(\frac{x-v}{h}\right) dv.$$

PROOF. Let P_{n-1} be the polynomial in Theorem 32.2a. Then

$$f(jh) = P_{n-1}(jh) + \varphi_n(f; jh), \quad j = 0, 1, \ldots, n,$$

and

$$f(x) - \sum_{j=0}^n f(jh) L_{n,j}\left(\frac{x}{h}\right)$$

$$= P_{n-1}(x) + \varphi_n(f;x) + \sum_{j=0}^n \frac{1}{h} \int_0^t \varphi_n(f; jh+v) L'_{n,j}\left(\frac{x-v}{h}\right) dv$$

$$- P_{n-1}(x) - \sum_{j=0}^n \varphi_n(f; jh) L_{n,j}\left(\frac{x}{h}\right).$$

The last equality and

$$L_{n,j}\left(\frac{x}{h}\right) = L_{n-1,j-1}(x/h - 1) + (-1)^{n-j}\binom{n}{j}L_{n,0}\left(\frac{x}{h}\right), \quad j = 1, 2, \ldots, n,$$

prove the theorem. □

THEOREM 32.2c. *The next relation holds*

$$\gamma_n = \max\left\{\sum_{j=0}^{n}\binom{n}{j}^{-1}|L_{n,j}(x)| : 0 \leqslant x \leqslant 1\right\} = 1.$$

PROOF. Since $\gamma_n = \max\{\gamma(t) : 0 \leqslant t \leqslant 1\}$, where

$$\gamma(t) = \frac{(1-t)(2-t)\cdots(n-t)}{n!} + \frac{t(1-t)(2-t)\cdots(n-t)}{n!}\sum_{j=1}^{n}\frac{1}{j-t},$$

the polynomial γ is of degree n and satisfies

$$\gamma(k) = (-1)^k\binom{n}{k}^{-1}$$

for $k = 0, 1, \ldots, n$. Therefore, γ' has no more than one zero in $[0, 1]$ and from

$$\gamma'(0) = 0, \quad \gamma''(0) = \sum_{j=0}^{n} j^{-2} - \left(\sum_{j=0}^{n} j^{-1}\right)^{-2} < 0$$

it follows that γ is monotonically decreasing in $[0, 1]$. In view of $\gamma(t) \leqslant \gamma(0) = 1$ the theorem is proved. □

THEOREM 32.2d. *Let*

$$\mu_{n,\nu} = \sum_{j=0}^{n}\binom{n}{j}^{-1}\max\{|L_{n,j}(x)| : \nu \leqslant x \leqslant \nu + 1\}, \tag{32.8}$$

then

$$\mu_{n,\nu} \leqslant (1 + \sigma_\nu + \sigma_{\nu+1})\binom{n}{\nu}^{-1}, \quad \nu = 0, 1, \ldots, (n-1)/2, \tag{32.9}$$

where $\sigma_\nu = 1 + 1/2 + 1/3 + \cdots + 1/\nu$, $\sigma_0 = 0$. *In particular*

$$\mu_{n,0} = 1 + \sum_{j=1}^{n}\binom{n}{j}^{-1}\max\{|L_{n,j}(x)| : 0 \leqslant x \leqslant 1\} \leqslant 2.$$

PROOF. Let $\nu \leqslant x \leqslant \nu + 1$, $x = \nu + t$, $0 \leqslant t \leqslant 1$. Then from $\nu \leqslant [(n-1)/2]$ it follows that

$$\mu_{n,\nu} = \frac{1}{n!}\sum_{j=0}^{n}\max\left\{\frac{(\nu+t)\cdots(1+t)t(1-t)\cdots(n-\nu-t)}{|\nu-j+t|} : 0 \leqslant t \leqslant 1\right\}$$

$$\leqslant \binom{n}{\nu}^{-1} + \frac{1}{n!}\sum_{j=0, j\neq\nu}^{n}\max\left\{\left|\frac{1+t/(\nu-j)}{1-t}\right|\right.$$

$$\left.\times\frac{(\nu+t)\cdots(1+t)t(1-t)\cdots(n-\nu-t)}{|\nu-j+t|} : 0 \leqslant t \leqslant 1\right\}$$

$$= \binom{n}{\nu}^{-1} + \frac{1}{n!} \max\{(\nu+t)\cdots(1+t)t(2-t)\cdots(n-\nu-t): 0 \leq t \leq 1\}$$

$$\times \sum_{j=0, j\neq \nu}^{n} \frac{1}{|\nu-j|}$$

$$= \binom{n}{\nu}^{-1} [1 + \max(q_{n,\nu}(t): 0 \leq t \leq 1)], \qquad (32.10)$$

where

$$q_{n,\nu}(t) = (\sigma_\nu + \sigma_{n-\nu})\left(1 + \frac{t}{\nu}\right)\cdots\left(1 + \frac{t}{1}\right)t\left(1 - \frac{t}{2}\right)\cdots\left(1 - \frac{t}{n-\nu}\right).$$

Let us show that

$$\max_{0 \leq t \leq 1} q_{n,\nu}(t) \leq \max_{0 \leq t \leq 1} q_{2\nu+1,\nu}(t)$$

$$= (\sigma_\nu + \sigma_{\nu+1}) \max_{0 \leq t \leq 1} t\left(1 - \frac{t(1-t)}{12}\right)\cdots\left(1 - \frac{t(1-t)}{\nu(\nu+1)}\right)$$

$$= (\sigma_\nu + \sigma_{\nu+1}). \qquad (32.11)$$

It is obvious that

$$q_{n,\nu}(0) = q_{n-1,\nu}(0) = 0,$$

$$q'_{n,\nu}(0) = \sigma_\nu + \sigma_{n-\nu} > \sigma_\nu + \sigma_{n-\nu-1} = q'_{n-1,\nu}(0), \qquad (32.12)$$

$$q_{n,\nu}(1) = \frac{\nu+1}{n-\nu}(\sigma_\nu + \sigma_{n-\nu}) < \frac{\nu+1}{n-\nu-1}(\sigma_\nu + \sigma_{n-\nu-1}) = q_{n-1,\nu}(1).$$

There is only one point $\tau'_n \in (0,1)$ such that $q_{n,\nu}(\tau'_n) = q_{n-1,\nu}(\tau'_n)$ and for this point $(\sigma_\nu + \sigma_{n-\nu})[1 - \tau'_n/(n-\nu)] = \sigma_\nu + \sigma_{n-\nu-1}$; i.e. $\tau'_n = 1/(\sigma_\nu + \sigma_{n-\nu})$.

The polynomial $q'_{n,\nu}$ has one zero $\tau''_n \in [0,1]$ and τ''_n is also a solution of the equation

$$\frac{1}{t} + \sum_{j=1}^{\nu} \frac{1}{j+t} - \sum_{j=2}^{n-\nu} \frac{1}{j-t} = 0,$$

from where it results that

$$\frac{1}{\tau''_n} < \sum_{j=2}^{n-\nu} \frac{1}{j-t} < \sigma_{n-\nu-1} < \sigma_{n-\nu}.$$

Hence

$$\tau''_n > \frac{1}{\sigma_{n-\nu}} \geq \tau'_n. \qquad (32.13)$$

The inequalities (32.12), (32.13) imply (32.11), and (32.8) and (32.9) follow from (32.10) and (32.11). □

THEOREM 32.2e. *For any function f that is integrable on $[0,1]$ the following inequality is fulfilled*

$$\left| f(x) - \sum_{j=1}^{n} f(jh) L_{n-1,j-1}(x/h - 1) \right| \leq \binom{n}{\nu}^{-1} [6 + 7\min(\sigma_\nu, \sigma_{n-\nu})] \omega_n(f; h)$$

for $x \in [\nu h, (\nu+1)h]$, $h = 1/(n+1)$, $\nu = 0, 1, \ldots, n$,

$$\sigma_\nu = 1 + \frac{1}{2} + \cdots + \frac{1}{\nu}, \quad \sigma_0 = 0.$$

PROOF. Since the knots of the interpolation polynomial

$$Q_{n-1}(x) = \sum_{j=1}^{n} f(jh) L_{n-1,j-1}(x/h - 1)$$

are symmetric with respect to the middle of the interval $[0, 1]$, it is sufficient to prove the theorem for $x \in [0, 1/2]$ or for $\nu = 0, 1, \ldots, [(n-1)/2]$. For $\nu = 0$, from Theorems 32.2b, 32.2c, and 32.2d, using the inequality

$$|\varphi_n(f; x)| \leq \binom{n}{\nu}^{-1} \omega_n(f; h)$$

it follows that

$$|f(x) - Q_{n-1}(x)| \leq \omega_n(f; h) \bigg(\max_{0 \leq t \leq 1} |L_{n,0}(t)| + 1 + \max_{0 \leq t \leq 1} \sum_{j=0}^{n} \binom{n}{j}^{-1} |L_{n,j}(t)|$$

$$+ \sum_{j=0}^{n} \binom{n}{j}^{-1} \int_0^t |L'_{n,j}(v)| \, dv \bigg)$$

$$\leq \omega_n(f; h) \bigg[3 + 1 + \sum_{j=1}^{n} \binom{n}{j}^{-1} \max_{0 \leq t \leq 1} |L_{n,j}(t)| \bigg] \leq 6 \omega_n(f; h).$$

For $\nu = 1, \ldots, [(n-1)/2]$ it follows analogously that

$$|f(x) - Q_{n-1}(x)| \leq \binom{n}{\nu}^{-1} \omega_n(f; h) \bigg[2 + \binom{n}{\nu} \max_{\nu \leq u \leq \nu+1} \sum_{j=0}^{n} \binom{n}{j}^{-1} |L_{n,j}(u)|$$

$$+ \binom{n}{\nu} \sum_{j=0}^{n} \binom{n}{j}^{-1} \int_0^1 |L'_{n,j}(\nu + v)| \, dv \bigg]$$

$$\leq \binom{n}{\nu}^{-1} \omega_n(f; h) \bigg[2 + 3 \binom{n}{\nu} \sum_{j=0}^{n} \binom{n}{j}^{-1} \max_{\nu \leq u \leq \nu+1} |L_{n,j}(u)| \bigg]$$

$$\leq \binom{n}{\nu}^{-1} [5 + 3(\sigma_\nu + \sigma_{\nu+1})] \omega_n(f; h)$$

$$\leq \binom{n}{\nu}^{-1} [6 + 7\sigma_\nu] \omega_n(f; h). \qquad \square$$

The proof of Theorem 32.2 follows immediately by Theorem 32.2e taking into account the inequality

$$\binom{n}{\nu}^{-1}[6+7\min(\sigma_\nu,\sigma_{n-\nu})]\leq 6 \quad \text{for } \nu=0,1,\ldots,n.$$

The problem for finding the exact Whitney constant remains unsolved. KRIAKIN [1989] using Sendov's approach proved the following theorem.

THEOREM 32.3. *Let the function f be defined and integrable on the interval $[0, 1]$ and the algebraic polynomial P of degree $n-1$ be defined by the conditions*

$$\int_0^{i/n}[f(t)-P(t)]\,dt=0, \quad i=1,2,\ldots,n;$$

then

$$\sup_{0\leq x\leq 1}|f(t)-P(t)|\leq 3\omega_n(f;n^{-1}).$$

THEOREM 32.4. *Let L be a bounded linear operator on $M_{[a,b]}$ and let $L(P) = P$ for every polynomial $P \in H_{k-1}$. Then for every function $f \in M_{[a,b]}$ the following inequality is fulfilled*

$$\|f-L(f)\|_{C_{[a,b]}} \leq (1+\|L\|_{M_{[a,b]}})W_k\omega_k\left(f;\frac{b-a}{k}\right),$$

where W_k is Whitney's constant.

PROOF. Let $P_k \in H_{k-1}$ be Whitney's polynomial for f; then

$$\|f-L(f)\|_C \leq \|f-P_k\|_C + \|P_k - L(P_k)\|_C + \|L(P_k)-L(f)\|_C$$

$$\leq W_k(1+\|L\|_M)\omega_k\left(f;\frac{b-a}{k}\right). \quad \square$$

The next theorem is similar to the previous theorem.

THEOREM 32.5. *Let F be a bounded linear functional on $M_{[a,b]}$ and $F(P) = 0$ for every $P \in H_{k-1}$. Then for every $f \in M_{[a,b]}$ the following relation is fulfilled*

$$|F(f)| \leq W_k\|F\|_{M_{[a,b]}}\omega_k\left(f;\frac{b-a}{k}\right).$$

33. On the order of the uniform approximation by polynomials

For a given continuous function f let us try to answer the question (c) in Section 24 about the behavior of the quantity

$$E_n^T(f) = \inf_{\varphi \in T_n}\max_{x\in[0,2\pi]}|\varphi(x)-f(x)|,$$

$$T_n = \left\{\varphi: \varphi(x) = b_0 + \sum_{i=1}^n(a_i\sin ix + b_i\cos ix),\ a_i, b_i \text{ are real numbers}\right\},$$

in the case of approximation by means of trigonometric polynomials. The main result is due to JACKSON [1911, 1912]. He proved that for every 2π-periodic function f the following estimate holds:

$$E_n^T(f) = c\omega(f; 1/n), \tag{33.1}$$

where c is an absolute constant.

KORNEICHUCK ([1962]; [1987], §6.2), obtained the relation

$$1 - \frac{1}{2n} \leq \sup_{f \in C} \frac{E_n^T(f)_C}{\omega(f; \pi/n)} < 1.$$

Jackson's estimation (33.1) has many generalizations. STECHKIN [1951] proved that if the function f is periodic in 2π, then

$$E_n^T(f)_{L_p} = \inf_{\varphi \in T_n} \|\varphi - f\|_{L_p} \leq c(k)\omega_{k+1}(f; 1/n)_{L_p}, \quad 1 \leq p \leq \infty, \tag{33.2}$$

for every natural number $k \geq 1$, where $E_n^T(f)_{L_\infty} = E_n^T(f)$.

If the 2π-periodic function f is smooth enough, then the inequality (33.2) gives

$$E_n^T(f)_{L_p} = O\left(\frac{1}{n^k} \omega(f^{(k)}; 1/n)_{L_p}\right), \quad 0 \leq p \leq \infty. \tag{33.3}$$

The last estimation shows how $E_n^T(f)_{L_p}$ tends to zero in the case of differentiable functions.

The estimation (33.2), the properties of $\omega_k(f; \delta)_{L_p}$ from Section 30 and the converse theorem of SALEM [1940] and STECHKIN [1951] (see also PETRUSHEV and POPOV [1987], Theorem 3.8)

$$\omega_k(f; 1/n)_{L_p} \leq \frac{c(k)}{n^k} \sum_{s=0}^{n} (s+1)^{k-1} E_s^T(f)_{L_p}, \quad 1 \leq p \leq \infty, \tag{33.4}$$

allow us to know in advance the approximation that can be achieved using the characteristics of the function f. For example, for $k > \alpha$,

$$E_n^T(f)_{L_p} = O(n^{-\alpha}) \Leftrightarrow \omega_k(f; \delta)_{L_p} = O(\delta^\alpha).$$

The estimations (33.1)–(33.4) are valid in the non-periodic case of approximation by means of algebraic polynomials in a given interval $[a, b]$. Unlike the periodic case NIKOLSKII [1946] observed that the algebraic approximation at the ends of the interval can be done better than the approximation in the middle of the interval—the so-called "effect of the ends"—keeping the estimation of the type (33.1)–(33.4) by the modulus of smoothness. For details see DZJADIK ([1977], Chapter VI), TIMAN ([1960], Chapter 5), PETRUSHEV and POPOV ([1987], Chapter 3.4). Some characterizations of the best algebraic approximation are given by DZAFAROV [1977], and POTAPOV [1977]. Their results are based on the modified translation concept. FUKSMAN [1965] characterizes the best uniform algebraic approximation in terms of the usual derivatives. Using new moduli IVANOV [1983a,b] complete the characterization of the best algebraic approximation in L_p, $1 \leq p \leq \infty$, obtaining results similar to (33.1)–(33.4).

SECTION 33. Uniform approximation

THEOREM 33.1 (IVANOV [1983b]). *If the function $f \in C_{[-1,1]}$, then*

$$E_m(f) = \inf_{\varphi \in H_m} \max_{x \in [-1,1]} |\varphi(x) - f(x)| = O\left(\tau\left(f; \frac{1}{m}\sqrt{1-x^2} + \frac{1}{m^2}\right)\right),$$

where

$$H_m = \left\{\varphi: \varphi(x) = \sum_{i=0}^{m} a_i x^i, \ a_i \text{ are real numbers}\right\},$$

$$\tau(f; \delta(x)) = \sup\{|f(x) - f(y)|: x, y \in [-1, 1], |x - y| \le \delta(x)\}.$$

PROOF. Consider the algebraic polynomial $Q \in H_{2n-2}$ of degree $2n - 2$, $n = [m/2] + 1$, where

$$Q(x) = J_n(f; \cos^{-1} x), \qquad J_n(f; x) = \int_{-\pi}^{\pi} f(\cos(x+t)) K_n(t) \, dt,$$

$$K_n(t) = \frac{3}{2\pi n(2n^2 + 1)} \left[\frac{\sin(nt/2)}{\sin(t/2)}\right]^4. \tag{33.5}$$

Since

$$\sin^2 \frac{nx}{2} = \frac{1 - \cos nx}{2} = \frac{1}{2} \sum_{i=0}^{n-1} [\cos ix - \cos(i+1)x] = \sin \frac{x}{2} \sum_{i=0}^{n-1} \sin \frac{(2i+1)x}{2}$$

$$= \sin \frac{x}{2} \sum_{i=0}^{n-1} \left[\sin \frac{x}{2} + \sum_{s=2}^{i+1} \sin \frac{(2s-1)x}{2} - \sin \frac{(2s-3)x}{2}\right]$$

$$= \sin \frac{x}{2} \sum_{i=0}^{n-1} \left[\sin \frac{x}{2} + 2 \sum_{s=2}^{i+1} \sin \frac{x}{2} \cos(s-1)x\right]$$

$$= \sin^2 \frac{x}{2} \sum_{i=0}^{n-1} \left[1 + 2 \sum_{s=2}^{i+1} \cos(s-1)x\right]$$

$$= \sin^2 \frac{x}{2} \left[n + 2 \sum_{k=1}^{n-1} (n-k) \cos kx\right], \tag{33.6}$$

it follows that

$$\left[\frac{\sin(nx/2)}{\sin(x/2)}\right]^2$$

is a trigonometric polynomial of degree $n - 1$ and therefore $K_n \in T_{2n-2}$.
Using the equalities

$$\int_{-\pi}^{\pi} \cos(kx) \, dx = \int_{-\pi}^{\pi} \sin(kx) \, dx = \int_{-\pi}^{\pi} \sin(kx) \cos(lx) \, dx$$

$$= \int_{-\pi}^{\pi} \cos(kx) \cos(lx) \, dx = \int_{-\pi}^{\pi} \sin(kx) \sin(lx) \, dx = 0,$$

$$\int_{-\pi}^{\pi} \sin^2(kx)\,dx = \int_{-\pi}^{\pi} \cos^2(kx)\,dx = \pi,$$

the relations (33.6) give

$$\int_{-\pi}^{\pi} \left[\frac{\sin(nt/2)}{\sin(t/2)}\right]^4 dt = \int_{-\pi}^{\pi} \left[n + 2\sum_{k=1}^{n-1}(n-k)\cos kt\right]^2 dt$$

$$= \pi\left[2n^2 + 4\sum_{k=1}^{n-1}(n-k)^2\right]$$

$$= \frac{2\pi n(2n^2+1)}{3}; \quad \text{i.e.} \int_{-\pi}^{\pi} K_n(t)\,dt = 1.$$

The estimation of $|f(x) - Q(x)|$ for $x \in [-1, 1]$ can be made, setting

$$x = \cos y, \quad h(t) = \frac{\pi}{4m}\operatorname{sgn} t, \quad r(t) = \frac{4m|t|}{\pi}.$$

Then

$$|f(x) - Q(x)| = |f(\cos y) - J_n(f; y)| \leq \int_{-\pi}^{\pi} |f(\cos y) - f(\cos(y+t))| K_n(t)\,dt$$

$$\leq \int_{-\pi}^{\pi} \left(|f(\cos(y + r(t)h(t))) - f(\cos(y+t))|\right.$$

$$\left. + \sum_{i=1}^{r(t)} |f(\cos(y + (i-1)h)) - f(\cos(y+ih))|\right) K_n(t)\,dt$$

$$\leq \int_{-\pi}^{\pi} \left(1 + \frac{4m|t|}{\pi}\right)\tau\!\left(f; \frac{1}{m}\sqrt{1-x^2} + \frac{1}{m^2}\right) K_n(t)\,dt,$$

using for the last inequality the fact that the relations

$$|\cos y - \cos(y+h)| = 2\sin\frac{|h|}{2}|\sin(y+h/2)| \leq 2\frac{|h|}{2}\left(|\sin y| + \frac{h}{2}\right)$$

$$\leq \frac{\pi}{4m}\left(\sqrt{1-\cos^2 y} + \frac{\pi}{8m}\right) \leq \left(\frac{1}{m}\sqrt{1-\cos^2 y} + \frac{1}{m^2}\right),$$

imply

$$|\cos(y+ih) - \cos(y+(i-1)h)| \leq \left(\frac{1}{m}\sqrt{1-\cos^2(y+(i-1)h)} + \frac{1}{m^2}\right),$$

$$|\cos(y + r(t)h(t)) - \cos(y+t)| = \left(\frac{1}{m}\sqrt{1-\cos^2(y+t)} + \frac{1}{m^2}\right),$$

or

$$|f(\cos(y+ih)) - f(\cos(y+(i-1)h))| \le \tau\left(f; \frac{1}{m}\sqrt{1-x^2} + \frac{1}{m^2}\right),$$

$$|f(\cos(y+r(t)h(t))) - f(\cos(y+t))| \le \tau\left(f; \frac{1}{m}\sqrt{1-x^2} + \frac{1}{m^2}\right).$$

On the other hand,

$$\int_0^\pi tK_n(t)\,dt = \sum_{k=0}^{n-1} \int_{k\pi/n}^{(k+1)\pi/n} tK_n(t)\,dt$$

$$= \frac{3}{2\pi n(2n^2+1)} \left(\int_0^{\pi/n} t\left(\frac{nt/2}{t/\pi}\right)^4 dt + \sum_{k=1}^{n-1} \int_{k\pi/n}^{(k+1)\pi/n} \frac{(k+1)\pi}{n} \left(\frac{1}{k/n}\right)^4 dt \right)$$

$$= \frac{3}{2\pi n(2n^2+1)} \left(\frac{\pi^6 n^2}{32} + \sum_{k=1}^{n-1} \pi^2 n^2 \frac{k+1}{k^4} \right)$$

$$\le \frac{3n^2}{2\pi n(2n^2+1)} \left(\frac{\pi^6}{32} + \sum_{k=1}^{\infty} \pi^2 \frac{k+1}{k^4} \right) \le \frac{c}{n}$$

and

$$\int_{-\pi}^{\pi} \left(1 + \frac{4m|t|}{\pi}\right) K_n(t)\,dt = 1 + \frac{8m}{\pi} \int_0^{\pi} tK_n(t)\,dt \le 1 + \frac{8cm}{\pi n}.$$

Consequently

$$E_m(f) = O\left(\tau\left(f; \frac{1}{m}\sqrt{1-x^2} + \frac{1}{m^2}\right)\right). \qquad \square$$

In Fig. 33.1 the graphs of the functions $|x| - J_{20}(|x|; \cos^{-1}x)$ and $|x| - P_{38}$ are given in the interval $[-1,1]$, where $E_{38}(|x|) = \max_{x\in[-1,1]} |P_{38}(x) - |x||$ and $J_{20}(|x|; \cos^{-1}x)$ is defined by (33.5).

For analytic functions the behaviors of $E_n^T(f)$ and $E_n(f)$ are quite different. BERNSTEIN [1913a,b] proved the next two theorems.

THEOREM 33.2. *A necessary and sufficient condition for the function f to satisfy $f \in A_{2\pi}$ is the inequality $E_n^T(f) \le Kq^n$, where $K>0$ and $q<1$ are constants and the set of functions $A_{2\pi}$ is defined as:*

$A_{2\pi} = \{f:$ *there exists a number $R>0$ such that for every x_0,*
$\sum_{k=0}^\infty c_k(x_0)(x-x_0)^k < \infty$ *for $|x-x_0|<R$ and*
$f(x) = \sum_{k=0}^\infty c_k(x_0)(x-x_0)^k$ *for such x, f is periodic in $2\pi\}$.*

An assertion similar to Theorem 33.2 holds in the algebraic case. Denote the set of analytic functions on the interval $[a,b]$ by

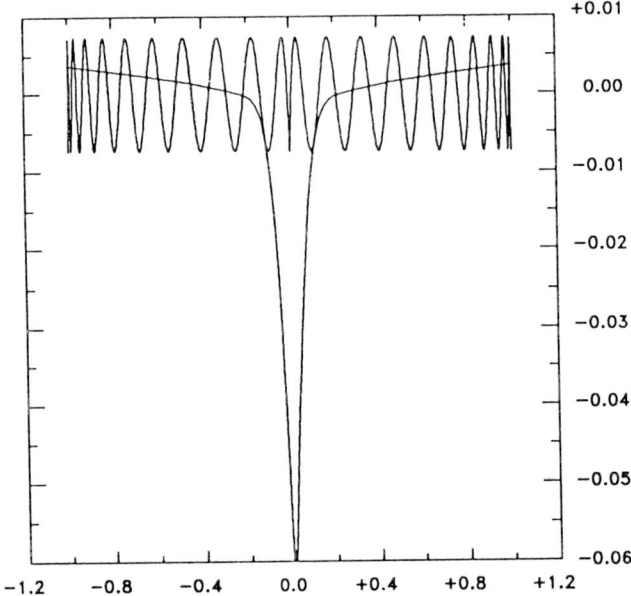

Fig. 33.1. Graphs of the functions $|x| - J_{20}(|x|; \cos^{-1}x)$ and $|x| - P_{38}$.

$$A_{[a,b]} = \{f: \text{there exists a number } R > 0 \text{ such that for every } x_0 \in [a, b] \text{ it follows that } \sum_{k=0}^{\infty} c_k(x_0)(x - x_0)^k < \infty \text{ for } |x - x_0| < R \text{ and for } x \in [a, b] \cap (x_0 - R, x_0 + R), f(x) = \sum_{k=0}^{\infty} c_k(x_0)(x - x_0)^k\},$$

the next theorem holds.

THEOREM 33.2a. *A necessary and sufficient condition for the function f to satisfy $f \in A_{[a,b]}$ is the inequality $E_n(f) \leq Kq^n$, where $K > 0$ and $q < 1$ are constants.*

As an illustration of the behavior of $E_n(f)$ as a function of the properties of f let us consider two functions, defined on the interval $[-1, 1]$, $f_1(x) = |x|$, $f_2(x) = e^x$ (Tables 33.1 and 33.2, respectively). The function f_1 is not differentiable at the point zero and this is the reason for its "bad" approximation by polynomials—see NATANSON ([1949], pp. 187, 215),

$$\frac{1}{2\pi(2n+1)} < E_n(f_1) = \max_{x \in [-1,1]} |P_{n_1}(x) - f_1(x)| \leq \frac{2}{\pi n}. \tag{33.7}$$

At the same time using (2.3) and (2.4) for the analytic function f_2 the following inequalities are fulfilled

$$E_n(f_2) = \max_{x \in [-1,1]} |P_{n_2}(x) - f_2(x)| \leq \max_{x \in [-1,1]} |f_2(x) - L_n(x)| \leq \frac{e}{2^n(n+1)!},$$

where L_n is the algebraic polynomial of nth degree that interpolates f_2 at the roots of the $(n+1)$th Chebyshev polynomial in the interval $[-1, 1]$. As a

TABLE 33.1. The function $E_n(|x|)$.

n	$E_n(|x|)$
4	$0.676209\ldots\times 10^{-1}$
10	$0.278451\ldots\times 10^{-1}$
50	$0.560198\ldots\times 10^{-2}$
100	$0.280152\ldots\times 10^{-2}$
150	$0.186774\ldots\times 10^{-2}$

TABLE 33.2. The function $E_n(e^x)$.

n	$E_n(e^x)$
2	$0.450174\ldots\times 10^{-1}$
4	$0.546668\ldots\times 10^{-3}$
6	$0.321088\ldots\times 10^{-5}$
8	$0.110643\ldots\times 10^{-7}$
11	$0.104093\ldots\times 10^{-11}$

numerical illustration see the Tables 33.1 and 33.2, where some of the best approximations of the functions $|x|$ and e^x by means of algebraic polynomials in the interval $[-1, 1]$ are given.

REMARK 33.1. The Jackson kernel

$$K_n(t) = \frac{3}{2\pi n(2n^2 + 1)} \left[\frac{\sin(nt/2)}{\sin(t/2)} \right]^4$$

plays an important role in approximation theory and the trigonometric polynomial of $(2n - 2)$th degree

$$G_n(f; x) = \int_{-\pi}^{\pi} f(x + t) K_n(t)\, dt$$

satisfies (NATANSON [1949], p. 117, LORENTZ [1986], p. 55)

$$E_{2n-2}^T(f) \le \max_{x \in [0, 2\pi]} |G_n(f; x) - f(x)| \le 6\omega(f; 1/n).$$

The last inequality leads to

$$E_n^T(f) \le E_{2[n+2/2]-2}^T(f) \le 6\omega\left(f; 1\bigg/\left[\frac{n+2}{2}\right]\right)$$

$$\le 6\omega\left(f; \frac{2}{n+1}\right) \le 12\omega\left(f; \frac{1}{n+1}\right).$$

34. Newman's results and approximation by means of rational functions

From the numerical point of view a very important step in the development of the rational approximations was the result of NEWMAN [1964] that for $n \ge 5$

$$e^{-\pi\sqrt{n+1}} \le E_{nn}(|x|)_{C_{[-1,1]}} \le 3 e^{-\sqrt{n}}, \tag{34.1}$$

where

$$E_{mn}(f)_{C_{[-1,1]}} = \inf_{\varphi \in R_{mn}} \max_{x \in [-1,1]} |f(x) - \varphi(x)|,$$

$$R_{mn} = \left\{\varphi\colon \varphi = \sum_{i=0}^{m} a_i x^i \bigg/ \sum_{i=0}^{n} b_i x^i,\ a_i, b_i \text{ are real numbers}\right\}.$$

VJACHESLAVOV [1975] gave the exact order of the best uniform approximation of $|x|$, obtaining the following result

$$c_1 e^{-\pi\sqrt{n}} \leq E_{nn}(|x|) \leq c_2 e^{-\pi\sqrt{n}}, \tag{34.2}$$

where c_1 and c_2 are constants.

A complete proof of the estimations (34.1) and (34.2) can be found in PETRUSHEV and POPOV ([1987], Chapter 4) and partially in LORENTZ ([1986], p. 81).

The latest result connected with the rational approximation of the function $|x|$ in the interval $[-1, 1]$ is obtained by STAHL [1991] (talk at the International Conference on Constructive Function Theory, Varna, Bulgaria)

$$\lim_{n\to\infty} [E_{nn}(|x|)/e^{-\pi\sqrt{n}}] = 8 .$$

Comparing the rational approximation (34.1) of the function $|x|$ with its polynomial approximation (33.7) it is clear that the estimation (33.7) cannot enter into competition with the estimation (34.1). Compare also the numerical results from the Tables 33.1 and 34.1.

Roughly speaking the estimation (34.1) shows that the approximation by the rational approximation of functions that are not smooth enough is much better than the approximation by polynomials. This fact was affirmed by the next basic theorem of POPOV [1977] in rational approximation of functions.

THEOREM 34.1. *Let the function* $f \in V_r M_{[a,b]}$, *where*

$$V_r M_{[a,b]} = \{f: f^{(r-1)} \text{ is absolutely continuous}, V_a^b f^{(r)} \leq M, r \geq 1\} .$$

Then for $n \geq r$,

$$E_{nn}(f)_{C_{[a,b]}} \leq D^r \frac{M(b-a)^r}{n^{r+1}} ,$$

where $D > 1$ *is an absolute constant.*

Let us mention that the estimations (33.3) and (33.4) give for $f \in V_r M_{[a,b]}$

TABLE 34.1.

n	k	$E_{n,k}(|x|)$
0	2	$0.268150\ldots$
2	2	$0.436890\ldots \times 10^{-1}$
2	4	$0.248222\ldots \times 10^{-1}$
4	4	$0.850148\ldots \times 10^{-2}$
4	6	$0.519820\ldots \times 10^{-2}$
6	6	$0.228211\ldots \times 10^{-2}$
6	8	$0.146705\ldots \times 10^{-2}$
8	8	$0.736567\ldots \times 10^{-3}$
8	10	$0.491254\ldots \times 10^{-3}$
15	16	$0.460365\ldots \times 10^{-4}$

Uniform approximation

TABLE 34.2.

n	k	$E_{n-1,k-1}(|x|)$	$\max_{-1\leq x\leq 1}||x|-N_k(x)|$
6	5	$0.850148\ldots\times 10^{-2}$	$0.742591\ldots\times 10^{-1}$
7	6	$0.427985\ldots\times 10^{-2}$	$0.450848\ldots\times 10^{-1}$
8	7	$0.228211\ldots\times 10^{-2}$	$0.261232\ldots\times 10^{-1}$
9	8	$0.127299\ldots\times 10^{-2}$	$0.166573\ldots\times 10^{-1}$
10	9	$0.736562\ldots\times 10^{-3}$	$0.105868\ldots\times 10^{-1}$
11	10	$0.439377\ldots\times 10^{-3}$	$0.706627\ldots\times 10^{-2}$
12	11	$0.267233\ldots\times 10^{-3}$	$0.475328\ldots\times 10^{-2}$
13	12	$0.107471\ldots\times 10^{-3}$	$0.329254\ldots\times 10^{-2}$
14	13	$0.697986\ldots\times 10^{-4}$	$0.249459\ldots\times 10^{-2}$
15	14	$0.460365\ldots\times 10^{-4}$	$0.207704\ldots\times 10^{-2}$
16	15	$0.307885\ldots\times 10^{-4}$	$0.174757\ldots\times 10^{-2}$
17	16	$0.208521\ldots\times 10^{-4}$	$0.146619\ldots\times 10^{-2}$

that $E_{n0}(f)_{C_{[a,b]}} = O(1/n^r)$, and so the class of functions $V_r M_{[a,b]}$ can be approximated better by rational functions than by polynomials.

It is interesting to compare $E_{mn}(|x|)_{C_{[-1,1]}}$ with the approximation given by Newman's rational function

$$N_n(x) = x\,\frac{p_n(x) - p_n(-x)}{p_n(x) + p_n(-x)}, \quad p_n(x) = \prod_{k=1}^{n-1}(x + e^{-k/\sqrt{n}}), \quad n \geq 5.$$

Some numerical results are given in Table 34.2, and Fig. 34.1 presents the graphs of the functions $|x| - N_8(x)$ and $|x| - R_{8,6}(x)$, where $E_{8,6}(|x|)_{C[-1,1]} = \||x| - R_{8,6}\|$.

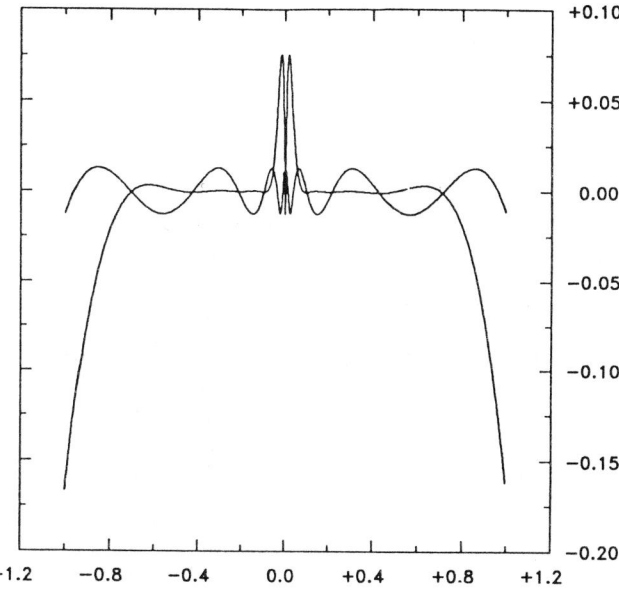

FIG. 34.1. Graphs of the functions $|x| - N_8(x)$ and $|x| - R_{8,6}(x)$.

The full survey of the rational approximation of functions in the one-dimensional case can be found in the book of PETRUSHEV and POPOV [1987].

35. Chebyshev polynomials

The algebraic polynomial of nth degree

$$C_n(x) = \cos(n \cos^{-1} x) \tag{35.1}$$

is called the Chebyshev polynomial of the first kind in the interval $[-1, 1]$. From the identity

$$\cos n\theta = 2 \cos \theta \cos(n-1)\theta - \cos(n-2)\theta$$

using the substitution $\theta = \cos^{-1} x$ the recursive relation follows

$$C_n(x) = 2x C_{n-1}(x) - C_{n-2}(x), \quad n = 2, 3, \ldots, \tag{35.2}$$

which gives $C_n \in H_n$, as $C_0(x) = 1$ and $C_1(x) = x$.

The explicit representation of C_n can be obtained with the help of de Moivre's formula

$$\cos n\theta \pm i \sin n\theta = (\cos \theta \pm i \sin \theta)^n$$

or

$$\cos n\theta = \tfrac{1}{2}[(\cos \theta + i \sin \theta)^n + (\cos \theta - i \sin \theta)^n].$$

Setting $\theta = \cos^{-1} x$ in the last identity it follows for $|x| \leq 1$ that

$$C_n(x) = \tfrac{1}{2}[(x + i\sqrt{1-x^2})^n + (x - i\sqrt{1-x^2})^n]. \tag{35.3}$$

The representation (35.3) is an algebraic polynomial of nth degree for all x because of

$$[(x + i\sqrt{1-x^2})^n + (x - i\sqrt{1-x^2})^n]$$

$$= \sum_{k=0}^{n} \binom{n}{k} i^k [1 + (-1)^k] x^{n-k} (\sqrt{1-x^2})^k;$$

i.e. the last sum does not contain imaginary terms.

For $|x| > 1$ the formula (35.3) can be used in the form

$$C_n(x) = \tfrac{1}{2}[(x + \sqrt{x^2 - 1})^n + (x - \sqrt{x^2 - 1})^n].$$

The main properties of the Chebyshev polynomials are the following.
(1) $C_n(x) = 2^{n-1} x^n + \cdots$.
The proof follows from (35.1) and (35.2);
(2) The polynomial C_n satisfies the differential equation

$$(1 - x^2) y'' - xy' + n^2 y = 0.$$

The proof is direct.
Representing C_n in the form $C_n(x) = \sum_{i=0}^{n} c_i x^{n-i}$ the above differential

equation allows us to obtain the coefficients c_i explicitly. Indeed from the equality

$$(1-x^2) \sum_{k=0}^{n-2} (n-k)(n-k-1)c_k x^{n-k-2} - x \sum_{k=0}^{n-1} (n-k)c_k x^{n-k-1}$$

$$+ n^2 \sum_{k=0}^{n} c_k x^{n-k} = 0,$$

it follows that

$$[n^2 - (n-1)^2]a_1 x^{n-1} + \sum_{k=2}^{n} \{(n-k+2)(n-k+1)c_{k-2}$$

$$+ [n^2 - (n-k)^2]c_k\} x^{n-k} = 0.$$

Hence

$$c_1 = 0, \quad c_k = -\frac{(n-k+2)(n-k+1)}{k(2n-k)} c_{k-2}; \tag{35.4}$$

i.e. all the $c_{2k+1} = 0$. As $c_0 = 2^{n-1}$, (35.4) gives

$$c_{2k} = (-1)^k \frac{n(n-1)\cdots(n-2k+1)}{k!(n-1)\cdots(n-k)} 2^{n-2k-1}$$

$$= (-1)^k \binom{n-k}{k} \frac{n}{n-k} 2^{n-2k-1}.$$

Finally,

$$C_n(x) = \sum_{k=0}^{[n/2]} (-1)^k \binom{n-k}{k} \frac{n}{n-k} 2^{n-2k-1} x^{n-2k}. \tag{35.5}$$

(3) $\min_{\{a_k\}} \max_{-1 \le x \le 1} \left| x^n - \sum_{k=0}^{n-1} a_k x^k \right| = \frac{1}{2^{n-1}} \max_{-1 \le x \le 1} |C_n(x)| = \frac{1}{2^{n-1}};$

i.e. the degree of approximation of x^n by polynomials of degree $n-1$ is $1/2^{n-1}$. This means that among all the polynomials of nth degree with leading coefficient one the polynomial $C_n/2^{n-1}$ deviates at least from zero in $[-1, 1]$. The proof follows immediately by Theorem 25.3 because

$$\max_{-1 \le x \le 1} |C_n(x)| = 1 \quad \text{and} \quad C_n\left(\cos \frac{k\pi}{n}\right) = (-1)^k, \quad k = 0, 1, \ldots, n.$$

Hence, every polynomial $P_n(x) = a_0 x^n + a_1 x^{n-1} + \cdots + a_{n-1} x + a_n$ satisfies

$$\max_{-1 \le x \le 1} |P_n(x)| \ge |a_0|/2^{n-1}. \tag{35.6}$$

After the substitution $x = \frac{1}{2}(a+b) + \frac{1}{2}(b-a)y$,

$$P_n(x) = P_n\left(\frac{a+b}{2} + \frac{b-a}{2} y\right) = a_0 \left(\frac{b-a}{2}\right)^n y^n + \cdots,$$

and (35.6) gives
$$\max_{a \leq x \leq b} |P_n(x)| \geq \frac{|a_0|}{2^{2n-1}} (b-a)^n .$$

(4) $\quad \displaystyle\int_{-1}^{1} \frac{C_n(x) C_m(x)}{\sqrt{1-x^2}} \, dx = \begin{cases} \pi, & n = m = 0, \\ \pi/2, & n = m \neq 0, \\ 0, & n \neq m. \end{cases}$

The integral can be easily calculated by setting $x = \cos t$;

(5) The zeros of C_n are the points
$$x_k = \cos \frac{2k-1}{2n} \pi, \quad k = 1, 2, \ldots, n.$$

So all the zeros of C_n are real, distinct and lie in $[-1, 1]$. They are symmetric with respect to the point 0.

(6) Let the polynomial $P_n(x) = a_0 x^n + a_1 x^{n-1} + \cdots + a_n$ satisfy
$$\max_{-1 \leq x \leq 1} |P_n(x)| = M .$$

Then for every $|x_0| > 1$
$$|P_n(x_0)| \leq M |C_n(x_0)| \leq M(|x_0| + \sqrt{x_0^2 - 1})^n .$$

PROOF. Assuming the inverse; i.e.
$$M < |P_n(x_0)| / |C_n(x_0)| , \tag{35.7}$$

then the polynomial
$$R_n(x) = P_n(x_0) C_n(x) / C_n(x_0) - P_n(x)$$
satisfies
$$R_n(x_i) = (-1)^i P_n(x_0) / C_n(x_0) - P_n(x_i), \quad x_i = \cos i\pi/n, \ i = 0, 1, \ldots, n.$$

Since $|P_n(x_i)| \leq M$ it follows that R_n changes the sign in every interval (x_i, x_{i+1}), $i = 0, 1, \ldots, n-1$. So the polynomial of nth degree R_n, has $n+1$ zeros $[R_n(x_0) = 0]$; i.e. $R_n \equiv 0$ and
$$P_n(x) = P_n(x_0) C_n(x) / C_n(x_0) . \tag{35.8}$$

Using $C_n(1) = 1$ the equality (35.8) gives $P_n(1) = P_n(x_0)/C_n(x_0)$, which contradicts (35.7);

(7) Let the integer numbers n and p, $p \leq n$, have the same evenness. Among all polynomials of the kind
$$a_0 x^n + \cdots + a_{n-p-1} x^{p+1} + x^p + a_{n-p+1} x^{p-1} + \cdots + a_n , \tag{35.9}$$

the polynomial $C_n/c_{p,n}$ deviates the least from zero in $[-1, 1]$, where the Chebyshev polynomial C_n is written as
$$C_n(x) = \sum_{i=0}^{n} c_{i,n} x^i .$$

If the evenness of n and p is different, then polynomial $C_{n-1}/c_{p,n-1}$ has such a property.

PROOF. Following NATANSON ([1949], p. 80) let us consider the case when n and p are even numbers. Assuming that there exists a polynomial P_n of the kind (35.9) such that for $x \in [-1, 1]$

$$|P_n(x)| < 1/|c_{p,n-1}|. \quad (35.10)$$

As p is an even number the polynomial $P_n(-x)$ is of the type (35.9) and it satisfies (35.10). Therefore,

$$|P_n(x) + P_n(-x)| < 2/|c_{p,n-1}|.$$

The polynomial of nth degree

$$R_n(x) = C_n(x)/c_{p,n} - [P_n(x) + P_n(-x)]/2$$

does not contain x^p and R_n has the form $R_n(x) = \sum_{k=0}^{n/2} a_k x^{2k}$, $a_{p/2} = 0$. Setting $Q_n(y) = \sum_{k=0}^{n/2} a_k y^k$ it follows that Q_n has at most $n/2$ terms. Hence Q_n has less than $n/2$ positive roots.

The last assertion follows from the fact that every function of the form $\sum_{i=1}^{s+1} b_i x^{\lambda_i}$, $\lambda_1 < \lambda_2 < \cdots < \lambda_{s+1}$, has at most s positive roots. The proof is trivial by induction using Rolle's theorem.

For $y_i = \cos^2 i\pi/n$,

$$Q_n(y_i) = R_n(\cos i\pi/n)$$
$$= C_n(\cos i\pi/n)/c_{p,n} - [P_n(\cos i\pi/n) + P_n(-\cos i\pi/n)]/2$$
$$= (-1)^i/c_{p,n} - [P_n(\cos i\pi/n) + P_n(-\cos i\pi/n)]/2 ,$$

i.e. $\operatorname{sgn} Q_n(y_i) = (-1)^i$. Hence Q_n changes its sign in the intervals (y_i, y_{i+1}), $i = 0, 1, \ldots, n/2 - 1$, or Q_n has $n/2$ positive zeros, which is impossible;

(8) If the algebraic polynomial P_n is of the kind (35.9), then

$$\max_{-1 \leq x \leq 1} |P_n(x)| \geq \begin{cases} \dfrac{p![(n-p)/2]!}{2^{p-1} n[(n+p)/2 - 1]!}, & n \text{ and } p \text{ have the same evenness}, \\ \dfrac{p![(n-p-1)/2]!}{2^{p-1}(n-1)[(n+p-3)/2]!}, & n \text{ and } p \text{ have different evenness}. \end{cases}$$

This property is a direct consequence of the property (7) and the representation of the coefficients of C_n in (35.5).

(9) If $P_n(x) = \sum_{i=0}^{n} a_i x^i$ then

$$|a_p| \leq \begin{cases} 2^{p-1} \dfrac{n[(n+p)/2 - 1]!}{p![(n-p)/2]!} \max_{-1 \leq x \leq 1} |P_n(x)|, & n - p \text{ is an even number}, \\ 2^{p-1} \dfrac{(n-1)[(n+p-3)/2]!}{p![(n-p-1)/2]!} \max_{-1 \leq x \leq 1} |P_n(x)|, & n - p \text{ is an odd number}. \end{cases}$$

The proof follows from the previous property.

(10) ERDÖS [1939] proved that the function cos nx has a maximal arc length in $[-\pi, \pi]$ among all the trigonometric polynomials of order n with a uniform norm equal to one. His conjecture that C_n satisfies

$$\sup\{l(f): f \in H_n, \max_{-1 \le x \le 1} |f(x)| \le 1\} = l(C_n),$$

was proved by BOIANOV [1982], where

$$l(f) = \int_{-1}^{1} [1 + f'^2(x)]^{1/2} \, dx$$

is the arc length of f in $[-1, 1]$.

For $|x| \le 1$ the algebraic polynomial of nth degree

$$U_n(x) = K_n \frac{\sin[(n+1)\cos^{-1} x]}{\sqrt{1 - x^2}}, \qquad (35.11)$$

is called the Chebyshev polynomial of the second kind.

The assertion that the expression (35.11) is indeed a polynomial of nth degree follows from the identity

$$\frac{\sin(n+1)\theta}{\sin \theta} = 2^n \cos^n \theta + \sum_{k=0}^{n-1} \lambda_k^{(n)} \cos^k \theta. \qquad (35.12)$$

The proof of (35.12) is based on

$$\sin(n+1)\theta = \sin n\theta \cos \theta + \cos n\theta \sin \theta,$$

$$\cos n\theta = 2^{n-1} \cos^n \theta + \sum_{k=0}^{n-1} \lambda_k^{(n)} \cos^k \theta.$$

The basic properties of the U_n are:
(1) for $K_n = \sqrt{2/\pi}$ the following relation is fulfilled:

$$\int_{-1}^{1} U_n(x) U_m(x) \sqrt{1 - x^2} \, dx = \begin{cases} 0, & n \ne m, \\ 1, & n = m. \end{cases}$$

(2) for $K_n = 2^{-n}$:
   (a) $U_n(x) = x^n + \cdots$;
   (b) $U_{n+2}(x) = x U_{n+1}(x) - U_n(x)/4$.
(3) for $K_n = 2^{-n}$ (KORKIN and ZOLOTAREV [1873])

$$\inf\left\{\int_{-1}^{1} |p(x)| \, dx: p(x) = x^n + \sum_{i=1}^{n} a_i x^{n-i}\right\} = \int_{-1}^{1} |U_n(x)| \, dx.$$

(4) $U_n[\cos k\pi/(n+1)] = 0$, $k = 1, 2, \ldots, n$.
(5) $C'_{n+1}(x) = K'_n U_n(x)$, where K'_n is a constant.
For details see NATANSON [1949].

36. Approximation of functions on a discrete point set

Let $K \subset [a, b]$ be a compact set and the functions $\{\varphi_i\}_{i=0}^{n}$ build a Chebyshev system on K. Theorem 25.3 shows that for every continuous function f on K the polynomial of the best uniform approximation

$$\varphi = \sum_{i=0}^{n} a_i \varphi_i, \qquad E_n(f)_K = \|\varphi - f\|_{C(K)},$$

satisfies

$$f(x_i) - \varphi(x_i) = \varepsilon(-1)^i \|f - \varphi\| = \varepsilon(-1)^i \max_{x \in K} |f(x) - \varphi(x)|,$$

$$i = 0, 1, \ldots, n+1, \quad \varepsilon = \pm 1,$$

where $x_0 < x_1 < \cdots < x_{n+1}$, $x_i \in K$.

This means that the polynomial φ is also the polynomial of the best approximation for f on the set $\{x_i\}_{i=0}^{n+1} \subset K$. If the points of alternation $\{x_i\}_{i=0}^{n+1}$ are known in advance, then the polynomial φ can be determined immediately by the linear system

$$\sum_{i=0}^{n} a_i \varphi_i(x_j) - \varepsilon(-1)^j E_n(f)_K = f(x_j), \quad 0, 1, \ldots, n+1, \qquad (36.1)$$

according to $n+2$ unknown quantities a_i, $i = 0, 1, \ldots, n$, and $\varepsilon E_n(f)_K$.

Unfortunately, the determination of the points of alternation in the system (36.1) can in many cases be done only numerically by successive approximations.

Let us consider the case when the compact $K = \{z_i\}_{i=0}^{m}$ consists of $m+1$ points in the complex plane. Assume that the functions $\{\varphi_i\}_{i=0}^{n}$ are linearly independent on K the problem is to find a polynomial $\sum_{i=0}^{n} a_i^* \varphi_i$ such that

$$E_n(f)_K = \min_{a_i} \max_{z \in K} \left| f(z) - \sum_{i=0}^{n} a_i \varphi_i(z) \right| = \max_{z \in K} \left| f(z) - \sum_{i=0}^{n} a_i^* \varphi_i(z) \right|. \qquad (36.2)$$

Setting $\varphi_k(z_i) = a_{ik}$, $a_k = u_k$, $f(z_i) = w_i$ the above problem reduces to finding an approximate solution $u^* = (u_0^*, u_1^*, \ldots, u_n^*)$ of the linear system

$$\begin{aligned}
(a_0, u) &= a_{00} u_0 + a_{01} u_1 + \cdots + a_{0n} u_n = w_0, \\
(a_1, u) &= a_{10} u_0 + a_{11} u_1 + \cdots + a_{1n} u_n = w_1, \\
&\vdots \\
(a_m, u) &= a_{m0} u_0 + a_{m1} u_1 + \cdots + a_{mn} u_n = w_m,
\end{aligned} \qquad (36.3)$$

$m = n + 1$, which satisfies

$$\rho^* = \min_{u} \max_{0 \le i \le m} |(a_i, u) - w_i| = \max_{0 \le i \le m} |(a_i, u^*) - w_i|.$$

The solution u^* is called the best approximation of the system (36.3). Every point $u^0 = (u_0^0, u_1^0, \ldots, u_n^0)$ that satisfies

$$A = |(a_0, u^0) - w_0| = |(a_1, u^0) - w_1| = \cdots = |(a_m, u^0) - w_m|$$

is called an *A*-equidistant point and *A* is the *A*-distance between the points u and w.

If in the system (36.3) $m = n + 1$, then the best approximation of the system (36.3) coincides with one of the equidistant points of this system and in this connection DZJADIK ([1974], p. 64), proved the following theorem.

THEOREM 36.1. *Let the system* (36.3) *be inconsistent and for every subsystem*

$$(a_k, u) = w_k, \quad k = 0, 1, \ldots, j-1, j+1, \ldots, n+1, \tag{36.4}$$

its determinant of coefficients satisfies $D^j \neq 0$ and let (36.4) *have a solution $u^j = (u_0^j, u_1^j, \ldots, u_n^j)$. Then:*

(1) *For $j = 0, 1, \ldots, n+1$ the following relation is fulfilled*

$$(a_j, u^j) - w_j = \frac{(-1)^{j+1}}{D^j} \sum_{\nu=0}^{n+1} (-1)^\nu w_\nu D^\nu ,$$

where

$$D^j = \begin{vmatrix} a_{00} & a_{01} & \cdots & a_{0n} \\ \vdots & \vdots & & \vdots \\ a_{j-1,0} & a_{j-1,1} & \cdots & a_{j-1,n} \\ a_{j+1,0} & a_{j+1,1} & \cdots & a_{j+1,n} \\ \vdots & \vdots & & \vdots \\ a_{n+1,0} & a_{n+1,1} & \cdots & a_{n+1,n} \end{vmatrix} ;$$

(2) *For all real numbers k_j, $j = 0, 1, \ldots, n+1$, that satisfy*

$$\sum_{\nu=0}^{n+1} |D^\nu| \exp(ik_\nu) \neq 0 ,$$

the point $u = (u_0, u_1, \ldots, u_n)$ defined by

$$u = \rho \sum_{j=0}^{n+1} \frac{u^j \exp(ik_j)}{|(a_j, u^j) - w_j|} = \rho \frac{\sum_{j=0}^{n+1} |D^j| u^j \exp(ik_j)}{|\sum_{j=0}^{n+1} (-1)^j D^j w_j|} , \tag{36.5}$$

where

$$\rho \equiv \left(\sum_{j=0}^{n+1} \frac{\exp(ik_j)}{|(a_j, u^j) - w_j|} \right)^{-1} = \frac{|\sum_{j=0}^{n+1} (-1)^j D^j w_j|}{\sum_{j=0}^{n+1} |D^j| \exp(ik_j)} , \tag{36.6}$$

is the equidistant point for the system (36.3) *and $|\rho|$ is the A-distance between the points u and w;*

(3) *Vice versa, every A-equidistant point u of the system* (36.3) *can be represented in the form* (36.5). *The numbers k_j, in particular, can take the form*

$$k_j = \arg[(a_j, u) - w_j] - \arg[(a_j, u^j) - w_j]$$

and the number ρ computed by these k_j using (36.6) *is positive.*

Uniform approximation

PROOF. As the coordinates u_k^j of the solution u^j are equal to

$$u_k^j = \frac{\begin{vmatrix} a_{00} & \cdots & a_{0,k-1} & w_0 & a_{0,k+1} & \cdots & a_{0n} \\ \vdots & & \vdots & \vdots & \vdots & & \vdots \\ a_{j-1,0} & \cdots & a_{j-1,k-1} & w_{j-1} & a_{j-1,k+1} & \cdots & a_{j-1,n} \\ a_{j+1,0} & \cdots & a_{j+1,k-1} & w_{j+1} & a_{j+1,k+1} & \cdots & a_{j+1,n} \\ \vdots & & \vdots & \vdots & \vdots & & \vdots \\ a_{n+1,0} & \cdots & a_{n+1,k-1} & w_{n+1} & a_{n+1,k+1} & \cdots & a_{n+1,n} \end{vmatrix}}{\begin{vmatrix} a_{00} & \cdots & a_{0,k-1} & a_{0,k} & a_{0,k+1} & \cdots & a_{0n} \\ \vdots & & \vdots & \vdots & \vdots & & \vdots \\ a_{j-1,0} & \cdots & a_{j-1,k-1} & a_{j-1,k} & a_{j-1,k+1} & \cdots & a_{j-1,n} \\ a_{j+1,0} & \cdots & a_{j+1,k-1} & a_{j+1,k} & a_{j+1,k+1} & \cdots & a_{j+1,n} \\ \vdots & & \vdots & \vdots & \vdots & & \vdots \\ a_{n+1,0} & \cdots & a_{n+1,k-1} & a_{n+1,k} & a_{n+1,k+1} & \cdots & a_{n+1,n} \end{vmatrix}}$$

$$= \frac{\sum_{\nu=0,\nu\neq j}^{n+1} w_\nu A_{\nu k}^j}{D^j} = \frac{\sum_{\nu=0,\nu\neq j}^{n+1} w_\nu (-1)^{\nu+k} \operatorname{sgn}(j-\nu) M_{\nu k}^j}{D^j},$$

where $A_{\nu k}^j$ and $M_{\nu k}^j$ are the cofactor and minor of the element $a_{\nu k}$ in the determinant D^j. Taking into account the fact that

$$M_{\nu k}^j = M_{jk}^\nu, \quad A_{\nu k}^j = (-1)^{\nu+k} \operatorname{sgn}(j-\nu) M_{\nu k}^j = -(-1)^{\nu+j} A_{jk}^\nu,$$

$$j = 0, 1, \ldots, n+1,$$

it follows that

$$(a_j, u^j) - w_j = \sum_{k=0}^n a_{jk} u_k^j - w_j = \sum_{k=0}^n a_{jk} \frac{\sum_{\nu=0,\nu\neq j}^{n+1} w_\nu A_{\nu k}^j}{D^j} - w_j$$

$$= \frac{1}{D^j} \sum_{k=0}^n a_{jk} \sum_{\nu=0,\nu\neq j}^{n+1} w_\nu (-1)^{\nu+j+1} A_{jk}^\nu - w_j$$

$$= \frac{(-1)^{j+1}}{D^j} \sum_{\nu=0,\nu\neq j}^{n+1} w_\nu (-1)^\nu \sum_{k=0}^n a_{jk} A_{jk}^\nu - w_j$$

$$= \frac{(-1)^{j+1}}{D^j} \sum_{\nu=0,\nu\neq j}^{n+1} (-1)^\nu w_\nu D^\nu - w_j = \frac{(-1)^{j+1}}{D^j} \sum_{\nu=0}^{n+1} (-1)^\nu w_\nu D^\nu$$

and the assertion (1) of the theorem is proved.

Let the point u be the equidistant point for the system (36.3). Because the system is inconsistent there exists a number $\rho > 0$ such that

$$(a_j, u) - w_j = \rho b_j, \quad j = 0, 1, \ldots, n+1, \tag{36.7}$$

where $b_j = \exp\{i \arg[(a_j, u) - w_j]\}$. The number b_j can be represented in the form

$$b_j = \frac{[(a_j, u^j) - w_j] \exp\{i \arg[(a_j, u) - w_j] - i \arg[(a_j, u^j) - w_j]\}}{|\arg[(a_j, u^j) - w_j]|}$$

$$= \frac{[(a_j, u^j) - w_j] \exp(ik_j)}{|\arg[(a_j, u^j) - w_j]|}.$$

From the system (36.7) it follows that

$$\rho = -\sum_{j=0}^{n+1} (-1)^j w_j D^j \bigg/ \sum_{j=0}^{n+1} (-1)^j b_j D^j$$

and therefore for $j = 0, 1, \ldots, n+1$,

$$b_j D^j = D^j \frac{[(a_j, u^j) - w_j] \exp(ik_j)}{|\arg[(a_j, u^j) - w_j]|}$$

$$= (-1)^{j+1} \sum_{\nu=0}^{n+1} (-1)^\nu w_\nu D^\nu \frac{\exp(ik_j)}{|(a_j, u^j) - w_j|}, \qquad (36.8)$$

$$\rho = \left(\sum_{j=0}^{n+1} \frac{\exp(ik_j)}{|(a_j, u^j) - w_j|} \right)^{-1}.$$

If some point u' has the form

$$u' = \rho \sum_{j=0}^{n+1} \frac{u^j \exp(ik_j)}{|(a_j, u^j) - w_j|}, \qquad (36.9)$$

then $u = u'$. Indeed the solution u^j satisfies

$$(a_j, u^i) = w_j, \quad i \neq j,$$

$$(a_j, u^j) \neq 0, \quad j = 0, 1, \ldots, n+1,$$

and the definition of u' is correct. From (36.8) and (36.9) it follows for all $j = 0, 1, \ldots, n+1$, that

$$(a_j, u') - w_j = \rho \sum_{\nu=0}^{n+1} \frac{(a_j, u^\nu) \exp(ik_\nu)}{|(a_\nu, u^\nu) - w_\nu|} - \rho \sum_{\nu=0}^{n+1} \frac{w_j^\nu \exp(ik_\nu)}{|(a_\nu, u^\nu) - w_\nu|}$$

$$= \rho \frac{[(a_j, u^j) - w_j] \exp(ik_j)}{|(a_j, u^j) - w_j|} = \rho b_j. \qquad (36.10)$$

Subtracting the equalities (36.10) from (36.7) the result is

$$(a_j, u - u') = a_{j0}(u_0 - u'_0) + a_{j1}(u_1 - u'_1) + \cdots + a_{jn}(u_n - u'_n) = 0,$$

$$j = 0, 1, \ldots, n+1.$$

Since $D^{n+1} \neq 0$ it follows that $u \equiv u'$ and the assertion (3) of the theorem is proved.

If the condition $\sum_{\nu=0}^{n+1}|D^\nu|\exp(ik_\nu)\neq 0$ is fulfilled, then the point u defined by (36.5) satisfies

$$(a_j, u) - w_j = \rho b_j, \quad \text{where } b_j = \frac{[(a_j, u^j) - w_j]\exp(ik_j)}{|(a_j, u^j) - w_j|}.$$

It leads to the equalities

$$|(a_0, u) - w_0| = |(a_1, u) - w_1| = \cdots = |(a_{n+1}, u) - w_{n+1}|;$$

i.e. the point u is the equidistant point of the system (36.3). □

The quantity

$$\rho = \left(\sum_{j=0}^{n+1} \frac{\exp(ik_j)}{|(a_j, u^j) - w_j|}\right)^{-1}$$

takes its minimum value when $\exp(ik_0) = \exp(ik_1) = \cdots = \exp(ik_{n+1})$. This means that under the conditions of Theorem 36.1 the best approximation ρ^* and the best solution u^* of the system (36.3) when $m = n+1$ are given by

$$u^* = \rho^* \sum_{j=0}^{n+1} \frac{u^j}{|(a_j, u^j) - w_j|} = \frac{\sum_{j=0}^{n+1}|D^j|u^j}{\sum_{j=0}^{n+1}|D^j|},$$

where

$$\rho^* \equiv \left(\sum_{j=0}^{n+1} \frac{1}{|(a_j, u^j) - w_j|}\right)^{-1} = \frac{|\sum_{j=0}^{n+1}(-1)^j D^j w_j|}{\sum_{j=0}^{n+1}|D^j|}.$$

Going back to the problem (36.2) the Theorem 36.1 takes the form (DZJADIK [1977], p. 72, Theorem 3)

THEOREM 36.2. *Let the function f be defined on the set $K = \{z_i\}_{i=0}^{n+1}$, where z_i are different points on the plane and the functions $\{\varphi_i\}_{i=0}^n$ build the Chebyshev system on K. If f is different from any polynomial $P_n = \sum_{i=0}^n a_i\varphi_i$ on K, then:*

(1) *The polynomial $P_n^* = \sum_{i=0}^n a_i^*\varphi_i$ that satisfies the conditions (36.2) can be determined by the equalities*

$$P_n^*(z) = E_n(f)_K \sum_{j=0}^{n+1} \frac{P_{nj}(z)}{|P_{nj}(z_j) - f(z_j)|} = \frac{\sum_{j=0}^{n+1}|D^j|P_{nj}(z)}{\sum_{j=0}^{n+1}|D^j|},$$

where the polynomial $P_{nj} = \sum_{i=0}^n a_{ni}\varphi_i$, $j = 0, 1, \ldots, n$, interpolates the function f at the points z_k, $k = 0, 1, \ldots, j-1, j+1, \ldots, n+1$, and

$$P_{nj}(z_j) - f(z_j) = \frac{(-1)^{j+1}}{D^j}\sum_{\nu=0}^{n+1}(-1)^\nu f(z_\nu)D^\nu, \qquad (36.11)$$

where

$$D^j = \begin{vmatrix} \varphi_0(z_0) & \varphi_1(z_0) & \cdots & \varphi_n(z_0) \\ \vdots & \vdots & & \vdots \\ \varphi_0(z_{j-1}) & \varphi_1(z_{j-1}) & \cdots & \varphi_n(z_{j-1}) \\ \varphi_0(z_{j+1}) & \varphi_1(z_{j+1}) & \cdots & \varphi_n(z_{j+1}) \\ \vdots & \vdots & & \vdots \\ \varphi_0(z_{n+1}) & \varphi_1(z_{n+1}) & \cdots & \varphi_n(z_{n+1}) \end{vmatrix};$$

(2) *The best approximation $E_n(f)_K$ can be computed by*

$$E_n(f)_K = \left(\sum_{j=0}^{n+1} \frac{1}{|P_{nj}(z_j) - f(z_j)|} \right)^{-1} = \frac{|\sum_{j=0}^{n+1} (-1)^j D^j f(z_j)|}{\sum_{j=0}^{n+1} |D^j|}.$$

From (36.11) it follows that if $Q_n = \sum_{i=0}^{n} b_i \varphi_i$ is an arbitrary polynomial, then

$$\frac{(-1)^{j+1}}{D^j} \sum_{\nu=0}^{n+1} (-1)^\nu Q_n(z_\nu) D^\nu = 0$$

and therefore

$$E_n(f)_K = \frac{|\sum_{j=0}^{n+1} (-1)^j D^j [f(z_j) - Q_n(z_j)]|}{\sum_{j=0}^{n+1} |D^j|}. \tag{36.12}$$

As an application of the results in this section let us consider the uniform approximation of the functions $f_1(z) = |z|$ and $f_2(z) = e^z$ by algebraic polynomials $p(f_1)$ and $p(f_2)$ of seventh degree on the discrete set K of 13 points, which are given in Fig. 36.1 by the symbol ∎.

Let $U = \{z: z = x + iy, -1 \leq x, y \leq 1\}$. Then

$$\max_{z \in K} |f_1(z) - p(f_1; z)| \leq 0.5414 \ldots, \quad \max_{z \in K} |f_2(z) - p(f_2; z)| \leq 0.00007 \ldots,$$

$$\max_{z \in U} |f_1(z) - p(f_1; z)| \leq 0.5547 \ldots, \quad \max_{z \in U} |f_1(z) - p(f_1; z)| \leq 0.00018 \ldots.$$

The graphs of the functions

$$|f_1(z) - p(f_1; z)|, \quad |f_2(z) - p(f_2; z)|$$

on the unit square U are given on the Figs. 36.2 and 36.3, respectively.

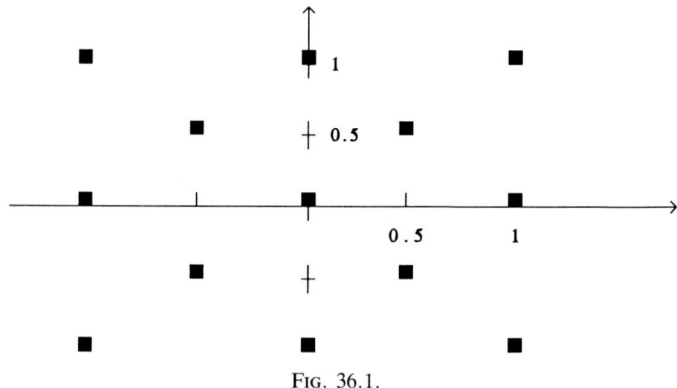

Fig. 36.1.

Section 36 Uniform approximation 353

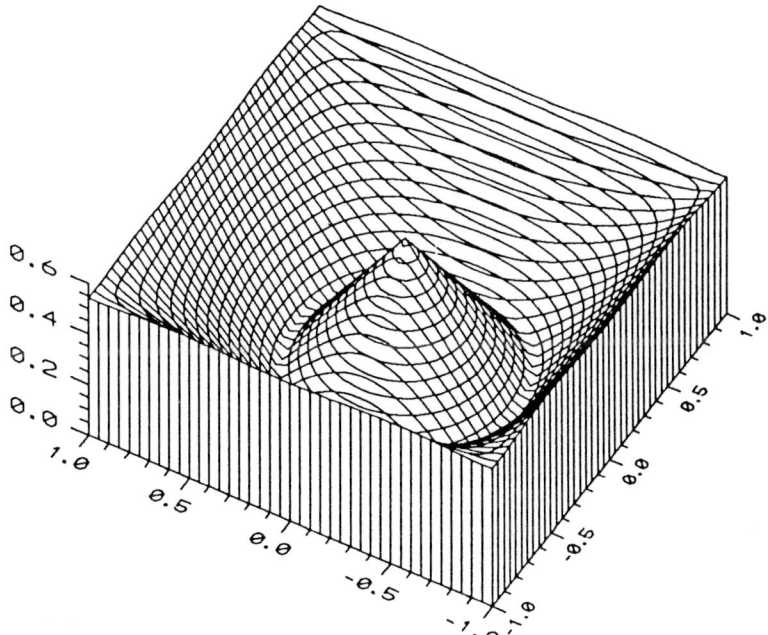

Fig. 36.2. Graph of the function $|f_1(z) - p(f_1; z)|$.

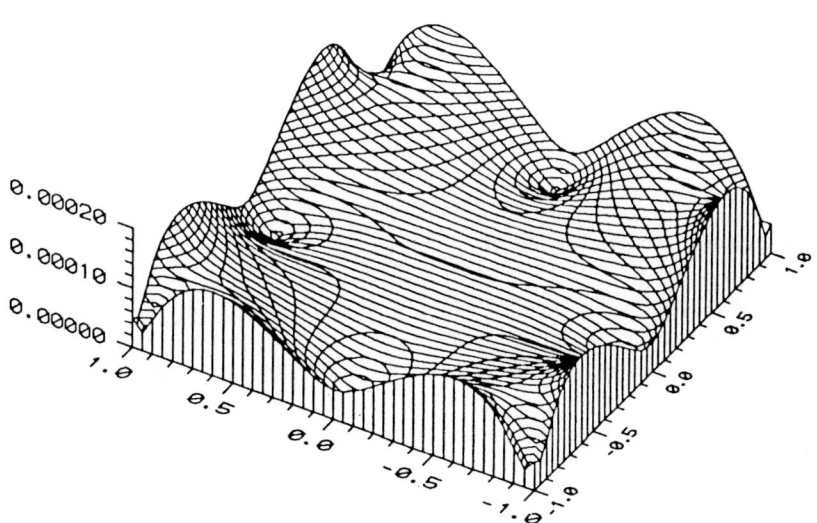

Fig. 36.3. Graph of the function $|f_2(z) - p(f_2; z)|$.

On the real axis, when $a \leq x_0 < x_1 < \cdots < x_{n+1} \leq b$, Theorem 25.5 gives that $\operatorname{sgn} D^j = \operatorname{sgn} D^i$ for $0 \leq i, j \leq n+1$. Using this fact the expression for the best approximation $E_n(f)_K$ in Theorem 36.2 takes the form

$$E_n(f)_K = \left(\sum_{j=0}^{n+1} \frac{1}{|P_{nj}(x_j) - f(x_j)|} \right)^{-1} = \frac{|\sum_{j=0}^{n+1} (-1)^j |D^j| f(x_j)|}{\sum_{j=0}^{n+1} |D^j|}. \qquad (36.13)$$

REMARK 36.1. In the case of algebraic polynomials $\varphi_i(x) = x^i$, $i = 0, 1, \ldots, n$,

$$D^j = \begin{vmatrix} 1 & x_0 & x_0^2 & \cdots & x_0^n \\ \vdots & \vdots & \vdots & & \vdots \\ 1 & x_{j-1} & x_{j-1}^2 & \cdots & x_{j-1}^n \\ 1 & x_{j+1} & x_{j+1}^2 & \cdots & x_{j+1}^n \\ \vdots & \vdots & \vdots & & \vdots \\ 1 & x_{n+1} & x_{n+1}^2 & \cdots & x_{n+1}^n \end{vmatrix} = \prod_{\substack{k > i \\ k, i \neq j}} (x_k - x_i).$$

Setting $d_{nj} = 1/\prod_{k=0, k \neq j}^{n+1} (x_j - x_k)$ and using the property

$$\operatorname{sgn} d_{nj} = -\operatorname{sgn} d_{n, j+1},$$

the best approximation $E_n(f)_K$ defined by (36.1) or (36.13) takes the form (see BEREZIN and JIDKOV [1966], p. 297)

$$E_n(f)_K = \left| \sum_{j=0}^{n+1} d_{nj} f(x_j) \right| \bigg/ \sum_{j=0}^{n+1} |d_{nj}|. \qquad (36.14)$$

If $\operatorname{sgn} f(x_i) = \varepsilon(-1)^i$, $\varepsilon = \pm 1$, $i = 0, 1, \ldots, n+1$, then from (36.14) it follows that

$$E_n(f)_K = \sum_{j=0}^{n+1} |d_{nj}| |f(x_j)| \bigg/ \sum_{j=0}^{n+1} |d_{nj}|$$

and

$$\min_{0 \leq i \leq n+1} |f(x_i)| \leq E_n(f)_K \leq \max_{0 \leq i \leq n+1} |f(x_i)|.$$

37. The discrete Remez algorithm

Using the ideas of VALLEE-POUSSIN [1919], REMEZ [1934] later gave an efficient algorithm for the numerical determination of the polynomial of the best uniform approximation. A discrete variant of this algorithm will be given below.

Let the function f be continuous on $K = [a, b]$ and the functions $\{\varphi_i\}_{i=0}^n$ build a Chebyshev system on K. Let the point set $K_{\delta(m)} = \{x_i\}_{i=0}^m$, $K_{\delta(m)} \subseteq K$, satisfy the condition

$$\operatorname{dist}(K, K_{\delta(m)}) = \max_{x \in K} \min_{y \in K_{\delta(m)}} |x - y| = \delta(m).$$

Let us denote by P_K and $P_{K_{\delta(m)}}$ the polynomials of the best approximation of the function f on K and $K_{\delta(m)}$; i.e.

$$E_n(f)_K = \min_{c_i} \max_{x \in K} \left| f(x) - \sum_{i=0}^n c_i \varphi_i(x) \right| = \max_{x \in K} |f(x) - P_K(x)|,$$

$$E_n(f)_{K_{\delta(m)}} = \min_{c_i} \max_{x \in K_{\delta(m)}} \left| f(x) - \sum_{i=0}^n c_i \varphi_i(x) \right| = \max_{x \in K_{\delta(m)}} |f(x) - P_{K_{\delta(m)}}(x)|.$$

If for the system $\{\varphi_i\}_{i=0}^n$ there exists a constant $\gamma = \gamma(n, K)$ such that every polynomial $\sum_{i=0}^n c_i \varphi_i$ satisfies

$$\left| \left(\sum_{i=0}^n c_i \varphi_i(x) \right)' \right| \leq \gamma(n, K) \max_{x \in K} \left| \sum_{i=0}^n c_i \varphi_i(x) \right|, \quad x \in K, \tag{37.1}$$

then

$$E_n(f)_K \leq \max_{x \in K} |f(x) - P_{K_{\delta(m)}}(x)|$$
$$\leq E_n(f)_K + \omega(f; \delta(m)) + \delta(m)\gamma[L + E_n(f)_K]/[1 - \delta(m)\gamma].$$
(37.2)

In particular, if

$$\varphi_i(x) = \begin{cases} x^i, & \text{then } \gamma = 2n^2/(b-a), \\ c_i \sin ix + d_i \cos ix, & \text{then } \gamma = n; \end{cases}$$

(37.1) is called Markov and Bernstein inequality in the first and second case, respectively.

The equality (37.2), proved below, shows that for small $\delta(m) > 0$ the polynomial $P_{K_{\delta(m)}}$ can be used instead of P_K. The second Remez algorithm (REMEZ [1969], Chapter 2, BEREZIN and JIDKOV [1966], p. 294) allows us to determine the polynomial $P_{K_{\delta(m)}}$ in finite steps. The algorithm is:

Step 1. Choose the set $K_0 \subseteq K_{\delta(m)}$, $K_0 = \{x_i^0\}_{i=0}^{n+1}$. Build the polynomial $P_{K_0}(x) = \sum_{i=0}^n a_i^0 \varphi_i(x_j)$ of the best approximation for f on K_0 and compute the best approximation $E_n(f)_{K_0}$, solving the linear system

$$\sum_{i=0}^n a_i^0 \varphi_i(x_j^0) - \varepsilon(-1)^j E_n(f)_{K_0} = f(x_j^0), \quad \varepsilon = \pm 1, \ j = 0, 1, \ldots, n+1.$$

Step 2. Compute $h_i = f(x_i) - P_{K_0}(x_i)$, $i = 0, 1, \ldots, m$.
Step 3. If $\max_{0 \leq i \leq m} |h_i| \leq E_n(f)_{K_0}$ then $P_{K_0} \equiv P_{K_{\delta(m)}}$. Stop.
Step 4. If $\max_{0 \leq i \leq m} |h_i| = |h_j| > E_n(f)_{K_0}$ then build the set $K_1 \subseteq K_{\delta(m)}$, $K_1 = \{x_i^1\}_{i=0}^{n+1}$, such that $x_i^0 \in K_1$ and for $i = 0, 1, \ldots, n$,

$$\text{sgn}[f(x_i^1) - P_{K_0}(x_i^1)] = -\text{sgn}[f(x_{i+1}^1) - P_{K_0}(x_{i+1}^1)].$$

Step 5. Go to Step 1, substituting K_0 by K_1.

The algorithm described generates the point sets $K_0, K_1, K_2, \ldots$, the polynomials $P_{K_0}, P_{K_1}, P_{K_2}, \ldots$ and the numbers $E_n(f)_{K_0}, E_n(f)_{K_1}, E_n(f)_{K_2}, \ldots$.

Let us prove the following inequalities:
$$E_n(f)_{K_0} < E_n(f)_{K_1} < E_n(f)_{K_2} < \cdots.$$

From (36.12), (36.13) it follows that

$$E_n(f)_{K_1} = \frac{|\sum_{i=0}^{n+1} (-1)^i D^i [f(x_i^1) - P_{K_0}(x_i^1)]|}{\sum_{i=0}^{n+1} |D^i|} = \frac{\sum_{i=0}^{n+1} |D^i| |f(x_i^1) - P_{K_0}(x_i^1)|}{\sum_{i=0}^{n+1} |D^i|}$$

$$> \frac{\sum_{i=0}^{n+1} |D^i| |f(x_i^0) - P_{K_0}(x_i^0)|}{\sum_{i=0}^{n+1} |D^i|} = E_n(f)_{K_0},$$

using the fact that the D^i do not change sign (see Theorem 25.5).

Using the monotonicity of the algorithm it is also proved that the algorithm stops after a finite number of steps because the number of the point sets K_i is finite.

Let us now prove the estimation (37.2). Let

$$\max_{x \in K} |f(x)| = L, \quad \max_{x \in K} |P_{K_{\delta(m)}}(x)| = |P_{K_{\delta(m)}}(x^*)| = M_{\delta(m)}.$$

There exists a point $y \in K_{\delta(m)}$ such that $|y - x^*| \leq \delta(m)$ and

$$P_{K_{\delta(m)}}(x^*) - P_{K_{\delta(m)}}(y) = (x^* - y) P'_{K_{\delta(m)}}(\xi), \qquad (37.3)$$

where ξ lies between x^* and y.

For $x_j \in K_{\delta(m)}$ the following relations are fulfilled:

$$|P_{K_{\delta(m)}}(x_j)| = |P_{K_{\delta(m)}}(x_j) - f(x_j) + f(x_j)| \leq E_n(f)_{K_{\delta(m)}} + L \leq E_n(f)_K + L$$

and from (37.1), (37.3) it follows that

$$M_{\delta(m)} - L - E_n(f)_K \leq P_{K_{\delta(m)}}(x^*) - P_{K_{\delta(m)}}(y) \leq \delta(m) \gamma M_{\delta(m)}.$$

So if $\delta(m)\gamma < 1$ then $M_{\delta(m)} \leq [L + E_n(f)_K]/[1 - \delta(m)\gamma]$ and for an arbitrary point $x \in K$ the last inequality and (37.3) give the result that there exists a point $y \in K_{\delta(m)}$ for which

$$|P_{K_{\delta(m)}}(x) - P_{K_{\delta(m)}}(y)| \leq \delta(m)\gamma [L + E_n(f)_K]/[1 - \delta(m)\gamma].$$

Finally, let

$$\max_{x \in K} |f(x) - P_{K_{\delta(m)}}(x)| = |f(\bar{x}) - P_{K_{\delta(m)}}(\bar{x})|$$

and $x_j \in K_{\delta(m)}$ is such that $|\bar{x} - x_j| \leq \delta(m)$. Then

$$E_n(f)_K \leq |f(\bar{x}) - P_{K_{\delta(m)}}(\bar{x})|$$
$$\leq |f(x_j) - P_{K_{\delta(m)}}(x_j)| + |f(\bar{x}) - f(x_j)| + |P_{K_{\delta(m)}}(\bar{x}) - P_{K_{\delta(m)}}(x_j)|$$
$$\leq E_n(f)_K + \omega(f; \delta(m)) + \delta(m)\gamma [L + E_n(f)_K]/[1 - \delta(m)\gamma]. \quad \square$$

38. The second Remez algorithm

In the case of approximation of a continuous function f on the compact set $K \subseteq [a, b]$ by means of polynomials $\Sigma_{i=0}^n c_i \varphi_i$ built by the Chebyshev system $\{\varphi_i\}_{i=0}^n$ on K, Theorem 25.3 plays an important role. Using this theorem, which characterizes the polynomial of the best uniform approximation in the linear case, REMEZ ([1934]; [1969], p. 49) suggested two algorithms for the approximate solution of the problem.

Following DZJADIK ([1977], p. 74), the second Remez algorithm will be given (see also CHENEY [1966], p. 95).

Step 1. Choose the point set $K_1 \subseteq K$, $K_1 = \{x_0^1 < x_1^1 < \cdots < x_{n+1}^1\}$. Using the linear system

$$\sum_{i=0}^n a_i^1 \varphi_i(x_j^1) - \varepsilon(-1)^j \underline{E}_n^{(1)} = f(x_j^1), \quad \varepsilon = \pm 1, \ j = 0, 1, \ldots, n+1,$$

compute the polynomial $P_n^{(1)} = \Sigma_{i=0}^n a_i^{(1)} \varphi_i$ of the best approximation of the function f on K_1. Set

$$r^1(x) = f(x) - P_n^{(1)}(x),$$

$$|r^1(x_k^{(1)})| = \underline{E}_n^{(1)}, \quad k = 0, 1, \ldots, n+1,$$

$$\max_{x \in K} |r^1(x)| = \bar{E}_n^{(1)}.$$

Step 2. If $\bar{E}_n^{(1)} = \underline{E}_n^{(1)}$ then by the Chebyshev Theorem 25.3 $P_n^{(1)}$ is the polynomial of the best approximation on K. Stop.

Step 3. If $\bar{E}_n^{(1)} > \underline{E}_n^{(1)}$ then there exists a point $x^* \in K$ such that $|r^1(x^*)| = \bar{E}_n^{(1)}$ and denote by $E_n(f)_K$ the best approximation of f on K

$$\underline{E}_n^{(1)} \leq E_n(f)_K < \bar{E}_n^{(1)}.$$

Step 4. Build a new point set $K_2 \subseteq K$, $K_2 = \{x_0^2 < x_1^2 < \cdots < x_{n+1}^2\}$ such that:

$$\operatorname{sgn} r^1(x_{k+1}^{(2)}) = -\operatorname{sgn} r^1(x_k^{(2)}), \quad k = 0, 1, \ldots, n,$$

$$|r^1(x_k^{(2)})| \geq \underline{E}_n^{(1)}, \quad \max_k |r^1(x_k^{(2)})| = \bar{E}_n^{(1)}, \quad k = 0, 1, \ldots, n+1.$$

These conditions can be satisfied by replacing in K_1 only one point by the point x^*. The algorithm works more effectively if the differences $|r^1(x_k^{(2)})| - \underline{E}_n^{(1)}$ are as large as possible—see the proof of Theorem 38.2.

Step 5. Go to Step 1 changing everywhere the index 1 by 2.

The described algorithm produces the following sequences:

of polynomials $\{P_n^{(i)}\}_{i=0,1,\ldots}$;

of functions $\{r^i = f - P_n^{(i)}\}_{i=0,1,\ldots}$;

of point sets $\{K_i = (x_0^i < x_1^i < \cdots < x_{n+1}^i)\}_{i=0,1,\ldots}$, $K_i \subseteq K$;

of numbers $\{\underline{E}_n^{(i)} = |r^i(x_k^{(i)})|\}_{i=0,1,\ldots}$, $\{\bar{E}_n^{(i)} = \max_{x \in K} |r^i(x)|\}_{i=0,1,\ldots}$.

They satisfy

$$\text{sgn } r^i(x_{k+1}^{(i+1)}) = -\text{sgn } r^i(x_k^{(i+1)}), \quad k = 0, 1, \ldots, n,$$

$$|r^i(x_k^{(i+1)})| \geq \underline{E}_n^{(i)}, \quad \max_k |r^i(x_k^{(i+1)})| = \bar{E}_n^{(i)}, \quad k = 0, 1, \ldots, n+1,$$

$$\underline{E}_n^{(i)} \leq E_n(f)_K < \bar{E}_n^{(i)}. \tag{38.1}$$

THEOREM 38.1. *Let f be a continuous function on the interval $[a, b]$ and $K = \{x_i\}_{i=0}^{n+1}$, $K \subseteq [a, b]$. Let*

$$E_n(f)_K = \min_{c_i} \max_{x \in K} \left| f(x) - \sum_{i=0}^n c_i \varphi_i(x) \right|$$

be the best approximation of f on K. Then for every $\varepsilon > 0$ there exists a $\delta > 0$ such that the inequality $\min_{i \neq j} |x_i - x_j| < \delta$ implies $E_n(f)_K < \varepsilon$.

PROOF. Assuming that the theorem is not true, then there exists a sequence of point sets $\{K_k = (x_i^{(k)})\}_{i=0}^{n+1}$, $k = 1, 2, \ldots$, for which

$$\lim_{k \to \infty} \min_{i \neq j} |x_i^{(k)} - x_j^{(k)}| = 0 \tag{38.2}$$

and $E_n(f)_{K^k} \geq \varepsilon$ for all $k = 1, 2, \ldots$. Choosing from the sequence $\{K^k\}_{k=1}^\infty$ the subsequence $\{K^{k_j}\}_{j=1}^\infty$ such that

$$\lim_{j \to \infty} x_i^{(k_j)} = x_i^0, \quad i = 0, 1, \ldots, n+1,$$

it follows from (38.2) that the different points among $\{x_i^0\}_{i=0}^{n+1}$ are less than $n + 2$. Suppose they are $K^0 = \{x_i^0\}_{i=0}^m$, $m \leq n + 1$. By Theorem 1.2 there is a polynomial $P_n^0 = \sum_{i=0}^n c_i^0 \varphi_i$, which interpolates the function f at the points K^0. By virtue of the continuity of f it follows that for large enough j

$$|P_n^0(x_i^{(k_j)}) - f(x_i^{(k_j)})| < \varepsilon, \tag{38.3}$$

because for every point $x_i^{(k_j)}$ there exists an arbitrarily close point from K^0. The inequality (38.3) contradicts the assumption. □

THEOREM 38.2 (REMEZ [1934]). *Let the function f be continuous on the compact $K \subseteq [a, b]$. Under the notation used for the description of the algorithm (Steps 1–5) there exist numbers $A > 0$, $0 < q < 1$, such that*

$$0 \leq \bar{E}_n^{(k)} - E_n(f)_K \leq \bar{E}_n^{(k)} - \underline{E}_n^{(k)} \leq Aq^k, \quad k = 1, 2, \ldots.$$

PROOF. By (36.13) and the inequalities (38.1) it follows that

$$\underline{E}_n^{(i)} = \frac{|\sum_{j=0}^{n+1} (-1)^j D_i^j [f(x_j^{(i)}) - P_n^{(i-1)}(x_j^{(i)})]|}{\sum_{j=0}^{n+1} |D_i^j|}$$

$$= \frac{|\sum_{j=0}^{n+1} (-1)^j D_i^j r^{i-1}(x_j^{(i)})|}{\sum_{j=0}^{n+1} |D_i^j|} = \frac{\sum_{j=0}^{n+1} |D_i^j| |r^{i-1}(x_j^{(i)})|}{\sum_{j=0}^{n+1} |D_i^j|},$$

where D_i^j is the determinant

$$D_i^j = \begin{vmatrix} \varphi_0(x_0^{(i)}) & \varphi_1(x_0^{(i)}) & \cdots & \varphi_n(x_0^{(i)}) \\ \vdots & \vdots & & \vdots \\ \varphi_0(x_{j-1}^{(i)}) & \varphi_1(x_{j-1}^{(i)}) & \cdots & \varphi_n(x_{j-1}^{(i)}) \\ \varphi_0(x_{j+1}^{(i)}) & \varphi_1(x_{j+1}^{(i)}) & \cdots & \varphi_n(x_{j+1}^{(i)}) \\ \vdots & \vdots & & \vdots \\ \varphi_0(x_{n+1}^{(i)}) & \varphi_1(x_{n+1}^{(i)}) & \cdots & \varphi_n(x_{n+1}^{(i)}) \end{vmatrix}.$$

Therefore

$$\underline{E}_n^{(i)} - \underline{E}_n^{(i-1)} = \frac{\sum_{j=0}^{n+1} |D_i^j| |r^{i-1}(x_j^{(i)})|}{\sum_{j=0}^{n+1} |D_i^j|} - \underline{E}_n^{(i-1)}$$

$$\geq \frac{\sum_{j=0}^{n+1} |D_i^j|[|r^{i-1}(x_j^{(i)})| - \underline{E}_n^{(i-1)}]}{\sum_{j=0}^{n+1} |D_i^j|}$$

$$\geq \frac{\min_j |D_i^j|(\bar{E}_n^{(i-1)} - \underline{E}_n^{(i-1)})}{\sum_{j=0}^{n+1} |D_i^j|}; \qquad (38.4)$$

i.e.

$$0 \leq \underline{E}_n^{(1)} < \underline{E}_n^{(2)} < \cdots < E_n(f). \qquad (38.5)$$

By Theorem 38.1 and (38.5) it follows that there exists a number $c > 0$ for which (note that $0 < \underline{E}_n^{(2)} < \underline{E}_n^{(i)}$ for $i > 2$)

$$x_{k+1}^{(i)} - x_k^{(i)} > c, \quad k = 0, 1, \ldots, n, \ i = 2, 3, \ldots, \qquad (38.6)$$

and since the points $\{x_k^{(1)}\}_{k=0}^{n+1}$ are different, (38.6) is also true for $i = 1$.

By virtue of the continuity of φ_k and the inequality (32.6) there exist numbers $m > 0$, $M > 0$ such that $m < |D_i^j| < M$, $j = 0, 1, \ldots, n+1$, $i = 1, 2, \ldots$, and from (38.5), (38.6) it follows that

$$\underline{E}_n^{(i+1)} - \underline{E}_n^{(i)} \geq \frac{m}{(n+2)M}(\bar{E}_n^{(i)} - \underline{E}_n^{(i)}),$$

$$E_n(f) - \underline{E}_n^{(i+1)} \leq E_n(f) - \underline{E}_n^{(i)} - \frac{m}{(n+2)M}[E_n(f) - \underline{E}_n^{(i)}] \qquad (38.7)$$

$$= q[E_n(f) - \underline{E}_n^{(i)}], \quad q = 1 - \frac{m}{(n+2)M}, \ 0 < q < 1.$$

The last inequality gives
$$E_n(f) - \underline{E}_n^{(i)} \leq q^{i-1}[E_n(f) - \underline{E}_n^{(1)}] \tag{38.8}$$
and from (38.7)
$$\bar{E}_n^{(i)} - \underline{E}_n^{(i)} \leq \frac{(n+2)M}{m}[E_n(f) - \underline{E}_n^{(1)}]q^{i-1}. \qquad \square$$

REMARK 38.1. It should be noted that in practice the rate of convergence of the Remez algorithm is better than given by (38.8). VEIDINGER [1960] proved that under some additional restrictions the inequality (38.8) can be written in the form
$$E_n(f) - \underline{E}_n^{(i)} \leq cq^{2^i}, \quad 0 < q < 1, \ c \text{ is a constant}; \tag{38.9}$$
i.e. the Remez algorithm has a quadratic rate of convergence. The main conditions for the validity of (38.9) are for the functions f and $\{\varphi_i\}_{i=0}^n$ to have second derivatives in $[a, b]$.

39. The Remez algorithm—Multidimensional case

The ideas of the second Remez algorithm described in Section 38 can be used for the numerical determination of the best approximation in the multidimensional case. Following LAURENT ([1972], Chapter 3.7), this algorithm will be given without proof for convergence. All details can be found in the cited book.

Let S be a compact, $C(S)$ is the set of continuous functions on S and $\{\varphi_i\}_{i=1}^n$ build a Chebyshev system on S. Setting
$$V = \left\{\varphi: \varphi = \sum_{i=1}^n a_i \varphi_i\right\},$$
for a given function $f \in C(S)$ the problem is to find the polynomial $g^* \in V$ of the best approximation
$$E_n(f)_S = \inf_{g \in V} \max_{x \in S} |f(x) - g(x)| = \max_{x \in S} |f(x) - g^*(x)|.$$
The algorithm is as follows.

Step 1. Choose $n+1$ points $M^\nu = \{x_i^\nu\}_{i=1}^{n+1}$, $M^\nu \subset S$. Setting $\lambda_{n+1}^\nu = 1$, solve the linear system
$$\sum_{i=1}^n \lambda_i^\nu \varphi_j(x_i^\nu) = -\lambda_{n+1}^\nu \varphi_j(x_{n+1}^\nu), \quad j = 1, 2, \ldots, n.$$
Because of Theorem 1.2 this system always has one solution.

Determine λ_{n+1}^ν such that $\sum_{i=1}^{n+1} |\lambda_i^\nu| = 1$ and $\sum_{i=1}^{n+1} \lambda_i^\nu f(x_i^\nu) < 0$. Set $\varepsilon_i^\nu = \text{sgn } \lambda_i^\nu$ and $\rho_i^\nu = \varepsilon_i^\nu \lambda_i^\nu$.

Step 2. Set $E_n^\nu = -\sum_{i=1}^{n+1} \varepsilon_i^\nu \rho_i^\nu f(x_i^\nu)$.

Step 3. Solve the linear system

$$\sum_{j=1}^{n} \alpha_j \varphi_j(x_i^\nu) = f(x_i^\nu) + \varepsilon_i^\nu E_n^\nu, \quad i = 1, 2, \ldots, n+1.$$

Set $g^\nu = \sum_{j=1}^{n} \alpha_j \varphi_j$.

Step 4. Find the point $x_0 \in S$ such that

$$\max_{x \in S} |f(x) - g^\nu(x)| = |f(x_0) - g^\nu(x_0)|$$

and set $\varepsilon_0 = \text{sgn}[g^\nu(x_0) - f(x_0)]$. If $E_n^\nu = |f(x_0) - g^\nu(x_0)|$ then $g^\nu = g^*$ and $E_n^\nu = E_n(f)_S$. Stop.

Step 5. Set $\omega_{n+1} = 0$, $\omega_0 = 1$ and solve the linear system

$$\sum_{i=1}^{n+1} \omega_i \varepsilon_i^\nu \varphi_j(x_i^\nu) + \omega_0 \varepsilon_0 \varphi_j(x_0) = 0, \quad j = 1, 2, \ldots, n.$$

Step 6. Determine the index i_0 from

$$\frac{\omega_{i_0}}{|\lambda_{i_0}^\nu|} = \min_{i=1,2,\ldots,n+1} \frac{\omega_i}{|\lambda_i^\nu|},$$

and set

$$M^{\nu+1} = \{x_1^\nu, \ldots, x_{i_0-1}^\nu, x_0, x_{i_0+1}^\nu, \ldots, x_{n+1}^\nu\} = \{x_i^{\nu+1}\}_{i=1}^{n+1},$$

$$\varepsilon_i^{\nu+1} = \begin{cases} \varepsilon_i^{\nu+1}, & \text{if } i \neq i_0, \\ \varepsilon_0, & \text{if } i = i_0, \end{cases}$$

$$\rho_i^{\nu+1} = \begin{cases} \rho_i^\nu(\omega_i/\rho_i^\nu - \omega_{i_0}/\rho_{i_0}^\nu)/k, & \text{if } i_0 \neq i, \\ \omega_0/k, & \text{if } i_0 = i, \end{cases}$$

where the positive number k must be determined from $\sum_{i=1}^{n+1} \rho_i^{\nu+1} = 1$. Go to Step 2, substituting ν by $\nu+1$ everywhere.

Unfortunately, the commonly used systems of multivariate functions $\{\varphi_i\}_{i=1}^{n}$, e.g., algebraic polynomials, do not build a Chebyshev system and Steps 3 and 5 in the algorithm described can sometimes fail because the determinants of the linear systems may happen to be equal to zero—see Sections 1 and 15. In this connection MAIRHUBER [1956] proved that if on the compact K it is possible to define a Chebyshev system $\{\varphi_i\}_{i=0}^{n}$, $n > 0$, then K is homeomorphic either to the circle or to some part of the circle.

The Theorem 3.7.9 in LAURENT [1972] proves the convergence of the algorithm, e.g., $\lim_{\nu \to \infty} E_n^\nu = E_n(f)_S$, $\lim_{\nu \to \infty} g^\nu = g^*$.

To illustrate the effectiveness of the Laurent method let us consider two numerical examples.

(1) For the function $f(x, y) = 2 - |x| - |y|$ in the domain

$$D = \{(x, y): -1 \leq x \leq 1, -1 \leq y \leq 1\} \tag{39.1}$$

the best uniform approximation has to be found by the polynomials

$$P_{2,2}(x, y) = a_{0,0} + a_{2,0}C_2(x) + a_{0,2}C_2(y) + a_{2,2}C_2(x)C_2(y),$$
$$P_{4,4}(x, y) = b_{0,0} + b_{1,0}C_1(x) + b_{2,0}C_2(x) + b_{3,0}C_3(x) + b_{4,0}C_4(x)$$
$$+ b_{0,1}C_1(y) + b_{0,2}C_2(y) + b_{0,3}C_3(y) + b_{0,4}C_4(y),$$

where $C_k(x) = \cos(n \cos^{-1} x)$. In Fig. 39.1 the graph of the function f is given. The graphs of $f - P_{2,2}$ and $f - P_{4,4}$ are given in Figs. 39.2 and 39.3, respectively. The approximations are $\max_{(x,y)\in D} |f(x, y) - P_{2,2}(x, y)| = 0.25$,

$$\max_{(x,y)\in D} |f(x, y) - P_{4,4}(x, y)| \approx 0.1351172 \ldots$$

and for the coefficients the algorithm gives

$a_{00} = 0.75$,	$b_{00} = 0.7337395$,	$b_{02} = -0.4323123$,
$a_{20} = -0.50$,	$b_{10} = -0.0000020$,	$b_{30} = -0.0000035$,
$a_{02} = -0.50$,	$b_{01} = 0.0001287$,	$b_{03} = 0.0002272$,
$a_{22} = 0.00$,	$b_{20} = -0.4323974$,	$b_{40} = 0.1331896$,
		$b_{04} = 0.1332440$.

(2) For the smooth function $g(x, y) = \exp(-x^2/4 - y^2)$ (see Fig. 39.4) in the domain D described in (39.1) let us try to obtain the polynomials of the best uniform approximation in the form

$$Q_{2,2}(x, y) = c_{0,0} + c_{2,0}C_2(x) + c_{0,2}C_2(y) + c_{2,2}C_2(x)C_2(y),$$

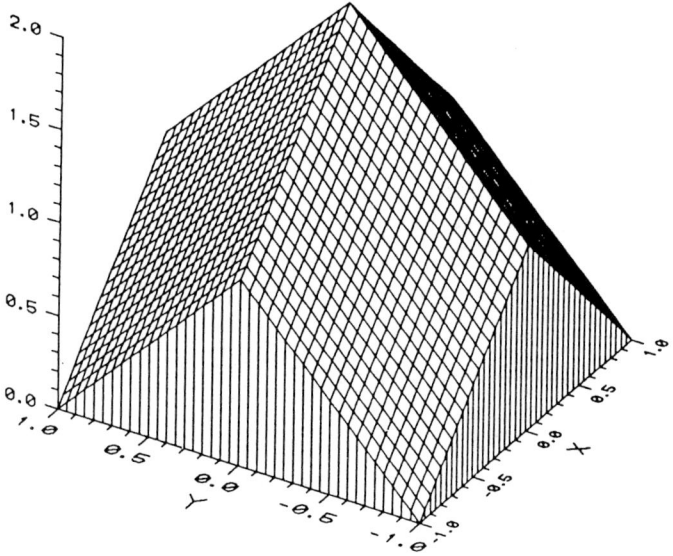

FIG. 39.1. Graph of the function f.

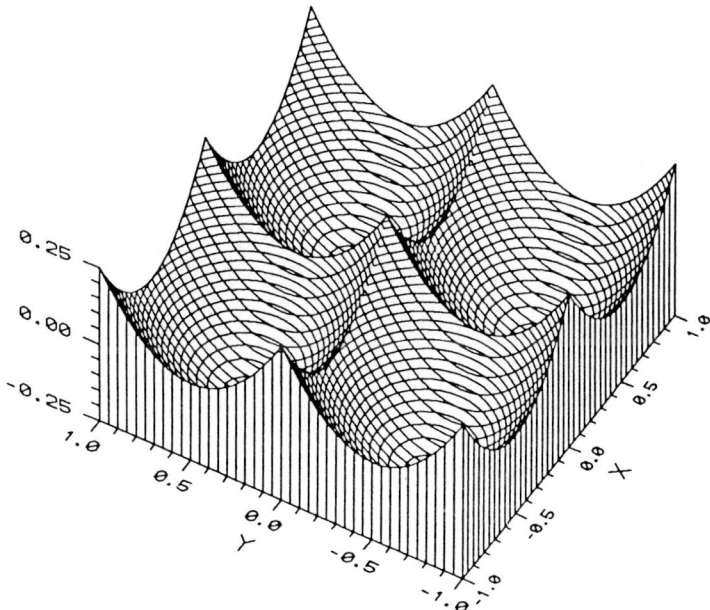

Fig. 39.2. Graph of the function $f - P_{2,2}$.

$$Q_{4,4}(x, y) = d_{0,0} + d_{2,0}C_2(x) + d_{4,0}C_4(x)$$
$$+ d_{0,2}C_2(y) + d_{0,4}C_4(y) + d_{2,2}C_2(x)C_2(y).$$

The graphs of $g - Q_{2,2}$ and $g - Q_{4,4}$ are given in Figs. 39.5 and 39.6, respectively. The approximations are

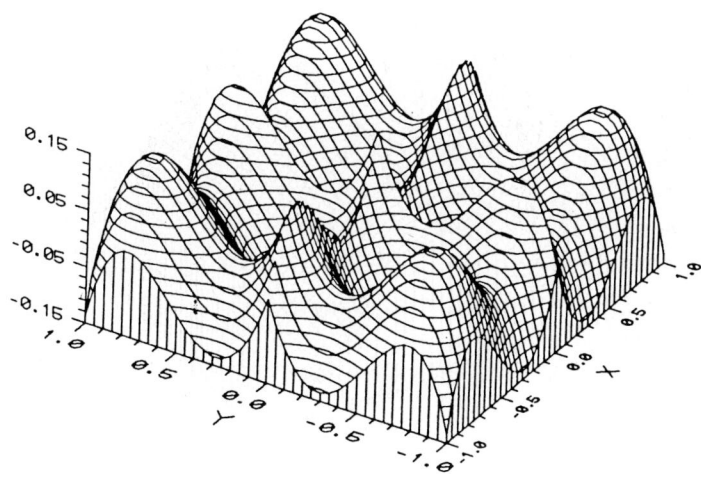

Fig. 39.3. Graph of the function $f - P_{4,4}$.

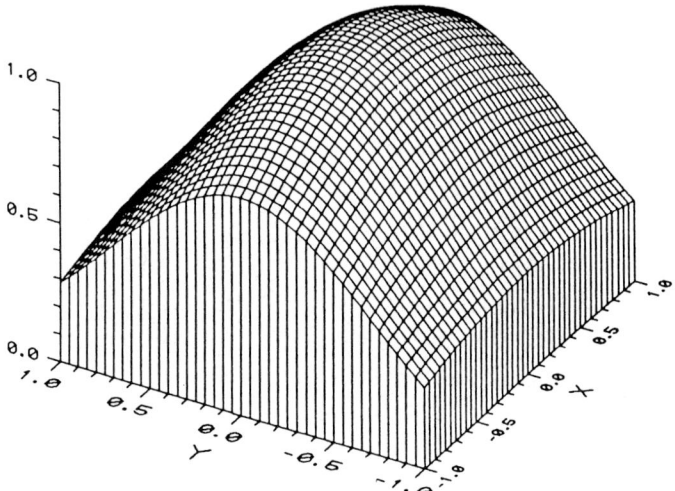

Fig. 39.4. Graph of the function $g(x, y) = \exp(-x^2/4 - y^2)$.

$$\max_{(x,y) \in D} |f(x, y) - Q_{2,2}(x, y)| \approx 0.03897367 \ldots,$$

$$\max_{(x,y) \in D} |f(x, y) - Q_{4,4}(x, y)| \approx 0.005613010 \ldots.$$

For the coefficients the algorithm gives

$$c_{00} = 0.5693226, \qquad c_{02} = -0.2811041,$$

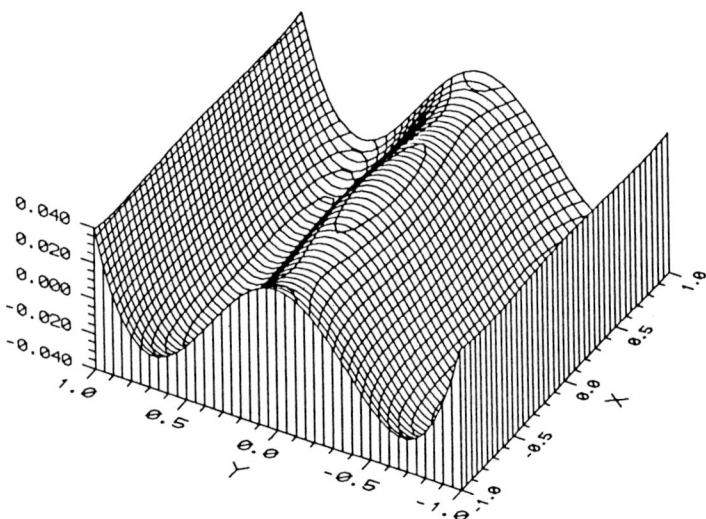

Fig. 39.5. Graph of the function $g - Q_{2,2}$.

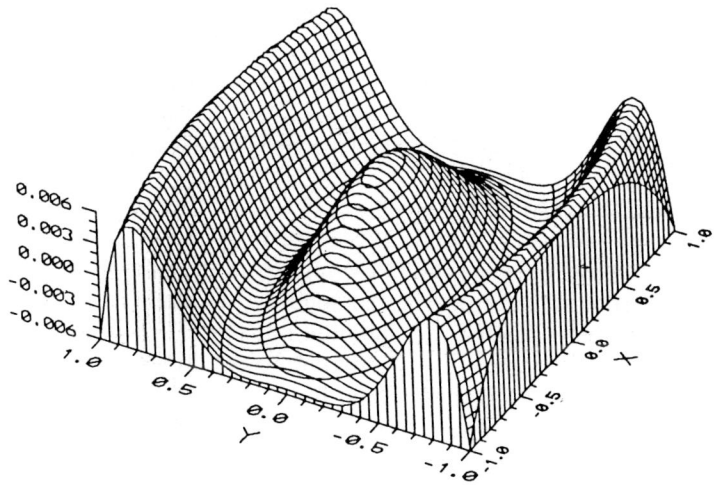

Fig. 39.6. Graph of the function $g - Q_{4,4}$.

Table 39.1. Points of maximal deviation between g and $Q_{4,4}$.

x	y	$g(x, y)$	$Q_{44}(x, y)$	$g(x, y) - Q_{44}(x, y)$
-0.64	-0.90	0.4016	0.3959	0.005613010
0.00	0.00	1.0000	0.9944	0.005613010
-0.34	-0.94	0.4015	0.3959	0.005613010
0.98	-0.22	0.7494	0.7550	-0.005613010
-1.00	-1.00	0.2865	0.2921	-0.005613010
0.98	-0.82	0.4015	0.3959	0.005613010
-0.27	-0.52	0.7493	0.7549	-0.005613010

$c_{20} = -0.0756435$, $c_{22} = 0.3495614$,

$d_{00} = 0.5714055$, $d_{02} = -0.2809077$,

$d_{20} = -0.0702269$, $d_{04} = 0.0348348$,

$d_{40} = 0.0021772$, $d_{22} = 0.0348348$.

It is interesting to consider the points of maximal deviation (alternation points in one-dimensional case)—see Theorem 25.6 and Table 39.1.

40. A second Remez algorithm for rational functions

Theorem 28.2 allows the second Remez algorithm to be applied for finding the rational function of best uniform approximation. Formally, the algorithm described below coincides with this in Section 38.

Let f be a continuous function on the compact $K \subseteq [a, b]$ and

$$L_{mn} = \left\{ \varphi \colon \varphi = w \sum_{i=0}^{m} a_i x^i \Big/ \sum_{i=0}^{n} b_i x^i, \ w(x) > 0 \text{ for } x \in [a, b] \right\},$$

$$E_{mn}(f)_K = \inf_{\varphi \in L_{mn}} \max_{x \in K} |f(x) - \varphi(x)| = \max_{x \in K} |f(x) - \varphi_{mn}(x)|.$$

By Theorem 28.2 the polynomial $\varphi_{mn} \in L_{mn}$ of the best uniform approximation of the function f attains the largest deviation from f at $N + 2 = m + n - d + 2$ points in $[a, b]$. The best case from the numerical point of view is when the number d is zero—see the stability theorems in Section 43.

RALSTON ([1965a], Chapter 7.9), pointed out that $d \neq 0$ occurs when f is an odd or an even function in $[a, b]$ and otherwise in exceptional cases. For example, the constant 0.5 is the rational function of the best approximation in $L_{1,1}$ for the function x^2 in the interval $[-1, 1]$. Here $d = 1$ and the points of alternation are $-1, 0, 1$.

Let us now assume that $d = 0$. The algorithm for the numerical determination of the rational function of the best approximation on the compact $K \subseteq [a, b]$ is the following.

Step 1. Take on K the point set $K_1 \subseteq K$, $K_1 = \{x_0^1 < x_1^1 < \cdots < x_{N+1}^1\}$. By the nonlinear system

$$f(x_i^1) - \sum_{j=0}^{m} a_j (x_i^1)^j \Big/ \sum_{j=0}^{n} b_j (x_i^1)^j = (-1)^i E_{mn}^{(1)}, \tag{40.1}$$

find the rational function

$$\varphi_{mn}^1(x) = \sum_{j=0}^{m} a_j x^j \Big/ \sum_{j=0}^{n} b_j x^j$$

and the number $|E_{mn}^{(1)}|$.

The system (40.1) can be solved iteratively by writing it in the form

$$\sum_{j=0}^{m} a_j (x_i^1)^j - [f(x_i^1) - (-1)^i E_{mn}^{1,k}] \sum_{j=1}^{n} b_j (x_i^1)^j = f(x_i^1) - (-1)^i E_{mn}^{1,k+1}.$$

Setting $E_{mn}^{1,k} = 0$ solve the above linear system with respect to $a_j, b_j, E_{mn}^{1,k+1}$, then substitute $E_{mn}^{1,k}$ by $E_{mn}^{1,k+1}$ and repeat this procedure again. Usually $\lim_{k \to \infty} E_{mn}^{1,k} = E_{mn}^{(1)}$.

Set

$$r^1(x) = \varphi_{mn}^1(x) - \sum_{j=0}^{m} a_j x^j \Big/ \sum_{j=0}^{n} b_j x^j$$

and compute $\max_{x \in K} |r^1(x)| = \bar{E}_{mn}^{(1)}$ (of course, approximately).

Step 2. If $\bar{E}_{mn}^{(1)} = |E_{mn}^{(1)}|$ then by the Chebyshev Theorem 28.2 the rational function φ_{mn}^1 is the element of best approximation in L_{mn}. Stop.

Step 3. If $\bar{E}_{mn}^{(1)} > |E_{mn}^{(1)}|$ then there exists a point $x^* \in K$ such that $|r^1(x^*)| = \bar{E}_{mn}^{(1)}$. Then $|E_{mn}^{(1)}| < E_{mn}(f)_K < \bar{E}_{mn}^{(1)}$.

Step 4. Build a new point set $K_2 \subseteq K$, $K_2 = \{x_0^2 < x_1^2 < \cdots < x_{N+1}^2\}$ such that

$$\operatorname{sgn} r^1(x_{k+1}^{(2)}) = -\operatorname{sgn} r^1(x_k^{(2)}), \quad k = 0, 1, \ldots, N+1,$$

$$|r^1(x_k^{(2)})| \geq |E_{mn}^{(1)}|, \quad \max_k |r^1(x_k^{(2)})| = \bar{E}_{mn}^{(1)}, \quad k = 0, 1, \ldots, N+1.$$

(These conditions can be satisfied by replacing in K_1 only one point by the point x^*. The algorithm works more effectively if the differences $|r^1(x_k^{(2)})| - |E_{mn}^{(1)}|$ are as large as possible.)

Step 5. Go to Step 1 substituting the point set K_1 by K_2.

The algorithm described produces the sequences of rational functions $\{\varphi_{mn}^i\}_{i=1,2,\ldots}$ and numbers $\{E_{mn}^{(i)}\}_{i=1,2,\ldots}$.

RALSTON [1965b] proved that under the conditions that the point set K_1 is enough close to the points of alternation of f on K from Theorem 28.2 and $||E_{mn}^1| - E_{mn}(f)_K|$ is a small number, then

$$\lim_{i \to \infty} \varphi_{mn}^i = \varphi_{mn}, \quad \lim_{i \to \infty} |E_{mn}^i| = E_{mn}(f)_K.$$

Ralston did not give the rate of convergence. More detailed investigations on the Remez algorithm can be found in WERNER [1962a,b, 1963, 1967], WATSON [1980], where the questions about the choice of initial approximation and the order of convergence (under additional assumptions for the smoothness of f) are considered.

41. The differential correction algorithm

This algorithm was first described by CHENEY and LOEB [1961]. The modified version of the algorithm given by the same authors a year later, CHENEY and LOEB [1962], is more popular than the original one, though it is known to be slower.

Let us use the notation

$$L_{mn} = \left\{ \varphi : \varphi = \sum_{i=0}^m a_i \varphi_i \Big/ \sum_{i=0}^n b_i \psi_i, \sum_{i=0}^n b_i \psi_i(x) > 0 \text{ for } x \in K, \max_{0 \leq i \leq n} |b_i| = 1 \right\},$$

$$\bar{L}_{mn} = \left\{ \varphi : \varphi = \sum_{i=0}^m a_i \varphi_i \Big/ \sum_{i=0}^n b_i \psi_i, \max_{0 \leq i \leq n} |b_i| = 1 \right\},$$

$$E_{mn}(f)_K = \inf_{\varphi \in L_{mn}} \max_{x \in K} |f(x) - \varphi(x)| = \max_{x \in K} |f(x) - r_{mn}(x)|,$$

$$\Delta(\varphi) = \max_{x \in K} |f(x) - \varphi(x)|,$$

where K is a finite compact point set and $\{\varphi_i\}_{i=0}^m$, $\{\psi_i\}_{i=0}^n$ are two Chebyshev systems on K.

The original differential correction algorithm for the determination of the rational functional r_{mn} of the best approximation for a given continuous function f on K consists of:

Step 1. Choose an initial approximation $r_0 \in L_{mn}$, $r_0 = p_0/q_0$.
Step 2. Set $k = 0$.
Step 3. Compute the number $\Delta_k = \Delta(r_k)$.
Step 4. Form the following function of $r = p/q$, $r \in \bar{L}_{mn}$,

$$\delta_k(r) = \max_{x \in K} \left(\frac{|f(x)q_k(x) - p(x)| - \Delta_k q(x)}{q_k(x)} \right).$$

Step 5. Select the function $r_{k+1} = p_{k+1}/q_{k+1}$, $r_{k+1} \in \bar{L}_{mn}$, from the condition

$$\delta_k(r_{k+1}) = \min\{\delta_k(r): r \in \bar{L}_{mn}\}.$$

Step 6. If $\delta_k(r_{k+1}) \geq 0$ then $r_k = r_{mn}$. Stop.
Step 7. Set $k = k + 1$ and go to Step 3.

The modified differential correction algorithm differs from the one represented above only at Step 4, where the functional is

$$\delta_k(r) = \max_{x \in K} (|f(x)q_k(x) - p(x)| - \Delta_k q(x)).$$

The proof of the convergence of the modified algorithm was given by CHENEY and LOEB [1962] by the next theorem.

THEOREM 41.1 (CHENEY [1966], p. 171). *In the modified differential correction algorithm*

$$\lim_{k \to \infty} \Delta_k = E_{mn}(f), \quad \Delta_k > \Delta_{k+1},$$

$$\Delta_{k+1} - E_{mn}(f) \leq \gamma[\Delta_k - E_{mn}(f)], \quad 0 < \gamma < 1.$$

For the existence of r_{mn} see Theorem 27.1.

Step 5 is the most difficult part of the algorithm. Fortunately, the minimization of the functional $\delta_k(r)$ is the problem of convex programming (note that $\delta_k(r)$ is a convex function with respect to the coefficients of r). One special feature of the algorithm is that $r_k = p_k/q_k$, $q_k > 0$, implies $r_{k+1} = p_{k+1}/q_{k+1}$ with $q_{k+1} > 0$; i.e. $r_{k+1} \in L_{mn}$.

For the original algorithm in the case $\varphi_i = \psi_i = x^i$, $i = 0, 1, \ldots$, the main result is the following.

THEOREM 41.2 (BARRODALE, POWELL and ROBERTS [1972]). *If K is a finite set, then*

$$\lim_{k \to \infty} \Delta_k = E_{mn}(f), \quad \Delta_k > \Delta_{k+1},$$

$$\Delta_{k+1} - E_{mn}(f) \leq \gamma[\Delta_k - E_{mn}(f)]^2;$$

i.e. the algorithm has a quadratic rate of convergence.

PROOF. Let us first prove that if $r_k = p_k/q_k$, $r_k \in L_{mn}$, $\Delta_k > E_{mn}(f)$, then $r_{k+1} = p_{k+1}/q_{k+1}$, $r_{k+1} \in \bar{L}_{mn}$, $\Delta_k > \Delta_{k+1}$. From $\Delta_k > E_{mn}(f)$ there exists a function $r = p/q$, $r \in L_{mn}$, such that $\Delta(r) < \Delta_k$. Setting $\eta = \min_{x \in K} |q(x)|$ then

$$\delta_k(r_{k+1}) = \max_{x \in K} \left(\frac{|f(x)q_{k+1}(x) - p_{k+1}(x)| - \Delta_k q_{k+1}(x)}{q_k(x)} \right)$$

$$\leq \max_{x \in K} \left(\frac{|f(x)q(x) - p(x)| - \Delta_k q(x)}{q_k(x)} \right)$$

$$= \max_{x \in K} \{[|f(x) - p(x)/q(x)| - \Delta_k] q(x)/q_k(x)\}$$

$$\leq -\min_{x \in K} [(\Delta_k - \Delta(r))q(x)/q_k(x)] \leq -\eta[\Delta_k - \Delta(r)] < 0. \quad (41.1)$$

If there exists a point $x_0 \in K$ for which $q_{k+1}(x_0) \leq 0$, then $\delta_k(r_{k+1}) > 0$, which contradicts (41.1). Moreover, if

$$\min_{x \in K} q_{k+1}(x)/q_k(x) = q_{k+1}(c)/q_k(c),$$

it follows that

$$\frac{-\Delta_k q_{k+1}(c)}{q_k(c)} \leq \frac{|f(c)q_{k+1}(c) - p_{k+1}(c)| - \Delta_k q_{k+1}(c)}{q_k(c)}$$

$$\leq \max_{x \in K} \left(\frac{|f(x)q_{k+1}(x) - p_{k+1}(x)| - \Delta_k q_{k+1}(x)}{q_k(x)} \right)$$

$$< -\eta[\Delta_k - \Delta(r)];$$

i.e.

$$q_{k+1}(x)/q_k(x) \geq \eta(\Delta_k - \Delta(r))/\Delta_k. \quad (41.2)$$

The inequality $\Delta_{k+1} < \Delta_k$ follows directly from

$$|f - p_{k+1}/q_{k+1}| = \Delta_k + \frac{q_k}{q_{k+1}} \cdot \frac{|fq_{k+1} - p_{k+1}| - \Delta_k q_{k+1}}{q_k}$$

$$\leq \Delta_k - \frac{q_k}{q_{k+1}} \eta[\Delta_k - \Delta(r)]. \quad (41.3)$$

So the sequence $\{\Delta_k\}_{k=0}^{\infty}$ decreases monotonically and is bounded from below. Let $\lim_{k \to \infty} \Delta_k = \tilde{\Delta}$. If $\tilde{\Delta} > E_{mn}(f)$ then there exists $r \in L_{mn}$, $r = p/q$, such that $\Delta(r) \leq \tilde{\Delta}$. Setting

$$\eta = \min_{x \in K} |q(x)|, \quad c = \min\{\tfrac{1}{2}, \eta[1 - \Delta(r)/\tilde{\Delta}]\},$$

it follows from (41.3) that

$$|f(x) - p_{k+1}(x)/q_{k+1}(x)| \leq \Delta_k \left(1 - c \frac{q_k(x)}{q_{k+1}(x)}\right). \quad (41.4)$$

By (41.4)

$$\Delta_{k+1} \leq \Delta_k \left(1 - c \min_{x \in K} \frac{q_k(x)}{q_{k+1}(x)}\right)$$

and since $\lim_{k\to\infty} \Delta_k = \tilde{\Delta}$ it follows that

$$\lim_{k\to\infty}\left(\min_{x\in K}\frac{q_k(x)}{q_{k+1}(x)}\right)=0.$$

This means that there exists a sequence $\{\xi_k\}_{k=1}^\infty$, $\xi_k \in K$, for which

$$\lim_{k\to\infty}\left(\frac{q_k(\xi_k)}{q_{k+1}(\xi_k)}\right)=0.$$

Since K is a finite point set, $K = \{x_k\}_{k=1}^N$, there is an integer k_0 such that

$$q_{k+1}(\xi_k) \geq c^{-N} q_k(\xi_k) \tag{41.5}$$

holds for all $k \geq k_0$.

Using the inequalities $\tilde{\Delta} \leq \Delta(r) \leq \Delta_k$, (41.2) can be rewritten as

$$q_{k+1}(x)/q_k(x) \geq \eta[\Delta_k - \Delta(r)]/\Delta_k \geq \eta[1 - \Delta(r)/\tilde{\Delta}] \geq c.$$

The last inequality and (41.5) give

$$\prod_{i=1}^N q_{k+1}(x_i) \geq \frac{c^{N-1}}{c^N}\prod_{i=1}^N q_k(x_i) \geq 2\sum_{i=1}^N q_k(x_i);$$

i.e. $\lim_{k\to\infty}(\prod_{i=1}^N q_k(x_i)) = \infty$, which contradicts $\max_{0\leq i\leq n}|b_i^k| = 1$, where $q_k = \sum_{i=0}^n b_i^k \psi_i$. This contradiction proves $\lim_{k\to\infty} \Delta_k = E_{mn}(f)$.

To prove the quadratic rate of convergence let us consider the rational function of the best approximation

$$r^* = p^*/q^*, \qquad r^* \in L_{mn}, \qquad \Delta(r^*) = E_{mn}(f).$$

By Theorem 43.4 there exists a constant c_1 such that for every function $r = p/q$, $r \in L_{mn}$, the following relation is fulfilled

$$\Delta(r) \geq \Delta(r^*) + c_1 \|q - q^*\|.$$

Suppose that the function r in (41.1) is r^*. Then

$$\min_{x\in K}\left(\frac{q^*(x)}{q_k(x)}\right) \geq \min_{x\in K}\left(\frac{q^*(x)}{q^*(x) + \|q^* - q_k\|}\right) \geq \frac{\eta}{\eta + [\Delta_k - \Delta(r^*)]/c_1}, \tag{41.6}$$

and taking into account the fact that $\Delta_{k+1} \leq \Delta_k$ similarly to (41.6) the next inequality holds

$$\min_{x\in K}\left(\frac{q_{k+1}(x)}{q_k(x)}\right) \geq \frac{\eta - [\Delta_k - \Delta(r^*)]/c_1}{\eta + [\Delta_k - \Delta(r^*)]/c_1}. \tag{41.7}$$

Substituting (41.6) in (41.1) it follows that

$$\left(\left|f(x) - \frac{p_{k+1}(x)}{q_{k+1}(x)}\right| - \Delta_k\right)\frac{q_{k+1}(x)}{q_k(x)} \leq -[\Delta_k - \Delta(r^*)]\frac{\eta}{\eta + [\Delta_k - \Delta(r^*)]/c_1}.$$

By multiplying the last expression by q_k/q_{k+1} and using (41.7) it follows that

$$\Delta_{k+1} - \Delta_k \leq -[\Delta_k - \Delta(r^*)]\frac{\eta}{\eta + [\Delta_k - \Delta(r^*)]/c_1}\frac{\eta - [\Delta_k - \Delta(r^*)]/c_1}{\eta + [\Delta_k - \Delta(r^*)]/c_1}.$$

Finally, adding $\Delta_k - \Delta(r^*)$ to both sides

$$\Delta_{k+1} - \Delta(r^*) \leq [\Delta_k - \Delta(r^*)]^2 - \frac{3\eta/c_1 + [\Delta_k - \Delta(r^*)]/c_1^2}{\{\eta + [\Delta_k - \Delta(r^*)]/c_1\}^2} \leq \frac{3}{\eta c_1}[\Delta_k - \Delta(r^*)]^2.$$

□

Numerical tests of the algorithm and codes have been given by many authors. For example, see KAUFMAN and TAYLOR [1975]. Their algorithm is initialized by the determination of $r_0 = p_0/q_0$ from

$$\begin{cases} \min_{p,q} \max_{x \in K} |f(x)q(x) - p(x)|, \\ q(x) = 1 + a_1 x + \cdots \end{cases}$$

providing that this yields q which does not change sign and is not too small; otherwise $p_0 \equiv 0$, $q \equiv 1$. One of their examples is an approximation of the function $f(x, y) = x^y$ by rational functions

$$r_{2,1}(x, y) = \sum_{i+j \leq 2} a_{ij} x^i y^j \Big/ \sum_{i+j \leq 1} a_{ij} x^i y^j$$

in the domain $K = \{0.5 \leq x \leq 1, 0 \leq y \leq 1\}$ using a 5×5 uniform grid in K. After two iterations the error on the grid is $\Delta_2 = 0.00307\ldots$ and

$$\max_{(x,y) \in K} |f(x, y) - r_{2,1}(x, y)| \leq 0.0036\ldots.$$

In Fig. 41.1 the graph of $f - r_{2,1}$ is given, where

$$r_{2,1}(x, y) = \frac{0.94622 + 0.19369x - 0.99133y - 0.10141x^2 + 1.4449xy - 0.03082y^2}{1 + 0.04170x + 0.42409y}.$$

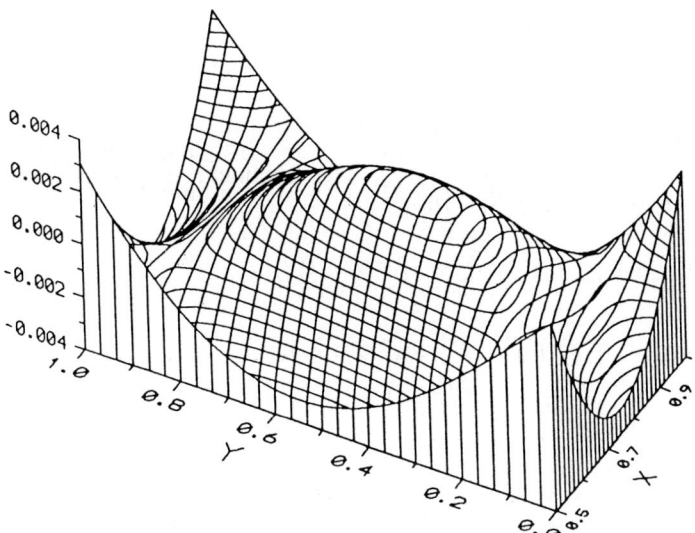

FIG. 41.1. Graph of the function $f - r_{2,1}$.

42. Algorithms for rational approximation

Let us use in this section the notation

$$L_{mn} = \left\{ \varphi : \varphi = \sum_{i=0}^{m} a_i \varphi_i \bigg/ \sum_{i=0}^{n} b_i \psi_i, \, b_0 = 1 \right\}.$$

where all the functions are defined on the compact K and $S \subset K$ is a finite point set.

LEE and ROBERTS [1973] reported eight numerical methods for the approximate determination of the rational function of the best uniform approximation for a given continuous function f defined on a compact K. They divide them into several classes.

(1) Methods based on the linear programming.

(a) The algorithm due to LOEB [1957] is an iterative scheme. At the kth stage the rational function $\varphi^{(k)} = p^{(k)}/q^{(k)} \in L_{mn}$ must be determined from

$$\min_{\varphi \in L_{mn}} \max_{x_i \in S} \left(\frac{1}{|q^{(k-1)}(x_i)|} |f(x_i)q(x_i) - p(x_i)| \right).$$

The term $1/|q^{(k-1)}(x_i)|$ can be considered as a weight factor and the minimization is a question of linear programming—see CHENEY ([1966], Chapter 5). BARRODALE and MASON [1970] gave numerical experiments changing the discrete metrics l_1, l_2, l_∞. For example in l_1 the problem is

$$\min_{\varphi \in L_{mn}} \sum_{x_i \in S} \frac{1}{|q^{(k-1)}(x_i)|} |f(x_i)q(x_i) - p(x_i)|.$$

(b) The linear inequality algorithm due to LOEB [1960], and ZUCHOVITZKII and AVDEEVA ([1967, p. 293]). The problem consists in the determination of the smallest value of w such that the problem

$$\min w, \tag{42.1a}$$

$$|f(x_i) - \varphi(x_i)| \leq w, \quad x_i \in S, \tag{42.1b}$$

$$-q(x_i) \leq 0, \tag{42.1c}$$

is consistent, where $\varphi = p/q \in L_{mn}$. The nonlinear system of inequalities in (42.1) may be written in the form

$$[f(x_i) - w] \sum_{k=1}^{n} b_k x_i^k - \sum_{k=0}^{n} a_k x_i^k \leq w - f(x_i),$$

$$[-f(x_i) - w] \sum_{k=1}^{n} b_k x_i^k - \sum_{k=0}^{n} a_k x_i^k \leq w + f(x_i),$$

$$-\sum_{k=1}^{n} b_k x_i^k \leq 1.$$

Since the smallest value of w satisfies $0 \leq w \leq \max_{x \in S} |f(x)|$ it may be located by the method of bisection.

(c) OSBORN and WATSON [1969/70], suggested an iterative process, which at the kth iteration determines $\varphi^k = p^k/q^k \in L_{mn}$ from the minimization of the expression

$$\max_{x \in S} f(x) - \varphi^{k-1}(x) + \frac{p^{k-1}(x)q(x) - q^{k-1}(x)p(x)}{q^{k-1}(x)}, \qquad (42.2)$$

and $\varphi^k = (p^{k-1} + \lambda^k p)/(q^{k-1} + \lambda^k q)$, where λ^k is chosen to minimize the expression

$$\max_{x \in S} f(x) - \frac{p^{k-1}(x) + \lambda p(x)}{q^{k-1}(x) + \lambda q(x)}. \qquad (42.3)$$

The minimization of (42.2) is a problem of linear programming and λ in (42.3) can be approximately determined in the set $\{0, 0.5, 1\}$.

(d) The differential correction algorithm (Difcor) described in Section 41. (In fact two variants of the algorithm are given. Let us call them I and II.) The third version, which can be used for the initial approximation of Difcor I and II is the determination of $\varphi = p/q \in L_{mn}$ from minimization of the expression

$$\max_{x \in S} |f(x)q(x) - p(x)|.$$

(2) The second Remez algorithm described in Section 40 and its modifications given in RICE ([1969], p. 109), FRASER and HART [1962], and WERNER [1962a,b].

(3) The combined Remez–Difcor algorithm (see KAUFMAN, LEEMING and TAYLOR [1978]) is a hybrid between the Remez and Difcor algorithms that differs from the classical Remez algorithm in that:

(a) the solution of the nonlinear system (40.1) is replaced by the Difcor algorithm;

(b) the exchange procedure, Step 4, in Section 40 is modified to eliminate cycles.

(4) The algorithm due to MAEHLY and WITZGALL [1963] assumes that the error function $r = f - \varphi$, ($\varphi \in L_{mn}$, $E_{mn}(f) = \|f - \varphi\|$), has exactly $m + n + 1$ zeros $\{z_i^*\}_{i=1}^{m+n+1}$; i.e.

$$r(x) = G(x) \prod_{k=1}^{m+n+1} (x - z_k^*),$$

where G is a positive (negative) function. Starting from some approximation of $\{z_i^*\}_{i=1}^{m+n+1}$ iteratively they must be corrected by solving the linear system of equations.

The conclusions of the numerical experiments are the following.

(1) Loeb's and Maehly's algorithms converge rapidly for smooth data. However, they often fail to converge or do not produce the best approximation. The Osborn–Watson algorithm has the same deficiencies, although the converge rate appears to be quadratic.

(2) The methods based on linear programming cannot compete with the Remez algorithm in terms of computer time. When the Remez algorithm

works, so does the Remez–Difcor algorithm, and with comparable speed. The Remez–Difcor algorithm usually still works when the Remez algorithm fails. The Difcor algorithm is more robust than the Remez–Difcor algorithm since it does not require an alternating theory.

43. Stability of numerical methods

The properties of the rational metric projection play an important role in numerical methods. Because of the approximate representation of the functions in the computer memory let us try to answer the question: let the functions f_1 and f_2 be close to each other. Is it true that their rational functions of the best approximations are also close.

Let f be a continuous function on the compact $K \subseteq [a, b]$ and

$$L_{mn} = \left\{ \varphi: \varphi(x) = \sum_{i=0}^{m} a_i x^i \bigg/ \sum_{i=0}^{n} b_i x^i \right\}, \quad (43.1)$$

$$E_{mn}(f)_K = \inf_{\varphi \in L_{mn}} \max_{x \in K} |f(x) - \varphi(x)| = \max_{x \in K} |f(x) - Pf(x)|.$$

The continuity of the operator P defined by (43.1) is the subject of the next theorems.

If $\varphi \in L_{mn}$ has the form

$$\varphi(x) = \sum_{i=0}^{m-\mu} a_i x^i \bigg/ \sum_{i=0}^{n-\nu} b_i x^i$$

then let us set

$$d(\varphi) = \begin{cases} \min(\mu, \nu), & \text{if } \varphi \neq 0, \\ n, & \text{if } \varphi \equiv 0. \end{cases}$$

THEOREM 43.1. *If $r = s/q \in L_{mn}$, $q(x) > 0$ for $x \in K$, then the set of functions $A = \{p + rg: p \in L_{m0}, g \in L_{n0}\}$ has a dimension $k = n + m + 1 - d(r)$. Every function $\varphi \in A$ has at most $k - 1$ zeros in K.*

PROOF. Evidently

$$\dim A = \dim L_{m0} + \dim rL_{n0} - \dim(L_{m0} \cap rL_{n0})$$

$$= m + n + 2 - \dim(L_{m0} \cap rL_{n0}),$$

where rL_{n0} denotes the function set $rL_{n0} = \{\varphi: \varphi = rt, t \in L_{n0}\}$. If $s \equiv 0$ then $d(r) = n$ and $\dim A = m + 1$. If $s \neq 0$ and $\varphi \in (L_{m0} \cap rL_{n0})$, then $\varphi = r\psi$, $\psi \in L_{n0}$, $\psi = qq_1$ and $sq \in L_{m0}$. The conditions $\psi \in L_{n0}$, $\psi = qq_1$ lead to $\deg(q_1) \leq \nu$, taking into account $\deg(q) = n - \nu$. From $sq_1 \in L_{m0}$ and $\deg(s) = m - \mu$ it follows that $\deg(q_1) \leq \mu$. So $q_1 \in L_{d(r),0}$ and consequently $\dim(L_{m0} \cap rL_{n0}) = d(r) + 1$; i.e. $\dim A = k$.

Suppose that $\varphi \in A$ has at least k zeros in K. Let $\varphi = p + rg$, $p \in L_{m0}$, $g \in L_{n0}$, $r = s/q \in L_{mn}$, $q(x) > 0$ for $x \in K$. Then the algebraic polynomial $pq + sg \in L_{n+m-d(r),0}$ has $k = m + n + 1 - d(r)$ zeros in K, which is impossible. □

THEOREM 43.2 (see PETRUSHEV and POPOV [1987], p. 30). *Let $f \in C[a, b]$ and for the operator P, defined by (43.1) it is fulfilled $d(Pf) = 0$. There exists a constant $c(f)$ such that for every function $g \in C_{[a,b]}$ the inequality*

$$\|Pf - Pg\| \le c(f)\|f - g\|$$

holds.

PROOF. Setting for $r \ne Pf$

$$\gamma(r) = \frac{\|f - r\| - \|f - Pf\|}{\|r - Pf\|}, \tag{43.2}$$

let us prove $\inf\{\gamma(r): r \in L_{mn}, r \ne Pf\} = \gamma > 0$. Suppose the contrary that $\gamma = 0$. Then there exists a sequence $\{r_k\}_{k=1}^{\infty}$ such that $r_k = p_k/q_k$, $r_k \ne Pf$, $p_k \in L_{m0}$, $q_k \in L_{n0}$,

$$\|p_k\| + \|q_k\| = 1, \qquad \lim_{k \to \infty} \gamma(r_k) = 0. \tag{43.3}$$

Let $Pf = p/q$, where $p \in L_{m0}$, $q \in L_{n0}$.

It follows from (43.3) that there exist subsequences for which

$$\lim_{s \to \infty} \|p_{k_s} - p^*\| = \lim_{s \to \infty} \|q_{k_s} - q^*\| = 0. \tag{43.4}$$

Note that $\|p^*/q^*\| < \infty$, because by (43.2) the opposite case leads to $\gamma = 1$.

Let us show that $p^*/q^* = r^* = p/q = Pf$. Indeed, if $r^* \ne p/q = Pf$ by (43.2) it follows that

$$0 = \gamma = \lim_{k \to \infty} \gamma(r_k) = \lim_{k \to \infty} \frac{\|f - r_k\| - \|f - Pf\|}{\|r_k - Pf\|}$$

$$= \frac{\|f - r^*\| - \|f - Pf\|}{\|r^* - Pf\|} > 0,$$

because $\|f - r^*\| > \|f - Pf\|$ if $r^* \ne Pf$ (Pf is a unique element of the best approximation). This is a contradiction.

Since $d(Pf) = 0$, $Pf = p/q$, either p has a degree of exactly m or q has a degree of exactly n.

Let

$$Y = \{x: |f(x) - Pf(x)| = \|f - Pf\|\}, \qquad \sigma(x) = \operatorname{sgn}\{f(x) - Pf(x)\}.$$

For every $y \in Y$ it is fulfilled that

$$\gamma(r_k)\|r_k - Pf\| = \|r_k - f\| - \|f - Pf\|$$
$$\ge \sigma(y)[f(y) - r_k(y)] - \sigma(y)[f(y) - Pf(y)]$$
$$= \sigma(y)[Pf(y) - r_k(y)]$$
$$= \frac{\sigma(y)[q_k(y)Pf(y) - p_k(y)]}{q_k(y)}. \tag{43.5}$$

By (43.4) and $|q(x)| > 0$ for $x \in [a, b]$ it follows that there exist $\varepsilon > 0$ and $N > 0$ such that for $k > N$, $|q_k(x)| \geq \varepsilon$.

Let

$$\inf\{\max_{y \in Y} \sigma(y)(\bar{q}Pf - \bar{p})(y): \bar{q} \in L_{n0}, \bar{p} \in L_{m0}, \|\bar{q}Pf - \bar{p}\| = 1\} = c > 0.$$

Assume the contrary, that $c = 0$. Since the set $\{\bar{p}, \bar{q}\}$, $\bar{q} \in L_{n0}$, $\bar{p} \in L_{m0}$, $\|\bar{q}Pf - \bar{p}\| = 1$, is a compact there are $\tilde{q} \in L_{n0}$, $\tilde{p} \in L_{m0}$, $\|\tilde{q}Pf - \tilde{p}\| = 1$, such that

$$\max_{y \in Y} \sigma(y)(\tilde{q}Pf - \tilde{p})(y) = 0. \tag{43.6}$$

By Theorem 28.2 the set Y contains $N = m + n + 2$ points $a \leq x_1 < x_2 < \cdots < x_N \leq b$ such that

$$\sigma(x_i) = \operatorname{sgn}[f(x_i) - Pf(x_i)] = \eta(-1)^i, \quad i = 1, 2, \ldots, N, \quad \eta = \pm 1. \tag{43.7}$$

The equalities (43.6), (43.7) give

$$\eta(-1)^i[\tilde{q}(x_i)Pf(x_i) - \tilde{p}(x_i)] \leq 0, \quad i = 1, 2, \ldots, N. \tag{43.8}$$

By Theorem 43.1 the function set

$$A = \{p + gPf: p \in L_{m0}, g \in L_{n0}\},$$

has a dimension $k = m + n + 1$ and every function $\varphi \in A$ has at most $k - 1$ zeros in $[a, b]$. It follows from (43.8) that $\tilde{q}Pf - \tilde{p} \in A$ has $k + 1$ zeros in $[a, b]$, i.e. $\tilde{q}Pf - \tilde{p} \equiv 0$, which contradicts $\|\tilde{q}Pf - \tilde{p}\| = 1$. Therefore $c > 0$.

From (43.5)–(43.7), and $\varepsilon \leq |q_k(x)| \leq 1$ for $k > N$, it follows that

$$\gamma(r_k)\|r_k - Pf\| \geq \max_{y \in Y} \frac{\sigma(y)[q_k(y)Pf(y) - p_k(y)]}{q_k(y)}$$

$$\geq \max_{y \in Y} \sigma(y)[q_k(y)Pf(y) - p_k(y)]$$

$$\geq c\|q_kPf - p_k\| \geq c\varepsilon\|Pf - r_k\|;$$

i.e. $\gamma(r_k) \geq c\varepsilon$, which contradicts $\lim_{k \to \infty} \gamma(r_k) = 0$.

By (43.2) for $r = Pg$ the existence of a constant $\gamma(f) > 0$ follows such that

$$\gamma(f)\|Pf - Pg\| \leq \|f - Pg\| - \|f - Pf\| \leq \|f - g\| + \|g - Pg\| - \|f - Pf\|$$

$$\leq \|f - g\| + \|g - Pf\| - \|f - Pf\|$$

$$\leq \|f - g\| + \|g - f\| + \|f - Pf\| - \|f - Pf\| = 2\|f - g\|;$$

that is

$$\|Pf - Pg\| \leq \frac{2}{\gamma(f)} \|f - g\|. \qquad \square$$

The situation for the function f, for which $d(Pf) > 0$, is quite different. The next theorem shows the possibility of an unstable numerical process.

Uniform approximation

THEOREM 43.3 (PETRUSHEV and POPOV [1987], p. 31). *Let $f \in C_{[0,1]}$ and $d(Pf) > 0$. There exists a $\delta > 0$ such that for every ε, $0 < \varepsilon < \delta$, there is a function $g \in C_{[0,1]}$ such that*

$$\|f - g\| \leq 2\varepsilon, \quad d(Pg) = d(Pf) - 1, \quad \|Pf - Pg\| \geq \delta.$$

PROOF. Let the points of alternation for $f - Pf$ be $0 \leq x_1 < x_2 < \cdots < x_k \leq 1$, $k = m + n + 2 - d(Pf)$. Without loss of generality let $f(x_1) - Pf(x_1) = E_{mn}(f)$ and therefore $f(x_2) - Pf(x_2) = -E_{mn}(f)$. The point x_1 can be determined by $x_1 = \max\{x: f(x) - Pf(x) = E_{mn}(f), x < x_2\}$. Let

$$z = \min\{x: f(x) - Pf(x) = 0, x_1 < x < x_2\},$$

$$I_1 = \{x: 0 \leq x \leq z\}, \quad I_2 = \{x: z \leq x \leq 1\}.$$

It is clear that there exists $\delta > 0$, $\delta < E_{mn}(f)$, such that

$$f(x) - Pf(x) - \delta > -E_{mn}(f) \quad \text{for } x \in I_1.$$

Let $0 < \varepsilon < \delta$, $y_1 = \max\{x: x \in [x_1, z], f(x) - Pf(x) = E_{mn}(f) - \varepsilon\}$, $Pf = p/q$, $q(x) \geq \mu > 0$ for $x \in [0, 1]$.

The function $\varphi_a(x) = \gamma(x - \alpha)/(x - \beta)$ satisfies the conditions $\varphi_a(0) = a$, $\varphi_a(y_1) = \min(\varepsilon\mu, a/2) \equiv b$, $\varphi_a'(x) < 0$ for $x \in [0, 1]$, if $\gamma > a > 0$ and

$$\alpha = ay_1(b - \gamma)/\gamma(b - a), \quad \beta = y_1(b - \gamma)/(b - a).$$

The function $\psi_a = \varphi_a/q$ satisfies

$$f(x_0) - [Pf(x) + \psi_a(x)] \geq -E_{mn}(f) \quad \text{for } x \in I_1 \text{ and } 0 < a \leq \delta\mu.$$

By continuity of φ_a as a function of a it follows that when a increases there exists a number a_1 and a point $x_0 \in [0, y_1)$ for which

$$f(x) - [Pf(x) + \psi_{a_1}(x_0)] = -E_{mn}(f)$$

and for every $x \in I_1$

$$|f(x) - [Pf(x_0) + \psi_{a_1}(x)]| \leq E_{mn}(f).$$

Obviously $a_1 \geq \delta$.

There is a point $y_2 \in [y_1, z)$ such that

$$f(y_2) - (Pf(y_2) + \psi_{a_1}(y_2)) = \max\{f(x) - (Pf(x) + \psi_{a_1}(x)): x \in [y_1, z)\}$$

$$= E_{mn}(f) - \xi,$$

where $0 < \xi < 2\varepsilon$. Define $Pg = Pf + \psi_{a_1}$, $Pg \in L_{m-d(Pf)+1, n-d(Pf)+1} \subset L_{m,n}$, where the function g is defined as

$$g(x) = \begin{cases} f(x) + \psi_{a_1}(x), & \text{for } x \in I_2, \\ f(x), & \text{for } x \in [0, x_0], \\ \text{to satisfy} \quad \begin{array}{l} g(y_1) = f(y_1) + \xi, \\ |f(x) - g(x)| \leq 2\varepsilon, \\ |g(x) - Pg(x)| \leq E_{mn}(f), \end{array} & \begin{array}{l} g \in C_{[0,1]}, \\ \text{for } x \in [x_0, z], \\ \text{for } x \in [y_1, z]. \end{array} \end{cases}$$

It follows from the above construction that the points $x_0 < y_2 < x_2 < x_3 < \cdots < x_k$ are the points of alternation for $g - Pg$ and consequently, by Theorem 28.2, $E_{mn}(g) = \|g - Pg\| = \|f - Pf\| = E_{mn}(f)$. Since $\|Pf - Pg\| \geq \|\psi_{a_1}\| \geq \delta$, $\|f - g\| \leq 2\varepsilon$, the theorem is proved. □

THEOREM 43.4 (BARRODALLE, POWELL and ROBERTS [1972]). *Let K be a finite point set and*

$$L_{mn} = \left\{ \varphi : \varphi = \sum_{i=0}^{m} a_i x^i \Big/ \sum_{i=0}^{n} b_i x^i, \sum_{i=0}^{n} b_i x^i > 0 \text{ for } x \in K, \max_{0 \leq i \leq n} |b_i| = 1 \right\}.$$

If $r^* = p^*/q^*$, $r^* \in L_{mn}$ is the rational function of the best uniform approximation of the continuous function f on K for which $d(Pf) = 0$ (see Theorem 43.2), then there exists a constant θ such that for every $r = p/q$, $r \in L_{mn}$, it is fulfilled that

$$\|q - q^*\| \leq \theta \|r - r^*\|.$$

PROOF. Let $\delta = \|r - r^*\|$ and $M = \max_{x \in K} \sum_{i=0}^{n} |x|^i$. Then

$$\max_{x \in K} |p(x)q^*(x) - q(x)p^*(x)| \leq M^2 \delta. \tag{43.9}$$

Denote

$$r(x) = \sum_{i=0}^{m} p_i x^i \Big/ \sum_{i=0}^{n} q_i x^i \quad \text{and} \quad r^*(x) = \sum_{i=0}^{m} p_i^* x^i \Big/ \sum_{i=0}^{n} q_i^* x^i.$$

The condition $d(Pf) = 0$ leads to $p_m^* q_n^* \neq 0$. Let $p_m^* \neq 0$ (otherwise the proof is similar). Determine $\alpha = p_m/p_m^*$ and

$$\bar{p}(x) = p(x) - \alpha p^*(x) = \sum_{i=0}^{m-1} \bar{p}_i x^i, \tag{43.10a}$$

$$\bar{q}(x) = q(x) - \alpha q^*(x) = \sum_{i=0}^{n} \bar{q}_i x^i. \tag{43.10b}$$

From (43.9) it follows that

$$\max_{x \in K} \left| \sum_{i=0}^{m-1} \bar{p}_i x^i q^*(x) - \sum_{i=0}^{n} \bar{q}_i x^i p^*(x) \right| \leq M \delta^2. \tag{43.11}$$

The functions $x^i q^*$, $i = 0, 1, \ldots, m - 1$, and $x^i p^*$, $i = 0, 1, \ldots, n$, are linearly independent on K. In the opposite case there exist polynomials $A \in H_{m-1}$ and $B \in H_n$ such that

$$A(x)q^*(x) - B(x)p^*(x) = 0 \quad \text{for } x \in K.$$

Let the number of points of K be $N \geq m + n + 1$. Then the polynomial $A(x)q^*(x) - B(x)p^*(x)$ is identically zero and therefore Aq^* vanishes at the m zeros of p^*. Because the degree of A is $m - 1$ it follows that p^* and q^* have at least one zero. This contradicts $d(Pf) = 0$. So the functions in (43.11) are linearly independent and therefore there exists a constant d such that the inequalities

$$\bar{p}_i \le d\delta, \quad i=0, 1, \ldots, m-1, \tag{43.12a}$$

$$\bar{q}_i \le d\delta, \quad i=0, 1, \ldots, n, \tag{43.12b}$$

are valid for all $r \in L_{mn}$.

Equations (43.10) give

$$\bar{q}_i = q_i - \alpha q_i^*, \quad i=0, 1, \ldots, n, \tag{43.13}$$

and if $|q_j| = 1$ then (43.12) and $|\bar{q}_i + \alpha q_i^*| = 1$ lead to $|\alpha| \ge 1 - d\delta$. Similarly if $|q_j^*| = 1$ in (43.13), then it follows that $|\alpha| \le 1 - d\delta$. So, $\lim_{\delta \to 0} \alpha = \pm 1$ and the condition $q(x) > 0$ for $x \in K$ gives $\lim_{\delta \to 0} \alpha = 1$.

The expressions (43.10) show that $0 < q(y) = \bar{q}(y) + \alpha q^*(y)$ for some $y \in K$ and using (43.12) the estimation

$$\|q^*\| \le Md\delta \tag{43.14}$$

follows. Hence, $\alpha > -Md\delta/q^*(y)$. The last inequality and $|\alpha| \ge 1 - d\delta$, $|\alpha| \le 1 - d\delta$ imply that the bounds

$$-d\delta \le 1 - \alpha \le d\delta[3 + 2M/q^*(y)] = \bar{d}\delta \tag{43.15}$$

hold for all $\delta > 0$. Combining (43.10), (43.14) and (43.15) it follows that

$$\|q - q^*\| \le \|\bar{q}\| + \|(\alpha - 1)q^*\| \le Md\delta + \bar{d}\delta\|q^*\|. \quad \square$$

REMARK 43.1. In the linear case Theorem 43.2 has the following form.

THEOREM 43.2' (NIKOLSKII [1947]). *Let there exist on the closed bounded set D for every continuous function f a unique polynomial $P(f; x) = \Sigma_{i=0}^n a_i \varphi_i(x)$ of the best uniform approximation, where $\{\varphi_i\}_{i=0}^n$ are linear independent continuous functions. Then for every $\varepsilon > 0$ there is a $\delta = \delta(f; \varepsilon) > 0$ such that*

$$\max_{x \in D} |f(x) - f_1(x)| < \delta \Rightarrow \max_{x \in D} |P(f; x) - P(f_1; x)| < \varepsilon.$$

GALKIN [1971] proved that the operator P of the best uniform approximation by algebraic polynomials is uniformly continuous in some cases. Let $f \in \text{Lip } 1$ on the interval $[a, b]$. Then

$$\sup_{f, g \in \text{Lip } 1, \rho(f,g) \le \delta} \rho(Pf, Pg) \le (\ge) c_1(c_2) \begin{cases} \delta^{1/(n+1)}, & \delta \le b-a, \\ \delta, & \delta > b-a, \end{cases}$$

where $\rho(f, g) = \max_{x \in [a,b]} |f(x) - g(x)|$.

CHAPTER III

Numerical Integration

In this chapter two main aspects for numerical integration are considered:
  (1) problems connected with existence and uniqueness of general quadrature formulas of Gaussian type of which classical ones are special cases. CHAKALOV'S [1954] investigations solve this problem in an elegant classical way;
  (2) as a rule the remainder terms of common used quadrature formulas are derived under some restrictions on the smoothness of the integrand function. At the same time quadrature formulas do not use the fact of existence of the derivatives of the integrand function. Using the so-called averaged moduli of smoothness it is possible for the remainder terms of a series of quadrature formulas to be obtained without any additional restrictions on the integrand, except those that are necessary for existence of the considered quadrature formulas. The well-known remainder terms can be obtained as a consequence if the integrand functions have a specific number of derivatives or some other smooth properties (bounded variation, Riemann integrable derivatives, etc.). Also in many cases a known order of convergence follows under weaker restrictions of the integrand functions.
  The optimal quadrature formulas are an important part of modern theory for numerical integration. Because of the big volume of problems in this field and interesting and useful obtained results the general statement of a question is considered in Section 52.
  This chapter also considers some recent results of Monte-Carlo methods for numerical integration. They are convenient in the multidimensional case, and for this aim useful approaches, quadrature formulas that use random variables as well as the probable errors of the considered methods can be found.

44. Quadrature formulas

Let us consider the problem of building a quadrature formula of the type

$$\int_a^b f(x)\,dx = \sum_{k=0}^m \sum_{\lambda=0}^{r_k} A_{k\lambda} f^{(\lambda)}(x_k) + R_N(f), \qquad (44.1)$$

for which $R_N(\varphi) = 0$ if φ is an algebraic polynomial of degree $N-1$, $N =$

$r_0 + r_1 + \cdots + r_m + m + 1$, where the coefficients $A_{k\lambda}$ do not depend on the function, the points $\{x_i\}_{i=0}^m$ are different and lie in the interval $[a, b]$ and to every knot x_k the positive number r_k is assigned.

A quadrature formula of the type (44.1) always exists and it is unique; i.e. the coefficients $A_{k\lambda}$ are defined in a unique way. Indeed, let P_{N-1} be the unique Hermite polynomial of degree $N-1$ that satisfies the interpolation conditions (see Section 12)

$$P_{N-1}^{(\lambda)}(x_k) = f^{(\lambda)}(x_k), \quad k = 0, 1, \ldots, m, \ \lambda = 0, 1, \ldots, r_k.$$

By Theorem 12.1 this polynomial can be written in the form

$$P_{N-1}(x) = \sum_{k=0}^{m} \sum_{\lambda=0}^{r_k} f^{(\lambda)}(x_k) L_{k\lambda}(x), \tag{44.2}$$

where $L_{k\lambda}$ are polynomials of degree $N-1$ for which

$$L_{k\lambda}^{(j)}(x_i) = 0 \quad \text{for } k \neq i \text{ and } j = 0, 1, \ldots, r_k,$$

$$L_{k\lambda}^{(j)}(x_k) = \begin{cases} 0 & \text{for } \lambda \neq j, \\ 1 & \text{for } \lambda = j. \end{cases} \tag{44.3}$$

From (44.2) it is evident that the quadrature

$$\int_a^b f(x)\,dx \approx \int_a^b P_{N-1}(x)\,dx$$

is of the type (44.1) with coefficients $A_{k\lambda} = \int_a^b L_{k\lambda}(x)\,dx$. Such a quadrature is called an interpolation one and by the remainder term of the Hermite polynomial (12.3) it follows that it is exact for polynomials of degree $N-1$.

Vice versa, if the formula (44.1) is exact for the polynomials of degree less than N, then

$$\int_a^b L_{k\lambda}(x)\,dx = \sum_{i=0}^{m} \sum_{j=0}^{r_i} A_{ij} L_{k\lambda}^{(j)}(x_i).$$

From the last equality and (44.3) it follows that $A_{k\lambda} = \int_a^b L_{k\lambda}(x)\,dx$; i.e. such a quadrature is an interpolation one.

Because of the often used formulae of the type (44.1) a detailed investigation of their properties and remainder term $R_N(f)$ will be given.

THEOREM 44.1 (PEANO [1914]). *Let L be a linear functional of the kind*

$$Lf = \int_a^b \left(\sum_{i=0}^{m-1} a_i(x) f^{(i)}(x) \right) dx + \sum_{j=0}^{m-1} \sum_{i=0}^{n_j} b_{ij} f^{(j)}(x_{ij}),$$

where the functions a_i are partially continuous and the points x_{ij} lie in the interval $[a, b]$. If $L\varphi = 0$ for every polynomial φ of degree less than m, then for every function f with integrable mth derivative the following relation is fulfilled,

$$Lf = \int_a^b K(t) f^{(m)}(t) \, dt,$$

where

$$K(t) = L[(x-t)_+^{m-1}/(m-1)!], \quad x_+ = \begin{cases} x, & \text{if } x \geq 0, \\ 0, & \text{if } x < 0. \end{cases}$$

PROOF. By Taylor's formula

$$f(x) = \sum_{k=0}^{m-1} \frac{f^{(k)}(x)}{k!} (x-a)^k + \frac{1}{(m-1)!} \int_a^b (x-t)_+^{m-1} f^{(m)}(t) \, dt$$

it follows that

$$Lf = L\left[\frac{1}{(m-1)!} \int_a^b (x-t)_+^{m-1} f^{(m)}(t) \, dt \right]$$

$$= \int_a^b f^{(m)}(t) \int_a^b \left[\sum_{i=0}^{m-1} \frac{a_i(x)(x-t)_+^{m-i-1}}{(m-i-1)!} \right] dx \, dt$$

$$= \int_a^b \left[\sum_{j=0}^{m-1} \sum_{i=0}^{n_j} \frac{b_{ij}(x_{ij}-x)_+^{m-j-1}}{(m-j-1)!} \right] f^{(m)}(t) \, dt$$

$$= \int_a^b L[(x-t)_+^{m-1}] f^{(m)}(t)/(m-1)! \, dt. \quad \square$$

From the remainder term of the Hermite interpolation polynomial (12.3) it follows that $R_N(f) = \text{const } f^{(N)}(\xi)/N!$, $\xi \in (a, b)$. Another approach for the determination of $R_N(f)$ and the coefficients $A_{k\lambda}$ in (44.1) was given by CHAKALOV ([1949]; [1983], p. 196) by the following theorem.

THEOREM 44.2. *Let $\{x_i\}_{i=1}^n$ be different points in $[a, b]$ and $r_1, r_2, \ldots, r_n$ be non-negative and integer numbers. Letting*

$$P(x) = (x-x_1)^{r_1+1}(x-x_2)^{r_2+1} \cdots (x-x_n)^{r_n+1},$$

$$R(z) = \frac{1}{P(z)} \int_a^b \frac{P(z) - P(x)}{z - x} \, dx,$$

a necessary and sufficient condition for the quadrature formula

$$\int_a^b f(x) \, dx = \sum_{k=1}^n \sum_{\lambda=0}^{r_k} A_{k\lambda} f^{(\lambda)}(x_k) + R_n(f) \tag{44.4}$$

to be exact for the polynomials of degree $N - 1$, $N = r_1 + r_2 + \cdots + r_n + n$, are the relations $\lambda! A_{k\lambda} = B_{k\lambda}$, where $B_{k\lambda}$ are the coefficients in the expansion

$$R(z) = \sum_{k=1}^{n} \sum_{\lambda=0}^{r_k} \frac{B_{k\lambda}}{(z - x_k)^{\lambda+1}}. \tag{44.5}$$

The remainder term has the form

$$R_n(f) = \int_a^b U(t) f^{(N)}(t)\, dt,$$

where

$$U(t) = \frac{(b - t)^N}{N!} - \sum_{k=1}^{n} \sum_{\lambda=0}^{r_k} A_{k\lambda} \frac{(x_k - t)_+^{N-\lambda-1}}{(N - \lambda - 1)!}.$$

PROOF. Let us denote

$$L[f] \equiv \sum_{k=1}^{n} \sum_{\lambda=0}^{r_k} A_{k\lambda} f^{(\lambda)}(x_k).$$

Let the quadrature (44.4) be exact for polynomials of degree less than N. For the polynomial $Q(x) \equiv [P(z) - P(x)]/(z - x)$ of degree $N - 1$ the following relation is fulfilled:

$$L[Q] = P(z) L[1/(z - x)] - L[P(x)/(z - x)] = P(z) \sum_{k=1}^{n} \sum_{\lambda=0}^{r_k} \frac{\lambda! A_{k\lambda}}{(z - x_k)^{\lambda+1}}.$$

The last equality and $L[Q] = \int_a^b Q(x)\, dx$ give

$$R(z) = \frac{1}{P(z)} \int_a^b \frac{P(z) - P(x)}{z - x}\, dx = \sum_{k=1}^{n} \sum_{\lambda=0}^{r_k} \frac{\lambda! A_{k\lambda}}{(z - x_k)^{\lambda+1}}. \tag{44.6}$$

Since the extension (44.6) of the rational function $R(z)$ is unique it follows that $\lambda! A_{k\lambda} = B_{k\lambda}$.

Let us now prove that if $\lambda! A_{k\lambda} = B_{k\lambda}$, then the quadrature (44.4) is exact for polynomials of degree less than N. Indeed let $B_{k\lambda}$ satisfy (44.5). From

$$L[f] \equiv \sum_{k=1}^{n} \sum_{\lambda=0}^{r_k} B_{k\lambda} f^{(\lambda)}(x_k)/\lambda!$$

it follows that

$$L\left[\frac{P(z) - P(x)}{z - x}\right] = P(z) L[1/(z - x)] - L[P(x)/(z - x)]$$

$$= P(z) \sum_{k=1}^{n} \sum_{\lambda=0}^{r_k} \frac{B_{k\lambda}}{(z - x_k)^{\lambda+1}}$$

$$= P(z) R(z) - \frac{1}{P(z)} \int_a^b \frac{P(z) - P(x)}{z - x}\, dx.$$

This means that for every z the quadrature (44.4) is exact for the polynomials
$$\frac{P(z) - P(x)}{z - x} = z^{N-1} + p_1(x)z^{N-2} + \cdots + p_{N-1}(x),$$
where
$$p_k(x) = x^k + a_{k1}x^{k-1} + \cdots + a_{k,k}.$$
Therefore,
$$\sum_{k=0}^{N-1} z^{N-k-1} \int_a^b p_k(x)\,dx = \sum_{k=0}^{N-1} z^{N-k-1} L[p_k].$$
Both sides of the last equality are polynomials of degree $N-1$ and therefore
$$\int_a^b p_k(x)\,dx = L[p_k], \quad k = 0, 1, \ldots, N-1.$$
If Q is an algebraic polynomial of degree less than N the equality
$$\int_a^b Q(x)\,dx = L[Q]$$
follows from the linear independence of the polynomials $\varphi_0, \varphi_1, \ldots, \varphi_{N-1}$.

The representation of the remainder term $R_n(f)$ in the theorem follows by applying Theorem 44.1 to the linear functional
$$R_n(f) = \int_a^b f(x)\,dx - L[f]. \qquad \square$$

In the case of equidistant knots, $x_k = a + k(b-a)/m$ and $r_k = 0$, $k = 0, 1, \ldots, m$, the interpolation quadrature formula (44.1) is called the Newton–Cotes formula. Examples of such simple formulas are:

(1) $m = 0$—the rectangle formula,
$$\int_a^b f(x)\,dx = (b-a)f\left(\frac{a+b}{2}\right) + \frac{(b-a)^3}{24} f''(\xi), \quad \xi \in (a,b);$$

(2) $m = 1$—the trapezoidal rule,
$$\int_a^b f(x)\,dx = \frac{b-a}{2}[f(a) + f(b)] - \frac{(b-a)^3}{12} f''(\xi), \quad \xi \in (a,b);$$

(3) $m = 2$—Simpson's rule,
$$\int_a^b f(x)\,dx = \frac{b-a}{6}\left[f(a) + 4f\left(\frac{a+b}{2}\right) + f(b)\right] - \frac{(b-a)^5}{2880} f^{(4)}(\xi),$$
$\xi \in (a,b)$;

(4) $m = 3$—the so-called $\frac{3}{8}$ rule,

$$\int_a^b f(x)\,dx = \frac{b-a}{8}\left[f(a) + 3f\left(\frac{2a+b}{3}\right) + 3f\left(\frac{a+2b}{3}\right) + f(b)\right] + R_3(f),$$

$$R_3(f) = -\frac{(b-a)^5}{6480} f^{(4)}(\xi), \quad \xi \in (a,b);$$

(5) $m = 4$,

$$\int_a^b f(x)\,dx = \frac{b-a}{90}\left[7f(a) + 32f\left(\frac{3a+b}{4}\right) + 12f\left(\frac{a+b}{2}\right)\right.$$

$$\left. + 32f\left(\frac{a+3b}{4}\right) + 7f(b)\right] + R_4(f),$$

$$|R_4(f)| = \frac{(b-a)^7}{1935360} |f^{(6)}(\xi)|, \quad \xi \in (a,b).$$

45. Optimal knots

It was shown in Section 44 that for every system of knots $a \leq x_1 < x_2 < \cdots < x_n \leq b$ and arbitrary non-negative integer numbers $r_1, r_2, \ldots, r_n$ it is possible to find numbers $A_{k\lambda}$ such that the quadrature

$$\int_a^b f(x)\,dx = \sum_{k=1}^n \sum_{\lambda=0}^{r_k} A_{k\lambda} f^{(\lambda)}(x_k) + R_n(f) \tag{45.1}$$

is exact for polynomials of degree less than N, $N = r_1 + r_2 + \cdots + r_n + n$. It is said that the quadrature has an algebraic degree of exactness (ADE) $N-1$.

The question is: does there exist points $a \leq x_1 < x_2 < \cdots < x_n \leq b$ for which the interpolation quadrature formula (45.1) has an ADE higher than $N-1$. The answer was given by CHAKALOV ([1954]; [1983], p. 203).

THEOREM 45.1. *For arbitrary non-negative even numbers $r_1, r_2, \ldots, r_n$ there exist n different points $a < x_1 < x_2 < \cdots x_n < b$ such that the polynomial*

$$P(x) = \prod_{k=1}^n (x - x_k)^{r_k + 1}$$

is orthogonal to every polynomial of degree less than n in $[a,b]$.

PROOF. The function

$$F(t_1, t_2, \ldots, t_n) = \int_a^b \prod_{k=1}^n (t - t_k)^{r_k + 2}\,dt \tag{45.2}$$

is positive for every t_k and has a minimum in the domain $D_n: -\infty < t_1 \leq t_2 \leq \cdots \leq t_n < \infty$ of n-dimensional space $\mathbb{R}^n$. Let $C_n \subseteq \mathbb{R}^n$, $C_n: a - \delta \leq t_k \leq b + \delta$, $k = 1, 2, \ldots, n$, where δ is a positive number. The set $E_n = C_n \cap D_n$ is compact and the function F attains its minimum value μ at some point $(x_1, x_2, \ldots, x_n) \in C_n$, $x_1 \leq x_2 \leq \cdots \leq x_n$. Let us show that the function F takes values larger than μ in every point of $D_n \backslash C_n$ for large enough δ. Indeed, if $t_j \not\in [a - \delta, b + \delta]$ then for every $x \in [a, b]$, $|x - t_j| \geq \delta$. Therefore,

$$\int_a^b \prod_{k=1}^n (t - t_k)^{r_k + 2} \, dt = \int_a^b (t - t_j)^2 \prod_{k=1}^n (t - t_k)^{r_k + 2} / (t - t_j)^2 \, dt$$

$$> \delta^2 \int_a^b \prod_{k=1}^n (t - t_k)^{r_k + 2} / (t - t_j)^2 \, dt .$$

Divide the interval $[a, b]$ into n equal parts. There are at most $n - 1$ points of $\{t_k\}_{k=1}^n$ in $[a, b]$. Therefore, there exists a subinterval $[a', b'] \subseteq [a, b]$ which does not contain a point from $\{t_k\}_{k=1}^n$. Divide the interval $[a', b']$ into three equal parts and let $[\alpha, \beta]$ lie in the middle. Evidently $\beta - \alpha = (b - a)/3n$ and

$$\int_a^b \prod_{k=1}^n (t - t_k)^{r_k + 2} / (t - t_j)^2 \, dt > \int_a^b \prod_{k=1}^n (\beta - \alpha)^{r_k + 2} / (\beta - \alpha)^2 \, dt = (\beta - \alpha)^{N + n - 2}.$$

So, if at least one coordinate of the point in $\mathbb{R}^n$ lies outside of the interval $[a - \delta, b + \delta]$, then the function F takes values larger than $\delta^2 (\beta - \alpha)^{N + n - 2}$. Let us choose δ to be sufficiently large that

$$\delta^2 (\beta - \alpha)^{N + n - 2} > F(c, c, \ldots, c), \quad c = (a + b)/2 .$$

Since the point $(c, c, \ldots, c) \in E_n$ it follows that $F(c, c, \ldots, c) \geq \mu$. Therefore, such a choice of δ ensures values of F larger than μ for every point outside of E_n. The conclusion is that the minimum of F in D_n is also μ and it attains for some end point of D_n

$$(x_1, x_2, \ldots, x_n), \quad x_1 \leq x_2 \leq \cdots \leq x_n .$$

Let us show that the coordinates x_k are different. Assuming the contrary $x_j = x_{j+1} = \cdots = x_m = d$, $x_{j-1} < x_j$, $x_m < x_{m+1}$ if $m < n$. Letting $r_k + 2 = p_k$, $k = 1, 2, \ldots, n$ and

$$Q(x) = (x - d)^{-p_j - p_m} \prod_{k=1}^n (x - x_k)^{p_k} ,$$

the function

$$\varphi(h) = \int_a^b Q(x)(x - d + p_m h)^{p_j} (x - d - p_j h)^{p_m} \, dx$$

takes the value μ for $h = 0$ and $\varphi'(0) = 0$,

$$\varphi''(0) = -p_m p_j \int_a^b Q(x)(x-d)^{p_j+p_m-2}\,dx < 0.$$

Hence, the function φ takes values of less than μ for sufficiently small and positive h. This is impossible because $\varphi(h)$ is equal to $F(t_1, t_2, \ldots, t_n)$ substituting t_k by x_k for $k \neq j, m$ and t_j, t_m by $d - p_m h$ and $d + p_j h$, respectively. This substitution does not disturb the ordering $t_1 \leq t_2 \leq \cdots \leq t_n$ for small enough h. So the points $\{x_k\}_{k=1}^n$ for which F attains its minimum in D_n are different. Therefore,

$$\left.\frac{\partial F}{\partial t_i}\right|_{t_k=x_k} = (r_i + 2) \int_a^b \prod_{k=1}^n (x-x_k)^{r_k+2}/(x_i-x)\,dx = 0, \quad i=1,2,\ldots,n.$$

From here $\int_a^b P(x)L_{i0}(x)\,dx = 0$, where L_{i0} are the basic Lagrange polynomials in the Lagrange interpolation polynomial for the knots $x_1, x_2, \ldots, x_n$, see Section 2. Since every polynomial of degree $n-1$ can be represented as a linear combination of $\{L_{k0}\}_{k=1}^n$ it follows that P is orthogonal to every polynomial of degree $n-1$.

Let us prove that the numbers $x_k \in (a, b)$. Assuming the contrary let at least one zero x_k of P lie outside of (a, b). Then the zeros $b_2, b_3, \ldots, b_\nu$ of P from (a, b) are of degree at most $n-1$. Therefore, $P_1(x) = (x-b_2)\cdots(x-b_\nu)$ is a polynomial of degree at most $n-1$ and

$$\int_a^b P(x)P_1(x)\,dx = 0.$$

The last equality is impossible because the function PP_1 does not change sign in the interval (a, b). This contradiction proves that all the zeros of P lie in the interval (a, b).

Conversely, if the polynomial P is orthogonal in (a, b) to every polynomial of degree $n-1$, then:
(1) all its zeros x_k are real, different and lie in (a, b);
(2) the multiplicities $r_k + 1$ of the zeros x_k are odd numbers;
(3) the function $F(t_1, t_2, \ldots, t_n)$ from (45.2) has a local minimum at $(x_1, x_2, \ldots, x_n)$.

The assertion (1) was proved from the orthogonality above. Assuming that $r_k + 1$ is an even number, the polynomial $P_2(x) = (x-x_1)\cdots(x-x_n)/(x-x_k)$ is of degree $n-1$ and

$$\int_a^b P(x)P_2(x)\,dx = 0,$$

which contradicts $PP_2 \geq 0$ in $[a, b]$. Finally, from

$$\frac{\partial F}{\partial x_j} = 0, \qquad \frac{\partial^2 F}{\partial x_j \partial x_i} = 0,$$

$$\frac{\partial^2 F}{\partial x_j^2} = (r_j + 2)(r_j + 1) \int_a^b \prod_{k=1}^n (x - x_k)^{r_k+2}/(x - x_j)^2 \, dt > 0,$$

it follows that the function F has a local minimum at the point $(x_1, x_2, \ldots, x_n)$. □

THEOREM 45.2. *For every n integer, non-negative numbers $r_1, r_2, \ldots, r_n$ there exist n real numbers $a < x_1 < x_2 < \cdots < x_n < b$ and N coefficients $A_{k\lambda}$, $k = 1, 2, \ldots, n$, $\lambda = 0, 1, \ldots, r_k$, $N = r_1 + r_2 + \cdots + r_n + n$, such that the quadrature (45.1) is exact for every polynomial of degree less than $N_1 = \sum_{k=1}^n (2[\frac{1}{2}r_k] + 2)$. Conversely, for arbitrary numbers x_k and $A_{k\lambda}$ the quadrature (45.1) cannot be exact for all polynomials of degree N_1.*

PROOF. Let us first prove the converse assertion. The polynomial $f(x) = \prod_{k=1}^n (x - x_k)^{2s_k}$ of degree N_1, $N_1 = 2(s_1 + s_2 + \cdots + s_n)$, $s_k = 1 + [\frac{1}{2}r_k]$, satisfies $\int_a^b f(x) \, dx > 0$ and at the same time the right-hand side of (45.1) vanishes because $r_k < 2s_k$. Therefore, the quadrature (45.1) is not exact for the polynomial f for arbitrary values of x_k and $A_{k\lambda}$.

Assuming that the numbers r_k are even, let the polynomial P of degree N with zeros $x_1^*, x_2^*, \ldots, x_n^*$ and with multiplicities $r_1 + 1, r_2 + 1, \ldots, r_n + 1$ be orthogonal to all polynomials of degree $n - 1$. By Theorem 45.1 such a polynomial exists. Let Q be an arbitrary polynomial of degree $N_1 - 1$. Representing Q in the form $Q = PQ_1 + R$, where Q_1 and R are polynomials of degree $n - 1$ and $N - 1$, set the knots x_k in (45.1) be equal to x_k^*. The coefficients $A_{k\lambda}$ can be taken as in Theorem 45.1; i.e. the quadrature (45.1) is exact for polynomials of degree $N - 1$. Denote by

$$L[f] = \sum_{k=1}^n \sum_{\lambda=0}^{r_k} A_{k\lambda} f^{(\lambda)}(x_k);$$

it follows that

$$L[R] = \int_a^b Q(x) \, dx = \int_a^b P(x) Q_1(x) \, dx + \int_a^b R(x) \, dx,$$

as P is orthogonal to Q_1. The equalities

$$R^{(\lambda)}(x_k) = Q^{(\lambda)}(x_k), \quad k = 1, 2, \ldots, n, \quad \lambda = 0, 1, \ldots, r_k,$$

imply that $L[R] = L[Q]$ and the quadrature (45.1) is exact for every polynomial of degree $N_1 - 1$.

Let us consider the case when there are odd numbers between the numbers $\{r_k\}_{k=1}^n$. For every r_k denote by r_k' the largest even number that satisfies $r_k' \leq r_k$; i.e. $r_k' = 2[\frac{1}{2}r_k]$. Since the numbers r_k' are even it is possible to build a quadrature formula

$$\int_a^b f(x) \, dx = \sum_{k=1}^n \sum_{\lambda=0}^{r_k'} A_{k\lambda} f^{(\lambda)}(x_k) + R_n'(f), \tag{45.3}$$

which is exact for the polynomials of degree $m = \sum_{k=1}^{n} (r'_k + 2) - 1$. The quadrature (45.3) is of the type (45.1) with coefficients $A_{kr_k} = 0$, for r_k an odd number and it is exact for every polynomial of degree $m - 1$,

$$m = \sum_{k=1}^{n} (2[\tfrac{1}{2}r_k] + 2) = N_1. \qquad \square$$

Theorem 44.2 shows that the quadrature formula of type (45.1) has a remainder term $R_n(f)$ of the form

$$R_n(f) = \int_a^b U(t) f^{(N_1)}(t)\, dt, \qquad U(t) = \frac{(b-t)^{N_1}}{N_1!} - L[(x-t)_+^{N_1-1}/(N_1-1)!]. \qquad (45.4)$$

Let x_k and $A_{k\lambda}$ be the knots and the coefficients in the quadrature (45.1). Letting $f = g'$ in (45.3) it follows that

$$g(b) - g(a) - \sum_{k=1}^{n} \sum_{\lambda=0}^{r_k} A_{k\lambda} g^{(\lambda+1)}(x_k) = \int_a^b U(t) g^{(N_1+1)}(t)\, dt.$$

The left-hand side of the last equality is a linear combination of $2 + \sum_{k=1}^{n}(r_k + 2) = N_1 + 2$ values

$$\{g^{(\lambda+1)}(x_k),\ k = 1, 2, \ldots, n,\ \lambda = 0, 1, \ldots, r_k + 1,\ g(a), g(b)\}$$

and vanishes for polynomials of degree less than $N_1 + 1$. On the other hand, it is different from zero for x^{N_1+1}. By Section 16 it follows that this linear combination is the divided difference

$$C \cdot D\!\left[f \,\bigg|\, \begin{matrix} a, b, x_1, \ldots, x_n \\ 1, 1, r_1 + I_2, \ldots, r_n + I_2 \end{matrix} \right],$$

where

$$C = \int_a^b U(t)(t^{N_1+1})^{(N_1+1)}\, dt. \qquad (45.5)$$

By Theorem 16.2 the divided difference $D[f]$ has a unique representation in the form

$$D[f] = \int_a^b U_1(t) f^{(N_1+1)}(t)\, dt$$

and U_1 is a positive function in (a, b). To evaluate the constant C let us substitute t^{N_1+1} in (45.5) by the polynomial (r_k are even numbers)

$$(N_1 + 1) \int_a^x \prod_{k=1}^{n} (t - x_k)^{r_k+2}\, dt = x^{N_1+1} + \varphi(x),$$

where φ is a polynomial of degree N_1. Therefore,

$$C = (N_1 + 1)! \int_a^b U(t)\,dt = (N_1 + 1) \int_a^b \prod_{k=1}^n (t - x_k)^{r_k+2}\,dt > 0.$$

By the positiveness of U and the mean-value theorem it follows that

$$R_n(f) = \int_a^b U(t) f^{(N_1)}(t)\,dt = f^{(N_1)}(\xi) \int_a^b U(t)\,dt$$

$$= \frac{f^{(N_1)}(\xi)}{N_1!} \int_a^b \prod_{k=1}^n (t - x_k)^{r_k+2}\,dt, \quad \xi \in (a, b). \tag{45.6}$$

REMARK 45.1. The quadrature (45.1) is an interpolation one and by Section 44 it is exact for polynomials of degree $\sum_{k=1}^n (r_k + 1) - 1$. By using a special choice of knots according to Theorem 45.2 the exactness of the interpolation quadrature (45.1) increases by an integer number G,

$$G = \sum_{k=1}^n \left(2\left[\frac{r_k}{2}\right] + 2\right) - \sum_{k=1}^n (r_k + 1) - 1.$$

It is evident that G is the number of the even numbers $r_1, r_2, \ldots, r_n$, i.e.:
 (1) odd numbers r_k are useless for the exactness of the quadrature (45.1);
 (2) if all numbers r_k are even the quadrature (45.1) has an algebraic degree of exactness $\sum_{k=1}^n r_k + 2n - 1$.

REMARK 45.2. GAUSS [1866] investigated the problem of optimal knots in the case $r_1 = r_2 = \cdots = r_n = 0$ for the first time. A detailed representation of the Gauss quadrature formula can be found, for example, in RALSTON [1965a], where the knots and the coefficients are given for different values of n.

The case $r_1 = r_2 = \cdots = r_n = \nu$ was studied by TURAN [1950]. If ν is an even number (see Remark 45.1), then Turan proved that the optimal knots are zeros of the unique polynomial $P_{n\nu}$ of degree n, which satisfies

$$\int_a^b [P_{n\nu}(x)]^{\nu+2}\,dx = \min_{x_k} \int_a^b [(x - x_1)(x - x_2) \cdots (x - x_n)]^{\nu+2}\,dx.$$

Only the uniqueness of the polynomial $P_{n\nu}$ is not a direct consequence of Theorem 45.2. If there are two such polynomials P_1 and P_2, then $P_1^{\nu+1}$ and $P_2^{\nu+1}$ are orthogonal to every polynomial of degree n and therefore

$$\int_a^b [P_2(x) - P_1(x)][P_2^{\nu+1}(x) - P_1^{\nu+1}(x)]\,dx$$

$$= \int_a^b [P_2(x) - P_1(x)]^2 \sum_{k=0}^\nu P_2^{\nu-k}(x) P_1^k(x)\,dx = 0.$$

The last equality is impossible, because

$$\frac{A^{\nu+1} - B^{\nu+1}}{A - B} = \sum_{k=0}^{\nu} A^{\nu-k} B^k > 0$$

implies $\sum_{k=0}^{\nu} P_2^{\nu-k}(x) P_1^k(x) > 0$ for all x, with a finite number of exceptions.

46. An estimate of the error of quadrature formulas

Let Lf be a quadrature formula in the interval $[0, 1]$

$$Lf = \sum_{i=0}^{m} \sum_{j=0}^{\alpha_i} A_{ij} f^{(j)}(x_i), \qquad (46.1)$$

where $0 \leq x_0 < x_1 < \cdots < x_m \leq 1$. Such a formula is determined uniquely by

$$A = \{A_{ij}: i = 0, 1, \ldots, m, \ j = 0, 1, \ldots, \alpha_i\},$$

$$\gamma = \{\gamma_i = (x_i, \alpha_i): i = 0, 1, \ldots, m\}.$$

The couple $\{A, \gamma\}$ determines the type of the quadrature formula Lf. From a quadrature formula Lf in the interval $[0, 1]$ one can obtain a quadrature formula for an arbitrary finite interval $[a, b]$ in the following way: multiply the coefficients A_{ij} by $(b - a)^{j+1}$; i.e. they become $(b - a)^{j+1} A_{ij}$, and the new knots y_i are determined by $y_i = a + x_i(b - a)$, $i = 0, 1, \ldots, m$. So for an arbitrary type $\{A, \gamma\}$ and for every finite interval $[a, b]$ a quadrature formula $L(\{A, \gamma\}, [a, b]) f$ of type $\{A, \gamma\}$ is given by

$$L(\{A, \gamma\}, [a, b]) f = \sum_{i=0}^{m} \sum_{j=0}^{\alpha_i} (b - a)^{j+1} A_{ij} f^{(j)}(y_i).$$

The quadrature formula $L_n(f)$ is called an n-composite quadrature formula in the interval $[a, b]$, generated by the quadrature formula Lf if

$$L_n(f) = \sum_{i=1}^{n} L(\{A, \gamma\}, [x_i, x_{i-1}]) f,$$

where $x_i = a + i(b - a)/n$, $i = 0, 1, \ldots, n$.

The quadrature formula Lf in the interval $[a, b]$ has a precision k if for every polynomial $f \in H_k$ the following relation is fulfilled

$$\int_a^b f(x) \, dx = Lf \quad \left(\text{or } \int_a^b p(x) f(x) \, dx = Lf, \text{ where } p \text{ is a weight function}\right).$$

Let us note that if Lf has a precision k, then $L(\{A, \gamma\}, [a, b]) f$ also has a precision k.

Let us consider the quadrature formula

$$Lf = \sum_{i=0}^{m} \sum_{j=0}^{\alpha_i} (b - a)^{j+1} A_{ij} f^{(j)}(y_i) \qquad (46.2)$$

in $[a, b]$ obtained in the way described above using (46.1).

THEOREM 46.1. *Let the quadrature formula (46.2) have precision k, i.e.,*

$$R(f) = \int_a^b f(x)\,dx - Lf = 0 \quad \text{for } f \in H_k.$$

Then for every function f, which has bounded derivatives up to the order $r = \max\{\alpha_i : 0 \leq i \leq m\}$, $k \geq r$, the following estimate holds:

$$|R(f)| \leq 6(b-a)^{r+1}\left(\frac{1}{r!} + \sum_{i=0}^{m}\sum_{j=0}^{\alpha_i} \frac{|A_{ij}|}{(r-j)!}\right)\omega_{k+1-r}(f^{(r)};[a,b]),$$

where $\omega_k(f;[a,b]) = \sup_{0 \leq \delta \leq (b-a)/k} \omega_k(f;\delta)$.

PROOF. Let P be the polynomial of the best uniform approximation of degree $k - r$ for the function $f^{(r)}$. By Whitney's Theorem 32.1 and Theorem 32.2 it follows that

$$\|P - f^{(r)}\|_{M[a,b]} \leq 6\omega_{k+1-r}(f;[a,b]). \tag{46.3}$$

The polynomial $Q \in H_k$,

$$Q(x) = f(a) + \frac{x-a}{1!}f'(a) + \cdots + \frac{(x-a)^{r-1}}{(r-1)!}f^{(r-1)}(a)$$

$$+ \frac{1}{(r-1)!}\int_a^x (x-t)^{r-1}P(t)\,dt, \tag{46.4}$$

and the identity

$$f(x) = f(a) + \frac{x-a}{1!}f'(a) + \cdots + \frac{(x-a)^{r-1}}{(r-1)!}f^{(r-1)}(a)$$

$$+ \frac{1}{(r-1)!}\int_a^x (x-t)^{r-1}f^{(r)}(t)\,dt, \tag{46.5}$$

together with (46.3) give

$$|f^{(j)}(y_i) - Q^{(j)}(y_i)| \leq 6\frac{(b-a)^{r-j}}{(r-j)!}\omega_{k+1-r}(f^{(r)};[a,b]), \tag{46.6}$$

for $i = 0, 1, \ldots, m$, $j = 0, 1, \ldots, \alpha_i$.

Since $Q \in H_k$, $R(Q) = 0$ and from (46.6)

$$|R(f)| \leq |R(f-Q)| + |R(Q)| = |R(f-Q)|$$

$$\leq \int_a^b |f(x) - Q(x)|\,dx + \sum_{i=0}^{m}\sum_{j=0}^{\alpha_i} |A_{ij}|(b-a)^{j+1}|f^{(j)}(y_i) - Q^{(j)}(y_i)|$$

$$\leq \int_a^b |f(x) - Q(x)|\,dx + 6(b-a)^{r+1}\omega_{k+1-r}(f^{(r)};[a,b])\sum_{i=0}^{m}\sum_{j=0}^{\alpha_i}\frac{|A_{ij}|}{(r-j)!}.$$

$$\tag{46.7}$$

From (46.3)–(46.5) it follows for every $x \in [a, b]$ that

$$|f(x) - Q(x)| \leq 6 \frac{(b-a)^r}{r!} \omega_{k+1-r}(f^{(r)}; [a, b]),$$

which together with (46.7) proves the theorem. □

THEOREM 46.2. *Let $L_n(f)$ be an n-composite quadrature formula for the interval $[a, b]$, generated by the quadrature formula (46.1). Let (46.1) have a precision k, $k \geq r$. Then the following estimate holds:*

$$|R_n(f)| = \left| \int_a^b f(x) \, dx - L_n(f) \right|$$

$$\leq 6 \left(\frac{b-a}{n} \right)^r \left(\frac{1}{r!} + \sum_{i=0}^m \sum_{j=0}^{\alpha_i} \frac{|A_{ij}|}{(r-j)!} \right) \tau_{k+1-r} \left(f^{(r)}; \frac{2(b-a)}{n(k+1-r)} \right)_L.$$

PROOF. Letting $L(\{a, \gamma\}, [a, b])f \equiv L(f; [a, b])$, from the definition it follows that

$$|R_n(f)| \leq \sum_{i=1}^n \left| \int_{x_{i-1}}^{x_i} f(x) \, dx - L(f; [x_i, x_{i-1}]) \right|. \tag{46.8}$$

Since $L(f; [x_i, x_{i-1}])$ has precision k and has the form (46.2), the Theorem 46.1 with $x_i - x_{i-1} = (b-a)/n$ gives

$$\left| \int_{x_{i-1}}^{x_i} f(x) \, dx - L(f; [x_i, x_{i-1}]) \right|$$

$$\leq 6 \left(\frac{b-a}{n} \right)^{r+1} \left(\frac{1}{r!} + \sum_{i=0}^m \sum_{j=0}^{\alpha_i} \frac{|A_{ij}|}{(r-j)!} \right) \omega_{k+1-r}(f^{(r)}; [x_i, x_{i-1}]).$$

If $x \in [x_i, x_{i-1}]$, then

$$\omega_{k+1-r}(f^{(r)}; [x_i, x_{i-1}]) \leq \omega_{k+1-r}\left(f^{(r)}, x; \frac{2(b-a)}{n(k+1-r)} \right).$$

The last two inequalities give

$$\left| \int_{x_{i-1}}^{x_i} f(x) \, dx - L(f; [x_i, x_{i-1}]) \right|$$

$$\leq 6 \left(\frac{b-a}{n} \right)^{r+1} \left(\frac{1}{r!} + \sum_{i=0}^m \sum_{j=0}^{\alpha_i} \frac{|A_{ij}|}{(r-j)!} \right) \int_{x_{i-1}}^{x_i} \omega_{k+1-r}\left(f^{(r)}, x; \frac{2(b-a)}{n(k+1-r)} \right) dx. \tag{46.9}$$

The assertion of the theorem follows from (46.8) and (46.9)

$$|R_n(f)|$$
$$\leq 6\left(\frac{b-a}{n}\right)^{r+1}\left(\frac{1}{r!} + \sum_{i=0}^{m}\sum_{j=0}^{\alpha_i}\frac{|A_{ij}|}{(r-j)!}\right)\int_a^b \omega_{k+1-r}\left(f^{(r)}, x; \frac{2(b-a)}{n(k+1-r)}\right) dx$$
$$\leq 6\left(\frac{b-a}{n}\right)^{r+1}\left(\frac{1}{r!} + \sum_{i=0}^{m}\sum_{j=0}^{\alpha_i}\frac{|A_{ij}|}{(r-j)!}\right)\tau_{k+1-r}\left(f^{(r)}; \frac{2(b-a)}{n(k+1-r)}\right)_L. \quad \square$$

47. Estimates for classical quadrature formulas

As a direct consequence of the Theorems 46.1 and 46.2 a series of error estimations follow for the well-known quadrature formulas.

(1) The composite Newton–Cotes quadrature formula is of the type

$$\int_a^b f(x)\,dx = \sum_{i=1}^{n}\int_{x_{i-1}}^{x_i} P_{i,k}(x)\,dx + R_n^k(f)$$

$$= \frac{b-a}{n}\sum_{i=1}^{n}\sum_{j=\varepsilon}^{k+\varepsilon} A_{kj} f(y_{i,j}) + R_n^k(f),$$

where $P_{i,k}$ is the interpolation polynomial for the function f of kth degree with knots at the points

$$y_{i,j} = \begin{cases} x_{i-1} + j(x_i - x_{i-1})/k, & j = 0, 1, \ldots, k \text{ (closed type—} \varepsilon = 0\text{)}, \\ x_{i-1} + j(x_i - x_{i-1})/(k+2), & j = 1, 2, \ldots, k+1 \text{ (open type—} \varepsilon = 1\text{)}, \end{cases}$$

and $x_i = a + i(b-a)/n$, $i = 0, 1, \ldots, n$.

It is well known that the quadrature formula

$$\int_{x_{i-1}}^{x_i} f(x)\,dx = \int_{x_{i-1}}^{x_i} P_{i,k}(x)\,dx + R_{i,k}(f)$$

has the precision k for odd k and the precision $k+1$ for even k. By Theorem 45.2

$$|R_n^k(f)| \leq 6\left(1 + \sum_{j=\varepsilon}^{k+\varepsilon}|A_{kj}|\right)\tau_{k+1}\left(f; \frac{2(b-a)}{n(k+1)}\right)_L \quad \text{for odd } k,$$

$$|R_n^k(f)| \leq 6\left(1 + \sum_{j=\varepsilon}^{k+\varepsilon}|A_{kj}|\right)\tau_{k+2}\left(f; \frac{2(b-a)}{n(k+2)}\right)_L \quad \text{for even } k.$$

(2) Let $L_n(f)$ be an n-composite quadrature formula in the interval $[a, b]$, generated by a Gaussian quadrature formula Lf of kth order with weight $p \equiv 1$

$$Lf = \sum_{i=1}^{k} A_i f(x_i),$$

which has precision $2k-1$ (see Remark 46.2 and note that $\sum_{i=1}^{k} A_i = 1$, $A_i > 0$). Hence

$$\left| \int_a^b f(x)\, dx - L_n(f) \right| \leq 12\tau_{2k}\left(f; \frac{b-a}{nk} \right)_L.$$

(3) The Hermite quadrature formulae $L_k f$ is obtained by replacing the integrand by its Hermite interpolation polynomial, which coincides with the values of the function and its derivatives at $k+1$ equidistant points. For the interval $[0, 1]$

$$L_k f = \sum_{j=0}^{k} \left\{ \left[\int_0^1 \left(1 - \frac{\varphi''(j/k)(x-j/k)}{\varphi'(j/k)} \right) \left(\frac{\varphi(x)}{(x-j/k)\varphi'(j/k)} \right)^2 dx \right] f(j/k) \right.$$

$$\left. + \left(\int_0^1 \frac{\varphi^2(x)}{(x-j/k)[\varphi'(j/k)]^2}\, dx \right) f'(j/k) \right\}$$

$$\equiv \sum_{j=0}^{k} [A_j f(j/k) + B_j f'(j/k)],$$

where $\varphi(x) = x(x-1/k)(x-2/k)\cdots(x-1)$. The above quadrature formula has a precision of $2k+1$ and the n-composite quadrature formula $L_n(f)$ in the interval $[a, b]$, generated by $L_k f$, satisfies

$$\left| \int_a^b f(x)\, dx - L_n(f) \right|$$

$$\leq 6 \frac{b-a}{n} \left[1 + \sum_{j=0}^{k} (|A_j| + |B_j|) \right] \tau_{2k+1}\left(f'; \frac{2(b-a)}{n(2k+1)} \right)_L.$$

(4) The Obreshkov–Chakalov quadrature formula for the interval $[0, 1]$ (see Section 12)

$$L_{l,m} f = \sum_{j=0}^{l} A_j f^{(j)}(0) + \sum_{j=0}^{m} B_j f^{(m)}(1),$$

has precision $l + m + 1$ and the n-composite quadrature formula $L_n(f)$ in the interval $[a, b]$ generated by $L_{l,m} f$ satisfies

$$\left| \int_a^b f(x)\, dx - L_n(f) \right| \leq 6 \left(\frac{b-a}{n} \right)^r \left(\frac{1}{r!} + \sum_{j=0}^{l} \frac{|A_j|}{(r-j)!} + \sum_{j=0}^{m} \frac{|B_j|}{(r-j)!} \right)$$

$$\times \tau_{l+m+2-r}\left(f^{(r)}; \frac{2(b-a)}{n(l+m+2-r)} \right)_L.$$

For the next formulae see SENDOV and POPOV ([1988], p. 41).

(1) The n-composite rectangle quadrature formula

$$\int_a^b f(x)\,dx = \frac{b-a}{n}\sum_{i=1}^n f(x_i) + R_n^0(f),$$

where $x_i = a + (b-a)(2i-1)/2n$, $i = 1, 2, \ldots, n$, has an estimate

$$|R_n^0(f)| \leq \tfrac{1}{2}\tau_2\!\left(f; \frac{b-a}{2n}\right)_L.$$

IVANOV [1980] proved that the above estimate is exact in the class of all infinitely differentiable functions; i.e. it is exact for the class of all bounded measurable functions.

(2) The n-composite trapezoidal quadrature formula

$$\int_a^b f(x)\,dx = \frac{b-a}{2n}\left(f(a) + 2\sum_{i=1}^{n-1} f(x_i) + f(b)\right) + R_n^1(f),$$

where $x_i = a + i(b-a)/n$, $i = 0, 1, \ldots, n$, has an estimate

$$|R_n^1(f)| \leq \tau_2\!\left(f; \frac{b-a}{n}\right)_L.$$

(3) The n-composite formula of Simpson

$$\int_a^b f(x)\,dx = \frac{b-a}{6n}\left[f(a) + 2\sum_{i=1}^{n-1} f(x_i) + 4\sum_{i=1}^n f\!\left(\frac{x_i + x_{i-1}}{2}\right) + f(b)\right] + R_n^2(f),$$

where $x_i = a + i(b-a)/n$, $i = 0, 1, \ldots, n$, has an estimate

$$|R_n^2(f)| \leq 6.485\,\tau_4\!\left(f; \frac{b-a}{2n}\right)_L.$$

48. Quadrature formulas with restrictions

Following BOIANOV ([1978], p. 36), let us consider the quadrature formulas of the type

$$\int_a^b f(x)\,dx = \sum_{i=1}^m B_i f(a_i) + \sum_{k=1}^n A_k f(x_k) + R_{mn}(f), \tag{48.1}$$

where $a \leq a_1 < \cdots < a_m \leq b$, $a \leq x_1 < \cdots < x_n \leq b$, and $a_i \neq x_j$ for every i and j. Fixing the numbers $\{a_i\}_{i=1}^m$ the problem is to determine the numbers $\{B_i\}_{i=1}^m$, $\{A_i\}_{i=1}^n$, $\{x_i\}_{i=1}^n$ such that $R_{mn}(f) = 0$ for $f \in H_{2n+m-1}$ (note that the number of parameters in (48.1) without $\{a_i\}_{i=1}^m$ is $2n + m$). Letting

$$\sigma(x) = (x - a_1)\cdots(x - a_m), \qquad \omega(x) = (x - x_1)\cdots(x - x_n),$$

the next theorem answers the above question.

THEOREM 48.1. *The necessary and sufficient conditions for the formula* (48.1) *to be exact for polynomials of degree* $2n + m - 1$ *are:*
  (1) *the formula* (48.1) *is an interpolation one;*

  (2) $\displaystyle\int_a^b \sigma(x)f(x)\omega(x)\,dx = 0$ *for all* $f \in H_{n-1}$.

PROOF. *Necessity.* Let (48.1) be exact for polynomials of degree $2n + m - 1$. From Section 44 it follows that (48.1) is an interpolation formula. If $q \in H_{n-1}$ then for $f = \sigma q \omega$

$$\int_a^b f(x)\,dx = \int_a^b \sigma(x)q(x)\omega(x)\,dx = \sum_{i=1}^m B_i f(a_i) + \sum_{k=1}^n A_k f(x_k) = 0.$$

Sufficiency. Let the conditions (1) and (2) in the theorem be fulfilled. Then every polynomial f of degree $2n + m - 1$ can be written in the form $f = \sigma \omega q + r$, where q and r are polynomials of degree $n - 1$ and $m + n - 1$, respectively. Since (48.1) is exact it follows for r that

$$\int_a^b r(x)\,dx = \sum_{i=1}^m B_i r(a_i) + \sum_{k=1}^n A_k r(x_k).$$

The last equality and

$$\int_a^b \sigma(x)q(x)\omega(x)\,dx = 0,$$

$$r(x_k) = f(x_k), \quad k = 1, \ldots, n, \qquad r(a_i) = f(a_i), \quad i = 1, \ldots, m,$$

proves that

$$\int_a^b f(x)\,dx = \sum_{i=1}^m B_i f(a_i) + \sum_{k=1}^n A_k f(x_k). \qquad \square$$

A detailed investigation of the formulas of type (48.1) was made by MARKOV [1910]. Two special cases are useful (for details see RALSTON [1965a], Chapter 4.10).

  (1) The case $m = 1$, $a_1 = a$ (or $a_1 = b$)—RADAU [1879]. Setting for simplicity $[a, b] = [-1, 1]$, then the knots $-1, x_1, x_2, \ldots, x_n$ are the roots of the equation

$$(n + 1)L_n(x) + (2n + 1)L_{n+1}(x) = 0,$$

where L_n is a Legendre polynomial. The coefficients are

$$B = \frac{2}{(n+1)^2},$$

$$A_k = \frac{2^{2n+2}(n+1)^2(n!)^4}{[(2n+1)!]^2(1+x_k)(1-x_k^2)[\omega'(x_k)]^2}, \quad k = 1, \ldots, n.$$

(2) The case $m = 2$, $a_1 = -1$, $a_2 = 1$—LOBATTO [1852]. The knots $-1, 1$, $x_1, \ldots, x_n$ are the roots of the equation

$$L_{n+2}(x) - \frac{(n+2)(n+1)}{(2n+3)(2n+1)} L_n(x) = 0$$

and

$$B_1 = B_2 = \frac{2}{(n+1)(n+2)},$$

$$A_k = \frac{8(n+1)[\omega(1)]^2}{(n+2)(1-x_k^2)^2[\omega'(x_k)]^2}, \quad k = 1, \ldots, n.$$

CHEBYSHEV [1874] considered the quadrature formulae of the type

$$\int_a^b f(x)\,dx = A \sum_{k=1}^n f(x_k) + R_n(f). \tag{48.2}$$

This formula is exact for the constants if $A = (b-a)/n$, and the expectation is that the different knots x_k can be chosen in such a way in the interval $[a, b]$ that $R_n(f) = 0$ for $f \in H_n$. The answer was given by BERNSTEIN [1936, 1937]. He proved that by substituting f by x^k in (48.2), $k = 1, 2, \ldots, n$, the corresponding system

$$\sum_{i=1}^n x_i^k = \frac{n}{b-a} \int_a^b x^k\,dx, \quad k = 1, 2, \ldots, n,$$

has a real and different solution $x_i \in [a, b]$, $i = 1, 2, \ldots, n$, only for $n = 1, 2, 3, 4, 5, 6, 7, 9$.

49. The Runge principle. Romberg's quadrature formulas

As the most commonly used quadrature formulas are of the type

$$\int_a^b f(x)\,dx = \sum_{i=1}^m A_i^{(m)} f(x_i) + \frac{cf^{(k)}(\xi)}{m^s},$$

letting for conciseness,

$$I = \int_a^b f(x)\,dx, \quad I_m = \sum_{i=1}^m A_i^{(m)} f(x_i),$$

let us assume that two computations of the integral I are performed with m_1, m_2:

$$I = I_{m_1} + \frac{cf^{(k)}(\xi_1)}{m_1^s}, \quad I = I_{m_2} + \frac{cf^{(k)}(\xi_2)}{m_2^s}.$$

If $f^{(k)}(\xi_1) \approx f^{(k)}(\xi_2)$, then from the above

$$I \approx I_{m_2} + m_1^s(I_{m_2} - I_{m_1})/(m_2^s - m_1^s).$$

Evidently $m_1^s(I_{m_2} - I_{m_1})/(m_2^s - m_1^s)$ can be used as an error of the approximation of I by I_{m_2}. Such an estimation is known as the Runge principle or Richardson's extrapolation—RICHARDSON and GAUND [1927], KOPAL [1955], DAVIS [1959], RALSTON ([1965a], Chapter 4.12-1), BACHVALOV ([1973], p. 167).

If the knots of the quadrature formula are equidistant, then

$$I = I_{2m} + (I_{2m} - I_m)/(2^s - 1)$$

and this method is convenient because the computed values of f for I_m can be used for I_{2m}.

Generalizing the Runge principle let us consider a quadrature formula of the type

$$I = I_m + \sum_{i=1}^{k} c_i m^{-s_i} + O(m^{-s_{k+1}}),$$

where $s_1 < s_2 < \cdots < s_k < s_{k+1}$ and c_i do not depend on the m. Eliminating c_i, $i = 1, 2, \ldots, k$, from the system

$$I = I_{m_j} + \sum_{i=1}^{k} c_i m_j^{-s_i} + O(m_j^{-s_{k+1}}), \quad j = 1, 2, \ldots, k,$$

the result is a formula of the type

$$I = \sum_{i=1}^{k} \alpha_i I_{m_j} + O(\min_j m_j^{-s_{k+1}}). \tag{49.1}$$

The quadrature formulas (49.1) are called the Romberg formulas. As an application of (49.1) let us consider the Euler–Maclaurin summation formula—RALSTON ([1965a], Chapter 4.15-1), HILDEBRAND ([1956], p. 149)—

$$\int_{x_0}^{x_0+nh} f(t)\,dt = h \sum_{j=0}^{n} f(x_0 + ih) - h[f(x_0 + nh) + f(x_0)]/2$$

$$- \sum_{k=1}^{m} \frac{h^{2k} B_{2k}}{(2k)!} [f^{(2k-1)}(x_0 + nh) + f^{(2k-1)}(x_0)] - hR_m,$$

where $R_m = nh^{2m+2} B_{2m+2} f^{(2m+2)}(\xi)/(2m+2)!$, $x_0 < \xi < x_0 + nh$, and the B_k are Bernoulli polynomials defined by

$$t(e^{xt} - 1)/(e^t - 1) = \sum_{k=0}^{\infty} B_k(x) t^k/k!.$$

Approximating $f^{(2k-1)}(x_0 + nh)$ and $f^{(2k-1)}(x_0)$ by finite differences and setting $f_i = f(x_0 + ih)$ the Euler–Maclaurin formula yields the Gregory formula

$$\int_{x_0}^{x_0+nh} f(t)\,dt = h(f_0/2 + f_1 + \cdots + f_{n-1} + f_n/2) + h(\Delta f_0 - \Delta f_{n-1})/12$$

$$- h(\Delta^2 f_0 - \Delta^2 f_{n-2})/24 + \cdots .$$

All these considerations show that the composite trapezoidal rule can be written in the form

$$\int_a^b f(t)\,dt = \frac{b-a}{m}(f_0/2 + f_1 + \cdots + f_{m-1} + f_m/2) + \sum_{i=1}^k c_i m_j^{-2i} + R_k m^{-2k-2},$$

with $j = 1, 2, \ldots, k$, where $f_i = f(a + i(b-a)/m)$, $i = 0, 1, \ldots, m$,

$$c_i = (b-a)^{2i} B_{2i}[f^{(2i-1)}(b) - f^{(2i-1)}(a)]/(2i)!\,,$$

$$R_k = -(b-a)^{2k+3} B_{2k+2} f^{(2k+2)}(\xi)/(2k+2)!\,, \quad a < \xi < b\,.$$

With the notation $m = 2^n$,

$$I_{0,n} = \frac{b-a}{2^n}(\tfrac{1}{2}f_0 + f_1 + \cdots + f_{2^n-1} + \tfrac{1}{2}f_{2^n})\,,$$

the next relation holds:

$$I_{1,n} = \tfrac{1}{3}(4 I_{0,n+1} - I_{0,n})$$

and this expression approximates I by the error $O(2^{-4n})$.

It follows that setting

$$I_{k,n} = \frac{1}{2^{2k}-1}(2^{2k} I_{k-1,n+1} - I_{k-1,n})\,,$$

$I_{k,n}$ approximates I with a precision of $O(2^{-2n(k+1)})$; i.e. the determination of $I_{k,n}$ is equivalent to the elimination of $c_1, c_2, \ldots, c_k$. The computation can be ordered in the table

$$
\begin{array}{cccc}
I_{0,0} & & & \\
I_{0,1} & I_{1,0} & & \\
\vdots & & \ddots & \\
I_{0,n} & I_{1,n-1} & \cdots & I_{n,0}\,.
\end{array}
$$

50. Integration of periodic functions

Let f be a 2π-periodic function. In a similar way to Section 44 let a quadrature formula of the type

$$\int_0^{2\pi} f(x)\,dx = \sum_{k=0}^{2n} A_k f(x_k) + R_n(f)\,, \tag{50.1}$$

be obtained by integration of the trigonometric polynomial (14.1) of nth degree

$$\tau_n(x) = \sum_{i=0}^{2n} f(x_i) \left(\prod_{s=0, s \neq i}^{2n} \sin \frac{x - x_s}{2} \bigg/ \prod_{s=0, s \neq i}^{2n} \sin \frac{x_i - x_s}{2} \right),$$

that satisfies $\tau_n(x_i) = f(x_i)$, $0 \leq x_0 < x_1 < \cdots < x_{2n} < 2\pi$, $i = 0, 1, \ldots, 2n$. The quadrature formula (50.1) determined in this way is exact for every trigonometric polynomial of degree n. The question of the optimal choice of the knots $\{x_i\}_{i=0}^{2n}$ (see Section 45) is answered by the following formula.

THEOREM 50.1. *The quadrature formula* (50.1) *with the coefficients*

$$A_i = \int_0^{2\pi} \left(\prod_{s=0, s \neq i}^{2n} \sin \frac{x - x_s}{2} \bigg/ \prod_{s=0, s \neq i}^{2n} \sin \frac{x_i - x_s}{2} \right) dx$$

is exact for trigonometric polynomials of degree $2n$ if and only if the knots $\{x_i\}_{i=0}^{2n} \in [0, 2\pi)$ are the roots of the trigonometric polynomial of half-integer order $n + \frac{1}{2}$, which is orthogonal to every trigonometric polynomial of half-integer order $n - \frac{1}{2}$.

Let us note that the expression

$$\sum_{k=0}^{n} [c_k \cos(k + \tfrac{1}{2})x + d_k \sin(k + \tfrac{1}{2})x]$$

is a trigonometric polynomial of half-integer order $n + \frac{1}{2}$.

An important implication of the Theorem 50.1 is given by the next theorem.

THEOREM 50.2. *The quadrature formula*

$$\int_0^{2\pi} f(x) \, dx = \frac{2\pi}{2n+1} \sum_{k=0}^{2n} f\left(x_0 + \frac{2\pi k}{2n+1}\right) + R_n(f)$$

is exact for every trigonometric polynomial of degree $2n$, where $x_0 \in (0, 2\pi/(2n + 1))$ is an arbitrary number.

For the proof of the above two theorems see BOIANOV ([1978], Chapter 1.8).

Theorem 46.2 shows that if the generating quadrature formula has a precision of k and the function f has the rth derivative of the bounded variation, then for the error $R_n(f)$ of the n-composite quadrature formula the next estimate holds,

$$R_n(f) = O(n^{-\min(k+1, r+1)});$$

i.e. the precision of the generating quadrature plays an important role. The situation is quite different for periodic functions. Keeping the notation of

Section 46 let $L_n(f)$ be an n-composite quadrature formula for the interval $[0, 2\pi]$ generated by a quadrature formula Lf of the type $\{A, \gamma\}$, which is exact for the constant function; i.e.

$$L_n(f) = \sum_{i=1}^{n} L(\{A, \gamma\}, [x_i, x_{i-1}])f = \sum_{i=1}^{n} \sum_{j=1}^{m} \frac{2\pi}{n} A_j f[x_{i-1} + \alpha_j(x_i - x_{i-1})],$$

where $x_i = 2\pi i/n$, $i = 0, 1, \ldots, n$, $\alpha_j \in [0, 1]$, $j = 0, 1, \ldots, m$.

THEOREM 50.3 (IVANOV [1979]). *Let f be a bounded 2π-periodic integrable function. Then for the error of the n-composite quadrature formula $L_n(f)$ the following inequality is fulfilled*

$$|R_n(f)| \leq \left| \int_a^b f(x)\,dx - L_n(f) \right| \leq c(r)\left(1 + \sum_{i=1}^{m} |A_i|\right) \tau_r(f; n^{-1})_L,$$

for every $r = 1, 2, \ldots$.

51. Obreshkov–Chakalov quadrature formulas

By Section 12 the polynomial P of degree $n = l + m + 1$ that satisfies

$$P^{(s)}(a) = f^{(s)}(a), \quad s = 0, 1, \ldots, l,$$

$$P^{(s)}(b) = f^{(s)}(b), \quad s = 0, 1, \ldots, m,$$

is the Obreshkov interpolation polynomial (OBRESHKOV [1940, 1942])

$$P(x) = \sum_{s=0}^{l} f^{(s)}(a) \frac{(x-b)^{m+1}(x-a)^s}{s!(a-b)^{m+1}} \sum_{i=0}^{l-s} \binom{m+i}{i} \frac{(x-a)^i}{(b-a)^i}$$

$$+ \sum_{s=0}^{m} f^{(s)}(b) \frac{(x-a)^{l+1}(x-b)^s}{s!(b-a)^{l+1}} \sum_{i=0}^{m-s} \binom{l+i}{i} \frac{(x-b)^i}{(a-b)^i}.$$

The remainder term $R(f)$ is

$$f(x) = P(x) + R(f; x)$$
$$= P(x) + (x-a)^{l+1}(x-b)^{m+1} f^{(l+m+2)}(\xi)/(l+m+2)!.$$

It follows from the above that

$$\int_a^b P(x)\,dx = \sum_{s=0}^{l} \frac{f^{(s)}(a)}{s!(a-b)^{m+1}} \sum_{i=0}^{l-s} \binom{m+i}{i} (b-a)^{-i} \int_a^b (x-b)^{m+1}(x-a)^{s+i}\,dx$$

$$+ \sum_{s=0}^{m} \frac{f^{(s)}(b)}{s!(b-a)^{l+1}} \sum_{i=0}^{m-s} \binom{l+i}{i} (b-a)^{-i} \int_a^b (x-b)^{s+i}(x-a)^{l+1}\,dx.$$

Since

$$\int_a^b (x-a)^\alpha (x-b)^\beta \, dx = (-1)^\beta (b-a)^{\alpha+\beta+1} \int_0^1 t^\alpha (1-t)^\beta \, dt$$

$$= (-1)^\beta (b-a)^{\alpha+\beta+1} \alpha! \beta! / (\alpha+\beta+1)!,$$

the final representation is

$$\int_a^b P(x) \, dx = \sum_{s=0}^l \frac{(-1)^{l+m} f^{(s)}(a)}{s! (b-a)^{m-l-s-1}} \sum_{i=0}^{l-s} \binom{m+i}{i} \frac{(l+1)!(s+i)!}{(l+s+i+2)!}$$

$$+ \sum_{s=0}^m \frac{(-1)^s f^{(s)}(b)}{s!(b-a)^{l-m-s-1}} \sum_{i=0}^{m-s} \binom{l+i}{i} \frac{(m+1)!(s+i)!}{(m+s+i+2)!}. \quad (51.1)$$

The interesting case $m = l$ leads to

$$\int_a^b P(x) \, dx = \sum_{s=0}^m \frac{(b-a)^{s+1} \binom{m+1}{s+1}}{(s+1)! \binom{2m+2}{s+1}} [f^{(s)}(a) + (-1)^s f^{(s)}(b)] \quad (51.2)$$

with the remainder term

$$\int_a^b R(f; x) \, dx = \frac{(-1)^{m+1}(b-a)^{2m+3}}{2m+3} \left(\frac{(m+1)!}{(2m+2)!}\right)^2 f^{(2m+2)}(\eta), \quad \eta \in (a, b).$$

The proof of (51.2) follows from (51.1) using the relations

$$\sum_{i=0}^{m-s} \binom{m+i}{i} \frac{(m+1)!(s+i)!}{(m+s+i+2)!}$$

$$= (m+1) \sum_{i=0}^{m-s} \frac{(i+1)(i+2) \cdots (i+s)}{(m+i+1)(m+i+2) \cdots (m+i+s+2)}$$

$$= \frac{1}{(s+1)!} \frac{\binom{m+1}{s+1}}{\binom{2m+2}{s+1}}.$$

CHAKALOV [1938, 1983] obtained (51.1) using another approach. Some investigations on the quadrature formulae of Obreshkov–Chakalov can be found in IONESCU [1952], MEIR and SHARMA [1968].

52. A concept for the best quadrature formulas

Let X be a set of functions and the functionals $L(f), L_1(f), \ldots, L_n(f)$ be defined in X. Every function S of n variables determines a method for the approximation of $L(f)$ by the formula

$$L(f) \approx S(L_1(f), \ldots, L_n(f)), \qquad (52.1)$$

where only the information $T(f) = \{L_1(f), \ldots, L_n(f)\}$ is used.
The quantity

$$R(S, T) = \sup_{f \in X} |L(f) - S(f)|$$

is the error of the method S in X using the information T.
Let $R(T) = \inf\{R(S, T): S\}$. The method S^* for which

$$R(S^*, T) = R(T)$$

is called the best method for the approximation of $L(f)$ in X using an information T. A general approach for building the best method S^* (not necessary unique) can be given following BOIANOV [1978]: let

$$X_f = \{g \in X: T(g) \equiv T(f)\}$$

and $\sup_{g \in X_f} L(g) < \infty$, $\inf_{g \in X_f} L(g) > -\infty$ for every $f \in X$. Then the method

$$S^*(f) = \tfrac{1}{2}(\sup_{g \in X_f} L(g) + \inf_{g \in X_f} L(g))$$

satisfies

$$R(T) = R(S^*, T) = \tfrac{1}{2} \sup_{f \in X} (\sup_{g \in X_f} L(g) - \inf_{g \in X_f} L(g)).$$

Indeed, let the method S be different from S^*; i.e. there is a function $f \in X$ such that $S(f) - S^*(f) = \varepsilon > 0$ (the case of $\varepsilon < 0$ can be considered similarly). There exists an $h \in X_f$ such that

$$L(h) < \inf_{g \in X_f} L(g) + \tfrac{1}{2}\varepsilon, \qquad S(h) = S(f),$$

and

$$S(h) - L(h) = S(f) - L(h) = S^*(f) + \varepsilon - L(h) > S^*(f) - \inf_{g \in X_f} L(g)$$

$$= \tfrac{1}{2}(\sup_{g \in X_f} L(g) - \inf_{g \in X_f} L(g)).$$

So for every $f \in X$ for which $S(f) \neq S^*(f)$ the following inequality is fulfilled

$$\sup_{g \in X_f} |S(g) - L(g)| \geq \tfrac{1}{2}(\sup_{g \in X_f} L(g) - \inf_{g \in X_f} L(g)).$$

If for $f \in X$, $S(f) = S^*(f)$ then

$$\sup_{g \in X_f} |S(g) - L(g)| = \tfrac{1}{2}(\sup_{g \in X_f} L(g) - \inf_{g \in X_f} L(g)).$$

Therefore,

$$\sup_{f \in X} |S(f) - L(f)| \geq \tfrac{1}{2} \sup_{f \in X} (\sup_{g \in X_f} L(g) - \inf_{g \in X_f} L(g))$$

and the assertion is proved.

The origin of this kind of investigation in the case of

$$L(f) = \int_a^b f(x)\,dx \qquad (52.2)$$

is due to SARD [1949, 1963]. A series of interesting best-quadrature formulas were built by NIKOLSKII [1950, 1952, 1974]. Sard and Nikolskii deal with linear best-quadrature methods. Later BACHVALOV [1967, 1970, 1971], considered the problem in its general statement of a question as it was described above.

Let us note that in the problem for numerical integration the functionals $L(f), L_1(f), \ldots, L_n(f)$ in (52.1), (52.2) are usually linear. Here a simple but useful result was proved by SMOLJAK [1965].

THEOREM 52.1. *Let the linear functionals $L(f), L_1(f), \ldots, L_n(f)$ be defined in the linear space H. Let $X \subseteq H$ be a convex body, centrally symmetric with respect to zero and*

$$\sup_{f \in X_0} L(f) < \infty,$$

where $X_0 = \{f \in X: L_k(f) = 0, k = 1, 2, \ldots, n\}$. Then there exist numbers $D_1, D_2, \ldots, D_n$ such that

$$\sup_{f \in X} \left| L(f) - \sum_{k=1}^{N} D_k L_k(f) \right| = R(T),$$

i.e. among the best methods there is a linear one.

53. Monte Carlo methods

Monte Carlo (MC) methods are numerical methods for solving problems via modeling random variables. Usually MC methods reduce the problems to the approximate calculation of mathematical expectation values. Let the scalar variable I be the desired solution of the problem or some desired linear functional of the solution. Then a random variable ξ with mathematical expectation equal to I must be constructed: $E\xi = I$. Then, using n independent values of $\xi, \xi_1, \xi_2, \ldots, \xi_n$, an approximation to I

$$I \approx \frac{1}{n}(\xi_1 + \xi_2 + \cdots + \xi_n), \qquad (53.1)$$

can be computed.

The year 1949 is regarded as the official birthday of MC methods, when the paper of METROPOLIS and ULAM [1949] was published, although some authors point to earlier dates. ERMAKOV [1975], for example, noticed that a solution of a problem by the MC method is contained in the Old Testament. The creation of the method is connected with the names of John von Neuman, E. Fermi, and H. Kahn, who worked at Los Alamos (USA) in the 1940s. The development of modern computers and especially of parallel computer systems, provided fast and specialized generators of random numbers and gave a new momentum to the development of these methods.

53.1. Convergence and error of the MC method

Let ξ be a random variable for which a mathematical expectation of $E\xi = I$ exists. Let us mention that

$$E\xi = \begin{cases} \int_{-\infty}^{\infty} \xi p(\xi) \, d\xi, \text{ where } \int_{-\infty}^{\infty} p(x) \, dx = 1, & \text{when } \xi \text{ is a continuous random variable,} \\ \sum_{\xi} \xi p(\xi), \text{ where } \sum_{x} p(x) = 1, & \text{when } \xi \text{ is a discrete random variable.} \end{cases}$$

By definition $E\xi$ exists if and only if $E|\xi|$ exists. The non-negative function $p(x)$ (continuous or discrete) is called the probability density function.

To approximate the variable I, a computation of the arithmetic mean value must usually be carried out,

$$\bar{\xi}_n = \frac{1}{n} \sum_{i=1}^{n} \xi_i.$$

Since for the sequence of uniformly distributed independent random variables, for which a mathematical expectation exists, the Hinchin theorem (the law of large numbers) holds. This means that the arithmetic mean value of these variables converges by probability to the mathematical expectation value when $n \to \infty$

$$\bar{\xi}_n \xrightarrow{P} I$$

(the sequence of the random variables $\eta_1, \eta_2, \ldots, \eta_n, \ldots$ converges by probability to the constant c if for every $h > 0$ it follows that

$$\lim_{n \to \infty} P\{|\eta_n - c| \geq h\} = 0).$$

Thus when n is sufficiently large

$$\bar{\xi}_n \approx I \tag{53.2}$$

and (53.1) can be used whenever $E\xi$ exists and $E\xi = I$.

Let us consider the problem for the error estimation of the method. Suppose that the random variable ξ has a finite dispersion

$$D\xi = E(\xi - E\xi)^2 = E\xi^2 - (E\xi)^2.$$

It is known that the sequences of the uniformly distributed independent random variables with finite dispersions satisfy the central limit theorem—see HAMMERSLEY and HAUDSCOMB [1964]. This means that for $x > 0$ it follows that

$$\lim_{n \to \infty} P\left\{\left|\frac{1}{n} \sum_{i=1}^{n} (\xi_i - I)\right| < x \sqrt{\frac{D\xi}{n}}\right\} = \Phi(x),$$

where

$$\Phi(x) = \frac{2}{\sqrt{2\pi}} \int_0^x \exp\left(-\tfrac{1}{2}t^2\right) dt$$

is the probability integral.

When n is sufficiently large

$$P\left\{|\bar{\xi}_n - I| < x\sqrt{\frac{D\xi}{n}}\right\} \approx \Phi(x). \tag{53.3}$$

Formula (53.3) gives a whole family of estimations, which depend on the parameter x. If a probability β is given, then the root $x = x_\beta$ of the equation $\Phi(x) = \beta$ can be found, e.g., approximately by the tables.

Then from (53.3) it follows that the probability of the inequality

$$|\bar{\xi}_n - I| < x_\beta \sqrt{D\xi/n} \tag{53.4}$$

is approximately equal to β.

The term in the right-hand side of the inequality (53.4) is called the probability error.

The probable error term, r_n, is used most often. This is the value r_n for which

$$P\{|\bar{\xi}_n - I| \leq r_n\} = \tfrac{1}{2} = P\{|\bar{\xi}_n - I| \geq r_n\}.$$

From (53.4) it follows that

$$r_n = x_{1/2} \sqrt{D\xi/n}, \tag{53.5}$$

where $x_{1/2} \approx 0.6745$.

54. Ordinary and geometric MC methods for integrals

54.1. Ordinary MC method

Let D be an arbitrary domain (bounded or unbounded, connected or not) and $x \in D \subset \mathbb{R}^d$ be a d-dimensional vector.

Let us consider the problem of the approximate computation of the integral

$$I = \int_D f(x)p(x)\, dx,$$

where the non-negative function $p(x)$, for which $\int_D p(x)\, dx = 1$, is called a density function.

Let x be a random point with probability density function $p(x)$. Introducing the random variable $\theta = f(x)$ with mathematical expectation equal to the value of the integral I, then

$$E\theta = \int_D f(x)\, dx .$$

For the calculation of I let us use (53.2).

Let $x_1, x_2, \ldots, x_n$ be independent realizations of the random point x with probability density function $p(x)$ and $\theta_1 = f(x_1), \ldots, \theta_n = f(x_n)$. Then an approximate value of I is

$$\bar{\theta}_n = \frac{1}{n} \sum_{i=1}^n \theta_i . \tag{54.1}$$

According to Section 53, if the integral (53.1) is absolutely convergent, then $\bar{\theta}_n$ is convergent by probability to I.

54.2. Geometric MC method

If the non-negative function f is bounded,

$$0 \leq f(x) \leq c \quad \text{for } x \in D , \tag{54.2}$$

let us consider the cylindrical domain $\tilde{D} = D \times [0, c]$ (Fig. 54.1) and the random point $\tilde{x} \equiv (x^{(1)}, x^{(2)}, z)$ in it with probability density function $\tilde{p}(\tilde{x}) = c^{-1} p(x^{(1)}, x^{(2)})$. Let $\tilde{x}_1, \ldots, \tilde{x}_n$ be independent realizations of the random point $\tilde{x}$. Introducing the random variable $\tilde{\theta}$, which depends on $\tilde{x}$ as it can be shown that

$$\tilde{\theta} = \begin{cases} c, & \text{if } z < f(x^{(1)}, x^{(2)}) , \\ 0, & \text{if } z \geq f(x^{(1)}, x^{(2)}) . \end{cases}$$

The random variable introduced is a meter of the points below the graph of f.

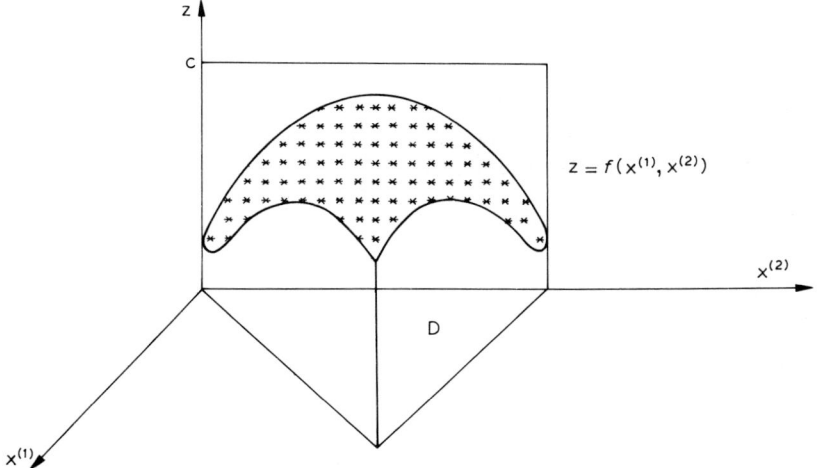

Fig. 54.1. The cylindrical domain $\tilde{D} = D \times [0, c]$.

Let us calculate $E\tilde{\theta}$:

$$E\tilde{\theta} = cP\{z' < f(x')\} = \int_D dx^{(1)} dx^{(2)} \int_0^{f(x^{(1)},x^{(2)})} \tilde{p}(x^{(1)}, x^{(2)}, z) \, dz = I.$$

The absolute convergence of the integral follows from (54.2). Therefore, as an approximate value of I

$$\tilde{\theta}_n = \frac{1}{n} \sum_{i=1}^{n} \tilde{\theta}_i$$

can be used, since $E\tilde{\theta}_n = I$ and $\tilde{\theta}_n \xrightarrow{P} I$.

Let us compare the accuracy of the geometric and the ordinary MC methods. Let $f \in L_2(D, p)$. This guarantees that the dispersion of the random variable

$$D\theta = \int_D f^2(x) p(x) \, dx - I^2 \tag{54.3}$$

in the ordinary MC method is finite.

For the geometric MC method the following equation holds:

$$E(\tilde{\theta}^2) = c^2 P\{z < f(x)\} = cI.$$

Hence the dispersion is

$$D\tilde{\theta} = cI - I^2 \tag{54.4}$$

Comparing (54.3) with (54.4) it follows that

$$\int_D f^2(x) p(x) \, dx \leq c \int_D f(x) p(x) \, dx = cI.$$

Therefore $D\theta \leq D\tilde{\theta}$.

The last inequality shows that the ordinary MC method is more accurate than the geometric one (except for the case when f is a constant). Nevertheless, the geometric method is often preferred from the algorithmic point of view, because it is less laborious—SOBOL [1973]. The problem of the cost of different MC algorithms is considered exhaustively in DIMOV and TONEV [1991].

55. Effective MC methods

As was shown in Section 53 the probable error in MC methods is

$$r_n = c\sqrt{D\xi/n}. \tag{55.1}$$

It is very important for such computation schemes and random variables that a value for ξ is chosen for which the dispersion is as small as possible. MC methods with reduced dispersion compared to simple MC method are usually called efficient MC methods. Let us consider several methods of this kind.

55.1. Separation of the principal part

Let us consider again the integral

$$I = \int_D f(x) p(x) \, dx, \qquad (55.2)$$

where $f \in L_2(D, p)$, $x \in D \subset \mathbb{R}^d$.

Let the function $h \in L_2(D, p)$ be "close" to f with respect to the L_2 norm; i.e. $\|f - h\|_{L_2(D,p)} \leq \varepsilon$, and the value of the integral

$$\int_D h(x) p(x) \, dx = I'$$

be known.

The random variable $\theta' = f(x) - h(x) + I'$ generates the following estimation for the integral (55.2):

$$\bar{\theta}'_n = c + \frac{1}{n} \sum_{i=1}^n [f(x_i) - h(x_i)].$$

Obviously $E\theta'_n = I$. One estimation of the dispersion of θ' is

$$D\theta' = \int_D [f(x) - h(x)]^2 p(x) \, dx - (I - I')^2 \leq \varepsilon^2.$$

This means that the dispersion and, respectively, the probable error can be quite small, if for the function h the integral I' can be calculated analytically. Very often a partially linear function is taken as h.

55.2. Symmetrization of the integrand

For a one-dimensional integral

$$I_0 = \int_a^b f(x) \, dx$$

on a finite interval $[a, b]$ let us consider the random variable ξ that is uniformly distributed in this interval and the random variable $\theta = (b-a)f(\xi)$. Since $E\theta = I_0$, the ordinary MC method leads to the following approximate estimation for I_0:

$$\bar{\theta}_n = \frac{b-a}{n} \sum_{i=1}^n f(\xi_i),$$

where ξ_i are independent realizations of ξ.

Let us consider the symmetric function

$$f_1(x) = \tfrac{1}{2}[f(x) + f(a + b - x)],$$

the integral from which is I_0 and let $\theta' = (b-a)f_1(x)$.

Since $E\bar{\theta}' = I_0$, the following symmetrized approximate estimation of the integral can be used

$$\bar{\theta}_n = \frac{b-a}{n} \sum_{i=1}^{n} [f(\xi_i) + f(a+b-\xi_i)].$$

THEOREM 55.1 (SOBOL [1973]). *If the partially continuous function f is monotonic when $a \leq x \leq b$, then*

$$D\bar{\theta}' \leq \tfrac{1}{2} D\bar{\theta}.$$

55.3. Important sampling method

Let us consider the problem of computing

$$I_0 = \int_D f(x)\,dx, \quad x \in D \subset \mathbb{R}^d,$$

where D_0 is the set of points x for which $f(x) - 0$ and $D_+ = D/D_0$.

Let us call the probability density function of a random point $p(x)$ permissible for $f(x)$, if $p(x) > 0$ for $x \in D_+$ and $p(x) \geq 0$ for $x \in D_0$.

For an arbitrary permissible probability density function $p(x)$ for $f(x)$ in D let

$$Z_0(x) = \begin{cases} f(x)/p(x), & x \in D_+, \\ 0, & x \in D_0. \end{cases}$$

There exists the following problem: what must be the permissible density $p(x)$ with a view for minimization of the dispersion of Z_0?

THEOREM 55.2 (KAHN [1950]). *The probability density function $\hat{p}(x) = c|f(x)|$ minimizes DZ_0 and the value of the minimal dispersion is*

$$D\hat{Z}_0 = \left(\int_D |f(x)|\,dx\right)^2 - I_0^2.$$

COROLLARY 55.1. *If f does not change its sign in D, then $D\hat{Z}_0 = 0$.*

This corollary is obvious.

For the practical algorithms this assertion allows random variables with very little dispersion (respectively, probable errors) to be built, using a more high random-point probability density in the domain, where the integrand has a large absolute value. It is intuitively clear that by using such an approach an increasing accuracy can be expected.

56. MC methods with increased rate of convergence

As was shown before, the probable error usually has the form (55.1) and the speed of convergence can be increased, if a method with probable error

$$r_n = cn^{-1/2-\varepsilon(d)}$$

can be constructed, where c is a constant, $\varepsilon(d)>0$ and d is the dimension of the space.

Monte Carlo methods with such a probable error are called MC methods with an overconvergent probable error.

Let us consider the problem of computing the integral

$$I = \int_D f(x)p(x)\,dx,$$

where $D \subset \mathbb{R}^d$, $f \in L_2(D;p)$, and p is a probability density function; i.e. $p(x) \geq 0$ and $\int_D p(x)\,dx = 1$.

Let D be separated to subdomains D_j, $j=1,2,\ldots,m$ (see, e.g., Fig. 56.1, where the unit cube

$$C^d = \{0 < x^{(1)} < 1, 0 < x^{(2)} < 1, \ldots, 0 < x^{(d)} < 1\}$$

with $p(x) \equiv 1$ is divided into $n = m^d$ equal cubes with edge $1/m$ (evidently $p_j = 1/n$ and $d_j = \sqrt{d}/m$)) such that the following conditions hold:

$$D = \bigcup_{j=1}^{m} D_j, \qquad D_i \cap D_j = \emptyset, \quad i \neq j,$$

$$p_j = \int_{D_j} p(x)\,dx \leq \frac{c_1}{n}, \tag{56.1}$$

$$d_j = \sup_{x_1, x_2 \in D_j} |x_1 - x_2| \leq \frac{c_2}{n^{1/d}}, \tag{56.2}$$

where c_1 and c_2 are constants.

Then $I = \sum_{j=1}^{m} I_j$, where $I_j = \int_{D_j} f(x)p(x)\,dx$ and obviously I_j is the mean of the random variable $p_j f(\xi_j)$, where ξ_j is a random point in D_j with probability

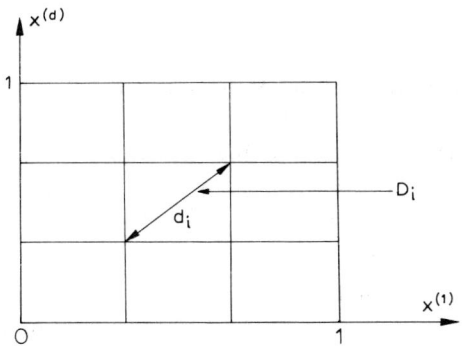

Fig. 56.1. Division of D into subdomains D_j.

density function $p(x)/p_j$. So it is possible to estimate I_j by the average of n_j observations

$$\bar{\theta}_{n_j} = \frac{p_j}{n_j} \sum_{s=1}^{n_j} f(\xi_j), \quad \sum_{j=1}^{m} n_j = n, \qquad (56.3)$$

and I by $\theta_n^* = \sum_{j=1}^{m} \bar{\theta}_{n_j}$.

THEOREM 56.1 (DUPAC [1956], HABER [1966, 1967]). *Let $n_j = 1$ for $j = 1, \ldots, m$ (so $m = n$), f has continuous and bounded derivatives ($|\partial f/\partial x^{(k)}| \leq L$ for every $k = 1, 2, \ldots, d$) and there exist constants c_1, c_2 such that the conditions (56.1) and (56.2) hold. Then for the variance of θ_n^* the following relation is fulfilled*

$$D\theta_n^* = (dc_1 c_2 L)^2 n^{-1-2/n}.$$

Using the inequality (53.5) it is possible to obtain

$$r_n = \sqrt{2} dc_1 c_2 L n^{-1/2-1/d}.$$

The MC method constructed above has an overconvergent probable error.

This problem was considered by DIMOV and TONEV [1985] with implementation of the τ-moduli. Their result is the estimation

$$r_n \leq \text{const} \cdot \tau(f; d)_{L_2} n^{-1/2-1/d}. \qquad (56.4)$$

Let us note that the best quadrature formula with fixed nodes in $\mathbb{R}^1$ in the meaning of NIKOLSKII [1988] for the class of functions $W^{(1)}(L; a, b)$ is the formula for rectangles with equidistant nodes, for which the error is about c/n. For the MC method given by (56.3) when $n_j = 1$ the rate of convergence is better with order $1/2$, which is based on the fact that the randomization of the quadrature formula (random nodes) increases the rate of convergence by 50%. At the same time, the estimation given by (56.4) for the rate of convergence reaches the lower bound estimation obtained by BACHVALOV [1959, 1961], for the error of an arbitrary random quadrature formula for the class of continuous functions in $[a, b]$.

57. Random interpolation quadrature formulas

If the quadrature formula for computing the integral

$$I = \int_D f(x) p(x) \, dx, \quad D \subset \mathbb{R}^d, \ p(x) \geq 0, \ \int_D p(x) \, dx = 1$$

is usually called the expression

$$I \approx \sum_{j=1}^{n} c_j f(x_j), \qquad (57.1)$$

where $x_1, \ldots, x_n \in D$ are random nodes and $c_1, \ldots, c_n$ are weights, then the random quadrature formula is called

$$I \approx \sum_{j=1}^{n} \kappa_j f(x_j), \qquad (57.2)$$

where $x_1, \ldots, x_n \in D$ are random nodes and $\kappa_1, \ldots, \kappa_n$ are random weights.

The random quadrature formulas considered above are a special case of (57.2) with fixed (non-random) weights.

All functions considered in this paragraph will be partially continuous and belong to $L_2(D)$.

Let $\varphi_0, \varphi_1, \ldots, \varphi_m$ be a system of orthonormal functions, such that

$$\int_D \varphi_k(x) \varphi_j(x) \, dx = \delta_{kj}.$$

For $p(x) = \varphi_0(x)$, an approximate solution for the integral

$$I = \int_D f(x) \varphi_0(x) \, dx \qquad (57.3)$$

has to be found using a quadrature formula of the type (57.1).

Let us fix arbitrary different nodes $x_0, x_1, \ldots, x_m$ and choose the weights $c_0, c_1, \ldots, c_m$ such that (57.1) is exact for the system of orthonormal functions $\varphi_0, \varphi_1, \ldots, \varphi_m$. In this case it is convenient to represent the quadrature formula (57.1) as a ratio of two determinants

$$I \approx \frac{W_f(x_0, x_1, \ldots, x_m)}{W_{\varphi_0}(x_0, x_1, \ldots, x_m)},$$

where

$$W_g(x_0, \ldots, x_m) = \begin{vmatrix} g(x_0) & \varphi_1(x_0) & \cdots & \varphi_m(x_0) \\ g(x_1) & \varphi_1(x_1) & \cdots & \varphi_m(x_1) \\ \vdots & \vdots & & \vdots \\ g(x_m) & \varphi_1(x_m) & \cdots & \varphi_m(x_m) \end{vmatrix}.$$

It is easy to check that if $W_{\varphi_0} \neq 0$ then the formula (57.3) is exact for every linear combination of the kind

$$f = a_0 \varphi_0 + \cdots + a_m \varphi_m.$$

THEOREM 57.1 (SOBOL [1973]). Let $\varphi_0, \varphi_1, \ldots, \varphi_m$ be an arbitrary set of orthonormal functions in D. Then

$$\int_D \cdots \int_D W_{\varphi_0}^2 \, dx_0 \cdots dx_m = (m+1)!.$$

THEOREM 57.2 (SOBOL [1973]). Let $\varphi_0, \varphi_1, \ldots, \varphi_m, \psi$ be an arbitrary set of orthonormal functions in D. Then

$$\int_D \cdots \int_D W_{\varphi_0} W_\psi \, dx_0 \cdots dx_m = 0.$$

Denote for brevity the $d(m+1)$-dimensional points of the domain $B \equiv D \times \cdots \times D$ by $t \equiv (x_0, \ldots, x_m)$ and $dt = dx_0 \cdots dx_m$, let B_0 be the set of points t, in which $W_{\varphi_0} = 0$ and $B_+ = B - B_0$. Let us consider the random points $\xi_0, \ldots, \xi_m$ in D and consider as an approximate value for (57.3) the random variable

$$\hat{\theta}[f] = \begin{cases} \dfrac{W_f(\xi_0, \xi_1, \ldots, \xi_m)}{W_{\varphi_0}(\xi_0, \xi_1, \ldots, \xi_m)}, & \text{if } (\xi_0, \ldots, \xi_m) \in B_+, \\ 0, & \text{if } (\xi_0, \ldots, \xi_m) \in B_0. \end{cases}$$

THEOREM 57.3 (ERMAKOV and ZOLOTUCHIN [1960], ERMAKOV [1967]). *If the joint probability density function of the random points $\xi_0, \xi_1, \ldots, \xi_m$ in B is*

$$p(x_0, \ldots, x_m) = \frac{1}{(m+1)!} [W_{\varphi_0}(x_0, \ldots, x_m)]^2,$$

then for every function $f \in L_2(D)$ the following relations are fulfilled

$$E\hat{\theta}[f] = \int_D f(x)\varphi_0(x) \, dx,$$

$$D\hat{\theta}[f] \leq \int_D f^2(x) \, dx - \sum_{j=0}^m \left(\int_D f(x)\varphi_j(x) \, dx \right)^2. \tag{57.4}$$

The inequality (57.4) turns into an equality if and only if $W_{\varphi_0} = 0$ only for a manifold with dimensions of less than $d(m+1)$.

58. Quasi-MC methods

The main point of the MC methods is the use of a random variable γ, uniformly distributed in the interval $(0, 1)$, the so-called ordinary random number. The concept of "real" random number is a mathematical abstraction. Numbers computed from specified formulas but satisfying an accepted set of tests just as though they were "real" random numbers, are called pseudorandom. Numbers that are being used instead of random numbers in some MC methods to imply their convergence are called quasi-random (SOBOL [1991]). Quasi-random numbers are connected with a certain class of algorithms and their applicability is more restricted than that of pseudorandom numbers (SOBOL [1991]). The reason in favor of quasirandom numbers is the possibility of increasing the rate of convergence: the usual rate of $n^{-1/2}$ is in some cases replaced by $n^{-1+\varepsilon}$, where $\varepsilon > 0$ is arbitrarily small.

Let $x \equiv (x^{(1)}, \ldots, x^{(d)})$ be a point that belongs to the d-dimensional cube $C^d = \{x : 0 \leq x^{(1)} \leq 1, \ldots, 0 \leq x^{(d)} \leq 1\}$ and $\xi = (\gamma^{(1)}, \ldots, \gamma^{(d)})$ be a random point, uniformly distributed in C^d.

A uniformly distributed sequence (u.d.s.) of non-random points was introduced by WEYL [1916].

Denote by $S_n(D)$ the number of points with $1 \leq i \leq n$ that fall into D, where $D \subset C^d$. The sequence $x_1, x_2, \ldots$ is called a u.d.s. if for arbitrary regions D

$$\lim_{n \to \infty} [S_n(D)/n] = V(D),$$

where $V(D)$ is the d-dimensional volume of D.

THEOREM 58.1 (H. Weyl, see SOBOL [1991]). *The relation*

$$\lim_{n \to \infty} \frac{1}{n} \sum_{i=1}^{n} f(\xi_j) = \int_{C^d} f(x) \, dx \qquad (58.1)$$

holds for all Riemann-integrable functions f if and only if the sequence $x_1, x_2, \ldots$, is u.d.s.

Comparing (54.1) with (58.1) one can conclude that if random points ξ_i are replaced by points x_i of a u.d.s., then for a wide class of functions f the averages converge. In this case the "i"th trial should be carried out using Cartesian coordinates $(x_i^{(1)}, \ldots, x_i^{(d)})$ of the point x_i rather than the random numbers $\gamma_1, \ldots, \gamma_n$. For practical purposes a u.d.s. must be found that satisfies three additional requirements (SOBOL [1973, 1989]):
 (i) the best asymptotic as $n \to \infty$;
 (ii) well distributed points for small n;
 (iii) a cheap calculation algorithm.

All Π_τ-sequences given in SOBOL [1989] satisfy the first requirement. The definition of Π_τ-sequences is as follows: binary estimates are called estimates of the kind $(j-1)2^{-m} \leq x < j2^{-m}$ when $j = 1, 2, \ldots, 2^m$, $m = 0, 1, \ldots$ (for $j = 2^m$ the right-hand end of the estimate is closed). A binary parallelepiped Π is a multiplication of binary estimates. A net in C^d, consisting of $n = 2^\nu$ points is called a Π_τ-sequence, if every binary Π with volume $2^\tau/n$ contains exactly 2^τ points of the net. It is supposed that $\nu > \tau$ are integers.

Subroutines to compute these points can be found in SOBOL [1979] and BRATLEY and FOX [1980]. More details are contained in LEVITAN, MARKOVICH, ROZIN and SOBOL [1988].

The problem of the error estimation of (58.1) arises.

If one uses the points $x_0, x_1, \ldots$ the answer is quite simple. Finite nets $x_0, \ldots, x_{n-1}$, $n = 2^m$ (m is a positive integer), have better uniform properties (SOBOL [1991]).

Non-random estimates of the error

$$\delta_n(f) = \frac{1}{n} \sum_{i=0}^{n-1} f(x_i) - \int_{C^d} f(x) \, dx \qquad (58.2)$$

are known (SOBOL [1991, 1989]).

Let us mention two results. First, assume that all partial derivatives of the function $f(x)$, $x \in C^d \subset \mathbb{R}^d$, that include no more than one differentiation with respect to each variable,

$$\frac{\partial^s f}{\partial x^{(i_1)} \cdots \partial x^{(i_s)}}, \quad 1 \leq i_1 < \cdots < i_s \leq d, \ s = 1, 2, \ldots, d,$$

are continuous. It follows from SOBOL [1991] that for $n = 2^m$

$$|\delta_n(f)| \leq A(f) n^{-1} \log^{d-1} n. \tag{58.3}$$

If in (58.2) arbitrary values of n are used then in (58.3) $\log^{d-1} n$ must be changed to $\log^d n$ (SOBOL [1991]).

Consider a class of functions $f(x)$, $x \in C^d \subset \mathbb{R}^d$ with continuous first partial derivatives. Denote

$$\sup \left| \frac{\partial f}{\partial x^{(i)}} \right| = L_i, \quad i = 1, \ldots, d.$$

It follows from SOBOL [1989] that when $n = 2^m$, then

$$|\delta_n(f)| \leq \max(s! L_{i_1} \cdots L_{i_s}/n),$$

where the maximum is extended over all groups satisfying $1 \leq i_1 < \cdots < i_s \leq d$ and $s = 1, \ldots, d$.

If, for example, several $L_i = 0$, the order of the last estimate is much better than $n^{-1/d}$. The orders of convergence in both cases are optimal for the corresponding classes of functions.

In DOROSHKEVICH and SOBOL [1987] a five-dimensional improper integral is evaluated by using the Π_τ-approximation and ordinary MC method.

59. MC methods for continual integrals, weight functions, splitting method

59.1. Continual integrals

Let μ be a measure that corresponds to the beginning from zero homogeneous process with independent increments $\xi(s)$, $0 \leq s \leq t < \infty$. Let us consider the MC method for the approximate computation of the continual integral from the functional F (ERMAKOV [1975], SOBOL [1973], LICHODED [1989])

$$\int F(\xi) \mu(d\xi).$$

First, the random process $\xi(s)$ is approximated by the process

$$\xi^{(m)}(s) = \sum_{k=1}^{m} i^{(k)}(s)[\xi(t_k) - \xi(t_{k-1})],$$

where $0 = t_0 < t_1 < \cdots < t_m = t$ is a splitting of $[0, t]$ into n parts and $i^{(k)}(s)$ is a function that determines the type of the approximation. If, e.g.,

$$i^{(k)}(s) = \frac{s - t_{k-1}}{t_k - t_{k-1}} \mathbb{1}_{[t_{k-1}, t_k)}(s) + \mathbb{1}_{[t_k, t]}(s),$$

where
$$\mathbb{1}_A(\tau) = \begin{cases} 1, & \text{if } \tau \in A, \\ 0, & \text{if } \tau \notin A, \end{cases}$$

then an approximation of the trajectory of the process is obtained by polygons with nodes at the points $(t_k, \xi(t_k))$, $k = 0, 1, \ldots, m$. The continual integral is approximated by

$$\int F(\xi)\mu(\mathrm{d}\xi) = EF(\xi) \approx EF(\xi^{(m)})$$

and $EF(\xi^{(m)})$ can be estimated by the formula

$$EF(\xi^{(m)}) \approx \frac{1}{n} \sum_{k=1}^{n} F(\xi_k^{(m)}), \tag{59.1}$$

where $\xi_k^{(m)}(s)$ are independent realizations of the process $\xi^{(m)}(s)$.

The necessity of the approximation of $\xi_k^{(m)}(s)$ with $\xi^{(m)}(s)$ is stipulated by the impossibility of obtaining a realization directly from the process $\xi(s)$.

Therefore (LICHODED [1989])

$$\int F(\xi)\mu(\mathrm{d}\xi) = \frac{1}{n} \sum_{k=1}^{n} F(\xi_k^{(m)}) + R^{(m)}(F) + r_n^m(F),$$

where $R^{(m)}(F) = \int F(\xi)\mu(\mathrm{d}\xi) - EF(\xi^{(m)})$ is the error arising from the replacement of the random process $\xi(s)$ by the random process $\xi^{(m)}(s)$. Here

$$r_n^m(F) = EF(\xi^{(m)}) - \frac{1}{n} \sum_{k=1}^{n} F(\xi_k^{(m)})$$

is the error of the computation of $EF(\xi^{(m)})$ using (59.1).

In LICHODED [1989] the formula (59.1) is made more precise by the approximate determination of the error $R^{(m)}(F)$. Of course, this procedure is meaningful only if $R^{(m)}(F) > r_n^m(F)$.

Let us suppose that an exact formula exists for generalized polynomials of degree $2m + 1$,

$$\int G(\xi)\mu(\mathrm{d}\xi) \approx \sum_{j=1}^{Q} A_j \int_0^{t_{(m)}} \cdots \int_0^{t} G\left(\sum_{\alpha=1}^{l} x_\alpha^{(j)} \mathbb{1}_{[s_\alpha, t)}(\cdot) + a(\cdot)\right) \mathrm{d}s_1 \cdots \mathrm{d}s_l,$$

where Q is an integer, A_j, $x_\alpha^{(j)}$, $1 \leq j \leq Q$, $1 \leq \alpha \leq m$ are coefficients and $a(s) = \int \xi_s \mu(\mathrm{d}\xi)$ is the mean value of the measure μ.

In LICHODED [1989] the following theorem is proved.

THEOREM 59.1. *The approximate equality*

$$R^{(m)}(F) \approx R_l^m(F) \equiv \sum_{j=1}^{Q} A_j \int_0^{t_{(m)}} \cdots \int_0^{t} F\left(\sum_{\alpha=1}^{l} x_\alpha^{(j)} \mathbb{1}_{[s_\alpha, t)}(\cdot) + a(\cdot)\right) \mathrm{d}s_1 \cdots \mathrm{d}s_l,$$

is exact for $(2m + 1)$-degree generalized polynomials.

It follows as a corollary that the approximate formula

$$EF(\xi) \approx EF(\xi^{(m)}) + R_l^{(m)}(F)$$

is exact for $(2m+1)$-degree generalized polynomials.

59.2. Weight functions

In SHAW [1988] MC quadratures with weight functions are considered for the computation of

$$S(q; m) = \int q(\theta) m(\theta) \, d\theta \, ,$$

where q is some function (possibly vector or matrix valued).

The unnormalized posterior density m is expressed as the product of two functions w and f, where w is called the weight function $m(\theta) = w(\theta)f(\theta)$. The weight function w is nonnegative and integrated to one; i.e. $\int w(\theta) \, d\theta = 1$, and it is chosen to have similar properties to m.

Most numerical integration methods then implicitly replace the function $m(\theta)$ by a discrete approximation in the form (SHAW [1988]):

$$\hat{m}(\theta) = \begin{cases} w_i f(\theta), & \theta = \theta_i, \ i = 1, 2, \ldots, n, \\ 0, & \text{elsewhere}, \end{cases}$$

so that the integral $S(q; m)$ may be estimated by

$$\hat{S}(q; m) = \sum_{i=1}^{n} w_i f(\theta_i) q(\theta_i) \, . \tag{59.2}$$

Integration methods use the weight function w as the kernel of the approximation of the integrand

$$S(q; m) = \int q(\theta) m(\theta) \, d\theta = \int q(\theta) w(\theta) f(\theta) \, d\theta = \int q(\theta) f(\theta) \, dW(\theta)$$
$$= E_w(q(\theta) f(\theta)) \, .$$

This suggests an MC approach to numerical integration (SHAW [1988]): generate nodes $\theta_1, \ldots, \theta_n$ independently from the distribution w and estimate $S(q; m)$ by $\hat{S}(q; m)$ in (59.2) with $w_i = 1/n$. If $q(\theta) f(\theta)$ is a constant, then $\hat{S}(q; m)$ will be exact. More generally $\hat{S}(q; m)$ is unbiased and its variance will be small if $w(\theta)$ has a similar shape to $|q(\theta) m(\theta)|$. The above procedure is known as important sampling (see Section 55.3).

In SHAW [1988] it is noted that the determination of the weight function can be done iteratively using posterior information.

MC quadratures which use posterior distributions are examined in VAN DIJK and KLOEK [1983, 1985], VAN DIJK, HOP and LOUTER [1987], STEWART [1983, 1985, 1987], STEWART and DAVIS [1986], KLOEK and VAN DIJK [1978].

59.3. Splitting method (MICHAILOV [1987])

Let us suppose that

$$I = \int_X \int_Y f(x, y)g(x, y)\,dx\,dy$$

has to be computed, where $f(x, y)$ is the density of the joint distribution of the random vectors ξ and η.

Following MICHAILOV [1987], let us introduce the notation:

$$\zeta = g(\xi, \eta), \qquad E[\zeta|x] = \int_Y f_2(y|x)\,d(x, y)\,dy, \qquad f_1(x) = \int_Y f(x, y)\,dy,$$

where $f_1(x)$ is the density of the absolute distribution of ξ, $f_2(y|x)$ is the density of the conditional distribution of η under the condition $\xi = x$; $E[\zeta|x]$ is the conditional mathematical expectation of the random variable ζ under the condition $\xi = x$.

So the problem is reduced to the computation of the integral

$$\int_X f_1(x)E[\zeta|x]\,dx.$$

Furthermore, the amount of dispersion decreases; i.e. $DE[\zeta|\xi] \leq D\zeta$, since $D\zeta = ED[\zeta|\xi] + DE[\zeta|\xi]$.

It is useful to use several values of η for one value of ξ.

In MICHAILOV [1987] a method for optimization of such an algorithm is proposed. Let ξ be distributed with density $f_1(x)$ and let $n(\xi)$ be an integer, which depends on ξ, $n(\xi) \geq 1$. The random variables $\eta_1, \ldots, \eta_{n(\xi)}$ are independent and equally conditionally distributed with density $f_2(y|x)$ under the condition $\xi = x$.

MICHAILOV [1987] used the following estimate:

$$\zeta_n = \frac{1}{n(\xi)} \sum_{k=1}^{n(\xi)} g(\xi, \eta_k),$$

and it is proved that

$$E\zeta_n = \int_X \int_Y f(x, y)g(x, y)\,dx\,dy, \qquad D\zeta_n = DE[\zeta|\xi] + E\left\{\frac{D[\zeta|\xi]}{n(\xi)}\right\}.$$

When $n(\xi) = \text{const} = n$, the optimal value of n is found (which minimizes the computational cost of the method $S_n = t_n D\zeta_n$, where $t_n = t_1 + E[n(\xi)t_2(\xi)]$, with t_1 the mean time for the computation of one value of ξ, and $t_2(x)$ the time for the computation of one value of η under the condition that $\xi = x$),

$$n = \sqrt{A_2 t_1/(A_1 t_2)},$$

where A_1 and A_2 are estimated by the result from special a priori calculations.

CHAPTER IV

Hausdorff Approximation

Many natural phenomena are subject to mathematical modeling by using discontinuous functions. However, the approximate representation of such functions by algebraic polynomials or spline functions with respect to the uniform distance is impossible with arbitrary accuracy. Usually the L_p metric is used as a measure of approximation for discontinuous functions. This metric does not ensure geometrical proximity between the graphs of the functions. For example, the well-known Gibbs effect takes place for the L_2 approximation of functions with jumps by means of trigonometric polynomials (Fourier series). It means that at the points of discontinuities the graph of the polynomial differs substantially from the graph of the approximated function, Section 65. Briefly, the proximity between two functions in the Hausdorff sense means the proximity between their graphs and that Gibbs effect is avoided.

In a way, the Hausdorff distance treats the coordinate axes equivalently while a neighborhood of a function, with respect to the uniform distance, is obtained by varying points of its graph in all directions in the plane.

This chapter gives basic theorems and facts for the Hausdorff approximation of bounded functions by polynomials and linear positive operators. The rate of convergence of the best Hausdorff polynomial approximation as well as the numerical methods for computation of the polynomial (or rational function) of the best Hausdorff approximation for a given bounded function are considered.

The multivariate case of the approximation of functions in Hausdorff metric is also a subject of investigation and series of numerical examples and figures illustrate the effectiveness of the suggested methods.

60. Segment functions and Hausdorff distance

Let $\mathbb{R}$ be the set of real numbers, and $\bar{\mathbb{R}} = \mathbb{R} \cup \{-\infty\} \cup \{\infty\}$. A segment $[a, b]$ with $a, b \in \bar{\mathbb{R}}$ is

$$[a, b] = \{x \in \bar{\mathbb{R}} : a \leq x \leq b\}.$$

The set of all such segments will be denoted by $S(\bar{\mathbb{R}})$.

Let $\Omega \subset \mathbb{R}$. The set of all segment functions defined on Ω will be denoted by $\mathbb{A}_\Omega$; i.e. every $f \in \mathbb{A}_\Omega$ is a certain mapping of Ω into $S(\bar{\mathbb{R}})$. By A_Ω will be denoted the set of all extended real (single-valued) functions defined on Ω; i.e. every $f \in \mathbb{A}_\Omega$ is a certain mapping of Ω onto $\bar{\mathbb{R}}$. Since $\bar{\mathbb{R}} \subset S(\bar{\mathbb{R}})$, it follows that $A_\Omega \subset \mathbb{A}_\Omega$.

To every $\delta > 0$ there correspond two operators defined on $\mathbb{A}_\Omega$ with values in $A_{\bar{\Omega}}$ (where $\bar{\Omega}$ is the closure of the set Ω), such that

$$I(\delta, f; x) = I(\Omega, \delta, f; x) = \inf\{y: y \in f(t), t \in [x - \delta, x + \delta] \cap \Omega\},$$

$$S(\delta, f; x) = S(\Omega, \delta, f; x) = \sup\{y: y \in f(t), t \in [x - \delta, x + \delta] \cap \Omega\}.$$

It is directly seen that for the modulus of continuity

$$\omega(f; \delta) = \sup\{|f(x') - f(x'')|: |x' - x''| \leq \delta, x', x'' \in \Omega\}$$

of every function $f \in A_\Omega$ the following equality holds:

$$\omega(f; \delta) = \sup\{S(\delta/2, f; x) - I(\delta/2, f; x): x \in \Omega\}.$$

The lower and upper Baire functions for $f \in \mathbb{A}_\Omega$ are

$$I(f; x) = I(\Omega, f; x) = \lim_{\delta \to +0} I(\delta, f; x),$$

$$S(f; x) = S(\Omega, f; x) = \lim_{\delta \to +0} S(\delta, f; x).$$

According to the definition of I and S, they are operators defined on $\mathbb{A}_\Omega$ with values in $A_{\bar{\Omega}}$.

The completed graph of a function $f \in \mathbb{A}_\Omega$ is the segment function $F(f) \in \mathbb{A}_{\bar{\Omega}}$ defined by

$$F(f; x) = F(\Omega, f; x) = [I(f; x), S(f; x)].$$

According to the definition F is an operator defined on $\mathbb{A}_\Omega$ with values in $\mathbb{A}_{\bar{\Omega}}$. Let us denote by $\mathbb{F}_\Omega$ the set of those functions f in $\mathbb{A}_\Omega$ for which $F(f; x) = f(x)$ for all $x \in \Omega$. Clearly, $\mathbb{F}_\Omega$ consists of all the fixed points of the operator F in $\mathbb{A}_\Omega$. As usual, C_Ω denotes all the continuous single-valued functions defined on Ω. Obviously, $C_\Omega \subset A_\Omega$ and for every $f \in C_\Omega$ the equality $F(f) = f$ holds; i.e. $C_\Omega \subset \mathbb{F}_\Omega$.

Let (M, ρ) be a metric space; i.e. to every pair $a, b \in M$ there corresponds a non-negative number $\rho(a, b)$ such that for all $a, b, c \in M$

$$\rho(a, b) = \rho(b, a) \geq 0, \tag{60.1}$$

$$\rho(a, b) = 0 \Leftrightarrow a = b, \tag{60.2}$$

$$\rho(a, b) \leq \rho(a, c) + \rho(c, b). \tag{60.3}$$

In his book, HAUSDORFF [1927] defined the distance between the subsets of a given metric space. Let $A \subset M$. Let us denote by $U(\alpha, A)$, where $\alpha \geq 0$, the set of all points $x \in M$ such that $\rho(x; A) \leq \alpha$; i.e.

$$U(\alpha, A) = \{x: x \in M \text{ and } \rho(x; A) \leq \alpha\}.$$

The infimimum of those α for which both $U(\alpha, A) \supset B$ and $U(\alpha, B) \supset A$ is called the Hausdorff distance. Let us denote this distance by $r(\rho; A, B)$. The distance $r(\rho; A, B)$ does not satisfy the condition (60.2) in the totality of non-empty subsets of the space M. For instance, if a is an arbitrary point of the line $\mathbb{R}$ with the usual metric, and $A = \{x: \rho(x, a) < 1\}$, $B = \{x: \rho(x, a) \leq 1\}$, then $A \neq B$, but $r(\rho; A, B) = 0$.

It is easy to see that if $\mathbb{F}(M)$ is the set of all closed subsets of the metric space M, then $r(\rho; A, B)$ is an infinite-valued metric of $\mathbb{F}(M)$, which satisfies the conditions (60.1)–(60.3). Clearly, $r(\rho; A, B)$ can become ∞, e.g., when A is bounded and B is unbounded. As a distance the symbol ∞ can also be admitted. Of course, it can be eliminated by considering only bounded sets, but this is inappropriate, since later on unbounded sets are involved. There are many cases when A and B are unbounded, yet the number $r(\rho; A, B)$ is finite, e.g., this happens when the sets are parallel lines in the plane.

In the sequel the following equivalent form of Hausdorff distance will often be more convenient:

$$r(\rho; A, B) = \max\{\sup_{a \in A} \inf_{b \in B} \rho(a, b), \sup_{b \in B} \inf_{a \in A} \rho(a, b)\} .$$

61. The metric space $\mathbb{F}_\Omega$ and H-distance in $\mathbb{A}_\Omega$

Let us define a distance in the set of functions $\mathbb{F}_\Omega$, which will be called the Hausdorff distance or H-distance.

Having in mind the definition of the Hausdorff distance between two subsets of a metric space, let us consider the plane $\mathbb{R}^2$ equipped with the usual metric as a metric space $(\mathbb{R}^2, \rho)$ and the graphs of two functions $f, g \in \mathbb{F}_\Omega$ as subsets of $\mathbb{R}^2$. Then identifying the segment functions with their graphs it follows that

$$r(\rho; f, g) = \max\{\sup_{A \in f} \inf_{B \in g} \rho(A, B), \sup_{A \in g} \inf_{B \in f} \rho(A, B)\} .$$

For our aims it is convenient to introduce a parametrized family of distances as follows: for each $\alpha > 0$

$$\rho_\alpha(A(x, y), B(\xi, \eta)) = \max\{\alpha^{-1}|x - \xi|, |y - \eta|\} .$$

With respect to each metric, the unit sphere is a rectangle with sides that are parallel to the coordinate axes and are in the ratio $1/\alpha$ (see Fig. 61.1).

The Hausdorff distance $r(\rho_\alpha; f, g)$ between two functions $f, g \in \mathbb{F}_\Omega$ will be denoted by $r(\Omega, \alpha; f, g)$. If Ω is understood, it can be abbreviated by $r(\alpha; f, g)$. The distance $r(\alpha; f, g)$ is called the Hausdorff distance (H-distance) with parameter α.

For $f, g \in \mathbb{F}_\Omega$,

$$r(\alpha; f, g) = \max\left\{\sup_{x \in \Omega} \sup_{y \in f(x)} \inf_{\xi \in \Omega} \inf_{\eta \in g(\xi)} \max\{\alpha^{-1}|x - \xi|, |y - \eta|\},\right.$$

$$\left.\sup_{x \in \Omega} \sup_{y \in g(x)} \inf_{\xi \in \Omega} \inf_{\eta \in f(\xi)} \max\{\alpha^{-1}|x - \xi|, |y - \eta|\}\right\} . \quad (61.1)$$

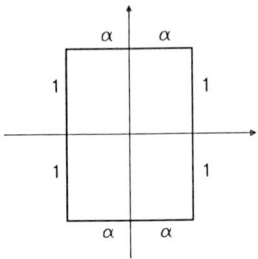

Fig. 61.1. The unit sphere of the metric ρ_α.

The H-distance was defined between functions that belong to $\mathbb{F}_\Omega$. If $f, g \in \mathbb{A}_\Omega$ then the H-distance between them is the H-distance between their completed graphs. If $f, g \in \mathbb{A}_\Omega$ then by definition

$$r(\Omega, \alpha; f, g) = r(\alpha; f, g) = r(\alpha; F(f), F(g)).$$

Of course, the H-distance in $\mathbb{A}_\Omega$ does not meet all the axioms of the metric. The condition $r(\alpha; f, g) = 0 \Rightarrow f = g$ is violated, since two different functions may have the same completed graphs. Let us consider some properties of the H-distance in A_Ω and $\mathbb{F}_\Omega$.

First, note that from the inclusion $\Delta_1 \subset \Delta_2$ for intervals, it does not follow that $r(\Delta_1, \alpha; f, g) \leq r(\Delta_2, \alpha; f, g)$. For example, if φ, ψ are the real functions

$$\varphi(x) = \begin{cases} |x|, & \text{if } |x| \leq 1, \\ 1, & \text{if } 1 \leq |x| \leq 2, \end{cases}$$

$$\psi(x) = \begin{cases} 0, & \text{if } |x| \leq 1, \\ |x| - 1, & \text{if } 1 \leq |x| \leq 2, \end{cases}$$

then it is directly verified (see Fig. 61.2) that $r([-1, 1], \alpha; \varphi, \psi) = 1$ whereas $r([-2, 2], \alpha; \varphi, \psi) = 1/(1 + \alpha) < 1$.

This example demonstrates one of the essential distinctions between the Hausdorff distance and the classical distances considered by analysis. It might happen that the sequence $\{f_n\}_{n=1}^\infty$ converges with regard to the Hausdorff distance on Δ_2, but it diverges on $A_1 \subset \Delta_2$. This property is illustrated in the next example. Let

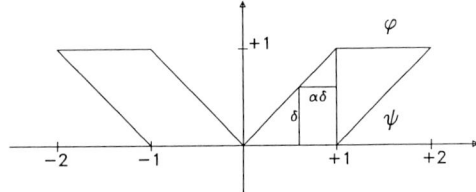

Fig. 61.2. The functions φ and ψ.

$$f_n(x) = \max\{0, 1 - |(-1)^n - nx|\}, \quad x \in [-1, 1], \quad n = 1, 2, 3, \ldots.$$

It is directly calculated that $r([-1, 1], \alpha; f_n, f_0) = 2/(1 + \alpha n)$, where

$$f_0(x) = \begin{cases} 0, & \text{if } 0 < |x| \leq 1, \\ [0, 1], & \text{if } x = 0, \end{cases}$$

and

$$\lim_{n \to \infty} r([-1, 1], \alpha; f_n, f_0) = 0;$$

i.e. the sequence $\{f_n\}_{n=1}^{\infty}$ converges to f_0 with respect to the Hausdorff distance on the closed interval $[-1, 1]$. On the other hand, for every n it follows that $r([0, 1], \alpha; f_n, f_{n+1}) = 1$ and, consequently, the sequence $\{f_n\}_{n=1}^{\infty}$ diverges with respect to the Hausdorff distance on the closed interval $[0, 1]$.

62. Relationships between the uniform distance and the Hausdorff distance

The uniform distance in the set C_Ω of all continuous functions on Ω is defined as follows:

$$R(f, g) = \|f - g\|_\Omega = \sup_{x \in \Omega} |f(x) - g(x)|.$$

It is possible to extend this definition to all the functions in $\mathbb{A}_\Omega$, where the expression $\sup_{x \in \Omega} |f(x) - g(x)|$ should be understood as

$$\sup_{x \in \Omega} |f(x) - g(x)| = \sup\{|y - \eta|: x \in \Omega, y \in f(x), \eta \in g(x)\}. \tag{62.1}$$

In the spirit of (62.1), let us recast the modulus of continuity of a function f in $\mathbb{A}_\Omega$ defined in Section 60 by

$$\omega(f; \delta) = \sup\{|y - \eta|: y \in f(x_1), \eta \in f(x_2), x_1, x_2 \in \Omega, |x_1 - x_2| \leq \delta\}. \tag{62.2}$$

For single-valued functions (62.2), of course, agrees with the usual definition.

In SENDOV ([1990], p. 35), the following theorem was proved.

THEOREM 62.1. *If $f, g \in \mathbb{A}_\Omega$ and $r(\Omega, \alpha; f, g) = r(\alpha; f, g)$ is the Hausdorff distance between f and g, then*

$$r(\alpha; f, g) \leq \|f - g\|_\Omega \leq r(\alpha; f, g) + \omega(\alpha r(\alpha; f, g)), \tag{62.3}$$

where $\omega(\delta) = \min\{\omega(f; \delta), \omega(g; \delta)\}$.

PROOF. The inequality of the left-hand side of (62.3) follows from the definition of the H-distance in (61.1), since $r(\alpha; f, g)$ is at most the Hausdorff distance between the graphs of f and g, and for $y \in f(x)$ and $\eta \in g(x)$, it follows that

$$\inf_{\xi \in \Omega} \inf_{\eta' \in g(\xi)} \max\{\alpha^{-1}|x - \xi|, |y - \eta'|\} \leq |y - \eta| \leq R(f, g).$$

To establish the inequality on the right-hand side of (62.3), let us assume that f and g are in $\mathbb{F}_\Omega$, as the Hausdorff distance between the segment functions is defined in terms of completed graphs, and the uniform distance is not decreased by replacing segment functions by their completed graphs. It is directly seen that for every $x \in \Omega$ and $y \in f(x)$ there exists an $\xi_x \in \Omega$ and an $\eta' \in g(\xi_x)$ such that

$$\inf_{\xi \in \Omega} \inf_{\eta \in g(\xi)} \max\{\alpha^{-1}|x - f|, |y - \eta|\} = \max\{\alpha^{-1}|x - \xi_x|, |y - \eta'|\}.$$

On the other hand, according to (62.1), for every $x \in \Omega$ and $y \in f(x)$, the inequalities

$$\alpha^{-1}|x - \xi_x| \leq r(\alpha; f, g), \qquad |y - \eta'| \leq r(\alpha; f, g)$$

hold. However, then, in view of

$$|y - \eta| \leq |y - \eta'| + |\eta' - \eta|,$$

the inequality

$$|y - \eta| \leq r(\alpha; f, g) + \omega(g; |x - \xi_x|) \leq r(\alpha; f, g) + \omega(g; \alpha r(\alpha; f, g)) \tag{62.4}$$

holds for every $x \in \Omega$. Similarly

$$|y - \eta| \leq r(\alpha; f, g) + \omega(f; \alpha r(\alpha; f, g)). \tag{62.5}$$

Taking the right-hand side of (62.3) from (62.4) and (62.5) the proof is completed. □

COROLLARY 62.1. *The uniform distance and the Hausdorff distance are topologically equivalent on every set of equicontinuous functions.*

Since $\omega(g; \delta) = 0$ for each δ when g is a constant function the next corollary is valid.

COROLLARY 62.2. *If $g(x) = c$, where c is a constant, then $r(\alpha; f, g) = R(f, g)$.*

Let us note that the ratio of the uniform distance to the Hausdorff distance for two given functions may be arbitrarily large. For instance, if f and g are defined on $\Delta = [0, 1]$ in the following manner

$$f(x) = \begin{cases} x/\lambda, & \text{if } 0 \leq x \leq \lambda, \\ 1, & \text{if } \lambda \leq x \leq 1, \end{cases}$$

$$g(x) = \begin{cases} 0, & \text{if } 0 \leq x \leq \lambda, \\ (x-\lambda)/\lambda, & \text{if } \lambda \leq x \leq 2\lambda, \\ 1, & \text{if } 2\lambda \leq x \leq 1, \end{cases}$$

then $r(\alpha; f, g) \leq \lambda/(\alpha + \lambda)$. On the other hand,

$$\|f - g\|_\Omega = R(f, g) \geq |f(\lambda) - g(\lambda)| = 1,$$

and hence

$$R(f, g)/r(\alpha; f, g) \geq 1/\alpha\lambda,$$

where λ can be chosen to be arbitrarily small.

COROLLARY 62.3. *If $f, g \in C_\Omega$ with Ω compact, then*

$$\lim_{\alpha \to +0} r(\alpha; f, g) = R(f, g).$$

PROOF. The proof follows directly from (62.3), letting $\alpha \to +0$. □

The last corollary says that the uniform distance may be considered as a limiting case of the Hausdorff distance with the parameter $\alpha = 0$; i.e. $r(0; f, g) = R(f, g)$.

The consideration of the Hausdorff distance as a generalization of the uniform distance enables us to obtain a series of classical theorems about the uniform approximation of continuous functions as corollaries of the corresponding theorems for the Hausdorff approximations of wider classes of functions.

63. Convergence of sequences of positive operators

Let $f \in \mathbb{A}_\Omega$. The modulus of H-continuity (with parameter α) of f is

$$\tau(\Omega, \alpha, f; \delta) = \tau(\alpha, f; \delta) = r(\alpha; S(\delta/2, f), I(\delta/2, f)).$$

Directly from the definition of H-continuity one obtains the following results.

(a) The modulus of H-continuity does not exceed the modulus of continuity $\tau(\alpha, f; \delta) \leq \omega(f; \delta)$, where $\omega(f; \delta)$ is the modulus of continuity of f. Indeed, by definition,

$$\begin{aligned} \tau(\alpha, f; \delta) &= r(\Omega, \alpha; S(\delta/2, f), I(\delta/2, f)) \\ &\leq \sup_{x \in \Omega} |S(\delta/2, f; x) - I(\delta/2, f; x)| \\ &= \sup_{x \in \Omega} \{|y - \eta|: y \in f(x_1), \eta \in f(x_2), x_1, x_2 \in \Omega, |x_1 - x_2| \leq \delta\} \\ &= \omega(f; \delta). \end{aligned}$$

(b) The modulus of H-continuity tends to the modulus of continuity as the parameter tends to zero:

$$\lim_{\alpha \to +0} \tau(\alpha, f; \delta) = \omega(f; \delta).$$

Indeed, $\lim_{\alpha \to +0} r(\Omega, \alpha; f, g) = \sup_{x \in \Omega} |f(x) - g(x)|$.

(c) The modulus of H-continuity is a monotone non-decreasing function of δ, i.e. if $\delta_1 < \delta_2$, then $\tau(\alpha, f; \delta_1) \leq \tau(\alpha, f; \delta_2)$.

An operator L, defined on $B_\Omega \subset A_\Omega$, is called linear if $L(\alpha f + \beta g; x) = \alpha L(f; x) + \beta L(g; x)$, for all $f, g \in B_\Omega$ and for all constants α, β and it is called positive if $L(f; x) \geq 0$ for all $x \in \Omega$ whenever $f(x) \geq 0$ for all $x \in \Omega$.

Let $\psi(\delta)$ be a non-decreasing continuous function such that $\psi(0) = 0$ and $0 \leq \psi(\delta) \leq 1$ for all $\delta > 0$. The convergence of the sequence of positive linear operators $\{L_n\}_{n=1}^\infty$ on $\Delta \subset \Omega$ will be considered, when the operators satisfy the conditions

$$\lim_{n \to \infty} r(\Delta, \alpha; L_n(1), 1) = 0, \qquad \lim_{n \to \infty} r(\Delta, \alpha; L_n(\psi(|x - t|); x), 0) = 0,$$

which, according to Corollary 62.2, are equivalent to

$$\lim_{n \to \infty} \sup_{x \in \Delta} |1 - L_n(1; x)| = 0, \qquad \lim_{n \to \infty} \sup_{x \in \Delta} |L_n(\psi(|x - t|); x)| = 0.$$

KOROVKIN ([1960], p. 21) proved that if for a sequence of positive linear operators $\{L_n\}_{n=1}^\infty$ the following three conditions

$$L_n(1; x) = 1 + \alpha_n(x), \qquad L_n(t; x) = x + \beta_n(x), \qquad L_n(t^2; x) = x^2 + \gamma_n(x),$$

all hold, where the functions $\alpha_n(x)$, $\beta_n(x)$ and $\gamma_n(x)$ tend uniformly to zero on the closed interval $\Delta = [a, b]$, then for each continuous function f on $[a, b]$ that is also bounded and continuous to the left at (a) and to the right at (b), the uniform convergence of $\{L_n\}_{n=1}^\infty$ to f follows. See also Theorem 27.1.

The natural class of functions in which to study the problem of approximation by positive linear operators with respect to the H-distance is the class of H-continuous functions. Of course, the estimates of approximation will be expressed in terms of the modulus of H-continuity. All estimates in what follows will be, in a certain sense, generalizations of the corresponding results for the uniform approximation, since the H-distance $r(\alpha; f, g)$ tends to the uniform distance $R(f, g) = \|f - g\|$, as $\alpha \to 0$ as well.

A general theorem on the order of approximation of functions by positive linear operators was given by Sendov.

THEOREM 63.1 (SENDOV [1990], p. 54). *Let the positive linear operator L be defined on $B_\Omega \subset A_\Omega$. Suppose $\Delta \subset \Omega$ and $f \in B_\Omega$. Let $M = \sup\{|f(x)|: x \in \Delta\}$, and write*

$$\omega(x, \delta, f; t) = \begin{cases} 0, & \text{if } t \in \Omega \cap [x - \delta, x + \delta], \\ \omega(f; |x - t| - \delta), & \text{if } t \in \Omega \setminus [x - \delta, x + \delta]. \end{cases}$$

Under the assumption $\omega(x, \delta, f; t) \in B_\Omega$, it follows that

$$r(\Delta, \alpha; L(f), f) \leq \tau(\Delta, \alpha, f; 2\delta) + \sup_{x \in \Omega} L(\omega(x, \delta, f); x)$$
$$+ M \sup_{x \in \Omega} |1 - L(1; x)| .$$

64. Approximation of periodic functions by positive integral operators

Let us consider a series of applications of Theorem 63.1 to the estimation of the order of approximation realized by the different operators that are encountered in analysis.

Let K be an even positive kernel that is square integrable on $[-\pi, \pi]$, i.e.:

$$K(t) \geq 0, \quad t \in [-\pi, \pi] ; \tag{64.1a}$$

$$K(t) = K(-t), \quad t \in [-\pi, \pi] ; \tag{64.1b}$$

$$\int_{-\pi}^{\pi} K(t) \, dt = 1 . \tag{64.1c}$$

Let us consider the operator

$$L(f; x) = \int_{-\pi}^{\pi} f(x + t) K(t) \, dt , \tag{64.2}$$

defined for all 2π-periodic functions that are square integrable. The operator (64.2) is linear and positive. It follows from (64.1c) that $L(1; x) \equiv 1$.

The set of real and 2π-periodic functions will be denoted by $A_{2\pi} \subset A_{[-\infty,\infty]}$. From Theorem 63.1 the following theorem arises.

THEOREM 64.1 (SENDOV [1990], p. 56). *If $f \in A_{2\pi}$ and f is square integrable, then for every $\delta > 0$, the estimation*

$$r(\alpha; f, L(f)) \leq \tau(\alpha, f; 2\delta) + 2 \int_\delta^\pi \omega(f; t - \delta) K(t) \, dt$$

holds true.

COROLLARY 64.1. *If $f \in A_{2\pi}$ and f is square integrable, then*

$$r(\alpha, f; L(f)) \leq \tau(\alpha, f; 2\delta) + 2\delta^{-1} \omega(f; \delta) \int_\delta^\pi t K(t) \, dt , \tag{64.3}$$

$$r(\alpha, f; L(f)) \leq \tau(\alpha, f; 2\delta) + 4M \int_\delta^\pi K(t) \, dt , \tag{64.4}$$

where $M = \sup_x |f(x)|$.

Inequality (64.3) is obtained with the help of the inequality

$$\omega(f; t-\delta) \leq \omega(f; \delta)\left(1 + \frac{t-\delta}{\delta}\right) = \frac{t\omega(f; \delta)}{\delta},$$

whereas (64.4) follows from the inequality $\omega(f; t-\delta) \leq 2M$.

Let us consider some applications of Theorem 64.1 and its corollaries for concrete operators.

The Fejer operator of the type (64.2) is defined by

$$\sigma_n(f; x) = \frac{1}{2\pi n} \int_{-\pi}^{\pi} f(x+t) \left(\frac{\sin(nt/2)}{\sin(t/2)}\right)^2 dt,$$

where

$$\frac{1}{2\pi n} \int_{-\pi}^{\pi} \left(\frac{\sin(nt/2)}{\sin(t/2)}\right)^2 dt = 1.$$

It should be pointed out that for every 2π-periodic square-integrable function, $\sigma_n(f; x)$ is a trigonometric polynomial of degree n.

THEOREM 64.2. *If $f \in A_{2\pi}$ and f is square integrable, then for $n \geq 2$, the inequalities*

$$r(\alpha; f, \sigma_n(f)) \leq \tau(\alpha, f; 2n^{-1} \ln n) + 2\pi\omega(f; n^{-1} \ln n)$$

and

$$r(\alpha; f, \sigma_n(f)) \leq \tau(\alpha, f; 2n^{-1/2}) + 2\pi M n^{-1/2}$$

hold, where $M = \sup|f(x)|$.

The classical Vallee-Poussin operator is defined by

$$V_n(f; x) = \frac{(2n)!!}{2\pi(2n-1)!!} \int_{-\pi}^{\pi} f(x+t) \cos^{2n}(t/2) dt,$$

where

$$\frac{(2n)!!}{2\pi(2n-1)!!} \int_{-\pi}^{\pi} \cos^{2n}(t/2) dt = 1.$$

Having in mind the inequality

$$\frac{(\pi/n)^{1/2}}{4} \leq \frac{(2n)!!}{2\pi(2n-1)!!} \leq (\pi/n)^{1/2},$$

it follows that

$$\frac{(2n)!!}{2\pi(2n-1)!!} \int_{\delta}^{\pi} t \cos^{2n}(t/2) dt \leq \frac{\pi^{3/2}}{2n^{1/2}} (1 - (\delta/\pi)^2)^n,$$

and

$$\frac{(2n)!!}{2\pi(2n-1)!!} \int_\delta^\pi \cos^{2n}(t/2)\,dt \leq (\pi n)^{1/2}(1-(\delta/\pi)^2)^n.$$

THEOREM 64.3. *If $f \in A_{2\pi}$ and f is square integrable, then*
$$r(\alpha; f, V_n(f)) \leq \tau(\alpha, f; 2\pi n^{-1/2}) + \pi\omega(f; \pi n^{-1/2}),$$
$$r(\alpha; f, V_n(f)) \leq \tau(\alpha, f; 2\pi(n^{-1}\ln n)^{1/2}) + 8Mn^{-1/2},$$
where $M = \sup_x |f(x)|$.

Let $x_0 < x_1 < x_2 < \cdots < x_n$ be $n+1$ points in the closed interval $\Delta = [a, b]$, and let $\{\varphi_i\}_{i=0}^n$ be $n+1$ non-negative continuous functions, defined on the closed interval Δ. Assume that the equality

$$\sum_{k=0}^n \varphi_k(x) = 1 \qquad (64.5)$$

holds for every $x \in \Delta$. Then

$$\Phi_n(f; x) = \sum_{k=0}^n f(x_k)\varphi_k(x) \qquad (64.6)$$

is a positive linear operator in B_Δ, and according to (64.5) it follows that

$$\Phi_n(1; x) \equiv 1. \qquad (64.7)$$

The operators of the form (64.6) are called summation formulas.

THEOREM 64.4. *If $f \in A_\Delta$, then for every $\delta > 0$, the inequality*

$$r(\Delta, \alpha; f, \Phi_n(f)) \leq \tau(\alpha, f; 2\delta) + \sup_{x \in \Delta} \sum_{k \in \Delta(x,\delta)} \omega(f; |x - x_k| - \delta)\varphi_k(x) \qquad (64.8)$$

holds, where $\Delta(x, \delta)$ is the set of those k for which $x_k \in \Delta\setminus[x - \delta, x + \delta]$.

PROOF. The inequality (64.8) follows directly from Theorem 62.3 and (64.7). □

Let us consider an example of a concrete summation formula. The well-known Bernstein polynomials

$$B_n(f; x) = \sum_{k=0}^n f(k/n)\binom{n}{k}x^k(1-x)^{n-k}$$

are summation formulas on the closed interval $[0, 1]$, since

$$\varphi_{n,k}(x) = \binom{n}{k}x^k(1-x)^{n-k} \geq 0 \quad \text{for } x \in [0, 1]$$

and

$$\sum_{k=0}^{n} \varphi_k(x) = \sum_{k=0}^{n} \binom{n}{k} x^k (1-x)^{n-k} = 1.$$

THEOREM 64.5 (VESELINOV [1972, 1974]). *If $f \in A_{[0,1]}$ then for sufficiently large n ($\ln n > 10$), the following relations are fulfilled:*

$$r([0,1], \alpha; f, B_n(f)) \leq \tau(\alpha, f; 2n^{-1/2}) + \omega(f; n^{-1/2})$$

and

$$r([0,1], \alpha; f, B_n(f)) \leq \tau(\alpha, f; 2(n^{-1} \ln n)^{1/2}) + 2O(Mn^{-3/4}),$$

where $M = \sup\{|f(x)|: x \in [0,1]\}$.

65. Approximation by partial sums of Fourier series

The partial sums of a Fourier series are a very important and classical means for the approximation of periodic functions. If f is a 2π-periodic integrable function, then the nth partial sum for its Fourier series is

$$S_n(f; x) = \frac{a_0}{2} + \sum_{\nu=1}^{n} (a_\nu \cos \nu x + b_\nu \sin \nu x),$$

where

$$a_\nu = \frac{1}{\pi} \int_{-\pi}^{\pi} f(t) \cos \nu t \, dt, \quad \nu = 0, 1, 2, \ldots,$$

$$b_\nu = \frac{1}{\pi} \int_{-\pi}^{\pi} f(t) \sin \nu t \, dt, \quad \nu = 1, 2, \ldots.$$

The integral representation of $S_n(f)$ by the singular Dirichlet integral is well known:

$$S_n(f; x) = \frac{1}{2\pi} \int_{-\pi}^{\pi} f(x+t) \frac{\sin[(2n+1)t/2]}{\sin(t/2)} \, dt. \qquad (65.1)$$

The kernel of the operator of (65.1), assumes negative values and therefore this operator is not a positive one. The continuity of f is necessary for the uniform convergence of $\{S_n(f)\}_{n=1}^{\infty}$ to the initial function f, but it is far from sufficient. A classical sufficient condition for the uniform convergence of the partial sums of the Fourier series is the Dini–Lipschitz condition: the modulus of continuity $\omega(\delta; f)$ satisfies

$$\lim_{\delta \to +0} \omega(\delta; f) \ln \delta = 0.$$

Let us investigate the Hausdorff convergence of the partial sums of the Fourier series, not only for continuous functions, but also for certain discontinuous functions as well. As a point of departure, let us look at a very simple 2π-periodic function, namely $\sigma(x) = \operatorname{sgn} \sin x$. The partial sums of its Fourier series are given by

$$S_{2n}(\sigma; x) = S_{2n-1}(\sigma; x) = \frac{4}{\pi} \sum_{\nu=0}^{n} \frac{\sin(2\nu + 1)x}{2\nu + 1}$$

$$= \frac{2}{\pi} \int_0^x \frac{\sin(2nt)}{\sin t} \, dt = \frac{1}{\pi n} \int_0^{2nx} \frac{\sin t}{\sin(t/2n)} \, dt. \qquad (65.2)$$

The last expression can be represented as a sum

$$S_{2n}(\sigma; x) = \frac{1}{n\pi} \left(\int_0^{\pi} + \int_{\pi}^{2\pi} + \cdots + \int_{(k-1)\pi}^{k\pi} + \int_{k\pi}^{2nx} \right) \frac{\sin t}{\sin(t/2n)} \, dt,$$

for $0 < x < \pi/2$, where $k = [2nx/\pi]$. Setting

$$v_\nu = \left| \int_{\nu\pi}^{(\nu+1)\pi} \frac{\sin t}{\sin(t/2n)} \, dt \right|,$$

it is obvious that for $\nu = 0, 1, 2, \ldots, n-1$,

$$v_\nu > 0, \quad v_{\nu+1} < v_\nu, \quad \nu = 0, 1, 2, \ldots, n-2.$$

Finally,

$$S_{2n}(\sigma; x) = S_{2n-1}(\sigma; x) = v_0 - v_1 + \cdots + (-1)^{k-1} v_{k-1} + (-1)^k v_k',$$

where $(-1)^k v_k'$ denotes the remaining summand with a sign of $(-1)^k$ and an absolute value of less than v_k. It follows from (65.2) that

$$S'_{2n}(\sigma; x) = \frac{2}{\pi} \frac{\sin(2nx)}{\sin x},$$

and, consequently, the function $S_{2n}(\sigma)$ attains its extreme values at the points $x_i = \pi i/2n$, $i = \pm 1, \pm 2, \ldots$.

Let us turn to the study of the Hausdorff convergence of $S_{2n}(\sigma; x)$ when n tends to infinity. The equality (65.2) shows that for every x it follows that $\lim_{n \to \infty} S_{2n}(\sigma; x) = \sigma(x)$, and this convergence is uniform on every segment $[a, b]$ that does not contain the points $k\pi$, $k = \pm 1, \pm 2, \ldots$. Since the uniform convergence is stronger than the Hausdorff convergence, it is necessary to examine the character of the convergence only in the neighborhoods of the discontinuities. Since $\sigma(x) = \operatorname{sgn} \sin x$ is a 2π-periodic odd function as is $S_{2n}(\sigma; x)$, it is sufficient to examine the nature of the graph of $S_{2n}(\sigma; x)$ to the right in a neighborhood of the point $x = 0$.

The first extremum of $S_{2n}(\sigma; x)$ on the right of the point $x = 0$ is attained for $x = \pi/2n$ and its value is

$$M_1(n) = S_{2n}(\sigma; \pi/2n) = \frac{1}{n\pi} \int_0^{\pi} \frac{\sin t}{\sin(t/2n)} \, dt.$$

It is easy to see that

$$\mu_1 = \lim_{n\to\infty} M_1(n) = \frac{2}{\pi} \int_0^\pi \frac{1}{t} \sin t \, dt = 1.179\ldots. \qquad (65.3)$$

On the other hand, $\sigma(+0) = 1 < 1.179\ldots$, and consequently $S_{2n}(\sigma)$ cannot tend to the completed graph of σ with respect to the Hausdorff distance. This is the so-called Gibbs effect: there is a pointwise convergence of the partial sums of the Fourier series, but the Hausdorff convergence to the completed graph of the initial function does not take place. This effect was noticed at the end of the last century and has been thoroughly studied.

Explaining the Gibbs effect in his famous text on calculus, FICHTENGHOLZ ([1960], Volume III, p. 490), states the following.

> It can be said that the limiting geometric image of the curves $y = S_{2n-1}(\sigma; x)$ as $n \to \infty$ is not the polygonal line in Fig. 65.1 (as it is natural to expect) but the polygonal line in Fig. 65.2 with correspondingly elongated (approximately 18%) upright segments.

The polygonal line in Fig. 65.1 is the completed graph of the function σ, and the polygonal line in Fig. 65.2 is the point set to which $\{S_{2n}(\sigma)\}_{n=1}^\infty$ converges with respect to the Hausdorff distance. This motivates us to introduce the following notation: let us denote by $D_{2\pi}$ the set of all 2π-periodic functions f without discontinuities of the second kind, such that at each point x the inequality

$$[f(x) - f(x-0)][f(x) - f(x+0)] \leq 0$$

holds.

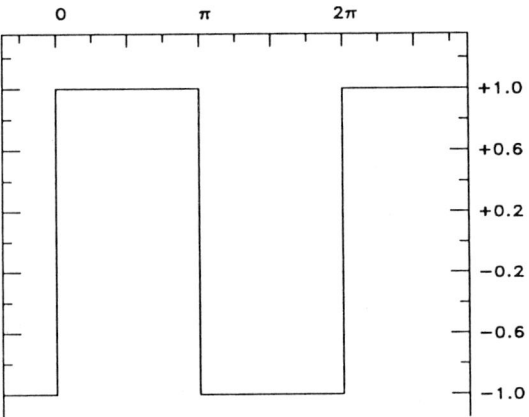

FIG. 65.1. The completed graph of the function σ.

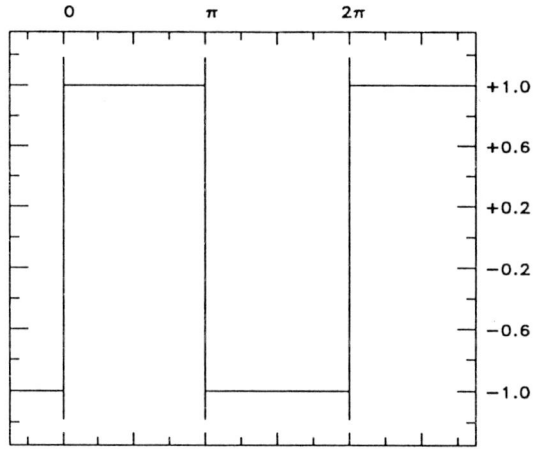

Fig. 65.2. The Gibbs completed graph of the function σ.

Obviously the set $D_{2\pi}$ consists of all the H-continuous 2π-periodic functions without discontinuities of the second kind. Let us denote by $H(f; x) = |f(x-0) - f(x+0)|$ the magnitude of the discontinuity of f at the point x. If $f \in D_{2\pi}$ then $H(f; x)$ is non-zero only at a countable set of values of x in $[0, 2\pi)$.

Let $f \in D_{2\pi}$. The Gibbs completed graph of f consists of the segment functions $\Phi(f) \in \mathbb{F}_{2\pi}$ defined by

$$\Phi(f; x) = [I(f; x) - \gamma H(f; x), S(f; x) + \gamma H(f; x)],$$

where $\gamma = \mu_1 - 1 = 0.179\ldots$, $I(f)$ and $S(f)$ are, respectively, the upper and lower Baire functions for the function f, and μ_1 is determined from (65.3).

Of course, Fig. 65.2 shows the Gibbs completed graph $\Phi(\sigma)$ of the function σ. From the above discussion with regards to the Hausdorff convergence of $\{S_{2n}(\sigma)\}_{n=1}^{\infty}$ the following theorem follows.

THEOREM 65.1. *Let $\sigma(x) = \operatorname{sgn} \sin x$. The relation*

$$\lim_{n \to \infty} r(\alpha; S_{2n}(\sigma), \Phi(\sigma)) = 0$$

holds; i.e. the partial sums of the Fourier series of the function σ converge to the Gibbs completed graph of the function σ with respect to the Hausdorff distance.

From the particular example analyzed above, it is natural to expect in a more general setting Hausdorff convergence of partial sums to the Gibbs completed graph and not to the completed graph of the initial function. It should be noted that the completed graph and the Gibbs completed graph of continuous functions coincide with the graph of the function itself.

Let f be an arbitrary 2π-periodic function. The modulus of non-monotonicity of f is

$$\mu(f;\delta) = \tfrac{1}{2} \sup_x \{|f(x_1) - f(x)| + |f(x_2) - f(x)| - |f(x_1) - f(x_2)|:$$
$$x_2 - x_1 \leq \delta\},$$

where $x_1 < x < x_2$. It is at once seen that

$$\mu(f;\delta) \leq \omega(f;\delta)$$

for every function f and $\delta > 0$. A function f, for which

$$\lim_{\delta \to +0} \mu(f;\delta) = 0$$

is called locally monotone.

THEOREM 65.2. *If for a function $f \in D_{2\pi}$ the condition $\lim_{\delta \to +0} \mu(f;\delta) \ln \delta = 0$ holds, then $\lim_{n \to \infty} r(\alpha; S_n(f), \Phi(f)) = 0$.*

66. The best Hausdorff approximation

Considering the problem for the best approximation of segment functions with regard to the Hausdorff distance let us confine ourselves to the consideration of functions defined on a finite interval.

Let $f \in \mathbb{A}_\Delta$ where Δ is a finite closed interval, and let W be a set of functions in $\mathbb{A}_\Delta$.

The best approximation of a function f by the elements of a set W with respect to the Hausdorff distance with parameter $\alpha > 0$ on the closed interval Δ is the following number:

$$E(W, \Delta, \alpha; f) = \inf_{\varphi \in W} r(\Delta, \alpha; f, \varphi).$$

Abbreviate this by $E(W, \Delta; f)$ when $\alpha = 1$, and if the closed interval Δ is understood, let us write $E(W, \alpha; f)$ or $E(W; f)$, respectively. For the class W, the classical means of approximation will be considered:

H_n, the set of algebraic polynomials of degree at most n;

T_n, the set of trigonometric polynomials of order at most n;

R_n, the set of rational functions that are quotients of two polynomials from H_n;

$S_{k,n}$, the set of spline functions of order (k, n).

Let us recall that f is a spline function of order (k, n) if $f \in C_\Delta^{k-1}$ (the function has a continuous derivative of $(k-1)$st order on the interval $\Delta = [a, b]$), and there exist $n+1$ points $a = x_0 < x_1 < \cdots < x_n = b$ such that for every interval $[x_{i-1}, x_i]$, $i = 1, 2, 3, \ldots, n$, the function f coincides with an algebraic polynomial of degree at most k.

If $\varphi^* \in W$ and $E(W, \Delta, \alpha; f) = r(\Delta, \alpha; f, \varphi^*)$, then φ^* is called the element of the best Hausdorff approximation of f from W.

The existence of an algebraic polynomial of the best Hausdorff approximation for every closed and bounded point set in the plane is established, as expected, using the compactness of the set of uniformly bounded algebraic polynomials from H_n (SENDOV [1962]).

The existence of a trigonometric polynomial of best approximation is established similarly. It turns out that the polynomial of the best Hausdorff approximation is not always unique.

Initially, let us give some examples for which it is possible to find the polynomial of the best Hausdorff approximation, or to compute the best Hausdorff approximation; i.e. the minimal possible Hausdorff distance.

Denote by $\delta(x)$ the delta function

$$\delta(x) = \begin{cases} [0,1], & \text{if } x=0, \\ 0, & \text{if } x \neq 0; \end{cases}$$

let us consider the problem of finding an algebraic polynomial of degree not higher than n, which approximates the function $M\delta(x)$ in the best way relative to the Hausdorff distance on $[-1, 1]$, where M is a positive constant. The ε-neighborhood of the function $M\delta(x)$ is shown in Fig. 66.1.

If for a certain polynomial $P \in H_n$ the inequality $r([-1,1], \alpha; M\delta, P) \leq \varepsilon$ holds, then the graph of the polynomial P on $[-1, 1]$ must be within the polygonal path $Aaa_2b_2bBB_1A_1$ as shown in the Fig. 66.1 and at least one point of the graph of P must belong to the rectangle $a_1a_2b_2b_1$. The minimal value of ε for which there exists a polynomial $P \in H_n$ with the above properties will be the best approximation of $M\delta$ by algebraic polynomials from H_n in the Hausdorff distance. Our task then reduces to finding the polynomial $P \in H_n$ satisfying these conditions for a minimal value of ε:

(a) $\max_{|x| \leq \alpha\varepsilon} P(x) \geq M - \varepsilon$;

(b) $\max_{\alpha\varepsilon \leq |x| \leq 1} |P(x)| \leq \varepsilon$.

An analogous problem arises in finding the algebraic polynomial of least deviation from zero on two closed intervals (AHIEZER [1965], p. 320, Problem 36).

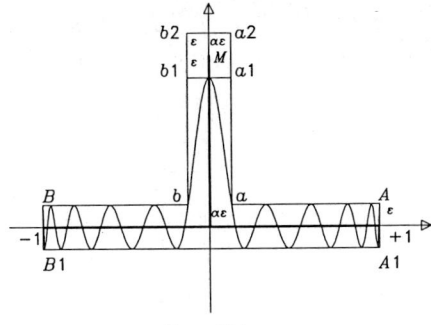

FIG. 66.1.

Here it is natural to use Chebyshev polynomials of degree $k = [n/2]$:

$$C_k(x) = \cos(k \cos^{-1} x) = \tfrac{1}{2}[(x + \sqrt{x^2 - 1})^k + (x - \sqrt{x^2 - 1})^k] \tag{66.1}$$

along with the change of variable

$$x = \frac{(2t^2 - 1 - \alpha^2 \varepsilon^2)}{(1 - \alpha^2 \varepsilon^2)}. \tag{66.2}$$

The transformation (66.2) maps both of the intervals $[-1, -\alpha\varepsilon]$ and $[\alpha\varepsilon, 1]$ into $[-1, 1]$. Consequently, the polynomial

$$P(x) = (-1)^k \varepsilon C_k\left(\frac{2x^2 - 1 - \alpha^2 \varepsilon^2}{1 - \alpha^2 \varepsilon^2}\right)$$

satisfies condition (b) above, since $|C_k(x)| \leq 1$ on the interval $[-1, 1]$. Moreover, $P \in H_n$ because $k = [n/2]$.

In order to satisfy the condition (a) for a minimal value of ε, it is necessary to take

$$P(0) = (-1)^k \varepsilon C_k\left(\frac{-1 - \alpha^2 \varepsilon^2}{1 - \alpha^2 \varepsilon^2}\right) = M - \varepsilon.$$

The last equality, in view of (66.1), can be written in the following form:

$$\left(\frac{1 + \alpha\varepsilon}{1 - \alpha\varepsilon}\right)^k + \left(\frac{1 - \alpha\varepsilon}{1 + \alpha\varepsilon}\right)^k + 2 = \frac{2M}{\varepsilon}. \tag{66.3}$$

It is not difficult to check that for given α, M and k, Equation (66.3) has only one positive root, since the left-hand side of (66.3) grows monotonically without bound as a function of ε, and the right-hand side decreases monotonically for $\varepsilon > 0$. Denote by ε_k the only positive root of (66.3), and let

$$P^*(x) = (-1)^k \varepsilon_k C_k\left(\frac{2x^2 - 1 - \alpha^2 \varepsilon_k^2}{1 - \alpha^2 \varepsilon_k^2}\right).$$

It is possible to show that P^* is the unique polynomial of best approximation of $M\delta$ among the polynomials in H_n, and that

$$E(H_n, [-1, 1], \alpha; M\delta) = \varepsilon_k.$$

In order to compute the best approximation ε_k in this case, it is necessary to solve the algebraic equation (66.3). Setting $\lambda = \alpha\varepsilon_k$ in (66.3), then

$$\left(\frac{1 + \lambda}{1 - \lambda}\right)^k + \left(\frac{1 - \lambda}{1 + \lambda}\right)^k + 2 = \frac{2\alpha M}{\lambda}. \tag{66.4}$$

It is interesting to study the asymptotic behavior of ε_k when k tends to infinity. From (66.4) it follows that when k tends to infinity, the only positive root λ of (66.4) must tend to zero, and hence ε_k must also tend to zero.

The following expansion is valid:

$$\left(\frac{1 + x}{1 - x}\right)^k - e^{2kx} = 4kx^3 + a_4 x^4 + a_5 x^5 + \cdots,$$

and consequently
$$\left(\frac{1+x}{1-x}\right)^k = e^{2kx} + O(kx^3) \tag{66.5}$$
for small x. By (66.4) and (66.5)
$$e^{2k\lambda} + e^{-2k\lambda} + 2 + O(k\lambda^3) = 2\alpha M/\lambda ;$$
that is
$$e^{n\lambda} + e^{-n\lambda} + 2 + O(n\lambda^3) = 2\alpha M/\lambda . \tag{66.6}$$
From (66.6) it follows that
$$\lambda = \frac{\ln n}{n} + \frac{\varphi(n)}{n} , \tag{66.7}$$
where $\varphi(n)$ is to be estimated. Insertion of λ into (66.6) gives
$$n\, e^{\varphi(n)} + n^{-1} e^{-\varphi(n)} + 2 + O(n^{-2} \ln n^3) = \frac{2\alpha M n}{\ln n + \varphi(n)} ,$$
and hence the function $\varphi(n)$ is bounded.

In this way, since (66.7), $\lambda = n^{-1} \ln n + O(n^{-1})$, or
$$\varepsilon_k = E(H_n, [-1, 1], \alpha; M\delta) = \alpha^{-1} n^{-1} \ln n + O(n^{-1}) .$$

Note that the main term does not depend on M.

Let us consider a related example in which it is possible to find the polynomial of best approximation and to estimate the asymptotic behavior of the best approximation. Let $\chi(x) = \delta(x-1)$; i.e.
$$\chi(x) = \begin{cases} 0, & \text{if } -1 \leq x < 1, \\ [0, 1], & \text{if } x = 1, \end{cases}$$
and let us consider the problem of finding the algebraic polynomial of degree no higher than n, which approximates the function $\chi(x)$ in the best way with respect to the Hausdorff distance, on the interval $[-1, 1]$. The ε-neighborhood of the function $\chi(x)$ with respect to the Hausdorff distance is shown in Fig. 66.2.

Proceeding in a way analogous to the delta function, let us consider the polynomial
$$P(x) = \varepsilon C_n\left(\frac{2x + \alpha\varepsilon}{2x - \alpha\varepsilon}\right), \tag{66.8}$$
where C_n is the Chebyshev polynomial. Obviously the polynomial of (66.8) satisfies the condition $|P(x)| \leq \varepsilon$ for $x \in [-1, 1 - \alpha\varepsilon]$. To obtain $r([-1, 1], \alpha; \chi, P) = \varepsilon$, it is necessary that
$$P(1) = \varepsilon C_n\left(\frac{2 + \alpha\varepsilon}{2 - \alpha\varepsilon}\right) = 1 - \varepsilon . \tag{66.9}$$

It is not difficult to see, using arguments similar to those of the previous

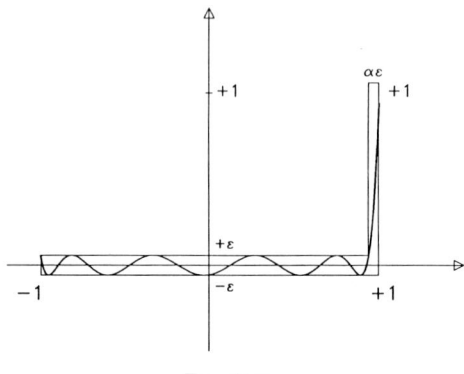

Fig. 66.2.

example, that if ε is determined from (66.9), then the polynomial (66.8) is the unique polynomial of the best Hausdorff approximation of χ among the polynomials in H_n.

Using (66.1), Equation (66.9) can be represented as follows:

$$\left(\frac{\sqrt{2}+\sqrt{\alpha\varepsilon}}{\sqrt{2}-\sqrt{\alpha\varepsilon}}\right)^n + \left(\frac{\sqrt{2}-\sqrt{\alpha\varepsilon}}{\sqrt{2}+\sqrt{\alpha\varepsilon}}\right)^n + 2 = 2\varepsilon^{-1},$$

which becomes, on setting $\alpha\varepsilon = 2\lambda^2$,

$$\left(\frac{1+\lambda}{1-\lambda}\right)^n + \left(\frac{1+\lambda}{1-\lambda}\right)^n + 2 = \frac{\alpha_-}{\lambda_2}. \qquad (66.10)$$

From (66.10), it is obvious that the only positive root λ tends to zero when n tends to infinity. By (66.10),

$$\lambda = n^{-1} \ln n + O(n^{-1}),$$

and consequently

$$\varepsilon = E(H_n, [-1, 1], \alpha; \chi) = 2\alpha^{-1}\left(\frac{\ln n}{n}\right)^2 + O\left(\frac{\ln n}{n^2}\right).$$

67. Universal estimates

Denote by $\mathbb{F}_{2\pi}$ the set of 2π-periodic segment functions in $\mathbb{F}_{(-\infty,\infty)}$.

THEOREM 67.1. *There exist absolute constants c_1 and c_2 such that for every $f \in \mathbb{F}_{2\pi}$, the inequality*

$$E(T_n, \alpha; f) \leq c_1 \frac{\ln n}{\alpha n} + c_2 \frac{M}{n}$$

holds, where $M = \max_x \{|y|: y \in f(x)\}$.

Let $f \in \mathbb{F}_\Delta$, where $\Delta = [a, b]$ and a and b are non-negative real numbers. By a linear change of variable it is possible to think of the domain as $[0, 2\pi]$. Let us extend f to an even periodic function on the entire real axis. Then the following theorem results from Theorem 67.1.

THEOREM 67.2. *There exist absolute constants c_3 and c_4 such that the inequality*

$$E(H_n, \Delta, \alpha; f) \leq \frac{b-a}{\alpha}\left(c_3 \frac{\ln n}{n} + c_4 \frac{M}{n}\right)$$

holds for every $f \in \mathbb{F}_\Delta$, $\Delta = [a, b]$, where $M = \max\{|y|: y \in f(x), x \in \Delta\}$.

The set of all functions $f \in \mathbb{F}_\Delta$ (resp., $f \in \mathbb{F}_{2\pi}$) such that

$$\max\{|y|: y \in f(x), x \in \Delta\} \leq M \quad (\text{resp.}, \max_x \{|y|: y \in f(x)\} \leq M)$$

will be denoted by $\mathbb{F}_\Delta^M$ (resp., $\mathbb{F}_{2\pi}^M$). The determination of the exact asymptotic behavior of the best Hausdorff approximation on such classes will be our goal in this section.

THEOREM 67.3 (SENDOV and POPOV [1972]). *The following equalities*

$$\lim_{n \to \infty} \frac{\alpha n}{\ln n} E(H_n, \Delta, \alpha; \mathbb{F}_\Delta^M) = \frac{b-a}{2},$$

$$\lim_{n \to \infty} \frac{\alpha n}{\ln n} E(T_n, \Delta, \alpha; \mathbb{F}_{2\pi}^M) = 1,$$

hold, where

$$E(H_n, \Delta, \alpha; \mathbb{F}_\Delta^M) = \sup\{E(H_n, \Delta, \alpha; f): f \in \mathbb{F}_\Delta^M\},$$

$$E(T_n, \Delta, \alpha; \mathbb{F}_{2\pi}^M) = \sup\{E(T_n, \Delta, \alpha; f): f \in \mathbb{F}_{2\pi}^M\}.$$

68. Numerical methods for calculating the polynomial of best Hausdorff approximation

A numerical algorithm of ANDREEV [1976a,b] will be presented for the approximate computation of the coefficients of the polynomial of the best one-sided Hausdorff approximation. This algorithm is a modification of one of the methods of REMEZ [1957].

The algorithm proceeds as follows.

Step 1. Construct a polynomial $P_{n,0} \in H_n$ such that there exist $n+2$ points $\{x_{k,0}\}_0^{n+1}$, for which $\text{sgn}[P_{n,0}(x_{k,0}) - f(x_{k,0})] = (-1)^k \varepsilon$, where $\varepsilon = \pm 1$, $k = 0, 1, 2, \ldots, n+1$. Set the index i equal to 0, and go to Step 2.

Step 2. Construct the function

$$\varphi_i(x) = \text{sgn}[f(x) - P_{n,i}(x)]\left(\min_{(\xi, \eta) \in f} \max\left\{\frac{1}{\alpha}|x - \xi|, |P_{n,i}(x) - \eta|\right\}\right).$$

Step 3. Find $n + 2$ points $\{z_{k,i}\}_{k=0}^{n+1}$ such that

$$\text{sgn } \varphi_i(z_{k,i}) = (-1)^k \varepsilon, \quad \text{where } \varepsilon = \pm 1, \ k = 0, 1, 2, \ldots, n+1.$$

Step 4. If $\max\{||\varphi_i(z_{\nu,i})| - |\varphi_i(z_{\mu,i})||: \nu, \mu = 0, 1, \ldots, n+1\} \leq \delta$, where $\delta > 0$ is a preassigned exactness, the polynomial $P_{n,i}$ is acceptable and the algorithm terminates. Otherwise go to Step 5.

Step 5. For the set of points $(z_{k,i}, \varphi_i(z_{k,i}))$, $k = 0, 1, 2, \ldots, n+1$, construct the polynomial $Q_{n,i} \in H_n$ of the best uniform approximation.

Step 6. Form the polynomial $P_{n,i+1}(x) = P_{n,i}(x) + Q_{n,i}(x)$; then set i equal to $i+1$, and return to Step 2.

ANDREEV [1976b] proved that the algorithm described above converges for functions f that are Lipschitz continuous. The next examples present this algorithm in action.

EXAMPLE 1. For the function

$$f_1(x) = \begin{cases} -1, & \text{if } -1 \leq x \leq -\tfrac{1}{3}, \\ 1, & \text{if } -\tfrac{1}{3} < x \leq 1, \end{cases}$$

the following inequalities are fulfilled:

$$0.2257 \leq e(H_5, [-1, 1], 1; f_1) = E(H_5, [-1, 1], 1; f_1) \leq 0.2266,$$

$$0.1413 \leq e(H_{10}, [-1, 1], 1; f_1) = E(H_{10}, [-1, 1], 1; f_1) \leq 0.1421,$$

and

$$P_5(f_1; x) = 0.22811x^5 + 3.18041x^4 - 1.07950x^3 - 3.96861x^2$$
$$+ 1.85136x + 1.01437,$$

$$P_{10}(f_1; x) = 1.17755x^{10} - 51.87041x^9 + 2.85984x^8 + 123.85465x^7$$
$$- 14.21173x^6 - 100.59484x^5 + 16.45178x^4$$
$$+ 30.42548x^3 - 7.39353x^2 - 0.95663x + 1.11606,$$

where $P_5(f_1)$ and $P_{10}(f_1)$ are polynomials of the best approximation of the fifth and tenth degree, respectively, with respect to the Hausdorff distance with parameter $\alpha = 1$. The graphs of f_1 along with $P_5(f_1)$ and $P_{10}(f_1)$ appear in Fig. 68.1.

EXAMPLE 2. For the function

$$f_2(x) = \begin{cases} -1, & \text{if } -1 \leq x \leq -\tfrac{1}{3}, \\ 0, & \text{if } -\tfrac{1}{3} < x < \tfrac{1}{3}, \\ 1, & \text{if } \tfrac{1}{3} \leq x \leq 1, \end{cases}$$

the estimates are

$$\varepsilon_1 = \varepsilon_2 = (\sqrt{73} - 7)/6 = 0.25733\ldots, \quad 0.1863 \leq \varepsilon_5 = \varepsilon_6 \leq 0.1871,$$

$$0.1481 \leq \varepsilon_7 = \varepsilon_8 \leq 0.1488, \quad 0.0985 \leq \varepsilon_{11} = \varepsilon_{12} \leq 0.0995.$$

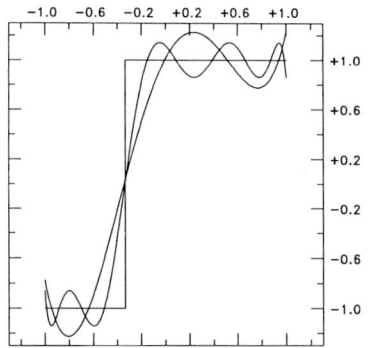 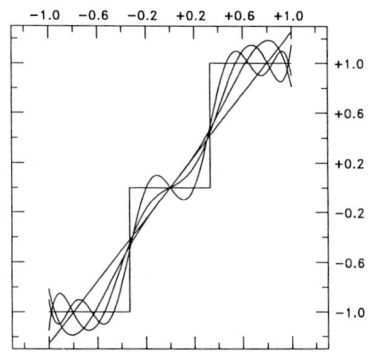

Fig. 68.1. Graphs of the functions f_1, $P_5(f_1)$ and $P_{10}(f_1)$.

Fig. 68.2. Graphs of the functions f_2 and $P_k(f_2)$ for $k = 1, 5, 7, 11$.

The graph of the function f_2 along with the graphs of its polynomials of the best Hausdorff approximation of degrees $1, 5, 7$ and 11 are shown in Fig. 68.2.

REMARK 68.1. ANDREEV [1980] considered the problem of the stability of the best approximations with respect to the Hausdorff distance. Numerical methods for finding the polynomials of the best uniform approximation of particular functions were considered by MARKOV and SENDOV [1968], KJURKCHIEV and SENDOV [1976], and KJURKCHIEV and MARKOV [1974]. MARINOV and ANDREEV [1987] considered one modification of the second algorithm of Remez producing rational functions of the best Hausdorff approximation in some important cases. The approximation by rational functions of the discontinuity functions in the Hausdorff metric is much better than the approximation by polynomials. For example, see Tables 68.1 and 68.2, where the best Hausdorff approximations of the functions

$$g_1(x) = \operatorname{sgn} x, \quad g_2(x) = \begin{cases} 0, & -1 \leq x < -0.5, \\ 1, & -0.5 \leq x < 0, \\ 1 - x, & 0 \leq x < 0.5, \\ 0.5, & 0.5 \leq x \leq 1, \end{cases}$$

are given for the interval $[-1, 1]$. Here, $\varepsilon_{m,k}(g)$ denotes (see Section 66)

$$\varepsilon_{m,k}(g) = E(R_{m,k}, [-1, 1], 1; g),$$

where

$$R_{m,k} = \left\{ \varphi \colon \varphi(x) = \sum_{i=0}^{m} a_i x^i \Big/ \sum_{i=0}^{k} b_i x^i \right\}.$$

In Fig. 68.3 the graphs of the function g_1 and its rational functions of the best Hausdorff approximation in $R_{10,0}$ and $R_{5,5}$ are given. In Fig. 68.4 similarly for g_2 the elements in $R_{14,0}$ and in $R_{7,6}$ are given.

TABLE 68.1.

m	k	$\varepsilon_{m,k}(g_1)$	m	k	$\varepsilon_{m,k}(g_1)$
2	0	0.414...	1	1	0.414...
2	0	0.271...	2	2	0.171...
6	0	0.208...	3	3	0.085...
8	0	0.172...	4	4	0.0470...
10	0	0.148...	5	5	0.0278...
12	0	0.130...	6	6	0.0175...
14	0	0.117...	7	7	0.0112...
16	0	0.106...	8	8	0.0077...
18	0	0.098...	9	9	0.0051...
20	0	0.091...	10	10	0.0034...
22	0	0.085...	11	11	0.0025...
24	0	0.080...	12	12	0.0018...
26	0	0.076...	13	13	0.0013...
28	0	0.072...	14	14	0.00098...
30	0	0.068...	15	15	0.00073...
32	0	0.065...	16	16	0.00055...
34	0	0.062...	17	17	0.00033...
36	0	0.060...	18	18	0.00018...
38	0	0.057...	19	19	0.00012...
48	0	0.048...			
98	0	0.028...			
148	0	0.020...			
198	0	0.016...			

TABLE 68.2.

m	k	$\varepsilon_{m,k}(g_2)$	m	k	$\varepsilon_{m,k}(g_2)$
13	0	0.0842...	6	7	0.0170...
14	0	0.0805...	7	6	0.0145...
70	0	0.0270...	7	7	0.0137...

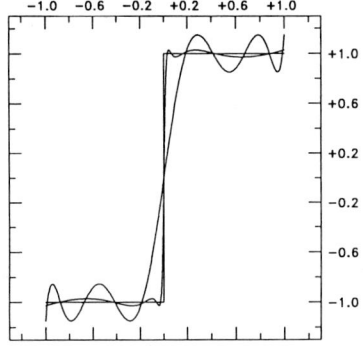

FIG. 68.3. Graphs of the functions g_1, $R_{10,0}(g_1)$ and $R_{5,5}(g_1)$.

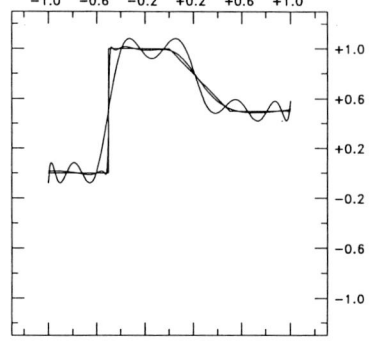

FIG. 68.4. Graphs of the functions g_2, $R_{14,0}(g_2)$ and $R_{7,6}(g_2)$.

69. Multidimensional Hausdorff approximation

SENDOV and POPOV [1970] considered the Hausdorff approximation by polynomials in the multidimensional case.

Let us denote the Hausdorff distance between two closed and bounded sets A and B in m-dimensional Euclidean space E^m by

$$r(A, B) = \max\{\max_{a \in A} \min_{b \in B} \rho(a, b), \max_{a \in B} \min_{b \in A} \rho(a, b)\},$$

where $\rho(a, b) = \max\{|a_1 - b_1|, |a_2 - b_2|, \ldots, |a_m - b_m|\}$, $a = (a_1, a_2, \ldots, a_m)$ and $b = (b_1, b_2, \ldots, b_m)$.

Let K be a compact set in E^m and F_K denotes the set of all bounded and closed point sets F in E^{m+1} for which:

(1) if $x = (x_1, x_2, \ldots, x_m, x_{m+1}) \in F$ then $x^* = (x_1, x_2, \ldots, x_m) \in K$ and for each point $x^* = (x_1, x_2, \ldots, x_m) \in K$ there exists a point $x = (x_1, x_2, \ldots, x_m, x_{m+1}) \in F$;

(2) F is a convex set according to the axis x_{m+1}; i.e. the inclusions $x' = (x_1', x_2', \ldots, x_{m+1}') \in F$ and $x'' = (x_1'', x_2'', \ldots, x_{m+1}'') \in F$ imply the inclusion $\alpha x' + (1 - \alpha) \in F$ for every $\alpha \in [0, 1]$.

For every function f, defined on K, denote by $\bar{f}$ the completed graph of f, as

$$\bar{f} = \bigcap_{G \in F_K, \tilde{f} \in G} G,$$

where $\tilde{f}$ is the graph of the function f; i.e. the point

$$(x_1, x_2, \ldots, x_m, f(x)) \in E^{m+1},$$

where $x = (x_1, x_2, \ldots, x_m)$.

Evidently, $\bar{f} \in F_K$ and if f is a continuous function then $\bar{f} = \tilde{f}$.

The Hausdorff distance between two functions f and g defined on K is the Hausdorff distance between their completed graphs

$$r(f, g) = r(\bar{f}, \bar{g}).$$

Let

$$H_n^m = \left\{ f \colon f(x_1, x_2, \ldots, x_m) = \sum_{0 \le i_s \le n} a_{i_1 i_2 \cdots i_m} x_1^{i_1} x_2^{i_2} \cdots x_m^{i_m} \right\},$$

and $F_{\Delta_m}^M$ is the set of all elements $F \in F_{\Delta_m}$, such that if $(x_1, x_2, \ldots, x_{m+1}) \in F$, then $|x_{m+1}| < M$, $M > 0$, where Δ_m is the unit cube in E^m.

The best Hausdorff approximation of the element $F \in F_{\Delta_m}^M$ by means of algebraic polynomials of nth degree is the number

$$E_{n,r}(F) = \inf_{p \in H_n^m} r(F, p). \tag{69.1}$$

THEOREM 69.1. *If* $F \in F_{\Delta_m}^M$, *then*

$$E_{n,r}(F) = 6m \frac{\ln n}{n} + O(n^{-1}).$$

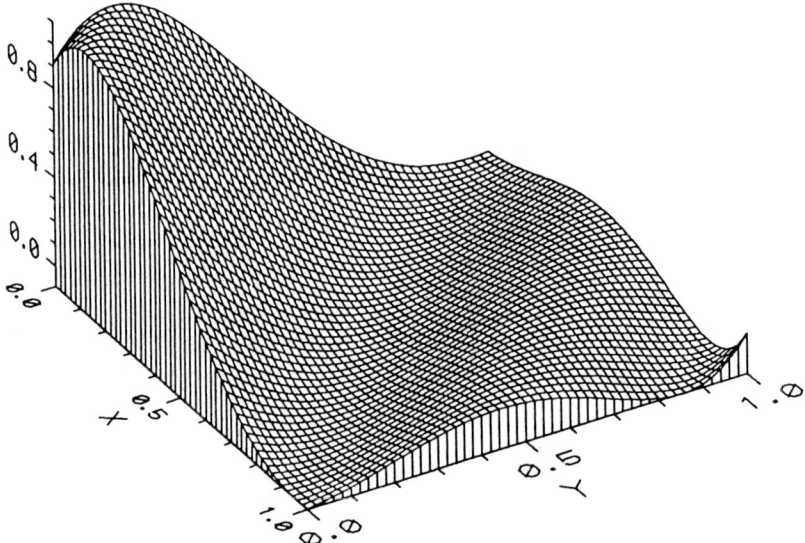

Fig. 69.1. Graph of the function $p \in R^2_{6,0}$.

Similarly to (69.1) the best Hausdorff approximation of the element $F \in F^M_{\Delta_m}$ by rational functions from $R^m_{n,s}$ can be defined as

$$R_{n,r}(F) = \inf_{p \in R^m_{n,s}} r(F, p),$$

where $R^m_{n,s} = \{\varphi: \varphi = f/g, f \in H^m_n, g \in H^m_s\}$.

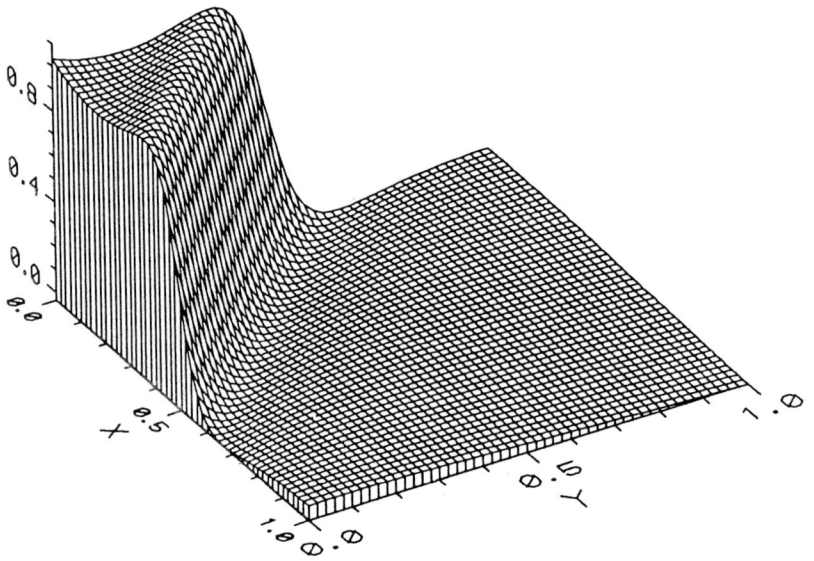

Fig. 69.2. Graph of the function $q \in R^2_{3,3}$.

As a numerical example let us consider the function
$$f(x, y) = \begin{cases} 1, & (x, y) \in D, \\ 0, & (x, y) \in \Omega \setminus D, \end{cases}$$
where $\Omega = \{(x, y): 0 \leq x \leq 1, 0 \leq y \leq 1\}$, $D = \{(x, y): (x, y) \in \Omega, x + y \leq \frac{1}{2}\}$.

The graphs of the functions $p \in R_{6,0}^2$ and $q \in R_{3,3}^2$ are given in Figs. 69.1 and 69.2. For them $r(f, p) \leq 0.090\ldots$ and $r(f, q) \leq 0.0120\ldots$.

References

AHIEZER, N. (1965), *Lectures on Approximation Theory* (Nauka, Moscow) in Russian.
AITKEN, A. (1932), On interpolation by iteration of proportional parts, without the use of differences, *Proc. Edinburgh Math. Soc.* **3** (2), 56–76.
ALPER, S. (1956), On the convergence of Lagrange interpolation polynomials in complex domain, *Uspekhi Mat. Nauk* **11** (5), 44–50 (in Russian).
ANDREEV, A. (1976a), Hausdorff approximations and spline interpolation, Ph.D. Thesis, Sofia University (in Bulgarian).
ANDREEV, A. (1976b), A numerical method for finding the polynomial of best Hausdorff approximation, *C.R. Acad. Bulgare Sci.* **29**, 163–166 (in Russian).
ANDREEV, A. (1980), On stability of the best approximation with respect to Hausdorff distance, *Serdica* **6**, 76–83 (in Russian).
ATKINSON, K. and A. SHARMA (1969), A partial characterization of poised Hermite–Birkhoff interpolation problems, *SIAM J. Numer. Anal.* **6**, 230–235.
BACHVALOV, N. (1959), On approximate computation of multiple integrals, *Vesnik of the Moscow University*, No. 4, 3–18 (in Russian).
BACHVALOV, N. (1961), Average estimation of the remainder term of quadrature formulas, *USSR Comput. Math. and Math. Phys.* **1** (1), 64–77 (in Russian).
BACHVALOV, N. (1967), On the optimal rate for integration of analytic functions, *USSR Comput. Math. and Math. Phys.* **7** (5), 1011–1020 (in Russian).
BACHVALOV, N. (1970), About optimization of numerical methods, *Actes of Congres Inter-math*, T.3, 289–295.
BACHVALOV, N. (1971), On the optimality of linear methods for approximation of operators on the convex sets of functions, *USSR Comput. Math. and Math. Phys.* **11** (4), 1014–1018 (in Russian).
BACHVALOV, N. (1973), *Numerical Methods*, I (Nauka, Moscow) in Russian.
BACHVALOV, N., N. JIDKOV and G. KOBELKOV (1987), *Numerical Methods* (Nauka, Moscow) in Russian.
BALAZS, J. and P. TURAN (1957, 1958), Notes on interpolation, II: Explicit formulae; III: Convergence; IV: Inequalities, *Acta Math. Acad. Sci. Hungar.* **8**, 201–215; **9**, 195–214, 243–258.
BARRODALE, I. and J. MASON (1970), Two simple algorithms for discrete rational approximation, *Math. Comp.* **24**, 877–891.
BARRODALE, I., M. POWELL and F. ROBERTS (1972), The differential correction algorithm for rational *l*-approximation, *SIAM J. Numer. Anal.* **9**, 493–504.
BEREZIN, I. and N. JIDKOV (1966), *Numerical Methods*, I (Nauka, Moscow).
BERNSTEIN, S. (1912), Demonstration du theoreme de Weierstrass fondee sur le calcul des probabilites, *Comm. of Charkov Math. Soc.* **13**, 1–2 (Coll. Works, T.I, 105, 1952, AN USSR).
BERNSTEIN, S. (1913a), On the asymptotic values of the best approximation of analytic functions, *Soobst. Math. Obstestva, Harkov* **2**, 76–90 (in Russian).
BERNSTEIN, S. (1913b), Sur le valeur asymptotique de la meilleure approximation des fonctions analytiques, admettant des singularites donnees, *Bull. Soc. Math. Belg. Ser. A* **2**, 76–90.
BERNSTEIN, S. (1916), Quelques remarques sur l'interpolation, *Soobst. Math. Obstestva, Harkov* **15** (2), 49–61 (in Russian).

BERNSTEIN, S. (1936), Sur la formule de quadraturee approchee de Tchebycheff, *Compt. Rendus Acad. Sci.* **203**, 1305–1306.
BERNSTEIN, S. (1937), Sur les formules de quadrature de Cotes et de Tchebycheff, *Dokl. Akad. Nauk Ukrain. SSR* **14**, 323–325.
BINEV, P. (1985), O(n) bounds of Whitney constants, *C.R. Acad. Bulgare Sci.* **38**, 1303–1305.
BIRKHOFF, G. (1906), General mean value and remainder theorems with applications to mechanical differentiation and quadrature, *Trans. Amer. Math. Soc.* **7**, 107–136.
BOIANOV, B. (1978), *Methods for Approximate Calculation of Integrals* (c/o Jusautor, Sofia) in Bulgarian.
BOIANOV, B. (1982), Proof of a conjecture of Erdös about the longest polynomial, *Proc. Amer. Math. Soc.* **84** (1), 99–103.
BOREL, E. (1905), Leçons sur les fonctions de variables réelles, Paris.
BORODIN, A. and I. MUNRO (1975), *The Computational Complexity of Algebraic and Numeric Problems* (Elsevier, New York).
BRATLEY, P. and B. Fox (1980), Implementing Sobol's quasi random sequence generator, *ACM Trans. Math. Software* **14** (1), 88–100.
BRUDNII, J. (1970), Approximation of functions of n-variable quasipolynomials, *Izv. Akad. Nauk SSSR, Ser. Math.* **34**, 564–583 (in Russian).
CAUCHY, A. (1840), *Oeuvres* (**1**).
CHAKALOV, L. (1938), On a representation of the Newtonian difference quotients and their applications, *God. Sofii. Univ. Mat. Fak.* **34** (1), 353–405.
CHAKALOV, L. (1949), On a general quadrature formula, *Dokl. Akad. Nauk SSSR* **68**, 233–236 (in Russian).
CHAKALOV, L. (1954), General quadrature formulae of Gauss type, *Izv. Math. Inst. BAS* **T.1** (2), 67–84.
CHAKALOV, L. (1957), Formules de cubature mecaniques a coefficients non negatifs, *Izv. Math. Inst. BAS* **81**, 123–134.
CHAKALOV, L. (1983), *Collected works*, Opera **2** (Publishing House of the Bulgarian Academy of Sciences, Sofia).
CHEBYSHEV, P. (1857–1859), On the smallest values connected with approximate representation of the function, *Collected works*, **T.II** (AN SSSR, Moscow–Leningrad, 1948, 146–150).
CHEBYSHEV, P. (1874), Sur les quadratures, *J. Math. Pures Appl.* **19**, 19–34.
CHENEY, W. (1966), *Introduction to Approximation Theory* (McGraw-Hill, New York).
CHENEY, W. and H. LOEB (1961), Two new algorithms for rational approximation, *Numer. Math.* **3**, 72–75.
CHENEY, W. and H. LOEB (1962), On Chebyshev rational approximation, *Numer. Math.* **4**, 124–127.
CHUNG, K. and T. YAO (1977), On lattices admitting unique Lagrange interpolations, *SIAM J. Numer. Anal.* **14** (4), 735–743.
CIARLET, P. (1978), *The Finite Element Method for Elliptic Problems* (North-Holland, Amsterdam).
CIARLET, P. and P. RAVIART (1972), General Lagrange and Hermite interpolation in $\mathbb{R}^n$ with applications to finite element methods, *Arch. Rational Mech. Anal.* **46** (3), 177–199.
CIARLET, P. and C. WAGSCHAL (1970), Multipoint Taylor formulas and applications to the finite element method, *Numer. Math.* **17**, 84–100.
COATMELEC, C. (1966), Approximation et interpolation des fonctions différentiables de plusieurs variables, *Ann. Sci. École Norm. Sup.* **83**, 271–341.
COOLEY, J.M. and J. TUKEY (1965), An algorithm for the machine calculation of complex Fourier series, *Math. Comp.* **19**, 297–301.
DAVIS, P. (1959), On the numerical integration of analytic functions, in: R. LANGER, ed., *On Numerical Approximation* (The University of Wisconsin Press, Madison, WI).
DAVYDOV, O. (1986), Lagrange interpolation polynomial over equidistant nodes that does not converge in measure to the function $|x|$ on $[-1, 1]$, in: *Investigations in Current Problems in Summation and Approximation of Functions and their Applications*, Dnepropetrovsk. Gos. Univ. **115**, 22–25.

DE-VORE, R., A. MEIR and A. SHARMA (1973), Strongly and weekly non-poised H–B interpolation problems, *Canad. J. Math.* **25**, 1040–1050.
DIMITROV, D. (1991), Recursion algorithm for Birkhoff interpolation problem, *Facta Univ. Ser. Math. Inform.* **6**, 75–86.
DIMOV, I. and O. TONEV (1985), Monte Carlo numerical methods with overconvergent probable error, in: *Proc. II Conference on Numerical Methods and Applications* (Publishing House of BAS, Sofia).
DIMOV, I. and O. TONEV (1991), Performance analysis of Monte Carlo algorithms for some models of computer architectures, in: BL. SENDOV and I. DIMOV, eds., *Monte Carlo Methods and Parallel Algorithms, International Workshop* (World Scientific, Singapore) 5–14.
DOLZENKO E. and E. SEVASTJANOV (1976), On the approximation of functions in a Hausdorff metric by means of piecewise monotone (in particular rational) functions, *Mat. Sb. (N.S.)* **101**, 503–541 (in Russian).
DOROSHKEVICH, A. and I. SOBOL (1987), Monte Carlo evaluation of integrals encountered in nonlinear theory of gravitational instability, *USSR Comput. Math. and Math. Phys.* **27** (10), 1577–1580.
DROLS, W. (1980), Zur Hermite–Birkhoff Interpolation: DMS-Matrizen, *Math. Z.* **72**, 179–194.
DUPAC, V. (1956), Stochasticke pocetni metody, *Časopis Pěst. Mat.* **81** (1), 55–68.
DZAFAROV, A. (1977), Averaged moduli of continuity and some of their connections with the best approximations, *Dokl. Akad. Nauk Ukrain SSR* **236** (2), 289–291 (in Russian).
DZJADIK, V. (1974), On the approximation of functions on the finite point sets, in: *Theory of Applications of Functions and its Application* (Inst. Mat., USSR, Kiev).
DZJADIK, V. (1977), *Introduction to the Theory of Uniform Approximation of Functions by Polynomials* (Nauka, Moscow).
ERDÖS, P. (1939), An extremum problem concerning trigonometric polynomials, *Acta Sci. Math. (Szeged)* **9**, 113–115.
ERDÖS, P. and P. VERTESI (1980), On the almost everywhere divergence of Lagrange interpolatory polynomials for arbitrary system of nodes, *Acta Math. Hungar.* **36**, 71–89.
ERMAKOV, S. (1967), On the admissibleness of Monte Carlo procedures, *Dokl. Akad. Nauk SSSR* **172** (2), 262–264.
ERMAKOV, S. (1975), *Monte Carlo Methods and Mixed Problems* (Moscow) in Russian.
ERMAKOV, S. and V. ZOLOTUCHIN (1960), Polynomial approximations and Monte Carlo method, *Teor. Veroyatnost. i Primenen.* **4** (4), 473–476.
FABER, G. (1914), Über die interpolatorische Darstellung stetiger Funktionen, *Jahresber. Deutsch. Math.-Verein.* **23**, 192–210.
FERGUSON, D. (1969), The question of uniqueness for G.D. Birkhoff interpolation problems, *J. Approx. Theory* **2**, 1–28.
FEYER, L. (1916), Über interpolation, *Gott. Nachr.*, 66–91.
FICHTENGHOLZ, G. (1960), A Course of Differential and Integral Calculus (Fizmatgiz, Moscow) in Russian.
FRASER, W. and J. HART (1962), On the computation of rational approximation to continuous functions, *Comm. ACM* **5**, 401–403.
FREUD, G. (1958), Bemerkung über die Konvergenz eines Interpolationsverfahrens von P. Turán, *Acta Math. Acad. Sci. Hungar.* **9**, 337–341.
FUKSMAN, A. (1965), The structure characteristic of the functions for which $E_n(f; -1, 1) \leq Mn^{-(k+\alpha)}$, *Uspekhi Mat. Nauk* **20** (4), 187–190 (in Russian).
GALKIN, P. (1971), On the modulus of continuity of the operator of the best approximation in the space of continuous functions, *Mat. Zametki* **10** (6), 601–613 (in Russian).
GASCA, M. and J. MAETZU (1982), On Lagrange and Hermite interpolation in $\mathbb{R}^k$, *Numer. Math.* **39**, 1–14.
GAUSS, C. (1866), Methodus nova integralium valores per approximationem inveniendi, *Ges. Werke*, **4** (Koniglichen Geselschaft der Wissenschaften, Gottingen) 163–196.
GEORGIEV, R. (1990), Asymptotically fast Hermite interpolation, *C.R. Acad. Bulgare Sci.* **43** (8), 27–30.

GERMAN, A. (1980), On the interpolation in complex domain, *Anal. Math.* **6** (2), 121–135 (in Russian).
GONTCHAROV, V. (1930), Recherches sur les derivees successives des fonctions analytiques, *Ann. Sci. École Norm.* **47**, 1–78.
GONTCHAROV, V. (1954), *Theory of Interpolation and Approximation of Functions* (Gos. Izd. Tech.-Theor. Liter., Moscow) in Russian.
GOOD, I. (1958), The interaction algorithm and practical Fourier series, *J. Roy. Statist. Soc. Ser. B* **20**, 361–370.
GRÜNWALD, G. (1936), Über Divergenzerscheinung der Lagrangeschen Interpolationspolynome stetiger Funktionen, *Ann. of Math.* **37**, 908–918.
HAAR, A. (1918), Die Minkowskische Geometrie und die Annahrung an stetige Funktionen, *Math. Ann.* **78**, 294–331.
HABER, S. (1966), A modified Monte Carlo quadrature, *Math. Comp.* **20** (95), 361–368.
HABER, S. (1967), A modified Monte Carlo quadrature, *Math. Comp.* **21** (99), 388–397.
HAKOPIAN, H. (1982), Multivariate divided differences and multivariate interpolation, *J. Approx. Theory* **34**, 286–305.
HAKOPIAN, A., D. GEVORGIAN and A. SAAKIAN (1990), On two-dimensional Hermite interpolation, *Mat. Zametki* **48** (6), 137–139.
HAMMERSLEY, J. and D. HANDSCOMB (1964), *Monte Carlo Methods* (Methuen, London).
HILDEBRANDT, F. (1956), *Introduction to Numerical Analysis* (McGraw-Hill, New York).
HOROWITZ, E. (1972), A fast method for interpolation using preconditioning, *Inform. Process. Lett.* **1** (4), 157–163.
HAUSDORF, F. (1927), *Mengenlehre* (Gruyter, Berlin).
IONESCU, D. (1952), Generalizarae formulei de cuadratura a lui Obreschkoff, *Studii de Cerc. St.* **3**, 1–10.
IVANOV, K. (1979), On the one-sided algebraic approximation in L_p. *C.R. Acad. Bulgare Sci.* **32** (8), 1037–1040.
IVANOV, K. (1980), New estimates of errors of quadrature formulae, formulae of numerical differentiation and interpolation, *Anal. Math.* **6**, 281–303.
IVANOV, K. (1983a), A constructive characteristic of the best algebraic approximation in $L_p[-1, 1]$ ($1 \leq p \leq \infty$), in: *Proc. Int. Conf. on Constr. Function Theory, Varna, 1981* (Publishing House of the Bulgarian Academy of Sciences, Sofia) 357–367.
IVANOV, K. (1983b), On a new characteristic of functions. II: Direct and converse theorems for best algebraic approximation in $C_{[-1,1]}$ and $L_{p[-1,1]}$, *Pliska* **5**, 151–163.
IVANOV, K. and M. TAKEV (1985), $O(n \ln n)$ bounds of Whitney constants, *C.R. Acad. Bulgare Sci.* **38**, 1129–1135.
IVANOV, V. (1951), The minimax problem for the system of linear functions, *Mat. Sb. (N.S.)* **28** (70), 3, 685–706 (in Russian).
IVANOV, V. (1952), On the uniform approximation of continuous functions, *Mat. Sb. (N.S.)* **30** (72), 3, 543–558 (in Russian).
JACKSON, D. (1911), Über die Genauigkeit der Annahrung stetiger Funktionen durch ganze rationale Funktionen, Dissertation, Gottingen.
JACKSON, D. (1912), On approximation by trigonometric sums and polynomials, *Trans. Amer. Math. Soc.* **14**, 491–515.
JETTER, K. (1983), Some contributions to bivariate interpolation and cubature, in: C. CHUI et al., eds., *Approximation Theory*, IV (Academic Press, New York) 533–538.
KAHN, H. (1950), Random sampling (Monte Carlo) techniques in neutron attenuation problems, *Nucelonics* **6** (5), 27–33; **6** (6), 60–65.
KARLIN, S. and W. STUDDEN (1966), *Tchebycheff Systems: With Applications in Analysis and Statistics* (Interscience Publishers, NY).
KAUFMAN, E., D. LEEMING and G. TAYLOR (1978), A combined Remez-differential correction algorithm for rational approximation, *Math. Comp.* **32** (141), 233–242.
KAUFMAN, E. and G. TAYLOR (1975), Uniform rational approximation of functions of several variables, *Internat. J. Numer. Methods Engrg.* **9**, 297–323.

KERGIN, P. (1980), A natural interpolation of C^k functions, *J. Approx. Theory* **29**, 278–293.
KJURKCHIEV, N. and S. MARKOV (1974), On the numerical approximation of the "cross" set, *God. Sofii. Univ. Mat. Fak.* **66**, 19–25 (in Bulgarian).
KJURKCHIEV, N. and BL. SENDOV (1976), Approximation of a class of functions by algebraic polynomials with respect to Hausdorff distance, *God. Sofii. Univ. Mat. Fak.* **67**, 573–579 (in Bulgarian).
KLOEK, T. and H. VAN DIJK (1978), Bayesian estimates of equation system parameter. An application of integration by Monte Carlo, *Econometrica* **46**, 1–19.
KOLMOGOROV, A. (1948), Remarks on the Chebyshev polynomials that deviate at least from a given function, *Uspekhi Mat. Nauk* **3** (1), 216–221.
KOPAL, Z. (1955), *Numerical Analysis* (Wiley, New York).
KORKIN, A. and E. ZOLOTAREV (1873), *Zolotarev Collected Works*, **T.I**, 138–153.
KORNEICHUCK, N. (1962), The best constant in the Jackson's theorem of the best uniform approximation of continuous periodic functions, *Dokl. Akad. Nauk Ukrain. SSR* **145**, 1218–1220 (in Russian).
KORNEICHUCK, N. (1987), *The Best Constants in Approximation Theory* (Nauka, Moscow) in Russian.
KOROVKIN, P. (1959), *Linear Operators in the Theory of Approximation* (Fizmatgiz, Moscow) in Russian.
KOROVKIN, P. (1960), *Linear Operators and Approximation Theory* (Hindustan, India).
KOROVKIN, P. (1969), An experience of axiomatic construction of some problems of the theory of approximation, *Uchen. Zap. Kalinin. Ped. Inst.* **69**, 91–109 (in Russian).
KRIAKIN, J. (1989), On Whitney constants, *Mat. Zametki* **46** (2), 155–157.
KRILOV, V., V. BOBKOV and P. MONASTIRNII (1972), *Numerical Methods of High Mathematic* (Wishaja Shkola, Minsk) in Russian.
LAGRANGE, J. (1795), Leçons élémentaires sur les mathématiques, *Oeuvres* **7**.
LAURENT, P.J. (1972), *Approximation et Optimization* (Hermann, Paris).
LEBESQUE, H. (1898), Sur l'approximation de fonctions, *Bull. Sci. Math.* **22**, 278–287.
LEE, C. and F. ROBERTS (1973), A comparison of algorithms for rational l_∞ approximation, *Math. Comp.* **27** (121), 111–121.
LERCH, M. (1903), Sur un point de la théorie des fonctions génératrices d'Abel, *Acta Math.* **27**, 339–352.
LEVITAN, Y., N. MARKOVICH, S. ROZIN and I. SOBOL (1988), On quasi-random sequences for numerical computations, *USSR Comput. Math. and Math. Phys.* **28** (5), 755–759.
LICHODED, H. (1989), *Precising of Monte Carlo Estimations for Continual Integrals* (Moscow) in Russian.
LOBATTO, R. (1852), *Lessen over de Integraal-Rekening*.
LOEB, H. (1957), On rational fraction approximations at discrete points, *Convair Astronautics Appl. Math.* **9**.
LOEB, H. (1960), Algorithms for Chebyshev approximations using the ratio of linear forms, *J. Soc. Indust. App. Math.* **8**, 458–465.
LORENTZ, G. (1966), *Approximation of Functions* (Holt, Rinehart and Winston, New York).
LORENTZ, G. (1975), The Birkhoff interpolation problem: New methods and results, in: P. BUTZER and B. SZ.-NAGY, eds., *Linear Operators and Approximation*, **II** (Birkhauser Verlag, Basel) 481–501.
LORENTZ, G. (1986), *Approximation of Functions* (Chelsea Publishing Company, New York).
LORENTZ, G., K. JETTER and S. RIEMANSCNEIDER (1983), Birkhoff interpolation, *Encyclopedia of Mathematics and its Applications*, **19** (Addison-Wesley, Reading, MA).
LORENTZ, G. and R. LORENTZ (1984), *Lecture Notes in Mathematics* **1105** (Springer Verlag, Berlin).
LORENTZ, G. and R. LORENTZ (1991), multivariate interpolation, *Numer. Math.* (in print).
LORENTZ, R. (1984), Some regular problems of bivariate interpolation, in: *Constructive Theory of Functions '84* (Publishing House of the Bulgarian Academy of Sciences, Sofia) 549–562.
MAEHLY, H. and C. WITZGALL (1963), Methods for finding rational approximations, II, III, *J. Assoc. Comput. Mach.* **10**, 257–277.

MAIRHUBER, J. (1956), On Haar's theorem concerning Chebysheff approximation problems having unique solutions, *Proc. Amer. Math. Soc.* **4**, 609–615.

MAMEDOV, R. (1959), On the order of approximation of functions by linear positive operators, *Dokl. Akad. Nauk SSSR* **128** (11), 674–676.

MARCINKIEWIEZ, I. (1937a), Quelques remarques sur l'interpolation, *Acta Literarum ac Scientiarum, Szeged* **8**, 127–130.

MARCINKIEWIEZ, I. (1937b), Sur la divergenze des polynomes d'interpolation, *Acta Literarum ac Scientiarum, Szeged* **8**, 131–135.

MARINOV, P. and A. ANDREEV (1987), A modified Remez algorithm for approximate determination of the rational function of best approximation in Hausdorff metric, *C.R. Acad. Bulgare Sci.* **40**, 13–16.

MARKOV, A. (1910), *Evaluation of Finite Differences* (Odessa) chapter 5 (in Russian).

MARKOV, S. and BL. SENDOV (1968), On the numerical evaluation of a class of polynomials of best approximation, *God. Sofii. Univ. Mat. Fak.* **61**, 17–27 (in Bulgarian).

MEIR, A. and A. SHARMA (1968), On extension of Obreshkov's formula, *SIAM J. Numer. Anal.* **5**, 488–490.

MERGELIAN, S. (1951), On the representation of functions by polynomials on the closed sets, *Dokl. Akad. Nauk Ukrain SSR* **78**, 405–408 (in Russian).

METROPOLIS, N. and S. ULAM (1949), The Monte Carlo method, *J. Amer. Statist. Assoc.* **44** (247), 335–341.

MICHAILOV, G. (1987), *Optimization of Weight Monte Carlo Methods* (Nauka, Moscow).

MITTAG-LEFFLER, G. (1900), Sur la réprésentation analytique des fonctions d'une variable réelle, *Rend. Circ. Mat. Palermo* **14**, 217–224.

MOENCK, R. and A. BORODIN (1972), Fast modular transformations via division, in: *Proc. 13th Annual IEEE Symp. on Switching and Automata Theory*.

MOROZOV, E. (1958), Convergence of a sequence of positive linear operators in the space of continuous 2π-periodic functions of two variables, *Kalinin Gos. Ped. Inst. Ucen. Zap.* **26**, 129–142 (in Russian).

MÜNTZ, C. (1914), Über den Approximationssatz von Weierstrass, H.A. Schwarz Festschrift, *Math. Abh., Berlin*, 303–312.

NATANSON, P. (1949), *Constructive Theory of Functions* (Gosizdat, Moscow, Leningrad).

NEFF, C. (1990), Specified precision polynomial root isolation is in NC, Res. Rept. RC 15653(#69571), IBM Research Div., T.J. Watson Res. Center, YH, New York.

NEVILLE, E. (1934), Iterative interpolation, *J. Indian Math. Soc.* **20**, 87–120.

NEWMAN, D. (1964), Rational approximation to $|x|$, *Michigan Math. J.* **11**, 11–14.

NICOLAIDES, R. (1972), On a class of finite elements generated by Lagrange interpolation, *SIAM J. Numer. Anal.* **9**, 435–445.

NIKOLSKII, S. (1946), On the best polynomial approximation of functions which satisfy the Lipschitz condition, *Izv. Akad. Nauk SSSR Ser. Mat.* **10**, 295–318 (in Russian).

NIKOLSKII, S. (1947), *Approximation Theory of Functions*, I: *Functional Analysis* (Dnepropetrovsk University, Dnepropetrovsk) in Russian.

NIKOLSKII, S. (1950), On the problem of estimations for approximation of quadrature formulas, *Uspekhi Mat. Nauk* **5**, 2(36), 165–177 (in Russian).

NIKOLSKII, S. (1952), Quadrature formulae, *Izv. Akad. Nauk SSSR, Ser. Mat.* **16**, 181–196.

NIKOLSKII, S. (1974), *Quadrature Formulas* (Nauka, Moscow).

NIKOLSKII, S. (1988), *Quadrature Formulas* (Nauka, Moscow).

OBRESHKOV, N. (1940), Neue Quadraturformeln, *Abh. der Preuss. Acad. der Wiss. Nat. Klasse* **5**, 1–20.

OBRESHKOV, N. (1942), On the mechanical quadratures, *J. Bulgar. Acad. Sci. and Arts* **LXV-8**, 191–289.

OSBORN, N. and G. WATSON (1969/70), An algorithm for minimax approximation in the nonlinear case, *Comput. J.* **12**, 64–68.

OSTROWSKI, A. (1954), On two problems in abstract algebra connected with Horner's rule, *Studies Presented to R. von Mises* (Academic Press, New York).

PAN, V. (1966), Methods of computing values of polynomials, *Uspekhi Mat. Nauk* **21** (1), 105–136.
PEANO, G. (1914), Residuo in formulas de quadratura. *Mathesis* (*4*) **34**, 5–10.
PETRUSHEV, P. and V. POPOV (1987), *Rational approximation of real functions* (Cambridge University Press, Cambridge).
PICARD, E. (1891), Sur la représentation approchée des fonctions, *C.R. Acad. Sci. Paris* **112**, 183–186.
POLYA, G. (1931), Bemerkung zur Interpolation und zur Nahrungstheorie der Balkonbiegung, *Z. Angew. Math. Mech.* **11**, 445–449.
POPOVICIU, T. (1934), Sur l'approximation des fonctions convexes d'ordre supérieur, *Mathematica* **10**, 49–54.
POPOV, V. (1977), Uniform rational approximation of the class V_r and its applications, *Acta Math. Acad. Sci. Hung.* **29**, 119–129.
POTAPOV, M. (1977), On approximation by Jacoby polynomials, *Vestnik Moskov. Univ. Ser. I Mat. Mekh.* **5**, 70–82.
RADAU, R. (1879), Etude sur les formules d'approximation qui servent *f* calculer la valeur numérique d'une intégrale définite, *J. Math. Pures Appl.* **3** (5), 283–336.
RADER, C. (1968), Discrete Fourier transforms when the number of data samples is prime, *Proc. IEEE* **56**, 1107–1108.
RADON, G. (1948), Zur mechanischen Kubatur, *Monatsh. Math.* **52** (4), 286–300.
RALSTON, A. (1965a), *A first course in numerical analysis* (McGraw-Hill, New York).
RALSTON, A. (1965b), Rational Chebyshev approximation by Remez' algorithms, *Numer. Math.* **7**, 322–330.
RAMOS, G. (1971), Roundoff error analysis of the fast Fourier transform, *Math. Comp.* **25**, 757–768.
REMEZ, E. (1934), Sur un procédé convergent d'approximations successives pour déterminer les polynomes d'approximation, *C.R. Acad. Sci. Paris* **T.198**, 2063–2065.
REMEZ, E. (1953), Some problems of the Chebyshev approximation on the complex plane, *Ukrainian Math. J.* **5** (1), 3–49 (in Russian).
REMEZ, E. (1957), On Chebyshev approximation in complex domain, *Dokl. Akad. Nauk Ukrain. SSR*, **77** (6), 965–968 (in Russian).
REMEZ, E. (1969), *Bases of Numerical Methods in Chebyshev Approximation* (Naukova Dumka, Kiev).
RICE, J. (1969), *The Approximation of Functions*, **2**: *Nonlinear and Multivariate Theory* (Addison-Wesley, Reading, MA).
RICHARDSON, L. and J. GAUND (1927), The deferred approach to the limit, *Trans. Roy. Soc. London, A* **226**, 299–361.
RUNGE, C. (1885a), Zur Theory der eindeutigen analytischen Funktionen, *Acta Math.* **6**, 229–245.
RUNGE, C. (1885b), Uber die Darstellung willkurlicher Funktionen, *Acta Math.* **7**, 387–392.
SALEM, R. (1940), *Essais sur les Series Trigonometriques: Actualites Sci. Indust.* (Herman, Paris).
SARD, A. (1949), Best approximative integration formulas, *Amer. J. Math.* **LXXI**, 80–91.
SARD, A. (1963), *Linear Approximation, Mathematical Surveys* **9** (American Mathematical Society, Providence, RI).
SCHOENBERG, I. (1966), On Hermite–Birkhoff interpolation, *J. Math. Anal. Appl.* **16**, 538–543.
SENDOV, BL. (1962), Approximation of functions by algebraic polynomials with respect to a metric of Hausdorff type, *God. Sofii, Univ. Mat. Fak.* **55**, 1–39 (in Bulgarian).
SENDOV, BL. (1967), Approximation with respect to the Hausdorff distance, Dissertation, Moscow.
SENDOV, BL. (1982), On the constants of H. Whitney, *C.R. Acad. Bulgare Sci.* **35**, 431–434.
SENDOV, BL. (1987), On the theorem and constants of H. Whitney, *Constr. Approx.* **3**, 1–11.
SENDOV, BL. (1990), *Hausdorff Approximation* (Kluwer, Dordrecht).
SENDOV, BL. and V. POPOV (1970), Approximation of functions of several variables by algebraic polynomials in a Hausdorff type metric, *God. Sofii. Univ. Mat. Fak.* **63**, 61–76 (in Bulgarian).
SENDOV, BL. and V. POPOV (1972), The exact asymptotic behavior of the best approximation by algebraic and trigonometric polynomials in the Hausdorff metric, *Mat. Sb. (N.S.)* **89**, 138–147 (*Math. USSR-Sb.* **18**, 1972, 139–149).

SENDOV, BL. and V. POPOV (1988), *The Averaged Moduli of Smoothness* (Wiley, New York).
SHAW, J. (1988), Aspects of numerical integration and summarization, *Bayesian Statistics* **3**, 411–428.
SHISHA, O. and B. MOND (1968), The degree of approximation to periodic functions by linear positive operators, *J. Approx. Theory* **1**, 335–339.
SMIRNOV, V. and N. LEBEDEV (1964), *Constructive Theory of Functions of Complex Variable* (Nauka, Moscow, Leningrad) in Russian.
SMOLJAK, S. (1965), On the optimal recovering of functions and their functionals, Ph.D. Thesis, Moscow.
SOBOL, I. (1973), *Monte Carlo Numerical Methods* (Nauka, Moscow) in Russian.
SOBOL, I. (1979), On the systematic search in a hypercube, *SIAM J. Numer. Anal.* **16**, 790–793.
SOBOL, I. (1989), On quadratic formulas for functions of several variables satisfying a general Lipschitz condition, *USSR Comput. Math. and Math. Phys.* **29** (6), 936–941.
SOBOL, I. (1991), Quasi-Monte Carlo methods, in: BL. SENDOV and I. DIMOV, eds., *Monte Carlo Methods and Parallel Algorithms, International Workshop* (World Scientific, Singapore) 75–81.
STAHL, H. (1991), *Int. Conf. on Constructive Function Theory*, Varna, Bulgaria.
STECHKIN, S. (1951), On the order of the best approximation of continuous functions, *Izv. Akad. Nauk SSSR Ser. Mat.* **15**, 219–241 (in Russian).
STEWART, L. (1983), Bayesian analysis using Monte Carlo integration—A powerful methodology for handling some difficult problems, *Statistician* **32**, 195–200.
STEWART, L. (1985), Multiparameter Bayesian inference using Monte Carlo integration—Some techniques for bivariate analysis, in: J.M. BERNARDO, M.H. DE GROOT, D.V. LINDLEY and A.F. SMITH, eds., *Bayesian Statistics* **2** (North-Holland, Amsterdam).
STEWART, L. (1987), Hierarchical Bayesian analysis using Monte Carlo integration computing posterior distributions when there are many possible models, *Statistician* **36**, 211–219.
STEWART, L. and W. DAVIS (1986), Bayesian posterior distribution over sets of possible models with inferences computed by Monte Carlo integration, *Statistician* **35**, 175–182.
STOUN, M. (1937), Applications of the theory of Boolean rings to general topology, *Trans. Amer. Math. Soc.* **41**, 375–481.
STOUN, M. (1948), The generalized Weierstrass approximation theory, *Math. Mag.* **21**, 167–184, 237–254.
TIMAN, A. (1960), *Theory of Approximation of Functions of Real Variable* (Fitzmatgis, Moscow).
TONELLI, L. (1908), J. polinomi d'approssimazione di Tchebychev, *Ann. di Math.* **15**, 47–119.
TURAN, P. (1950), On the theory of the mechanical quadrature, *Acta Sci. Math. (Szeged)* **XII**, 30–37.
VALLEE-POUSSIN, CH.-J. (1910), Sur les polynômes d'approximation et la représentation approchée d'un angle, *Bull. Soc. Math. Belg.* 808–844.
VALLEE-POUSSIN, CH.-J. (1919), *Leçons sur l'Approximation des Fonctions d'une Variable Réelle* (Gautie-Villars, Paris).
VAN DIJK, H., J. HOP and A. LOUTER (1987), An algorithm for the computation of posterior moments and densities using simple importance sampling, *Statistician* **37**, 83–90.
VAN DIJK, H. and T. KLOEK (1983), Monte Carlo analysis of skew posterior distributions: An illustrative econometric example, *Statistician* **32**, 216–223.
VAN DIJK, H. and T. KLOEK (1985), Experiments with some alternatives for simple importance sampling in Monte Carlo integration, in: J. BERNARDO, M. DE GROOT, D. LINDLEY and A. SMITH, eds., *Bayesian Statistics* **2** (North-Holland, Amsterdam).
VEIDINGER, L. (1960), On the numerical determination of the best approximation in the Chebyshev sense, *Numer. Math.* **2**, 99–105.
VERTESI, P. (1982), Divergence of Lagrange interpolation (complex and trigonometric cases), *Acta Math. Acad. Sci. Hungar.* **39**, 367–377.
VESELINOV, V. (1972), On the exact order of approximation by Bernstein polynomials in Hausdorff metric, *Mat. Zametki* **12**, 501–510 (in Russian).
VESELINOV, V. (1974), The exact constants in the theory of approximation by Bernstein polynomials in the Hausdorff metric, *C.R. Acad. Bulgare Sci.* **30**, 1019–1021 (in Russian).

VIDENSKII, V. (1956), On the uniform approximation on the complex plane, *Uspekhi Mat. Nauk* **11** 5(71), 169–175 (in Russian).
VIDENSKII, V. (1960), Qualitative problems of the best uniform approximation of functions of complex variable, in: *Investigations on Current Problems in the Theory of Functions of Complex Variable* (Fizmatgis, Moscow) in Russian.
VJACHESLAVOV, N. (1975), On the uniform approximation of $|x|$ by rational functions, *Dokl. Akad. Nauk SSSR* **220**, 512–515.
VOLKOV, V. (1957), On the convergence of sequences of linear positive operators in the space of continuous functions of two variables, *Dokl. Akad. Nauk SSSR* **115**, 17–19 (in Russian).
VOLTERRA, V. (1897), Sul principio di Dirichlet, *Rend. Circ. Mat. Palermo* **11**, 83–86.
WALSH, J. (1960a), *Interpolation and Approximation by Rational Functions in the Complex Domain* (American Mathematical Society, New York, 2nd ed.).
WALSH, J. (1960b), *Interpolation and Approximation by Rational Functions in the Complex Domain* (American Mathematical Society, New York, 2nd ed.); Russian translation (1961) with supplement by Mergelian.
WATSON, J. (1980), *Approximation Theory and Numerical Methods* (Wiley, New York).
WEIERSTRASS, K. (1885), Über die analytische Darstellung sogenannter willkurlicher Funktionen einer reelen Veranderlichen, *Sitzungsber. der Akad. zu Berlin*, 633–639, 789–805.
WELCH, P. (1969), a fixed-point fast Fourier transform error analysis, *IEEE Trans. Audio and Electroacoustics* **AU-17**, 151–157.
WERNER, H. (1962a), Die konstruktive Ermittlung der Tschebyscheff-Approximierenden im Bereich der rationalen Funktionen, *Arch. Rational Mech. Anal.* **11** (4), 368–384.
WERNER, H. (1962b), Tschebyscheff-Approximation im Bereich der rationalen Funktionen bei Vorliegen einer guten Ausgang Nahrung, *Arch. Rational Mech. Anal.* **10**, 205–219.
WERNER, H. (1963), Rationale Tschebyscheff-Approximation, Eigenwerttheorie und Differenzenrechnung, *Arch. rational Mech. Anal.* **13** (5), 330–347.
WERNER, H. (1967), Die Bedeutung der Normalität bei rationaler Tschebyscheff-Approximation, *Computing* **2**, 34–52.
WERNER, H. (1980), Remarks on Newton type multivariate interpolation for subsets of grids, *Computing* **25**, 181–191.
WEYL, H. (1916), Über die Gleichverteilung von Zahlen mod Eins, *Math. Ann.* **77** (3), 313–352.
WHITNEY, H. (1957), On functions with bounded nth difference, *J. Math. Pures Appl.* **36**, 67–95.
WHITNEY, H. (1959), On bounded functions with bounded nth difference, *Proc. Amer. Math. Soc.* **10**, 480–481.
WINOGRAD, S. (1978), On computing the discrete Fourier transform, *Math. Comp.* **32**, 175–199.
WHITTAKER, J. (1935), *Interpolation Function Theory* (Cambridge University Press, Cambridge).
ZLAMAL, M. (1968), On the finite element method, *Numer. Math.* **12**, 394–409.
ZLAMAL, M. (1969), On some finite element procedures for solving second order boundary value problems, *Numer. Math.* **14**, 42–48.
ZUCHOVITZKII, S. and L. AVDEEVA (1967), *Linear and Convex Programming* (Nauka, Moscow) in Russian.

Subject Index

A-distance, 348
A-equidistant point, 348
Abel–Gontcharov interpolation, 248, 252
Aitken's scheme, 238
Algebraic degree of exactness (ADE), 386
Atkinson and Sharma, 251
Averaged moduli, 320

Backward finite difference, 239
Baire functions, 424
Basic Lagrange polynomials, 232
Bernoulli polynomials, 400
Bernstein inequality, 355
Bernstein polynomial, 323
Bessel interpolation, 243
Best approximation, 301
Best quadrature formulas, 404

Central finite difference, 239
Central limit theorem, 407
Chakalov's approach, 270
Chebyshev alternation, 307
Chebyshev polynomials, 342
Chebyshev system, 231
Chebyshev theorem, 306
Completed graph, 447
Complex functions, 266
Continual integrals, 418
Cooley–Tukey algorithm, 291
Cyclic convolution, 295

Differential correction algorithm, 367
Dini–Lipschitz condition, 434
Dirichlet integral, 434
Discrete Fourier transforms, 289
Divided differences, 234, 257, 270
Division of polynomials, 297

Effect of the ends, 334
Effective MC methods, 410
Erdös conjecture, 346
Error of quadrature formulas, 392
Error of the MC method, 407
Euler–Maclaurin summation formula, 400
Everett interpolation, 244

Fast Fourier transforms, 290

Fejer, 256
Fejer operator, 432
Finite-difference table, 239
Finite differences, 239
Fourier series, 434
Frazer's diagram, 245

Gauss backward interpolation, 242
Gauss forward interpolation, 242
Gauss quadrature formula, 391
Gaussian quadrature formula, 395
GC condition, 277
General interpolation, 229
Geometric characterization (GC), 276
Geometric MC method, 409
Gibbs completed graph, 437
Gibbs effect, 436
Good's algorithm, 293
Gregory formula, 400

H-continuity, 429
Hausdorff approximation, 447
Hausdorff distance, 423
Hermite interpolation, 248, 254, 268
Hermite quadrature formula, 396
Hermite–Birkhoff interpolation, 248
Hinchin theorem, 407
Horner's scheme, 298

Important sampling method, 412
Incidence matrix, 248
Infinite-valued metric, 425
Integral moduli, 319
Interpolation processes, 284
Inverse interpolation, 247

Jackson's estimation, 334

k-dimensional DFT, 295
Kolmogorov's criteria, 306

Lagrange coefficient, 233
Lagrange interpolation, 230, 284
Lagrange polynomials, 230
Laurent method, 361
Law of large numbers, 407
Linear inequality algorithm, 372

Linear operators, 323
Loeb's algorithm, 373
Loran series, 269
Lozenge diagram, 245

Maehly's algorithm, 373
Markov inequality, 355
MC, *see* Monte Carlo,
Metric space, 424
Moduli of functions, 317
Moduli of smoothness, 318
Modulus of continuity, 427
Modulus of nonmonotonicity, 438
Moivre's formula, 342
Monte Carlo (MC) methods, 406
Multivariate interpolation, 274, 281

n-composite quadrature formula, 392
Natural lattice, 277
Newman's rational function, 341
Newman's results, 339
Newton backward interpolation, 242
Newton forward interpolation, 241
Newton interpolation, 234, 279
Newton–Cotes formula, 385
Newton–Cotes quadrature formula, 395
Non-random points, 417
Norm, 302

Obreshkov interpolation polynomial, 403
Obreshkov–Chakalov interpolation, 255
Obreshkov–Chakalov quadrature, 403
Obreshkov–Chakalov quadrature formula, 396
Optimal knots, 386
Ordinary MC method, 408
Overconvergent probable error, 414

Points of alternation, 307
Poised matrix, 249
Pólya condition, 249, 283
Polynomial multiplication, 297
Popov theorem, 340
Positive integral operators, 431
Positive operators, 429
Possibility for approximation, 316
Probability density function, 407
Probability error, 408
Probability integral, 408
Probable error, 408
Pseudorandom numbers, 416

Quadrature formula, 381, 392
Quadrature with restrictions, 397
Quasi-MC methods, 416
Quasi-random numbers, 416

Random nodes, 414
Random points, 417
Random quadrature formula, 415
Random variable, 406
Random weights, 415
Rational approximation, 311
Rectangle formula, 385
Rectangle quadrature formula, 397
Regular sequence, 241
Remainder term, 232, 236, 237
Remez algorithm, 360
  discrete, 354
  second, 357, 365
Remez–Difcor algorithm, 373
Repeating knots, 257
Richardson's extrapolation, 400
Romberg formulas, 400
Romberg quadrature formulas, 399
3/8 rule, 386
Runge principle, 399

Segment functions, 423
Separation of the principal part, 411
Simpson's formula, 397
Simpson's rule, 385
Smoljak's result, 406
Splitting method, 421
Stability, 374
Steffensen interpolation, 244
Stirling formula, 233
Stirling interpolation, 242
Stoun algebra, 317
Strongly normed space, 304
Summation formulas, 433
Symmetrization of the integrand, 411

Taylor formula, 248
Taylor interpolation, 265
Trapezoidal quadrature formula, 397
Trapezoidal rule, 385

Uniform approximation, 301
Uniform distance, 301
Unit sphere, 425
Universal estimates, 442
Universal matrix, 285

Vallee-Poussin operator, 432
Vallee-Poussin theorem, 313

Weierstrass theorem, 317
Weight functions, 420
Whitney's constant, 325
Whitney's theorem, 325
Winograd algorithm, 295

Numerical Methods for Solids
(Part 1)

Numerical Methods for Nonlinear Three-dimensional Elasticity

Patrick Le Tallec

Université de Paris Dauphine,
F-75775 Paris Cedex 16, France

Contents

Preface	469
Chapter I. Mechanical Models	471
1. Kinematics	471
2. Deformation invariants and special cases	473
3. The equations of equilibrium	474
4. Constitutive laws	476
4.1. Hyperelastic compressible materials	477
4.2. Hyperelastic incompressible materials	481
4.3. Nearly incompressible materials	483
Chapter II. Mathematical Analysis	485
5. Definition of the boundary value problem	487
6. Examples of solutions	488
7. Weak formulations of equilibrium problems	490
7.1. The compressible case	490
7.2. The incompressible case	491
8. The minimization approach	493
9. Existence results by minimization arguments	498
10. Existence results by differential calculus	501
Chapter III. Approximation Theory	507
11. Approximation of compressible problems	508
12. Approximation of incompressible problems	511
13. Approximation of nearly incompressible problems	513
14. Linearization and compatibility condition	515
15. Existence and convergence results	519
16. Convergence in the compressible case	526
17. Additional remarks on the convergence theorems	527
Chapter IV. Numerical Solution Techniques	529
18. The system to solve	530
19. The basic Newton's method	533
20. Newton's method with incremental loading	535
21. Arc-length continuation	539
21.1. General presentation	539
21.2. Arclength continuation: Detailed algorithm	541
21.3. Extended Newton's algorithm	543
22. On the solution of the linear system (S)	544
23. On the choice of the stored energy function $\hat{W}$	545
24. Conclusion	546

CHAPTER V. Augmented Lagrangian Methods 549

    25. Introduction of a new discrete formulation 549
    26. Basic iterative method 553
    27. The problems in displacements 554
    28. The local problems in deformation gradients 556
        28.1. Formulation and preliminary lemma 556
        28.2. Solution procedure 557
    29. Numerical results 560
        29.1. Stretching of a cracked rectangular bar 561
        29.2. Postbuckling solution of a three-dimensional beam 561

CHAPTER VI. Equilibrium Problems with Frictionless Contact 565

    30. Formulation of a contact problem 566
    31. Existence results 570
    32. Finite-element discretization 572
    33. A first numerical algorithm 573
    34. The nonlinear programming approach 575
    35. Extensions to self-contact 577

CHAPTER VII. Extension to Viscoelasticity 579

    36. The rheological model 580
    37. Thermodynamical model 581
    38. Mathematical formulation 584
        38.1. The complete nonlinear model 584
        38.2. Choosing the free energy potential 585
        38.3. Linearization 586
    39. Approximation in space 588
        39.1. Galerkin approximation 588
        39.2. Linearized problems 589
        39.3. Transformation of the linearized problems 590
        39.4. Main result 591
        39.5. Technical theorems 593
        39.6. Proof of the main result 598
    40. Discretization in time 601
        40.1. Approximation in time 601
        40.2. Convergence theory 601
    41. Numerical solution 603
        41.1. Basic algorithm 603
        41.2. Numerical implementation 605
        41.3. Numerical tests 606
    42. Conclusion 607

REFERENCES 611

LIST OF SYMBOLS 617

SUBJECT INDEX 621

Preface

The main object of three-dimensional finite elasticity is to predict changes in the geometry of solid bodies. In standard solid mechanics, these changes are very small: the deformation of most classical structures under working loads are not detectable by the human eye. Thus, it makes sense to consider their configuration as fixed once and for all and to neglect any changes in their geometry. This small-strain assumption is the starting point of the classical theory of linear elasticity as described in the literature (LOVE [1927], TIMOSHENKO [1951]), and successfully used in structural mechanics and many other engineering applications. In contrast, many modern situations involve large deformations. The thermoviscoelastic response of solid propellants, the postbuckling behavior of flexible structures, the use of inflatable structures, the nonlinear behavior of polymers and synthetic rubbers are such examples. The situation is even more critical in biomechanics where many vital organs such as the eye, the heart or the trachea fulfill their functions only because of their large deformations.

In this framework of large deformations, finite elasticity covers the simplest case where internal forces (stresses) only depend on the present deformation of the body and not on its history. While this assumption is sufficiently general to allow the description of phenomena like buckling, cavitation or change of phases, it excludes all situations involving plasticity, damage or forming processes. Despite this weakness, the assumption of elasticity is very interesting from the modeling point of view and it has led to the introduction of a general theory of large deformation (TRUESDELL and NOLL [1965], WANG and TRUESDELL [1973] or GURTIN [1981b]). As a result, explicit tools are now available for describing in detail the changes of shape of the domain of study. These tools of elementary differentiable geometry are both simple and general: for example, they can be used for generating structured grids around complex obstacles in computational fluid dynamics. Nonlinear elasticity is also the starting point of the nonlinear theories of viscoelasticity which are proposed in the literature (ERINGEN [1966]), and establishes guiding principles for deriving more elaborate constitutive laws in large deformations (TRUESDELL and NOLL [1965]).

Because of the large deformations and hence the large rotations which are involved, the mathematical models used in finite elasticity are always nonlinear (FOSDICK and SERRIN [1979]). Their study has motivated the introduction of new mathematical concepts. These mathematical treatments of nonlinear elasticity have been pioneered by STOPPELLI [1954], MORREY [1952] and BALL [1977], and are described at length in the books of MARSDEN and HUGHES [1983], CIARLET

[1988] and VALENT [1990]. Because of their inherent nonlinearity, the numerical solution of the resulting mathematical equations also requires a careful approximation strategy and powerful algorithms as described in the early book of ODEN [1972] and developed on many occasions since then.

The purpose of the present work is to give a general description of three-dimensional finite elasticity and of its approximation. We want first to describe the models which are used in this field. We want then to give qualitative information on their mathematical structure, not by considering particular solutions to specific problems but by studying the existence and nonuniqueness of solutions. Finally, we want to describe at length the main strategies which can be used for their numerical treatment. This description tries to be relevant to definition of a handbook. Its goal is therefore to be short but complete and to indicate specific references to the reader interested in more detailed developments.

The text is organized in two parts. The first part gives a complete presentation of the central problem in finite elasticity which consists in finding the equilibrium position of an elastic body when it is subjected to given applied forces. This begins with the introduction of the mechanical model (Chapter I), continues with the study of the basic variational formulations of the equilibrium problems (Chapter II), with the definition and analysis of different mixed finite-element approximations (Chapter III), and concludes with a detailed description of the algorithms which are now available for the numerical solution of these problems (Chapter IV).

The second part presents different possible developments. The first extension considers an alternative numerical strategy based on augmented Lagrangians (Chapter V). The second one (Chapter VI) adds contact forces to the model. Indeed, in their large deformations, elastic bodies are very likely into enter into contact with neighboring obstacles and therefore both the mathematical formulation and the numerical algorithm must be modified to take these phenomena into account. The last development introduces time-dependence in the models. Equilibrium problems in elasticity are time-independent. But in practice time plays a role not so much because of inertia but because of viscous effects. The extension of existing elastic models in order to take into account these viscous effects is explained in Chapter VII.

Each chapter begins with a brief introduction explaining the problem to be considered, what is known on this problem, what is to be described in the chapter, and what are the relevant references.

CHAPTER I

Mechanical Models

This chapter introduces the main equations which are used in three-dimensional elasticity. These equations describe first the kinematics of the motion, that is the changes of geometry which occur during the motion of a continuous body. As soon as large displacements or large deformations become involved, monitoring these changes of geometry becomes a delicate matter and requires specific variables. The next step in the mathematical modeling is to relate the kinematic variables introduced above to the external loads applied on the continuum. This is achieved by the fundamental stress principle of Euler and Cauchy as used universally in mechanics. Finally, these equations of equilibrium must be complemented by constitutive relations that specify the nature of the constitutive material which is under consideration. As seen in the last section of this chapter, these constitutive relations take a simple form in finite elasticity.

This mathematical modeling of three-dimensional elasticity is general and very widely accepted. A detailed exposition is given in TRUESDELL and NOLL [1965], following an earlier work of GREEN and ADKINS [1960]. More mathematically oriented presentations of these models are also found in GURTIN [1981b], MARSDEN and HUGHES [1983], and CIARLET [1988].

1. Kinematics

Kinematics describes the change of geometry undergone by continuous bodies during their evolution (Fig. 1.1). Denoting by $\mathbb{E}$ the three-dimensional Euclidian space, a *continuous body* is a compact domain B of $\mathbb{E}$. It is made of particles, or *material points*, whose positions at a time t define the configuration of the body.

More precisely, a configuration is a smooth mapping of B onto a region of $\mathbb{E}$. Among all configurations, we will choose one, once and for all, which will not vary in time, as a *reference configuration*. We will then identify each particle of the body with its position x in the reference configuration. As a consequence, the interior of the body is identified as an open, bounded, connected subset Ω of $\mathbb{E}$ with boundary Γ. We will assume that Γ is Lipschitz-continuous; in particular a unit normal vector n exists almost everywhere along Γ.

A *deformation* of the body is a one-to-one, orientation-preserving vector field,

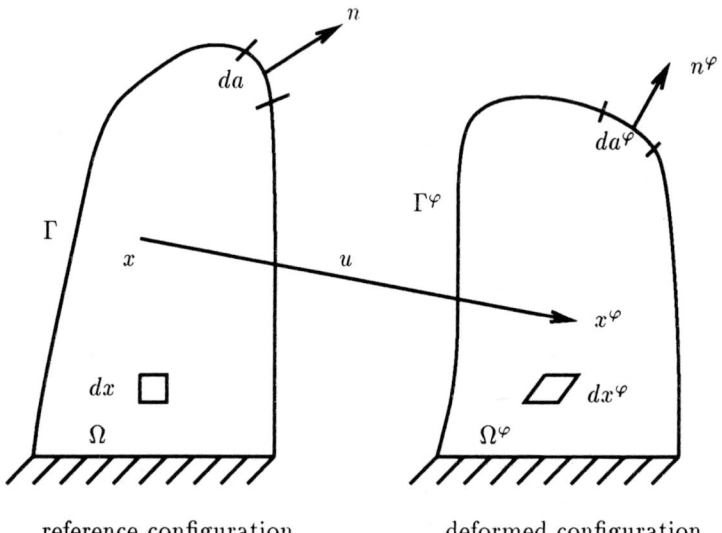

FIG. 1.1. Kinematics. Description of the different kinematic variables. For simplicity, this picture is drawn in two dimensions but the variables and the problem under consideration are actually three-dimensional.

defined on the reference configuration, with values in $\mathbb{E}$; in other words, it is a map

$$\varphi : \bar{\Omega} \to \mathbb{E},$$

with

$$\det \nabla \varphi > 0 \quad \text{on } \Omega,$$

and such that φ is injective on Ω (the reason a deformation need not be injective on $\bar{\Omega}$ is that self contact must be allowed). The spatial point $x^\varphi = \varphi(x)$ corresponds to the place occupied by the particle x in the deformation φ. The displacement field will then be the field defined by

$$u(x) = \varphi(x) - x.$$

When needed, we relate both u and x to a fixed orthonormal basis (e_i) chosen once for all in $\mathbb{E}$.

Changes of length, area and volume in the deformation φ are governed by the *deformation gradient*

$$F = \nabla \varphi$$

or, componentwise in the basis (e_i),

$$F_{ij} = \frac{\partial \varphi^i}{\partial x^j}.$$

Indeed, if δx is an elementary vector engraved on the body at the point x in the reference configuration (i.e a vector following the material points in their deformation), then, after deformation, this vector is transformed within the first order into the vector $\delta x^\varphi = F \delta x$, whose length is given by

$$|\delta x^\varphi|^2 = \delta x^\varphi \cdot \delta x^\varphi$$

$$= (F \delta x) \cdot (F \delta x)$$

$$= \delta x (F^T F) \delta x$$

$$= \delta x C \delta x.$$

The tensor $C = F^T F$, which measures the length of an elementary vector after deformation in terms of its definition in the reference configuration, is called the *right Cauchy–Green tensor*. It is symmetric positive definite by construction.

Similarly, a volume element dx located at the point x in the reference configuration is transformed, after deformation, into the volume element

$$dx^\varphi = \det(F(x)) \, dx.$$

Finally, an area element $n \, da$ (with da the area of the considered element and n its unit normal vector) is transformed into

$$n^\varphi \, da^\varphi = (\det F) F^{-T} n \, da = (\operatorname{cof} F) n \, da.$$

2. Deformation invariants and special cases

To the right Cauchy–Green strain tensor

$$C = F^T F \text{ in } \mathbb{M}^3 = \mathbb{E} \otimes \mathbb{E}$$

corresponds the *left Cauchy–Green strain tensor*

$$B = FF^T.$$

By construction, C is a symmetric positive definite tensor in $\mathbb{E} \otimes \mathbb{E}$, which implies that C has three strictly positive eigenvalues $(\lambda_i^2(C))_{i=1}^3$. From these, we define the *invariants* of C by

$$I_1(C) = \operatorname{tr}(C) = \lambda_1^2 + \lambda_2^2 + \lambda_3^2,$$

$$I_2(C) = \tfrac{1}{2}\{(\operatorname{tr} C)^2 - \operatorname{tr}(C^2)\}$$

$$= \operatorname{tr}(\operatorname{cof}(C)) = \lambda_1^2 \lambda_2^2 + \lambda_2^2 \lambda_3^2 + \lambda_3^2 \lambda_1^2,$$

$$I_3(C) = \det(C) = (\det F)^2 = \lambda_1^2 \lambda_2^2 \lambda_3^2 = J^2.$$

Among all possible deformations, we find two important special cases corresponding to rigid and isochoric deformations, respectively.

A deformation is called a *rigid* deformation if and only if there exists a rotation Q and a translation of vector a such that

$$\varphi(x) = Qx + a \quad \forall x \in \Omega.$$

By construction such deformations do not induce any change of shape in $\mathbb{E}$. Moreover, they are easy to characterize since we have (see, for example, CIARLET [1988], p. 44):

THEOREM 2.1. *Let Ω be open connected in $\mathbb{E}$. Then a deformation $\varphi \in C^1(\Omega, \mathbb{E})$ is a rigid deformation if and only if its right Cauchy–Green strain tensor C satisfies*

$$C(x) = \mathrm{Id} \quad \forall x \in \Omega.$$

A deformation is *isochoric* if and only if it preserves volumes ($\mathrm{d}x^\varphi = \mathrm{d}x$). From the previous section, it follows that such deformations are characterized by deformation gradients F which satisfy the *incompressibility constraint*

$$\det F(x) = 1 \quad \forall x \in \Omega.$$

In particular, rigid deformations are isochoric.

REMARK 2.1. Strictly speaking, the tensors $F(x)$ and $C(x)$ belong to the spaces $\mathcal{T}_{\varphi(\Omega)}(\varphi(x)) \otimes (\mathcal{T}_\Omega(x))'$ and $(\mathcal{T}_\Omega(x))' \otimes (\mathcal{T}_\Omega(x))'$, with $\mathcal{T}_\Omega(x)$ denoting the tangent space to Ω at x. Such a distinction is important in shell theory, but is of little interest in three-dimensional elasticity since here the set $\mathcal{T}_\Omega(x)$ is equal to $\mathbb{E}$.

3. The equations of equilibrium

In classical continuum mechanics, the forces acting on a continuous body in its actual configuration $\Omega^\varphi = \varphi(\Omega)$ consist of:

- *body forces* f^φ measured by unit volume of Ω^φ, which describe the action exerted on the body at 'long range';
- *contact forces* $t^\varphi(n^\varphi)\,\mathrm{d}a^\varphi$ which represent the contact forces exerted by one part of the body on its other part through the surface $n^\varphi\,\mathrm{d}a^\varphi$;
- *surface tractions* g^φ, measured by unit area of Γ^φ, which describe the tractions exerted on the body through Γ^φ.

For instance, the gravity field corresponds to a density of body forces $f^\varphi = \rho^\varphi g$ with g the gravitational vector and ρ^φ the mass density of the body in its present configuration. Similarly, a pressure load corresponds to a density $g^\varphi = -\pi n^\varphi$ where the scalar π denotes the pressure intensity.

When the body is in static equilibrium, the vector fields f^φ, g^φ and t^φ satisfy the stress principle of Euler and Cauchy (also called the principle of balance of momentum), which implies Cauchy's theorem and the *principle of virtual work* (CIARLET [1988], SALENÇON [1988], MARSDEN and HUGHES [1983]). This axiom

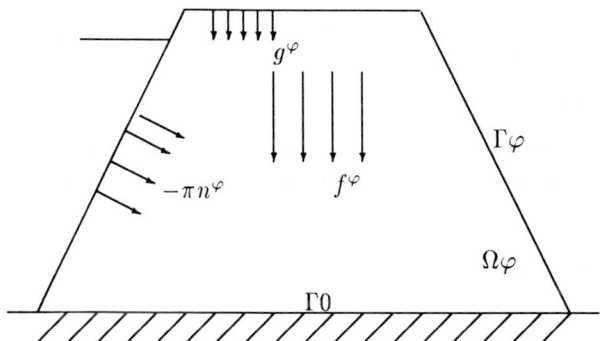

FIG. 3.1. Description of the Different Forces. A pressure force $-\pi n^\varphi$ is applied on the left, a surface traction g^φ is applied on the top, body forces f^φ are exerted inside.

and these resulting theorems can be summarized in the following classical weak equations of equilibrium:

THEOREM 3.1. *There exists a symmetric tensor T^φ, called the Cauchy stress tensor such that*

$$t^\varphi(n^\varphi) = T^\varphi n^\varphi,$$

$$\int_{\Omega^\varphi} T^\varphi : \frac{\partial v^\varphi}{\partial x^\varphi}\, dx^\varphi = \int_{\Omega^\varphi} f^\varphi \cdot v^\varphi\, dx^\varphi + \int_{\Gamma^\varphi} g^\varphi \cdot v^\varphi\, da^\varphi,$$

for all test functions $v^\varphi: \bar{\Omega}^\varphi \to \mathbb{E}$.

The notation above is taken from CIARLET [1988] (in other texts, the Cauchy stress tensor is often denoted by σ). The notation $T : \partial v/\partial x$ and $f \cdot v$ denote the usual dot product of tensors and vectors as explained in the glossary of symbols. This weak formulation of the equilibrium equations is very convenient and does not require any differentiability on the stress field T^φ (ANTMAN and OSBORN [1979]).

Unfortunately, in finite elasticity, Ω^φ is unknown and may be very different from the known reference configuration Ω. Therefore, it is more convenient to rewrite the equilibrium equations on Ω, through the change of variables

$$x^\varphi = x + u(x).$$

Doing this, we get

$$0 = \int_{\Omega^\varphi} T^\varphi : \frac{\partial v^\varphi}{\partial x^\varphi}\, dx^\varphi - \int_{\Omega^\varphi} f^\varphi \cdot v^\varphi\, dx^\varphi - \int_{\Gamma^\varphi} g^\varphi \cdot v^\varphi\, da^\varphi$$

$$= \int_\Omega T^\varphi : \frac{\partial v^\varphi}{\partial x} \frac{\partial x}{\partial x^\varphi} \left|\frac{dx^\varphi}{dx}\right| dx - \int_\Omega f^\varphi \cdot v^\varphi \left|\frac{dx^\varphi}{dx}\right| dx$$

$$- \int_\Gamma g^\varphi \cdot v^\varphi \frac{da^\varphi}{da} da$$

$$= \int_\Omega \left[T^\varphi \left(\frac{\partial x}{\partial x^\varphi}\right)^T \left|\frac{dx^\varphi}{dx}\right|\right] : \frac{\partial v^\varphi}{\partial x} dx - \int_\Omega \left(f^\varphi \left|\frac{dx^\varphi}{dx}\right|\right) \cdot v^\varphi \, dx$$

$$- \int_\Gamma \left(g^\varphi \frac{da^\varphi}{da} \right) \cdot v^\varphi \, da.$$

By setting

$F(x) = (\partial x^\varphi / \partial x)(x)$

$\quad = \mathrm{Id} + \nabla u(x) =$ deformation gradient,

$T(x) = T^\varphi(x^\varphi(x)) F(x)^{-T} \det(F(x))$

$\quad =$ first Piola–Kirchhoff stress tensor,

$v(x) = v^\varphi(x^\varphi(x))$,

$f(x) = f^\varphi(x^\varphi(x)) \det(F(x))$

$\quad =$ density of body forces in the reference configuration,

$g(x) = g^\varphi \, da^\varphi / da$

$\quad =$ density of surface tractions in the reference configuration,

we finally obtain the following equilibrium equations in the reference configuration:

$$\int_\Omega T : \nabla v \, dx = \int_\Omega f \cdot v \, dx + \int_\Gamma g \cdot v \, da \quad \forall v : \bar{\Omega} \to \mathbb{E}. \tag{3.1}$$

Once integrated by parts, (3.1) reduces to the strong form

$\operatorname{div} T + f = 0 \quad$ in Ω,

$Tn = g \quad$ on Γ,

with div T denoting the divergence of the stress tensor T.

4. Constitutive laws

In order to compute the equilibrium positions of the considered body as a function of the external loads f and g, it is necessary to complement the above equilibrium equations by adequate constitutive laws. These laws relate the stress tensor T to characteristic kinematic variables and characterize the mechanical properties of the material of which the continuum is composed.

A material is said to be *elastic* if and only if its stress tensor T at a point x is a function of x and of the deformation gradient F at x. In other words, elastic materials are characterized by the existence at each point x of a response function

$$\hat{T} : (x, F) \in \Omega \times \mathbb{M}^3_+ \mapsto T(x) = \hat{T}(x, F) \in \mathbb{M}^3.$$

Here we have used the notation

$$\mathbb{M}^3_+ = \{F \in \mathbb{M}^3 = \mathbb{E} \otimes \mathbb{E},\ \det F > 0\}.$$

The relation

$$T(x) = \hat{T}(x, F)$$

is called the *constitutive equation* of the material. It has to be defined at each point x of $\bar{\Omega}$ and for each orientation-preserving deformation gradient $F \in \mathbb{M}^3_+$. The material is said to be *homogeneous* when this relation is independent of the particle x.

Such constitutive laws are essentially determined by experiments. Unfortunately, the experiments made on given elastic materials only cover a narrow range of possible values of the variable F, which means that our knowledge of the constitutive relations is quite imperfect. Moreover, important experimental phenomena occurring in plasticity and in fracture are time-dependent and do not enter into the framework of elastic constitutive laws. Despite these imperfections, elastic models are nevertheless very useful and lead to quite accurate predictions in many engineering applications. These models are also getting very popular in biomechanics and we refer to HANNA, JOUVE and CIARLET [1990] for an application of these models in opthalmology.

In addition to elasticity, it is usually assumed that homogeneous elastic materials do not dissipate energy during cyclic homogeneous deformations. This means that for any admissible deformation field $\varphi(x, t) = F(t)x + c(t)$ which is τ periodic in time, the work

$$W_{\text{cycle}} = \int_0^\tau \int_\Omega \hat{T}(F) : \dot{F}\ \mathrm{d}x\ \mathrm{d}t$$

developed by the stresses T during one time period must be equal to zero. Materials satisfying this additional assumption are said to be *hyperelastic* and are the only elastic materials considered in practice.

4.1. Hyperelastic compressible materials

For a compressible material, an admissible homogeneous deformation is an arbitrary map $\varphi(x, t) = F(t)x + c(t)$ such that $\det F > 0$. Then, by the change of variables $t \mapsto F(t)$, the nullity of W_{cycle} reads

$$0 = W_{\text{cycle}}$$

$$= \int_0^\tau \int_\Omega \hat{T}(F) : \dot{F} \, dx \, dt$$

$$= \text{vol}(\Omega) \int_{F(0)}^{F(\tau)=F(0)} \hat{T}(F) : dF,$$

this for any closed path $t \mapsto F(t)$ defined in $\mathbb{M}_+^3$. From an elementary result in differential calculus, this identity implies that there exists a function $\hat{W}(F)$ whose gradient is equal to $\hat{T}$. In other words, we must have

$$\hat{T}(F) = \frac{\partial \hat{W}}{\partial F}(F). \tag{4.1}$$

The function $\hat{W}(F)$ is the material *stored energy* function, and corresponds to the density of elastic energy locally stored in the body during the deformation φ. Since the material properties might vary from one particle to another, $\hat{W}$ is in general a function of x and F. Thus (4.1) is to be read pointwise in x as

$$T(x) = \frac{\partial}{\partial F} \hat{W}(x, F).$$

Any function $\hat{W}$ will not be suitable for defining the internal elastic energy. From the *axiom of frame indifference*, $\hat{W}$ must not depend on the frame in which the deformation φ is observed; in other words, for any rotation Q of $\mathbb{E}$, the change of φ into $Q\varphi$ must not affect the value of $\hat{W}$. In terms of deformation gradients, this is equivalent to

$$\hat{W}(x, QF) = \hat{W}(x, F) \quad \forall Q \ \forall F \in \mathbb{M}_+^3.$$

With the choice

$$Q = \sqrt{C} F^{-1},$$

which is a rotation since

$$Q^T Q = F^{-T} C F^{-1} = F^{-T} F^T F F^{-1} = \text{Id},$$

the axiom of frame indifference reduces to

$$\hat{W}(x, F) = \hat{W}(x, \sqrt{C}) = \tilde{W}(x, C).$$

In other words, the axiom of frame indifference expresses that the internal elastic energy is only a function of the right Cauchy–Green tensor.

As a consequence, from the chain rule and from the symmetry of the tensor C, we may write

$$\frac{\partial \hat{W}}{\partial F} : dF = dW$$

$$= \frac{\partial \tilde{W}}{\partial C} : dC$$

$$= \frac{\partial \tilde{W}}{\partial C} : (dF^T F + F^T dF)$$

$$= \left(\frac{\partial \tilde{W}}{\partial C}\right)^T : (dF^T F)^T + \frac{\partial \tilde{W}}{\partial C} : (F^T dF)$$

$$= 2\frac{\partial \tilde{W}}{\partial C} : F^T dF$$

$$= 2F\frac{\partial \tilde{W}}{\partial C} : dF.$$

By identification, the constitutive law (4.1) reduces then to

$$T = \frac{\partial \tilde{W}}{\partial F} = 2F\frac{\partial \tilde{W}}{\partial C}. \tag{4.2}$$

In particular, the Cauchy stress tensor T^φ is now given by

$$T^\varphi = (\det F)^{-1} T F^T$$

$$= 2(\det F)^{-1} F \frac{\partial \tilde{W}}{\partial C} F^T, \tag{4.3}$$

and is automatically symmetric.

The constitutive law (4.2) is much simpler for isotropic materials, that is materials which are invariant in any local rotation of the body. Indeed, such materials verify the Rivlin–Eriksen representation theorem:

THEOREM 4.1. *For any isotropic hyperelastic material, the elastic potential $\hat{W}$ satisfies*

$$\hat{W}(x, F) = W(x, I_1(C), I_2(C), I_3(C)). \tag{4.4}$$

PROOF. Since isotropic materials are invariant in any local rotation Q of the body, their energy potential satisfies

$$\hat{W}(x, FQ) = \hat{W}(x, F),$$

for all Q, and for all F in $\mathbb{M}_+^3$. Equivalently, in terms of C, we have

$$\tilde{W}(x, Q^T C Q) = \tilde{W}(x, C) \quad \forall Q.$$

Taking for Q the matrix built with the eigenvectors of the matrix C (put in any order), we deduce from the above identity that $\tilde{W}$ is a symmetric function of the eigenvalues of the matrix C, that is a function of the invariants of C. This concludes the proof. □

As a consequence of the Rivlin–Eriksen theorem, the stress tensors T and T^φ are easy to compute in isotropic elasticity and are given by

$$T(x) = 2F\left[\left(\frac{\partial W}{\partial I_1} + I_1\frac{\partial W}{\partial I_2}\right) \mathrm{Id} - \frac{\partial W}{\partial I_2}C + I_3\frac{\partial W}{\partial I_3}C^{-1}\right],$$

$$T^{\varphi}(x) = 2I_3^{-1/2}\left[\left(\frac{\partial W}{\partial I_1} + I_1\frac{\partial W}{\partial I_2}\right)B - \frac{\partial W}{\partial I_2}B^2 + I_3\frac{\partial W}{\partial I_3}\text{Id}\right].$$

Observe now that in any orthonormal basis, the Cauchy stress tensor T^{φ} and the left Cauchy–Green strain tensor B have the same principal directions. Observe also that since all compressible materials are sensitive to volume changes, the stored energy function W will always depend on I_3 and that therefore the stress tensor T is always a nonlinear function of the deformation gradient F.

EXAMPLE 4.1. There are well-known classical examples of such compressible hyperelastic isotropic materials. They are characterized by the associated internal elastic energy $\hat{W}(F)$ which will be given as a symmetric function of the invariants I_i of C. The real numbers C_{ij}, μ_i or α_j which appear below are material constants.

The simplest law uses a quadratic isotropic function of the Green–Saint-Venant strain tensor $E = \frac{1}{2}(C - \text{Id})$. It was proposed by SAINT-VENANT [1844] and Kirchhoff [1852]. A *Saint-Venant–Kirchhoff material* is characterized by the stored energy

$$\hat{W}(F) = \frac{\lambda}{2}(\text{tr}\,E)^2 + \mu\,\text{tr}(E^2),$$

where λ and μ are the so-called Lamé constants classically introduced in linear elasticity. Because of their simplicity, these Saint-Venant–Kirchhoff materials are very popular in actual computations (ODEN [1972], WASHIZU [1975]). Unfortunately, such materials can reach infinite compression rates with finite energy and do not satisfy the polyconvexity assumptions used in the existence theory. These remarks have led CIARLET and GEYMONAT [1982] to propose a slightly more complicated stored energy function correcting these drawbacks and given by

$$\hat{W}(F) = C_1(I_1 - 3) + C_2(I_2 - 3) + a(I_3 - 1) - (C_1 + 2C_2 + a)\ln I_3.$$

In another direction, OGDEN [1976] has introduced a different expression of $\hat{W}$ in order to fit experimental results obtained for rubbers. His new expression is given as a function of the eigenvalues λ_j^2 of the strain tensor C by

$$\hat{W}(F) = \sum_{i=1}^{3}\frac{\mu_i}{\alpha_i}\sum_j \lambda_j^{\alpha_i} + \mu_4\alpha_4^{-2}J^{-\alpha_4} + \left(\mu_4\alpha_4^{-1} - \sum_{i=1}^{3}\mu_i\right)\ln J$$
$$+\mu_5 J^{2/3}(J-1)\sum_j \lambda_j^{-2}.$$

For all the above examples, the second Piola–Kirchhoff stress tensor

$$\tilde{\Sigma} = F^{-1}T$$

satisfies a constitutive relation of the type

$$\tilde{\Sigma} = \lambda(\text{tr}\,E)\,\text{Id} + 2\mu E + o(\|E\|^2).$$

This means that all these examples correspond to a stress-free reference configuration (zero stress for zero deformation) and reduce to the standard linearly elastic materials (Hooke's law) when the deformations are small ($\|E\| \ll 1$).

4.2. Hyperelastic incompressible materials

For incompressible materials, any deformation is volume-preserving, and therefore an arbitrary admissible deformation is an arbitrary map $\varphi(x,t) = F(t)x + c(t)$ such that $\det F = 1$. Then the nullity of the dissipated energy W_{cycle} for any closed path $[F(0), F(\tau) = F(0)]$ defined in the admissible set

$$M_1^3 = \{F \in \mathbb{E} \otimes \mathbb{E}, \ \det F = 1\}$$

classically implies that there exists a function $\hat{W}$ and an arbitrary scalar p (the *hydrostatic pressure*) such that

$$\hat{T}(F) = \frac{\partial \hat{W}}{\partial F}(F) - p\frac{\partial \det F}{\partial F} = \frac{\partial \hat{W}}{\partial F}(F) - pF^{-\text{T}}. \tag{4.5}$$

As for compressible materials, the axiom of frame indifference implies that $\hat{W}$ is a function of the right Cauchy–Green strain tensor only. The constitutive law (4.5) therefore becomes

$$T = 2F\frac{\partial \tilde{W}}{\partial C} - pF^{-\text{T}},$$

$$T^\varphi = 2F\frac{\partial \tilde{W}}{\partial C}F^{\text{T}} - p\,\text{Id}.$$

Similarly, for isotropic materials, $\tilde{W}$ is again a function of the invariants of C only. Thus, in this case we have simply

$$\frac{\partial \tilde{W}}{\partial C} = \left(\frac{\partial W}{\partial I_1} + I_1\frac{\partial W}{\partial I_2}\right)\text{Id} - \frac{\partial W}{\partial I_2}C,$$

$$T = 2\left(\frac{\partial W}{\partial I_1} + I_1\frac{\partial W}{\partial I_2}\right)F - 2\frac{\partial W}{\partial I_2}FC - pF^{-\text{T}}.$$

In all these constitutive laws, the hydrostatic pressure p is an additional unknown, and is the Lagrange multiplier associated with the additional nonlinear kinematic constraint

$$J = \det F = 1.$$

EXAMPLE 4.2. There are several popular examples of hyperelastic incompressible isotropic materials. They are characterized by the associated stored energy function $\hat{W}(F)$ which is given as a symmetric function of the first two invariants I_1 and I_2 of the strain tensor C. In our examples, the real numbers C_{ij}, μ_i or α_j denote material constants.

The simplest example is the neo-Hookean material (TRELOAR [1975]) corresponding to the choice

$$\hat{W}(F) = C_{10}(I_1 - 3).$$

If we add a linear term in I_2 to this function, we get the well-known Mooney–Rivlin materials (MOONEY [1940], RIVLIN [1948]) whose energy is given by

$$\hat{W}(F) = C_{10}(I_1 - 3) + C_{01}(I_2 - 3).$$

For rubbers, the numerical values of the above constants are typically

$$\begin{cases} C_{10} = 0.183 \, \text{MPa}, \\ C_{01} = 0.0034 \, \text{MPa}. \end{cases}$$

This last expression was further generalized by HAINES and WILSON [1979] who have proposed a third-order polynomial in I_i which fits well to numerous experimental data, and which is given by

$$\hat{W}(F) = C_{10}(I_1 - 3) + C_{01}(I_2 - 3)$$

$$+ C_{20}(I_1 - 3)^2 + C_{02}(I_2 - 3)^2$$

$$+ C_{11}(I_1 - 3)(I_2 - 3) + C_{30}(I_1 - 3)^3.$$

Another possibility is to use explicitly the eigenvalues λ_j^2 of the tensor C as proposed by OGDEN [1972]:

$$\hat{W}(F) = \sum_{i=1}^{n} \mu_i \alpha_i^{-1} \left(\sum_j \lambda_j^{\alpha_i} - 3 \right).$$

The numerical values proposed by Ogden were:

$$\begin{cases} n = 3, \quad \alpha_1 = 1.3, \quad \alpha_2 = 5, \quad \alpha_3 = 2, \\ \mu_1 = 0.63 \, \text{MPa}, \quad \mu_2 = 0.0012 \, \text{MPa}, \\ \mu_3 = -0.01 \, \text{MPa}, \end{cases}$$

and mainly correspond to rubbers.

A last example was introduced by KNOWLES and STERNBERG [1980] to study a possible loss of ellipticity in the equilibrium equations of finite elasticity. They proposed the stored energy function

$$\hat{W}(F) = \frac{\mu}{2\alpha} \left\{ \left[1 + \frac{\alpha}{n}(I_1 - 3) \right]^n - 1 \right\}.$$

A more complete list and description of hyperelastic materials is given in OGDEN [1984], in DAVET [1985], or in VAN DEN BOGERT [1991].

REMARK 4.1. The above constitutive laws can be updated to take into account possible reinforcing fibers embedded in the material. For example, for a Mooney–Rivlin material reinforced by fibers parallel to the direction e_α, we will propose an energy function given by

$$\hat{W}(F) = C_{10}(I_1 - 3) + C_{01}(I_2 - 3) + \mu(C_{\alpha\alpha} - 1)^2,$$

with $C_{\alpha\alpha} = |Fe_\alpha|$ measuring the material dilatation along the direction e_α.

4.3. Nearly incompressible materials

To any incompressible material with stored energy $\hat{W}_{\text{inc}}(x, F)$, one can always associate a nearly incompressible material with constitutive law

$$T = \frac{\partial \hat{W}_\varepsilon}{\partial F}(x, \text{Id} + \nabla u) \tag{4.6}$$

and with stored energy

$$\hat{W}_\varepsilon(x, F) = \hat{W}_{\text{inc}}(x, (\det F)^{-1/3} F) + \frac{1}{2\varepsilon}(\det F - 1)^2 \tag{4.7}$$

$$= \hat{W}_0(x, F) + \frac{1}{2\varepsilon}(\det F - 1)^2.$$

For example, to a Mooney–Rivlin material, one would associate a compressible material with energy

$$\hat{W}_\varepsilon(x, F) = C_{10}(\det F)^{-2/3}|F|^2 + C_{01}(\det F)^{-4/3}|\text{cof} F|^2$$
$$+ \frac{1}{2\varepsilon}(\det F - 1)^2.$$

The terms $(\det F)^{-2/3}|F|^2$ and $(\det F)^{-4/3}|\text{cof} F|^2$ are the so-called reduced invariants of the deformation gradient F.

These new materials formally reduce to the corresponding incompressible materials for the choice $\varepsilon = 0$ and $p = -\varepsilon^{-1}(\det F - 1)$. They are often preferred to the original incompressible materials for two reasons:

- they take into account the small compressibility effects that are experimentally observed for many hyperelastic materials (OGDEN [1976]);
- they lead to equilibrium problems whose solutions are very close to the solutions of the corresponding incompressible problems but which are simpler to compute. Indeed they do not involve the hydrostatic pressure p or the incompressibility constraint.

REMARK 4.2. In (4.7), the compressible term $(1/2\varepsilon)(\det F - 1)^2$ can be replaced by a more complicated function of $\det F$, depending on the available experimental data. What is critical, however, is the expression

$$\hat{W}_0(x, F) = \hat{W}_{\text{inc}}(x, (\det F)^{-1/3} F)$$

which ensures that stresses in the reference configuration are zero. The choice

$$W_0(x, F) = \hat{W}_{\text{inc}}(x, F)$$

will not correspond in general to a stress-free reference configuration.

REMARK 4.3. The simplicity of the equilibrium problems in the nearly incompressible case has a price: the finite-element approximation is more delicate and the condition number of the resulting discrete algebraic problem is much higher.

CHAPTER II

Mathematical Analysis

As stated earlier, the central problem in nonlinear three-dimensional elasticity consists in finding the equilibrium position of an elastic body when it is subjected to applied forces. The corresponding mathematical model is obtained by writing the equilibrium equations introduced in Section 3 and defined on the reference configuration by

$$\text{div}\,\hat{T}(x,F) + f = 0 \text{ in } \Omega,$$
$$\hat{T}(x,F)n = g \text{ on } \Gamma.$$

Here, $\hat{T}(x,F)$ is the elastic nonlinear constitutive equation defining the first Piola–Kirchhoff stress tensor T as a known function of the deformation gradient

$$F = \nabla\varphi = \text{Id} + \nabla u.$$

This model is complemented by boundary conditions which are of two possible types:

(i) displacements: the displacement $u(x)$ is imposed to a prescribed value $u_0(x)$ on a part Γ_0 of the boundary Γ;
(ii) traction: the traction force g is prescribed on the part Γ_1 of the boundary Γ.

In general, the applied tractions g are prescribed as a given function of the point x and displacement $u(x)$. For example, for an applied pressure of intensity π, we have

$$g(x) = -\pi(x)[\det F(x)]F(x)^{-T}n.$$

More complex boundary conditions can also be considered and will be discussed later.

In any case, we obtain a nonlinear boundary value problem, defined on Ω, whose unknown is the displacement field u. In the terminology of partial differential equations, this resulting problem is a second-order quasilinear equation, whose higher-order terms are nonlinear functions of the gradient of u. Such quasilinear partial differential equations are hard to analyze mathematically. Multiple solutions can be produced easily, as we will see later in simple examples.

The existence of solutions to such problems can be approached in two ways. The more general approach is due to BALL [1977] and treats the hyperelastic case with conservative loading (loads deriving from a potential V). This approach writes the initial boundary value problem as the problem of finding the stationary points of the total energy

$$J(u) = \int_\Omega \hat{W}(x, \text{Id} + \nabla u) \, dx + V(u)$$

when u varies on a set $\mathbb{U}$ of admissible displacement fields. Because of frame indifference, the function $\hat{W}$ cannot be convex. Nevertheless, we will see that $\hat{W}$ can be assumed to be polyconvex. Minimizing sequences of J can then be constructed which, because of polyconvexity, converge weakly in an adequate product space towards global minimizers of J. The existence results of Ball, although very general, lead to two major unsolved problems:

(i) there is no known result of continuity of the global minimizer u as a function of the data;
(ii) the minimizers are found in $W^{1,s}(\Omega)$ for some $\infty > s > 3/2$, and cannot be proved to satisfy the original boundary value problem even in a weak sense. This would require more regularity than is presently guaranteed.

The second approach to existence results is based on the implicit function theorem. It was first used by STOPPELLI [1954] and VAN BUREN [1968]. A complete proof of existence using the implicit function theorem was then given by VALENT [1978], MARSDEN and HUGHES [1978] and CIARLET and DESTUYNDER [1979]. Unfortunately, this approach can only prove the existence of solutions for special problems, such as the pure displacement problem ($\Gamma_0 = \Gamma$) and for small data. Indeed, the application of the implicit function theorem is always local and requires the differentiability of the operator $\mathcal{A}$ of nonlinear elasticity and the surjectivity of the derivative $\mathcal{A}'(0)$. This cannot be satisfied if we define $\mathcal{A}$ on $W^{1,p}(\Omega)$ (VALENT and ZAMPIERI [1977]); this is satisfied if we define $\mathcal{A}$ on $W^{2,p}(\Omega)$ but then the surjectivity of $\mathcal{A}'(0)$ requires the H^2 regularity of the solutions of the linearized problems and hence pure Dirichlet data, or very special distributions of boundary conditions.

All this analysis is detailed in the present chapter. We first define the boundary value problem to be considered and describe formally several simple examples to illustrate its nonlinear structure. Next, this boundary value problem is written in a weak form which will be used for its numerical solution. The existence theory of J. Ball is then described in two steps: introduction of the minimization formulation and construction of a minimizer. We conclude this chapter by a brief description of the existence results which can be obtained with the implicit function theorem.

The reader interested in further details should refer to the fundamental paper of BALL [1977] and to the recent books of CIARLET [1988] and VALENT [1990].

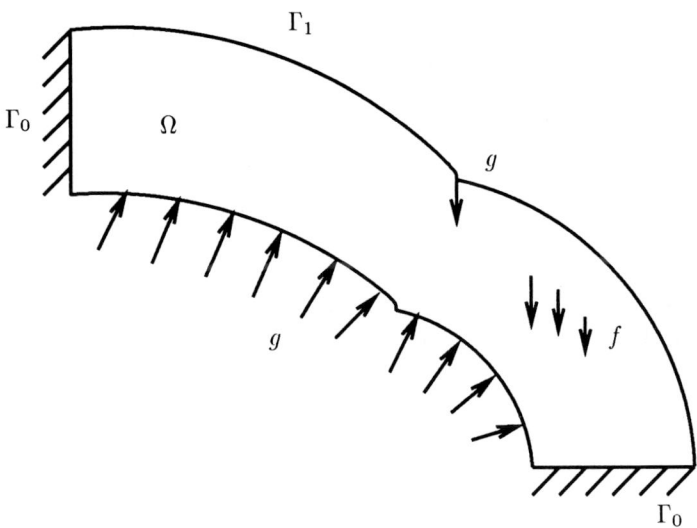

FIG. 5.1. Description of the boundary value problem. The body is fixed on Γ_0, surface tractions g are applied on Γ_1, body forces f are exerted inside.

5. Definition of the boundary value problem

Equilibrium problems in finite elasticity consist in determining the final equilibrium position $\varphi(x) = x + u(x)$ of any particle x of an elastic body which occupies a known domain Ω in its reference configuration and which is subjected to large deformations due to the application of given external loads and imposed displacements (Fig. 5.1). In a typical equilibrium problem in finite elasticity, the reference configuration Ω, the stored energy function $\hat{W}(x, F)$ and the body forces f are given. Moreover, given surface tractions g are imposed on the part Γ_1 of the boundary Γ and a prescribed displacement u_0 is imposed on the remaining part Γ_0 of Γ. In a general setting, the forces f and g are given functions of the displacement field u.

In such a problem, the unknowns are the displacement field u and the stress field T. They satisfy the weak equation of equilibrium (3.1)

$$\int_\Omega T : \nabla v \, dx = \int_\Omega f \cdot v \, dx + \int_\Gamma g \cdot v \, da \quad \forall v \colon \bar{\Omega} \to \mathbb{E},$$

the constitutive law

$$T(x) = \frac{\partial \hat{W}}{\partial F}(x, \mathrm{Id} + \nabla u) \quad \text{(compressible case)},$$

$$T(x) = \frac{\partial \hat{W}}{\partial F}(x, \text{Id} + \nabla u) - p(\text{Id} + \nabla u)^{-T},$$

$\det(\text{Id} + \nabla u) = 1$ (incompressible case),

and the boundary conditions

$u = u_0$ on Γ_0,

g given on Γ_1.

6. Examples of solutions

We briefly describe below three simple situations which illustrate the nonlinear structure of the considered problem of equilibrium. The first situation considers the buckling of an elastic bar as described in Fig. 6.1. For small compressions, there is only one stable symmetric solution with small transversal displacements. When the imposed compression increases, a bifurcation occurs leading to the appearance of two types of solutions. The first one stays symmetric, corresponds

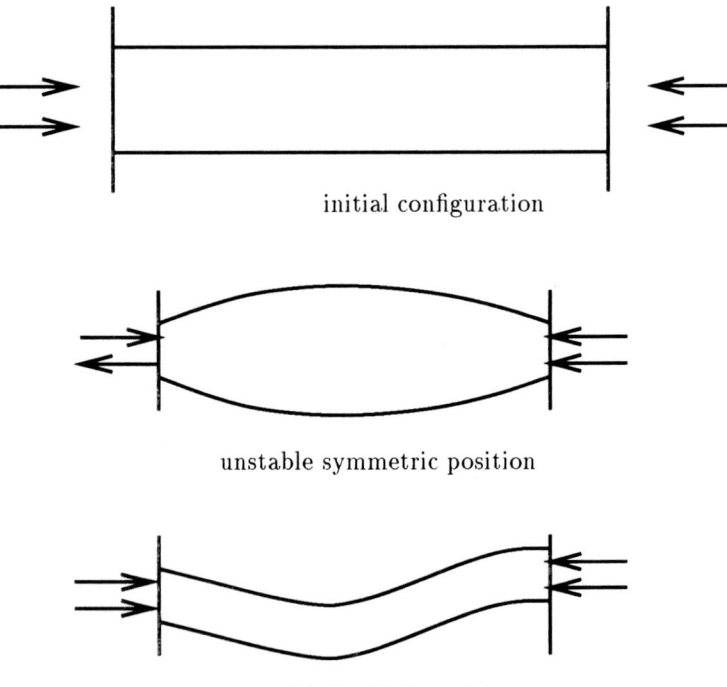

Fig. 6.1. A physical situation leading to buckling. An elastic bar under compression with its unstable symmetric solution and its stable buckled solution with large lateral displacements.

to a small transversal motion, and is unstable. Then, for each transversal direction e_y, there is a stable solution associated with a large transversal displacement along the direction e_y. Such a situation is described in detail in ANTMAN and KENNEY [1981] in the framework of one-dimensional elasticity. It is also illustrated in the numerical examples to be given in Section 28. Bifurcation can also be observed when considering elastic rotating bodies (see ODEN and RABIER [1989]).

The second example corresponds to the cavitation of an elastic sphere under traction as described in Fig. 6.2 and studied in BALL [1982]. For sufficiently large tractions, the stable equilibrium position of the sphere has a hole in its center.

The last example is the pure traction problem proposed by RIVLIN [1948] and described in Fig. 6.3, GURTIN [1981a]. It considers a cube made of a neo-Hookean material. A given normal traction $g = -\pi n$ is exerted on each face, and it stays constant during the deformation (dead loading). Assuming the resulting deformation to be homogeneous and F given by

$$F = \begin{pmatrix} \lambda_1 & 0 & 0 \\ 0 & \lambda_2 & 0 \\ 0 & 0 & \lambda_3 \end{pmatrix}$$

we can reduce the boundary value problem to the solution of the algebraic system

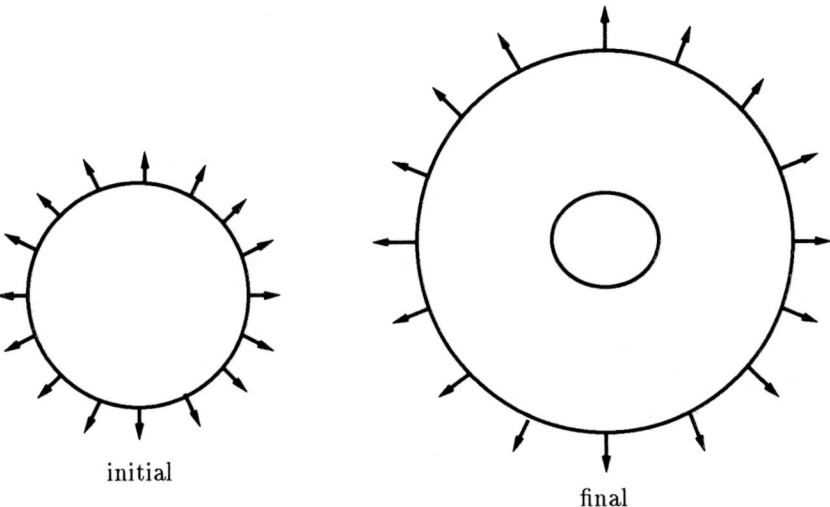

FIG. 6.2. A physical situation leading to cavitation. Under the action of traction, the stable equilibrium position of the sphere can be a position having a hole in its center.

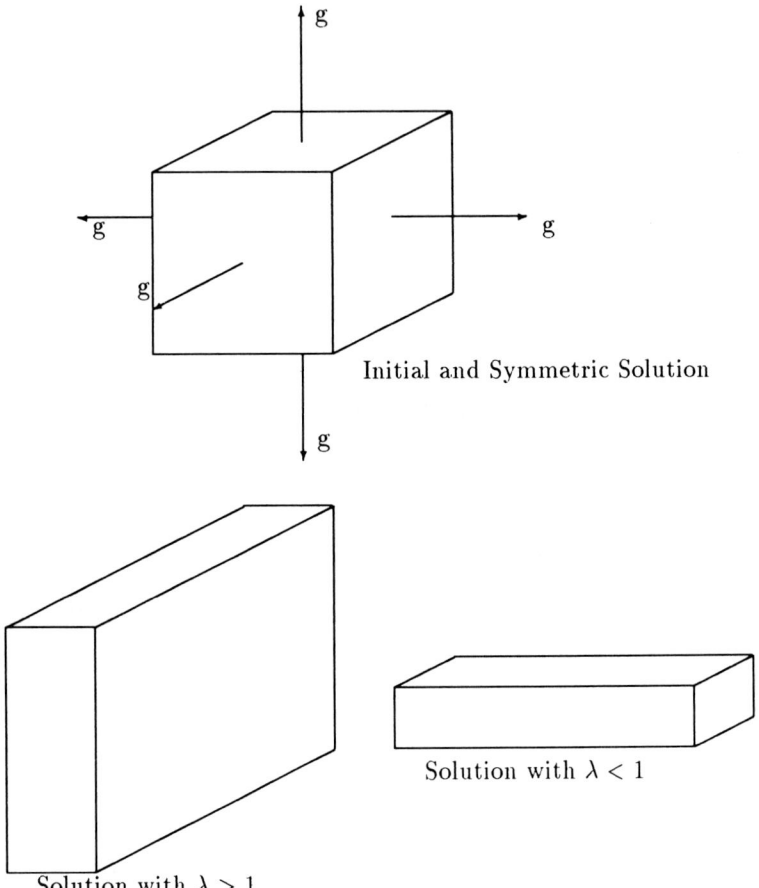

FIG. 6.3. The Rivlin cube. Loading and three different solutions. For $\lambda > 1$, two sides are elongated. For $\lambda < 1$, the same sides are shortened. For $\lambda = 1$, all sides keep the same length.

$$2C_{10}\lambda_1^2 - p = \pi\lambda_1,$$
$$2C_{10}\lambda_2^2 - p = \pi\lambda_2,$$
$$2C_{10}\lambda_3^2 - p = \pi\lambda_3,$$
$$\det F = \lambda_1\lambda_2\lambda_3 = 1.$$

For $\pi > 3(2)^{1/3}C_{10}$, there are seven different solutions to this system, given by

$$\lambda_i = \lambda_j = \lambda,$$
$$\lambda_k = \lambda^{-2},$$

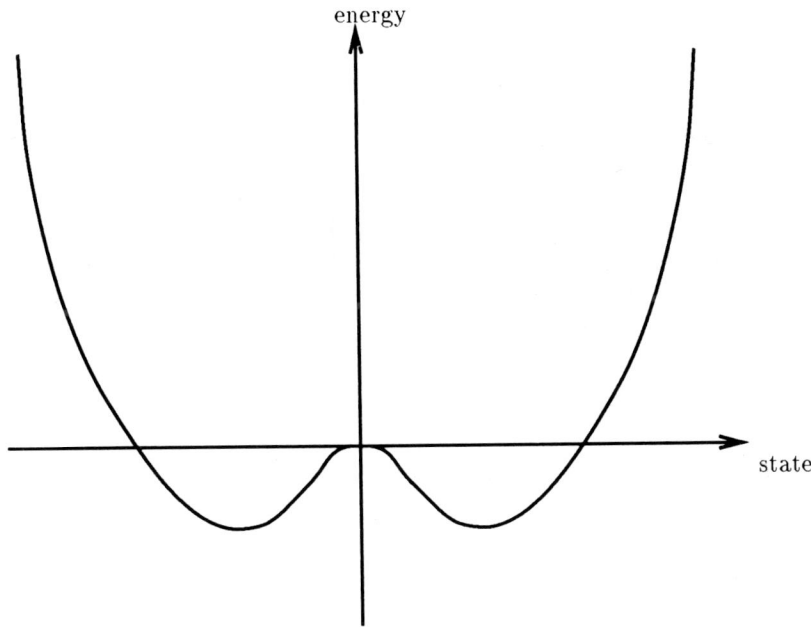

Fig. 6.4. An energy curve with dimples.

with $\lambda = 1$ or λ solution of the cubic equation

$$\lambda^3 - \frac{\pi}{2C_{10}}\lambda^2 + 1 = 0.$$

Replacing the neo-Hookean material by a Mooney–Rivlin material leads to an even larger set of solutions (BALL and SCHAEFFER [1982]). An even more complex situation is obtained for nonconvex energy functions with dimples (Fig. 6.4). Such dimples are used to model phase transitions in solids (JAMES [1985]) but will not be considered here.

7. Weak formulations of equilibrium problems

7.1. The compressible case

In the compressible case, the elimination of the stress tensor T between the principle of virtual power (3.1) and the constitutive law (4.1) characterizes the displacement field u at equilibrium as solution of the weak problem

$$\int_\Omega \frac{\partial \hat{W}}{\partial F}(x, \mathrm{Id} + \nabla u) : \nabla v \, dx = \int_\Omega f \cdot v \, dx + \int_{\Gamma_1} g \cdot v \, da, \qquad (7.1)$$

$$\forall v \in \mathbb{V}, \ (u - u_0) \in \mathbb{V},$$

where the space $\mathbb{V}$ of test functions is of the form

$$\mathbb{V} = \{v \in W^{1,s}(\Omega; \mathbb{E}), \ v|_{\Gamma_0} = 0\}. \qquad (7.2)$$

The number $s \geqslant 1$ is such that the integrals of (7.1) make sense for any choice of v and u. In view of the existence results of BALL [1977], the definition of $\mathbb{V}$ will in fact be slightly modified, but such a change will not affect our numerical strategy.

7.2. The incompressible case

In the incompressible case, the elimination of the stress tensor T yields

$$\int_\Omega \left[\frac{\partial \hat{W}}{\partial F}(x, \mathrm{Id} + \nabla u) - p \frac{\partial \det}{\partial F}(\mathrm{Id} + \nabla u) \right] : \nabla v \, dx$$

$$= \int_\Omega f \cdot v \, dx + \int_{\Gamma_1} g \cdot v \, da \quad \forall v \in \mathbb{V}, \ (u - u_0) \in \mathbb{V},$$

$$\det(\mathrm{Id} + \nabla u) = 1.$$

Writing the above incompressibility condition in a weak form leads then to the following weak formulation of equilibrium problems in incompressible finite elasticity:

$$\int_\Omega \frac{\partial \hat{W}}{\partial F}(x, \mathrm{Id} + \nabla u) : \nabla v \, dx - \int_\Omega p \frac{\partial \det}{\partial F}(\mathrm{Id} + \nabla u) : \nabla v \, dx$$

$$= \int_\Omega f \cdot v \, dx + \int_{\Gamma_1} g \cdot v \, da \quad \forall v \in \mathbb{V}, \ (u - u_0) \in \mathbb{V}, \qquad (7.3)$$

$$\int_\Omega q[\det(\mathrm{Id} + \nabla u) - 1] \, dx = 0 \quad \forall q \in \mathbb{P}, \ p \in \mathbb{P}. \qquad (7.4)$$

Above, $\mathbb{V}$ is as defined in (7.2) and $\mathbb{P}$ is of the form

$$\mathbb{P} = L^{s^*}(\Omega; \mathbb{R}), \quad \frac{1}{3s} + \frac{1}{s^*} = 1. \qquad (7.5)$$

REMARK 7.1. Formulations (7.1) and (7.3)–(7.4) do not impose any restrictions on the mechanical model. They allow for any type of hyperelastic constitutive law, the reference configuration Ω may be of arbitrary shape and does not have to be stress-free, and the external loads f and g may depend on the displacement field u. Unfortunately, no general existence theory is available for such formulations. In fact, the existence theory of Ball deals with minimization problems which are a bit more restrictive and are equivalent to (7.1) and (7.3)–(7.4) in a formal sense only.

REMARK 7.2. As written (7.1) and (7.3)–(7.4) correspond to genuine three-dimensional situations ($\mathbb{E} = \mathbb{R}^N, N = 3, \Omega \subset \mathbb{R}^3$). They will also model *plane-strain* situations (situations which are invariant along x_3) simply by setting $N = 2$, defining $\Omega \subset \mathbb{R}^2$ as the section of the reference configuration by the plane $x_3 = 0$ and by considering only functions $v(x_1, x_2)$ and $u(x_1, x_2)$ defined over Ω with values in $\mathbb{R}^2$ to represent respectively the virtual and the real in-plane displacements of the particle $\{x_1, x_2, 0\}$ of the body. As for plane-stresses situations, they can be reduced to plane-strain problems by an adequate change of the energy potential $\hat{W}$ (ODEN [1972]).

REMARK 7.3. The weak formulation (7.3)–(7.4) can easily handle hyperelastic bodies whose part Ω_1 is incompressible and whose part $\Omega - \Omega_1$ is compressible. In such a case, the integrals involving p and q will have to be taken over the incompressible part Ω_1 only and not over the whole domain Ω.

REMARK 7.4. The proposed formulations do not guarantee the global injectivity of the transformation $x + u$ at the solution. The solution of the compressible problem is not even guaranteed to correspond to an orientation preserving mapping $x + u$. Such an omission is standard in numerical computations: in most cases it is much easier to verify that the numerical solution obtained satisfies these physical restrictions than to impose these restrictions during the whole numerical process. The case with a global injectivity constraint is studied in BALL [1981] for the pure displacement problem and by CIARLET and NEČAS [1987] in the general case. They showed that injectivity is ensured if the constraint

$$\int_\Omega \det F \, \mathrm{d}x \leqslant \mathrm{vol}(\varphi(\Omega)),$$

is imposed in the set of admissible deformations (with $\varphi(x) = x + u(x)$).

8. The minimization approach

In conservative loading, the imposed external loads f and g represent the gradient in $L^{s^*}(\Omega) \times L^{s^*}(\Gamma_1)$ of a given potential energy $[-V(u)]$ (with $s^* = (1 - 1/s)^{-1}$). For example, when f and g are independent of the displacement field u (dead loading), we simply have

$$V(u) = -\int_\Omega f \cdot u \, \mathrm{d}x - \int_{\Gamma_1} g \cdot u \, \mathrm{d}a.$$

For a pressure force of a fixed intensity π applied between two fixed boundaries (Fig. 8.1), we similarly have (CIARLET [1988], p. 83)

$$V(u) = -\frac{\pi}{3} \int_{\Gamma_1} (\text{cof}(\text{Id}+\nabla u)n) \cdot (x+u) \, da.$$

For such conservative loadings and hyperelastic materials, we can define the total *potential energy* of the body by

$$J(u) = \int_\Omega \hat{W}(x, \text{Id}+\nabla u) \, dx + V(u). \tag{8.1}$$

We then introduce the set $\mathbb{U}$ of *kinematically admissible* displacement fields as

$$\mathbb{U} = \Big\{ v, v - u_0 \in \mathbb{V}, \; H = \text{cof}(\text{Id}+\nabla v) \in L^q(\Omega; \mathbb{M}^3), \\ \delta = \det(\text{Id}+\nabla v) \in L^r(\Omega), \det(\text{Id}+\nabla v) > 0 \text{ a.e. on } \Omega \Big\}, \tag{8.2}$$

in the compressible case and

$$\mathbb{U} = \Big\{ v, v - u_0 \in \mathbb{V}, \; H = \text{cof}(\text{Id}+\nabla v) \in L^q(\Omega; \mathbb{M}^3), \\ \delta = \det(\text{Id}+\nabla v) = 1 \text{ a.e. on } \Omega \Big\}, \tag{8.3}$$

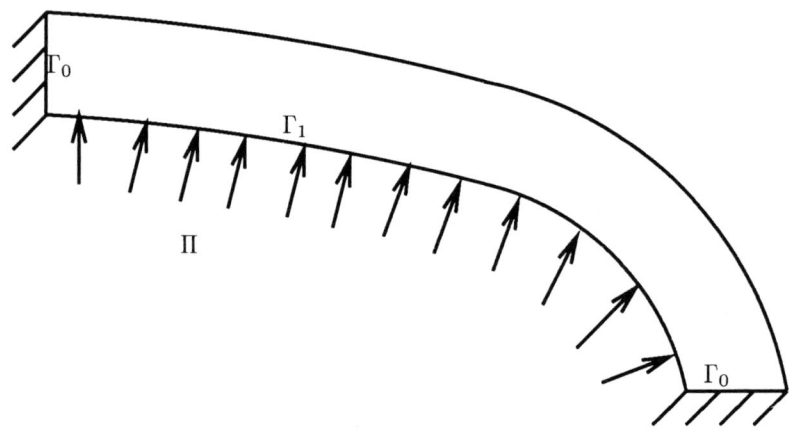

FIG. 8.1. Example of a conservative loading. A constant pressure of intensity π is applied between two parts of the boundary Γ_0.

in the incompressible case. The above definitions take into account all the kinematic constraints imposed locally on u and all the regularity assumptions to be used in the existence theory. The exponents s, q and r are deduced from coerciveness assumptions on the elastic potential $\hat{W}$. In any case, in order for $\mathbb{U}$ to be a weakly closed subset of

$$\mathbb{H} = W^{1,s}(\Omega; \mathbb{E}) \times L^q(\Omega; \mathbb{M}^3) \times L^r(\Omega),$$

we impose that these exponents satisfy

$$s > \frac{3}{2}, \qquad \frac{4}{3} > \frac{1}{q} + \frac{1}{s}, \qquad r > 1.$$

Under this assumption we have (BALL [1977]):

THEOREM 8.1. *The set $\mathbb{U}$ defined by (8.3) and the set*

$$\mathbb{U}_a = \{(v, H, \delta) \in \mathbb{H}, \ v = u_0 \text{ on } \Gamma_0, \ H = \mathrm{cof}(\mathrm{Id} + \nabla v), \ \delta = \det(\mathrm{Id} + \nabla v)\}$$

are weakly closed in $\mathbb{H}$.

PROOF. For smooth functions ψ, we have the identity

$$(\mathrm{cof}\ \nabla \psi)_{ij} = \frac{\partial}{\partial x_{i+2}} \left(\psi_{i+2} \frac{\partial}{\partial x_{i+1}} \psi_{i+1} \right) - \frac{\partial}{\partial x_{i+1}} \left(\psi_{i+2} \frac{\partial}{\partial x_{i+2}} \psi_{i+1} \right),$$

$$\det \nabla \psi = \sum_{j=1}^{3} \frac{\partial}{\partial x_j} \left(\psi_1 (\mathrm{cof}\ \nabla \psi)_{1j} \right).$$

Hence, for all ψ in $W^{1,s}(\Omega, \mathbb{E})$ with $\mathrm{cof}(\nabla \psi)$ in $L^q(\Omega; \mathbb{M}^3)$, we can define $(\mathrm{cof}\ \nabla \psi)_{ij}$ and $\det \nabla \psi$ in $\mathcal{D}'(\Omega)$ by

$$\langle (\mathrm{cof}\ \nabla \psi)_{ij}, v \rangle = - \int_\Omega \psi_{i+2} \frac{\partial \psi_{i+1}}{\partial x_{i+1}} \frac{\partial v}{\partial x_{i+2}} \, dx$$

$$+ \int_\Omega \psi_{i+2} \frac{\partial \psi_{i+1}}{\partial x_{i+2}} \frac{\partial v}{\partial x_{i+1}} \, dx \quad \forall v \in \mathcal{D}(\Omega),$$

$$\langle \det \nabla \psi, v \rangle = - \int_\Omega \sum_{j=1}^{3} \psi_1 (\mathrm{cof}\ \nabla \psi)_{1j} \frac{\partial v}{\partial x_j} \, dx \quad \forall v \in \mathcal{D}(\Omega).$$

Let us now consider a sequence (u^l) in $\mathbb{U}_a$ (respectively in $\mathbb{U}$) such that the sequence $\{\psi^l = x + u^l, \mathrm{cof}\ \nabla \psi^l, \det \nabla \psi^l\}$ weakly converges towards $\{\psi, H, \delta\}$ in $\mathbb{H}$. In particular, ψ^l converges towards ψ strongly in $L^{s^*}(\Omega)$ and we then have for all v in $\mathcal{D}(\Omega)$

$$0 = \lim \langle (\mathrm{cof}\ \nabla \psi^l - H)_{ij}, v \rangle$$

$$= \lim \left(- \int_\Omega \psi^l_{i+2} \frac{\partial \psi^l_{i+1}}{\partial x_{i+1}} \frac{\partial v}{\partial x_{i+2}} \, dx + \int_\Omega \psi^l_{i+2} \frac{\partial \psi^l_{i+1}}{\partial x_{i+2}} \frac{\partial v}{\partial x_{i+1}} \, dx \right)$$

$$-\int_\Omega H_{ij} v \, dx$$

$$= -\int_\Omega \lim \left(\psi_{i+2}^l \frac{\partial \psi_{i+1}^l}{\partial x_{i+1}} \right) \frac{\partial v}{\partial x_{i+2}} \, dx + \int_\Omega \lim \left(\psi_{i+2}^l \frac{\partial \psi_{i+1}^l}{\partial x_{i+2}} \right) \frac{\partial v}{\partial x_{i+1}} \, dx$$

$$-\int_\Omega H_{ij} v \, dx$$

$$= -\int_\Omega \psi_{i+2} \frac{\partial \psi_{i+1}}{\partial x_{i+1}} \frac{\partial v}{\partial x_{i+2}} \, dx + \int_\Omega \psi_{i+2} \frac{\partial \psi_{i+1}}{\partial x_{i+2}} \frac{\partial v}{\partial x_{i+1}} \, dx$$

$$-\int_\Omega H_{ij} v \, dx$$

$$= \langle (\operatorname{cof} \nabla \psi - H)_{ij}, v \rangle.$$

This implies that $H = \operatorname{cof}(\nabla \psi)$ and therefore $\operatorname{cof}(\nabla \psi^l)$ converges weakly in L^q towards $\operatorname{cof}(\nabla \psi)$. We can now write

$$0 = \lim \langle \det \nabla \psi^l - \delta, v \rangle$$

$$= \lim \left(-\int_\Omega \sum_{j=1}^3 \psi_1^l (\operatorname{cof} \nabla \psi^l)_{1j} \frac{\partial v}{\partial x_j} \, dx \right) - \int_\Omega \delta v \, dx$$

$$= -\int_\Omega \sum_{j=1}^3 \lim (\psi_1^l (\operatorname{cof} \nabla \psi^l)_{1j}) \frac{\partial v}{\partial x_j} \, dx - \int_\Omega \delta v \, dx$$

$$= -\int_\Omega \sum_{j=1}^3 \psi_1 (\operatorname{cof} \nabla \psi)_{1j} \frac{\partial v}{\partial x_j} \, dx - \int_\Omega \delta v \, dx$$

$$= \langle \det \nabla \psi - \delta, v \rangle.$$

Therefore, we have $\det \nabla \psi = \delta$ and thus the limit of the weakly converging sequence (u^l) still belongs to $\mathbb{U}_a$ (respectively to $\mathbb{U}$). □

The above theorem is actually a special case of the general phenomenon of compensated compactness extensively introduced by TARTAR [1979] and MURAT [1978].

We are now ready to introduce variational characterizations of the solutions of our equilibrium problem.

THEOREM 8.2. *Stable equilibrium positions of hyperelastic bodies under conservative loading formally correspond to those displacement fields that minimize the total energy $J(\cdot)$ over the set $\mathbb{U}$ of kinematically admissible displacement fields.*

PROOF. This result is formal in the sense that its proof requires more regularity than is available. With this added regularity, the energy potential $J(v)$ is differentiable. From standard results of calculus and from our definition of V, its gradient $\nabla J(u)$ is such that

$$\nabla J(u) \cdot v = \int_\Omega \frac{\partial \hat{W}}{\partial F}(x, \text{Id} + \nabla u) : \nabla v \, dx$$
$$- \int_\Omega f \cdot v \, dx - \int_{\Gamma_1} g \cdot v \, da \quad \forall v \in \mathbb{V}.$$

Moreover, if we consider the compressible case and if we endow $\mathbb{V}$ with a stronger topology than the one used in its definition, the set $\mathbb{U}$ defined in (8.2) becomes an open subset of $\mathbb{V}$. Thus, by definition, the stationary points u of J on $\mathbb{U}$ are characterized by

$$\nabla J(u) \cdot v = 0 \quad \forall v \in \mathbb{V},$$

which is exactly (7.1).

In the incompressible case, if $\mathbb{V}$ keeps the same strong topology, the set $\mathbb{U}$ introduced in (8.3) is the smooth submanifold of $\mathbb{V}$ defined by the equation

$$\det(\text{Id} + \nabla u) = 1 \text{ on } \Omega.$$

Its tangent set $T_\mathbb{U}(u)$ at u to $\mathbb{U}$ is then given by

$$T_\mathbb{U}(u) = \{v \in \mathbb{V}, \frac{\partial \det(\text{Id} + \nabla u)}{\partial \nabla u} : \nabla v = 0 \text{ on } \Omega\}$$
$$= \text{Ker } B,$$

under the notation

$$Bv = \frac{\partial \det(\text{Id} + \nabla u)}{\partial \nabla u} : \nabla v.$$

The normal set $N_\mathbb{U}(u)$ at u to $\mathbb{U}$ is then

$$N_\mathbb{U}(u) = (T_\mathbb{U}(u))^\perp$$
$$= \text{Ker } B^\perp$$
$$= \text{Im } B^T$$
$$= \{L \in \mathbb{V}', \exists p \text{ with } L(v) = \langle p, Bv \rangle\}$$
$$= \{L \in \mathbb{V}', L(v) = \int_\Omega p \frac{\partial \det(\text{Id} + \nabla u)}{\partial \nabla u} : \nabla v \, dx\}.$$

Now, by definition, the stationary points u of J on $\mathbb{U}$ are points where the gradient of J is normal to $\mathbb{U}$. This reads

$$\nabla J(u) \in N_\mathbb{U}(u), \quad u \in \mathbb{U},$$

which is precisely (7.3)–(7.4).

In summary, we have just proved that any equilibrium position u of the body is a stationary point of J on $\mathbb{U}$. We then conclude our proof by observing that if this equilibrium position u were not a minimizer, stability could be violated for an adequate smooth perturbation of this position. □

This *formal* theorem is the basis of the energetic formulation of equilibrium problems in finite elasticity which, for conservative loading, is

Minimize the total potential energy $J(\cdot)$

over the set $\mathbb{U}$ of admissible displacement fields. (8.4)

9. Existence results by minimization arguments

Under adequate assumptions on the energy potential $\hat{W}$, BALL [1977] was able to prove existence results for the energetic formulations. In the compressible case, he proved

THEOREM 9.1. *Let Ω be open, bounded connected in $\mathbb{E}$, and satisfy a strong Lipschitz condition (in the sense of NEČAS [1967]). Let its boundary Γ be such that $\Gamma = \bar{\Gamma}_0 \cup \bar{\Gamma}_1, \Gamma_0 \cap \Gamma_1 = \emptyset, \mathrm{meas}(\Gamma_0) > 0$. Let u_0 be measurable, f and g be given independently of u in $L^{s^*}(\Omega)$ and $L^{s^*}(\Gamma_1)$, and suppose that there exists an element w in $\mathbb{U}$ with $J(w) < +\infty$.*

Suppose in addition that the energy potential $\hat{W}(x, F)$ satisfies

$\hat{W}(x, F) = \mathscr{G}(x, F, \mathrm{cof}\ F, \det F),$

$\mathscr{G}(x, \cdot, \cdot, \cdot)$ *is continuous and convex on* $\mathbb{M}^3 \times \mathbb{M}^3 \times (0, +\infty)$,

$\mathscr{G}(\cdot, F, H, \delta)$ *is measurable on* Ω,

$\mathscr{G}(x, F, H, \delta) \geq a(x) + C_1 |F|^s + C_2 |H|^q + C_3 \delta^r$ *(coercivity),*

$C_i > 0, i = 1, 3, \quad a \in L^1(\Omega),$

$\lim_{\det F \to 0} \hat{W}(x, F) = +\infty.$

Then there exists a solution to the energy minimization problem (8.4).

PROOF. We briefly outline the proof which is based on the Weierstrass-theorem, and which we will later adapt to the study of the finite-element approximation problem. First, introduce

$\mathbb{H} = W^{1,s}(\Omega; \mathbb{E}) \times L^q(\Omega; \mathbb{M}^3) \times L^r(\Omega),$

$\mathbb{U}_a = \{(v, H, \delta) \in \mathbb{H},\ v = u_0 \text{ on } \Gamma_0,\ H = \mathrm{cof}(\mathrm{Id} + \nabla v),\ \delta = \det(\mathrm{Id} + \nabla v)\},$

$\mathscr{G}_a(x, F, H, \delta) = \begin{cases} \mathscr{G}(x, F, H, \delta) & \text{if } \delta > 0, \\ +\infty & \text{if not,} \end{cases}$

$$J_a(v, H, \delta) = \int_\Omega \mathcal{G}_a(x, \mathrm{Id} + \nabla v, H, \delta) \, dx - \int_\Omega f \cdot v \, dx - \int_{\Gamma_1} g \cdot v \, da.$$

We have already seen in the previous paragraph that $\mathbb{U}_a$ is weakly sequentially closed in $\mathbb{H}$. To prove the sequentially weak lower semicontinuity of J_a on $\mathbb{U}_a$, we consider a sequence (u^l) in $\mathbb{U}_a$ with $\{\psi^l = x + u^l,\ \mathrm{cof}\,\nabla\psi^l,\ \det\nabla\psi^l\}$ weakly converging in $\mathbb{H}$ and with $(J_a(u^l))$ converging in $\mathbb{R}$. Since $[J_a(u^l)]_l$ converges to a real number, it is bounded when l is large. By construction of $\mathcal{G}_a$, this implies that $\det\nabla\psi^l(x)$ is strictly positive for almost all x on Ω and for all l greater than a certain number l_0. On the other hand, since $\mathbb{U}_a$ is weakly closed, we have

$u^l \rightharpoonup u \quad \text{in } W^{1,s}(\Omega),$

$\mathrm{cof}(\nabla\psi^l) \rightharpoonup \mathrm{cof}(\nabla\psi) \quad \text{in } L^q(\Omega),$

$\det(\nabla\psi^l) \rightharpoonup \det(\nabla\psi) \quad \text{in } L^r(\Omega).$

From Mazur's theorem, there exists for each $l > l_0$ integers $i(l) \geq l$ and numbers $(\lambda_k^l)_{l \leq k \leq i(l)}$ such that

$$\lambda_k^l \geq 0, \quad \sum_{k=l}^{i(l)} \lambda_k^l = 1,$$

$$\sum_{k=l}^{i(l)} \lambda_k^l (\nabla\psi^k, \mathrm{cof}(\nabla\psi^k), \det(\nabla\psi^k))$$

$$\to (\nabla\psi, \mathrm{cof}(\nabla\psi), \det(\nabla\psi)) \quad \text{a.e. on } \Omega.$$

Since we have $\det(\nabla\psi^k) > 0$ for almost all x in Ω, the above relation implies that at the limit we have $\det(\nabla\psi) \geq 0$ for almost all x in Ω. Suppose now that there exists a subset A of Ω with strictly positive measure such that $\det(\nabla\psi) = 0$ for almost all x in A. Then, from the weak convergence of $\det(\nabla\psi^k)$ towards $\det(\nabla\psi)$ in $L^r(\Omega)$, it follows that $\det(\nabla\psi^s)$ converges to 0 in $L^1(A)$. As a consequence, there exists a subsequence (u^m) of (u^l) such that $\det(\nabla\psi^m)$ converges to 0 for almost all x in A. From our assumption on $\hat{W}$, this implies

$$\lim_{m \to \infty} \mathcal{G}_a(x, \nabla\psi^m, \mathrm{cof}\,\nabla\psi^m, \det\nabla\psi^m)$$

$$= \lim_{\det(\nabla\psi^m) \to 0} \hat{W}(x, \mathrm{Id} + \nabla u^m) = +\infty.$$

From Fatou's lemma, we would deduce

$$\lim_{m \to \infty} J_a(u^m) \geq \int_A \lim_{m \to \infty} \hat{W}(x, \mathrm{Id} + \nabla u^m) \, dx - \beta = +\infty,$$

which contradicts the assumption that $(J_a(u^l))$ converges to a real number. Hence, $\det(\nabla\psi)$ is strictly positive for almost all x in Ω. From the continuity of $\mathcal{G}$ on $\mathbb{M}^3 \times \mathbb{M}^3 \times (0, +\infty)$, Fatou's lemma and the convexity of $\mathcal{G}$, we then have

$$\int_\Omega \mathcal{G}_a(x, \nabla\psi, \operatorname{cof} \nabla\psi, \det \nabla\psi) \, dx$$

$$= \int_\Omega \lim_{l\to\infty} \mathcal{G}_a(x, \sum_{k=l}^{i(l)} \lambda_k^l \nabla\psi^k, \sum_{k=l}^{i(l)} \lambda_k^l \operatorname{cof} \nabla\psi^k, \sum_{k=l}^{i(l)} \lambda_k^l \det \nabla\psi^k) \, dx$$

$$\leq \liminf \left(\int_\Omega \mathcal{G}_a(x, \sum_{k=l}^{i(l)} \lambda_k^l \nabla\psi^k, \sum_{k=l}^{i(l)} \lambda_k^l \operatorname{cof} \nabla\psi^k, \sum_{k=l}^{i(l)} \lambda_k^l \det \nabla\psi^k) \, dx \right)$$

$$\leq \liminf \left(\int_\Omega \sum_{k=l}^{i(l)} \lambda_k^l \mathcal{G}_a(x, \nabla\psi^k, \operatorname{cof} \nabla\psi^k, \det \nabla\psi^k) \, dx \right).$$

By addition, using the weak continuity of the linear mapping

$$L(v) = -\int_\Omega f \cdot v \, dx - \int_{\Gamma_1} g \cdot v \, da,$$

and the convergence of the sequence $(J_a(u^l))$, we deduce

$$J_a(u) = \int_\Omega \mathcal{G}_a(x, \nabla\psi, \operatorname{cof} \nabla\psi, \det \nabla\psi) \, dx - L(u)$$

$$\leq \liminf \left\{ \sum_{k=l}^{i(l)} \lambda_k^l \left(\int_\Omega \mathcal{G}_a(x, \nabla\psi^k, \operatorname{cof} \nabla\psi^k, \det \nabla\psi^k) \, dx - L(u^k) \right) \right\}$$

$$\leq \lim_{l\to\infty} \left(\int_\Omega \mathcal{G}_a(x, \nabla\psi^l, \operatorname{cof} \nabla\psi^l, \det \nabla\psi^l) \, dx - L(u^l) \right)$$

$$\leq \lim_{l\to\infty} J_a(u^l).$$

This means precisely that J_a is weakly sequentially lower semicontinuous on $\mathbb{H}$.

Finally, the coercivity of $\mathcal{G}_a$ implies the coercivity of J_a on $\mathbb{U}_a$. Moreover $\mathbb{U}_a$ is not empty because it contains $\{w, \operatorname{cof}(\operatorname{Id}+\nabla w), \det(\operatorname{Id}+\nabla w)\}$.

The Weierstrass theorem can now be applied (minimization of a coercive lower semicontinuous function on a nonempty closed set using the weak topology of $\mathbb{H}$). Therefore, there exists $\{u, \operatorname{cof}(\operatorname{Id}+\nabla u), \det(\operatorname{Id}+\nabla u)\}$ in $\mathbb{U}_a$ which minimizes J_a on $\mathbb{U}_a$. Since $J_a(w, \operatorname{cof}(\operatorname{Id}+\nabla w), \det(\operatorname{Id}+\nabla w)) = J(w)$ is finite, $J_a(u, \operatorname{cof}(\operatorname{Id}+\nabla u), \det(\operatorname{Id}+\nabla u))$ is also finite which implies, by construction of J_a, that u belongs to $\mathbb{U}$ and therefore minimizes J over $\mathbb{U}$. □

REMARK 9.1. The same technique yields a similar existence result for the incompressible case. In such a case, the assumptions on $\hat{W}$ take the form

$\hat{W}(x, F) = \mathcal{G}(x, F, \operatorname{cof} F),$

$\mathcal{G}(x, \cdot, \cdot)$ is continuous and convex on $\mathbb{M}^3 \times \mathbb{M}^3$,

$\mathcal{G}(\cdot, F, H)$ is measurable on Ω,

$\mathcal{G}(x, F, H) \geqslant a(x) + C_1|F|^s + C_2|H|^q$ (coercivity),

$C_i > 0, i = 1, 2, \quad a \in L^1(\Omega).$

REMARK 9.2. The assumption $J(w) < \infty$ will often be satisfied for very simple choices of piecewise linear displacement fields w. Moreover, some of the assumptions of the existence theorem can be slightly relaxed (BALL [1977]); however, in Ball's theory, the energy potential $\hat{W}$ must always be polyconvex (i.e. $\mathcal{G}$ convex) and coercive, as are, for example, the potentials introduced in Section 4.

REMARK 9.3. The main limitation in the above existence theorem lies in the fact that it cannot be proved that the minimizers of J on $\mathbb{U}$ do satisfy some sort of weak equation of equilibrium such as (7.1) or (7.3). The topology taken for $\mathbb{U}$ is too weak to prove such a result (BALL [1977], LE TALLEC and ODEN [1981], LE DRET [1985]). For the $\mathbb{H}$ topology, the total energy $J(v)$ is not Gâteaux-differentiable and $\mathbb{U}$ is not a manifold.

10. Existence results by differential calculus

Under restrictive regularity conditions and severe limitations on the type of boundary conditions that can be considered, local existence results can also be obtained by differential calculus. For this purpose, we introduce some additional notation and assumptions.

NOTATION 10.1. We introduce

$E(u) = \frac{1}{2}(C - \operatorname{Id}) = \frac{1}{2}(\nabla u + \nabla u^T + \nabla u^T \cdot \nabla u),$

$e(v) = \dfrac{\partial E(0)}{\partial u} \cdot v = \frac{1}{2}(\nabla v + \nabla v^T) = $ linearized strain tensor,

$\tilde{\Sigma}(E) = F^{-1}T(F) = 2\dfrac{\partial \tilde{W}(C)}{\partial C} = $ second Piola–Kirchhoff stress tensor,

$\mathcal{A}(u) = -\operatorname{div}(T(F)) = -\operatorname{div}[(\operatorname{Id} + \nabla u)\tilde{\Sigma}(E)],$

together with the space

$\mathbb{V}^r = \{v \in W^{2,r}(\Omega; \mathbb{E}), \ v = 0 \text{ on } \Gamma\}.$

ASSUMPTIONS 10.1. We now suppose that the boundary Γ is of class $\mathcal{C}^2$, that the displacement is imposed everywhere on Γ, ($\Gamma_0 = \Gamma$), that the load f is dead and that the constitutive law $\tilde{\Sigma}(E)$ is of class $\mathscr{C}^2$ and satisfies

$$\tilde{\Sigma}(E) = \lambda(\operatorname{tr} E) \operatorname{Id} + 2\mu E + O(\|E\|^2), \tag{10.1}$$
$$\lambda > 0, \quad \mu > 0.$$

The above assumptions will guarantee that the solution u will have the regularity required for our analysis ($u \in W^{2,r}(\Omega)$ with $r > 3$). They are rather restrictive, especially the one imposing Dirichlet conditions on the whole boundary Γ. Nevertheless, from (4.4), (10.1) is satisfied by any compressible homogeneous isotropic material at rest in its reference configuration since we have

$$\frac{\partial I_1}{\partial C} = \operatorname{Id},$$

$$\frac{\partial I_2}{\partial C} = (\operatorname{tr} C) \operatorname{Id} - C = 2(1 + \operatorname{tr} E) \operatorname{Id} - 2E,$$

$$\frac{\partial I_3}{\partial C} = (\det C) C^{-1} = (1 + 2 \operatorname{tr} E) \operatorname{Id} - 2E + O(\|E\|^2).$$

With these assumptions, we can now prove the following results.

THEOREM 10.1. *If $r > 3$, the mapping $\tilde{\Sigma}$ defined from $W^{1,r}(\Omega; \mathbb{M}^3)$ into $W^{1,r}(\Omega; \mathbb{M}^3)$, which to E associates $\tilde{\Sigma}(E)$ is of class $\mathscr{C}^2$ with bounded derivatives:*

$$\sup_{\|E\| < \rho} \left\| \frac{\partial^2 \tilde{\Sigma}}{\partial E^2} \right\| = C_\rho < +\infty \quad \forall \rho.$$

PROOF. The proof is based on the Lebesgue dominated convergence theorem and can be found in CIARLET ([1988], p. 303). A similar proof will be given later in the analysis of the finite element approximation (Theorem 15.1, Step 1). □

THEOREM 10.2. *If $r > 3$, the mapping $\mathscr{A}'(0)$ defined by*

$$\mathscr{A}'(0) \cdot u := -\operatorname{div}\left(\lambda(\operatorname{tr} e(u)) \operatorname{Id} + 2\mu e(u)\right)$$

is an isomorphism from $\mathbb{V}^r$ into $L^r(\Omega; \mathbb{E})$.

PROOF. This mapping is linear by construction. Moreover, we have

$$\|\operatorname{div}(\lambda(\operatorname{tr} e(u)) \operatorname{Id} + 2\mu e(u))\|_{0,r} \leqslant \|\lambda(\operatorname{tr} e(u)) \operatorname{Id} + 2\mu e(u)\|_{1,r}$$

$$\leqslant C \|\nabla u\|_{1,r}$$

$$\leqslant C \|u\|_{2,r},$$

and hence the mapping is continuous. Now, from the closed graph theorem, it is an isomorphism if and only if it is invertible, that is if and only if the problem

$$-\operatorname{div}\left(\lambda(\operatorname{tr} e(u)) \operatorname{Id} + 2\mu e(u)\right) = f \tag{10.2}$$

has a unique solution u in $\mathbb{V}^r$ for any f in $L^r(\Omega;\mathbb{E})$.

But (10.2) is the standard problem of linearized elasticity which is proved to have a unique solution u in $H_0^1(\Omega;\mathbb{E})$ by the Lax–Milgram lemma. From the strong ellipticity of the operator of linearized elasticity, this solution u belongs to $H^2(\Omega)$ if f belongs to $L^2(\Omega)$ (NEČAS [1967], p. 260). Thus $\mathcal{A}'(0)$ is an isomorphism from $\mathbb{V}^2$ into $L^2(\Omega;\mathbb{E})$.

The theorem is therefore proved for $r = 2$. This in turn guarantees that the theorem is true for any $r \geqslant 2$ because, from a result of GEYMONAT [1965], the index of $\mathcal{A}'(0)$ defined by

$$\operatorname{Ind} \mathcal{A}'(0) = \dim(\operatorname{Ker} \mathcal{A}'(0)) - \dim(\operatorname{Coker} \mathcal{A}'(0))$$

is independent of r. □

THEOREM 10.3. *The mapping $\mathcal{A}$ from $\mathbb{V}^r$ into $L^r(\Omega;\mathbb{E})$ defined by*

$$\mathcal{A}(v) = -\operatorname{div} T(F(v))$$

is of class $\mathscr{C}^2$. Moreover, there exists a closed ball B_ρ^r of radius ρ in $\mathbb{V}^r$ on which the mapping $\mathcal{A}'(v)^{-1}$ exists and is Lipschitz continuous in v.

PROOF. As observed in CIARLET ([1988], p. 310), the mapping $\mathcal{A}$ is obtained by composition of the mappings

$$v \in \mathbb{V} \longmapsto \nabla v \in W^{1,r}(\Omega, \mathbb{M}^3),$$

$$\nabla v \in W^{1,r}(\Omega; \mathbb{M}^3) \longmapsto E = \tfrac{1}{2}(\nabla v + \nabla v^T + \nabla v^T \nabla v) \in W^{1,r}(\Omega; \mathbb{M}^3),$$

$$E \in W^{1,r}(\Omega; \mathbb{M}^3) \longmapsto \tilde{\Sigma}(E) \in W^{1,r}(\Omega; \mathbb{M}^3),$$

$$(\nabla v, \tilde{\Sigma}) \in (W^{1,r}(\Omega; \mathbb{M}^3))^2 \longmapsto (\operatorname{Id} + \nabla v)\tilde{\Sigma} \in W^{1,r}(\Omega; \mathbb{M}^3),$$

$$(\operatorname{Id} + \nabla v)\tilde{\Sigma} \in W^{1,r}(\Omega; \mathbb{M}^3) \longmapsto -\operatorname{div}[(\operatorname{Id} + \nabla v)\tilde{\Sigma}] \in L^r(\Omega; \mathbb{E}).$$

Since $r > 3$, $W^{1,r}(\Omega)$ is an algebra and hence the second and fourth mappings above are of class $\mathscr{C}^\infty$. The first and fifth mappings are linear continuous and, from our previous result, the third mapping is of class $\mathscr{C}^2$ with bounded derivatives. By composition, the mapping $\mathcal{A}$ is of class $\mathscr{C}^2$ with bounded derivatives. We can therefore apply the mean value theorem to $\mathcal{A}'(v)$ which yields

$$\|\mathcal{A}'(v) - \mathcal{A}'(w)\| \leqslant \|v - w\| \sup\nolimits_{t \in]v,w[} \|\mathcal{A}''(t)\|$$

$$\leqslant C_{\rho_0}\|v - w\| \quad \forall (v, w) \in B_{\rho_0}^r.$$

Hence, there exists a smaller ball B_ρ^r on which we have

$$\|\mathcal{A}'(v) - \mathcal{A}'(0)\| \leqslant \rho C_{\rho_0} \leqslant \tfrac{1}{2}\|\mathcal{A}'(0)^{-1}\|^{-1} \quad \forall v \in B_\rho^r.$$

We observe that the map $\mathcal{A}'(0)^{-1}$ is well-defined from Theorem 10.2.

After multiplication by $\mathcal{A}'(0)^{-1}$, this implies that the mapping

$$x \to x - \mathcal{A}'(0)^{-1}(\mathcal{A}'(v)x - f)$$

is strictly contracting with a Lipschitz constant $\|L\|$ such that
$$\|L\| \leq \|\mathcal{A}'(0)^{-1}\| \, \|\mathcal{A}'(0) - \mathcal{A}'(v)\| \leq \tfrac{1}{2}.$$
From the fixed point theorem, it has a unique fixed point $\hat{x} = \mathcal{A}'(v)^{-1}f$ in the ball B_ρ^r such that
$$\|\hat{x}\| = \|L^\infty(0)\| \leq \sum_{n=0}^{\infty} \|L^{n+1}(0) - L^n(0)\|$$
$$\leq \sum_{n=0}^{\infty} \|L\|^n \|L(0) - 0\|$$
$$\leq 2\|\mathcal{A}'(0)^{-1}\| \, \|f\|.$$
It then follows that $\mathcal{A}'(v)$ is also invertible on B_ρ^r with
$$\|\mathcal{A}'(v)^{-1}\| \leq 2\|\mathcal{A}'(0)^{-1}\| \quad \forall v \in B_\rho^r.$$
And finally, we have
$$\|\mathcal{A}'(v)^{-1} - \mathcal{A}'(w)^{-1}\| = \|\mathcal{A}'(v)^{-1}(\mathcal{A}'(v) - \mathcal{A}'(w))\mathcal{A}'(w)^{-1}\|$$
$$\leq \|\mathcal{A}'(v)^{-1}\| \cdot \|\mathcal{A}'(v) - \mathcal{A}'(w)\| \cdot \|\mathcal{A}'(w)^{-1}\|$$
$$\leq \|\mathcal{A}'(v)^{-1}\| \cdot \|\mathcal{A}'(w)^{-1}\| C_{\rho_0} \|v - w\|$$
$$\leq 4 C_{\rho_0} \|\mathcal{A}'(0)^{-1}\|^2 \|v - w\| \quad \forall (v, w) \in (B_\rho^r)^2,$$
which proves the Lipschitz continuity of $\mathcal{A}'(v)^{-1}$ on B_ρ^r. $\square$

THEOREM 10.4. *Introducing a smooth loading path $f(s)$ with $f(0) = 0$ and $f(1) = f$, the equilibrium problem (7.1) is equivalent to the differential equation*
$$\begin{cases} \dfrac{du}{ds} = \mathcal{A}'(u)^{-1} \dfrac{df}{ds} & \forall s \in [0, 1], \\ u(0) = 0. \end{cases} \tag{10.3}$$

PROOF. By integration between 0 and 1, we get
$$\mathcal{A}(u(1)) - \mathcal{A}(u(0)) = \int_0^1 \frac{d}{ds}[\mathcal{A}(u(s))] \, ds$$
$$= \int_0^1 \mathcal{A}'(u) \frac{du}{ds} \, ds$$
$$= \int_0^1 \frac{df}{ds} \, ds$$
$$= f(1) - f(0) = f,$$

which is the strong form of (7.1). □

THEOREM 10.5. *Assuming $f(s) = sf$, the differential equation (10.3) (and hence the equilibrium problem (7.1)) has a unique solution in B_ρ^r if f is sufficiently small, i.e. if*

$$\|f\|_{0,r} < \frac{\rho}{2}\|\mathcal{A}'(0)^{-1}\|.$$

PROOF. The differential equation (10.3) is locally well-posed since from Theorem 10.3, $\mathcal{A}'(u)^{-1}(df/ds)$ is locally Lipschitz continuous in u. Moreover, if the solution blows up at $s = s_0$, this means that

$$\mathcal{A}'(u(s_0))^{-1}\frac{df}{ds}$$

is no longer Lipschitz continuous, which implies that $u(s_0)$ is no longer in B_ρ^r. But at the point s_1 where $u(s)$ leaves B_ρ^r for the first time, we have

$$\rho = \|u(s_1)\| \leqslant \int_0^{s_1} \|\mathcal{A}'(u)^{-1}f\|\,ds$$

$$\leqslant s_1\|f\| \sup_{v\in B_\rho^r} \|\mathcal{A}'(v)^{-1}\|$$

$$\leqslant 2s_1\|f\| \cdot \|\mathcal{A}'(0)^{-1}\|$$

$$< \rho s_1.$$

Hence we have $s_0 \geqslant s_1 > 1$, which implies that the solution of the differential equation is defined on the whole interval $[0, 1]$. □

REMARK 10.1. The solution curve of the differential equation (10.3) will be followed step by step in the numerical strategy in order to arrive safely to the solution of the original problem (7.1).

CHAPTER III

Approximation Theory

In view of their numerical approximations, the variational formulations introduced in the preceding chapter must first be approximated by problems having a finite number of unknowns. In finite elasticity, because of the complex geometries which are involved, this approximation is usually achieved by *finite-element methods*.

Finite-element methods have been used in solid mechanics for more than thirty years (ARGYRIS [1954], CLOUGH [1960]) and are now commonly used in many fields of engineering. In particular, most practical problems of linear elasticity are presently solved by this method. The reader is referred to the books of ZIENKIEWICZ [1971] or of HUGHES [1987] for a complete description of the possible applications of finite-elements. In addition, a detailed mathematical presentation of the finite-element method can be found in CIARLET [1978] or in Volume II of this Handbook.

The approximation of unconstrained variational problems like (7.1) simply amounts to the replacement of the fundamental space $\mathbb{V}$ in which it is posed by a finite-dimensional subspace $\mathbb{V}_h$ made of finite-elements. For uniformly convex problems, the error between the solution of the approximate problem and the exact solution u is proved to be proportional to the distance between u and the subspace $\mathbb{V}_h$ (CÉA [1964], FALK [1974]). The finite-element space $\mathbb{V}_h$ can then be adapted in order to reduce this distance (JOHNSON [1987]) and hence the corresponding error.

The approximation of constrained problems such as (7.3)–(7.4) is more delicate and was first considered by BABUSKA [1973] and by BREZZI [1974]. As described in GIRAULT and RAVIART [1986] and in BREZZI and FORTIN [1991], two compatible finite-element subspaces are needed for such constrained problems: one for the constrained variable v, one for the Lagrange multiplier p. With this technique, the approximation results obtained in the unconstrained problems can be extended to the linearly constrained problems.

The application of the finite-element method to nonlinear elasticity was initiated by ODEN [1972] and analyzed in LE TALLEC [1982]. In the polyconvex framework used in the existence theory of J. Ball, one can prove the strong convergence of the finite-element solutions towards global minimizers of the potential energy. Unfortunately, no information is available on the rate of convergence of these solutions as function of the discretization step h; this remains a major unsolved problem.

The present chapter will first describe the finite-element approximation of the compressible equilibrium problem (7.1) and of the incompressible problem (7.3)–(7.4). It will then concentrate on the analysis of the incompressible problem which is more significant from both the mathematical and the engineering points of view. This analysis will consider first the linearized problem, then derive a general convergence result, and conclude by some remarks on the consistency of the proposed approximation.

11. Approximation of compressible problems

As recalled above, the finite-element approximation of the original problem (7.1) is simply obtained by replacing the space $\mathbb{V}$ by a finite-dimensional subspace $\mathbb{V}_h$. Its formulation is therefore

Find $(u_h - u_0) \in \mathbb{V}_h$ satisfying, for all $v_h \in \mathbb{V}_h$,

$$\int_\Omega \frac{\partial \hat{W}}{\partial F}(x, \mathrm{Id} + \nabla u_h) : \nabla v_h \, dx = \int_\Omega f \cdot v_h \, dx + \int_{\Gamma_1} g \cdot v_h \, da. \tag{11.1}$$

In elasticity, in order to achieve accuracy at low cost, the construction of the approximate space $\mathbb{V}_h$ is usually done with quadrilateral (respectively hexahedral if $\Omega \subset \mathbb{R}^3$) isoparametric finite-elements. More precisely, we suppose that Ω is a polygonal (respectively polyhedral) domain in $\mathbb{R}^2$ (respectively $\mathbb{R}^3$) which can be decomposed into a finite number N_h of quadrilaterals (respectively hexahedra) Ω_l such that:

(i) $\overline{\Omega} = \bigcup_{l=1, N_h} \overline{\Omega_l}$,
(ii) the diameter of any Ω_l is bounded by h,
(iii) any Ω_l contains a ball of radius αh, α given once for all and independent of h,
(iv) two different elements Ω_l have either nothing, a vertex, an edge or a face in common.

By extension, we will still refer to such families of partitions $\mathcal{T}_h$ of Ω as regular families of 'triangulations' of Ω. Once $\mathcal{T}_h$ is constructed (see Fig. 11.1), the space $\mathbb{V}_h$ is simply given by

$$\mathbb{V}_h = \Big\{ v_h \colon \bar{\Omega} \to \mathbb{E}, \ v_h \text{ continuous}, \ v_h = 0 \text{ on } \Gamma_0,$$

$$v_{h|\Omega_l} = v_l \circ \varphi_l^{-1}, \ v_l \in [Q_1(\hat{\Omega})]^N, \ \forall l = 1, \ldots, N_h \Big\}. \tag{11.2}$$

Here φ_l is the mapping from the reference element $\hat{\Omega} = (-1, +1)^N$ into Ω_l

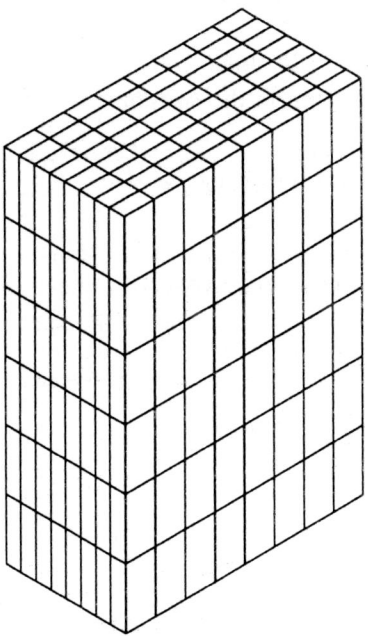

Fig. 11.1. Three-dimensional triangulation. The domain Ω is partitioned into hexahedra. Each hexahedron is the image of a reference cube $\hat{\Omega}$.

defined by

$$\varphi_l(\hat{x}) = \sum_{\alpha=1}^{2^N} x^{\alpha l} \hat{\varphi}^\alpha(\hat{x}),$$

where the $x^{\alpha l}$ are the coordinates of the vertex M_α of the element Ω_l and where $\hat{\varphi}^\alpha$ is the function of $Q_1(\hat{\Omega})$ with values 1 at vertex α and 0 at all other vertices. The space $Q_1(\hat{\Omega})$ is the usual space of tensorial products of linear polynomials defined over $\hat{\Omega}$, that is

$$Q_1(\hat{\Omega}) = \{\hat{q}, \hat{q}(\hat{x}) = a_0 + \sum_{i=1}^{N} a_i \hat{x}_i + \sum_{i \neq j} a_{ij} \hat{x}_i \hat{x}_j + \sum_{i \neq j \neq k} a_{ijk} \hat{x}_i \hat{x}_j \hat{x}_k\}.$$

With this construction, the elements of $\mathbb{V}_h$ are then simply characterized by their values v^α at the vertices of the triangulation since we have (CIARLET [1991], p. 78)

$$v_h(\varphi_l(\hat{x}))_{|\Omega_l} = \sum_{\alpha=1}^{2^N} v^\alpha \hat{\varphi}^\alpha(\hat{x}).$$

The above choice of finite-element $\mathbb{V}_h$ is very simple but a bit too crude. The local approximation of u by bilinear polynomials is too coarse to reproduce accurately the displacement fields u observed in structural analysis. Therefore, it is advisable to replace in the above construction of $\mathbb{V}_h$ the space $Q_1(\hat{\Omega})$ by the larger space $Q'_2(\hat{\Omega})$ defined in the two-dimensional case by

$$Q'_2(\hat{\Omega}) = \{\hat{q} \in Q_2(\hat{\Omega}), 4\hat{q}(M_9) + \sum_{\alpha=1}^{4} \hat{q}(M_\alpha) - 2\sum_{\beta=5}^{8} \hat{q}(M_\beta) = 0\},$$

and with a similar definition for the three-dimensional case (Figs. 11.2 and 11.3). Here, $(M_\alpha)_{\alpha=1,4}$ denotes the vertices, $(M_\beta)_{\beta=5,8}$ the midsides and M_9 the center of $\hat{\Omega}$, respectively. Moreover, $Q_2(\hat{\Omega})$ denotes the space of biquadratic polynomials

$$Q_2(\hat{\Omega}) = \{\hat{q}, \hat{q}(\hat{x}) = \sum_{i=0}^{2} \sum_{j=0}^{2} a_i a_j \hat{x}_1^i \hat{x}_2^j\}.$$

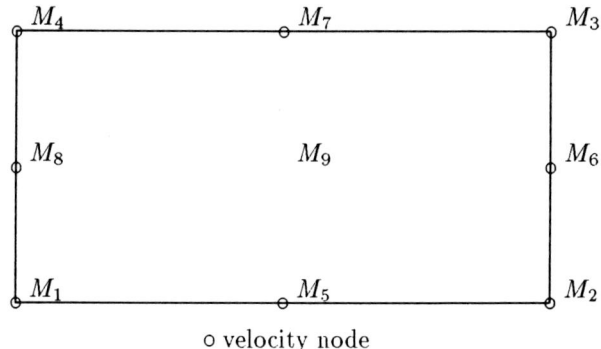

○ velocity node

FIG. 11.2. Description of the serendipity element in two dimensions. The dots indicate the nodes of the element. The values of v_h at these nodes characterize v_h in the approximation space.

This new finite-element is the widely used *serendipity element* (ZIENKIEWICZ [1971], p. 108) and it has two main characteristics which motivate its choice:

(i) the local space $Q'_2(\hat{\Omega})$ contains the space of second-order polynomials which implies that the local truncation error is small (CIARLET [1978]);

(ii) the elements of $\mathbb{V}_h$ are simply characterized by their values at the vertices and mid-edges of the triangulation, that is

$$v_h(\varphi_l(\hat{x})) = \sum_{\alpha=1}^{m} v^\alpha \hat{\varphi}^\alpha(\hat{x}),$$

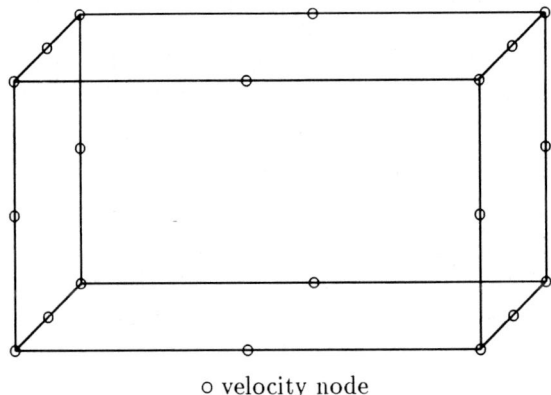

o velocity node

FIG. 11.3. Description of the serendipity element in three dimensions. The dots indicate the nodes of the element. The values of v_h at these nodes characterize v_h in the approximation space.

with $m = 8$ (respectively $m = 20$) in the two-dimensional (respectively three-dimensional) case.

12. Approximation of incompressible problems

In the incompressible case, the finite-element approximation of the original equilibrium problem (7.3)–(7.4) is simply obtained by replacing the spaces V and P by finite-dimensional subspaces V_h and P_h. Its formulation is therefore

Find $(u_h - u_0) \in V_h$ and $p_h \in P_h$ such that

$$\int_\Omega \frac{\partial \hat{W}}{\partial F}(x, \mathrm{Id} + \nabla u_h) : \nabla v_h \, dx - \int_\Omega p_h \frac{\partial \det}{\partial F}(\mathrm{Id} + \nabla u_h) : \nabla v_h \, dx$$

$$= \int_\Omega f \cdot v_h \, dx + \int_{\Gamma_1} g \cdot v_h \, da \quad \forall v_h \in V_h, \tag{12.1}$$

$$\int_\Omega q_h [\det(\mathrm{Id} + \nabla u_h) - 1] \, dx = 0 \quad \forall q_h \in P_h. \tag{12.2}$$

As our first choice of discrete spaces, we construct the approximation spaces V_h and P_h using quadrilateral (respectively hexahedral if $\Omega \subset \mathbb{R}^3$) isoparametric finite-elements, the displacements of V being interpolated at each vertex, the elements of P being interpolated at the center of each element. More precisely, for a given regular triangulation $\mathcal{T}_h$ of Ω (see Fig. 11.1), the spaces V_h and P_h

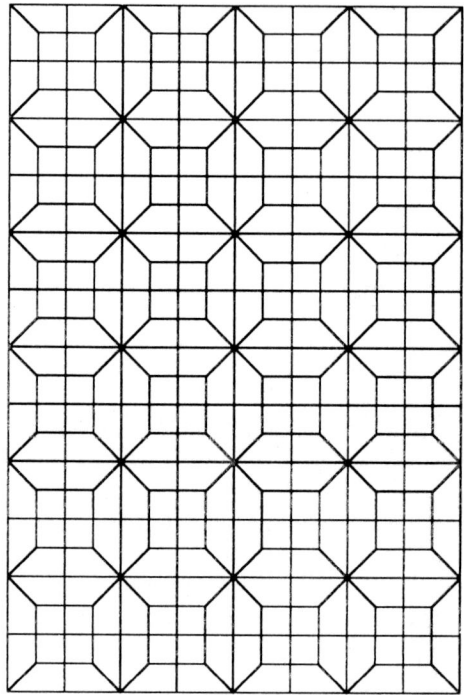

FIG. 12.1. Special two-dimensional triangulation. With this partition, the incompressible problem is well-posed when approximated by $Q2 - P1$ finite-elements.

are respectively defined by (11.2) and by

$$\mathbb{P}_h = \{q_h \colon \Omega \to \mathbb{R}, \ q_{h|\Omega_l} = \text{constant}, \ \forall l = 1, \ldots, N_h\}. \tag{12.3}$$

The above choice of finite-elements leads in certain specific situations to local numerical instabilities: the computed displacement field u_h and pressure p_h may oscillate next to Γ_0 for irregular loadings. For $\Omega \subset \mathbb{R}^2$, these oscillations can be suppressed either by considering triangulations of the type of Fig. 12.1 or by choosing asymmetric triangular finite-elements (RUAS [1981]).

In the latter case, the domain Ω is divided into triangles (this triangulation being regular in the sense described in Section 11), the displacements are interpolated at each vertex and at one mid-side, and the elements of $\mathbb{P}$ are interpolated at the center of each triangle (Fig. 12.2). More precisely, we have

$$\mathbb{P}_h = \{q_h \colon \Omega \to \mathbb{R}, \ q_{h|\Omega_l} = \text{constant}, \ \forall l = 1, \ldots, N_h\}, \tag{12.4}$$

$\mathbb{V}_h = \{v_h \colon \bar{\Omega} \to \mathbb{E}, \ v_h \text{ continuous}, \ v_h = 0 \text{ on } \Gamma_0,$

$v_{h|\Omega_l}$ is a second-order polynomial whose restriction

to two sides of Ω_l is a first-order polynomial,
$$\forall l = 1, \ldots, N_h\}. \tag{12.5}$$

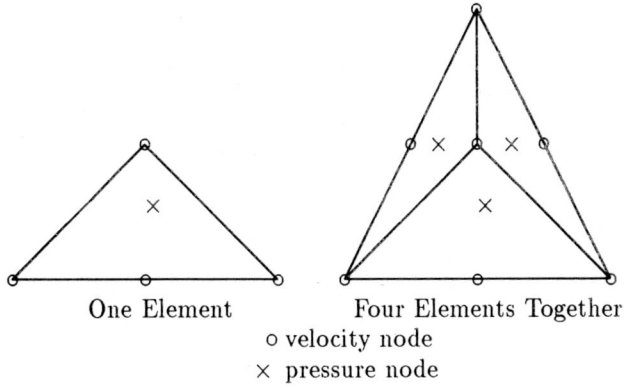

One Element   Four Elements Together
○ velocity node
× pressure node

Fig. 12.2. The Ruas finite-element. This is a triangle with four velocity nodes (not symmetric) and one pressure node.

Yet another example of finite-element spaces is given in Fig. 12.3. It is defined on the triangulation $\mathcal{T}_h$ of Section 11 through the choice

$$\mathbb{P}_h = \{q_h \colon \Omega \to \mathbb{R}, \ q_{h|\Omega_l} \in P_1(\Omega_l), \ \forall l = 1, \ldots N_h\}, \tag{12.6}$$

$$\mathbb{V}_h = \{v_h \colon \bar{\Omega} \to \mathbb{E}, \ v_h \text{ continuous}, \ v_h = 0 \text{ on } \Gamma_0,$$
$$v_{h|\Omega_l} = v_l \circ \varphi_l^{-1}, \ v_h \in [Q_2(\hat{\Omega})]^N, \ \forall l = 1, \ldots, N_h\}. \tag{12.7}$$

At first sight, many other choices exist for $\mathbb{V}_h$ and $\mathbb{P}_h$. Nevertheless, we will see later that they cannot be chosen independently and they must satisfy a compatibility condition which restricts the choice to a few finite-elements.

13. Approximation of nearly incompressible problems

The nearly incompressible materials are compressible, but must be treated as incompressible materials in their finite-element approximation.

Let us develop this last point. Since such materials are compressible, the associated variational formulation is (7.1), that is

$$\int_\Omega \frac{\partial \hat{W}_0}{\partial F}(x, \mathrm{Id} + \nabla u) : \nabla v \, dx$$

$$+ \int_\Omega \frac{1}{\varepsilon}[\det(\mathrm{Id} + \nabla u) - 1] \frac{\partial \det}{\partial F}(\mathrm{Id} + \nabla u) : \nabla v \, dx$$

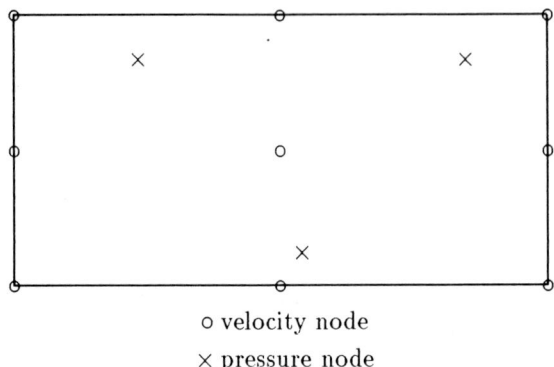

○ velocity node
× pressure node

FIG. 12.3. The two-dimensional $Q2 - P1$ finite-element. It has nine nodes for velocity (vertices, mid-sides and center) and three internal nodes for pressure.

$$= \int_\Omega f \cdot v \, dx + \int_{\Gamma_1} g \cdot v \, da \quad \forall v \in \mathbb{V}, \ (u - u_0) \in \mathbb{V}. \tag{13.1}$$

Now, a correct finite-element approximation of (13.1) cannot be simply obtained by replacing $\mathbb{V}$ by a given finite-element subspace $\mathbb{V}_h$. Indeed, the term $-\varepsilon^{-1}(\det(\mathrm{Id} + \nabla u) - 1)$ can be identified with a pressure. Therefore, at the incompressible limit, the single replacement of $\mathbb{V}$ by $\mathbb{V}_h$ in (13.1) amounts to a finite-element approximation of the incompressible problem by the spaces $\mathbb{V}_h$ and $\mathbb{P}_h = \operatorname{div} \mathbb{V}_h$. For such a choice, the consistency condition (14.6) to be introduced later will not be satisfied in general, and the discrete incompressible problem will be overconstrained. For nearly incompressible materials, this overconstraint will result in an artificially large stiffness of the considered body. There will be "locking".

To avoid locking, one must proceed as in the incompressible case and introduce a pair of finite-element spaces $\mathbb{V}_h$ and $\mathbb{P}_h$ which are compatible in the sense indicated in Section 14. Then one introduces a reduced gradient field

$$\nabla_h v = L^2 \text{ projection of } \nabla v \text{ on } (\mathbb{P}_h)^{N \times N}$$

and defines the finite-element approximation of (13.1) as follows:

Find $u_h \in \mathbb{V}_h + u_0$ such that

$$\int_\Omega \frac{\partial \hat{W}_0}{\partial F}(x, \mathrm{Id} + \nabla u_h) : \nabla v_h \, dx$$

$$+ \int_\Omega \frac{1}{\varepsilon}[\det(\mathrm{Id} + \nabla_h u_h) - 1] \frac{\partial \det}{\partial F}(\mathrm{Id} + \nabla_h u_h) : \nabla_h v_h \, dx$$

$$= \int_\Omega f \cdot v_h \, dx + \int_{\Gamma_1} g \cdot v_h \, da \quad \forall \, v_h \in \mathbb{V}_h. \tag{13.2}$$

REMARK 13.1. The reduced integration techniques fall within the framework of (13.2). As described in ZIENKIEWICZ [1971], such techniques use a direct finite-element approximation of (13.1), but the term

$$\int_\Omega \frac{1}{\varepsilon} [\det(\mathrm{Id} + \nabla u_h) - 1] \frac{\partial \det}{\partial F}(\mathrm{Id} + \nabla u_h) : \nabla v_h \, dx$$

is numerically integrated with fewer points than normally required. For example, on each finite-element, one would use a one-point quadrature formula for the space $\mathbb{V}_h$ given by (11.2) and an (2^N)-point quadrature formula for the space $\mathbb{V}_h$ given by (12.7). Such a strategy is equivalent to (13.2): it simply amounts to choosing a space $\mathbb{P}_h$ of piecewise constant functions (to each integration point corresponds a cell on which the functions of $\mathbb{P}_h$ are constant).

14. Linearization and compatibility condition

The analysis of the finite-element approximation of equilibrium problems in compressible finite elasticity is a simple variant of the analysis of the incompressible case (Section 16) and does not introduce any practical restriction on the choice of the finite-element space $\mathbb{V}_h$.

The situation is quite different for incompressible or nearly incompressible problems. These problems are very frequently encountered in practice, and their approximation involves an auxiliary pressure space $\mathbb{P}_h$ which must be chosen with care. These problems are therefore more delicate to handle numerically. That is why we now concentrate our analysis on the incompressible case.

Before solving the full discrete problem (12.1)–(12.2), it is always useful to study its linearization around a solution. This linearized problem consists in finding the elementary variation $\{\dot{u}_h \, dt, \dot{p}_h \, dt\}$ of the known solution corresponding to an elementary variation $\{\dot{f} \, dt, \dot{g} \, dt\}$ of the external loads. Writing with obvious notation Problem (12.1)–(12.2) as

$$\mathscr{F}(u_h, p_h, f, g) = 0 \quad \text{in } \mathbb{V}'_h \times \mathbb{P}'_h,$$

we obtain $\{\dot{u}_h, \dot{p}_h\}$ by solving

$$\frac{\partial \mathscr{F}}{\partial u} \dot{u}_h + \frac{\partial \mathscr{F}}{\partial p} \dot{p}_h + \frac{\partial \mathscr{F}}{\partial f} \dot{f} + \frac{\partial \mathscr{F}}{\partial g} \dot{g} = 0 \quad \text{in } \mathbb{V}'_h \times \mathbb{P}'_h. \tag{14.1}$$

All computations done, the linearized problem is finally

$$a(\dot{u}_h, v_h) + b(\dot{p}_h, v_h) = L(v_h) \quad \forall v_h \in \mathbb{V}_h, \ \dot{u}_h \in \mathbb{V}_h, \tag{14.2}$$

$$b(q_h, \dot{u}_h) = 0 \quad \forall q_h \in \mathbb{P}_h, \ \dot{p}_h \in \mathbb{P}_h, \tag{14.3}$$

where the bilinear forms $a(\cdot,\cdot)$ and $b(\cdot,\cdot)$ and the linear form $L(\cdot)$ are respectively given by

$$a(w_h, v_h) = \int_\Omega \left(\frac{\partial^2 \hat{W}}{\partial F^2}(x, \mathrm{Id} + \nabla u_h) : \nabla w_h\right) : \nabla v_h \, dx$$

$$- \int_\Omega p_h \left(\frac{\partial^2 \det}{\partial F^2}(\mathrm{Id} + \nabla u_h) : \nabla w_h\right) : \nabla v_h \, dx, \qquad (14.4)$$

$$b(q_h, v_h) = -\int_\Omega q_h \frac{\partial \det}{\partial F}(\mathrm{Id} + \nabla u_h) : \nabla v_h \, dx, \qquad (14.5)$$

$$L(v_h) = \int_\Omega \dot{f} \cdot v_h \, dx + \int_{\Gamma_1} \dot{g} \cdot v_h \, dx,$$

and where $\partial^2 \hat{W}/\partial F^2$ denotes as usual the second derivative of $\hat{W}$ with respect to the variable $F = \mathrm{Id} + \nabla u$.

As written, (14.2)–(14.3) is a so-called *mixed variational problem*. Such problems have been extensively studied (BREZZI [1974], BABUSKA [1973] among others). They have proved the following theorem (the so-called Ladyzenskaya–Babuska–Brezzi theorem):

THEOREM 14.1. *Consider the mixed problem*

$$a(v, w) + b(p, w) = L_v(w) \quad \forall w \in \mathbb{V}, \; v \in \mathbb{V},$$
$$b(q, v) = L_p(q) \quad \forall q \in \mathbb{P}, \; p \in \mathbb{P},$$

with $\mathbb{V}$ and $\mathbb{P}$ given Hilbert spaces, L_v and L_p belonging to $\mathbb{V}'$ and $\mathbb{P}'$ respectively. Moreover, a and b are continuous bilinear forms defined on $\mathbb{V} \times \mathbb{V}$ and $\mathbb{P} \times \mathbb{V}$, respectively. Define the operators

$$\mathscr{B} : \mathbb{V} \to \mathbb{P}'$$
$$v \mapsto \mathscr{B}v \text{ such that } \langle \mathscr{B}v, q \rangle = b(q, v) \quad \forall q \in \mathbb{P},$$
$$\mathscr{A} : \mathrm{Ker}\,\mathscr{B} \to (\mathrm{Ker}\,\mathscr{B})'$$
$$v \mapsto \mathscr{A}v \text{ such that } \langle \mathscr{A}v, w \rangle = a(v, w) \quad \forall w \in \mathrm{Ker}\,\mathscr{B}.$$

Then, the operator $\mathscr{B}$ is onto if and only if the spaces $\mathbb{V}$ and $\mathbb{P}$ satisfy the following fundamental compatibility condition:

$$\inf_{q \in \mathbb{P}, \|q\|=1} \left\{ \sup_{v \in \mathbb{V}, \|v\|=1} \{b(q, v)\} \right\} = \beta > 0.$$

Moreover, the mixed problem is well-posed if and only if $\mathscr{B}$ is onto and $\mathscr{A}$ is invertible.

PROOF. We begin by proving the first statement. Let $\mathscr{B}$ be onto. Then, from the closed range theorem (YOSIDA [1978], p. 105), there is a continuous inverse $\mathscr{B}^{-1}$

from $\mathbb{P}'$ to $\mathbb{V}$. By identifying $\mathbb{P}$ to its dual, we then have for all $q \neq 0$

$$\sup_{v \in \mathbb{V}, \|v\|=1} \{b(q,v)\} = \sup_{v \in \mathbb{V}} \{\frac{b(q,v)}{\|v\|}\}$$

$$\geqslant \frac{b(q, \mathscr{B}^{-1}q)}{\|\mathscr{B}^{-1}q\|}$$

$$\geqslant \frac{\|q\|^2}{\|\mathscr{B}^{-1}q\|}$$

$$\geqslant \frac{\|q\|}{\|\mathscr{B}^{-1}\|}.$$

This is the desired inf-sup condition with $\beta = 1/\|\mathscr{B}^{-1}\|$.

Conversely, from the inf-sup condition, we first have for all $q \neq 0$

$$\|\mathscr{B}^T q\| = \sup_{w \in \mathbb{V}} \{\frac{\langle \mathscr{B}^T q, w \rangle}{\|w\|}\}$$

$$= \sup_{w \in \mathbb{V}} \{\frac{b(q,w)}{\|w\|}\}$$

$$\geqslant \beta \|q\|.$$

Hence, the image of $\mathscr{B}^T$ is closed and thus, from the closed range theorem, the image of $\mathscr{B}$ is also closed. Moreover, using the inf-sup condition again, we find that the orthogonal of the image of $\mathscr{B}$ satisfies

$$(\text{Image } \mathscr{B})^\perp := \{q \in \mathbb{P}, \ b(q,w) = 0, \ \forall w \in \mathbb{V}\} = \{0\}.$$

Being closed and having the null space as orthogonal, Image $\mathscr{B}$ is therefore equal to the whole space $\mathbb{P}'$, which then implies that $\mathscr{B}$ is onto.

This achieves the proof of the first part of the theorem. To study its second part, that is the well-posedness of the mixed problem, we begin by observing that if $\mathscr{B}$ were not onto, the second equation of this mixed problem would not be solvable as soon as L_p were not in Image $\mathscr{B}$. Hence, the solvability of the mixed problem requires $\mathscr{B}$ to be onto.

Assuming now that this is the case, we can split $\mathbb{V}$ into

$$\mathbb{V} = \text{Ker } \mathscr{B} \oplus \text{Image } \mathscr{B}^{-1},$$

and infer as in the first part of the proof that $\mathscr{B}$ (resp. $\mathscr{B}^T$) is an isomorphism from Image $\mathscr{B}^{-1}$ onto $\mathbb{P}'$ (resp. from $\mathbb{P}$ onto Ker $\mathscr{B}^\perp$). By decomposing v into

$$v = v^0 + v^1, \quad v^0 \in \text{Ker } \mathscr{B}, \quad v^1 \in \text{Image } \mathscr{B}^{-1},$$

the second equation of the mixed problem takes the form

$$\mathscr{B} v^1 = L_p$$

which is equivalent to

$$v^1 = \mathscr{B}^{-1} L_p.$$

Using this value of v^1 in the first equation, we obtain
$$a(v^0, w) + b(p, w) = L_v(w) - a(\mathcal{B}^{-1}L_p, w) \quad \forall w \in \mathbb{V}.$$
By restricting ourselves to test functions w belonging to $\operatorname{Ker}\mathcal{B}$, and introducing the notation
$$L_k(w) = L_v(w) - a(\mathcal{B}^{-1}L_p, w) \quad \forall w \in \operatorname{Ker}\mathcal{B},$$
we finally obtain
$$\langle \mathcal{A}v^0, w\rangle = L_k(w) \quad \forall w \in \operatorname{Ker}\mathcal{B}, \ v^0 \in \operatorname{Ker}\mathcal{B}.$$

Obviously, this new equation is well-posed if and only if $\mathcal{A}$ is invertible. Assuming that this is also the case, we can then explicitly solve the mixed problem. Indeed, from above, we have first
$$v = \mathcal{A}^{-1}(L_k) + \mathcal{B}^{-1}(L_p)$$
which implies by construction
$$a(v, \cdot) - L_v(\cdot) \in \operatorname{Ker}\mathcal{B}^{\perp}.$$

But, $\mathcal{B}^{\mathrm{T}}$ is invertible on $\operatorname{Ker}\mathcal{B}^{\perp}$ and thus the above property implies the existence of a unique element p in $\mathbb{P}$ such that
$$\mathcal{B}_p^{\mathrm{T}}(\cdot) = b(p, \cdot) = a(v, \cdot) - L_v(\cdot) \in \mathbb{V}'.$$
This equality, combined with the property
$$\mathcal{B}v^1 = L_p,$$
implies that the pair (v, p) constructed above is the solution of the original mixed problem. This achieves the proof of the Ladyzenskaya–Babuska–Brezzi theorem. $\square$

For the present problem (14.2)–(14.3), replacing $b(\cdot, \cdot)$ by its definition, we find that the above inf-sup condition takes the form
$$\inf_{q_h \in \mathbb{P}_h, \|q_h\|=1} \left\{ \sup_{v_h \in \mathbb{V}_h, \|v_h\|=1} \left\{ \int_\Omega q_h \frac{\partial \det}{\partial F}(\operatorname{Id} + \nabla u_h) : \nabla v_h \, dx \right\} \right\}$$
$$= C_0(h) > 0. \tag{14.6}$$

The Ladyzenskaya–Babuska–Brezzi theorem now states that, for the linearized problem to be well-posed, which is certainly in general a minimal requirement to impose on the discrete problem, *the spaces $\mathbb{V}_h$ and $\mathbb{P}_h$ and the desired solution u_h must satisfy the above compatibility condition.* This condition causes the following remarks:

(i) Although (14.6) appears as an important and realistic condition to satisfy, it is very difficult to verify (14.6) in practice. Nevertheless, in any case, this forbids $\mathbb{P}_h$ to be too large, otherwise (14.6) would be obviously violated.

(ii) If we introduce the function $\varphi_h(x) = u_h(x) + x$ and suppose that φ_h is injective, then, from the identity

$$\frac{\partial \det}{\partial F}(F) : G = (\operatorname{cof} F) : G = \operatorname{tr}(GF^{-1})\det(F), \tag{14.7}$$

the condition (14.6) can be written as follows:

$$\inf_{q_h \in \mathbb{P}_h, \|q_h\|=1} \left\{ \sup_{v_h \in \mathbb{V}_h, \|v_h\|=1} \left\{ \int_{\varphi_h(\Omega)} (q_h \circ \varphi_h^{-1}) \operatorname{div}(v_h \circ \varphi_h^{-1}) \, dx^{\varphi} \right\} \right\} > 0. \tag{14.8}$$

In other words, (14.6) is a linear compatibility condition associated with the divergence operator on the deformed configuration.

(iii) For a given pair of spaces $\mathbb{V}_h$ and $\mathbb{P}_h$, (14.6) may or may not be satisfied depending on the value of the discrete solution u_h.

(iv) Condition (14.6), which appears here as a necessary condition to be satisfied by $\mathbb{V}_h$ and $\mathbb{P}_h$, is in fact sufficient to guarantee the existence of solutions for the full discrete problem and, for a given u_h, the uniqueness of the associated pressure field p_h (LE TALLEC [1981]).

In view of the above remarks, a practical strategy for choosing spaces $\mathbb{V}_h$ and $\mathbb{P}_h$ which are likely to satisfy (14.6), that is which are *likely* to lead to a reasonable discrete problem, can be the following:

Choose $\mathbb{V}_h$ and $\mathbb{P}_h$ satisfying (14.6) for $u_h = 0$. In other words, from (14.8), choose a pair of finite-element spaces that is well adapted to the mixed finite-element discretization of the Stokes problem. Such pairs, among which we find the elements of Section 12, are well known and can be found for example in GIRAULT and RAVIART [1986].

Verify that at the computed solution u_h, the spaces $\varphi_h(\mathbb{V}_h)$ and $\varphi_h(\mathbb{P}_h)$ keep the same structure so that (14.8), that is (14.6), is likely to hold.

15. Existence and convergence results

For completeness we give a brief survey of existence and convergence results for the incompressible discrete problem in the case of dead loading. The reader can find more details in LE TALLEC [1982].

First, let us recall our notation:

$$L(v) = \int_{\Omega} f \cdot v \, dx + \int_{\Gamma_1} g \cdot v \, da, \tag{15.1}$$

$$J(v) = \int_{\Omega} \hat{W}(x, \operatorname{Id} + \nabla v) \, dx - L(v), \tag{15.2}$$

$$\mathbb{H} = W^{1,s}(\Omega; \mathbb{E}) \times L^q(\Omega; \mathbb{M}^3),$$

$$\mathbb{U} = \{v, (v, \operatorname{cof}(\operatorname{Id} + \nabla v)) \in \mathbb{H}, \quad v = u_0 \text{ on } \Gamma_0,$$

$$\det(\mathrm{Id}+\nabla v) = 1 \text{ a.e in } \Omega\}, \tag{15.3}$$

$$\mathbb{U}_h = \{v_h, v_h - u_0 \in \mathbb{V}_h,$$

$$\int_\Omega q_h[\det(\mathrm{Id}+\nabla v_h) - 1] \, dx = 0, \quad \forall q_h \in \mathbb{P}_h\}, \tag{15.4}$$

$$d_{s,q}(u,v) = \|u - v\|_{1,s} + \|\operatorname{cof}(\mathrm{Id}+\nabla u) - \operatorname{cof}(\mathrm{Id}+\nabla v)\|_{0,q}, \tag{15.5}$$

$$B_{s,q}(u,r_0) = \{v, (v, \operatorname{cof}(\mathrm{Id}+\nabla v)) \in \mathbb{H}, \; d_{s,q}(u,v) \leqslant r_0\}. \tag{15.6}$$

Under this notation, we make the following assumptions:

(1) The stored energy function $\hat{W}$ satisfies

$$\hat{W}(x,\cdot) \text{ is continuously differentiable on } \mathbb{M}^3; \tag{15.7}$$

$$\hat{W} \text{ sends } L^r(\Omega; \mathbb{M}^3) \text{ into } L^1(\Omega); \tag{15.8}$$

$$\left|\frac{\partial \hat{W}}{\partial F}(x,F) : G\right| \leqslant K(x) + \lambda |F|^{r-1}|G|, \tag{15.9}$$

$$\forall \{F, G\} \in (\mathbb{M}^3)^2, \; K(x) \in L^1(\Omega), \; \lambda > 0 ;$$

$$\hat{W}(x,F) = a_1 |F|^s + a_2 |\operatorname{cof} F|^q + \hat{W}_0(x, F, \operatorname{cof} F), \tag{15.10}$$

$$s \geqslant \frac{3}{2}, \; q \geqslant \frac{s}{s-1}, \; a_1 > 0, \; a_2 > 0;$$

$$\hat{W}_0(x,\cdot,\cdot) \text{ is convex and } \hat{W}_0(\cdot, F, G) \text{ is measurable}; \tag{15.11}$$

$$\hat{W}_0(x, F, G) \geqslant a(x), \quad \forall \{F, G\} \in (\mathbb{M}^3)^2, \; a(x) \in L^1(\Omega). \tag{15.12}$$

(2) The loading $\{f, g\}$ is independent of u (dead loading) and

$$L(\cdot) \in [W^{1;s}(\Omega; \mathbb{E})]'.$$

(3) The displacement field u is an isolated minimizer of J over $\mathbb{U}$:

there exists a number r_0 such that

$$J(u) < J(v) \quad \forall v \in \mathbb{U} \cap B_{s,q}(u, r_0). \tag{15.13}$$

(4) The discrete spaces satisfy

$$\mathbb{V}_h \subset W^{1,r}(\Omega; \mathbb{E}), \tag{15.14}$$

$$\mathbb{P}_h \subset L^\infty(\Omega), \tag{15.15}$$

$$\mathcal{D}(\Omega) \text{ is included in the } L^\infty \text{ closure of } \bigcup_h \mathbb{P}_h ; \tag{15.16}$$

$$\forall h < h_0, \; \forall u_h \in \mathbb{U}_h \cap B_{s,q}(u, r_0),$$

the compatibility condition (14.6) is satisfied . \quad (15.17)

(5) The displacement field u can be approximated in $\mathbb{U}_h$, which means that there exists a field w_h in $\mathbb{U}_h \cap B_{s,q}(u, r_0)$ such that

$$\lim_{h \to 0} J(w_h) = J(u) \quad \text{(consistency)}. \tag{15.18}$$

Under the above assumptions, we can *prove* that any stable solution of the continuous problem can be approximated by a sequence of solutions of the discrete problems. More precisely, we have:

THEOREM 15.1. *For any isolated minimizer u satisfying (15.13)–(15.18), we can construct a sequence $\{u_h, p_h\}_h$ of solutions of the discrete incompressible problem (12.1)–(12.2) strongly converging towards u in the sense*

$$\lim_{h \to 0} d_{s,q}(u, u_h) = 0. \tag{15.19}$$

PROOF. The proof of this result follows closely the existence proof of BALL [1977] and is based on compactness arguments. It uses in fact two different topologies. For the continuous problem, as in BALL [1977], it uses the $\mathbb{H}$ topology in which we have coerciveness, convexity and weak compactness. As for the discrete space $\mathbb{V}_h + u_0$, it is endowed with the $W^{1,r}$ norm for which we will have continuous differentiability of the functional and of the constraints.

Step 1. J is of class $\mathscr{C}^1$ on $W^{1,r}(\Omega; \mathbb{E})$.

From a lemma due to KRASNOL'SKII [1964], any function Φ of the type

$$\Phi(y)(x) = \rho(x, y(x))$$

is continuous from $L^p(\Omega)$ into $L^q(\Omega)$ if ρ is Caratheodory and if Φ sends $L^p(\Omega)$ into $L^q(\Omega)$. If we apply this lemma successively for $\rho(x, y) = \hat{W}(x, F)$ and for $\rho(x, y) = (\partial \hat{W} / \partial F)(x, F)$, then from (15.8) and (15.9), we find that $\hat{W}$ and $(\partial \hat{W} / \partial F)$ are continuous from $L^r(\Omega; \mathbb{M}^3)$ into $L^1(\Omega)$ and $L^{r/(r-1)}(\Omega; \mathbb{M}^3)$, respectively. Hence, the functions $J(v)$ and $\nabla J(v)$ defined by (15.2) and by

$$\nabla J(v) \cdot w = \int_\Omega \frac{\partial \hat{W}}{\partial F}(x, \mathrm{Id} + \nabla v) : \nabla w \, dx - L(w) \tag{15.20}$$

are continuous from $W^{1,r}(\Omega; \mathbb{E})$ into $\mathbb{R}$ and $(W^{1,r}(\Omega; \mathbb{E}))'$, respectively.

We must now prove that ∇J is the gradient of J. For that purpose, for v and w in $W^{1,r}(\Omega; \mathbb{E})$, let us consider the function

$$\sigma(t, x) = \frac{1}{t}[\hat{W}(x, \mathrm{Id} + \nabla(v + tw)(x)) - \hat{W}(x, \mathrm{Id} + \nabla v(x))].$$

Since $\hat{W}$ is $\mathscr{C}^1$ on $\mathbb{M}^3$, we have

$$\forall x \in \Omega, \quad \lim_{t \to 0} \sigma(t, x) = \frac{\partial \hat{W}}{\partial F}(x, \mathrm{Id} + \nabla v) : \nabla w,$$

and

$$\sigma(t, x) = \frac{\partial \hat{W}}{\partial F}(x, \mathrm{Id} + \nabla v + \theta \nabla w) : \nabla w.$$

From (15.9), the above equation implies

$$|\sigma(t,x)| \leqslant K(x) + \lambda(|\operatorname{Id}+\nabla v| + |\nabla w|)^{r-1}|\nabla w|. \tag{15.21}$$

In summary, the functions $\sigma(t,x)$ are L^1 functions, dominated by (15.21) and converging pointwise. From the Lebesgue dominated convergence theorem, there is convergence of the integrals, which means that

$$\lim_{t \to 0} \frac{1}{t} [J(v+tw) - J(v)]$$

$$= \int_{\Omega} \lim_{t \to 0} \frac{1}{t} [\hat{W}(x, \operatorname{Id}+\nabla(v+tw)) - \hat{W}(x, \operatorname{Id}+\nabla v)] \, dx - L(w)$$

$$= \int_{\Omega} \frac{\partial \hat{W}}{\partial F}(x, \operatorname{Id}+\nabla v) : \nabla w \, dx - L(w)$$

$$= \nabla J(v) \cdot w.$$

Therefore, the continuous function J has for gradient the continuous function ∇J. Hence, it is of class $\mathscr{C}^1$ on $W^{1,r}(\Omega;\mathbb{E})$.

Step 2. $\mathbb{U}_h \cap B_{s,q}$ is closed.

Let us first recall that $\mathbb{V}_h + u_0$ is endowed once for all with the $W^{1,r}$ topology. From (15.10) and (15.12), we have

$$|\operatorname{Id}+\nabla u|^s + |\operatorname{cof}(\operatorname{Id}+\nabla u)|^q \leqslant \hat{W}(x, \operatorname{Id}+\nabla u) - a(x).$$

Since $\hat{W}$ sends continuously $L^r(\Omega;\mathbb{M}^3)$ into $L^1(\Omega)$ (step 1), this implies that the mappings $(\operatorname{Id}+\nabla v)$ and $\operatorname{cof}(\operatorname{Id}+\nabla v)$ are continuous from $W^{1,r}(\Omega,\mathbb{E})$ into $L^s(\Omega;\mathbb{M}^3)$ and $L^q(\Omega;\mathbb{M}^3)$, respectively. As a first consequence, this implies that $B_{s,q}(u,r_0) \cap (\mathbb{V}_h + u_0)$ is closed in $\mathbb{V}_h + u_0$ as the reciprocal image of a closed interval by a continuous function.

As a second consequence, this implies that the application $\det(\operatorname{Id}+\nabla v) = (\operatorname{Id}+\nabla v)_{i1} \operatorname{cof}(\operatorname{Id}+\nabla v)_{i1}$ is continuously differentiable from $W^{1,r}(\Omega;\mathbb{E})$ into $L^1(\Omega)$. Since $\mathbb{P}_h$ is included in $L^\infty(\Omega)$, this in turn implies that for any ψ_i in $\mathbb{P}_h$, the map

$$\mathscr{G}_i(v) = \int_{\Omega} \psi_i[\det(\operatorname{Id}+\nabla v) - 1] \, dx \tag{15.22}$$

is continuously differentiable on $\mathbb{V}_h + u_0$ with gradient

$$\nabla \mathscr{G}_i(v) \cdot w = \int_{\Omega} \psi_i \frac{\partial \det}{\partial F}(\operatorname{Id}+\nabla v) : \nabla w \, dx. \tag{15.23}$$

Let now $(\psi_i)_{i=1,M_h}$ be a given basis of $\mathbb{P}_h$. By construction, we have

$$\mathbb{U}_h = \left\{ v_h \in \mathbb{V}_h + u_0, \int_{\Omega} q_h[\det(\operatorname{Id}+\nabla v_h) - 1] \, dx = 0, \forall q_h \in \mathbb{P}_h \right\}$$

SECTION 15   *Approximation theory*   523

which by linearity yields

$$\mathbb{U}_h = \left\{ v_h \in \mathbb{V}_h + u_0, \int_\Omega \psi_i [\det(\mathrm{Id} + \nabla v_h) - 1] \, dx = 0, \forall i = 1, M_h \right\}. \quad (15.24)$$

In other words, $\mathbb{U}_h$ is the intersection of the reciprocal images of 0 by the continuous functions $\mathcal{G}_i$. It is therefore closed. Then $\mathbb{U}_h \cap B_{s,q}(u, r_0)$ is closed in $\mathbb{V}_h + u_0$ as the intersection of two closed subsets.

Step 3. Construction of u_h.

Let u be any isolated minimizer of J satisfying (15.13)–(15.18). For u given, let u_h be a minimizer of J over $\mathbb{U}_h \cap B_{s,q}(u, r_0)$. From the Weierstrass theorem, such a minimizer exists since $\mathbb{U}_h \cap B_{s,q}(u, r_0)$ contains w_h and is therefore not empty, $\mathbb{U}_h \cap B_{s,q}(u, r_0)$ is bounded and closed in the finite-dimensional space $\mathbb{V}_h + u_0$ (step 2), and J is continuous on $(\mathbb{V}_h + u_0)$ (step 1).

Moreover, since all these minimizers $(u_h)_h$ belong to $B_{s,q}(u, r_0)$ by construction, the sequences (u_h) and $(\mathrm{cof}(\nabla u_h + \mathrm{Id}))$ are bounded in the spaces $W^{1,s}(\Omega; \mathbb{E})$ and $L^q(\Omega; \mathbb{M}^3)$ respectively.

Step 4. Convergence of $(u_h)_h$.

From the above boundedness of $(u_h)_h$ and $(\mathrm{cof}(\mathrm{Id} + \nabla u_h))_h$, we can extract a subsequence $\{u_{hn}, \mathrm{cof}(\mathrm{Id} + \nabla u_{hn})\}_{hn}$ weakly converging towards $\{\overline{u}, \overline{G}\}$ in $\mathbb{H}$.

From BALL [1977], the application $\mathrm{cof}(\mathrm{Id} + \nabla \cdot)$ is weakly continuous from $W^{1,s}(\Omega; \mathbb{E})$ in $\mathcal{D}'(\Omega)$. By uniqueness of the limit in $\mathcal{D}'(\Omega)$, we have first

$$\overline{G} = \mathrm{cof}(\mathrm{Id} + \nabla \overline{u}) \in L^q(\Omega; \mathbb{M}^3). \quad (15.25)$$

Let now q be any element of $\mathcal{D}(\Omega)$. By assumption, there is a sequence $\{q_h\}_h$ of elements of $\mathbb{P}_h$ strongly converging towards q in $L^\infty(\Omega)$. The boundedness of the sequence $\{u_h, \mathrm{cof}(\mathrm{Id} + \nabla u_h)\}_h$ in $\mathbb{H}$ then yields

$$\lim_{h \to 0} \int_\Omega q[\det(\mathrm{Id} + \nabla u_h) - 1] \, dx$$

$$= \lim_{h \to 0} \int_\Omega q[(\mathrm{Id} + \nabla u_h)_{i1} \mathrm{cof}(\mathrm{Id} + \nabla u_h)_{i1} - 1] \, dx$$

$$= \lim_{h \to 0} \int_\Omega q_h[(\mathrm{Id} + \nabla u_h)_{i1} \mathrm{cof}(\mathrm{Id} + \nabla u_h)_{i1} - 1] \, dx$$

$$= \lim_{h \to 0} \int_\Omega q_h[\det(\mathrm{Id} + \nabla u_h) - 1] \, dx$$

$$= 0 \quad \text{because } u_h \in \mathbb{U}_h.$$

But, from BALL [1977], the weak convergence of $\{u_{hn}, \mathrm{cof}(\mathrm{Id} + \nabla u_{hn})\}$ towards $\{\overline{u}, \mathrm{cof}(\mathrm{Id} + \nabla \overline{u})\}$ in $\mathbb{H}$ implies the convergence of $\det(\mathrm{Id} + \nabla u_{hn})$ towards $\det(\mathrm{Id} + \nabla \overline{u})$ in $\mathcal{D}'(\Omega)$. Combining with the above inequality, we have

$$0 = \lim_{h_n \to 0} [\det(\mathrm{Id} + \nabla u_{hn}) - 1]$$

$$= \det(\mathrm{Id} + \nabla \bar{u}) - 1 \quad \text{in } \mathcal{D}'(\Omega), \tag{15.26}$$

which implies that $\bar{u}$ is in $\mathbb{U}$.

From (15.25), (15.26) and from the fact that closed balls are weakly closed in $\mathbb{H}$, we finally deduce that

$$\bar{u} \in \mathbb{U} \cap B_{s,q}(u, r_0). \tag{15.27}$$

Step 5. Characterization of $\bar{u}$.

By construction, u_h is a minimizer of J over $\mathbb{U}_h \cap B_{s,q}(u, r_0)$. In particular, we have

$$J(u_h) \leqslant J(w_h) \quad \forall h,$$

where w_h is the element introduced in (15.18). Let us now go to the limit as h goes to zero. From (15.12) and Fatou's lemma, the function

$$J_a(v, G) = \int_\Omega \{a_1 |\mathrm{Id} + \nabla v|^s + a_2 |G|^q + \hat{W}_0(x, \mathrm{Id} + \nabla v, G)\} \, dx - L(v)$$

is lower-semicontinuous on $\mathbb{H}$ (BALL [1977]). Since J_a is also convex, it is then sequentially weakly lower-semicontinuous on $\mathbb{H}$. Hence we have

$$J(\bar{u}) = J_a(\bar{u}, \mathrm{cof}(\mathrm{Id} + \nabla \bar{u}))$$
$$\leqslant \liminf J_a(u_{hn}, \mathrm{cof}(\mathrm{Id} + \nabla u_{hn}))$$
$$\leqslant \limsup J(u_{hn})$$
$$\leqslant \lim J(w_{hn})$$
$$\leqslant J(u).$$

Since u is the unique minimizer of J on $\mathbb{U} \cap B_{s,q}(u, r_0)$, this implies

$$\bar{u} = u \quad \text{and} \quad \lim_{hn \to 0} J(u_{hn}) = J(u).$$

By repeating Steps 4 and 5 for any converging subsequence $\{u_{hn}, \mathrm{cof}(\mathrm{Id} + \nabla u_{hn})\}_{hn}$, we deduce that the whole sequence $\{u_h, \mathrm{cof}(\mathrm{Id} + \nabla u_h)\}_h$ converges weakly towards $\{u, \mathrm{cof}(\mathrm{Id} + \nabla u)\}$ in $\mathbb{H}$ and that

$$J(u) = \lim_{h \to 0} J(u_h). \tag{15.28}$$

Step 6. Strong convergence.

From (15.10), J can be written

$$J(v) = J_0(v, \mathrm{cof}(\mathrm{Id} + \nabla v)) + J_1(v) + J_2(\mathrm{cof}(\mathrm{Id} + \nabla v))$$

with J_0 weakly lower-semicontinuous on $\mathbb{H}$ and J_1 and J_2 given by

$$J_1(v) = a_1 \|\mathrm{Id} + \nabla v\|_{0,s}^s,$$
$$J_2(G) = a_2 \|G\|_{0,q}^q,$$

respectively. From (15.28), we must have

$$\lim_{h \to 0} J_i(u_h, \mathrm{cof}(\mathrm{Id} + \nabla u_h)) = J_i(u, \mathrm{cof}\,\mathrm{Id} + \nabla u)),$$

otherwise the weak lower semi-continuity of one of the functions J_i would be violated. But J_1 and J_2 define norms on $W^{1,s}(\Omega;\mathbb{E})$ and $L^q(\Omega,\mathbb{M}^3)$, respectively. Therefore $\{u_h, \mathrm{cof}(\mathrm{Id}+\nabla u_h)\}_h$ converges weakly and in norm towards $\{u, \mathrm{cof}(\mathrm{Id}+\nabla u)\}$ in $W^{1,s}(\Omega;\mathbb{E}) \times L^q(\Omega;\mathbb{M}^3)$. This implies strong convergence, which means that we have

$$\lim_{h \to 0} d_{s,q}(u, u_h) = 0. \tag{15.29}$$

Step 7. u_h corresponds to a solution of the discrete problem.

Since $d_{s,q}(u, \cdot)$ is continuous on $\mathbb{V}_h + u_0$, (15.29) implies that, for h sufficiently small, u_h is in the interior of $B_{s,q}(u, r_0)$. It is therefore by construction a local minimizer of J on $\mathbb{U}_h$. From the characterization of $\mathbb{U}_h$ given in (15.24), this means that u_h is a local solution of the problem

Minimize $J(v_h)$
subject to $v_h \in \mathbb{V}_h + u_0$
$\mathcal{G}_i(v_h) = 0 \quad \forall i = 1, M_h$.

From the Lagrange multiplier theory, since J and $\mathcal{G}_i$ are $\mathscr{C}^1$ real functions defined on $\mathbb{V}_h + u_0$, there exist numbers r_0 and r_i, not all zero, such that

$$r_0 \nabla J(u_h) \cdot v_h + \sum_{i=1}^{M_h} r_i \nabla \mathcal{G}_i(u_h) \cdot v_h = 0 \quad \forall v_h \in \mathbb{V}_h. \tag{15.30}$$

Suppose now that $r_0 = 0$. From (15.23), the above equation will then be

$$\int_\Omega \left(\sum_{i=1}^{M_h} r_i \psi_i\right) \frac{\partial \det}{\partial F}(\mathrm{Id}+\nabla u_h) : \nabla v_h \, dx = 0 \quad \forall v_h \in \mathbb{V}_h,$$

which clearly violates (14.6). Therefore, r_0 must be different from zero. Then, after division by r_0, (15.30) yields

$$\nabla J(u_h) \cdot v_h - \int_\Omega p_h \frac{\partial \det}{\partial F}(\mathrm{Id}+\nabla u_h) : \nabla v_h \, dx = 0 \quad \forall v_h \in \mathbb{V}_h,$$

with ∇J given by (15.20) and where we have denoted

$$p_h = -\left(\sum_{i=1}^{M_h} r_i \psi_i\right) r_0^{-1}.$$

This is exactly (12.1), and since u_h belongs to $\mathbb{U}_h$ by construction, $\{u_h, p_h\}$ is a solution of the discrete problem (12.1)–(12.2).

This completes our proof. Observe in addition that for a given u_h, there can only be one associated pressure field p_h. If there were two, their difference would violate (14.6). □

16. Convergence in the compressible case

With few modifications, the above proof of convergence can be applied to the compressible case as well. More precisely, in the compressible case, the definitions of $\mathbb{U}_h$ and $d_{s,q}$ are changed into

$$\mathbb{U}_h = \left\{ v_h, v_h - u_0 \in \mathbb{V}_h, \det(\mathrm{Id} + \nabla v_h) > 0 \text{ a.e. on } \Omega \right\},$$

$$d_{s,q}(u,v) = \|u - v\|_{1,s} + \|\operatorname{cof}(\mathrm{Id} + \nabla u) - \operatorname{cof}(\mathrm{Id} + \nabla v)\|_{0,q}$$
$$+ \|\det(\mathrm{Id} + \nabla u) - \det(\mathrm{Id} + \nabla v)\|_{0,r}.$$

Then the assumptions (15.7) and (15.10) are replaced by

$$\hat{W}(x,F) = a_1 |F|^s + a_2 |\operatorname{cof} F|^q + a_3 |\det F|^r$$
$$+ W_0(x, F, \operatorname{cof} F, \det F),$$

$$\lim_{\det F \to 0} \hat{W}(x,F) = +\infty,$$

$$W_0(x, F, G, \delta) \in C^1(\bar{\Omega} \times \mathbb{M}^3 \times \mathbb{M}^3 \times \mathbb{R}^+)$$

$$s \geq \frac{3}{2}, \quad q \geq \frac{s}{s-1}, \quad r > 1, \quad a_1 > 0, \quad a_2 > 0, \quad a_3 > 0, \tag{16.1}$$

the conditions on the discrete spaces become

$$\mathbb{V}_h \subset \left\{ v_h \in C^0(\bar{\Omega}), v_{h|\Omega_l} \in C^1(\bar{\Omega}_l), \forall l = 1, \ldots, N_h \right\},$$

and the other assumptions are unchanged. We then have

THEOREM 16.1. *For any isolated minimizer u satisfying the above assumptions, we can construct a sequence $\{u_h\}_h$ of solutions of the discrete compressible problem (11.1) strongly converging towards u in the sense*

$$\lim_{h \to 0} d_{s,q}(u, u_h) = 0. \tag{16.2}$$

PROOF. We briefly sketch the proof which follows the steps of the incompressible case.

First, as for the continuous problem, we associate with the energy potential J the auxiliary function J_a equal to J on $\mathbb{U}$ and to $+\infty$ elsewhere. This functional is easily proved to be lower-semicontinuous on $\mathbb{V}_h + u_0$. Hence, by the Weierstrass theorem, it has a minimizer u_h on $(\mathbb{V}_h + u_0) \cap B_{s,q}(u, r_0)$. By weak compactness argument, it follows as in Theorem 8.1 that the sequence $\{u_h\}_h$ weakly converges to elements $\bar{u} \in \mathbb{U}$. From the weak lower-semicontinuity of J_a on $\mathbb{U}$, it also follows that we have

$$\bar{u} = u, \quad J(u) = \lim_{h \to 0} J(u_h).$$

As in the incompressible case, this convergence result implies the strong convergence of u_h towards u in $\mathbb{H}$. As a consequence, u_h is a local minimizer of J_a

on ($\mathbb{V}_h + u_0$). But $J_a(u_h)$ is finite, thus u_h belongs to $\mathbb{U}_h$. Since u_h is also piecewise continuously differentiable, we have by continuity

$$\det(\mathrm{Id} + \nabla u_h)(x) \geq \delta_{\min} > 0 \quad \forall x \in \Omega.$$

From (16.1), it follows that u_h belongs to the interior of $\mathbb{U}_h$ for the $W^{1,\infty}$ topology and that J_a is differentiable at u_h in $\mathbb{V}_h$. Being also a minimizer of J_a, it satisfies

$$\nabla J_a(u_h) \cdot v_h = 0 \quad \forall v_h \in \mathbb{V}_h,$$

which is precisely (11.1). □

17. Additional remarks on the convergence theorems

Among the assumptions of the above convergence theorems, the conditions (15.7)–(15.12) on the stored energy function are not restrictive. They are satisfied for example by Mooney–Rivlin materials and by different classes of Ogden-type materials.

The conditions (15.17) and (15.18) are much more restrictive. We have already discussed the implications of (15.17) in Section 14. We will now state a consistency result, which proves (15.18) under additional regularity assumptions on the solution u (LE TALLEC [1982]).

For this purpose, we will *assume* that u belongs to $W^{1,3r}(\Omega)$. We also *assume* that the spaces $\mathbb{V}_h$ and $\mathbb{P}_h$ satisfy the compatibility condition (14.6) uniformly around u, that is there exists $\varepsilon_0 > 0$ and $C_0(h) > 0$ such that for any w_h verifying

$$w_h \in \mathbb{V}_h + u_0, \quad \|w_h - u\|_{1,r} \leq \varepsilon_0,$$

$$\int_\Omega q_h (\det(\mathrm{Id} + \nabla w_h) - 1)\, \mathrm{d}x \leq \varepsilon_0 \|q_h\|_{0,r^*} \quad \forall q_h \in \mathbb{P}_h,$$

we have

$$\inf_{q_h \in \mathbb{P}_h} \left\{ \sup_{v_h \in \mathbb{V}_h} \left\{ \frac{\int_\Omega q_h (\partial \det / \partial F)(\mathrm{Id} + \nabla w_h) : \nabla v_h \, \mathrm{d}x}{\|q_h\|_{0,r^*} \|v_h\|_{1,r}} \right\} \right\} \geq C_0(h).$$

Finally, we *suppose* that the spaces $\mathbb{V}_h$ and $\mathbb{P}_h$ are such that

$$\lim_{h \to 0} \left\{ C_0(h)^{-2} h^{-2/r} \inf_{w_h \in \mathbb{V}_h + u_0} \left(\|u - w_h\|_{1,3r} \right) \right\} = 0.$$

Under the above assumptions, it is then possible to *prove* that for any h, there exists w_h in $\mathbb{U}_h$ such that

$$\|u - w_h\|_{1,r} \leq C(u) C_0(h)^{-1} \inf_{z_h \in \mathbb{V}_h + u_0} \|u - z_h\|_{1,3r}. \tag{17.1}$$

To prove this, we construct an element w_h of $\mathbb{U}_h$ by solving the equation

$$\int_\Omega q_h [\det(\mathrm{Id} + \nabla w_h) - 1] \, \mathrm{d}x = 0 \quad \forall q_h \in \mathbb{P}_h,$$

by a Newton's method taking as initial guess the best approximation of u in $\mathbb{V}_h + u_0$.

REMARK 17.1. From the continuity of J on $W^{1,r}(\Omega;\mathbb{E})$, (15.18) becomes a direct consequence of (17.1). Observe that the additional regularity required on u for proving (17.1) will not be needed if one could prove the following conjecture:

$$\forall u \in \mathbb{U}, \ \exists u_\varepsilon \in \mathbb{U} \cap W^{m,p}(\Omega;\mathbb{E}) \text{ such that}$$
$$\lim_{\varepsilon \to 0} d_{s,q}(u, u_\varepsilon) = 0.$$

In other words, are there regular volume-preserving approximations of any given volume-preserving map?

CHAPTER IV

Numerical Solution Techniques

After introduction of the mathematical formulation of equilibrium problems in finite elasticity (Chapter II) and their approximation by finite-elements (Chapter III), we are facing the problem of numerically solving nonlinear variational problems with a finite number of unknowns. After development of the unknown fields on an adequate nodal basis of the finite-element spaces, these discrete problems take the form of algebraic systems of N_h nonlinear equations with N_h scalar unknowns. These systems are large (typical values range from $N_h = 10^3$ to $N_h = 10^6$), but sparse and somewhat easy to linearize. They can be efficiently solved numerically by Newton's type techniques.

The Newton–Raphson method replaces the nonlinear equation $\mathscr{F}(X) = 0$ by its first-order expansion around the point X^n

$$\mathscr{F}(X^n) + \frac{\mathrm{D}\mathscr{F}(X^n)}{\mathrm{D}(X)}(X^{n+1} - X^n) = 0.$$

The resulting linear system can then be solved, leading to an approximate solution X^{n+1} which is used as a starting value for another step in the iteration process. This method has very nice local convergence properties as explained in detail in ORTEGA and RHEINBOLDT [1970]. It has been applied with success in finite elasticity as described in ODEN [1972].

Unfortunately, Newton's method has three drawbacks. First, the tangent matrix is often difficult to compute. Second, the method is expensive because of the large number of algebraic operations involved in the construction and factorisation of the tangent matrix. Finally, the method often fails to converge if not properly initialized. In finite elasticity, the calculation of the tangent matrix is technical but is done locally at each quadrature point of each finite-element. Furthermore, its calculation is greatly simplified by the use of computer algebra software like MAPLE. The computing cost stays high but is now affordable due to the increased power of modern computers. Initialization is therefore the main problem when applying Newton's techniques to finite elasticity.

The initialization strategy classically used in finite elasticity is the method of incremental loading described in ODEN ([1972], p. 284). In this method, the load acting on the body is considered to be applied in small increments. The equilibrium position of the body is calculated at the end of each load increment using the position at previous increment as initial guess. This strategy therefore computes a whole path of solutions between the initial configuration and the final equilibrium position. This strategy has a long history (FICKEN [1951]), but is very sensitive to the choice of the load increment. Arclength continuation methods introduced in KELLER [1983] overcome this difficulty by replacing the arbitrary choice of the load increment by an arclength constraint imposed on the solution curve. This results in an automatic procedure which is only marginally different from a standard Newton's method but which is far more robust. Overall, the best numerical strategy is therefore to use the basic Newton's method when it works and, in case of convergence problems, to switch directly to an arclength continuation procedure.

The present chapter describes such an application of Newton's techniques to the numerical solution of equilibrium problems in finite elasticity. We first recall the algebraic system we have to solve (Section 18). Newton's method is then introduced, first in its original version (Section 19), then in conjunction with incremental loading (Section 20) and finally within an arclength continuation framework (Section 21). The chapter concludes with a brief overview of some implementation aspects.

More details on the numerical solution of nonlinear problems can be found in ORTEGA and RHEINBOLDT [1970], FLETCHER [1980], GILL, MURRAY and WRIGHT [1981] or DENNIS and SCHNABEL [1983]. For a first description of the application of the Newton's method to finite elasticity problems, we refer to ODEN [1972].

18. The system to solve

In the incompressible case, the finite-element approximation of the original equilibrium problem (7.3)–(7.4) is simply:

Find $(u - u_0)$ in $\mathbb{V}_h$ and p_h in $\mathbb{P}_h$ such that:

$$\int_\Omega \frac{\partial \hat{W}}{\partial F}(x, \mathrm{Id} + \nabla u_h) : \nabla v_h \, dx - \int_\Omega p_h \frac{\partial \det}{\partial F}(\mathrm{Id} + \nabla u_h) : \nabla v_h \, dx$$

$$= \int_\Omega f \cdot v_h \, dx + \int_{\Gamma_1} g \cdot v_h \, da \quad \forall v_h \in \mathbb{V}_h,$$

$$\int_\Omega q_h [\det(\mathrm{Id} + \nabla u_h) - 1] \, dx = 0 \quad \forall q_h \in \mathbb{P}_h.$$

Let us choose a basis $\{\varphi_i\}_{i=1,N_h}$ of $\mathbb{V}_h$ and a basis $\{\psi_i\}_{i=1,M_h}$ of $\mathbb{P}_h$. The most natural choice is obviously to take for φ_i and ψ_i the shape functions associated with the i-nodal degree of freedom of $\mathbb{V}_h$ and $\mathbb{P}_h$, respectively (CIARLET [1991]). If we expand the above system in these basis, our finite-element problem takes the form of the algebraic system:

Find $\{U, P\} \in \mathbb{R}^{N_h} \times \mathbb{R}^{M_h}$ such that

$$\mathcal{F}(U, P, f, g) = 0 \quad \text{in } \mathbb{R}^{N_h} \times \mathbb{R}^{M_h}, \tag{18.1}$$

with the notation

$$\mathscr{F}_i(U,P,f,g) = \int_\Omega \frac{\partial \hat{W}}{\partial F}(x, \mathrm{Id}+\nabla u_h) : \nabla \varphi_i \, dx$$

$$- \int_\Omega p_h \frac{\partial \det}{\partial F}(\mathrm{Id}+\nabla u_h) : \nabla \varphi_i \, dx$$

$$- \int_\Omega f \cdot \varphi_i \, dx - \int_{\Gamma_1} g \cdot \varphi_i \, da \text{ for } i = 1, N_h, \tag{18.2}$$

$$\mathscr{F}_{i+N_h}(U,P,f,g) = - \int_\Omega \psi_i [\det(\mathrm{Id}+\nabla u_h) - 1] \, dx \text{ for } i = 1, M_h, \tag{18.3}$$

$$u_h(x) = u_0(x) + \sum_{i=1}^{N_h} U_i \varphi_i(x), \tag{18.4}$$

$$p_h(x) = \sum_{i=1}^{M_h} P_i \psi_i(x). \tag{18.5}$$

The gradient of $\mathscr{F}$ has already been computed in Section 14 and has value:

$$\frac{\partial \mathscr{F}_i}{\partial U}(U,P,f,g) V = a_{u_h,p_h}(v_h, \varphi_i) \quad \text{for } 1 \leqslant i \leqslant N_h, \tag{18.6}$$

$$\frac{\partial \mathscr{F}_{i+N_h}}{\partial U}(U,P,f,g) V = b_{u_h}(\psi_i, v_h) \quad \text{for } 1 \leqslant i \leqslant M_h, \tag{18.7}$$

$$\frac{\partial \mathscr{F}_i}{\partial P}(U,P,f,g) Q = b_{u_h}(q_h, \varphi_i) \quad \text{for } 1 \leqslant i \leqslant N_h, \tag{18.8}$$

$$\frac{\partial \mathscr{F}_{i+N_h}}{\partial P}(U,P,f,g) Q = 0 \quad \text{for } 1 \leqslant i \leqslant M_h, \tag{18.9}$$

with the notation

$$v_h = \sum_{i=1}^{N_h} V_i \varphi_i, \tag{18.10}$$

$$q_h = \sum_{i=1}^{M_h} Q_i \psi_i, \tag{18.11}$$

$$a_{u_h,p_h}(v_h, w_h) = \int_\Omega \left(\frac{\partial^2 \hat{W}}{\partial F^2}(x, \mathrm{Id}+\nabla u_h) : \nabla v_h \right) : \nabla w_h \, dx$$

$$- \int_\Omega p_h \left(\frac{\partial^2 \det}{\partial F^2}(\mathrm{Id}+\nabla u_h) : \nabla v_h \right) : \nabla w_h \, dx, \tag{18.12}$$

$$b_{u_h}(q_h, v_h) = -\int_\Omega q_h \frac{\partial \det}{\partial F}(\mathrm{Id} + \nabla u_h) : \nabla v_h \, dx. \tag{18.13}$$

In the nearly incompressible case, the finite-element formulation (13.2) also takes the form (18.1) but then we have $M_h = 0$, and

$$\mathcal{F}_i(U, f, g) = \int_\Omega \frac{\partial \hat{W}_0}{\partial F}(x, \mathrm{Id} + \nabla u_h) : \nabla \varphi_i \, dx$$

$$+ \int_\Omega \frac{1}{\varepsilon} [\det(\mathrm{Id} + \nabla_h u_h) - 1] \frac{\partial \det}{\partial F}(\mathrm{Id} + \nabla_h u_h) : \nabla_h \varphi_i \, dx$$

$$- \int_\Omega f \cdot \varphi_i \, dx - \int_{\Gamma_1} g \cdot \varphi_i \, da \quad \text{for } 1 \leqslant i \leqslant N_h, \tag{18.14}$$

$$a_{u_h}(v_h, w_h) = \int_\Omega \left(\frac{\partial^2 \hat{W}_0}{\partial F^2}(x, \mathrm{Id} + \nabla u_h) : \nabla v_h \right) : \nabla w_h \, dx$$

$$+ \int_\Omega \frac{1}{\varepsilon} [\det(\mathrm{Id} + \nabla_h u_h) - 1]$$

$$\times \left[\frac{\partial^2 \det}{\partial F^2}(\mathrm{Id} + \nabla_h u_h) : \nabla_h v_h \right] : \nabla_h w_h \, dx$$

$$+ \int_\Omega \frac{1}{\varepsilon} \left[\frac{\partial \det}{\partial F}(\mathrm{Id} + \nabla_h u_h) : \nabla_h v_h \right]$$

$$\times \left[\frac{\partial \det}{\partial F}(\mathrm{Id} + \nabla_h u_h) : \nabla_h w_h \right] dx. \tag{18.15}$$

Finally, the truly compressible case is obtained by suppressing the terms involving ε in (18.14)–(18.15). In any case, we face a nonlinear system (18.1) whose linearized form is explicitly known. We now proceed to describe its numerical solution by Newton's type methods.

In what follows, the numerical algorithms will be described in the incompressible case, which is the more complicated one. The compressible case is then simply obtained by setting $M_h = 0$ or, equivalently, by erasing the variable P everywhere in the algorithms.

REMARK 18.1. From the constitutive relation introduced in the earlier sections

$$\hat{W}(F) = \tilde{W}(C)$$

with

$$C = \mathrm{Id} + 2E = F^T F,$$

we have
$$\frac{\partial \hat{W}}{\partial F} = 2F \frac{\partial \tilde{W}}{\partial C}.$$

Thus, if we introduce the notation
$$\tilde{\Sigma}_c = 2\frac{\partial \tilde{W}}{\partial C} = \frac{\partial \tilde{W}}{\partial E},$$

the bilinear form (18.12) can also be rewritten
$$a_{u_h,p_h}(v_h, w_h) = \int_\Omega \left\{ \left(\frac{\partial^2 \tilde{W}}{\partial E^2} : F^T \nabla v_h\right) : F^T \nabla w_h + \tilde{\Sigma}_c : \nabla v_h^T \nabla w_h \right\} dx$$
$$- \int_\Omega p_h \left(\frac{\partial^2 \det}{\partial F^2}(\mathrm{Id} + \nabla u_h) : \nabla v_h\right) : \nabla w_h \, dx.$$

This last form is often used in practice.

19. The basic Newton's method

The basic Newton's method replaces iteratively in the equation $\mathscr{F} = 0$ the function $\mathscr{F}$ by its first-order expansion around the point $\{U^n, P^n\}$. In other words, the basic Newton's method solves iteratively the linear equation (Fig. 19.1)

$$\mathscr{F}(U^n, P^n, f, g) + \frac{\mathrm{D}\mathscr{F}(U^n, P^n, f, g)}{\mathrm{D}(U, P)}(U^{n+1} - U^n, P^{n+1} - P^n) = 0.$$

More precisely, the numerical solution of problem (18.1) by the basic Newton's method corresponds to the algorithm:

Step 0. Initialization.
With $\{U^0, P^0\}$ in $\mathbb{R}^{N_h} \times \mathbb{R}^{M_h}$ specified arbitrarily, calculate
$$R_i^0 = \mathscr{F}_i(U^0, P^0, f, g), \quad 1 \leqslant i \leqslant N_h + M_h.$$

Step 1. Iterative loop.
Then, for $n \geqslant 0$, with U^n, P^n, R^n known, compute $U^{n+1}, P^{n+1}, R^{n+1}$ by

(i) solving the linear system (S)
$$\frac{\mathrm{D}\mathscr{F}(U^n, P^n, f, g)}{\mathrm{D}(U, P)}(V^n, Q^n) = R^n \quad \text{in } \mathbb{R}^{N_h} \times \mathbb{R}^{M_h},$$

(ii) setting $U^{n+1} = U^n - V^n$ and $P^{n+1} = P^n - Q^n$,
(iii) computing $R_i^{n+1} = \mathscr{F}_i(U^{n+1}, P^{n+1}, f, g), 1 \leqslant i \leqslant N_h + M_h$.

The algorithm is stopped as soon as the error
$$\text{error} = a_1 \|R^{n+1}\| + a_2 \|V^n\| + a_3 \|Q^n\|$$

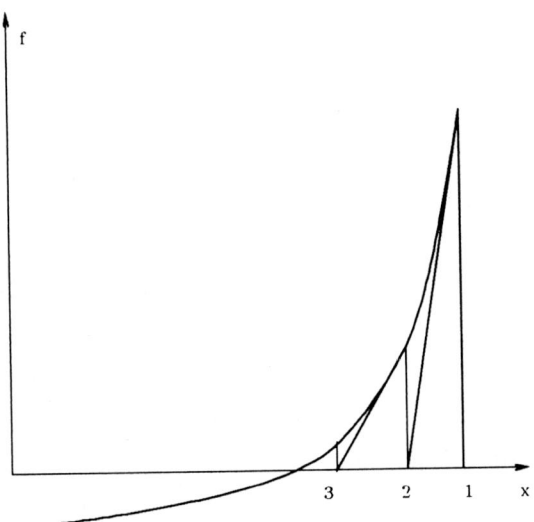

FIG. 19.1. Newton's method. We iteratively replace the curve $f(x)$ by its tangent at point i and compute the intersection $i+1$ of this tangent with the plane $f = 0$.

is sufficiently small.

This algorithm is known to converge fast if we are in a neighborhood of a solution:

THEOREM 19.1. *Let (U, P) be a solution of $\mathcal{F}(U, P) = 0$, with $D\mathcal{F}(U, P, f, g)/D(U, P)$ invertible and locally Lipschitz continuous. Then, if (U^0, P^0) is sufficiently close to (U, P), we have*

$$\|(U^{n+1}, P^{n+1}) - (U, P)\| \leqslant \beta \|(U^n, P^n) - (U, P)\|^2.$$

The above convergence theorem, proved in ORTEGA and RHEINBOLDT [1970], guarantees the quadratic convergence of the Newton's method only if we are in a neighborhood of the desired solution. Therefore, the choice of the initial guess $\{U^0, P^0\}$ is critical.

Moreover, the theorem requires the invertibility of the gradient

$$\frac{D\mathcal{F}(U, P, f, g)}{D(U, P)},$$

which means that we must be able to solve the linear system (S). By construction, this system is

$$\frac{\partial \mathcal{F}_i}{\partial U} V^n + \frac{\partial \mathcal{F}_i}{\partial P} Q^n + \left(\frac{\partial \mathcal{F}_i}{\partial f} \frac{\partial f}{\partial U} + \frac{\partial \mathcal{F}_i}{\partial g} \frac{\partial g}{\partial U} \right) V^n = R_i^n,$$

$1 \leqslant i \leqslant N_h + M_h.$

By using the values of the gradient of $\mathcal{F}$, this system takes the matricial form

$$\begin{pmatrix} (\mathcal{A} + C) & B^T \\ B & 0 \end{pmatrix} \begin{pmatrix} V^n \\ Q^n \end{pmatrix} = \begin{pmatrix} R_U^n \\ R_P^n \end{pmatrix} \quad \text{in } \mathbb{R}^{N_h} \times \mathbb{R}^{M_h}, \tag{19.1}$$

with

$$\mathcal{A}_{ij} = a_{u_h^n, p_h^n}(\varphi_j, \varphi_i), \quad 1 \leqslant i, j \leqslant N_h,$$

$$C_{ij} = \int_\Omega \frac{\partial f}{\partial U_j} \cdot \varphi_i \, dx + \int_{\Gamma_1} \frac{\partial g}{\partial U_j} \cdot \varphi_i \, da, \quad 1 \leqslant i, j \leqslant N_h,$$

$$B_{ij} = b_{u_h^n}(\psi_i, \varphi_j), \quad 1 \leqslant i \leqslant M_h, \ 1 \leqslant j \leqslant N_h.$$

From the Ladyzenskaya–Babuska–Brezzi theorem, for (19.1) to be well-posed, it is first necessary that the application $\mathcal{B}$ of matrix B defined in Section 14 from $\mathbb{V}_h$ onto $\mathbb{P}'_h$ by

$$\langle \mathcal{B} v_h, q_h \rangle = b(q_h, v_h) \quad \forall q_h \in \mathbb{P}_h, \ \forall v_h \in \mathbb{V}_h,$$

be onto. As seen in Section 14, this means equivalently that the compatibility condition (14.6) must be satisfied. If $\mathcal{B}$ is onto, then the same theorem states that (19.1) will be well-posed if and only if $(\mathcal{A} + C)$ is invertible on the kernel of $\mathcal{B}$, which is the case if we are away from limit points or bifurcation points.

In summary, the linear system (19.1) is well posed (and hence the Newton's algorithm is well defined) away from limit points and bifurcation points and if the discrete spaces $\mathbb{V}_h$ and $\mathbb{P}_h$ are compatible in the sense of condition (14.6).

20. Newton's method with incremental loading

We have just seen how critical a good initial guess was for ensuring the convergence of the Newton's method. Incremental loading is a computing strategy which provides such initial guesses. In incremental loading, instead of directly computing the final solution, we follow the differential curve

$$\mathcal{A}'(u) \frac{du}{ds} = \frac{df}{ds},$$

$$u(0) = u^0,$$

introduced in Section 10 (Fig. 20.1). In our present notation, we have

$$u = (U, P), \quad \mathcal{A}'(u) = \frac{D\mathcal{F}}{D(U, P)},$$

$$f(s) = \lambda(s)\{f, g\}, \quad \lambda(s) = s.$$

The construction of the solution curve is then done step by step, each step being solved by the following algorithm:

(i) Predict the solution $u(\lambda^n + \Delta\lambda)$ by the explicit Euler scheme

$$u(\lambda^n + \Delta\lambda) \approx \tilde{u}^{n+1} = u(\lambda^n) + \Delta\lambda \, (\mathcal{A}'(u(\lambda^n)))^{-1} \frac{df}{ds}.$$

(ii) Correct this first-order prediction by solving

$$\mathcal{A}\,(u(\lambda^n + \Delta\lambda)) = f(\lambda^n + \Delta\lambda)$$

by a Newton's method taking as initial guess the prediction $\tilde{u}^{n+1}$.

Such a guess $\tilde{u}^{n+1}$ will indeed be close to the corresponding equilibrium solution if the load increment is not too large. As a consequence, the second step of the above algorithm will converge fast in most cases.

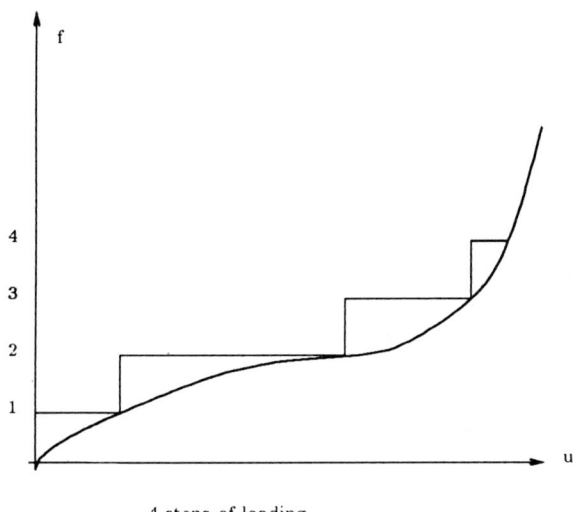

4 steps of loading

FIG. 20.1. Incremental loading. Instead of directly computing the solution for a given value of f, we compute the solution for different values i equally distributed between 0 and the final loading. With this, we get intermediate solutions u_i which can be used to initiate the calculation of the next step $i + 1$.

To further enhance the convergence of the Newton's method, one must also avoid the kind of divergent behavior which is described in Fig. 20.2, and which might occur if the initial guess is not sufficiently close to the solution.

Line damping avoids this divergent behavior by imposing a decrease in the residual at each iteration: if the residual at the proposed new iterate (U^n +

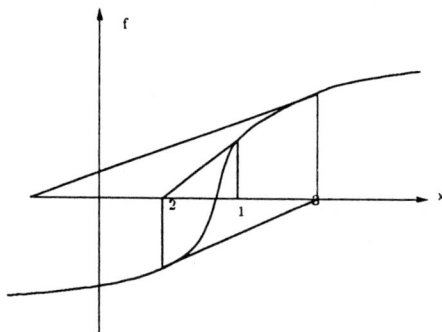

FIG. 20.2. Diverging Newton's sequence. Starting from the point 1, Newton's algorithm generates a diverging sequence.

ΔU, $P^n + \Delta P$) is bigger than the residual at step n, one decreases the increment by a factor α until one reaches a point $(U^n + \alpha * \Delta U, P^n + \alpha * \Delta P)$ with a lower residual (or with a lower energy).

With these two convergence enhancements, it is then possible to freeze the tangent operator. Recall that the update and the factorization of the tangent operator

$$\frac{\partial \mathscr{F}}{\partial (U, P)}$$

often account for more than 80% of the computing time when dealing with three-dimensional situations on sequential machines. Keeping the same operator for several consecutive iterations might save some computing time without jeopardizing the overall convergence, at least if one uses incremental loading and line damping. The simultaneous use of incremental loading, line damping and "frozen" tangential operators leads to the most popular algorithm in finite elasticity. This algorithm has been described in many places, starting with ODEN [1972], and is used in many physical situations.

NEWTON WITH INCREMENTAL LOADING AND LINE DAMPING: DETAILED ALGORITHM

Initialization
We start with $U^0 = 0$, P^0 equal to the hydrostatic pressure at rest, $\lambda = 0$ and with a given load increment $\Delta \lambda$. Then, we increase the value of λ by increments of $\Delta \lambda$ until we reach the value $\lambda = 1$. For each value of λ, starting with the solution (U^0, P^0) obtained at the previous increment, we compute the solution values of (U, P) by a Newton's procedure. More precisely:

Newton's procedure
Step 0. Initialization.
   We compute the residual: $R^0 = \mathscr{F}(U^0, P^0, \lambda f, \lambda g)$.
Step 1. Iterative loop.

Then, for $n \geqslant 0$ and until satisfied, with U^n, P^n, R^n known, we compute $U^{n+1}, P^{n+1}, R^{n+1}$ by

(i) computing and factoring the tangent operator (if needed):
$$K = \frac{\partial \mathcal{F}(U^n, P^n, \lambda f, \lambda g)}{\partial (U, P)},$$

(ii) solving the linear system (S):
$$K(\Delta U, \Delta P) = -R^n,$$

(iii) setting $(U^{n+1}, P^{n+1}) = (U^n, P^n) + (\Delta U, \Delta P)$,
(iv) correcting this value by line damping,
(v) and computing the residual: $R^{n+1} = \mathcal{F}(U^{n+1}, P^{n+1}, \lambda f, \lambda g)$.

REMARK 20.1. For many materials, the hydrostatic pressure field is different from zero at rest. For example, for a Mooney–Rivlin material at rest, the hydrostatic pressure field has for value
$$p = 2C_{10} + 4C_{01},$$
which corresponds to a zero stress field
$$T = \frac{\partial \hat{W}}{\partial F}(x, \mathrm{Id}) - p\,\mathrm{Id}.$$

REMARK 20.2. Since at the step 0, $\{U, P\}$ satisfies the equilibrium equations at the previous load increment, we have simply
$$\begin{aligned} R^0 &= \frac{\partial \mathcal{F}_i(U, P, \lambda f, \lambda g)}{\partial \lambda} \Delta \lambda \\ &= \int_\Omega \Delta \lambda f \cdot \varphi_i \, \mathrm{d}x + \int_{\Gamma_1} \Delta \lambda g \cdot \varphi_i \, \mathrm{d}a \quad \text{if } 1 \leqslant i \leqslant N_h, \\ &= 0 \quad \text{if not.} \end{aligned}$$

REMARK 20.3. Newton's loop is stopped if the error
$$\text{error} = \alpha \|R\| + \beta \|\Delta U\| + \gamma \|\Delta P\|$$
is sufficiently small.

REMARK 20.4. Three main options exist for updating the tangent operator within the Newton's loop: there might be no update, one update at the first iteration, one update every p iterations.

In choosing an option, one has to compromise between computing cost and convergence speed. The optimal choice is problem- and machine-dependent.

REMARK 20.5. In our notation, $\mathcal{F}$ is considered as a function of $u = (U, P)$ and λ, the loads f and g being treated as parameters.

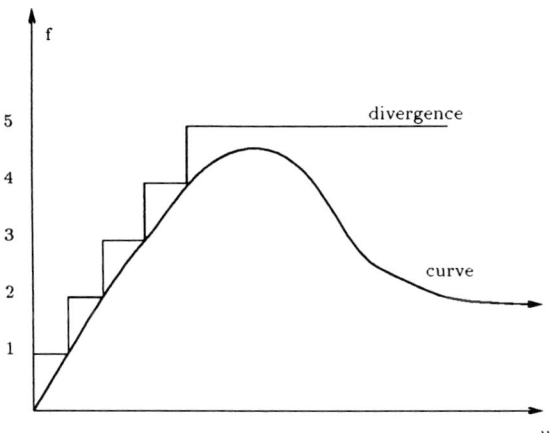

FIG. 21.1. Limit points and incremental loading. In the above situation, there is no solution when the loading factor λ is greater than 4.5. At this limit point, we will obtain no additional solution by trying to impose a value $\lambda = 5$. On the other hand, we will find additional solutions by decreasing the values of λ and increasing the values of u.

REMARK 20.6. There are many line-damping procedures. They can be upgraded by using apriori estimates on the local nonlinearity of $\mathscr{F}$. Introducing as in DEUFLHARD [1990] the Lipschitz constant ω defined by

$$\|D\mathscr{F}(w)^{-1}\left(D\mathscr{F}(u) - D\mathscr{F}(v)\right)(u-v)\| \leqslant \omega\|u-v\|^2,$$

it is then easy to observe that the Newton's update Δu is accurate in the ball $B(u, 1/\omega)$. Hence, one is led to use the following line damping procedure

$$u = u + \min\left(1, (\omega\|\Delta u\|)^{-1}\right) \Delta u.$$

We refer to DEUFLHARD [1990] for more details on such affine-invariant strategies.

21. Arc-length continuation

21.1. General presentation

The preceding algorithm, although of very general use, is not able to treat limit points, that is situations where the relation $u = \mathscr{G}(\lambda)$ is not monotone (Fig. 21.1). Moreover, it might be unstable even for reasonable load increments.

Arclength continuation methods, described in detail in KELLER [1983], overcome this difficulty by replacing the arbitrary choice of $\Delta\lambda$ by an arclength constraint of the type

$$\|\Delta U\|^2 + \|\Delta P\|^2 + \|\Delta\lambda\|^2 = \text{given value}.$$

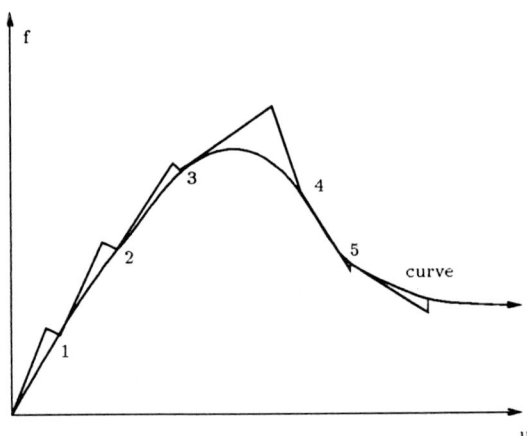

FIG. 21.2. Arclength continuation. An arclength continuation procedure follows the solution curve by trying to compute solutions which are at a constant distance one from another. This procedure is unaffected by the presence of limit points.

The arclength continuation method is in fact looking for a map

$$s \longmapsto \{U(s), P(s), \lambda(s)\}$$

defined on the solution curve

$$\mathcal{F}(U, P, \lambda f, \lambda g) = 0, \tag{21.1}$$

and satisfying the additional differential equation

$$\left\| \frac{dU}{ds} \right\|^2 + \left\| \frac{dP}{ds} \right\|^2 + \left\| \frac{d\lambda}{ds} \right\|^2 = 1.$$

In other words, it solves the differential system

$$\frac{d}{ds} \mathcal{F}(U(s), P(s), \lambda(s)f, \lambda(s)g) = 0, \tag{21.2}$$

$$\left\| \frac{dU}{ds}(s), \frac{dP}{ds}(s), \frac{d\lambda}{ds}(s) \right\| = 1, \tag{21.3}$$

$$\{U, P, \lambda\}(0) = \{U^0, P^0, \lambda^0\}, \tag{21.4}$$

where $\{U^0, P^0, \lambda^0\}$ is a given point of the solution curve (21.1).

This differential system is of prime interest because it is well-posed, because its solution generates the solution curve (21.1) that we want to compute and, above all, because its solution can be easily computed by the Euler–Newton algorithm introduced in the previous section and described below.

EULER–NEWTON ALGORITHM
Let $\{U^0, P^0, \lambda^0\}$ be given. Then, for $n = 0$ and as long as $\lambda^n \leqslant 1$,

(i) compute the "velocity" at step n, that is the solution of

$$\frac{D\mathcal{F}(U^n, P^n, \lambda^n f, \lambda^n g)}{D(U, P, \lambda)}(\dot{U}^n, \dot{P}^n, \dot{\lambda}^n) = 0, \tag{21.5}$$

$$\|(\dot{U}^n, \dot{P}^n, \dot{\lambda}^n)\| = 1; \tag{21.6}$$

(ii) set the solution at step $(n+1)$ to the value of the Euler predictor
$$\{U_0^{n+1}, P_0^{n+1}, \lambda_0^{n+1}\} = \{U^n, P^n, \lambda^n\} + \Delta s \{\dot{U}^n, \dot{P}^n, \dot{\lambda}^n\};$$

(iii) project this solution back to the solution curve (21.1) by a Newton's method (corrector step), that is, iteratively compute the solution of the nonlinear extended system

$$\mathcal{F}(U^{n+1}, P^{n+1}, \lambda^{n+1} f, \lambda^{n+1} g) = 0, \tag{21.7}$$

$$\dot{U}^n \cdot (U^{n+1} - U_0^{n+1}) + \dot{P}^n \cdot (P^{n+1} - P_0^{n+1})$$
$$+ \dot{\lambda}^n (\lambda^{n+1} - \lambda_0^{n+1}) = 0. \tag{21.8}$$

REMARK 21.1. In a simpler variant, one can replace the definition (21.5)–(21.6) of the velocity by the explicit definition

$$\dot{U}^n = -\frac{(U^{n-1} - U^n)}{\Delta s},$$

$$\dot{P}^n = -\frac{(P^{n-1} - P^n)}{\Delta s},$$

$$\dot{\lambda}^n = -\frac{(\lambda^{n-1} - \lambda^n)}{\Delta s}.$$

REMARK 21.2. In a more elaborate version, one can replace the orthogonality condition (21.8) by a dynamic orthogonality condition given by
$$\dot{U}^{n+1}{}_k \cdot (U_{k+1}^{n+1} - U_k^{n+1}) + \dot{P}^{n+1}{}_k \cdot (P_{k+1}^{n+1} - P_k^{n+1}) + \dot{\lambda}^{n+1}{}_k (\lambda_{k+1}^{n+1} - \lambda_k^{n+1}) = 0,$$
where $\{U_k^{n+1}, P_k^{n+1}, \lambda_k^{n+1}\}$ denotes the solution of the nonlinear system after k iterations. This variant is detailed in the next paragraphs.

The implementation of the above arclength continuation procedure requires a practical definition of the norm $\|\cdot\|$ and an adaptive strategy for choosing the incremental step Δs. The algorithm detailed below describes a typical implementation.

21.2. Arclength continuation: Detailed algorithm

Initialization
We start with $U^0 = 0$, P^0 equal to the hydrostatic pressure at rest, $\lambda^0 = 0$ and Δs given. We choose $\Delta \lambda^0$ and set $\lambda^1 = \Delta \lambda^0$. We then solve the nonlinear problem

$$\mathcal{F}(U^1, P^1, \lambda^1 f, \lambda^1 g) = 0,$$

by a regular Newton's method (Section 19) and set

$$\Delta U^1 = U^1 - U^0,$$
$$\omega_p = \|\Delta U^1\|_{l^2}^2 / \|P^1 - P^0\|_{l^2}^2,$$
$$\omega_\lambda = \|\Delta U^1\|_{l^2}^2 / \|\Delta \lambda^0\|^2,$$
$$\|\dot{U}, \dot{P}, \dot{\lambda}\| = \|\dot{U}\|_{l^2}^2 + \omega_p \|\dot{P}\|_{l^2}^2 + \omega_\lambda \|\dot{\lambda}\|_{l^2}^2,$$
$$\Delta s_1 = \sqrt{3} \|\Delta U^1\|_{l^2}.$$

Continuation loop
Then, for $p \geq 0$, with U^p, P^p, λ^p and Δs^p known and as long as $\lambda^p \leq 1$,

(i) we compute the velocity $(\dot{U}^p, \dot{P}^p, \dot{\lambda}^p)$ by solving the system (21.5)–(21.6);
(ii) we set $\{U_0^{p+1}, P_0^{p+1}, \lambda_0^{p+1}\} = \{U^p, P^p, \lambda^p\} + \Delta s_p \{\dot{U}^p, \dot{P}^p, \dot{\lambda}^p\}$;
(iii) we solve the extended nonlinear system in $\{U^{p+1}, P^{p+1}, \lambda^{p+1}\}$

$$\mathscr{F}(U^{p+1}, P^{p+1}, \lambda^{p+1} f, \lambda^{p+1} g) = 0, \tag{21.9}$$

$$\dot{U}^{p+1}{}_k \cdot (U_{k+1}^{p+1} - U_k^{p+1}) + \omega_p \dot{P}^{p+1}{}_k \cdot (P_{k+1}^{p+1} - P_k^{p+1})$$
$$+ \omega_\lambda \dot{\lambda}^{p+1}{}_k (\lambda_{k+1}^{p+1} - \lambda_k^{p+1}) = 0; \tag{21.10}$$

(iv) we set $\Delta s_{p+1} = \nu_p \Delta s_p$ with ν_p a function of the number of Newton's iterations required in Step (iii).

REMARK 21.3. The parameters ω_p and ω_λ have been added to scale the ratio between $(U^{p+1} - U_k^{p+1})$, $(P^{p+1} - P_k^{p+1})$ and $(\lambda^{p+1} - \lambda_k^{p+1})$ which can otherwise be of several orders of magnitude. These parameters are defined automatically. The choice of the adaptive strategy for Δs is more problem-dependent, but a generic choice is

$$\nu_p = 2^{(a-n)/b}$$

with a and b two fixed parameters and n the number of Newton's iterations needed at the previous step.

REMARK 21.4. When the velocity is defined by (21.5)–(21.6), it can be computed by the following block Gaussian elimination strategy:

$$\text{compute } \mathscr{F}_{,\lambda} = \frac{\partial \mathscr{F}(U, P, \lambda f, \lambda g)}{\partial \lambda}; \tag{21.11}$$

$$\text{solve } \frac{\partial \mathscr{F}(U, P, \lambda f, \lambda g)}{\partial (U, P)} (\Delta U, \Delta P) = -\mathscr{F}_{,\lambda}; \tag{21.12}$$

$$\text{set } \dot{\lambda} = [\omega_\lambda + \|\Delta U\|_{l^2}^2 + \omega_p \|\Delta P\|_{l^2}^2]^{-1/2}; \tag{21.13}$$

$$\text{set } (\dot{U}, \dot{P}) = \dot{\lambda}(\Delta U, \Delta P). \tag{21.14}$$

21.3. Extended Newton's algorithm

We now explain how to solve the nonlinear system (21.9)–(21.10) by an extended Newton's algorithm. This algorithm is in fact a Newton's method in which the linearized system

$$\frac{\partial \mathcal{F}(U,P,\lambda f,\lambda g)}{\partial(U,P)}(\Delta U, \Delta P) + \frac{\partial \mathcal{F}(U,P,\lambda f,\lambda g)}{\partial \lambda}\Delta\lambda = -R,$$

$$\dot{U}\cdot\Delta U + \omega_p \dot{P}\cdot\Delta P + \omega_\lambda \dot{\lambda}\Delta\lambda = 0,$$

is solved as in the above remark by a block Gaussian elimination of the variables $(\Delta U, \Delta P)$. We finally obtain the following iterative process, called the bordering algorithm (KELLER [1983]):

EXTENDED NEWTON'S ALGORITHM

For $n \geq 0$, with (U^n, P^n, λ^n) and $(\dot{U}, \dot{P}, \dot{\lambda})$ known and until the residual R is small, we update $(\dot{U}, \dot{P}, \dot{\lambda})$ and compute $(U^{n+1}, P^{n+1}, \lambda^{n+1})$ by

(i) computing the residual $R = \mathcal{F}(U^n, P^n, \lambda^n f, \lambda^n g)$,
(ii) computing and factoring the tangent operator:

$$K = \frac{\partial \mathcal{F}(U^n, P^n, \lambda^n f, \lambda^n g)}{\partial(U,P)},$$

(iii) computing the line derivative

$$\mathcal{F}_{,\lambda} = \frac{\partial \mathcal{F}(U^n, P^n, \lambda^n f, \lambda^n g)}{\partial \lambda},$$

(iv) solving the linear systems (S):

$$K(\Delta U_0, \Delta P_0) = -R,$$
$$K(\Delta U_1, \Delta P_1) = -\mathcal{F}_{,\lambda},$$

(v) setting

$$\dot{\lambda} = \frac{\text{sgn}[\dot{U}\cdot\Delta U_1 + \omega_p\dot{P}\cdot\Delta P_1 + \omega_\lambda \dot{\lambda}]}{[\omega_\lambda + \|\Delta U_1\|^2 + \omega_p\|\Delta P_1\|^2]^{1/2}},$$

$$(\dot{U}, \dot{P}) = \dot{\lambda}(\Delta U_1, \Delta P_1),$$

$$\Delta\lambda = -(\dot{U}\cdot\Delta U_0 + \omega_p\dot{P}\cdot\Delta P_0)\dot{\lambda},$$

$$\{U^{n+1}, P^{n+1}\} = \{U^n + \Delta U_0 + \frac{\Delta\lambda}{\dot{\lambda}}\dot{U}, P^n + \Delta P_0 + \frac{\Delta\lambda}{\dot{\lambda}}\dot{P}\}.$$

Each iteration of the above algorithm involves one (costly) calculation of the tangent matrix and two (cheap) solutions of linear systems, compared to one calculation of the tangent matrix and one linear-system solution for the original Newton's method. Therefore, from the numerical point of view, the difference between the standard Newton's method (with incremental loading) and arclength continuation is very small. Since arclength continuation performs far better, it should always be preferred to incremental loading.

22. On the solution of the linear system (S)

In any one of the above algorithms, one has to solve linear systems of the form
$$\frac{\partial \mathcal{F}(U,P,\lambda f,\lambda g)}{\partial(U,P)}(\Delta U, \Delta P) = R. \tag{22.1}$$

Such systems are associated with large, sparse matrices with rather large condition numbers. The question then arises: what algorithm to choose for solving these systems? The answer to this question arises in two different situations.

(i) For compressible and nearly incompressible materials, as indicated in (18.14) and (18.6), the linear system (22.1) takes the matrix form
$$(\mathcal{A} + C)(\Delta U) = R \quad \text{in } \mathbb{R}^{N_h}, \tag{22.2}$$
with

$$\mathcal{A}_{ij} = a_{u_h}(\varphi_j, \varphi_i),$$

$$C_{ij} = \int_\Omega \frac{\partial f}{\partial U_j} \varphi_i \, dx + \int_{\Gamma_1} \frac{\partial g}{\partial U_j} \cdot \varphi_i \, da,$$

and $a_{u_h}(v_h, w_h)$ as defined in (18.15). If we neglect the contribution of C and if we are before any limit point, then the matrix $\mathcal{A}$ is symmetric definite positive and the best choice is to factor and solve the linear system (22.2) by a Cholesky method. If we want to keep the full matrix $(\mathcal{A}+C)$ and if we are away from any limit or bifurcation point, then a Gauss elimination technique without pivoting is the best choice. In any case, the ordering of the unknowns is unimportant, provided the bandwidth of the resulting matrix is not too large.

(ii) For incompressible materials, we have already seen that the linear system (22.1) can be written as follows:
$$\begin{pmatrix} (\mathcal{A}+C) & B^T \\ B & 0 \end{pmatrix} \begin{pmatrix} \Delta U \\ \Delta P \end{pmatrix} = \begin{pmatrix} R_U \\ R_P \end{pmatrix} \quad \text{in } \mathbb{R}^{N_h} \times \mathbb{R}^{M_h}.$$

Away from limit points, this system can again be solved by a Gauss elimination technique without pivoting. But now the solution procedure is more expensive (the order of the system is $N_h \times M_h$) and, due to the presence of zero terms on the diagonal, the order of the unknowns cannot be arbitrary. A good solution strategy is to order the unknowns node by node, starting with the degrees of freedom in displacements. In such an ordering, one must ensure that even in the presence of Dirichlet boundary conditions, every pressure unknown is related to at least one unknown in displacement of lower rank (Fig. 22.1).

An alternative method for solving (19.1) is the following augmented Lagrangian algorithm:
solve
$$[(\mathcal{A}+C)+rB^T B]\Delta U = R_U - B^T(\Delta P - rR_P);$$

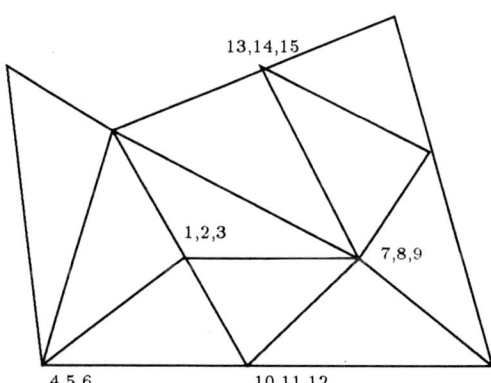

Fig. 22.1. Unknown ordering. Pressures are multiple of 3. This ordering ensures that every pressure unknown is related to an internal displacement unknown of lower rank. Hence, such an ordering of the unknowns avoids the presence of zero pivots on the diagonal.

If $(B\Delta U - R_P)$ is not sufficiently small, set

$$\Delta P = \Delta P + r(B\Delta U - R_P)$$

and reiterate.

For large values of r, this algorithm "converges" in less than 3 iterations (see FORTIN and GLOWINSKI [1982, 1983] and GLOWINSKI and LE TALLEC [1989] for further details). This algorithm is of particular interest, and should be preferred to any other algorithm, in the case where there are no pressure nodes on the interelement boundaries. In this situation, which includes all the finite-elements described in Section 12, the matrix $B^T B$ has the simple form

$$B^T B = \sum_l B_{|\Omega_l}^T B_{|\Omega_l}.$$

This means that adding $rB^T B$ to $(A + C)$ does not change its profile and thus does not change the cost of the solution of the linear system in U.

23. On the choice of the stored energy function $\hat{W}$

If in the compressible case the choice of $\hat{W}$ is only dictated by physical considerations, the situation is slightly different in the incompressible or nearly incompressible case where two options are possible.

The first option is *penalization* . There, one ignores the incompressibility constraint and takes as stored energy the stored energy function $\hat{W}_\varepsilon$ of the associated nearly incompressible material (4.7). In this option, the choice of the penalization factor ε must be taken in the range

$$10^2 C_s \leqslant \frac{1}{\varepsilon} \leqslant 10^6 C_s,$$

where C_s is a characteristic shear modulus of the material. For larger ε, there is a loss in accuracy; for smaller ε, the condition number becomes too large. Moreover, the linear system (22.1) takes the form (22.2) and is therefore simpler and cheaper to solve. But, due to the increase of the condition number, Newton's method loses in robustness and accuracy.

The second option is *dualization*. There, one solves the full incompressible problem (12.1)–(12.2). But even in this case, it is useful to take for $\hat{W}$ the stored energy function $\hat{W}_\varepsilon$ of the associated nearly incompressible material. This obviously has no effect on the final solution, but modifies the tangent operator K. For reasonable values of ε, the tangent operator will have a better condition number and will be more compatible with the incompressibility constraint. This will speed up the convergence of Newton's method. In this option, the linear system takes the form (19.1) and is rather expensive to solve, but the condition number is smaller and hence Newton's method gains in speed and accuracy.

REMARK 23.1. The use of $\hat{W}_\varepsilon$ in the truly incompressible approach can be interpreted as an augmented Lagrangian technique. Such techniques regularize the energy away from the set of admissible solutions in order to improve the speed of convergence without affecting the final result.

24. Conclusion

To conclude this presentation of the application of Newton's method to finite elasticity, one should remember three facts:

(i) First, the most popular numerical method in finite elasticity involves compressible or nearly incompressible materials (the penalization approach), uses the first-order isoparametric finite-elements of Section 12 and solves the resulting nonlinear problem by the Newton-incremental loading algorithm of Section 20 (Fig. 24.1).

(ii) Secondly, the most sophisticated methods involve incompressible models, and use second-order finite-elements (Section 12) and arclength continuation methods (Section 21).

(iii) Thirdly and last, these methods are very expensive in three-dimensional situations. In such situations, an alternative is to use augmented Lagrangian techniques as described in Chapter 7 of GLOWINSKI and LE TALLEC [1989] and reviewed in the following sections.

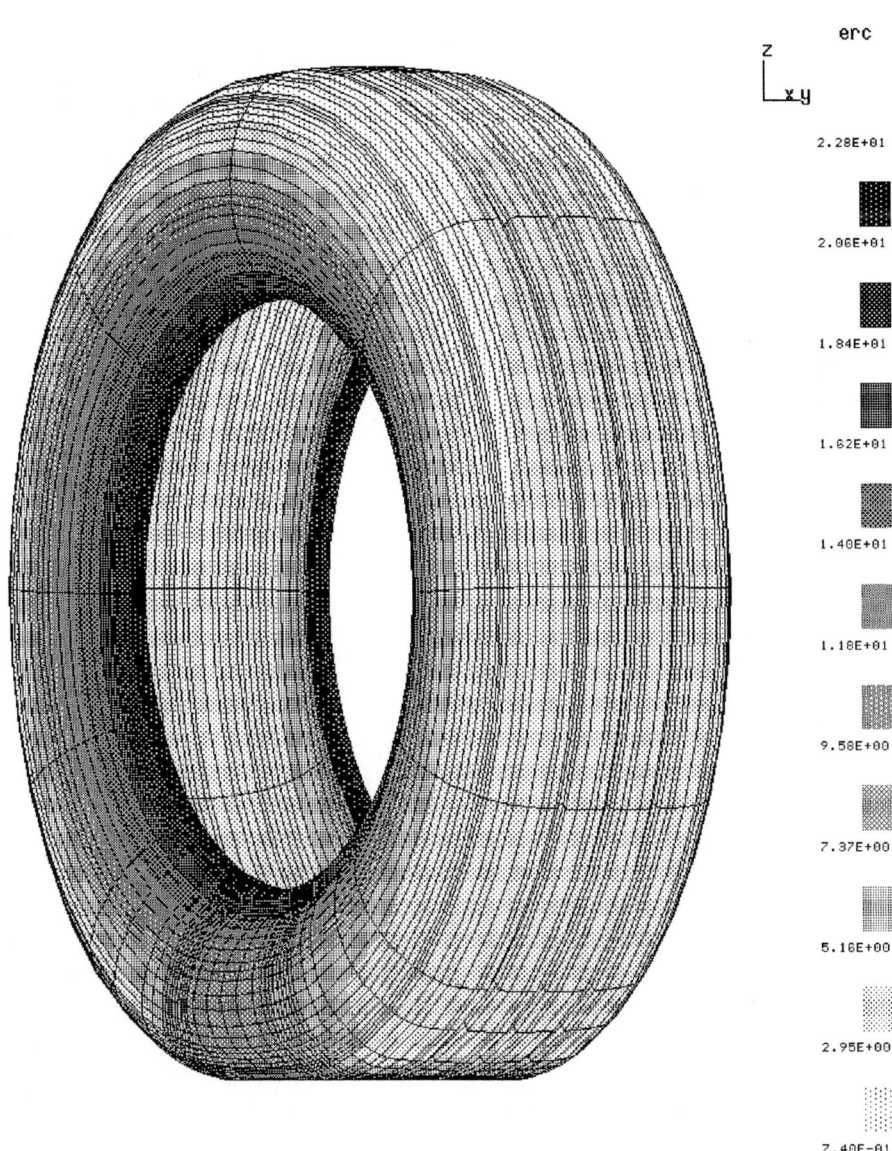

FIG. 24.1. A 3-D tire calculation in finite elasticity (courtesy of Société MICHELIN).

CHAPTER V

Augmented Lagrangian Methods

Augmented Lagrangian methods were first introduced to improve the performance of the numerical algorithms used in contrained optimization (HESTENES [1969], POWELL [1969]). These methods mainly consist of introducing an augmented Lagrangian formulation and an associated dual formulation of the original minimization problem. The problems are then numerically solved by descent methods operating on this dual formulation, that is on the Lagrange multipliers (GLOWINSKI and LE TALLEC [1989], Chapter 3). During the seventies, it was realized (GLOWINSKI and MARROCCO [1975], POLYAK [1979]) that these methods were ideally suited to take advantage of the decomposition principles that often appear in practical applications. Actually, these decomposition principles can be used to transform a very large class of minimization problems into problems that have a primal–dual structure and which therefore can be solved by augmented Lagrangian methods. These techniques have then been applied to many different situations, some of them being described in FORTIN and GLOWINSKI ([1982, 1983]) and in GLOWINSKI and LE TALLEC [1989]. In particular, they have been applied to problems in finite elasticity in an attempt to reduce the computing cost compared to the more traditional numerical techniques described in the previous chapter.

We describe below the application of these techniques to the numerical solution of equilibrium problems in finite elasticity. The starting point is the introduction of a new formulation of these discrete equilibrium problems (Section 25) which is proved to be equivalent to the original one. This new formulation can then be solved by a very simple algorithm which is introduced in Section 26. The last part of this chapter details the different steps of the algorithm (Sections 27 and 28) and illustrates its application in several numerical examples. Further details on the subject can be found in GLOWINSKI and LE TALLEC ([1982, 1989]), or in LE TALLEC and VIDRASCU [1984].

25. Introduction of a new discrete formulation

Let us go back to our original finite-element approximation of equilibrium problems in incompressible finite elasticity, which was

   Find $\{u_h, p_h\} \in (\mathbb{V}_h + u_0) \times \mathbb{P}_h$ such that

$$\int_\Omega \frac{\partial \hat{W}}{\partial F}(x, \mathrm{Id}+\nabla u_h) : \nabla v_h \, dx - \int_\Omega p_h \frac{\partial \det}{\partial F}(\mathrm{Id}+\nabla u_h) : \nabla v_h \, dx$$

$$= \int_\Omega f \cdot v_h \, dx + \int_{\Gamma_1} g \cdot v_h \, da \quad \forall v_h \in \mathbb{V}_h, \tag{25.1}$$

$$\int_\Omega q_h [\det(\mathrm{Id}+\nabla u_h) - 1] = 0 \quad \forall q_h \in \mathbb{P}_h. \tag{25.2}$$

We will now suppose that the space $\mathbb{P}_h$ is made up of piecewise constant functions, i.e.

$$\mathbb{P}_h = \left\{ q_h \colon \Omega \to \mathbb{R}, \, q_{h|\Omega_l} = \text{constant}, \forall l \text{ with } \overline{\Omega} = \bigcup_{l=1}^{M_h} \Omega_l \right\}, \tag{25.3}$$

that the integrals

$$\int_{\Omega_l} p_h \frac{\partial \det}{\partial F}(\mathrm{Id}+\nabla u_h) : \nabla v_h \, dx \quad \text{and} \quad \int_{\Omega_l} q_h [\det(\mathrm{Id}+\nabla u_h) - 1] \, dx$$

are computed by a one-point numerical quadrature rule, and that $\hat{W}$ splits into two parts $\hat{W} = \hat{W}_1 + \hat{W}_2$, with $\hat{W}_1$ a "simple" function of F, and where the integral

$$\int_{\Omega_l} \frac{\partial \hat{W}_2}{\partial F}(x, \mathrm{Id}+\nabla u_h) : \nabla v_h \, dx$$

is also computed by a one-point numerical integration rule.

Under these approximations, the discrete problem (25.1)–(25.2) takes the form

Find $\{u_h, p_h\} \in (\mathbb{V}_h + u_0) \times \mathbb{P}_h$ such that

$$\int_\Omega \frac{\partial \hat{W}_1}{\partial F}(x, \mathrm{Id}+\nabla u_h) : \nabla v_h \, dx$$

$$+ \int_\Omega \left\{ \frac{\partial \hat{W}_2}{\partial F}(x, \mathrm{Id}+\nabla_h u_h) - p_h \frac{\partial \det}{\partial F}(\mathrm{Id}+\nabla_h u_h) \right\} : \nabla_h v_h \, dx$$

$$= \int_\Omega f \cdot v_h \, dx + \int_{\Gamma_1} g \cdot v_h \, da \quad \forall v_h \in \mathbb{V}_h, \, (u_h - u_0) \in \mathbb{V}_h, \tag{25.4}$$

$$\int_\Omega q_h [\det(\mathrm{Id}+\nabla_h u_h) - 1] \, dx = 0 \quad \forall v_h \in \mathbb{V}_h, \, (u_h - u_o) \in \mathbb{V}_h. \tag{25.5}$$

Here, $\nabla_h v_h$ is the piecewise constant function defined by

$$\nabla_h v_{h|\Omega_l} = \frac{1}{\mathrm{meas}(\Omega_l)} \int_{\Omega_l} \nabla v_h \, dx \quad \forall l = 1, M_h. \tag{25.6}$$

We now observe that all the complicated terms in the above problem (those involving $\hat{W}_2$ or $\det(\cdot)$) only involve the variable

$$F_h = \mathrm{Id} + \nabla_h u_h. \tag{25.7}$$

Hence, we are led to the idea of considering F_h as a *local independent variable* (i.e. as a variable whose variations are independent of those of u_h) and of imposing the constraint (25.7) at the solution only. This linear constraint can then be imposed by *augmented Lagrangian techniques* (FORTIN and GLOWINSKI [1982], GLOWINSKI and LE TALLEC [1989]), that is combining *penalization* (one adds a term $(r/2)\|F_h - \mathrm{Id} - \nabla_h u_h\|^2$ to the energy) and *dualization* (one introduces a multiplier λ_h of the linear constraint (25.7)).

Putting this idea to work leads to the following system of equations:
Equations in u_h (no variation in F_h or in λ_h):

$$\int_\Omega \frac{\partial \hat{W}_1}{\partial F}(x, \mathrm{Id} + \nabla u_h) : \nabla v_h \, dx + \frac{\partial}{\partial u}\left[\frac{r}{2}\|F_h - \mathrm{Id} - \nabla_h u_h\|^2\right] \cdot v_h$$

$$+ \frac{\partial}{\partial u}[\langle \lambda_h, \mathrm{Id} + \nabla_h u_h - F_h \rangle] \cdot v_h$$

$$= \int_\Omega f \cdot v_h \, dx + \int_{\Gamma_1} g \cdot v_h \, da \quad \forall v_h \in \mathbb{V}_h; \tag{25.8}$$

Equation in F_h (no variation in u_h or in λ_h):

$$\int_\Omega \left[\frac{\partial \hat{W}_2}{\partial F}(x, F_h) - p_h \frac{\partial \det F_h}{\partial F}\right] : G_h \, dx + \frac{\partial}{\partial F}\left[\frac{r}{2}\|F_h - \mathrm{Id} - \nabla_h u_h\|^2\right] : G$$

$$+ \frac{\partial}{\partial F}[\langle \lambda_h, \mathrm{Id} + \nabla_h u_h - F_h \rangle] : G_h = 0 \quad \forall G_h \in (\mathbb{P}_h)^{N \times N}, \tag{25.9}$$

$$\int_\Omega q_h(\det F_h - 1) \, dx = 0 \quad \forall q_h \in \mathbb{P}_h; \tag{25.10}$$

Equation in λ_h (no variation in u_h or in F_h):

$$\langle \mu_h, \mathrm{Id} + \nabla_h u_h - F_h \rangle = 0 \quad \forall \mu_h \in (\mathbb{P}_h)^{N \times N}. \tag{25.11}$$

System (25.8)–(25.11) can be more properly written by introducing the scalar product

$$\langle \mu_h, G_h \rangle = \int_\Omega \eta(x) \mu_h : G_h \, dx \quad \forall \mu_h, G_h \in (\mathbb{P}_h)^{N \times N}, \tag{25.12}$$

the augmented Lagrangian

$$\mathscr{L}_r^h(v_h, G_h; \mu_h) = \int_\Omega \hat{W}_1(x, \mathrm{Id} + \nabla v_h)\,\mathrm{d}x + \int_\Omega \hat{W}_2(x, G_h)\,\mathrm{d}x$$

$$+ \frac{r}{2} \int_\Omega \eta(x) |\mathrm{Id} + \nabla_h v_h - G_h|^2 \,\mathrm{d}x$$

$$+ \int_\Omega \eta(x) \mu_h : (\mathrm{Id} + \nabla_h v_h - G_h)\,\mathrm{d}x, \qquad (25.13)$$

and the spaces

$$\mathbb{H}_h = (\mathbb{P}_h)^{N \times N}, \qquad (25.14)$$

$$Y = \{G: \Omega \to \mathbb{R}^{N \times N},\ \det G = 1 \text{ a.e. on } \Omega\}, \qquad (25.15)$$

$$\mathrm{d}Y(F) = \{G: \Omega \to \mathbb{R}^{N \times N}, \frac{\partial \det}{\partial F}(F) : G = 0 \text{ a.e. on } \Omega\}. \qquad (25.16)$$

Above, r and $\eta(x)$ are given arbitrary strictly positive numbers. With the notation (25.12)–(25.16), the Lagrangian system (25.8)–(25.11) takes the final form:

Find $\{u_h - u_0, F_h, \lambda_h\} \in \mathbb{V}_h \times (Y \cap \mathbb{H}_h) \times \mathbb{H}_h$ such that

$$\frac{\partial \mathscr{L}_r^h}{\partial v}(u_h, F_h; \lambda_h) \cdot v_h = \int_\Omega f \cdot v_h\,\mathrm{d}x + \int_{\Gamma_1} g \cdot v_h\,\mathrm{d}a \quad \forall v_h \in \mathbb{V}_h, \qquad (25.17)$$

$$\frac{\partial \mathscr{L}_r^h}{\partial F}(u_h, F_h; \lambda_h) \cdot G_h = 0 \quad \forall G \in \mathrm{d}Y(F_h) \cap \mathbb{H}_h, \qquad (25.18)$$

$$\frac{\partial \mathscr{L}_r^h}{\partial \lambda}(u_h, F_h; \lambda_h) \cdot \mu_h = 0 \quad \forall \mu_h \in \mathbb{H}_h. \qquad (25.19)$$

REMARK 25.1. The choice of $\hat{W}_1$, r and η plays no role from the theoretical point of view, but will be critical in ensuring a good convergence of the numerical algorithms to be used later.

We can now prove the following equivalence result:

THEOREM 25.1. *The augmented Lagrangian formulation (25.17)–(25.19) and the original discrete problem (25.4)–(25.5) are equivalent, through the identification*

$$F_h = \mathrm{Id} + \nabla_h u_h, \qquad (25.20)$$

$$\eta \lambda_h = \frac{\partial \hat{W}_2}{\partial F}(x, F_h) - p_h \frac{\partial \det}{\partial F}(F_h). \qquad (25.21)$$

PROOF. Let $\{u_h, p_h\}$ be a solution of (25.4)–(25.5). Writing (25.5) with $q_h = 0$ everywhere except on Ω_l, we get, since q_h and $\nabla_h u_h$ are constant on Ω_l,

$$\mathrm{meas}(\Omega_l) q_l [\det(\mathrm{Id} + \nabla_h u_{h|\Omega_l}) - 1] = 0 \quad \forall q_l \in \mathbb{R},$$

hence
$$\det(\mathrm{Id}+\nabla_h u_h)_{|\Omega_l} = \det(\mathrm{Id}+\nabla_h u_{h_{|\Omega_l}}) = 1.$$

In other words $(\mathrm{Id}+\nabla_h u_h)$ belongs to Y. If we now define F_h and λ_h by (25.20) and (25.21), then (25.17) is satisfied from (25.4) and (25.21), (25.18) is a direct consequence of (25.21), and (25.19) is a rewriting of (25.20). Thus, $\{u_h, F_h; \lambda_h\}$ as constructed is a solution of the Lagrangian problem (25.17)–(25.19).

Conversely, let $\{u_h, F_h; \lambda_h\}$ be a solution of (25.17)–(25.19). From (25.19), we must then have
$$F_h = \mathrm{Id}+\nabla_h u_h.$$
Therefore, since F_h belongs to Y by construction, we have
$$\det(\mathrm{Id}+\nabla_h u_h) = 1,$$
which clearly implies (25.5). On the other hand, let us write (25.18) with an element G_h equal to zero everywhere except on Ω_l. Since λ_h, G_h and $\nabla_h u_h$ are constant over Ω_l, this yields
$$\mathrm{meas}(\Omega_l) A_{h|\Omega_l} : G = 0 \quad \forall G \in \mathrm{Ker}(\nabla\mathscr{G}_l), \tag{25.22}$$
with A_h and $\nabla\mathscr{G}_l$ defined by
$$A_h = \frac{\partial \hat{W}_2}{\partial F}(x, \mathrm{Id}+\nabla_h u_h) - \eta\lambda_h,$$

$$\nabla\mathscr{G}_l : \mathbb{R}^{N\times N} \to \mathbb{R},$$
$$G \longmapsto \frac{\partial \det}{\partial F}(\mathrm{Id}+\nabla_h u_{h_{|\Omega_l}}) : G,$$
respectively. From (25.22), $A_{h_{|\Omega_l}}$ belongs to the orthogonal space to $\mathrm{Ker}(\nabla\mathscr{G}_l)$. Therefore, there exists $p_l \in \mathbb{R}$ such that
$$A_{h_{|\Omega_l}} = \nabla\mathscr{G}_l^T(p_l) = p_l \frac{\partial \det}{\partial F}(\mathrm{Id}+\nabla_h u_{h_{|\Omega_l}}). \tag{25.23}$$
Using now (25.23) in (25.17), we obtain (25.4) and our proof is complete. □

26. Basic iterative method

In the previous section, we introduced an augmented Lagrangian formulation which is equivalent to the standard mixed finite-element approximation of the original equilibrium problem. The major interest of this new formulation is that, as written, it can be solved numerically by one of the many algorithms existing for solving saddle-point problems. In finite elasticity, the algorithm that we have used in practice and which appears to be the most stable is that of Uzawa (ARROW, HURWICZ and UZAWA [1958]). Combined with block relaxation and applied to the discrete problem (25.17)–(25.19) this algorithm is
$$\lambda^0 \in \mathbb{H}_h \quad \text{and} \quad F^0 \in Y \cap \mathbb{H}_h \quad \text{given}; \tag{26.1}$$

then for $n \geq 0$, λ^n being known, determine u^n, F^n, λ^{n+1} by setting

$$F^{n,0} = F^{n-1}, \tag{26.2}$$

by solving sequentially, for $1 \leq k \leq K$,

$$\frac{\partial \mathscr{L}_r^h}{\partial v}(u^{n,k}, F^{n,k-1}, \lambda^n) \cdot v = \int_\Omega f \cdot v \, dx + \int_{\Gamma_1} g \cdot v \, da \tag{26.3}$$

$$\forall v \in \mathbb{V}_h, \quad (u^{n,k} - u_0) \in \mathbb{V}_h,$$

$$\frac{\partial \mathscr{L}_r^h}{\partial G}(u^{n,k}, F^{n,k}, \lambda^n) \cdot G = 0 \tag{26.4}$$

$$\forall G \in \mathbb{H}_h \cap dY(F^{n,k}), \quad F^{n,k} \in \mathbb{H}_h \cap Y,$$

and finally by setting

$$u^n = u^{n,K}, \quad F^n = F^{n,K}, \tag{26.5}$$

$$\lambda^{n+1} = \lambda^n + r(\mathrm{Id} + \nabla_h u^n - F^n). \tag{26.6}$$

Algorithm (26.1)–(26.6) is very simple: it reduces the solution of (25.17)–(25.19) mainly to a sequence of problems (26.3) posed in terms of *displacements*, to be studied in Section 27, and of problems (26.4) posed in terms of *deformation gradients*, to be studied in Section 28. In practice, the good values of K appear to be between 1 and 5 and the algorithm is stopped as soon as we have

$$\frac{\|F^n - \mathrm{Id} - \nabla_h u^n\|_{0,2}}{\|F^n\|_{0,2}} + \frac{\|u^n - u^{n-1}\|_{0,2}}{\|u^n\|_{0,2}} \leq \varepsilon \quad (\approx 10^{-4}).$$

27. The problems in displacements

From the definition of the augmented Lagrangian $\mathscr{L}_r^h$, problem (26.3) is

Find $(u - u_0) \in \mathbb{V}_h$ such that

$$\int_\Omega \frac{\partial \hat{W}_1}{\partial F}(x, \mathrm{Id} + \nabla u) : \nabla v \, dx$$

$$+ \int_\Omega \eta(x)(r(\mathrm{Id} + \nabla_h u - F) + \lambda) : \nabla_h v \, dx$$

$$= \int_\Omega f \cdot v \, dx + \int_{\Gamma_1} g \cdot v \, da \quad \forall v \in \mathbb{V}_h,$$

where, for simplicity, we have dropped the subscript and the superscripts n and k from all variables. If we did choose $\hat{W}_1$ as a convex function of F, then, except for the possible dependence of f and g on u, (26.3) corresponds to the variational formulation of an unconstrained convex minimization problem on

$\mathbb{V}_h$, to be solved by one of the many numerical techniques existing for such problems (POLAK [1971], GLOWINSKI [1984]).

But, in fact, problem (26.3) can be even more simplified. If we choose $\hat{W}_1$ as a quadratic function of F, which is legitimate since the choice of $\hat{W}_1$ can be rather arbitrary, and if we approximate the external loads $f(u)$ and $g(u)$ by their values $f(u^{n,k-1})$ and $g(u^{n,k-1})$ at the previous iterate, then (26.3) reduces to the linear system

$$\text{Find } u = u_0 + \sum_{j=1}^{\dim V_h} U^j \varphi_j \text{ such that}$$

$$\sum_{j=1}^{\dim V_h} a_{ij} U^j = b_i \quad \forall 1 \leqslant i \leqslant \dim \mathbb{V}_h. \tag{27.1}$$

Above, $(\varphi_i)_{i=1,\dim V_h}$ is a known basis of $\mathbb{V}_h$ and the coefficients a_{ij} and b_j are given by

$$a_{ij} = \int_\Omega \left\{ \left(\frac{\partial^2 \hat{W}_1}{\partial F^2} : \nabla \varphi_i \right) : \nabla \varphi_j + r\eta(x) \nabla_h \varphi_i : \nabla_h \varphi_j \right\} dx,$$

$$b_i = -\int_\Omega \left\{ \left(\frac{\partial^2 \hat{W}_1}{\partial F^2} : (\text{Id} + \nabla u_0) \right) : \nabla \varphi_i \right.$$

$$\left. + \eta(x)(r(\text{Id} + \nabla_h u_0 - F) + \lambda) : \nabla_h \varphi_i \right\} dx$$

$$+ \int_\Omega f(u^{n,k-1}) \cdot \varphi_i \, dx + \int_{\Gamma_1} g(u^{n,k-1}) \cdot \varphi_i \, da.$$

By construction, the linear system (27.1) is associated with a sparse, symmetric, positive definite matrix which does not change during the iterations. This matrix being computed and factorized once for all, the solution of (27.1) is then a standard, cheap and stable operation.

In our numerical experiments, we did solve the problems (26.3) (posed in terms of displacement) by solving the associated linear systems (27.1) either by a standard *Cholesky method* or by an *incomplete Cholesky conjugate gradient* (ICCG) method. This last method, developed by MEIJERINK and VAN DER VORST [1977] and AJIZ and JENNINGS [1984], consists in multiplying the linear system (27.1) by the inverse of an incomplete Cholesky factorization of the matrix $\mathcal{A}$ and in solving the resulting system by a conjugate gradient method; this saves computer storage and running time when dealing with large systems ($\dim \mathbb{V}_h \geqslant 1000$).

28. The local problems in deformation gradients

28.1. Formulation and preliminary lemma

We now turn to the study of the most specific step of algorithm (26.1)–(26.6), that is the solution of problem (26.4) posed in terms of deformation gradients. From the definition of $\mathscr{L}_r^h$, (26.4) is given by

Find $F \in \mathbb{H}_h \cap Y$ such that

$$\int_\Omega \left\{ \frac{\partial \hat{W}_2}{\partial F}(x, F) - \eta(x)(r(\mathrm{Id} + \nabla_h u - F) + \lambda) \right\} : G \, dx = 0$$

$$\forall G \in \mathbb{H}_h \cap dY(F), \tag{28.1}$$

where, for simplicity, we have dropped the subscript h and the superscripts n and k from all variables. Recall that $\mathbb{H}_h$ is a given finite-dimensional approximation of $(L^\infty(\Omega))^{N \times N}$, that $\nabla_h v$ denotes the L^2 projection of ∇v on $\mathbb{H}_h$, that $\hat{W}_2(x, \cdot)$ represents the part of the stored energy which is not taken into account in the problem in displacements, that r and $\eta(x)$ are given positive numbers, and that at this step the values of u and λ are known.

Moreover, we have

$$Y \cap \mathbb{H}_h = \{G \in \mathbb{H}_h, \det G = 1 \text{ in } \Omega\},$$

$$dY(F) \cap \mathbb{H}_h = \left\{ G \in \mathbb{H}_h, \frac{\partial \det}{\partial F}(F) : G = 0 \right\}.$$

To study (28.1), we recall that the *singular values* $G_1 \geqslant G_2 \cdots \geqslant G_N$ of a real 3×3 matrix $G \in \mathbb{M}^3$ are the square roots of the eigenvalues of GG^T and that a real function $\hat{W}(F)$ defined on $\mathbb{M}^3$ is said to be *isotropic* if and only if it is a symmetric function of the singular values of F. With this definition, we can now prove

THEOREM 28.1. *Let $\hat{W}: \mathbb{M}^3 \to \mathbb{R}$ be differentiable and isotropic. Then for any choice $\{D, G, Q, R\}$ of 3×3 matrices with D diagonal, Q and R orthogonal, we have:*

$$\frac{\partial \hat{W}}{\partial F}(D) \text{ is diagonal,} \tag{28.2}$$

$$\frac{\partial \hat{W}}{\partial F}(QGR) = Q \frac{\partial \hat{W}}{\partial F}(G) R. \tag{28.3}$$

PROOF. To get (28.2), we simply observe that, for D diagonal,

$$\det((D + tH)(D + tH)^T - \mu \, \mathrm{Id})$$

$$= \det(DD^T - \mu \, \mathrm{Id}) + 2t \sum_{i=1}^3 H_{ii} D_{ii} \prod_{j \neq i} (D_{jj}^2 - \mu) + o(t)$$

$\forall t, \mu \in \mathbb{R}, \ \forall H \in \mathbb{M}^3.$

In other words, if H has all its components equal to zero on the diagonal, then, at the first order in t, the singular values of D and of $(D+tH)$ are identical. Since $\hat{W}$ is isotropic, this implies

$$\hat{W}(D+tH) = \hat{W}(D) + o(t) \quad \forall H \in \mathbb{M}^3 \text{ with } H_{ii} = 0. \tag{28.4}$$

From (28.4) we then deduce

$$\frac{\partial \hat{W}}{\partial F}(D) : H = \lim_{t \to 0} \frac{1}{t}(\hat{W}(D+tH) - \hat{W}(D)),$$
$$= 0 \quad \forall H \in \mathbb{M}^3 \text{ with } H_{ii} = 0.$$

By definition of a partial derivative, this implies

$$\frac{\partial \hat{W}}{\partial F}(D)_{ij} = 0 \quad \forall i \neq j,$$

which is precisely (28.2).

Similarly, to get (28.3), we observe that, for *orthogonal matrices* Q and R, we have

$$\det((QGR)(QGR)^{\mathrm{T}} - \mu\,\mathrm{Id}) = \det(QGG^{\mathrm{T}}Q^{\mathrm{T}} - \mu\,\mathrm{Id})$$
$$= \det(GG^{\mathrm{T}} - \mu\,\mathrm{Id}) \quad \forall G \in \mathbb{M}^3.$$

In other words G and QGR have the same singular values and thus

$$\hat{W}(QGR) = \hat{W}(G) \quad \forall G \in \mathbb{M}^3. \tag{28.5}$$

From (28.5) applied to G and $G+tQ^{\mathrm{T}}HR^{\mathrm{T}}$, we then get

$$\frac{\partial \hat{W}}{\partial F}(QGR) : H = \lim_{t \to 0} \frac{1}{t}(\hat{W}(QGR+tH) - \hat{W}(QGR))$$
$$= \lim_{t \to 0} \frac{1}{t}(\hat{W}(G+tQ^{\mathrm{T}}HR^{\mathrm{T}}) - \hat{W}(G))$$
$$= \frac{\partial \hat{W}}{\partial F}(G) : Q^{\mathrm{T}}HR^{\mathrm{T}}$$
$$= Q\frac{\partial \hat{W}}{\partial F}(G)R : H \quad \forall H \in \mathbb{M}^3,$$

which is (28.3) and our proof is complete. □

28.2. Solution procedure

With the above lemma, problem (26.4) reduces to the solution in parallel of M_h nonlinear equations set on $\mathbb{R}^2$. Indeed, defining the map T from $\mathbb{R}^2$ into $\mathbb{M}^3$ by

$$T(t_1, t_2) = \begin{pmatrix} t_1 & 0 & 0 \\ 0 & t_2 & 0 \\ 0 & 0 & 1/(t_1 t_2) \end{pmatrix}, \tag{28.6}$$

we have the following:

THEOREM 28.2. *If $\hat{W}_2$ is isotropic and if $\mathbb{H}_h$ is a space of piecewise constant functions defined by*

$$\mathbb{H}_h = \{G \colon \Omega \to \mathbb{R}^{N \times N}, G_{|\Omega_l} = \text{constant}, \forall l = 1, \ldots, M_h\},$$

then a solution F of (28.1) can be obtained by the following sequence of computations:

For $l = 1, \ldots, M_h$,

$$\text{compute} A_l = \eta[r(\text{Id} + \nabla_h u) + \lambda]_{|\Omega_l}, \tag{28.7}$$

$$\text{diagonalize } A_l \text{ into } A_l = Q_l D_l R_l, \text{with } Q_l \text{ and} \tag{28.8}$$

R_l orthogonal, $(D_l)_{11} \geqslant \cdots \geqslant (D_l)_{33}$, and $\det D_l = \det A_l$,

$$\text{solve } \frac{\partial J_l}{\partial t}(t_{il}) = 0 \quad \text{in } \mathbb{R}^2, \tag{28.9}$$

$$\text{set} F_{|\Omega_l} = Q_l T(t_{il}) R_l. \tag{28.10}$$

The function J_l introduced above is defined by

$$J_l(t_i) = \hat{W}_2(x, T(t_i))_{|\Omega_l} + \frac{r}{2}\eta |T(t_i)|^2 - D_l : T(t_i). \tag{28.11}$$

PROOF. Let F be given by (28.10) with T as defined in (28.6). We first have

$$\det(F)_{|\Omega_l} = \det(Q_l) \det(T) \det(R_l) = \det(T) \det(A_l)/\det(D_l) = 1,$$

and thus F belongs to $\mathbb{H}_h \cap Y$.

Let us then compute $\mathbb{H}_h \cap dY(F)$. By definition, this is

$$\mathbb{H}_h \cap dY(F) = \left\{G \in \mathbb{H}_h, \frac{\partial \det}{\partial F}(F_{|\Omega_l}) : G_{|\Omega_l} = 0, \forall l = 1, \ldots M_h\right\}. \tag{28.12}$$

But, F being constructed by (28.10) and the function $\det(\cdot)$ being isotropic and therefore satisfying (28.3), we have

$$\frac{\partial \det}{\partial F}(F_{|\Omega_l}) = Q_l \frac{\partial \det}{\partial F}(T(t_{il})) R_l = Q_l(\text{cof}(T(t_{il}))) R_l.$$

Thus, (28.12) can be rewritten

$$\mathbb{H}_h \cap dY(F) = \{G \in \mathbb{H}_h, [\text{cof}(T(t_{il}))] :$$
$$(Q_l^T G_{|\Omega_l} R_l^T) = 0, \forall l = 1, \ldots, M_h\},$$

which, by construction of T, finally yields

$$\mathbb{H}_h \cap dY(F) = \Bigg\{G \in \mathbb{H}_h, \sum_{i=1}^{2}(Q_l^T G_{|\Omega_l} R_l^T)_{ii}/t_{il} \tag{28.13}$$

$$+ (Q_l^T G_{|\Omega_l} R_l^T)_{33} t_{1l} t_{2l} = 0, \forall l = 1, \ldots, M_h\Bigg\}.$$

We are now ready to compute the quantity

$$q = \int_\Omega \left\{ \frac{\partial \hat{W}_2}{\partial F}(x, F) + r\eta F - \eta[r(\mathrm{Id} + \nabla_h u) + \lambda] \right\} : G \, dx,$$

with F given by (28.10) and G arbitrary in $\mathbb{H}_h \cap dY(F)$. Since all functions appearing in the above integral are constant over Ω_l, we have

$$q = \sum_{l=1}^{M_h} \mathrm{meas}(\Omega_l) \, Q_l \left\{ \frac{\partial \hat{W}_2}{\partial F}(x, T(t_{il}))_{|\Omega_l} + r\eta T(t_{il}) - D_l \right\} R_l : G_{|\Omega_l}. \quad (28.14)$$

But, T and D_l are diagonal by construction, $(\partial \hat{W}_2/\partial F)(x, T)$ is diagonal from Theorem 28.1 and thus (28.14) takes the explicit form

$$q = \sum_{l=1}^{M_h} \mathrm{meas}(\Omega_l) \sum_{i=1}^{3} \left\{ \frac{\partial \hat{W}_2}{\partial F}(x, T)_{|\Omega_l} + r\eta T - D_l \right\}_{ii} (Q_l^T G_{|\Omega_l} R_l^T)_{ii}.$$

From the characterization (28.13) of $\mathbb{H}_h \cap dY(F)$, this implies

$$q = \sum_{l=1}^{M_h} \mathrm{meas}(\Omega_l) \left(\sum_{i=1}^{2} (Q_l^T G_{|\Omega_l} R_l^T)_{ii} \left[\left\{ \frac{\partial \hat{W}_2}{\partial F}(x, T)_{|\Omega_l} + r\eta T - D_l \right\}_{ii} \right.\right.$$
$$\left.\left. - \left\{ \frac{\partial \hat{W}_2}{\partial F}(x, T)_{|\Omega_l} + r\eta T - D_l \right\}_{33} t_{il}^{-2}(t_{jl})^{-1} \right] \right)$$

$$= \sum_{l=1}^{M_h} \mathrm{meas}(\Omega_l) \left(\sum_{i=1}^{2} (Q_l^T G_{|\Omega_l} R_l^T)_{ii} \frac{\partial J_l}{\partial t_i}(t_{1l}, t_{2l}) \right).$$

Therefore, from (28.9), $q = 0$, which means that $F \in Y \cap \mathbb{H}_h$ is a solution of (28.1), which completes our proof. $\square$

To illustrate the feasibility and the performances of the solution procedure described in the theorem above, it is useful to make the following remarks.

REMARK 28.1. The diagonalization of A_l in $\mathbb{M}^3$ can be achieved by a direct method which proceeds as follows:
- computation of $A_l A_l^T$;
- tridiagonalization of $A_l A_l^T$;
- computation of the eigenvalues $\mu_1 \geq \mu_2 \geq \mu_3$ of the tridiagonal matrix by computing the roots of the associated characteristic polynomial (by Cardan's formulas for example) ;
- computation of the corresponding normalized eigenvectors (g_i) by solving

$$A_l A_l^T g_j = \mu_j g_j, \quad |g_j|^2 = 1;$$

- computation of

$$(D_l)_{11} = \sqrt{\mu_1}, \quad (D_l)_{22} = \sqrt{\mu_2},$$
$$(D_l)_{33} = \sqrt{\mu_3}\,\text{sgn}(\det A_l);$$

- computation of $(Q_l)_{ij} = (g_i)_j$;
- computation of $R_l = D_l^{-1} Q_l^T A_l$.

REMARK 28.2. The nonlinear equation (28.9) always has a solution corresponding to the absolute minimum of J_l over $\mathbb{R}^2$. Indeed, (28.9) consists in finding a critical point of the "potential" energy J_l over the set of admissible diagonal matrices, a set which is parametrized on $\mathbb{R}^2$ by the map T. By construction, J_l is coercive and continuous on this set, and thus attains its minimum. This minimal point is a critical point of J_l and thus corresponds to a solution of (28.9).

REMARK 28.3. The nonlinear equation (28.9) in $\mathbb{R}^2$ is solved numerically by Newton's method with line search, the initial guess being the solution (t_{il}) at the previous resolution of (26.4). In that respect, it is interesting to choose r sufficiently large in order to guarantee the local convexity of J_l around the computed solution. Indeed, there will then be local uniqueness of the solution, local convergence of Newton's method, and thus consistency of algorithm (26.1)–(26.6) which in the same neighborhood will always pick the same solution of (28.9).

REMARK 28.4. The above solution procedure for (28.1) respects and uses at best the isotropy and the incompressibility of the considered material. Indeed, it reduces the problem posed in terms of deformation gradients to local problems (28.9) whose only unknowns are the independent singular values (t_{il}) of F with the exclusion of any rotational component of F.

REMARK 28.5. The solution procedure for compressible materials will be completely similar within the replacement of the map T by

$$T(t_1, t_2, t_3) = \begin{pmatrix} t_1 & 0 & 0 \\ 0 & t_2 & 0 \\ 0 & 0 & t_3 \end{pmatrix}.$$

29. Numerical results

In all our numerical tests, we have implemented algorithm (26.1)–(26.6) in the case of quadratic potentials $\hat{W}_1$, of isotropic potentials $\hat{W}_2$, and of spaces $\mathbb{H}_h$ made of piecewise constant functions.

For a given problem, the practical choice of r, η and $\hat{W}_1$ is not so clear. Due to the lack of convexity of the original problems, there are no theoretical results on the convergence of the algorithm which could help us in this choice. The only numerical evidence is that algorithm (26.1)–(26.6) diverges if r is too small and converges very slowly if r is too large.

For heterogeneous materials of Ogden type, whose stored energy potential $\hat{W}$ is given by

$$\hat{W}(x,F) = C_{10}(x)(|F|^2 - 3) + C_{01}(x)(|\operatorname{cof} F|^2 - 3)$$
$$+ a(x)[(\det F)^2 - 1]$$
$$- [2a(x) + 2C_{10}(x) + 4C_{01}(x)] \ln(\det F), \qquad (29.1)$$

and which reduces to the energy of an incompressible Mooney–Rivlin material when $a(x) = +\infty$, the choice that we have used with good success is

$$\hat{W}_1(x,F) = C_{10}(x)(|F|^2 - 3), \qquad (29.2)$$
$$\eta(x) = 2C_{10}(x), \qquad (29.3)$$
$$2 \leqslant r \leqslant 20.$$

In this range, the choice of r was usually not critical but could nevertheless, if properly done, accelerate the convergence by a factor of 2. As an additional verification of our choice of r, we were monitoring the local convexity of J_l in (28.9).

29.1. Stretching of a cracked rectangular bar

We consider a thick rectangular slab of Mooney–Rivlin material, with a non-propagating crack in its middle, and subjected to vertical stretching forces at its extremities. Under the action of the external loads, this bar is stretched and its equilibrium position, computed under the plane-strains assumption, is shown in Fig. 29.1.

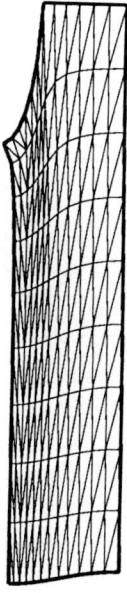

FIG. 29.1. Deformed cracked bar. The top left part corresponds to the open crack, and is horizontal in the initial configuration. There is a very large change of shape at this location.

This solution was obtained after 20 iterations of algorithm (26.1)–(26.6) with $K = 1, \mathbb{H}_h$ and $\mathbb{V}_h$ respectively given by (12.3) and (11.2), $\hat{W}_1$ and η given by (29.2) and (29.3) and $r = 4$. The relative difference between the stresses computed at the boundary and the applied tension was less than 10^{-4}.

29.2. Postbuckling solution of a three-dimensional beam

This example illustrates the capability for algorithm (26.1)–(26.6) to compute stable postbuckling equilibrium positions of elastic bodies even in a three-dimensional situation. It considers a 0.2 m × 0.2 m × 2 m beam, compressed along its axis and subjected to a pressure of 10^{-4} MPa on one of its lateral faces. The beam is made of a compressible hyperelastic material, whose energy potential is given by (29.1), with $C_{10} = 0.5$ MPa, $C_{01} = 0.125$ MPa and $a = 25$ MPa. The compression is achieved by an imposed displacement of 0.2 m of its upper extremity, the lower one remaining fixed.

For symmetry reasons, we only compute the upperhalf of the beam, using the spaces $\mathbb{H}_h$ and $\mathbb{V}_h$ defined in (12.3) and (11.2) with $N = 3$. On this problem, algorithm (26.1)–(26.6) yields two solutions, one unstable, symmetric, and characterized by small lateral displacements and the other one, stable and characterized by large lateral displacements (Fig. 29.2).

On this example, it is very interesting to monitor the quantity

$$\log[\| \operatorname{Id} + \nabla_h u^n - F^n \|_{0,2}^2]$$

during the iterations (Fig. 29.3). This quantity, measuring the lack of convergence of our algorithm, first decreases to a minimum corresponding to the unstable symmetric solution, then automatically diverges for a few steps, and finally

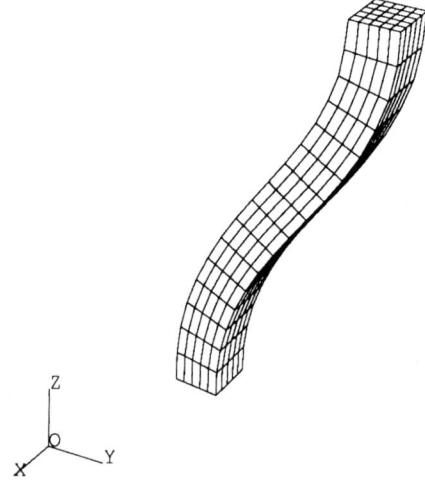

FIG. 29.2. Three-dimensional beam after buckling. The actual shape of the upper half of the beam after deformation is depicted.

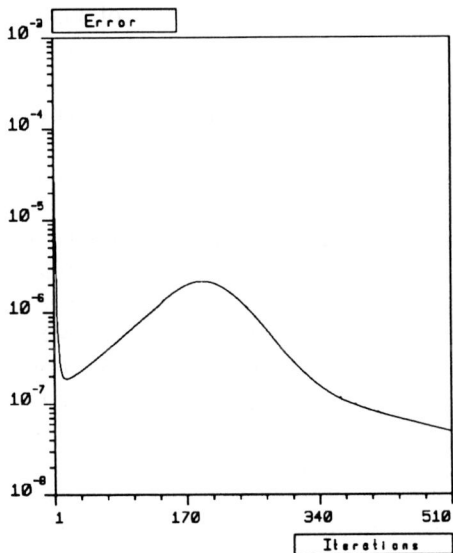

FIG. 29.3. Convergence history. This curve shows the evolution of the residual during the iterations. The residual reaches a minimum, then increases, and then converges to zero.

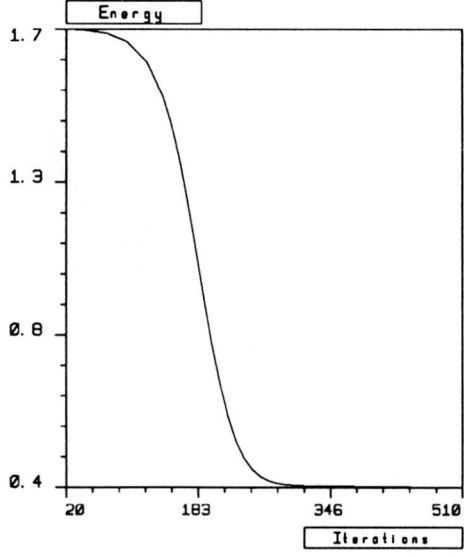

FIG. 29.4. Energy vs iterations. This curve shows the evolution of the total energy during the iterations.

converges to zero while we approach the stable buckled solution. Parallel to this graph, we have also shown in Fig. 29.4 the evolution of the total potential energy during the iterations.

Numerical comparisons between the above augmented Lagrangian methods and Newton's techniques of Chapter IV lead to different conclusions depending on the physical problem under consideration.

For three-dimensional bodies made of isotropic quasi-homogeneous materials and subjected to very large deformations, augmented Lagrangian techniques appear to work faster. More precisely, on typical problems of this kind solved without incremental loading on a sequential machine, Newton's method will converge in around 10 iterations while the augmented Lagrangian algorithm (26.1)–(26.6) will require 50 iterations for a total computing time three times smaller. Moreover, the rate of growth of the cost as a function of the number of unknowns is superlinear for Newton and linear for algorithm (26.1)–(26.6).

When the condition number of the problem increases (because of nonconservative loading, or because of strong anisotropy or heterogeneity), the performances of Newton's method stay the same, while the convergence of algorithm (26.1)–(26.6) experiences a significant slow-down. In those situations, it is clear that the preconditioning strategy now available for the augmented Lagrangian algorithm (i.e. the choice of r, η and $\hat{W}_1$) lacks efficiency and that therefore Newton's method is presently more competitive.

CHAPTER VI

Equilibrium Problems with Frictionless Contact

The boundary value problems that we have considered up to now were dealing with boundary conditions imposing a given displacement, traction or pressure on the boundary. These conditions do not cover all the situations found in practice. Other boundary conditions that are very important are those encountered in contact problems. In such problems, the deformable body under consideration is constrained to stay outside different obstacles existing in its neighborhood. For example, for a tire rolling on a road, the tire must stay above the road and cannot penetrate the road surface.

The objective of the present chapter is to describe equilibrium problems involving such contact problems. We first introduce their mathematical formulation, introducing the case of a plane rigid obstacle, then the case of a curved rigid obstacle, and finally the case with self-contact. In doing so, we will make the simplifying assumption of frictionless contact. The existence theory of Chapter II can then be extended to these new mathematical problems, thanks to the results of CIARLET and NEČAS ([1985, 1987]) (Section 31). After approximation by finite elements (Section 32) and excluding self-contact, we are faced with nonlinear variational inequalities, which can be numerically solved either by a simple predictor–corrector approach (Section 33) or by a nonlinear programming approach (Section 34). We conclude this brief chapter with a few indications of the numerical strategies which presently exist for treating the case with self-contact.

From the mathematical point of view, the problem of frictionless contact in finite elasticity is clearly understood (CIARLET and NEČAS [1987], CIARLET [1988]). The existing numerical algorithms can still be improved, especially when considering self-contact or contact with geometrically complex obstacles (BELYTSCHKO and YEH [1992]). But the major unsolved problems involve contact with friction, whose physical, mathematical and numerical aspects are not clearly understood (ODEN and PIRES [1983], ODEN and KIKUCHI [1988]).

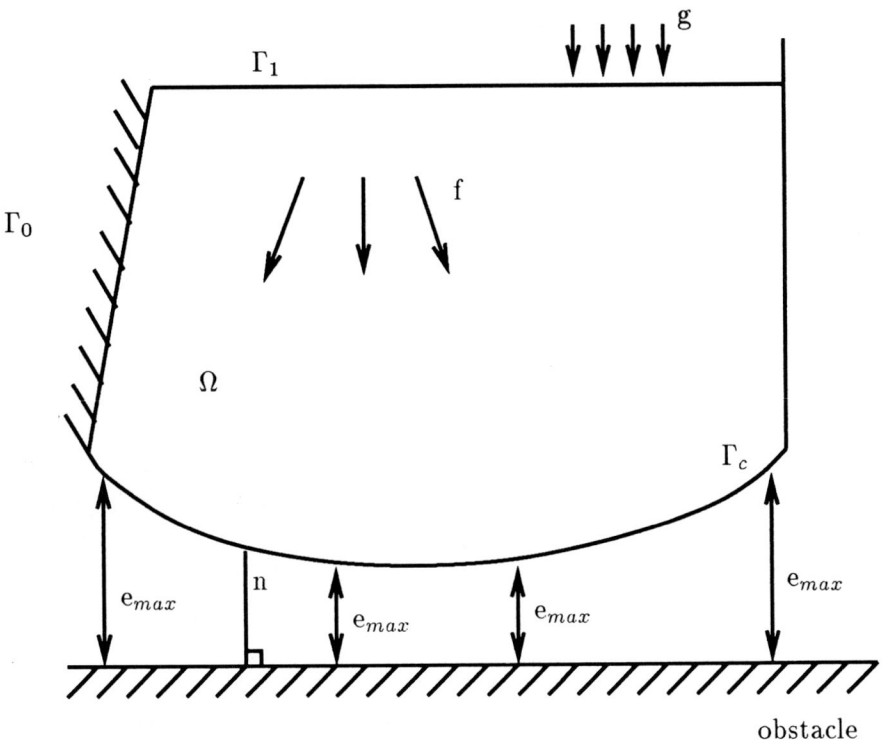

FIG. 30.1. Plane obstacle. Under vertical loading, the body will move downwards. When the displacement reaches the value $e_{\max}$, the body enters into contact with the obstacle.

30. Formulation of a contact problem

Let us first consider situations involving contact with a plane rigid obstacle. The corresponding physical problem is the same as in Section 5, but now the boundary Γ of Ω contains a part Γ_c (Fig. 30.1) where, due to the presence of a *plane rigid obstacle* in the neighborhood of the considered body, the displacement $u \cdot n$ of the body perpendicularly to the obstacle cannot exceed a given value, that is

$$u(x) \cdot n \leqslant e_{\max}(x) \quad \forall x \in \Gamma_c. \tag{30.1}$$

To impose this constraint, the obstacle exerts a reaction force on the points of Γ_c where contact has occurred. In the case of a *contact without friction*, the reaction is normal to the obstacle and oriented towards the body. In other words the contact force is of the form:

$$g = g_c n, \quad g_c \leqslant 0, \quad g_c(u \cdot n - e_{\max}) = 0. \tag{30.2}$$

In this framework, the variational formulation of the corresponding equilibrium problem is obtained as in the contact-free case but, in addition, one must take into account the reaction g_c in the virtual work theorem (3.1) and impose the kinematic constraint (30.1) to the real displacement field. Then, using the definitions and notation of Section 7, the variational formulation of equilibrium problems in incompressible finite elasticity with frictionless contact becomes:

$$\int_\Omega \left\{ \frac{\partial \hat{W}}{\partial F}(x, \mathrm{Id} + \nabla u) - p \frac{\partial \det}{\partial F}(\mathrm{Id} + \nabla u) \right\} : \nabla v \, dx$$

$$= \int_\Omega f \cdot v \, dx + \int_{\Gamma_1} g \cdot v \, da + \int_{\Gamma_c} g_c n \cdot v \, da$$

$$\forall v \in \mathbb{V}, \ (u - u_0) \in \mathbb{V}, \tag{30.3}$$

$$\int_\Omega q[\det(\mathrm{Id} + \nabla u) - 1] \, dx = 0 \quad \forall q \in \mathbb{P}, \ p \in \mathbb{P}, \tag{30.4}$$

$$(u \cdot n - e_{\max}) \leqslant 0, g_c \leqslant 0 \text{ and } g_c(u \cdot n - e_{\max}) = 0 \text{ on } \Gamma_c. \tag{30.5}$$

We now consider the general case of frictionless contact problems involving a rigid curved obstacle (Fig. 30.2). This obstacle may be made of several disconnected pieces and will be characterized by the equation of its boundary

$$e(y) = 0, \tag{30.6}$$

with e a given function from $\mathbb{E}$ into $\mathbb{R}$. For example, a plane obstacle would be characterized by the function

$$e(y) = y \cdot n - c.$$

Once e is given, the unilateral contact constraint (30.1) takes the form

$$e(x + u(x)) \leqslant 0 \quad \forall x \in \Gamma_c. \tag{30.7}$$

In the absence of friction forces, the associated reaction force exerted by the obstacle on Γ_c is again normal to the obstacle and is therefore given by

$$g(x) = g_c(x) \frac{\partial e}{\partial y}(x + u(x)), \tag{30.8}$$

with $n = n^o(x) = \partial e / \partial y$ the unit normal vector to the obstacle (oriented towards the obstacle) and

$$g_c(x) \leqslant 0 \quad \text{and} \quad g_c(x) e(x + u(x)) = 0 \quad \forall x \in \Gamma_c. \tag{30.9}$$

Then, the variational formulation of the corresponding equilibrium problem is simply

$$\int_\Omega \frac{\partial \hat{W}}{\partial F}(x, \mathrm{Id} + \nabla u) : \nabla v \, dx - \int_\Omega p \frac{\partial \det}{\partial F}(\mathrm{Id} + \nabla u) : \nabla v \, dx$$

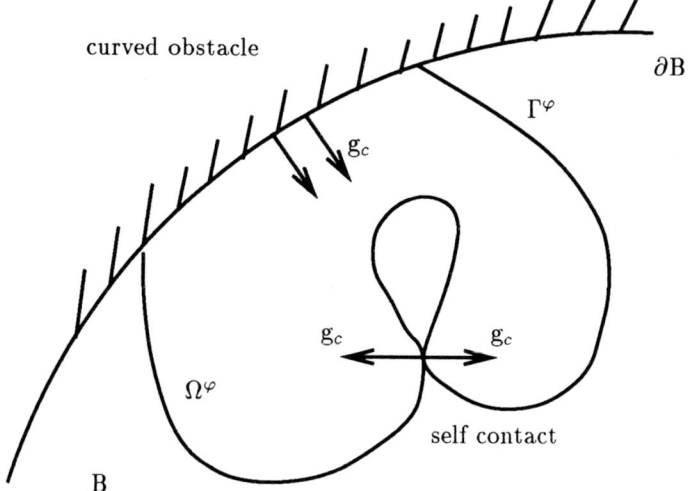

FIG. 30.2. General contact problem. After deformation, the body Ω enters into contact with the obstacle ∂B and with itself. When contact occurs, a reaction force g_c is applied at the contact points to prevent interpenetration.

$$= \int_\Omega f \cdot v \, dx + \int_{\Gamma_1} g \cdot v \, da + \int_{\Gamma_c} g_c \frac{\partial e}{\partial y}(x + u(x)) \cdot v \, da \qquad (30.10)$$

$\forall v \in \mathbb{V}, \ (u - u_0) \in \mathbb{V},$

$$\int_\Omega q[\det(\mathrm{Id} + \nabla u) - 1] \, dx = 0, \quad \forall q \in \mathbb{P}, \ p \in \mathbb{P}, \qquad (30.11)$$

$$g_{c|\Gamma_c} \leqslant 0, \ e(x + u(x))_{|\Gamma_c} \leqslant 0, \ g_c e(x + u(x))_{|\Gamma_c} = 0. \qquad (30.12)$$

The formulation (30.10)–(30.12) of equilibrium problems in finite elasticity is quite general but does not guarantee the physical admissibility of the solution u. The local incompressibility condition $\det(\mathrm{Id} + \nabla u) = 1$ (or the orientation-preserving condition $\det(\mathrm{Id} + \nabla u) > 0$ in the compressible case) does not guarantee the global injectivity of the mapping $\varphi = x + u$ (Remark 7.4). As indicated in Fig. 30.3, for large loads, the solution of these equilibrium problems may cease to be globally injective on Ω and may thus correspond to interpenetrating configurations.

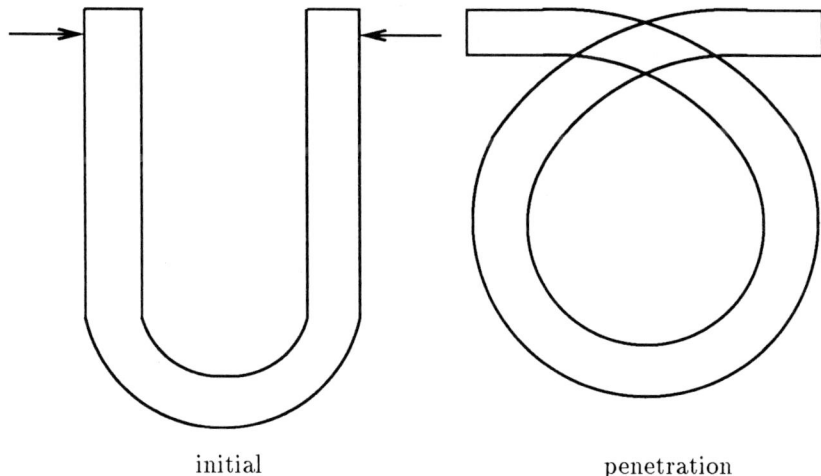

FIG. 30.3. Interpenetration. We show here a forbidden situation with a noninjective deformation.

In practice, this unphysical situation is prevented by the existence of reaction forces which appear as soon as the considered body reaches a condition of self-contact. Then, two different points x and y of its boundary come into contact with each other and a reaction force develops at these points of contact. In the absence of friction, the reaction force acts on x along the normal $n^\varphi(x)$ and acts on y along $n^\varphi(y)$. In addition, these forces are self-equilibrated (Fig. 30.2), which means that we have

$$g_c(x)n^\varphi(x) = -g_c(y)n^\varphi(y),$$

where $g_c(x)$ denotes the intensity (negative in value) of the contact force exerted at x on the body, and measured per unit surface of the reference configuration.

These new conditions of self-contact can still be handled by the previous variational formulation (30.10)–(30.12). Let Γ_c denote the part of the boundary of Ω that can enter into contact either with itself or with the boundary ∂B of a rigid obstacle. Let B denote the exterior of the obstacle. By writing the virtual work Theorem (3.1) and the local incompressibility constraint $\det(\text{Id} + \nabla u) = 1$, and by taking into account the hyperelastic constitutive laws and the special form of the frictionless contact forces $g = g_c n^\varphi$, we first get

$$\int_\Omega \frac{\partial \hat{W}}{\partial F}(x, \mathrm{Id} + \nabla u) : \nabla v \, dx - \int_\Omega p \frac{\partial \det}{\partial F}(\mathrm{Id} + \nabla u) : \nabla v \, dx$$

$$= \int_\Omega f \cdot v \, dx + \int_{\Gamma_1} g \cdot v \, da + \int_{\Gamma_c} g_c n^\varphi \cdot v \, da \qquad (30.13)$$

$$\forall v \in \mathbb{V}, \ (u - u_0) \in \mathbb{V},$$

$$\int_\Omega q[\det(\mathrm{Id} + \nabla u) - 1] \, dx = 0 \quad \forall q \in \mathbb{P}, \ p \in \mathbb{P}. \qquad (30.14)$$

To these variational equations, we must now add the contact condition (30.12) and the above conditions on global injectivity and self-contact. Putting all these constraints together, we get

$$\varphi(x) \in \bar{B} \quad \forall x \in \bar{\Omega}, \qquad (30.15)$$

φ injective on Ω, $\qquad (30.16)$

$g_{c|\Gamma_c} \leq 0$, $\qquad (30.17)$

$g_c(x) = 0 \quad$ if φ injective at x and $\varphi(x) \notin \partial B$, $\qquad (30.18)$

$g_c(x)n^\varphi(x) = -g_c(y)n^\varphi(y) \quad$ if $\varphi(x) = \varphi(y)$. $\qquad (30.19)$

The variational system (30.13)–(30.19) is the most general formulation of equilibrium problem in finite elasticity and it covers all possible cases of frictionless contact.

REMARK 30.1. Equation (30.12) is a particular case of the constitutive equation

$$-g_c \in \partial \left[\frac{1}{3\varepsilon} \sup[0, e(x + u(x))]^3\right], \qquad (30.20)$$

corresponding to the choice $\varepsilon = 0$. Above $\partial(\cdot)$ denotes the subgradient with respect to u of the convex function $(1/3\varepsilon) \sup[0, e(x+u)]^3$ (ROCKAFELLAR [1970], EKELAND and TEMAM [1975]), and reduces to its classical gradient if $\varepsilon \neq 0$. The regularized constitutive equation (30.20) plays the role here of the nearly incompressible law introduced in Section 4.

31. Existence results

The analysis of the above variational system (30.13)–(30.19) is based on the variational theory of J. BALL [1977], and uses the following improved definition of the set $\mathbb{U}$ of admissible displacement fields (CIARLET and NEČAS [1987]):

$$\mathbb{U} = \left\{v, v - u_o \in \mathbb{V}, H = \mathrm{cof}(\mathrm{Id} + \nabla v) \in L^q(\Omega; \mathbb{M}^3),\right.$$

$$\delta = \det(\mathrm{Id} + \nabla v) = 1 \text{ a.e. on } \Omega, \int_\Omega \det(\mathrm{Id} + \nabla v)\, dx \leqslant \mathrm{vol}(\varphi(\Omega)),$$

$$\varphi(\bar{\Omega}) \subset \bar{B}, \text{ with } \varphi(x) = x + v(x) \Big\}. \tag{31.1}$$

More precisely, the mathematical analysis of the variational system (30.13)–(30.19) relies on the following four theorems.

THEOREM 31.1 (Sufficient condition of injectivity). *Let $\varphi \in C^1(\bar{\Omega}, \mathbb{E})$ be such that*

$$\det(\nabla \varphi) > 0 \quad \text{on } \Omega,$$

$$\int_\Omega \det(\nabla \varphi)\, dx \leqslant \mathrm{vol}(\varphi(\Omega)).$$

Then the mapping φ is injective on Ω.

PROOF. If φ were not injective, there would exist an open ball B^φ in $\varphi(\Omega)$ whose elements were the image of at least two points of Ω, that is such that

$$\mathrm{card}(\varphi^{-1}(x^\varphi)) \geqslant 2 \quad \forall x^\varphi \in B^\varphi.$$

This would in turn imply

$$\mathrm{vol}(\varphi(\Omega)) = \int_{\varphi(\Omega)} dx^\varphi < \int_{\varphi(\Omega)} \mathrm{card}(\varphi^{-1}(x^\varphi))\, dx^\varphi = \int_\Omega \det(\nabla \varphi(x))\, dx,$$

and would therefore contradict our initial assumption on φ. □

THEOREM 31.2 (Energetic formulation). *In the case of dead loading, a smooth enough solution of the minimization problem*

Minimize the total potential energy

$$J(v) = \int_\Omega \hat{W}(x, \mathrm{Id} + \nabla v)\, dx - \int_\Omega f \cdot v\, dx - \int_{\Gamma_1} g \cdot v\, dx \tag{31.2}$$

over the set $\mathbb{U}$ of admissible displacement fields,

is solution of the variational problem (30.13)–(30.19).

PROOF. The proof is outlined in CIARLET ([1988], p. 324). For smooth fields u, the contact reaction $g_c n^\varphi$ can be identified as Lagrange multipliers of the nonpenetration conditions (30.15)–(30.16). □

THEOREM 31.3. *For $s > 3$, the set $\mathbb{U}$ of admissible displacement fields defined in (31.1) is weakly closed in $\mathbb{H} = W^{1,s}(\Omega, \mathbb{E}) \times L^q(\Omega, \mathbb{M}^3)$.*

PROOF. For $s > 3$, the injection of $W^{1,s}(\Omega, \mathbb{E})$ in $C(\bar{\Omega}, \mathbb{E})$ is compact. Hence, any sequence $(\varphi_l)_l$ of $\mathbb{U}$ weakly converging towards φ in $W^{1,s}(\Omega, \mathbb{E})$ is uniformly converging towards φ in $\bar{\Omega}$. In particular, since $\bar{B}$ is closed, and since φ_l belongs to $\mathbb{U}$, we have

$$\lim_{l \to \infty} \varphi_l(x) = \varphi(x) \in \bar{B} \quad \forall x \in \bar{\Omega}.$$

Similarly, the uniform convergence of $(\varphi_l)_l \in \mathbb{U}$ towards φ in $C(\bar{\Omega}, \mathbb{E})$ guarantees that at the limit we have (CIARLET and NEČAS [1987], CIARLET [1988], p. 390):

$$\int_{\Omega} \det(\nabla \varphi) \, dx \leq \text{vol}(\varphi(\Omega)).$$

The rest of the proof then follows the steps of Theorem 8.1. □

THEOREM 31.4. *Let the set $\mathbb{U}$ of admissible displacement fields be given by* (31.1) *with $s > 3$. Let Ω be open, bounded connected in $\mathbb{E}$, and satisfy a strong Lipschitz condition (in the sense of NEČAS [1967]). Let its boundary Γ be such that $\Gamma = \bar{\Gamma}_o \cup \bar{\Gamma}_1, \Gamma_o \cap \Gamma_1 = \emptyset, \text{meas}(\Gamma_o) > 0$. Let u_o be measurable, f and g be given independently of u in $L^{s*}(\Omega)$ and $L^{s*}(\Gamma_1)$ (dead loading), and suppose that there exists an element w in $\mathbb{U}$ with $J(w) < +\infty$.*

Suppose in addition that the energy potential $\hat{W}(x, F)$ satisfies

$\hat{W}(x, F) = \mathcal{G}(x, F, \text{cof } F)$,

$\mathcal{G}(x, \cdot, \cdot, \cdot)$ *is continuous and convex on* $\mathbb{M}^3 \times \mathbb{M}^3$,

$\mathcal{G}(\cdot, F, H)$ *is measurable on* Ω,

$\mathcal{G}(x, F, H) \geq a(x) + C_1 |F|^s + C_2 |H|^q$ *(coercivity)*,

$C_i > 0, i = 1, 3, \quad a \in L^1(\Omega)$.

Then there exists a solution to the energy minimization problem (31.2).

PROOF. Under the above assumptions, it was proved in Theorem 9.1 that the energy potential J is coercive and weakly lower semicontinuous on $\mathbb{U}$ for the $\mathbb{H}$ topology. But, we have just seen in the above theorem that $\mathbb{U}$ is weakly closed for the $\mathbb{H}$ topology. Hence, by the Weierstrass theorem, the minimization problem (31.2) has a solution. □

32. Finite-element discretization

To approximate problem (30.3)–(30.5) or (30.10)–(30.12), the spaces $\mathbb{V}, \mathbb{P}$ and $L^s(\Gamma_c)$ must first be replaced by finite-dimensional subspaces $\mathbb{V}_h, \mathbb{P}_h$ and $\mathbb{H}_{ch}$. The introduction of $\mathbb{V}_h$ and $\mathbb{P}_h$ has already been done in Section 12. As for the space $\mathbb{H}_{ch}$, let us introduce a regular triangulation of Γ_c:

$$\bar{\Gamma}_c = \bigcup_{l=1}^{M_c} \bar{\Gamma}_l$$

and simply define

$$\mathbb{H}_{ch} = \{q_h : \Gamma_c \to \mathbb{R}, \; q_{h|\Gamma_l} = \text{constant}, \; \forall l = 1, \ldots, M_c\}, \tag{32.1}$$

$$s_h : L^s(\Gamma_c) \to \mathbb{H}_{ch},$$

$$q \longmapsto s_h(q)_{|\Gamma_l} = \frac{1}{\text{meas}(\Gamma_l)} \int_{\Gamma_l} q \, da. \tag{32.2}$$

For example, we can triangulate Ω into quadrilaterals (respectively hexahedrals if $N = 3$), construct $\mathbb{V}_h$ and $\mathbb{P}_h$ by (11.2) and (12.3) and use as triangulation of Γ_c the trace on Γ_c of the triangulation of Ω. Alternatively, for $N = 2$, one can triangulate Ω into triangles, construct $\mathbb{P}_h$ and $\mathbb{V}_h$ by (12.4)–(12.5), use as initial triangulation of Γ_c the trace on Γ_c of the triangulation of Ω, and divide into two pieces any segment Γ_l where $v_h \in \mathbb{V}_h$ is a second-order polynomial (Fig. 32.1). A third possible choice is also indicated in Fig. 32.1, and uses the finite-element spaces introduced in (12.6)–(12.7).

A final choice is described by Fig. 32.1, where the segments Γ_l are now associated with the nodes of the triangulation.

In any case, one would need to satisfy the compatibility condition (14.6), and, by analogy, a condition of the type (ODEN and KIKUCHI [1988])

$$\inf_{q_h \in \mathbb{H}_{ch}, \|q_h\|=1} \sup_{v_h \in \mathbb{V}_h, \|v_h\|=1} \left[\int_{\Gamma_c} q_h s_h(v_h \cdot n) \, da \right] = C_0(h) > 0. \tag{32.3}$$

Then, the discrete equivalent of (30.10)–(30.12) simply becomes

$$\int_\Omega \frac{\partial \hat{W}}{\partial F}(x, \text{Id} + \nabla u_h) : \nabla v_h \, dx - \int_\Omega p_h \frac{\partial \det}{\partial F}(\text{Id} + \nabla u_h) : \nabla v_h \, dx$$

$$= \int_\Omega f \cdot v_h \, dx + \int_{\Gamma_1} g \cdot v_h \, da + \int_{\Gamma_c} g_c \frac{\partial e}{\partial y}(s_h(x + u_h(x))) \cdot s_h(v_h) \, da \tag{32.4}$$

$$\forall v_h \in \mathbb{V}_h, \; (u_h - u_0) \in \mathbb{V}_h,$$

$$\int_\Omega q_h [\det(\text{Id} + \nabla u_h) - 1] \, dx = 0 \quad \forall q_h \in \mathbb{P}_h, \; p_h \in \mathbb{P}_h, \tag{32.5}$$

$$g_{c|\Gamma_l} \leq 0, \; e[s_h(x + u_h(x))_{|\Gamma_l}] \leq 0, \; g_{c|\Gamma_l} e[s_h(x + u_h(x))_{|\Gamma_l}] = 0 \tag{32.6}$$

$$\forall l = 1, M_c, \; g_c \in \mathbb{H}_{ch}.$$

33. A first numerical algorithm

The most popular algorithm for solving (32.4)–(32.6) in the case of a plane obstacle is of predictor–corrector type. One predicts the subset of Γ_c where the constraint (30.1) will be active, eliminates the corresponding degrees of freedom

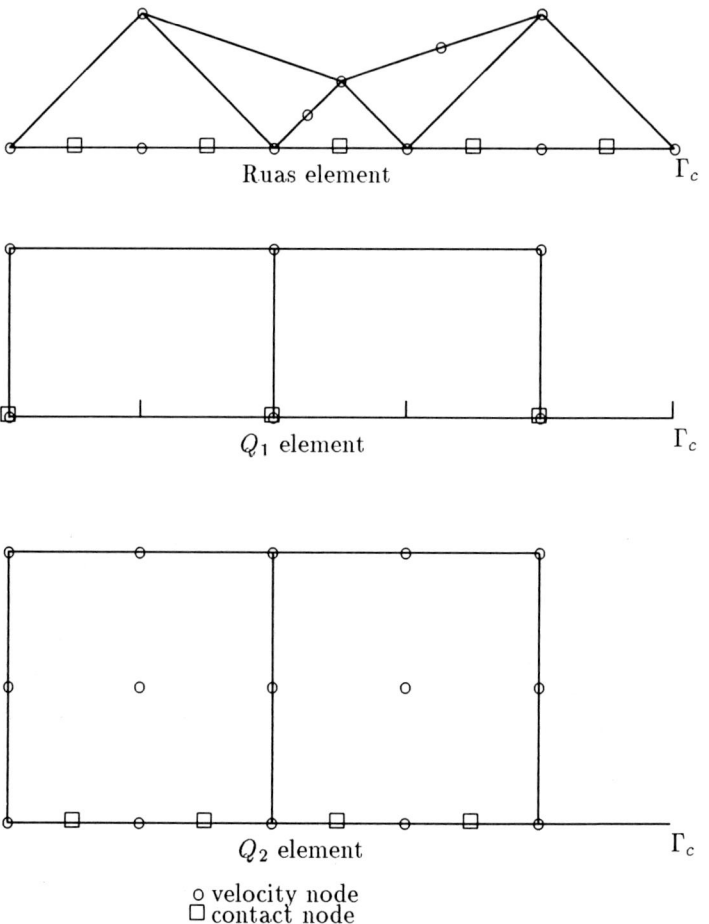

FIG. 32.1. Finite elements with contact nodes. The squares indicate the locations where we verify the contact constraint and impose the reaction force.

from $\mathbb{V}_h$, solves the resulting contact-free equilibrium problem, and updates the subset of active constraints by monitoring the points where (30.5) is violated. This leads to the following algorithm.

We predict

$$\Gamma_c^+ = \{l, s_h(u_h \cdot n) = e_{\max} \text{ on } \Gamma_l\},$$

and define

$$\mathbb{V}_h^+ = \{v_h \in \mathbb{V}_h, s_h(v_h \cdot n)_{|\Gamma_l} = 0 \quad \forall l \in \Gamma_c^+\}.$$

With $\mathbb{V}_h^+$ given, we solve the equilibrium problem

$$\int_\Omega \frac{\partial \hat{W}}{\partial F}(x, \mathrm{Id}+\nabla u_h) : \nabla v_h \, dx - \int_\Omega p_h \frac{\partial \det}{\partial F}(\mathrm{Id}+\nabla u_h) : \nabla v_h \, dx$$

$$= \int_\Omega f \cdot v_h \, dx + \int_{\Gamma_1} g \cdot v_h \, da \quad \forall v_h \in \mathbb{V}_h^+, \tag{33.1}$$

$(u_h - u_0) \in \mathbb{V}_h$, $(s_h(u_h \cdot n) - e_{\max})_{|\Gamma_l} = 0$, $\forall l \in \Gamma_c^+$,

$$\int_\Omega p_h[\det(\mathrm{Id}+\nabla u_h) - 1] \, dx = 0 \quad \forall q_h \in \mathbb{P}_h, \; p_h \in \mathbb{P}_h. \tag{33.2}$$

We then compute g_c from (32.4) and check for the contact condition (30.5) on any element Γ_l:

if $(s_h(u_h \cdot n) - e_{\max})_{|\Gamma_l} > 0$, we add l to Γ_c^+,

if $(g_c)_{|\Gamma_l} > 0$, we remove l from Γ_c^+.

The above process is reiterated with Γ_c^+ replaced by its new updated value until the contact boundary Γ_c^+ stays invariant between two successive iterations.

In this algorithm, the solution of (33.1)–(33.2) is simply obtained by one of the numerical methods described in chapter IV or V. The whole algorithm then appears as a simple and easy-to-implement extension of the methods used for the contact-free problem. It turns out to be an efficient solver of the full contact problem in situations where the contact surface Γ_c^+ can be correctly predicted and where the contact constraints are not too severe.

34. The nonlinear programming approach

With the notation of Chapter IV, the discrete system (32.4)–(32.6) can also be rewritten as the algebraic system

Find $\{U, P, G_c\} \in \mathbb{R}^{N_h} \times \mathbb{R}^{M_h} \times \mathbb{R}^{M_c}$ such that

$$\mathscr{F}(U, P, f, g) - G_c \cdot \frac{\partial \mathscr{G}(U)}{\partial U} = 0 \quad \text{in } \mathbb{R}^{N_h} \times \mathbb{R}^{M_h}, \tag{34.1}$$

$$G_c \leqslant 0, \quad \mathscr{G}(U) \leqslant 0, \quad G_c \cdot \mathscr{G}(U) = 0 \quad \text{in } \mathbb{R}^{M_c}. \tag{34.2}$$

Here, we have set

$$G_c^l = \mathrm{meas}(\Gamma_l) g_{c|\Gamma_l} \quad \forall l = 1, M_c, \tag{34.3}$$

$$\mathscr{G}_l(U) = e(s_h(x + u_h(x))_{|\Gamma_l}) \quad \forall l = 1, M_c, \tag{34.4}$$

and we have kept the definitions (18.2)–(18.5) for $\mathscr{F}, u_h$ and p_h.

But now, systems like (34.1)–(34.2) have been extensively studied in nonlinear programming, and a general algorithm exists for their solution. This algorithm is an extension of Newton's method and, when applied to (34.1)–(34.2), it takes the form:

Initialization (Penalization).
For ε given (not too small), we solve the nonlinear system (S_0):

$$\mathcal{F}(U,P,f,g) + \frac{1}{\varepsilon} \sum_{l=1}^{M_c} \sup(0, \mathcal{G}_l(U))^2 \frac{\partial \mathcal{G}_l(U)}{\partial U} = 0 \quad \text{in } \mathbb{R}^{N_h} \times \mathbb{R}^{M_h},$$

and set

$$G_c^l = -\frac{1}{\varepsilon} \sup(0, \mathcal{G}_l(U))^2,$$

$$R = \mathcal{F}(U,P,f,g) - G_c \cdot \frac{\partial \mathcal{G}(U)}{\partial U},$$

$$\Gamma_c^+ = \{l, G_c^l < 0\}.$$

Correction loop.
These first values of (U, P, G_c) and Γ_c^+ are then updated iteratively by solving the linearized complementary system (S_L):

$$\left[\frac{\partial \mathcal{F}(U,P,f,g)}{\partial (U,P)} - G_c \cdot \frac{\partial^2 \mathcal{G}_l(U)}{\partial U^2} \right](\Delta U, \Delta P) - \sum_{l \in \Gamma_c^+} \Delta G_c^l \frac{\partial \mathcal{G}_l(U)}{\partial U} = R,$$

$$\frac{\partial \mathcal{G}_l}{\partial U} \Delta U = \mathcal{G}_l(U) \quad \forall l \in \Gamma_c^+,$$

by setting $(U, P, G_c) = (U, P, G_c) - (\Delta U, \Delta P, \Delta G_c)$, by computing the residual

$$R = \mathcal{F}(U,P,f,g) - G_c \cdot \frac{\partial \mathcal{G}(U)}{\partial U},$$

and by updating Γ_c^+:

if $G_c^l > 0$, set $G_c^l = 0$ and suppress l from Γ_c^+, (34.5)

if $\mathcal{G}_l(U) > 0$, add l to Γ_c^+. (34.6)

This correction loop is repeated until a stationary solution (U, P, G_c, Γ_c^+) is reached.

This algorithm is very general and very expensive. It calls for the following remarks.

REMARK 34.1. The penalized nonlinear system (S_0) is to be solved by one of the Newton's methods described in Chapter IV. Few iterations will be sufficient here since its solution is only used as an initial guess. Then, the linearized system (S_L), of order $N_h + M_h + \dim \Gamma_c^+$, is very expensive to solve. A block Gaussian elimination of the variables (U, P) appears to be the most reasonable strategy for its solution. As for Γ_c^+, its updating at each step might not be the best choice. Experiments and developments are still required to determine the optimal updating strategy.

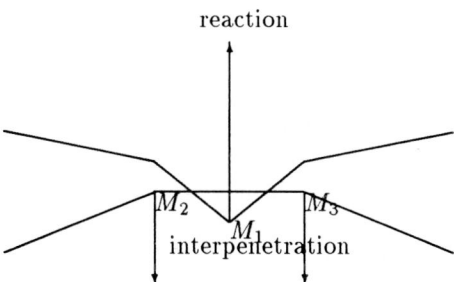

FIG. 35.1. Slave and masters. The slave node M_1 is checked against the master surface M_2M_3. If interpenetration occurs, reaction forces are applied.

REMARK 34.2. For nonlinear constraints $\mathscr{G}_l$, it is not possible to work in the kernel of $\mathscr{G}_l$ as we did in Section 33 for a plane obstacle. Nevertheless, the solution of the penalized system (S_0) may be sufficiently accurate for many engineering applications, so that the costly correction loop is not always necessary.

REMARK 34.3. In any case, the physical meaning of the solution obtained might be questionable. Indeed, for curved obstacles, there may be a large number of equilibrium positions and the correct physical one can only be picked by tracking the past history of the body. This tracking is even more critical if one deals with friction forces.

REMARK 34.4. The solution of (34.1)–(34.2) can also be achieved by using the recently developed interior point algorithms (see KRANISH [1991]).

35. Extensions to self-contact

The development of algorithms for the treatment of self-contact has been pioneered by HALLQUIST, GOUDREAU and BENSON [1987] and BENSON and HALLQUIST [1987]. They have introduced the so-called single surface contact algorithms based on the notion of slave nodes and master segments. In our previous notation, the slave nodes play the role of the surfaces Γ_c where contact may occur, and the master elements play the role of the potential obstacles. The difference is that the obstacles are part of the deformable body. Once these slave nodes and master elements are defined, interpenetration is checked on each slave node M_1 by comparing the deformed position of the line M_1M_2 with the deformed position of the corresponding master element (Fig. 35.1). Above M_2 is the nearest neighbor of M_1 among the nodes of all possible master elements, the master element is a predefined element associated with the node M_2 and penetration is declared when M_1M_2 is on the wrong side of the master element. A contact force is applied to the different nodes (slave and masters) whenever penetration has been detected, and the new equilibrium position corresponding to this updated reaction force is then computed as in the contact-free problem. This method is used in many industrial codes, such as DYNACODE, but it has three drawbacks: it is computationally expensive, it involves many special cases, and the definition of reliable master elements is technical and problem-dependent.

BELYTSCHKO and NEAL [1991] have introduced a very simple contact–impact method which overcomes these difficulties. Their proposed pinball algorithm embeds a sphere (a pinball) in each finite element at the surface of the body and checks interpenetration simply by determining whether the pinballs have overlapped. This check is very simple: it first classifies the different pinballs in separate boxes, depending on their present positions, and for each pair of pinballs within each box it compares the current distance between the centers with the sum of the radii. When overlap of pinballs is detected, a contact reaction is applied to the centers of the overlapping pinballs and then transferred to the nodes of the elements where the pinballs are embedded. In terms of the nonlinear programming approach described in the previous paragraph, this pinball algorithm both detects the surface Γ_c^+ and computes the contact reaction g_c. It is simple, of general use, and its accuracy can be improved at will by introducing a hierarchy of splitting pinballs as described in BELYTSCHKO and YEH [1992].

CHAPTER VII

Extension to Viscoelasticity

Hyperelasticity is a constitutive model which does not take memory effects or energy dissipation into account. Unfortunately, such nonlinear viscoelastic phenomena can be observed in the behavior of many real materials such as rubber or biological tissues (LOCKETT [1972], ODEN and LIN [1986], HANNA, JOUVE and CIARLET [1990] and HANNA, JOUVE and WARING [1989]). The purpose of this chapter is to indicate how the previous hyperelastic numerical models can be modified in order to take viscoelasticity into account. The difficulty is to stay consistent with the second law of thermodynamics, to preserve incompressibility, and to obtain a well-posed three-dimensional model which stays close to the initial hyperelastic model.

This chapter is based on a recent paper of LE TALLEC, RAHIER and KAISS [1993]. It first introduces a rheological and thermodynamical model of the viscoelastic behavior of incompressible solids in large deformations (Sections 36 and 37). There are two classes of possible models: those of integral type (LOCKETT [1972], CHRISTENSEN [1980], SALENÇON [1983]), which express the viscoelastic stress as an integral in time of a function of the deformation field, and those of differential type (LUBLINER [1985], SIDOROFF [1974], SIMO [1987]). We will concentrate on this latter class which introduces an additional internal variable governed by a differential equation in time.

Combining such thermodynamical models with the equations of static equilibrium, we obtain a mathematical formulation of equilibrium problems in large strains viscoelasticity (Section 38). The resulting problem is now time-dependent: with respect to the internal variable, it is a first-order evolution equation in time with constraints. The equation in time is the constitutive relation associated with the internal variable, the constraints are the equilibrium equations and the incompressibility condition which must be satisfied at all times. Two forms of this constrained evolution problem are interesting in practice: Cauchy problems where a given initial distribution of internal variables is given and which model situations involving creeping or relaxation, and problems periodic in time which model vibration problems with internal damping. Both forms will be considered, approximated in space by finite-element techniques (Section 39), in time by an implicit Euler scheme (Section 40), and their linearized version will be completely analyzed. After discretization, the viscoelastic variable can be eliminated, reducing each discrete problem to a standard hyper-

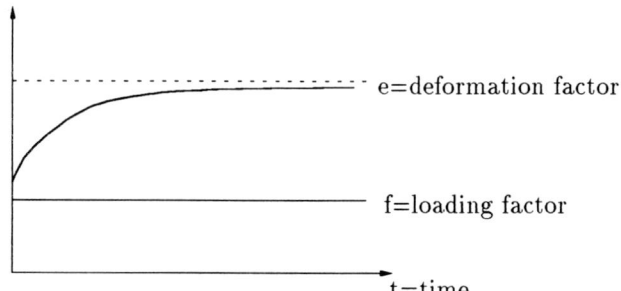

FIG. 36.1. Step loading. History of the loading and of the deformation of a viscoelastic material during a creep test.

elastic problem which can be easily solved numerically by the Newton's method already introduced in finite elasticity (Section 41).

36. The rheological model

Let us consider a step loading, that is a loading where the external forces jump instantaneously from zero to their final values. When a viscoelastic material is subjected to such a step loading (Fig. 36.1), one observes two different types of response: there is first an instantaneous reaction and then the material progressively reaches a long-term equilibrium state in large strains.

The first problem therefore consists in finding a rheological model which can handle this type of behavior. Such a model is classically obtained by combining springs and dapshots as described below (Fig. 36.2).

Here, $(k + K)$ measures the instantaneous elastic stiffness, K represents the long-term elastic stiffness,

$$\tau = \frac{\nu}{K}\left(1 + \frac{k}{K}\right)$$

is a characteristic relaxation time which indicates how long it takes for the material to reach its long-term equilibrium state. More precisely, after integration of the constitutive laws of Fig. 36.2, the response of the above model to a step loading is given by

$$e(t) = e_\mathrm{e} + e_\mathrm{v} = \frac{f}{K}\left[1 + \left(\frac{K}{K+k} - 1\right)\mathrm{e}^{-t/\tau}\right]. \tag{36.1}$$

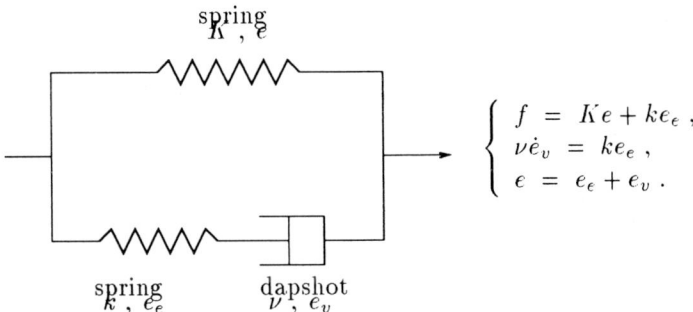

FIG. 36.2. Rheological model. The viscoelastic material is supposed to react as this combination of springs and dapshots.

37. Thermodynamical model

The next step is to generalize this simple model to general three-dimensional situations involving isochoric large deformations. To do that, we use the framework of the theory of standard materials, which is of very general use and which automatically respects the second law of thermodynamics. In viscoelasticity, this theory introduces (MANDEL [1978], SIDOROFF [1974]) internal state variables, a specific free energy W, and a dissipation function ϕ.

(i) By analogy with the rheological model, we choose as internal variables
- the right Cauchy–Green tensor measuring the total deformation of the body and given by

$$C = F^T F \qquad (37.1)$$

with $F = \text{Id} + \nabla u$ the deformation gradient;
- the viscous strain tensor C_v measuring the deformation of a fictitious dapshot embedded in the material.

We also need to introduce the elastic strain tensor of the viscous branch. If we were allowed to formally decompose the deformation at microscopic level into

$$\varphi = \varphi_e \circ \varphi_v,$$

the deformation gradient F and right Cauchy–Green strain tensor C would be given by

$$F = \frac{\partial \varphi}{\partial x} = \frac{\partial \varphi_e}{\partial \varphi_v} \cdot \frac{\partial \varphi_v}{\partial x} = F_e F_v,$$
$$C = F^T F = F_v^T C_e F_v.$$

Putting all rotation effects in the map φ_e, we would have from the polar decomposition theorem

$$F_v = \sqrt{C_v},$$
$$C = \sqrt{C_v} C_e \sqrt{C_v}.$$

To be consistent with these formal results, we *define* the elastic deformation of the viscous branch by

$$C_e = \sqrt{C_v^{-1}} C \sqrt{C_v^{-1}}. \tag{37.2}$$

This multiplicative splitting is the natural generalization of the additive splitting introduced in small strains (SIMO [1988])

$$e = e_e + e_v, \tag{37.3}$$

and indeed reduces to (37.3) by linearization around the reference configuration. Above, e_e stands for the elastic part of the deformation and e_v stands for its viscous part.

If we assume in addition that the considered material is incompressible in its elastic and in its viscoelastic evolution, then these internal variables are also constrained by the incompressibility conditions

$$\det F = \det F_v = 1. \tag{37.4}$$

(ii) Still by analogy with the rheological model, we propose a free energy potential of the form

$$\tilde{W}(C, C_v) = \tilde{W}_0(C) + \tilde{W}_e(C_e). \tag{37.5}$$

Above, $\tilde{W}_0(C)$ measures the stored energy of the elastic branch, that is the stored energy associated to the long term behavior of the material. This is the energy which is usually taken into account in the existing hyperelastic models. The other component $\tilde{W}_e$ measures the stored energy of the viscous branch which disappears progressively during relaxation. This part of the energy must be identified by specific experiments such as dynamic shear loading or relaxation tests.

(iii) Finally, we introduce a dissipation function $\phi(\dot{C}_v)$, which acts as a generalized friction force and which predicts the energy dissipated in a given variation dC_v of the fictitious dapshot via the formula

$$\text{dissipated energy} = \phi(\dot{C}_v) : dC_v. \tag{37.6}$$

The second law of thermodynamics then takes the form

$$\phi(\dot{C}_v) : \dot{C}_v \geq 0 \quad \forall \dot{C}_v. \tag{37.7}$$

It is automatically satisfied for suitable choices of ϕ, such as for example

$$\phi(\dot{C}_v) = -\nu \dot{C}_v^{-1}. \tag{37.8}$$

Indeed, introducing the viscous deformation rate tensor

$$D_v = (\dot{F}_v F_v^{-1})_{\text{sym}} = \sqrt{C_v^{-1}} \dot{C}_v \sqrt{C_v^{-1}},$$

we will have, as for any Newtonian fluid,

$$\phi(\dot{C}_v) : \dot{C}_v = \nu D_v : D_v \geqslant 0.$$

The choice (37.8) is very interesting in practice because it fits well to experiments, because its parameter ν is easily identified and because it leads to very simple constitutive laws (WEBER [1975]).

In this thermodynamical framework (37.1)–(37.7), the viscoelastic constitutive laws are simply obtained by imposing that the energy dissipated in any mechanical evolution of the material is equal to the postulated value $\phi(\dot{C}_v) : \mathrm{d}C_v$. In other words, we must have

$$\tfrac{1}{2}\tilde{\Sigma} : \mathrm{d}C - \mathrm{d}\tilde{W} = \phi(\dot{C}_v) : \mathrm{d}C_v, \tag{37.9}$$

for any $\mathrm{d}C$ and $\mathrm{d}C_v$ satisfying the incompressibility relations

$$\det(C) = \det(C + \mathrm{d}C) = \det(C_v) = \det(C_v + \mathrm{d}C_v) = 1.$$

Introducing the Lagrange multipliers p and q associated with these constraints, (37.9) takes the equivalent form

$$\begin{cases} \tilde{\Sigma} = 2\dfrac{\partial \tilde{W}(C, C_v)}{\partial C} - pC^{-1}, \\[2mm] \phi(\dot{C}_v) = -\dfrac{\partial \tilde{W}(C, C_v)}{\partial C_v} + qC_v^{-1}, \\[2mm] \det(C) = 1, \\[2mm] \det(C_v) = 1. \end{cases} \tag{37.10}$$

The above equations are our desired viscoelastic constitutive laws. The first equation is a standard hyperelastic constitutive law relating as in Section 4 the second Piola–Kirchhoff stress tensor $\tilde{\Sigma} = F^{-1}T$ to the right Cauchy–Green strain tensor, with C_v acting as a constitutive parameter. The second equation is a first-order differential equation in time and introduces (via the variable C_v) a time-dependence in this model. In the general case dealing with heterogeneous incompressible materials, the free energy potential $\tilde{W}(x, C, C_v)$ depends on the particle x as well as on the strain tensor C or C_v.

REMARK 37.1. The above constitutive laws (37.10) are intrinsic since they are written independently of any choice of basis in the Euclidian space $\mathbb{E}$. Moreover, they are frame-indifferent. Indeed, they are written in a fixed Lagrangian framework and the tensors C or C_v and functions $\tilde{W}$ or ϕ which are defined on this configuration are defined independently of any observer in the deformed configuration.

REMARK 37.2. By construction of ϕ, the second law of thermodynamics is automatically satisfied as soon as ϕ satisfies (37.7).

REMARK 37.3. Memory effects are present in the equation in C_v which introduces a certain inertia in the evolution of the considered material. Modeling such effects is the purpose of viscoelasticity. These effects could also be modeled by integral constitutive laws such as

$$\tilde{\Sigma}(t) = 2\frac{\partial \tilde{W}_0}{\partial C} - pC^{-1} + \int_{-\infty}^{t} m(t-s)\phi(C(s))\,ds.$$

These laws usually lead to different mathematical models, but these models can be solved by the same numerical techniques through the identification

$$C_v = \int_{-\infty}^{t} m(t-s)\phi(C(s))\,ds.$$

REMARK 37.4. If we no longer assume elastic incompressibility, the constraint $\det(C) = 1$ must be dropped from (37.10). The variation of C can then be arbitrary and the first line of (37.10) becomes

$$\tilde{\Sigma} = 2\frac{\partial \tilde{W}}{\partial C}(x, C, C_v).$$

38. Mathematical formulation

38.1. The complete nonlinear model

By writing the weak form of the equilibrium equations (3.1) (in a fixed reference configuration Ω, with $\partial\Omega = \Gamma_0 \cup \Gamma_1$) together with the above constitutive laws, we obtain

$$\begin{cases} \int_\Omega T : \nabla v \, dx = \int_\Omega f \cdot v \, dx + \int_{\Gamma_1} g \cdot v \, da \quad \forall v : \Omega \to \mathbb{E}', \\ T = F\tilde{\Sigma} = F\left(2\frac{\partial \tilde{W}}{\partial C}(x, C, C_v) - pC^{-1}\right), \\ \frac{\partial \tilde{W}}{\partial C_v}(x, C, C_v) + \phi(\dot{C}_v) - qC_v^{-1} = 0, \\ \det F = 1, \\ \det(C_v) = 1. \end{cases} \quad (38.1)$$

By elimination of the stress tensor T, by introducing the new variable $A = C_v^{-1}$ and by multiplying the differential equation on both sides by C_v, we obtain the final variational formulation

$$\int_\Omega F(2\frac{\partial \tilde{W}}{\partial C}(x,C,A) - pC^{-1}) : \nabla v \, dx$$

$$= \int_\Omega f \cdot v \, dx + \int_{\Gamma_1} g \cdot v \, da \quad \forall v \in \mathbb{V}, \tag{38.2}$$

$$\int_\Omega \hat{p}(\det F - 1) \, dx = 0 \quad \forall \hat{p} \in \mathbb{P}, \tag{38.3}$$

$$-\frac{\partial \tilde{W}}{\partial A}(x,C,A) + \nu A^{-1} - qA^{-1} = 0 \quad \forall x \in \Omega, \tag{38.4}$$

$$\det(A) = 1. \tag{38.5}$$

Above, the spaces $\mathbb{V}$ and $\mathbb{P}$ are as defined in Section 7, that is

$$\mathbb{V} = \{v \in W^{1,s}(\Omega; \mathbb{E}),\ v|_{\Gamma_0} = 0\},$$

$$\mathbb{P} = L^{s^*}(\Omega; \mathbb{R}), \quad \frac{1}{3s} + \frac{1}{s^*} = 1.$$

The unknowns are the displacement field $u(\cdot, t)$ in $(\mathbb{V} + u_0)$ and the internal variable $A = C_v^{-1}(x,t)$ at any positive time and at each point of the material. The above formulation uses the special form of dissipation that we have selected, namely

$$\phi(\dot{C}_v) = -\nu \dot{C}_v^{-1}.$$

Moreover, since (38.4) is a first-order differential equation in time, this formulation must be completed by an initial condition on the viscoelastic variable A. In practice, we are interested either by Cauchy problems

$$A(\cdot, t_0) = \text{given value}$$

or by periodic solutions in time

$$A(\cdot, t) = A(\cdot, t + \tau).$$

REMARK 38.1. For elastically compressible materials (including nearly incompressible materials), the incompressibility constraint

$$\int_\Omega \hat{p}(\det F - 1) \, dx = 0$$

and the Lagrange multiplier p disappear from (38.2)–(38.5).

38.2. Choosing the free energy potential

A simple but basic construction of the free energy potential proceeds by choosing three smooth functions $\tilde{W}_1$, $\tilde{W}_2$ and $\tilde{W}_0$ satisfying (38.7) below and by setting

$$\begin{cases} \tilde{W}(x,C,A) = \tilde{W}_0(x,E) + \tilde{W}_e(x,C_e), \\ \tilde{W}_e(x,C_e) = \tilde{W}_1(x, \operatorname{tr} C_e) + \tilde{W}_2(x, \det C_e). \end{cases} \tag{38.6}$$

Here, we use our previous notation

$E = \frac{1}{2}(C - \text{Id})$ = Green–Lagrange strain tensor,

$C_e = \sqrt{C_v^{-1}} C \sqrt{C_v^{-1}} = \sqrt{A} C \sqrt{A}.$

Easy algebraic manipulations then yield (since $\det A = 1$)

$\text{tr } C_e = A : C,$

$\det C_e = \det C,$

$\frac{\partial \tilde{W}}{\partial C}(x, C, A) = \frac{\partial \tilde{W}_1}{\partial y}(x, A : C)A + \frac{\partial \tilde{W}_2}{\partial y}(x, \det C)\text{cof } C + \frac{1}{2}\frac{\partial \tilde{W}_0}{\partial E}(x, E),$

$\frac{\partial \tilde{W}}{\partial A}(x, C, A) = \frac{\partial \tilde{W}_1}{\partial y}(x, A : C)C.$

The functions $\tilde{W}_i(x, \cdot)$ are generally such that the stress tensor $\tilde{\Sigma}$ is zero in the elastic and in the viscoelastic branch when $E = 0$ and $C_e = \text{Id}$. In other words, we must have

$$\frac{\partial \tilde{W}_0}{\partial E}(x, 0) = 0, \quad \frac{\partial \tilde{W}_1}{\partial y}(x, 3) + \frac{\partial \tilde{W}_2}{\partial y}(x, 1) = 0. \tag{38.7}$$

Moreover, the function $\tilde{W}_0$ measures the stored energy of the elastic branch. The best choice is here to use existing hyperelastic potentials such as (CIARLET [1988]) the quadratic Saint-Venant–Kirchhoff potential given by

$$\tilde{W}_0(E) = \frac{\lambda}{2}(\text{tr } E)^2 + \mu E : E, \tag{38.8}$$

where λ and μ are the usual Lamé constants, the isotropic Mooney–Rivlin potential given as a function of the invariants of C by

$$\tilde{W}(E) = aI_1(C) + bI_2(C) + cI_3(C) - (a + 2b + c)\text{Log}(I_3(C)), \tag{38.9}$$

or transversally isotropic quadratic potentials involving five elasticity coefficients.

All these choices of $\tilde{W}_0$ can be used both for compressible and for incompressible materials.

38.3. Linearization

Let us consider a nonlinear compressible isotropic model with $\tilde{W}$ given by (38.6) and satisfying (see Section 4 and (38.7))

$$\begin{cases} \frac{\partial \tilde{W}_0}{\partial E} = \lambda(\text{tr } E)\,\text{Id} + 2\mu E + O(\|E\|^2), \\ \frac{\partial \tilde{W}_1}{\partial y}(\cdot, 3) = -\frac{\partial \tilde{W}_2}{\partial y}(\cdot, 1) = k_1, \\ \frac{\partial^2 \tilde{W}_1}{\partial y^2}(\cdot, 3) = k_2, \\ \frac{\partial^2 \tilde{W}_2}{\partial y^2}(\cdot, 1) = k_3. \end{cases} \tag{38.10}$$

Extension to viscoelasticity

We wish to linearize the constitutive law (37.10) around the reference state $E = 0$ and $A = \mathrm{Id}$. For this purpose, we introduce the notation

$$e = \frac{\partial E}{\partial u}(0) \cdot v = \tfrac{1}{2}(\nabla v + \nabla v^{\mathrm{T}}) = \text{linearized strain tensor}, \tag{38.11}$$

$$e_{\mathrm{v}} = \tfrac{1}{2}(\mathrm{Id} - A) = \text{viscoelastic strain tensor}. \tag{38.12}$$

Assuming e_{v} and E to be small, we obtain at a first order approximation

$$E = e, \tag{38.13}$$

$$A^{-1} = \mathrm{Id} + 2e_{\mathrm{v}}. \tag{38.14}$$

If we replace in (37.10) E and A^{-1} by these approximate values, if we linearize around the reference state, and if we take (38.7) into account, we get at first order

$$\begin{aligned}\tilde{\Sigma} &= 2k_1(-2e_{\mathrm{v}}) - 2k_1((2\operatorname{tr} e)\,\mathrm{Id} - 2e)\\ &\quad + 4k_2(\operatorname{tr} e - \operatorname{tr} e_{\mathrm{v}})\,\mathrm{Id} + 4k_3(\operatorname{tr} e)\,\mathrm{Id}\\ &\quad + \lambda(\operatorname{tr} e)\,\mathrm{Id} + 2\mu e,\end{aligned} \tag{38.15}$$

$$2v\dot{e}_{\mathrm{v}} = k_1(\mathrm{Id} + 2e) + 2k_2(\operatorname{tr} e - \operatorname{tr} e_{\mathrm{v}})\,\mathrm{Id} + q(\mathrm{Id} + 2e_{\mathrm{v}}), \tag{38.16}$$

$$\operatorname{tr} e_{\mathrm{v}} = 0. \tag{38.17}$$

Then, by taking the trace of (38.16), we obtain

$$q = -k_1(1 + \tfrac{2}{3}\operatorname{tr} e) - 2k_2 \operatorname{tr}(e - e_{\mathrm{v}}). \tag{38.18}$$

If we replace q by this value, if we neglect the second-order term $e_{\mathrm{v}} \operatorname{tr} e$, we can then rewrite the linearized constitutive laws (38.15)–(38.17) in the final form

$$\begin{aligned}\tilde{\Sigma} &= T = \tilde{\lambda}(\operatorname{tr} e)\,\mathrm{Id} + 2\mu e + 4k_1(e - e_{\mathrm{v}}),\\ v\dot{e}_{\mathrm{v}} &= k_1(e_{\mathrm{D}} - e_{\mathrm{v}}),\\ \operatorname{tr} e_{\mathrm{v}} &= 0,\end{aligned} \tag{38.19}$$

with

$$e_{\mathrm{D}} = e - \tfrac{1}{3}(\operatorname{tr} e)\,\mathrm{Id} \tag{38.20}$$

the deviatoric part of e. We recognize in (38.19) the usual Kelvin linear viscoelastic law.

REMARK 38.2. For an incompressible material, (38.10) is replaced by

$$\tilde{\Sigma} = 2\mu E + 2\frac{\partial \tilde{W}_1}{\partial y}(x, A : C)A + 2\frac{\partial \tilde{W}_2}{\partial y}(x, \det C)\operatorname{cof} C - pC^{-1} + O(\|E\|^2),$$

$$\det C = 1 + 2\operatorname{tr} E + O(\|E\|^2) = 1.$$

Once linearized, the corresponding constitutive laws reduce to

$$\begin{cases}\tilde{\Sigma} = 2\mu e + 4k_1(e - e_{\mathrm{v}}) - p\,\mathrm{Id},\\ v\dot{e}_{\mathrm{v}} = k_1(e - e_{\mathrm{v}}),\\ \operatorname{tr} e = \operatorname{tr} e_{\mathrm{v}} = 0.\end{cases} \tag{38.21}$$

39. Approximation in space

39.1. Galerkin approximation

In addition to the finite-element spaces $\mathbb{V}_h$ and $\mathbb{P}_h$ already introduced in the elastic case (Section 12), the approximation of the viscoelastic problem (38.2)–(38.5) requires the introduction of an additional space Σ_h for computing the viscoelastic internal variable A. The simplest choice uses piecewise constant functions belonging to the space

$$\Sigma_h = \{H: \Omega \to (\mathbb{M}^3)_{\text{sym}}, H|_{C_i} = \text{constant}\}$$

with $(C_i)_{i \in I}$ a given partition of Ω. A natural way of defining this partition is to associate a cell C_{jl} with every integration point x_j^l of a given quadrature rule

$$\int_{\Omega_l} f(x)\,dx \simeq \sum_{j=1}^{NG} \omega_j f(x_j^l)$$

defined on each finite-element Ω_l.

We also need a space $\mathbb{Q}_h$ where to compute the viscoelastic Lagrange multiplier q. With the above choice of Σ_h, we take

$$\mathbb{Q}_h = \{q_h: \Omega \to \mathbb{R}, q_h|_{C_i} = \text{constant}\}.$$

Once $\mathbb{V}_h$, $\mathbb{P}_h$ and Σ_h are defined, the variational problem (38.2) is approximated as before by replacing the spaces $\mathbb{V}$ and $\mathbb{P}$ by $\mathbb{V}_h$ and $\mathbb{P}_h$ and by restricting the differential equation to the dual of Σ_h. Hence, the discrete problem is:

Find $(u_h(t), p_h(t), A_h(t), q_h(t)) \in \mathbb{V}_h \times \mathbb{P}_h \times \Sigma_h \times \mathbb{Q}_h$ verifying at each time t the following variational system:

$$\int_\Omega F_h \left(2 \frac{\partial \tilde{W}}{\partial C} - p_h C_h^{-1}\right) : \nabla v_h \, dx$$

$$= \int_\Omega f \cdot v_h \, dx + \int_{\Gamma_1} g \cdot v_h \, da \quad \forall v_h \in \mathbb{P}_h,$$

$$\int_\Omega \hat{p}_h (\det F_h - 1)\, dx = 0, \forall \hat{p}_h \in \mathbb{P}_h, \qquad (39.1)$$

$$\int_\Omega \left(-\frac{\partial \tilde{W}}{\partial A} + \nu \dot{A}_h^{-1} - q_h A_h^{-1}\right) : H_h \, dx = 0 \quad \forall H_h \in \Sigma_h,$$

$$\int_\Omega \hat{q}_h (\det A_h - 1)\, dx = 0 \quad \forall \hat{q}_h \in \mathbb{Q}_h.$$

REMARK 39.1. When H_h and $\hat{q}_h$ are defined as piecewise constants, the last equations of (39.1) take the simpler form

$$-\frac{1}{\operatorname{meas} C_i} \int_{C_i} \frac{\partial \tilde{W}}{\partial A} \, dx + \nu \dot{A}_h^{-1}|_{C_i} - q_h|_{C_i} A_h^{-1}|_{C_i} = 0 \quad \forall i,$$

$$\det A_h|_{C_i} = 1 \quad \forall i.$$

39.2. Linearized problems

Before solving (39.1), we need to know under what conditions on the spaces $\mathbb{V}_h$, $\mathbb{P}_h$ and Σ_h it will be well-posed. We can guess that $\mathbb{V}_h$ and $\mathbb{P}_h$ will be subjected to the restrictions already encountered in elasticity (Section 14). But what about Σ_h? Because of the complexity of (39.1), a general answer is out of reach. We do not even know in general if u_h and p_h are continuous functions of the viscoelastic variable A_h. Nevertheless, a practical answer can be obtained by looking at the linearized model derived in Section 38. Indeed, using the linearized law (38.21) in the variational problem (38.2)–(38.5) and in its discrete counterpart (39.1) and using the symmetry of $e(u)$ and e_v, we obtain the following continuous and discrete linear systems, to be satisfied at each time t:

$$\begin{cases} \int_\Omega \{2\mu e(u) + 4k_1(e(u) - e_v) - p \operatorname{Id}\} : e(v) \, dx \\ \quad = \int_\Omega f \cdot v \, dx + \int_{\Gamma_1} g \cdot v \, dx \quad \forall v \in \mathbb{V}, \ (u(t) - u_0) \in \mathbb{V}, \\ \int_\Omega \hat{p} \operatorname{tr} e(u) \, dx = \int_\Omega \hat{p} \operatorname{div} u \, dx = 0 \quad \forall \hat{p} \in \mathbb{P}, \ p(t) \in \mathbb{P}, \\ \nu \dot{e}_v + k_1(e_v - e(u)) = 0 \quad \forall x, \\ \operatorname{tr} e_v = 0, \end{cases} \quad (39.2)$$

$$\begin{cases} \int_\Omega \{2\mu e(u_h) + 4k_1(e(u_h) - e_v h) - p_h \operatorname{Id}\} : e(v_h) \, dx \\ \quad = \int_\Omega f \cdot v_h \, dx + \int_{\Gamma_1} g \cdot v_h \, dx \quad \forall v \in \mathbb{V}_h, \ (u_h(t) - u_0) \in \mathbb{V}_h, \\ \int_\Omega \hat{p}_h \operatorname{div} u_h \, dx = 0 \quad \forall \hat{p}_h \in \mathbb{P}_h, \ p_h(t) \in \mathbb{P}_h, \\ \int_\Omega (\nu \dot{e}_{vh} + k_1(e_{vh} - e(u_h)) - q_h \operatorname{Id}) : H_h \, dx = 0 \\ \quad \forall H_h \in \Sigma_h, \ e_{vh}(t) \in \Sigma_h, \\ \int_\Omega \hat{q}_h \operatorname{tr} e_{vh} \, dx = 0 \quad \forall \hat{q}_h \in \mathbb{Q}_h, \ q_h(t) \in \mathbb{Q}_h. \end{cases} \quad (39.3)$$

39.3. Transformation of the linearized problems

The above linearized problems can be reduced to standard first-order ordinary differential equations with unknown $e_v(t)$. For this purpose we introduce the solution $z(t)$ and $u(\varepsilon)$ of the following linear Stokes problems:

$$\begin{cases} \int_\Omega \left((2\mu + 4k_1)e(z) - p_z \operatorname{Id} \right) : e(v) \, dx \\ \quad = \int_\Omega f(t) \cdot v \, dx + \int_{\Gamma_1} g(t) \cdot v \, dx \quad \forall v \in \mathbb{V}, \ (z(t) - u_0) \in \mathbb{V}, \\ \int_\Omega \hat{p} \operatorname{div} z \, dx = 0 \quad \forall \hat{p} \in \mathbb{P}, \ p_z \in \mathbb{P}, \end{cases} \quad (39.4)$$

$$\begin{cases} \int_\Omega [(2\mu + 4k_1)e(u(\varepsilon)) - p_\varepsilon \operatorname{Id}] : e(v) \, dx = \int_\Omega 4k_1 \varepsilon : e(v) \, dx, \\ \quad \forall v \in \mathbb{V}, \ u(\varepsilon) \in \mathbb{V}, \\ \int_\Omega \hat{p} \operatorname{div}(u(\varepsilon)) \, dx = 0 \quad \forall \hat{p} \in \mathbb{P}, p_\varepsilon \in \mathbb{P}. \end{cases} \quad (39.5)$$

We then define their discrete equivalent $z_h(t)$ in $(\mathbb{V}_h + u_0)$ and $u_h(\varepsilon) \in \mathbb{V}_h$ by solving the finite-element versions of the above variational problems.

We also introduce the reduced spaces

$$\mathbb{V}_{hD} = \{ v_h \in \mathbb{V}_h, \int_\Omega \hat{p}_h \operatorname{div} v_h \, dx = 0, \forall \hat{p}_h \in \mathbb{P}_h \}, \quad (39.6)$$

$$\mathbb{M}_D^3 = \{ H \in (\mathbb{M}^3)_{\text{sym}}, \operatorname{tr} H = 0 \}, \quad (39.7)$$

$$\Sigma_{hD} = \{ H_h \in \Sigma_h, \int_\Omega \hat{q}_h \operatorname{tr} H_h \, dx = 0, \forall \hat{q}_h \in \mathbb{Q}_h \}. \quad (39.8)$$

The L^2 projection on Σ_{hD} will be denoted by Π_Σ. With the above notation, we easily observe that the first lines of (39.2) are equivalent to the relation $u = u(e_v) + z$, and that therefore the linearized problem (39.2) reduces to

$$\nu \dot{e}_v + k_1[e_v - e(u(e_v) + z)] = 0 \text{ in } L^2(\Omega, \mathbb{M}_D^3).$$

Under the additional notation

$$F(e_v) = k_1[e_v - e(u(e_v))], \quad (39.9)$$

this problem takes the final form

$$\nu \dot{e}_v + F(e_v) = k_1 e(z) \text{ in } L^2(\Omega, \mathbb{M}_D^3). \quad (39.10)$$

For the discrete problem, we have in a similar fashion $u_h = u_h(e_{vh}) + z_h(t)$ and here the discrete linearized problem (39.3) reduces to

$$\begin{cases} \Pi_\Sigma \left(\nu \dot{e}_{vh} + k_1(e_{vh} - e(u_h(e_{vh})) + z_h) \right) = 0, \\ e_{vh} \in \Sigma_{hD}. \end{cases}$$

If we assume in addition that the multiplication by ν or k_1 sends Σ_{hD} into itself, the projection Π_Σ and the multiplication by ν or by k_1 commute. Therefore, the above problem takes the final form

$$\nu \dot{e}_{vh} + F_h(e_{vh}) = k_1 \Pi_\Sigma(e(z_h)) \text{ in } \Sigma_{hD}, \tag{39.11}$$

with the notation

$$F_h(e_{vh}) = k_1 \left[e_{vh} - \Pi_\Sigma(e(u_h(e_{vh}))) \right]. \tag{39.12}$$

REMARK 39.2. Above, ν, k_1 and μ were defined as real numbers. But in fact they can be defined more generally as fourth-order tensors. In the analysis to come, we will treat them as general fourth-order tensors $\nu(x), k_1(x)$ and $\mu(x)$ defined on $\mathbb{E}$.

39.4. Main result

In the following, the space $C_\tau^q(X)$ denotes the space of functions of time, with values in X which are τ periodic and of class $\mathscr{C}^q$, that is

$$C_\tau^q(X) = \{ v \in \mathscr{C}^q(\mathbb{R}; X), v(t + \tau) = v(t), \forall t \}.$$

This space is endowed with the standard norm

$$\|v\|_{q,\tau,X} = \sup_{i \leqslant q} \sup_t \|v^{(i)}(t)\|_X.$$

We also introduce the space

$$Y = H^{-1}(\Omega; \mathbb{E}) \times H^{-1/2}(\Gamma_1; \mathbb{E}) \times H^{1/2}(\Gamma_0, \mathbb{E})$$

which will be the space for the external loads $\{f; g\}$ and for the imposed displacement u_0. In addition, a uniformly elliptic tensor will denote a tensor field $k(x)$ of symmetric fourth-order tensors defined on $\mathbb{E}$ such that there exist real numbers $|k|$ and α_k with

$$\begin{cases} (k(x) : C) : C \geqslant \alpha_k \|C\|^2 \quad \forall C \in \mathbb{M}^3, \\ (k(x) : C) : H \leqslant |k| \cdot \|C\| \cdot \|H\| \quad \forall C \text{ and } H \in \mathbb{M}^3. \end{cases} \tag{39.13}$$

Finally, the solution interpolation error denotes the quantity

$$i_{h,q}(t) = \|(\Pi_\Sigma e_v - e_v)^{(q)}(t)\|_{0,2} + \|(\Pi_\Sigma e(u) - e(u))^{(q)}(t)\|_{0,2}$$
$$+ \inf_{w_h \in V_h} \|z^{(q)}(t) - w_h\|_{1,2} + \inf_{w_h \in V_h} \|u^{(q)}(e_v)(t) - w_h\|_{1,2}$$
$$+ \inf_{q_h \in \mathbb{P}_h} \|p_z^{(q)}(t) - q_h\|_{0,2} + \inf_{q_h \in \mathbb{P}_h} \|p_\varepsilon^{(q)}(t) - q_h\|_{0,2},$$

with e_v the solution of the continuous problem (39.10) and z and $u(e_v)$ the solutions of the auxiliary problems (39.4) and (39.5). We then have the following convergence theorem which is proved at the end of this section.

THEOREM 39.1. *Assume that $\mathbb{P}_h$ and $\mathbb{V}_h$ satisfy the classical* inf-sup *condition*

$$\inf_{p_h \in \mathbb{P}_h} \sup_{w_h \in \mathbb{V}_h} \int_\Omega p_h \, \text{div} \, w_h \, dx \geq \beta \|p_h\|_{0,2} \|w_h\|_{1,2}$$

with $\beta > 0$ independent of h. Assume that k_1, ν and μ are uniformly elliptic tensors and that k_1 and ν send Σ_{hD} into itself. Then, for (f, g, u_0) in $L^2(0, T; Y)$, the Cauchy problems defined by the system (39.2) and by the initial data $e_v(\cdot, 0)$ in $L^2(\Omega; \mathbb{M}_D^3)$ (resp. by (39.3) and by $e_{vh}(\cdot, 0)$ in Σ_{hD}) have unique solutions (u, p, e_v) (resp. (u_h, p_h, e_{vh})) which satisfy

$$\|(u - u_h)(t)\|_{1,2} + \|(p - p_h)(t)\|_{0,2} + \|(e_v - e_{vh})(t)\|_{0,2}$$
$$\leq i_{h,0}(t) + i_{h,0}(0) \exp(-\alpha t) + C \int_0^t i_{h,0}(s) \exp[-\alpha(t-s)] \, ds.$$

Similarly, for (f, g, u_0) in $C_\tau^q(Y)$, the continuous and the discrete problems (39.2) and (39.3) have unique periodic solutions (u, p, e_v) and (u_h, p_h, e_{vh}) which belong to the spaces $C_\tau^q(\mathbb{V}) \times C_\tau^q(\mathbb{P}) \times C_\tau^{q+1}(L^2(\Omega; \mathbb{M}_D^3))$ and $C_\tau^q(\mathbb{V}_h) \times C_\tau^q(\mathbb{P}_h) \times C_\tau^{q+1}(\Sigma_{hD})$, respectively and which satisfy

$$\|u^{(q)} - u_h^{(q)}\|_{0,\tau,V} + \|p^{(q)} - p_h^{(q)}\|_{0,\tau,L^2} + \|e_v^{(q)} - e_{vh}^{(q)}\|_{1,\tau,L^2} \leq C \|i_{h,q}\|_{0,\tau}.$$

This theorem does not require any compatibility between Σ_h and the other finite-element spaces. This means that the space Σ_h of viscoelastic internal variables can be chosen independently of the spaces $\mathbb{V}_h$ and $\mathbb{P}_h$ of discrete displacements and pressures, at least for the incompressible Kelvin linear model. The only restriction is that Σ_{hD} must be stable by multiplication by k_1 or ν and must be such that

$$\lim_{h \to 0} \sup_{H \in L^2(\Omega; \mathbb{M}^3)} \|H - \Pi_\Sigma H\|_{0,2} = 0.$$

Such restrictions are easy to satisfy. In particular, any space of piecewise constants can be chosen, provided that k_1 and ν are also piecewise constant.

REMARK 39.3. The above result is not true in the limiting case of a Maxwell material with $\alpha_\mu = 0$. In this case, as proved in LE TALLEC [1990], convergence can only be achieved if we satisfy the additional inf-sup condition

$$\inf_{w_h \in \mathbb{V}_h} \sup_{H_h \in \Sigma_h} \frac{\int_\Omega H_h : e(v_h) \, dx}{\|H_h\|_{0,2} \|v_h\|_{1,2}} \geq \beta > 0.$$

39.5. Technical theorems

Before proving the convergence theorem, we introduce three technical theorems, to be proved under the same assumptions as above.

THEOREM 39.2. *The operators F and F_h introduced in (39.9) and (39.12) are well-defined, linear, continuous and elliptic with an ellipticity constant which only depends on the tensors k_1, ν and μ.*

PROOF. (i) *Continuity.* Since k_1 and μ are uniformly elliptic, we have by Korn's inequality

$$a(v,v) := \int_\Omega [(4k_1 + 2\mu) : e(v)] : e(v) \, dx$$

$$\geq (4\alpha_k + 2\alpha_\mu) \int_\Omega \|e(v)\|^2 \, dx$$

$$\geq C_0(4\alpha_k + 2\alpha_\mu)\|v\|_{1,2}^2 \quad \forall v \in \mathbb{V}.$$

Since $a(\cdot, \cdot)$ is also continuous, the Lax–Milgram lemma then implies that a is invertible on any closed subspace of $\mathbb{V}$, with $\|a^{-1}\|$ bounded independently of the subspace. Moreover, the bilinear form

$$b(p,v) := \int_\Omega p \operatorname{div} v \, dx$$

satisfies the inf-sup condition (uniformly in h) both at the continuous level (div is onto from $H_0^1(\Omega; \mathbb{E})$ into $L^2(\Omega)/\mathbb{R}$) and at the discrete level (by assumption). Therefore, by the Ladyzenskaya–Babuska–Brezzi theorem (Section 14), problem (39.5) and its finite-element counterpart have unique solutions $(u, p)(\varepsilon)$ and $(u_h, p_h)(\varepsilon)$ depending linearly on the right-hand side

$$L_v(w) := \int_\Omega [4k_1 : \varepsilon] : e(w) \, dx$$

and such that

$$\|u(\varepsilon)\|_{1,2} \leq C\|L_v\|_{V'} \leq 4|k_1|C\|\varepsilon\|_{0,2},$$
$$\|u_h(\varepsilon)\|_{1,2} \leq C\|L_v\|_{V'_h} \leq 4|k_1|C\|\varepsilon\|_{0,2},$$

with C a constant independent of h. By composition, and since the projection Π_Σ is a linear contraction on L^2, the maps

$$F(e_v) := k_1 : (e_v - e(u(e_v)))$$
$$F_h(e_{vh}) := k_1 : (e_{vh} - \Pi_\Sigma [e(u(e_{vh}))])$$

are therefore linear continuous from $L^2(\Omega; \mathbb{M}_D^3)$ into itself and from Σ_{hD} into itself, respectively.

(ii) *Ellipticity*. In order to have a proof of ellipticity valid for both the continuous and the discrete case, we introduce the notation

$\mathbb{V}_{\text{div}} = \{v \in \mathbb{V},\ \text{div}\, v = 0\}$ in the continuous case,

$\phantom{\mathbb{V}_{\text{div}}} = \mathbb{V}_{hD}$ in the discrete case,

$\Sigma = L^2(\Omega; \mathbb{M}_D^3)$ in the continuous case,

$ = \Sigma_{hD}$ in the discrete case.

Moreover, we drop all subscripts h from the discrete variables and denote $u(e_v)$ by u_e. We also endow $L^2(\Omega; \mathbb{M}^3)$ with the scalar products

$$\langle C, H \rangle_k := \int_\Omega (k_1 : C) : H \, dx,$$

$$\langle C, H \rangle_\mu := \int_\Omega (\mu : C) : H \, dx.$$

From the uniform ellipticity of k_1 and μ, the associated norms satisfy

$$\|C\|_k^2 \leqslant |k_1| \|C\|_{0,2}^2 \leqslant \frac{|k_1|}{\alpha_\mu} \|C\|_\mu^2, \tag{39.14}$$

$$\|C\|_\mu^2 \leqslant |\mu| \|C\|_{0,2}^2 \leqslant \frac{|\mu|}{\alpha_k} \|C\|_k^2. \tag{39.15}$$

We use the scalar product $\langle \cdot, \cdot \rangle_k$ to decompose any element H of $L^2(\Omega; \mathbb{M}^3)$ into the orthogonal sum

$$H = \hat{H} + H^\perp,$$
$$\hat{H} = e(\hat{w}) \in e(\mathbb{V}_{\text{div}}),$$
$$H^\perp \in e(\mathbb{V}_{\text{div}})_k^\perp.$$

In particular, we have

$$e_v = e(\hat{w}) + e_v^\perp.$$

We can then write

$$\begin{aligned}
\langle F e_v, e_v \rangle &= \int_\Omega [k_1 : (e_v - e(u_e))] : e_v \, dx \\
&= \langle e_v - e(u_e), e_v \rangle_k \\
&= \langle e(\hat{w}) + e_v^\perp - e(u_e), e(\hat{w}) + e_v^\perp \rangle_k \\
&= \|e_v^\perp\|_k^2 + \langle e(\hat{w}) - e(u_e), e(\hat{w}) \rangle_k \\
&= \left(\|e_v^\perp\|_k^2 + \|e(\hat{w}) - e(u_e)\|_k^2 + \langle e(\hat{w}) - e(u_e), e(u_e) \rangle_k \right).
\end{aligned}$$

Moreover, writing (39.5) (or its discrete equivalent) with $w = u_e$, we get

$$\begin{aligned} 4\langle e(\hat{w}) - e(u_e), e(u_e)\rangle_k &= 4\langle e_v - e(u_e), e(u_e)\rangle_k \\ &= 2\langle e(u_e), e(u_e)\rangle_\mu \\ &= 2\|e(u_e)\|_\mu^2. \end{aligned} \qquad (39.16)$$

Writing then (39.5) (or its discrete equivalent) with $w = \hat{w}$, we also have

$$4\langle e(\hat{w}) - e(u_e), e(\hat{w})\rangle_k = 2\langle e(u_e), e(\hat{w})\rangle_\mu.$$

From the Cauchy–Schwarz inequality and (39.14)–(39.15), this implies

$$\|e(\hat{w})\|_k^2 \leqslant \|e(u_e)\|_k \|e(\hat{w})\|_k + \|e(u_e)\|_\mu \|e(\hat{w})\|_\mu / 2$$

$$\leqslant \left(\frac{|k_1|}{\alpha_\mu}\right)^{1/2} \|e(u_e)\|_\mu \|e(\hat{w})\|_k + \frac{1}{2}\left(\frac{|\mu|}{\alpha_k}\right)^{1/2} \|e(u_e)\|_\mu \|e(\hat{w})\|_k.$$

From this, we deduce

$$\|e(\hat{w})\|_k \leqslant \alpha \|e(u_e)\|_\mu \qquad (39.17)$$

with

$$\alpha = \left[\left(\frac{|k_1|}{\alpha_\mu}\right)^{1/2} + \frac{1}{2}\left(\frac{|\mu|}{\alpha_k}\right)^{1/2}\right].$$

Using (39.17) in (39.16), we then obtain

$$\langle e(\hat{w}) - e(u_e), e(u_e)\rangle_k \geqslant \tfrac{1}{2}\alpha^{-2}\|e(\hat{w})\|_k^2$$

which, combined with our previous calculation of $\langle F e_v, e_v\rangle$, implies

$$\begin{aligned} \langle F e_v, e_v\rangle &\geqslant \left[\|e_v^\perp\|_k^2 + \tfrac{1}{2}\alpha^{-2}\|e(\hat{w})\|_k^2\right] \\ &\geqslant \min\left(1, \tfrac{1}{2}\alpha^{-2}\right) \|e_v\|_k^2 \\ &\geqslant \tfrac{1}{2}\alpha_k \min(2, \alpha^{-2}) \|e_v\|_{0,2}^2. \end{aligned}$$

Hence the desired ellipticity of F and F_h follows with constant

$$\alpha_0 = \frac{\alpha_k}{2} \min\left(2, \left[\left(\frac{|k_1|}{\alpha_\mu}\right)^{1/2} + 1/2 \left(\frac{|\mu|}{\alpha_k}\right)^{1/2}\right]^{-2}\right).$$

Our proof is therefore complete. □

THEOREM 39.3. *Let F be a continuous linear elliptic operator defined on the Hilbert space X. Let v be a self-adjoint continuous elliptic operator defined on X. Let $f(t)$ be in $C_\tau^q(X)$. Then the differential equation*

$$v\dot{u} + Fu = f$$

has a unique periodic solution, belonging to $C_\tau^{q+1}(X)$.

PROOF. Through the change of variables

$$u_\nu = \nu^{1/2}u, \qquad F_\nu = \nu^{-1/2}F\nu^{-1/2}, \qquad f_\nu = \nu^{-1/2}f,$$

and after multiplication by $\nu^{-1/2}$, the above differential equation takes the form

$$\dot{u}_\nu + F_\nu u_\nu = f_\nu.$$

We know that the solutions of such a linear first-order differential equation satisfy

$$u_\nu(t) = \exp(-tF_\nu)u_\nu(0) + \int_0^t \exp(-(t-s)F_\nu)f_\nu(s)\,ds.$$

In a periodic problem, $u_\nu(0)$ is then determined by the periodicity condition

$$u_\nu(0) = u_\nu(\tau) = \exp(-\tau F_\nu)u_\nu(0) + \int_0^\tau \exp(-(\tau-s)F_\nu)f_\nu(s)\,ds,$$

which gives

$$u_\nu(0) = [\mathrm{Id} - \exp(-\tau F_\nu)]^{-1} \int_0^\tau \exp(-(\tau-s)F_\nu)f_\nu(s)\,ds.$$

The above relation completely determines the solution of the differential equation, with the desired regularity in time, provided that the operator $[\mathrm{Id} - \exp(-\tau F_\nu)]$ is invertible. But this invertibility is a consequence of the ellipticity of this operator, which we deduce from the ellipticity of F. Indeed, from the ellipticity of F, we have

$$\frac{1}{2}\frac{d}{dt}\|\exp(-tF_\nu)w\|^2$$
$$= -\langle F_\nu \exp(-tF_\nu)w, \exp(-tF_\nu)w\rangle,$$
$$= -\langle F\nu^{-1/2}\exp(-tF_\nu)w, \nu^{-1/2}\exp(-tF_\nu)w\rangle,$$
$$\leqslant -\alpha_F\|\nu^{-1/2}\exp(-tF_\nu)w\|^2,$$
$$\leqslant -\alpha_F\alpha_\nu\|\exp(-tF_\nu)w\|^2,$$
$$\leqslant -\alpha\|\exp(-tF_\nu)w\|^2.$$

After integration in time, this implies

$$\|\exp(-tF_\nu)w\|^2 \leqslant \exp(-2\alpha t)\|w\|^2.$$

From this, we deduce the desired ellipticity condition

$$\langle w - \exp(-tF_\nu)w, w\rangle \geqslant \|w\|^2 - \exp(-\alpha t)\|w\|^2$$
$$\geqslant (1 - \exp(-\alpha t))\|w\|^2,$$

and our proof is complete. □

THEOREM 39.4. *Let (v, p) be the solution of the mixed problem (39.5) with arbitrary right-hand side and let (v_h, p_h) be the corresponding finite-element solution. Then, we have*

$$\|v - v_h\|_{1,2} \leqslant C(\inf_{w_h \in \mathbb{V}_h} \|v - w_h\|_{1,2} + \inf_{q_h \in \mathbb{P}_h} \|p - q_h\|_{0,2}).$$

PROOF. This is a classical result for mixed problems (GIRAULT and RAVIART [1986]). For completeness, we outline the proof.

Let $\hat{w}_h$ be such that

$$\|v - \hat{w}_h\|_{1,2} = \inf_{w_h \in \mathbb{V}_h} \|v - w_h\|_{1,2},$$

and set

$$\hat{w}_{hD} = \hat{w}_h - B_h^{-1} B_h \hat{w}_h.$$

Here, B_h is the discrete operator associated with the bilinear form b. Since b satisfies the discrete inf-sup condition, the Ladyzenskaya–Babuska–Brezzi theorem (Section 14) implies that

$$B_h^{-1}: \mathbb{P}_h' \to \operatorname{Ker} B_h^{\perp}$$

is well-defined with

$$\|B_h^{-1}\| \leqslant 1/\beta.$$

By construction, we then have

$$\begin{aligned}
\|v - \hat{w}_{hD}\|_{1,2} &\leqslant \|v - \hat{w}_h\|_{1,2} + \|\hat{w}_h - \hat{w}_{hD}\|_{1,2} \\
&\leqslant \|v - \hat{w}_h\|_{1,2} + \|B_h^{-1}\| \|\operatorname{div} \hat{w}_h\|_{0,2} \\
&\leqslant \|v - \hat{w}_h\|_{1,2} + \|B_h^{-1}\| \|\operatorname{div}(v - \hat{w}_h)\|_{0,2} \\
&\leqslant \|v - \hat{w}_h\|_{1,2} + \beta^{-1} \|\operatorname{div}(v - \hat{w}_h)\|_{0,2} \\
&\leqslant (1 + \beta^{-1}) \|v - \hat{w}_h\|_{1,2}.
\end{aligned} \tag{39.18}$$

Let us now write (39.5) and its discrete equivalent with $w = \hat{w}_{hD} - v_h$ and subtract one equality from another. We get

$$a(\hat{w}_{hD} - v_h, \hat{w}_{hD} - v_h)$$
$$= a(\hat{w}_{hD} - v, \hat{w}_{hD} - v_h) + b(q_h - p, \hat{w}_{hD} - v_h),$$

this for all q_h belonging to $\mathbb{P}_h$. From the ellipticity and continuity of a, this yields

$$\alpha_a \|\hat{w}_{hD} - v_h\|_{1,2} \leqslant |a| \|\hat{w}_{hD} - v\|_{1,2} + \|q_h - p\|_{0,2}.$$

Adding $\alpha_a \|\hat{w}_{hD} - v\|_{1,2}$ on both sides and using (39.18), we finally obtain

$$\|v - v_h\|_{1,2} \leqslant \left(1 + \frac{|a|}{\alpha_a}\right)(1 + \beta^{-1}) \inf_{w_h \in \mathbb{V}_h} \|v - w_h\|_{1,2}$$
$$+ \frac{1}{\alpha_a} \inf_{q_h \in \mathbb{P}_h} \|p - q_h\|_{0,2}. \tag{39.19}$$

□

39.6. Proof of the main result

We are now ready to prove the convergence theorem. We will prove it at the order $(q) = 0$, the other estimates being obtained by differentiation of the original problems with respect to time. Since F and F_h are continuous linear elliptic operators, existence and uniqueness of solutions follow directly from the Cauchy–Lipschitz theorem in the case of the Cauchy problem and from Theorem 39.3 in the periodic case. The error estimates are then obtained by classical algebraic manipulations. To simplify the notation, the norm $\|\cdot\|_{0,\tau}$ and interpolation error $i_{h,0}$ will be written $\|\cdot\|_\tau$ and i_h respectively, and positive constants independent of h will be denoted by C or by α. Moreover, we set

$\|e\|_\nu = (\langle \nu : e, e \rangle)^{1/2},$

$\Pi_\Sigma e_v = L^2$ projection of e_v onto Σ_{hD},

$\delta e = \Pi_\Sigma e_v - e_{vh},$

$u_e = u(e_v) =$ solution of (39.5) with $\varepsilon = e_v$,

$u_{eh} = u_h(e_v) =$ discrete solution of (39.5) with $\varepsilon = e_v$,

$u_{\Sigma h} = u_h(\Pi_\Sigma e_v) =$ discrete solution of (39.5) with $\varepsilon = \Pi_\Sigma e_v$.

If we subtract the discrete equation (39.11) from the continuous one (39.10) and multiply the result by δe, we first get

$$\frac{1}{2}\frac{d}{dt}\|\delta e\|_\nu^2 = \langle \nu : \delta\dot{e}, \delta e \rangle$$
$$= \langle \nu : (\Pi_\Sigma \dot{e}_v - \dot{e}_{vh}), \delta e \rangle$$
$$= \langle \nu : (\dot{e}_v - \dot{e}_{vh}), \delta e \rangle$$
$$= -\langle F(e_v) - F_h(e_{vh}), \delta e \rangle \qquad (39.20)$$
$$+ \langle k_1 : e(z - z_h), \delta e \rangle$$
$$= -\langle F_h \delta e, \delta e \rangle + \langle F_h(\Pi_\Sigma e_v) - \Pi_\Sigma F(e_v), \delta e \rangle$$
$$+ \langle k_1 : e(z - z_h), \delta e \rangle.$$

Using the ellipticity of F_h and the Cauchy–Schwarz inequality we deduce:

$$\|\delta e\|_\nu \frac{d}{dt}\|\delta e\|_\nu + \alpha \|\delta e\|_{0,2}^2$$
$$\leq (\|F_h(\Pi_\Sigma e_v) - \Pi_\Sigma F(e_v)\|_{0,2} + |k_1|\|z - z_h\|_{1,2})\|\delta e\|_{0,2}.$$

But, from our assumption on ν, we have

$$\frac{1}{|\nu|}\|\delta e\|_\nu^2 \leq \|\delta e\|_{0,2}^2 \leq \frac{1}{\alpha_\nu}\|\delta e\|_\nu^2,$$

and thus, after division by $\|\delta e\|_\nu$, we obtain

$$\frac{d}{dt}\|\delta e\|_\nu + \frac{\alpha}{|\nu|}\|\delta e\|_\nu$$

$$\leqslant \alpha_\nu^{-1/2} \left(\|F_h(\Pi_\Sigma e_v) - \Pi_\Sigma F(e_v)\|_{0,2} + |k_1| \|z - z_h\|_{1,2} \right). \tag{39.21}$$

But from Theorem 39.4, the continuous and the discrete solutions z and z_h of the mixed problem (39.4) satisfy

$$\|z - z_h\|_{1,2}(t) \leqslant C i_h(t). \tag{39.22}$$

Moreover, by definition of F and of F_h, we have

$$\|\Pi_\Sigma F(e_v) - F_h(\Pi_\Sigma e_v)\|_{0,2} = \|k_1 : \Pi_\Sigma e(u_e - u_{\Sigma h})\|_{0,2}$$
$$\leqslant |k_1| \|u_e - u_{\Sigma h}\|_{1,2}$$
$$\leqslant |k_1| (\|u_e - u_{eh}\|_{1,2} + \|u_{eh} - u_{\Sigma h}\|_{1,2}). \tag{39.23}$$

In addition, by construction of u_{eh} and $u_{\Sigma h}$, we have after subtraction

$$\int_\Omega [(2\mu + 4k_1) : e(u_{eh} - u_{\Sigma h})] : e(u_{eh} - u_{\Sigma h}) \, dx$$
$$= \int_\Omega [4k_1 : (e_v - \Pi_\Sigma e_v)] : e(u_{eh} - u_{\Sigma h}) \, dx.$$

By the uniform ellipticity of μ and k_1, this implies after division by $\|u_{eh} - u_{\Sigma h}\|_{1,2}$

$$(2\alpha_k + \alpha_\mu) \|u_{eh} - u_{\Sigma h}\|_{1,2} \leqslant 2|k_1| \cdot \|e_v - \Pi_\Sigma e_v\|_{0,2}$$
$$\leqslant 2|k_1| i_h(t). \tag{39.24}$$

Using (39.24) in (39.23) and using Theorem 39.4 to estimate the difference $(u_e - u_{eh})$, we obtain

$$\|\Pi_\Sigma F(e_v) - F_h(\Pi_\Sigma e_v)\|_{0,2} \leqslant C i_h(t).$$

Hence the inequality (39.21) finally implies

$$\frac{d}{dt} \|\delta e\|_\nu + \alpha \|\delta e\|_\nu \leqslant C i_h(t),$$

or equivalently after integration in time

$$e^{\alpha t} \|\delta e(t)\|_\nu \leqslant \|\delta e(0)\|_\nu + C \int_0^t e^{\alpha s} i_h(s) \, ds. \tag{39.25}$$

This is the estimate needed for the Cauchy problem. To derive the estimate needed in the periodic case, we write (39.25) at time τ. In the periodic case, we have $\delta e(0) = \delta e(\tau)$ and thus (39.25) implies

$$\|\delta e(0)\|_\nu \leqslant C \|i_h\|_\tau \int_0^\tau e^{\alpha s} [e^{\alpha \tau} - 1]^{-1} \, ds$$
$$\leqslant (C/\alpha) \|i_h\|_\tau.$$

Once $\delta e(0)$ is replaced by this upper bound in (39.25), we deduce

$$e^{\alpha t}\|\delta e(t)\|_\nu \leq \frac{C}{\alpha}\|i_h\|_\tau [1 + e^{\alpha t} - 1] \quad \forall t$$

which yields

$$\|\delta e\|_{0,\tau,L^2} \leq \frac{C}{\alpha}\|i_h\|_\tau. \tag{39.26}$$

Since the map $u_h(\varepsilon)$ defined by the discrete counterpart of (39.5) is linear and continuous (uniformly in h), (39.26) implies in particular

$$\|u_{\Sigma h} - u_h(e_{vh})\|_{\tau,V} = \|u_h(\delta e)\|_{\tau,V} \leq C_1\|i_h\|_\tau. \tag{39.27}$$

From the triangular inequality, the definition of i_h, (39.26), (39.24), (39.27) and (39.22), we finally obtain

$$\|e_v - e_{vh}\|_{\tau,L^2} + \|u - u_h\|_{\tau,V} \leq \|e_v - \Pi_\Sigma e\|_{\tau,L^2}$$
$$+ \|\delta e\|_{\tau,L^2} + \|u_e - u_{eh}\|_{\tau,V}$$
$$+ \|u_{eh} - u_{\Sigma h}\|_{\tau,V}$$
$$+ \|u_{\Sigma h} - u_h(e_{vh})\|_{\tau,V} + \|z - z_h\|_{\tau,V}$$
$$\leq C\|i_h\|_\tau. \tag{39.28}$$

Moreover, subtracting (39.11) from (39.10) we get

$$\left\|\frac{d}{dt}(e_v - e_{vh})\right\| \leq |\nu^{-1}||k_1| \Big[\|e_v - e_{vh}\| + \|e(u) - \Pi_\Sigma e(u)\|$$
$$+ \|\Pi_\Sigma e(u) - \Pi_\Sigma e(u_h)\| \Big],$$

and thus (39.28) also implies

$$\|e_v - e_{vh}\|_{1,\tau,L^2} \leq C\|i_h\|_\tau. \tag{39.29}$$

The convergence result is then completely proved if we can estimate $(p - p_h)$. But, from the inf-sup condition, we have

$$\beta\|p_h - q_h\|_{0,2} \leq \sup_{w_h \in V_h} \frac{b(p_h - q_h, w_h)}{\|w_h\|_{1,2}}$$
$$\leq \sup_{w_h \in V_h} \frac{b(p_h - p, w_h) + b(p - q_h, w_h)}{\|w_h\|_{1,2}}$$
$$\leq \sup_{w_h \in V_h} \frac{1}{\|w_h\|_{1,2}} \Big(2\langle e(u - u_h), e(w_h)\rangle_\mu$$
$$+ 4\langle e(u - u_h) - e_v + e_{vh}, e(w_h)\rangle_k + b(p - q_h, w_h)\Big)$$
$$\leq (2|\mu| + 4|k_1|)\|u - u_h\|_{1,2} + 4|k_1|\|e_v - e_{vh}\|_{0,2}$$
$$+ \|p - q_h\|_{0,2}.$$

This is so for any q_h in $\mathbb{P}_h$. This is the missing estimate which completes the proof.

40. Discretization in time

40.1. Approximation in time

The present viscoelastic problem ((38.2)–(38.5) or (39.1)) is an evolution problem in time. In its approximation in time either by an explicit or by an implicit scheme, the main cost will be associated with the solution of the first equation giving u as a function of the viscoelastic variables. Therefore both schemes have a similar cost per time step. In this framework, an implicit scheme is much better because it is unconditionally stable which is very important in viscoelastic situations which involve time scales of different orders of magnitude, and because it has very nice long-term convergence properties for problems involving energy dissipation (LE TALLEC [1990]).

Let $\Delta t > 0$ be a given time-discretization step. Then the implicit Euler scheme applied to the viscoelastic problem (38.2)–(38.5) leads to the following sequence of problems:
For each $n \geq 0$, solve

$$\int_\Omega F^{n+1} \left(2\frac{\partial \tilde{W}}{\partial C}(x, C^{n+1}, A^{n+1}) - p^{n+1}(C^{n+1})^{-1} \right) : \nabla v \, dx$$

$$= \int_\Omega f \cdot v \, dx + \int_{\Gamma_1} g \cdot v \, da \quad \forall v \in \mathbb{V}, \ u^{n+1} - u_0 \in \mathbb{V}, \tag{40.1}$$

$$\int_\Omega \hat{p}(\det F^{n+1} - 1) \, dx = 0 \quad \forall \hat{p} \in \mathbb{P}, \ p^{n+1} \in \mathbb{P}, \tag{40.2}$$

$$\nu \frac{(A^{n+1})^{-1} - (A^n)^{-1}}{\Delta t} - \frac{\partial \tilde{W}}{\partial A}(x, C^{n+1}, A^{n+1}) - q(A^{n+1})^{-1} = 0, \tag{40.3}$$

$$\det A^{n+1} = 1. \tag{40.4}$$

In view of Remark 39.1, the discrete problem in space and time takes the same form with the addition of the subscript h to each variable and space. Of course, this system has to supplemented by initial data. For a Cauchy problem, we impose

$$A^o = \text{given value},$$

and for a periodic problem in time, we impose (with $N = \tau/\Delta t$)

$$A^N = A^o.$$

40.2. Convergence theory

As before, the approximation error can only be studied in the linear case. Under the notation of Section 39, the implicit Euler scheme applied to the linearized viscoelastic model of Section 38 leads to the sequence of problems:

For $n \geqslant 0$, solve

$$\nu \frac{e_v^{n+1} - e_v^n}{\Delta t} + F(e_v^{n+1}) = k_1 : e(z^{n+1}) \text{ in } L^2(\Omega; \mathbb{M}_D^3). \tag{40.5}$$

For the finite-element approximation of the linearized model, we obtain instead:
For $n \geqslant 0$, solve

$$\nu \frac{e_{vh}^{n+1} - e_{vh}^n}{\Delta t} + F_h(e_{vh}^{n+1}) = k_1 : \Pi_\Sigma e(z_h^{n+1}) \text{ in } \Sigma_{hD}. \tag{40.6}$$

We then have the standard result.

THEOREM 40.1. *Under the notation and assumption of Section 39, and considering either the Cauchy or the time-periodic problem, the discrete problem* (40.5) *has a unique solution* $(e_v^n)_{n>0}$. *It satisfies*

$$\|e_v^n - e_v(n\Delta t)\|_{0,2} + \|u^n - u(n\Delta t)\|_{1,2} \leqslant \frac{C}{\alpha} \Delta t, \tag{40.7}$$

with a similar estimate for the corresponding finite-element approximations.

PROOF. By construction, the sequence e_v^n satisfies the recurrence formula

$$(\text{Id} + \Delta t \nu^{-1/2} : F : \nu^{-1/2}) \nu^{1/2} : e_v^{n+1}$$
$$= \nu^{1/2} : e_v^n + \Delta t \nu^{-1/2} : k_1 : e(z^{n+1}), \tag{40.8}$$

or equivalently

$$\nu^{1/2} : e_v^{n+1} = (\text{Id} + \Delta t F_\nu)^{-1} : \left(\nu^{1/2} : e_v^n + \Delta t \nu^{-1/2} : k_1 : e(z^{n+1})\right). \tag{40.9}$$

We have already proved that the ellipticity of F and ν implies the ellipticity of $(\text{Id} + \Delta t F_\nu)$ with constant $(1 + \alpha \Delta t)$. Hence, $(\text{Id} + \Delta t F_\nu)$ is invertible with

$$\|(\text{Id} + \Delta t F_\nu)^{-1}\| \leqslant (1 + \alpha \Delta t)^{-1}. \tag{40.10}$$

Thus, the recurrence (40.9) (or (40.5)) is well-defined and uniquely determines $(e_v^n)_{n>0}$ as soon as e_v^o is known. For the Cauchy problem, this is indeed the case. For the periodic problem, e_v^o has to be computed by the periodicity condition

$$\nu^{1/2} : e_v^N = \nu^{1/2} : e_v^o.$$

Coupled with (40.9), this condition takes the form

$$0 = \nu^{1/2} : e_v^o - \nu^{1/2} : e_v^N$$
$$= \nu^{1/2} : e_v^o - (\text{Id} + \Delta t F_\nu)^{-N} : \nu^{1/2} : e_v^o$$
$$- \Delta t \sum_{i=0}^{N-1} [(\text{Id} + \Delta t F_\nu)^{i-N} : \nu^{-1/2} : k_1 : e(z^{i+1})]. \tag{40.11}$$

From (40.10), we have

$$\|(\text{Id} + \Delta t F_\nu)^{-N}\| \leqslant (1 + \alpha \Delta t)^{-N} < 1$$

hence $\text{Id} - (\text{Id} + \Delta t F_\nu)^{-N}$ is continuously invertible, which implies that (40.11) has a unique solution e_v^o. Hence the existence and uniqueness result holds for the periodic problem as well as for the Cauchy problem.

The estimate (40.7) is then standard for ordinary differential equations with Lipschitz-continuous operators. More precisely, by Taylor expansion, we have

$$\Delta t \dot{e}_v((n+1)\Delta t) = e_v((n+1)\Delta t) - e_v(n\Delta t) - \Delta t^2 \varepsilon_n,$$

$$\|\varepsilon_n\|_{0,2} \leqslant \|e_v\|_{2,\tau,L^2} = C_0.$$

Subtracting from (40.5) and eliminating $\dot{e}_v$ by the differential equation (39.10), we then obtain

$$(\text{Id} + \Delta t F_\nu) \delta e^{n+1} = \delta e^n + \Delta t^2 \nu^{-1/2} : \varepsilon_n$$

under the notation

$$\delta e^{n+1} = \nu^{1/2} : \left(e_v(n\Delta t) - e_v^n \right).$$

From (40.10), this implies

$$\|\delta e^{n+1}\|_{0,2} \leqslant (1+\alpha\Delta t)^{-1} (\|\delta e^n\|_{0,2} + \Delta t^2 C_0).$$

By induction, this gives

$$\|\delta e^n\|_{0,2} \leqslant (1+\alpha\Delta t)^{-n} \|\delta e^o\|_{0,2}$$

$$+ C_0 \Delta t \sum_{i=0}^{n-1} \Delta t (1+\alpha\Delta t)^{i-n}. \tag{40.12}$$

In (40.12), the value of δe^o is either given (Cauchy problem) or obtained by writing (40.12) at $n = N$ and using the periodicity of δe, which yields

$$\|\delta e^o\|_{0,2} \leqslant C_0 \Delta t \sum_{i=0}^{N-1} \Delta t (1+\alpha\Delta t)^{i-N} [1 - (1+\alpha\Delta t)^{-N}]^{-1}. \tag{40.13}$$

The result (40.7) then follows from (40.12), (40.13) and from the inequalities

$$(1+\alpha\Delta t)^{-n} \leqslant C \exp(-\alpha n \Delta t),$$

$$\sum_{i=0}^{N-1} \Delta t (1+\alpha\Delta t)^{i-N} \leqslant C \int_0^\tau \exp(-\alpha s) \, ds$$

$$\leqslant \frac{C}{\alpha} (1 - \exp(-\alpha\tau)). \qquad \square$$

41. Numerical solution

41.1. Basic algorithm

After discretization in time, the viscoelastic variable can be easily eliminated, reducing the evolution problem to the solution of a sequence of standard problems of static elasticity. Indeed, at each time step, we can calculate locally $A^{n+1}(C)$ by solving the differential equation (40.3). For this purpose, we first observe that the system (40.3)–(40.4) can be written as the minimization problem

$$A^{n+1} = \arg \min_{H \in \mathbb{U}_{ad}} \left(\tilde{W}(x, C^{n+1}, H) + \frac{\nu}{\Delta t}(A^n(x))^{-1} : H \right), \tag{41.1}$$

with

$$\mathbb{U}_{ad} = \{H \in (\mathbb{M}^3)_{\text{sym}}, \ \det H = 1\}.$$

Let now a mapping $A : \mathbb{R}^5 \to \mathbb{U}_{ad}$ be given. A typical example would be

$$A(Y) = Y_1 e_1 \otimes e_1 + Y_2 e_2 \otimes e_2$$
$$+ \frac{(1 + Y_1 Y_3^2 - 2Y_3 Y_4 Y_5 + Y_2 Y_4^2)}{(Y_1 Y_2 - Y_5^2)} e_3 \otimes e_3$$
$$+ Y_3(e_2 \otimes e_3 + e_3 \otimes e_2) + Y_4(e_1 \otimes e_3 + e_3 \otimes e_1)$$
$$+ Y_5(e_1 \otimes e_2 + e_2 \otimes e_1).$$

With respect to Y, the above minimization problem becomes, if we omit the dependence on x,

$$Y = \arg \min_{Z \in \mathbb{R}^5} \left\{ \tilde{W}(C^{n+1}, A(Z)) + \frac{\nu}{\Delta t}(A^n)^{-1} : A(Z) \right\}$$

or equivalently

$$F_{\Delta t}(Y) = \left\{ \frac{\partial \tilde{W}}{\partial A}(C^{n+1}, A(Y)) + \frac{\nu}{\Delta t}(A^n)^{-1} \right\} : \frac{\partial A}{\partial Y} = 0.$$

This nonlinear equation defines an implicit function $A^{n+1} = \mathscr{G}(C^{n+1})$ which is computed when needed by a standard Newton's method operating in $\mathbb{R}^5$. After elimination of A, the discrete viscoelastic system (40.1)–(40.4) reduces simply to the standard hyperelastic problem

$$\begin{cases} \int_\Omega F_h^{n+1} \tilde{\Sigma}_h^{n+1} : \nabla v_h \, dx = \int_\Omega f \cdot v_h \, dx + \int_{\Gamma_1} g \cdot v_h \, da, \\ \forall v_h \in \mathbb{V}_h, \ u_h^{n+1} - u_0 \in \mathbb{V}_h, \\ \int_\Omega \hat{p}_h(\det F_h^{n+1} - 1) \, dx = 0 \quad \forall \hat{p}_h \in \mathbb{P}_h, \ p^{n+1} \in \mathbb{P}_h, \end{cases} \tag{41.2}$$

with the notation

$$\tilde{\Sigma} = 2 \frac{\partial \tilde{W}}{\partial C}(C, \mathscr{G}(C)) - p C^{-1}, \tag{41.3}$$

$$C = F^T F, \tag{41.4}$$

$$F = \text{Id} + \nabla u. \tag{41.5}$$

With this elimination, the numerical solution of the viscoelastic problem (39.1) with a given initial data $A_h^0 = A_h(\cdot, 0)$ (Cauchy problem) proceeds at each time step n as follows: for $n > 0$ and A_h^n known, we solve the hyperelastic problem (41.2) with unknown (u_h^{n+1}, p_h^{n+1}) by a standard Newton's procedure such as the one described in Section 19.

To obtain the numerical solution of the periodic viscoelastic problem, we can either solve the Cauchy problem with arbitrary initial data and proceed until we reach a periodic solution or we can solve the equation

$$A_h^N(A_h^o) = A_h^o$$

by a nonlinear solver such as the Generalized Minimal Residual algorithm (GM-RES). These solvers will only have to compute the values of A_h^N corresponding to given values of A_h^o, which is achieved by using the algorithm above.

REMARK 41.1. The proposed elimination strategy preserves the symmetry of the linearized operator and eliminates the incompressibility constraint

$$\det A = 1.$$

Because A_h is piecewise constant, the elimination is done locally at each Gauss point. The new problem (41.2) obtained after elimination has therefore the same Jacobian matrix as the usual hyperelastic problem (same number of unknowns, same symmetry, same sparsity). The only difference is that part of the stored energy is now defined in an implicit way.

REMARK 41.2. In the case of an integral constitutive law, the discrete viscoelastic problem keeps the form (41.2), but there the function $\mathcal{G}$ will correspond to an explicit integration along the history of C.

REMARK 41.3. When one keeps the variable A in the algebraic system, which is unavoidable if one uses continuous high-order elements as in CROCHET and KEUNINGS [1982], this system becomes very large (six extra variables per viscoelastic node) and is almost impossible to solve in three-dimensional situations.

41.2. Numerical implementation

With the choice of energy described in Section 38, the equation in Y, to be solved on each cell C_i, becomes

$$F_{\Delta t}(Y) = \left(\frac{\partial \tilde{W}_1}{\partial y} C + \frac{\nu}{\Delta t}(A^n)^{-1}\right) : \frac{\partial A}{\partial Y} = 0.$$

The linearized operator to be inverted at each local Newton's iteration is then given by the symmetric expression

$$K = \frac{\partial F_{\Delta t}}{\partial Z} = \frac{\partial^2 \tilde{W}_1}{\partial y^2} \left(C : \frac{\partial A}{\partial Y}\right) \otimes \left(C : \frac{\partial A}{\partial Z}\right)$$

$$+ \left(\frac{\partial \tilde{W}_1}{\partial y} C + \frac{\nu}{\Delta t}(A^n)^{-1}\right) : \frac{\partial^2 A}{\partial Y \partial Z}.$$

Once $A = \mathcal{G}(C)$ is computed, the constitutive law (41.3) becomes (in a compressible or nearly incompressible case)
$$\tilde{\Sigma} = \frac{2\partial \tilde{W}_1}{\partial y} A + \frac{2\partial \tilde{W}_2}{\partial y} \text{cof}(C) + \frac{\partial \tilde{W}_0(E)}{\partial E}.$$

The linearization of this relation uses the implicit function theorem to compute
$$\frac{\partial A}{\partial E} = 2\frac{\partial \mathcal{G}}{\partial C}(C).$$

All calculation done, we obtain
$$\frac{\partial \tilde{\Sigma}}{\partial E} = 4\frac{\partial^2 \tilde{W}_1}{\partial y^2}(A \otimes A) + 4\frac{\partial^2 \tilde{W}_2}{\partial y^2}\text{cof}\,C \otimes \text{cof}\,C + 4\frac{\partial \tilde{W}_2}{\partial y}\frac{\partial \text{cof}\,C}{\partial C}$$
$$- B \cdot K^{-1} \cdot B^{\text{T}} + \frac{\partial^2 \tilde{W}_0(E)}{\partial E^2}$$
$$= \frac{\partial^2 \tilde{W}_e}{\partial E^2} + \frac{\partial^2 \tilde{W}_0}{\partial E^2},$$

with
$$B = 2\frac{\partial^2 \tilde{W}_1}{\partial y^2}A(C : \frac{\partial A}{\partial Y}) + 2\frac{\partial \tilde{W}_1}{\partial y}\frac{\partial A}{\partial Y}.$$

The tangential stiffness matrix $\mathcal{A}$ of the resulting linearized system in U is simply given as in Remark 18.1 by
$$\mathcal{A}_{ij} = a_{u_h}(\varphi_j, \varphi_i)$$
$$= \int_\Omega \left\{\left[\left(\frac{\partial^2 \tilde{W}_0}{\partial E^2} + \frac{\partial^2 \tilde{W}_e}{\partial E^2}\right) : F^{\text{T}}\nabla\varphi_j\right] : F^{\text{T}}\nabla\varphi_i + \tilde{\Sigma} : \nabla\varphi_j^{\text{T}}\nabla\varphi_i\right\} dx$$

and is clearly symmetric. Compared to a standard hyperelastic code, the addition of viscoelastic effects just requires a specific subroutine which, for each cell and for C given, solves (41.1) in Y by a standard Newton's method, with matrix K, updates the stress tensor $\tilde{\Sigma}$ by adding $\partial \tilde{W}_e/\partial E$, updates the local stiffness matrix by adding $\partial^2 \tilde{W}_e/\partial E^2$ to $\partial^2 \tilde{W}_0/\partial E^2$.

41.3. Numerical tests

As a test of this viscoelastic approach, we study the deformation of a rectangular block made of a soft material whose energy is given by
$$\tilde{W}_1(y) = k_1 y$$
$$\tilde{W}_2(y) = -k_1 \ln(y),$$
that is which corresponds to the constitutive laws
$$\tilde{\Sigma} = \lambda(\text{tr}(E))\,\text{Id} + 2\mu E + 2k_1 \left(A - \frac{1}{\det(C)}\text{Cof}(C)\right)$$

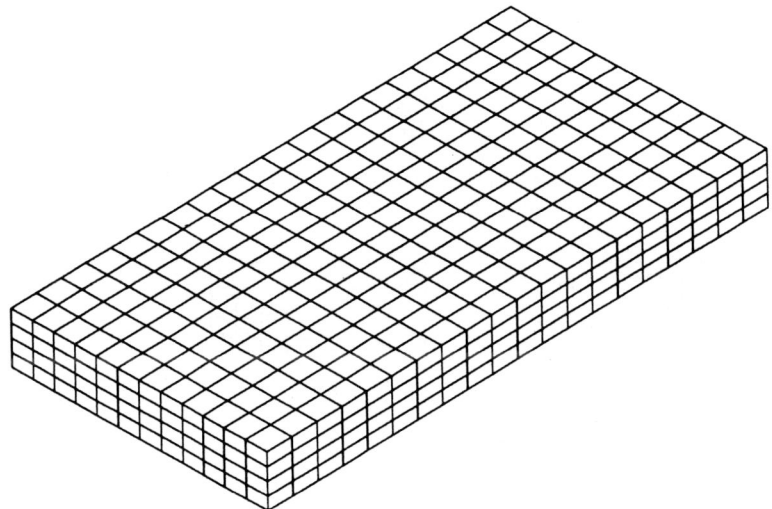

Fig. 41.1. Initial configuration of the block.

$$\begin{cases} \nu \dot{A}^{-1} = k_1 C - q A^{-1}, \\ \det A = 1. \end{cases}$$

The face $z = 0.0$ is submitted to a pressure load. The plate is fixed on its lateral faces. For symmetry reasons, only one quarter of this membrane is considered. The symmetry conditions then impose a zero displacement U_x on the

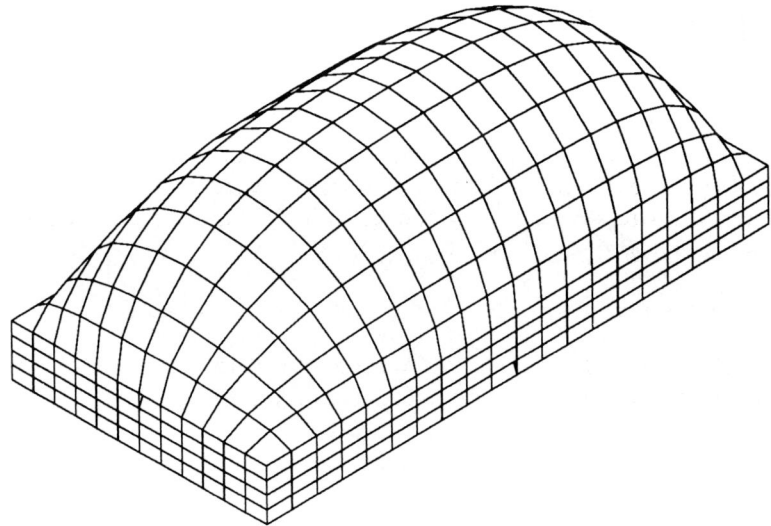

Fig. 41.2. Totally relaxed (elastic) deformed configuration of the block, under the action of a uniform pressure applied on its lower face.

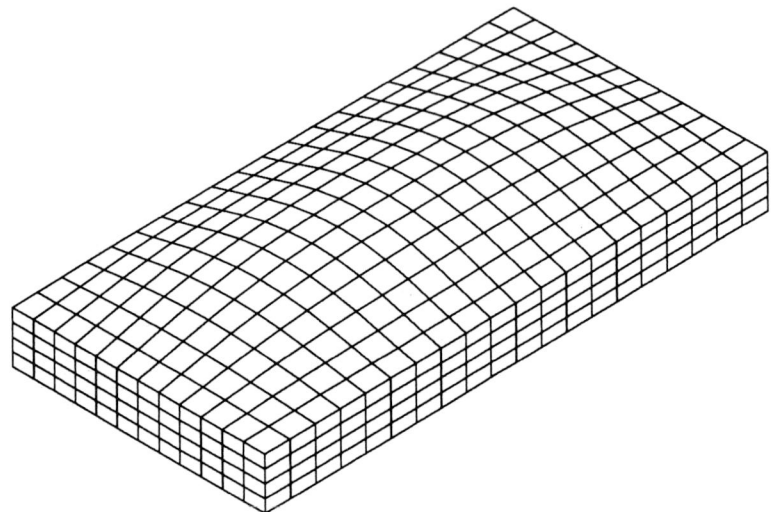

Fig. 41.3. Deformed block after the first time step.

face $x = 0$, a zero displacement U_y on the face $y = 0$. We present the initial configuration (before and just after loading) (Figs. 41.1 and 41.3), the totally relaxed configuration (Fig. 41.2) (which can be directly obtained by an elastic computation neglecting the viscoelastic branch), and a time history of the displacement observed at the center of the membrane (Fig. 41.5). The finite-element mesh consists of 120 elements of order 2 and of 1365 nodes. As expected, we ob-

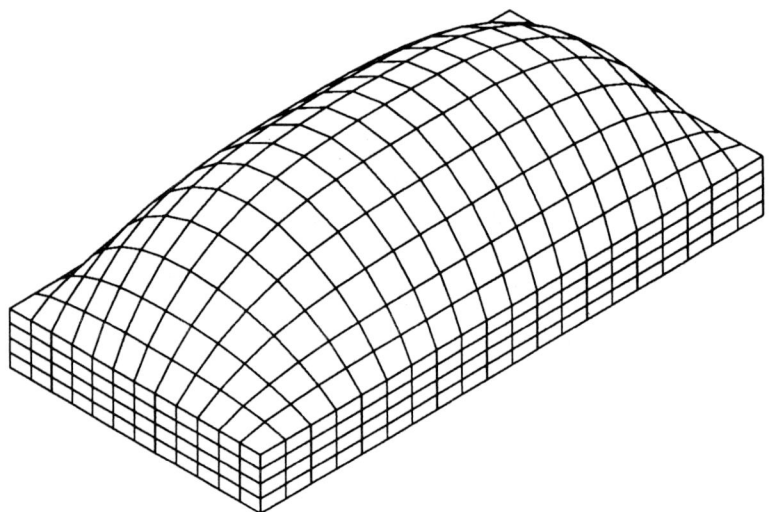

Fig. 41.4. Deformed block after the 100th time step.

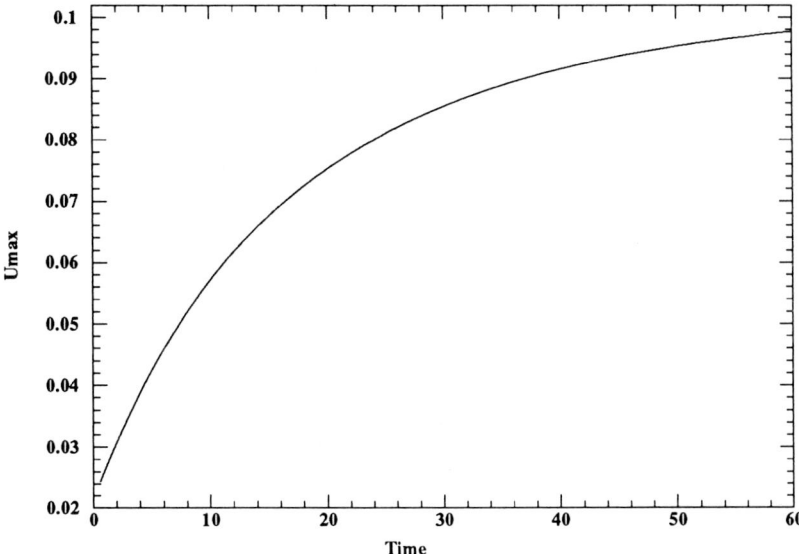

FIG. 41.5. Time history of the displacement at the center of the block.

serve a smooth transition in time from a stiff instantaneous response to a softer long-term behavior.

42. Conclusion

To conclude our presentation, we give a brief overview of the performances of the existing models in three-dimensional finite elasticity.

From the mechanical point of view, the constitutive models are well established. Unfortunately, the constitutive parameters and the different energy functions are very hard to identify, especially for viscoelastic materials. Moreover, the modeling of friction forces is still very imperfect.

From the mathematical point of view, the situation is less satisfactory. The general existence and (finite-element) approximation theory only applies to situations where the equilibrium problems can be written as minimization problems. This result can be extended to situations with frictionless contact but cannot be applied in large-strains viscoelasticity. Moreover, no existence theory is available for the weak form of the equilibrium equations except in the case of small Dirichlet data. The possible continuity of the solutions as functions of the data is also an unsolved problem.

From the numerical point of view, the existing numerical algorithms are efficient, robust (with arclength continuation), but costly. The present effort is trying to adapt the existing industrial finite-element codes to the new parallel and vector architectures.

References

AJIZ, M.A. and A. JENNINGS (1984), A robust incomplete Cholesky conjugate gradient algorithm, *Internat. J. Numer. Methods Engrg.* **20**, 946–966.

ANTMAN, S.S. and C.S. KENNEY (1981), Large buckled states of nonlinear elastic rods under tension, thrust and gravity, *Archive for Rational Mechanics and Analysis* **76** (4), 289–338.

ANTMAN, S.S. and J.E. OSBORN (1979), The principle of virtual work and integral laws of motion, *Archive for Rational Mechanics and Analysis* **69**, 231–262.

ARGYRIS, J.H. (1954), Energy theorems and structural analysis. Part I: General theory, *Aircraft Engrg.* **26**, 347–356, 383–387, 394.

ARROW, K.J., L. HURWICZ and H. UZAWA (1958), *Studies in Nonlinear Programming* (Stanford University Press, Stanford, CA).

BABUSKA, I. (1973), The finite-element method with Lagrangian multipliers, *Numerische Mathematik* **20**, 179–192.

BALL, J.M. (1977), Convexity conditions and existence theorems in nonlinear elasticity, *Arch. Rat. Mech. Anal.* **63**, 337–403.

BALL, J.M. (1981), Global invertibility of Sobolev functions and the interpenetration of matter, *Proc. Roy. Soc. Edinburgh* **88A**, 315–328.

BALL, J.M. (1982), Discontinuous equilibrium solutions and cavitation in nonlinear elasticity, *Philos. Trans. Roy. Soc. London Ser. A* **306**, 557–611.

BALL, J.M. and D. SCHAEFFER (1982), Bifurcation and stability of homogeneous equilibrium configurations of an elastic body under dead load tractions, Report, Heriott-Watt University.

BELYTSCHKO, T. and M.O. NEAL (1991), Compact-impact by the pinball algorithm with penalty and Lagrangian methods, *Internat. J. Numer. Meth. Engrg.* **31**, 547–572.

BELYTSCHKO, T. and I.S. YEH (1992), The splitting pinball method for general contact, in: R. GLOWINSKI, ed., *Computing Methods in Applied Sciences and Engineering* (Nova Science Publishers, New York).

BENSON, D.J. and J.O. HALLQUIST (1987), A single surface contact algorithm for the postbuckling analysis of shell structures, Report to the University of California at San Diego, CA.

BREZZI, F. (1974), On the existence, uniqueness and approximation of saddle-point problems arising from Lagrangian multipliers, *RAIRO Analyse Numérique, Série Rouge* **8**, 129–151.

BREZZI, F. and M. FORTIN (1991), *Mixed and Hybrid Finite Element Methods* (Springer, Berlin).

CÉA, J. (1964), Approximation variationnelle des problèmes aux limites, *Annales Institut Fourier* **14**, 345–444.

CHRISTENSEN, R.M. (1980), A nonlinear theory of viscoelasticity for application to elastomers, *J. Appl. Mech.* **762–768**, 129–151.

CIARLET P.G. (1978), *The Finite Element Method for Elliptic Problems* (North-Holland, Amsterdam, New York).

CIARLET P.G. (1988), *Mathematical Elasticity* (North-Holland, Amsterdam).

CIARLET P.G. (1991), Finite Element Methods I, in: P.G. CIARLET and J.L. LIONS, eds., *Handbook of Numerical Analysis*, Vol. II (North-Holland, Amsterdam, New York).

CIARLET, P.G. and P. DESTUYNDER (1979), A justification of a nonlinear model in plate theory, *Comp. Meth. Appl. Mech. Engrg.* **17/18**, 227–258.

CIARLET, P.G. and G. GEYMONAT (1982), Sur les lois de comportement en elasticité nonlinéaire, *C.R.A.S., Série II* **295**, 423–426.

CIARLET, P.G. and J. NEČAS (1985), Unilateral problems in nonlinear, three-dimensional elasticity, *Arch Rat. Mech. Anal.* **87**, 319–338.

CIARLET, P.G. and J. NEČAS (1987), Injectivity and self-contact in nonlinear elasticity, *Arch. Rat. Mech. Anal.* **89**, 171–188.

CLOUGH, R.W. (1960), The finite-element method in plane stress analysis, *Proceedings Second ASCE Conference on Electronic Computation*, Pittsburgh, PA.

CROCHET, M. and R. KEUNINGS (1982), Finite element analysis of die swell of a highly elastic fluid, *J. Non-Newtonian Fluid Mech.* **10**, 339–356.

DAVET, J.L. (1985), Sur les densités d'énergie en élasticité nonlinéaire: confrontation de modèles et de travaux expérimentaux, *Annales des Ponts et Chaussées, 3eme trimestre*, 2–33.

DENNIS, J.E. and R.B. SCHNABEL (1983), *Numerical Methods for Unconstrained Opimization and Nonlinear Equations* (Prentice-Hall, Englewood Cliffs, NJ).

DEUFLHARD, P. (1990), Global inexact Newton methods for very large scale nonlinear problems, in: *Proceedings of the Copper Mountain Conference*, Copper Mountain, April 1990.

EKELAND, I. and R. TEMAM (1975), *Convex Analysis and Variational Problems* (North-Holland, Amsterdam).

ERINGEN, A.C. (1966), A unified theory of thermomechanical materials, *Int J. Engrg. Sci.* **4**, 179–202.

FALK, R.S. (1974), Error estimates for the approximation of a class of variational inequalities, *Math. Comp.* **28**, 963–971.

FICKEN, F. (1951), The continuation method for nonlinear functional equations, *Comm. Pure Appl. Math.* **4**, 435–456.

FLETCHER, R. (1980), *Practical Methods of Opimization* (Wiley, New York).

FORTIN, M. and R. GLOWINSKI (1982), *Méthodes de Lagrangien Augmenté* (Dunod–Bordas, Paris); English translation: *Augmented Lagrangian Methods* (North-Holland, Amsterdam, 1983).

FORTIN, M. and R. GLOWINSKI, eds. (1983), *Augmented Lagrangian Methods* (North-Holland, Amsterdam, New York).

FOSDICK, R.L. and J. SERRIN (1979), On the impossibility of linear Cauchy and Piola–Kirchhoff constitutive theories for stress in solids, *J. Elasticity* **9**, 83–89.

GEYMONAT, G. (1965), Sui problemi ai limiti per i sistemi lineari elliptic004, *Ann. Mat. Pura Appl.* **69**, 207–284.

GILL, P.E., W. MURRAY and M.H. WRIGHT (1981), *Practical Opimization* (Academic Press, New York).

GIRAULT, V. and P.G. RAVIART (1986), *Finite Element Approximation of the Navier Stokes Equations* (Springer, Berlin).

GLOWINSKI, R. (1984), *Numerical Methods for Nonlinear Variational Problems* (Springer Verlag, Berlin, New York).

GLOWINSKI, R. and P. LE TALLEC (1982), Numerical solution of problems in incompressible finite elasticity by augmented Lagrangian methods, *SIAM J. Applied Maths* **42** (2), 400–425.

GLOWINSKI, R. and P. LE TALLEC (1989), *Augmented Lagrangian and Operator Splitting Methods in Nonlinear Mechanics* (SIAM, Philadelphia).

GLOWINSKI, R. and A. MARROCCO (1975), Sur l'approximation par éléments finis d'ordre un et la résolution par pénalité dualité d'une classe de problèmes de Dirichlet nonlinéaires, *RAIRO Analyse Numérique, Série Rouge* **9** (R2), 41–76.

GREEN, A.E and ADKINS J.E. (1960), *Large Elastic Deformations* (Clarendon Press, Oxford); 2nd edition in 1970.

GURTIN, M.E. (1981a), *Topics in Finite Elasticity*, CBMS-NSF Regional Conferences Series in Applied Mathematics, SIAM, Philadelphia.

GURTIN, M.E. (1981b), *An Introduction to Continuum Mechanics* (Academic Press, New York).

HAINES, D.Q. and W.D. WILSON (1979), Strain energy density of rubber-like materials, *J. Mech. Phys. Sol.* **27**, 345–360.

HALLQUIST, J.O, G.L. GOUDREAU and D.J. BENSON (1987), Sliding interface with contact-impact in large scale Lagrangian computation, *Comp. Meth. Appl. Mech. Engrg.* **51**, 107–137.
HANNA, K., F. JOUVE and G. WARING (1989), Preliminary computer simulation of the effects of radial keratotomy, *Archives of Ophthalmology* **107**, 911–918 .
HANNA, K., F. JOUVE and P. CIARLET (1990), Computer simulation of arcuate keratotomy for astigmatism, in: G. WARING, ed., *Keratotomy for Myopia and Astigmatism* (Mosby Co., St Louis, MO).
HESTENES, M. (1969), Multiplier and gradient methods *J. Opt. Theory Apl.* **4**, 303–320.
HUGHES, T.J.R. (1987), *The Finite Element Method: Linear Static and Dynamic Finite Element Analysis* (Prentice-Hall, Englewood Cliffs, NJ).
JAMES, R.D. (1985), Displacive Phase Transformation in Solids. Report of Brown University, Division of Engineering, Providence.
JOHNSON, C. (1987), *Numerical Solution of Partial Differential Equations by the Finite Element Method* (Cambridge University Press, Cambridge).
KELLER, H.B. (1983), The bordering algorithm and path following near singular points of higher nullity, *SIAM J. Sci. Stat. Comput.* **4**, 573–582.
KIRCHHOFF, G. (1852), Uber die Gleichungen des Gleichgewichts eines elastischeen Korpers bei nicht unendlich kleinen Verschiebungen seiner Theile, *Sitzungsber. Akad. Wiss. Wien* **9**, 762–773.
KNOWLES, J.K and E. STERNBERG (1980). Discontinuous gradient near the tip of a crack in finite antiplane shear, *J. of Elasticity* **10**, 81–110.
KRANISH, E. (1991), Interior points methods for mathematical programming: A bibliography, Diskussionsbeitrag No. 171, Fern Universität Hagen, Germany.
KRASNOL'SKII, M.A. (1964), *Topological Methods in the Theory of Nonlinear Integral Equations* (Pergamon Press, New York).
LE DRET, H. (1985), Constitutive laws and existence questions in incompressible nonlinear elasticity, *J. of Elasticity* **15**, 369–387.
LE TALLEC, P. (1981), Compatibility condition and existence results in discrete finite incompressible elasticity, *Comp. Meth. Appl. Mech. Eng.* **27**, 239–259.
LE TALLEC, P. (1982), Existence and approximation results for nonlinear mixed problems, *Numerische Mathematik* **38**, 365–382.
LE TALLEC, P. (1990), *Numerical Analysis of Viscoelastic Problems* (Masson, Paris; Springer, Berlin).
LE TALLEC, P. and J.T. ODEN (1981), Existence and characterizaton of hydrostatic pressure in finite deformations of incompressible elastic bodies, *J. Elasticity* **11**, 341–358.
LE TALLEC, P., C. RAHIER, and A. KAISS (1993), Three-dimensional incompressible viscoelasticity in large strains: Formulation and numerical approximation, *Comput. Methods Appl. Mech. Engrg.* (to appear).
LE TALLEC, P. and M. VIDRASCU (1984), Une méthode numérique pour les problèmes d'équilibre de corps hyperélastiques compressibles en grandes déformations, *Numer. Math.* **43**, 199–224.
LOCKETT, F.J. (1972), *Nonlinear Viscoelastic Solids* (Academic Press, New York).
LOVE, A.E.H. (1927), *A Treatise on the Mathematical Theory of Elasticity* (Cambridge University Press, Cambridge); reprinted by Dover Publications, New York 1944.
LUBLINER, J. (1985), A model of rubber viscoelasticity, *Mechanics Research Comm.* **12**, 93–99.
MANDEL, J. (1978), *Propriétés Mécaniques des Matériaux* (Eyrolles, Paris).
MARSDEN, J.E. and T.J.R. HUGHES (1978), Topics in the mathematical foundations of elasticity, in: *Nonlinear Analysis and Mechanics: Heriot-Watt Symposium* **2**, 30–285 (Pitman, London).
MARSDEN, J.E. and T.J.R. HUGHES (1983), *Mathematical Foundation of Elasticity* (Prentice-Hall, Englewood Cliffs, NJ).
MEIJERINK, J.A. and H.A. VAN DER VORST (1977), An iterative solution method for linear systems of the coefficient matrix is a symmetric M. matrix, *Math. Comp.* **31**, 148–162.
MOONEY, M. (1940), A theory of large elastic deformation, *J. Appl. Phys.* **11**, 582–592.
MORREY, C.B. (1952), Quasi-convexity and the lower semicontinuity of multiple integrals, *Pacific J. Math.* **2**, 25–53.
MURAT, F. (1978), Compacité par compensation, *Annali Scu. Norm. Sup. Pisa, Ser. IV* **5**, 489–507.
NEČAS, J. (1967), *Les Méthodes Directes en Théorie des Equations Elliptiques* (Masson, Paris).

ODEN, J.T. (1972), *Finite Elements for Nonlinear Continua* (McGraw Hill, New York).
ODEN, J.T. and N. KIKUCHI (1988), *Contact Problems in Elasticity: a Study of Variational Inequalities and Finite Element Methods* (SIAM, Philadelphia).
ODEN, J.T. and T.L. LIN (1986), On the general rolling contact problem for finite deformations of a viscoelastic cylinder, *Comp. Meth. Appl. Mech. Eng.* **57**, 297–367.
ODEN, J.T. and E. PIRES (1983), Numerical analysis of certain contact problems with nonclassical friction laws, *Comput. & Structures* **16**, 481–500.
ODEN, J.T. and P. RABIER (1989), *Bifurcation in Rotating Bodies* (Masson, Paris).
OGDEN, R.W. (1972), Large deformation isotropic elasticity. On the correlation of theory and experiment for incompressible rubber-like solids, *Proceedings Roy. Society London* **A328**, 567–583.
OGDEN, R.W. (1976), Volume changes associated with the deformation of rubber-like solids, *J. Mech. Phys. Solids* **24**, 323–338.
OGDEN, R.W. (1984), *Nonlinear Elastic Deformations* (Ellis Horwood, Chichester and J. Wiley).
ORTEGA, J.M. and E. RHEINBOLDT (1970), *Iterative Solution of Nonlinear Equations in Several Variables* (Academic Press, New York).
POLAK, E. (1971), *Computational Methods in Optimization* (Academic Press, New York).
POLYAK, B.T. (1979), On the Betsekas minimization method of composite functions, in: A. BENSOUSSAN and J.L. LIONS, eds., *International Symposium on Systems Optimization and Algorithms*, Lecture Notes in Control and Information Sciences, (Springer, Berlin).
POWELL, M.J.D. (1969), A method for nonlinear constraints in minimization problems, in: R. FLETCHER, ed., *Optimization* (Academic Press, London).
RIVLIN, R.S. (1948), Large elastic deformations of isotropic materials. II Some uniqueness theorems for pure homogeneous deformation, *Philos. Trans. Roy. Soc. London Ser. A* **240**, 491–508.
ROCKAFELLAR, R.T. (1970), *Convex Analysis* (Princeton University Press, Princeton, NJ).
RUAS, V. (1981), A class of asymmetric finite element method for solving finite incompressible elasticity problems, *Comp. Meth. Appl. Mech. Eng.* **27**, 319–343.
SAINT-VENANT, A.J.C.B. DE (1844), Sur les pressions qui se développent à l'intérieur des corps solides lorsque les déplacements de leurs points, sans altérer l'élasticité, ne peuvent cependant pas être considérés comme très petits, *Bull. Soc. Philomath.* **5**, 26–28.
SALENÇON, J. (1983), *Cours de Calcul des Structures Anélastiques* (Presses de l'Ecole Nationale des Ponts et Chaussées, Paris).
SALENÇON, J. (1988), *Mécanique des Milieux Continus* (Ellipses Editeur, Paris).
SIDOROFF, F. (1974), Un modèle viscoélastique nonlinéaire avec configuration intermédiaire, *J. Mécanique* **13**, 679–713.
SIMO, J. (1987), On a fully three-dimensional finite-strain viscoelastic damage model: Formulation and computational aspects, *Comp. Meth. Appl. Mech. Eng.* **66**, 199–219.
SIMO, J. (1988), A framework for finite strain elastoviscoplasticity based on maximum plastic dissipation and the multiplicative decomposition: 1 Continuum formulation, *Comp. Meth. Appl. Mech. Eng.* **60**, 153–173.
STOPPELLI, F. (1954), Un teorema di existenza e di unicita relativo alle equazioni dell'elastostatica isoterma per deformazioni finite, *Ricerce Math.* **3**, 247–267.
TARTAR, L. (1979), Compensated compactness and partial differential equations, in: R.J. KNOPS, ed., *Nonlinear Analysis and Mechanics, Heriot–Watt Symposium*, Pitman, **IV**, 136–212.
TIMOSHENKO, S. (1951), *Theory of Elasticity* (McGraw Hill, New York).
TRELOAR, L.R.G. (1975), *The Physics of Rubber Elasticity* (Oxford University Press, Oxford).
TRUESDELL C. and W. NOLL (1965), The nonlinear field theories of mechanics theory of elasticity, *Handbuch der Physik*, **III/3** (Springer, Berlin) 1–602.
VALENT, T. (1978), Local theorems of existence and uniqueness in finite elastostatics, in: D.E. CARLSON and R.T SHIELDS, eds., *Finite Elasticity* (Nijhoff, The Hague) 401–421.
VALENT, T. (1990), *Boundary Value Problems of Finite Elasticity* (Springer, Heidelberg).
VALENT, T. and G. ZAMPIERI (1977), Sulla differenziabilità di un operatore legato a una classe di sistemi differenziali quasi-lineari, *Rend. Sem. Mat. Univ. Padova* **57**, 311–322.
VAN BUREN, M. (1968), On the existence and uniqueness of solutions to boundary value problems in finite elasticity, Thesis, Carnegie-Mellon University, Pittsburgh, PA.

VAN DEN BOGERT, J. (1991), Computational modelling of rubberlike materials, Thesis, Technische Universiteit Delft, Netherlands.
WANG, C.C. and C. TRUESDELL (1973), *Introduction to Rational Elasticity* (Noordhoff, Groningen).
WASHIZU, K. (1975), *Variational Methods in Elasticity and Plasticity* (2nd edition, Pergamon, Oxford).
WEBER, J.D. (1975), Elasticité non-lineaire: étude du cas particulier d'une seule variable interne tensorielle. in: J. HULT, ed., *Mechanics of Viscoelastic Media and Bodies*, 147–155, IUTAM Symposium, Göteborg, Sweden, 1974 (Springer, Berlin).
YOSIDA, K. (1978), *Functional Analysis* (Springer, Berlin).
ZIENKIEWICZ, O. (1971), *The Finite Element Method in Engineering Science* (McGraw-Hill, New York, Toronto, London).

List of Symbols

Matrices and tensors

We denote as usual:

$\mathbb{R}$ the set of real numbers,

$\mathbb{E}$ the three-dimensional Euclidian space, which we identify with its dual,

$(e_i)_{i=1,3}$ a given orthonormal basis of $\mathbb{E}$,

$A = A_{ij} e_i \otimes e_j$ an element of $\mathbb{M}^3 = \mathbb{E} \otimes \mathbb{E} = \mathscr{L}(\mathbb{E}, \mathbb{E})$,

tr A the trace of A.

Moreover, $u \cdot v$ denotes the scalar product in $\mathbb{E}$ and AB is the usual tensor product of tensors A and B. If $A = A_{ij} e_i \otimes e_j$ and $B = B_{jk} e_j \otimes e_k$, then

$$AB = A_{ij} B_{jk} e_i \otimes e_k,$$

with an implicit summation on repeated indices. Finally, $A:B$ represents the double dot product of the tensors A and B, that is

$$A:B = \operatorname{tr}(A^T B) = \langle A, B \rangle = A_{ij} B_{ij}.$$

Also of interest is the cofactor cof A of A, defined for $A \in \mathbb{M}^3$ by:

$$\operatorname{cof}(A) = \det(A) A^{-T} \text{ if } A \text{ is invertible,}$$
$$= \frac{\partial \det(A)}{\partial A}.$$

Differential calculus

For $f(x,t)$ a function of particle x and time t (defined on $\mathbb{E} \times \mathbb{R}$), we denote:

∇f or $\dfrac{\partial f}{\partial x}$ the gradient of f with respect to x,

$e(f) = \frac{1}{2}(\nabla f + \nabla f^t)$ its symmetric part,

div $f = \operatorname{tr} \nabla f$ its divergence,

$\dot{f}$ the derivative of f with respect to time.

Mechanics

(a) scalars. We introduce

τ a given period in time,

p the hydrostatic pressure,

$\hat{W}(F) = \tilde{W}(C)$ the material elastic potential,

λ and μ the Lamé constants,

k_1 the elastic stiffness in a viscoelastic branch,

ν the viscosity of this viscoelastic branch.

(b) vectors. We have as usual :

$f =$ body forces (in the reference configuration),

$g =$ surface tractions (imposed on Γ_1 in the reference configuration),

$\lambda(s) =$ loading factor,

$\varphi =$ deformation,

$u =$ displacement field,

$u_o =$ imposed displacement field on Γ_o,

$v =$ velocity field or test function.

(c) second-order tensors on $\mathbb{E}$. We denote :

F the deformation gradient,

E the Green–Lagrange strain tensor,

e the linearized strain tensor,

e_D its deviatoric part,

T the first Piola–Kirchhoff stress tensor,

$\tilde{\Sigma}$ the second Piola–Kirchhoff stress tensor,

$\mathcal{A} = -\text{div } T$.

In viscoelasticity, we also introduce

C_v the viscous strain tensor,

$\phi(C_v)$ a dissipation function,

$A = C_v^{-1}$ the fundamental viscoelastic variable,

e_v the linearized viscous strain tensor,

C_e the elastic strain tensor of the viscoelastic branch.

Usually, G will denote any test function in $\mathbb{M}^3$.

Functional spaces

We introduce the following spaces :

$\mathbb{V}$ the space of velocity fields,

$\mathbb{V}_h$ the corresponding finite-element space (of dimension N_h),

$\mathbb{P}$ the space of pressure fields,

$\mathbb{P}_h$ the corresponding finite-element space (of dimension M_h),

$\mathbb{U}$ the set of kinematically admissible displacement fields,

$\mathbb{U}_h$ the corresponding finite-element set,

Σ_h the finite-element space of viscous strain tensors,

$\Sigma_{h\mathrm{D}}$ the subspace of weakly deviatoric viscous strain tensors,

Π_Σ the L^2 projection on $\Sigma_{h\mathrm{D}}$.

In addition, we will use the space $C_\tau^q(X)$ of τ periodic functions of time, of class q, with values in X, and the product of Sobolev space

$$\mathbb{H} = W^{1,s}(\Omega; \mathbb{E}) \times L^q(\mathbb{M}^3).$$

with norm $\|v, F\| = \|v\|_{1,s} + \|F\|_{0,q}$.

Vector notations

We finally introduce:

$J(v)$ the total potential energy,

$\mathscr{F}$ the algebraic system to solve after discretization,

U the set of nodal values of u_h,

P the set of nodal values of p_h,

$\mathscr{R}$ the residual,

$K = \dfrac{\mathrm{D}\mathscr{F}(U,P)}{\mathrm{D}(U,P)}$ the stiffness matrix.

In general, $a(\cdot,\cdot)$ and $b(\cdot,\cdot)$ will be bilinear forms related to the Hessian of J and to the gradient of the incompressibility constraint, respectively. The numerical analysis of the linearized viscoelastic problem will also introduce a linear operator F operating on the strain tensor e_V.

Tensorial calculus

The present text extensively uses tensorial notations. Such a notation is very convenient in mechanics because it is the natural framework in which to define all the kinematic variables independently of any frame of reference. Generally speaking, a tensor is an n-multilinear form operating on the product of n copies of $\mathbb{E}$ (or of its dual). More precisely,

$$T \in \mathbb{E} \otimes \mathbb{E}' \otimes \cdots \otimes \mathbb{E} \Leftrightarrow T \in \mathscr{L}(\mathbb{E}' \times \mathbb{E} \times \cdots \times \mathbb{E}', \mathbb{R}).$$

In particular, elements of $\mathbb{E}$ or of its dual are (first order) tensors. Addition, multiplication by a scalar, tensor product and dot product are the different possible operations on tensors.

Among all possible tensors, the positive symmetric tensors of $\mathbb{E}' \otimes \mathbb{E}'$ play a special role. By definition, $C \in \mathbb{E}' \otimes \mathbb{E}'$ is symmetric positive if and only if

(i) $u \cdot C \cdot v = v \cdot C \cdot u \quad \forall u \in \mathbb{E}, \ \forall v \in \mathbb{E}$,
(ii) $u \cdot C \cdot u \geq 0 \quad \forall u \in \mathbb{E}$.

The metric tensor G defined from the scalar product $\langle \cdot, \cdot \rangle$ of $\mathbb{E}$ by

$$u \cdot G \cdot v = \langle u, v \rangle \quad \forall u \in \mathbb{E}, \ \forall v \in \mathbb{E},$$

is an example of such tensors. Through this tensor, we can identify $\mathbb{E}$ with its dual.

After this identification, the invariants of a symmetric tensor C of $\mathbb{E}' \otimes \mathbb{E}'$ are

$$I_1(C) = \operatorname{tr}(C),$$
$$I_2(C) = \tfrac{1}{2}\{(\operatorname{tr}(C))^2 - \operatorname{tr}(C^2)\},$$
$$I_3(C) = \det(C),$$
$$dI_1 = \operatorname{tr}(dC) = \operatorname{Id} : dC,$$
$$dI_2 = \operatorname{tr}(C)\operatorname{Id} : dC - C : dC$$
$$dI_3 = I_3 C^{-1} : dC$$
$$\frac{\partial I_1}{\partial C} = \operatorname{Id}$$
$$\frac{\partial I_2}{\partial C} = I_1 \operatorname{Id} - C,$$
$$\frac{\partial I_3}{\partial C} = I_3 C^{-1},$$
$$\frac{\partial^2 I_1}{\partial C^2} = 0,$$
$$\frac{\partial^2 I_2}{\partial C^2} : dC = \operatorname{Id} : dC \operatorname{Id} - dC,$$
$$\frac{\partial^2 I_3}{\partial C^2} : dC = I_3 C^{-1} : dC C^{-1} - I_3 C^{-1} \cdot dC \cdot C^{-1}.$$

Subject Index

Arclength continuation, 530, 539, 541, 543, 546
Augmented Lagrangian, 544, 546, 549, 551, 552, 554, 562

Body forces, 474
Bordering algorithm, 543
Buckling, 488, 561

Cauchy problem, 585, 592, 598, 599, 601, 602, 605
Cauchy stress tensor, 475, 479
Cauchy–Green tensor, 473, 474, 478, 480, 481, 581, 583
Closed range theorem, 516
Compatibility condition, 516, 527, 535
Conservative loading, 493
Consistency, 527
Constitutive law, 476, 477, 479, 481, 483, 487, 490, 492, 502, 532, 583, 584, 587, 606
Contact, 565
Contact forces, 474, 566
Contact–Impact, 578
Continuous body, 471
Convex minimization, 554

Dead loads, 493, 520
Deformation, 471
Deformation gradient, 472, 477, 483, 581
Deformed configuration, 519, 583
Deviatoric, 587
Dissipation, 581, 582, 585, 601
Dominated convergence, 502, 522
Dualization, 546

Elastic, 477
Equations of equilibrium, 475, 476, 487, 492, 501, 511, 515, 530, 538, 549, 561, 565, 567, 570, 575, 584
Euler, 536, 601

Euler–Newton, 540
Extended Newton's algorithm, 543
Extended system, 541, 542

Fatou's lemma, 499, 524
Finite element, 508, 511, 512, 514, 530, 532, 573, 588, 590, 592, 593, 597, 602, 607
Frame indifference, 478, 481
Free energy, 581–583, 585
Friction forces, 577
Frictionless contact, 565, 570

Galerkin, 511, 588
Gaussian elimination, 542, 544
Green–Lagrange, 618
Green–Saint-Venant tensor, 480

Homogeneous, 477, 502
Hydrostatic pressure, 481, 483, 538
Hyperelastic, 477, 479, 481, 494, 579, 582, 586, 604–606

Implicit function theorem, 486
Incompressibility, 474, 492, 582, 585, 605
Incremental loading, 535, 537
Inf–sup condition, 517, 518, 592, 597, 600
Internal variables, 579, 581, 585, 588, 592
Interpenetration, 569, 577
Interpolation error, 591, 598
Invariants, 473, 481, 586, 620
Isochoric, 474
Isolated minimizer, 520, 521, 523, 526
Isotropic, 502, 556, 560, 586

Kelvin's model, 587, 592
Kinematically admissible, 494, 496
Kinematics, 471

Ladyzenskaya–Babuska–Brezzi theorem, 516, 518, 535, 593, 597
Lagrange multiplier, 525, 549, 571, 583, 585, 588
Lamé constants, 480, 586
Lax–Milgram, 593
Limit points, 539
Line damping, 536, 539
Linearization, 515, 589
Linearized law, 587, 602
Linearized strain tensor, 501, 587
Loading path, 504
Locking, 514

Material points, 471
Memory effects, 579, 584
Mixed problem, 516, 517, 597, 599
Mooney–Rivlin, 482, 483, 527, 538, 561, 586

Nearly incompressible, 483, 513, 532, 546, 585, 606
Neo-Hookean, 481
Newton's method, 528, 529, 533, 535, 536, 543, 546, 560, 562, 576, 604, 606
Nodal basis, 529
Nonlinear programming, 575

Ogden's materials, 480, 482, 527, 561

Penalization, 545, 576
Piola–Kirchhoff stress tensor, 476, 480, 485, 501, 583, 618
Plane obstacle, 566
Plane strain, 493
Polyconvexity, 486, 501, 507
Predictor–corrector, 573
Pressure, 474, 485, 494, 565

Reaction forces, 567, 578

Reduced invariants, 483
Reference configuration, 471, 475, 481, 483, 487, 492, 502, 582
Reference element, 508
Relaxation, 580
Rheological model, 580
Rigid deformation, 474
Rigid obstacle, 566, 567
Rivlin–Eriksen theorem, 479

Saint-Venant–Kirchhoff, 480, 586
Self-contact, 565, 569, 570, 577
Serendipity element, 510
Singular values, 556, 557, 560
Standard materials, 581
Step loading, 580
Stokes problem, 519, 590
Stored energy, 478, 483, 487, 498, 520, 527, 582, 586
Strain tensor, 586
Stress-free configuration, 483
Surface tractions, 474, 487

Total energy, 486, 494, 496, 498, 562, 571
Triangulation, 508

Uniformly elliptic, 591–594
Uzawa, 553

Variational formulation, 490, 493, 513, 585, 588, 590
Viscoelastic, 579, 583, 587, 601, 603, 606
Viscous strain tensor, 581, 587

Weakly closed, 495, 499, 524, 572
Weierstrass theorem, 498, 500, 523, 526, 572

Solution of Equations in $\mathbb{R}^n$ (Part 2)

Numerical Solution of Polynomial Equations

Bl. Sendov, A. Andreev and N. Kjurkchiev

Institute of Mathematics
Bulgarian Academy of Sciences
Acad. G. Bonchev bl. 8
1113 Sofia, Bulgaria

HANDBOOK OF NUMERICAL ANALYSIS, VOL. III
Techniques of Scientific Computing (Part 1)
Numerical Methods for Solids (Part 1)
Solutions of Equations in $\mathbb{R}^n$ (Part 2)
Edited by P.G. Ciarlet and J.L. Lions
© 1994 Elsevier Science B.V. All rights reserved

Contents

PREFACE	629
CHAPTER I. Properties of Algebraic Equations	631
1. Existence of the roots	631
2. Newton's formula and symmetric functions	635
3. Resolvent and discriminant of polynomials	637
4. Algebraic equations from first till fourth degree	639
5. Number of roots in an interval	640
6. Number of roots in a domain	645
7. Algebraic equations with a negative real part of the roots	648
8. Number of roots in a disc	650
9. The Gauss–Lucas theorem and Sendov's conjecture	651
10. Distribution of the roots on the plane	654
CHAPTER II. Localization Bounds	657
11. Elementary bounds	657
12. Estimations of the unique positive root	673
13. Sendov's method for localization of all positive roots	683
CHAPTER III. Local and Global Methods	687
14. Bernoulli's iteration	687
15. Graeffe's method	689
16. The method of Laguerre	693
17. The Lehmer–Schur method	697
CHAPTER IV. Iterative Methods for Computation of All Roots	699
18. Iterative methods without derivatives	699
19. Iterative methods with derivatives	710
20. Simultaneous approximation of multiple roots	724
21. Multi-point methods for simultaneous approximation	733
22. Factorization of a polynomial	735
23. Interval methods for polynomial root determining	739
CHAPTER V. Computational Complexity (Renegar and Neff Approach)	747
24. Definitions and notation	747
25. The lower bound (Renegar approach)	748
26. Algorithm for the upper bound (Neff approach)	752
27. Approximate factorization	754

28. q-Splittings of the complex plane   756
29. Approximating the factors by contour integration   759
30. Finding a balanced splitting point   762

REFERENCES   767

SUBJECT INDEX   777

Preface

Today, the tendency in developing numerical methods is oriented exclusively to the use of computers. The character of these methods is naturally influenced to be easily performed by computers. Many of the classical numerical methods were discovered long before the existence of the computers, but still represent a practical interest.

One very basic and classical problem in the numerical methods and numerical analysis is the approximate solution of polynomial equations. The polynomials as mathematical objects have been studied extensively for a long time, and the knowledge collected about them is enormous. The problem for finding the roots of a polynomial equation gives rise to modern algebra, starting with the fact of non-existence of an algebraic formula for the roots of a polynomial equation of fifth and higher degree.

For the purpose of the numerical solution of polynomial equations we need some classical results, presented in Chapter I. In this chapter we present theorems for the number of the roots in an interval, in a domain and the distribution of the roots of a polynomial and its derivative. This material in general comes from the last century, but still has some fresh and unsolved problems.

A polynomial equation has as many roots as its degree. To start the numerical calculation of a given root, this root has to be localized. In Chapter II a rich variety of theorems for the estimation of the values and for localizing the roots of a polynomial is given.

The methods for the numerical solution of a polynomial equation may be divided into two types: methods for calculating one separate root, previously localized or distinguished, methods for calculating all the roots together. Such methods are presented in Chapters III and IV.

Chapter V is devoted to the problem of the computational complexity of approximating roots of polynomials.

In this paper we include many theorems and statements without proof or analysis, just for information and practical use.

We are thankful to our colleagues P. Marinov and R. Georgiev for the help during the preparation of the book.

We are partially supported by Contract MM-208/92 with Ministry of Education and Science in Bulgaria.

CHAPTER I

Properties of Algebraic Equations

Solution of algebraic equations is a subject of long investigations starting with exact formulas for the zeros of equations of degree less than five. One can say that a series of classical results that are due to Fourier, Descartes, Newton, Lagrange, Gauss and other famous mathematicians build a separate part of mathematics: *'Zeros of polynomials'*. All these theoretical results lie in the base of the modern numerical iterative methods applied on the powerful computers.

This chapter presents basic properties and theorems for algebraic equations. Together with theorems for existence and localizing the roots, the number of the roots within a specified region, there exist old, but still unsolved problems connected with polynomials. An example of such a problem is *Sendov's conjecture* for the distribution of the zeros of the derivative of an algebraic polynomial. This conjecture can be considered as a quantitative continuation of the Gauss–Lucas theorem for the distribution of the zeros of the derivative and is a subject of intensive investigations.

1. Existence of the roots

Let us consider the algebraic equation or algebraic polynomial of nth degree

$$f(z) = \sum_{i=0}^{n} a_i z^{n-i} = 0, \qquad (1.1)$$

where the a_i are complex numbers. The basic theorem of algebra states that there exists at least one complex number $z_0 = a+ib, i^2 = -1$, such that $f(z_0) = 0$. A first proof was given in 1746 by D'Alambert with some incompleteness. The strict proof is due to Gauss in 1799.

Let us prove that Eq. (1.1) has a root using Cauchy's approach. Note that, the inequality $|f(z_0)| > 0$ implies $|f(z_0 + h)| < |f(z_0)|$ for some complex number h (this is the so called D'Alambert's lemma). Indeed, from

$$f(z_0 + h) = \sum_{i=0}^{n} \frac{h^i}{i!} f^{(i)}(z_0),$$

under the assumption $f^{(i)}(z_0) = 0$ for $i = 1, 2, \ldots, m-1$ and $f^{(m)}(z_0) \neq 0$, it follows that

$$\frac{f(z_0 + h)}{f(z_0)} = 1 + \sum_{i=m}^{n} \frac{h^i}{i!} \frac{f^{(i)}(z_0)}{f(z_0)}.$$

Denote

$$h = \rho(\cos \varphi + i \sin \varphi),$$

$$\frac{1}{s!} \frac{f^{(s)}(z_0)}{f(z_0)} = R_s(\cos \varphi_s + i \sin \varphi_s), \quad s = m, m+1, \ldots, n.$$

We obtain

$$\frac{f(z_0 + h)}{f(z_0)} = 1 + \sum_{s=m}^{n} R_s \rho^s [\cos(s\varphi + \varphi_s) + i \sin(s\varphi + \varphi_s)].$$

Determine φ and ρ such that $m\varphi + \varphi_m = \pi$, $R_m \rho^m < 1$, then

$$\left| \frac{f(z_0 + h)}{f(z_0)} \right| \leqslant 1 - \rho^m (R_m - R_{m+1}\rho - \cdots - R_n \rho^{n-m}).$$

For sufficiently small ρ, the last inequality gives $|f(z_0 + h)| < |f(z_0)|$.

The proof of the basic theorem of algebra now follows from the previous assertion and the facts that:

(a) $|f(z)| > 0$ for $|z| > R$, where

$$R = \max\{1, 1 + \rho\}, \quad \rho = \max\{|a_i|/|a_0| : i = 1, \ldots, n\}.$$

Indeed,

$$|f(z)| \geqslant |a_0||z|^n - |a_1||z|^{n-1} - \cdots - |a_n|$$
$$\geqslant |a_0||z|^n \left\{ 1 - \rho \sum_{i=0}^{\infty} |z|^{-i} \right\}$$
$$= |a_0||z|^n \left(1 - \frac{\rho}{|z|-1} \right) > 0;$$

(b) the continuous function $|f(z)|$ achieves its minimum in the compact $|z| \leqslant R$.

As a consequence of the basic theorem of algebra, it follows that every polynomial of the kind (1.1) can be represented in a unique way as

$$f(z) = a_0 \prod_{i=1}^{n} (z - z_i). \tag{1.2}$$

There exists at least one number z_1 such that $f(z_1) = 0$. Then, $f(z) = (z - z_1)f_1(z) + R$, where f_1 is a polynomial of degree $n - 1$ and R is a constant. Since $f(z_1) = 0$, it follows that $R = 0$ and consequently

$$f(z) = (z - z_1)f_1(z). \tag{1.3}$$

The representation (1.2) follows applying Eq. (1.3) recursively and taking into account the fact that $f_n(z) = a_0$.

Every polynomial (1.1) can have at most n roots. Some of them can be equal. If the factor $z - z_s$ repeats k-times in (1.2), the root z_s is called k-multiple. One-multiple roots are called simple roots.

Several simple properties of the polynomials follow from the above considerations:

(a) if the polynomial $f(z)$ has more than n different zeros, then $f(z) \equiv 0$;
(b) if two polynomials $f(z)$ and $g(z)$ of nth degree coincide at $n+1$ different points, then $f(z) \equiv g(z)$;
(c) comparing the representations (1.1) and (1.2), the dependence between the coefficients and roots can be obtained in the form

$$\begin{aligned} z_1 + z_2 + \cdots + z_n &= -\frac{a_1}{a_0}, \\ z_1 z_2 + \cdots + z_1 z_n + \cdots + z_{n-1} z_n &= \frac{a_2}{a_0} \\ z_1 z_2 z_3 + \cdots + z_{n-2} z_{n-1} z_n &= -\frac{a_3}{a_0}, \\ &\vdots \\ z_1 z_2 \cdots z_n &= (-1)^n \frac{a_n}{a_0}; \end{aligned} \tag{1.4}$$

(d) if the coefficients of the polynomial (1.1) are real numbers and $f(\alpha+i\beta) = 0$, then $f(\alpha - i\beta) = 0$. Indeed, $f(\alpha + i\beta) = P(\alpha, \beta) + iQ(\alpha, \beta)$, where P and Q are polynomials of α and β such that P contains only even degrees of β and Q contains only odd degrees of β. Therefore,

$$P(\alpha, -\beta) = P(\alpha, \beta), \quad Q(\alpha, -\beta) = -Q(\alpha, \beta).$$

The last equalities give (note that $f(\alpha + i\beta) = 0$ implies $P(\alpha, \beta) = Q(\alpha, \beta) = 0$)

$$f(\alpha + i\beta) = P(\alpha, \beta) - iQ(\alpha, \beta) = P(\alpha, -\beta) + iQ(\alpha, -\beta) = f(\alpha - i\beta);$$

(e) if the polynomial (1.1) has real coefficients, then

$$f(z) = a_0 \prod_{s=1}^{k} (z^2 + p_s z + q_s) \prod_{s=1}^{m} (z - r_s),$$

where p_s, q_s, r_s are real numbers and $2k + m = n$. The proof is a direct consequence of (1.2) and property (d);

(f) we say that the polynomial Q divides the polynomial P if there exists a polynomial R such that $P = QR$. If a polynomial C divides the polynomials A and B, then the polynomial C is called the common divisor of A and B. The polynomial D of highest degree which divides the polynomials A and B is called the greatest common divisor.

If the polynomials A and B are in the form (1.2),

$$A(z) = a_0 \prod_{i=1}^{n}(z - \alpha_i), \qquad B(z) = b_0 \prod_{i=1}^{m}(z - \beta_i),$$

then the greatest common divisor C is the product of common linear factors that take place in both right parts. If A and B are given in the form (1.1), then the well-known *Euclidean algorithm* works:

$$\begin{aligned} A &= BQ + R_1, \\ B &= R_1 Q_1 + R_2, \\ R_1 &= R_2 Q_2 + R_3, \\ &\vdots \\ R_{s-2} &= R_{s-1} Q_{s-1} + R_s. \end{aligned} \qquad (1.5)$$

The degrees of the polynomials $R_i, i = 1, 2, \ldots, s$, decrease and $R_s = \text{const}$. Every common divisor of A and B divides $R_i, i = 1, 2, \ldots, s$. This means that if $R_s \neq 0$, then A and B do not have a common divisor, otherwise R_{s-1} is the greatest common divisor;

(g) if A and B are two polynomials, then there exist polynomials X and Y such that $XA - YB = \text{const}$. If A and B have a common divisor, $XA - YB = 0$. The proof follows from the representation of R_s in (1.5).

Elimination of multiple roots is a part of some numerical methods for determining the zeros of polynomials. Let u be an m-multiple root of the equation $f(z) = 0$. Then $f(z) = (z - u)^m \varphi(z)$, where $\varphi(u) \neq 0$. From

$$\begin{aligned} f'(z) &= (z - u)^{m-1} [m\varphi(z) + (z - u)\varphi'(z)] \\ &= (z - u)^{m-1} \varphi_1(z), \quad \varphi_1(u) \neq 0, \end{aligned}$$

it follows that $f'(u) = 0$. Continuing the above process, the conclusion is that the number u is an m-multiple, $(m-1)$-multiple,..., 1-multiple (simple) root of $f, f', \ldots, f^{(m-1)}$, respectively, and $f^{(m)}(u) \neq 0$. Following the Euclidean algorithm, if

$$\begin{aligned} f(z) &= a_0 \left(\prod_{i=1}^{n_1}(z - \alpha_i) \right) \left(\prod_{i=1}^{n_2}(z - \beta_i) \right)^2 \left(\prod_{i=1}^{n_3}(z - \gamma_i) \right)^3 \cdots \\ &= X_1(z) X_2^2(z) X_3^3(z) \cdots, \end{aligned}$$

then the common greatest divisor of f and f' is $D_1 = X_2 X_3^2 X_4^3 \cdots$. Similarly the greatest common divisor of D_1 and D_1' is $D_2 = X_3 X_4^2 \cdots$, the greatest common divisor of D_2 and D_2' is $D_3 = X_4 \cdots$. This process stops at some polynomial D such that D and D' are coprime. Obviously,

$$f_1(z) = f(z)/D_1(z) = X_1(z) X_2(z) X_3(z) X_4(z) \cdots,$$
$$f_2(z) = D_1(z)/D_2(z) = X_2(z) X_3(z) X_4(z) \cdots,$$
$$f_3(z) = D_2(z)/D_3(z) = X_3(z) X_4(z) \cdots,$$
$$\vdots$$

and $X_1(z) = f_1(z)/f_2(z), X_2(z) = f_2(z)/f_3(z), X_3(z) = f_3(z)/f_4(z), \ldots$. The equations $X_1(z) = 0, X_2(z) = 0, X_3(z) = 0, \ldots$ give all the roots of $f(z) = 0$ (as simple roots).

2. Newton's formula and symmetric functions

The functions on the left-hand side of Eq. (1.4) are called elementary symmetric functions of the variables $z_1, z_2, \ldots, z_n$. Other commonly used symmetric functions of $z_1, z_2, \ldots, z_n$ are:

(a) power sums $S_i = z_1^i + z_2^i + \cdots + z_n^i$, $i = \pm 1, \pm 2, \ldots$;
(b) simple symmetric functions: homogeneous symmetric functions consisting of terms with the same degree of variables. Depending on the number of variables, the simple symmetric functions are divided into two-form functions of the kind $\sum z_1^\alpha z_2^\beta$, three-form functions of the kind $\sum z_1^\alpha z_2^\beta z_3^\gamma$, etc.

It is clear that every symmetric function $f(z_1, z_2, \ldots, z_n)$ can be represented by simple symmetric functions.

Newton's formulas give the connection between the coefficients of the equation $f(z) = \sum_{i=0}^{n} a_i z^{n-i} = \prod_{i=1}^{n}(z - z_i) = 0, a_0 = 1$, and the power sums

$$S_1 + a_1 = 0,$$
$$S_2 + a_1 S_1 + 2a_1 = 0,$$
$$S_3 + a_1 S_2 + a_2 S_1 + 3a_3 = 0, \qquad (2.1)$$
$$\vdots$$
$$S_{n-1} + a_1 S_{n-2} + a_2 S_{n-3} + \cdots + a_{n-2} S_1 + (n-1) a_{n-1} = 0.$$

The proof follows by comparing the expressions

$$f'(z) = \sum_{k=1}^{n} \frac{f(z)}{z - z_k} = \sum_{k=1}^{n} \frac{f(z) - f(z_k)}{z - z_k}$$
$$= \sum_{k=1}^{n} \left[z^{n-1} + (z_k + a_1) z^{n-2} + (z_k^2 + a_1 z_k + a_2) z^{n-3} + \cdots \right.$$

$$+(z_k^{n-1} + a_1 z_k^{n-2} + \cdots + a_{n-1})\Big]$$
$$= nz^{n-1} + (S_1 + na_1)z^{n-2} + (S_2 + a_1 S_1 + na_2)z^{n-3} + \cdots$$
$$+ (S_{n-1} + a_1 S_{n-2} + \cdots + a_{n-2} S_1 + na_{n-1})$$

and
$$f'(z) = nz^{n-1} + (n-1)a_1 z^{n-2} + (n-2)a_2 z^{n-3} + \cdots + a_{n-1}.$$

For the power sums $S_n, S_{n+1}, S_{n+2}, \ldots$, the formulas similar to Eq. (2.1) are

$$\begin{aligned} S_n + a_1 S_{n-1} + a_2 S_{n-2} + \cdots + a_{n-1} S_1 + na_n &= 0, \\ S_{n+1} + a_1 S_n + a_2 S_{n-1} + \cdots + a_{n-1} S_2 + a_n S_1 &= 0, \\ S_{n+2} + a_1 S_{n+1} + a_2 S_n + \cdots + a_{n-1} S_3 + a_n S_2 &= 0, \\ &\vdots \end{aligned} \qquad (2.2)$$

The proof follows directly from

$$\sum_{k=1}^{n} z_k^s f(z_k) = \sum_{k=1}^{n} z_k^s \left[\sum_{i=0}^{n} a_i z_k^{n-i}\right] = 0, \quad s = 0, 1, \ldots.$$

The equalities (2.1) and (2.2) give

$$S_1 = -a_1,$$
$$S_2 = a_1^2 - 2a_2,$$
$$S_3 = -a_1^3 + 3a_1 a_2 - 3a_3,$$
$$S_4 = a_1^4 - 4a_1^2 a_2 + 4a_1 a_3 + 2a_2^2 - 4a_4,$$
$$\vdots$$

$$S_i = - \begin{vmatrix} 1 & 0 & 0 & \cdots & a_1 \\ a_1 & 1 & 0 & \cdots & 2a_2 \\ a_2 & a_1 & 1 & \cdots & 3a_3 \\ \vdots & \vdots & \vdots & & \vdots \\ a_{i-1} & a_{i-2} & a_{i-3} & \cdots & ia_i \end{vmatrix}.$$

Negative power sums $S_{-i}, i = 1, 2, \ldots$, are S_i for the equation $f(1/z) = 0$, which has roots $1/z_s, s = 1, 2, \ldots, n$.

Any k-form simple symmetric function can be represented by power sums. Indeed, the two-form symmetric function $\sum z_1^\alpha z_2^\beta$ satisfies for $\alpha \neq \beta$

$$S_\alpha S_\beta = \sum z_1^\alpha z_2^\beta + S_{\alpha+\beta}, \quad \sum z_1^\alpha z_2^\alpha = \tfrac{1}{2}(S_\alpha^2 - S_{2\alpha}). \qquad (2.3)$$

For three-form symmetric functions $\sum z_1^\alpha z_2^\beta z_3^\gamma$, we have

$$\left(\sum z_1^\alpha z_2^\beta\right) S_\gamma = \sum z_1^\alpha z_2^\beta z_3^\gamma + \sum z_1^{\alpha+\gamma} z_2^\beta + \sum z_1^\alpha z_2^{\beta+\gamma}$$

and by Eq. (2.3)

$$\sum z_1^\alpha z_2^\beta z_3^\gamma = S_\alpha S_\beta S_\gamma - S_{\alpha+\gamma} S_\beta - S_{\alpha+\beta} S_\gamma - S_{\beta+\gamma} S_\alpha + 2S_{\alpha+\beta+\gamma}.$$

This process can continue further.

3. Resolvent and discriminant of polynomials

Let the equations

$$f(z) = \sum_{i=0}^{n} a_i z^{n-i} = 0, \quad \varphi(z) = \sum_{i=0}^{m} b_i z^{m-i} = 0, \tag{3.1}$$

have a common root. A necessary and sufficient condition for this is the equality

$$S(\alpha_1, \alpha_2, \ldots, \alpha_n, \beta_1, \beta_2, \ldots, \beta_m) = \prod_{i=1}^{n}\prod_{j=1}^{m}(\alpha_i - \beta_j) = 0, \tag{3.2}$$

where $\{\alpha_i\}_{i=1}^{n}$ and $\{\beta_i\}_{i=1}^{m}$ are the roots of the Eq. (3.1). The function S in (3.2) is a symmetric function of its arguments and by the results in Section 2, S is a function of $\{a_i/a_0\}_{i=1}^{n}$ and $\{b_i/b_0\}_{i=1}^{m}$ of degree m and n, respectively. The expression

$$R = a_0^m b_0^n S(a_1, a_2, \ldots, a_n, b_1, b_2, \ldots, b_m)$$

is called a resolvent. From

$$f(z) = a_0 \prod_{i=1}^{n}(z - \alpha_i), \quad \varphi(z) = b_0 \prod_{i=1}^{m}(z - \beta_i),$$

follows the simple representation of the resolvent R in the form

$$R = a_0^m \varphi(\alpha_1)\varphi(\alpha_2)\cdots\varphi(\alpha_n) = (-1)^{mn} b_0^n f(\beta_1)f(\beta_2)\cdots f(\beta_m). \tag{3.3}$$

If f and φ have a common root, $\alpha_1 = \beta_1$, then the last equality gives

$$\frac{\partial R}{\partial b_i} = a_0^m \alpha_1^{m-i}\varphi(\alpha_2)\cdots\varphi(\alpha_n) + a_0^m \alpha_2^{m-i}\varphi(\alpha_1)\varphi(\alpha_3)\cdots\varphi(\alpha_n) + \cdots$$

$$+ a_0^m \alpha_n^{m-i}\varphi(\alpha_1)\cdots\varphi(\alpha_{n-1})$$

$$= a_0^m \alpha_1^{m-i}\varphi(\alpha_2)\cdots\varphi(\alpha_n).$$

Similarly,

$$\frac{\partial R}{\partial b_{i-1}} = a_0^m \alpha_1^{m-i+1}\varphi(\alpha_2)\cdots\varphi(\alpha_n)$$

and

$$\alpha_1 = \frac{\partial R}{\partial b_{i-1}} \bigg/ \frac{\partial R}{\partial b_i}, \tag{3.4}$$

i.e. α_1 is a root of the equation

$$\left(\frac{\partial}{\partial b_i} x - \frac{\partial}{\partial b_{i-1}}\right) R = 0.$$

All the above considerations show that the necessary and sufficient condition for Eq. (3.1) to have only one common root is

$$R = 0, \quad \frac{\partial R}{\partial b_i} \neq 0,$$

for some $i \in [1, m]$. This common root is given by Eq. (3.4).

In a similar way, the necessary and sufficient conditions for Eq. (3.1) to have k common roots are

$$R = 0, \quad \frac{\partial R}{\partial b_i} = 0, \quad \frac{\partial^2 R}{\partial b_i^2} = 0, \ldots, \quad \frac{\partial^{k-1} R}{\partial b_i^{k-1}} = 0, \quad \frac{\partial^k R}{\partial b_i^k} \neq 0$$

and they are given by the equation

$$\left(\frac{\partial}{\partial b_i} x - \frac{\partial}{\partial b_{i-1}}\right)^k R = 0.$$

The discriminant $D = D(a_0, a_1, \ldots, a_n)$ of the polynomial (1.1) is an arithmetic expression of its coefficient such that nullification of D is the necessary and sufficient condition for Eq. (1.1) to have multiple roots. If $\{z_i\}_{i=1}^n$ are the roots of the equation $f(z) = \sum_{i=0}^n a_i z^{n-i} = 0$, then using the symmetric function $P(z_1, z_2, \ldots, z_n) = \prod_{i>j}(z_i - z_j)^2$, the discriminant is $D = a_0^{2n-2} P$. Two other representations of D follow from:

(a)

$$D = (-1)^{n(n-1)/2} a_0^{n-2} \left[a_0 \prod_{i \neq 1}(z_1 - z_i)\right] \left[a_0 \prod_{i \neq 2}(z_2 - z_i)\right]$$

$$\cdots \left[a_0 \prod_{i \neq n}(z_n - z_i)\right]$$

$$= (-1)^{n(n-1)/2} a_0^{n-2} f'(z_1) f'(z_2) \cdots f'(z_n);$$

(b) denote by Δ, the Wandermond determinant

$$\Delta = \begin{vmatrix} 1 & 1 & \cdots & 1 \\ z_1 & z_2 & \cdots & z_n \\ \vdots & \vdots & & \vdots \\ z_1^{n-1} & z_2^{n-1} & \cdots & z_n^{n-1} \end{vmatrix} = \prod_{i>j}(z_i - z_j).$$

Then

$$D = a_0^{2n-2} \Delta^2 = a_0^{2n-2} \Delta^T \Delta = a_0^{2n-2} \begin{vmatrix} S_0 & S_1 & S_2 & \cdots & S_{n-1} \\ S_1 & S_2 & S_3 & \cdots & S_n \\ \vdots & \vdots & \vdots & & \vdots \\ S_{n-1} & S_n & S_{n+1} & \cdots & S_{2n-2} \end{vmatrix}.$$

Let R be the resolvent of f and f'. Then from (3.3) it follows that

$$R = a_0^{n-1} f'(z_1) f'(z_2) \cdots f'(z_n)$$

and therefore $R = (-1)^{n(n-1)/2} a_0 D$.

For the quadratic equation $a_0 x^2 + a_1 x + a_2 = 0$ the discriminant is

$$D = a_0^2 (z_1 - z_2)^2 = a_0^2 [(z_1 + z_2)^2 - 4 z_1 z_2] = a_1^2 - 4 a_0 a_2,$$

and for the cubic equation $f(z) = z^3 + pz + q = 0$,

$$D = -f'(z_1) f'(z_2) f'(z_3)$$

$$= -27(z_1 z_2 z_3)^3 - 9p(z_1^2 z_2^2 + z_1^2 z_3^2 + z_2^2 z_3^2) - p^3 - 3p^2(z_1^2 + z_2^2 + z_3^2)$$

$$= -27 q^2 - 4 p^3.$$

4. Algebraic equations from first till fourth degree

For $a \neq 0$, the linear equation $az = b$ has a solution $z_1 = b/a$ and the quadratic equation $az^2 + bz + c = 0$ has two roots

$$z_{1,2} = \frac{-b \pm \sqrt{b^2 - 4ac}}{2a}.$$

The substitution $z = u - a/3$ transforms the cubic equation $z^3 + az^2 + bz + c = 0$ into

$$u^3 + pu + q = 0, \tag{4.1}$$

where $p = -a^2/3 + b, q = 2a^3/27 - ab/3 + c$.

Cardano's formula for the solution of (4.1) is $u = A + B$, where

$$A = \sqrt[3]{-\frac{q}{2} + \sqrt{\Delta}}, \quad B = \sqrt[3]{-\frac{q}{2} - \sqrt{\Delta}}, \quad \Delta = \frac{q^2}{4} + \frac{p^3}{27}.$$

Note that separately A and B can take three values and therefore $A + B$ can have nine values. Choosing A and B to satisfy the condition $AB = -p/3$, the solution of (4.1) is

$$u_1 = A + B, \quad u_{2,3} = -\frac{A + B}{2} \pm i \frac{A - B}{2} \sqrt{3}, \quad i^2 = -1.$$

For the equation of the fourth degree, $z^4 + az^3 + bz^2 + cz + d = 0$, the substitution $z = u - a/4$ transforms it into the incomplete type

$$u^4 + pu^2 + qu + r = 0. \tag{4.2}$$

Let $\alpha_1^2, \alpha_2^2, \alpha_3^2$ be the roots of the cubic equation

$$\alpha^3 + 2p\alpha^2 + (p^2 - 4r)\alpha - q^2 = 0.$$

Then the roots of Eq. (4.2) are

$$u_{1,2} = \frac{-\alpha_1 \pm (\alpha_2 + \alpha_3)}{2}, \quad u_{3,4} = \frac{\alpha_1 \pm (\alpha_2 - \alpha_3)}{2}.$$

Detailed investigation of the roots of Eqs. (4.1) and (4.2) can be found in OBRESHKOV [1962].

For the first time, in 1799, the Italian mathematician Paolo Ruffini proved (with some incompletenesses) that it is not possible to find algebraic expressions for the roots of Eq. (1.1) when $n > 4$ (*Teoria generale delle Equazioni, in cui si dimonstra impossibile la soluzione algebraica delle equazioni generali di grado superiore al quarto, Bologna*). ABEL [1826] gave a strong proof of the problem. Galoa's theory solves the problem for conditions under which the roots of Eq. (1.1) can be expressed explicitly.

5. Number of roots in an interval

Let us consider the question of determining the number of roots of the equation with real coefficients,

$$f(x) = \sum_{i=0}^{n} a_i x^{n-i} = 0 \tag{5.1}$$

in a given interval $[a, b]$. In 1690, in his paper *Traite d'Algebre*, Rolle proved that, between consecutive real zeros of (5.1), the derivative f' has a root. An immediate corollary to this is that if Eq. (5.1) has m zeros in $[a, b]$, then the equation $f'(x) = 0$ has at least $m - 1$ roots in $[a, b]$.

THEOREM 5.1 (HERMITE [1866], POULAIN [1867]). See OBRESHKOV [1963a], HOUSEHOLDER [1970]. *If the polynomial* (5.1) *has real coefficients and the polynomial*

$$g(x) = \sum_{i=0}^{n} c_i x^{n-i}, \quad c_0 c_n \neq 0,$$

has only real roots, then the polynomial

$$h(x) = c_0 f^{(n)}(x) + c_1 f^{(n-1)}(x) + \cdots + c_n f(x)$$

has at least as many real zeros as the polynomial f. If f has only real zeros, then each multiple root of $h(x) = 0$ is also a multiple root of f.

The Hermite–Poulain theorem is an important tool for proving the reality of the roots in some cases. For example:

(a) Let $\sum_{i=0}^{n} a_i x^{n-i} = 0$ have only real roots. This means that the equation $\sum_{i=0}^{n} a_i x^i = 0$ also has only real roots. Letting $f(x) = x^n$ we obtain $h(x) = n!a_0 + (n-1)!a_1 x + \cdots + n a_{n-1} x^{n-1} + a_n x^n$. Therefore, $\sum_{i=0}^{n} a_i x^i / i! = 0$ has only real roots.

(b) Let us denote $Df = f'$. Then the polynomial h in the Hermite–Poulain theorem can be written as

$$h(x) = c_0 D^n f(x) + c_1 D^{n-1} f(x) + \cdots + c_n f(x) = g(D) f(x).$$

If $g(0) \neq 0$, the expansion $1/g(x) = b_0+b_1x+b_2x^2+\cdots$ shows that the polynomial
$$\varphi(x) = b_0 f(x) + b_1 f'(x) + \cdots + b_n f^{(n)}(x)$$
has less or equal real roots than the polynomial f. Indeed, it is enough for the Hermite–Poulain theorem to be applied to φ and to use the equality $f(x) = g(D)\varphi(x)$.

(c) For an arbitrary real number $\alpha \notin (-n, 0)$, the polynomial $\alpha f(x) + xf'(x)$ does not have less real roots than the n-degree polynomial f with real coefficients; as a consequence of the Hermite–Poulain theorem, the next result of Laguerre follows: if the m-degree polynomial $g(x)$ with real coefficients has only real zeros, none of which lies on the interval $(0, n)$, then $h(x) = \sum_{i=0}^{n} a_i x^i g(i)$ does not have less real zeros than $\sum_{i=0}^{n} a_i x^i$.

THEOREM 5.2 (OBRESHKOV [1963a]). *If $f(x)$ and $g(x)$ are real polynomials of degrees differing by at most 1 and having no common zero, then a necessary and sufficient condition for their zeros to be real and distinct and to separate each other is that $h(x) = \lambda f(x) + \mu g(x)$ has only distinct real zeros for all real λ and μ.*

Descartes gave a method (*Descartes' rule of signs*) for determining the upper bound of the number of positive zeros of real polynomials.

Given a real n-degree polynomial (suppose that the terms with zero coefficients are omitted), it is said that between two consecutive coefficients there is a variation of their signs if these two coefficients, have opposite signs. For example, the number of variations in the polynomial $x^5 + x^3 - 5x^3 + 2 = 0$ is 2.

THEOREM 5.3 (Descartes' rule of signs). *The number N of positive roots of Eq. (5.1) is less than or equal to the number V of variations in the sequence of its coefficients. If $V - N > 0$, then $V - N$ is an even number.*

THEOREM 5.4. *If all the roots of Eq. (5.1) are real, then the number of positive roots is equal to the number of variations of coefficients of $f(x)$ and the number of negative roots is equal to the number of variations of coefficients of $f(-x)$.*

THEOREM 5.5. *Let $\alpha > 0$. The number N of positive roots of (5.1) greater than α is not greater than the number V of variations in the sequence*
$$f_0(\alpha) = \alpha,$$
$$f_1(\alpha) = a_0\alpha + a_1,$$
$$f_2(\alpha) = a_0\alpha^2 + a_1\alpha + a_2,$$
$$\vdots$$
$$f_n(\alpha) = f(\alpha) = a_0\alpha^n + a_1\alpha^{n-1} + \cdots + a_n,$$
and $V - N$ is an even number.

Applying the last theorem to the equation $x^n f(1/x)$, it follows that the number of roots N of the equation $f(x) = 0$ in $(0, \alpha), \alpha > 0$, is not greater than the number of variations V in the sequences

$$a_n,$$
$$a_n + a_{n-1}\alpha,$$
$$a_n + a_{n-1}\alpha + a_{n-2}\alpha^2,$$
$$\vdots$$
$$a_n + a_{n-1}\alpha + a_{n-2}\alpha^2 + \cdots + a_0\alpha^n,$$

and $V - N$ is an even number.

Let Eq. (5.1) have real coefficients. The sequence

$$f(x), f'(x), \ldots, f^{(n)}(x), \qquad (5.2)$$

is called the Fourier sequence. Let $V(x)$ denote the number of variations in (5.2).

THEOREM 5.6 (BUDAN [1826] and FOURIER [1831]). *For arbitrary real numbers α and β, $\alpha < \beta$, the number of roots N of (5.1) that lie in (α, β) satisfies the condition $N \leqslant V(\alpha) - V(\beta)$. If $V(\alpha) - V(\beta) - N > 0$, then the difference $V(\alpha) - V(\beta) - N$ is an even number.*

Theorem 5.3 is a corollary of Theorem 5.6. Indeed, the sequence (5.2) for $x = 0$ is

$$a_n, a_{n-1}, 2!a_{n-2}, 3!a_{n-3}, \ldots, (n-1)!a_1, n!a_0,$$

and for $x = \infty$, all terms in (5.2) have the sign of a_0, i.e. $V(\infty) = 0$ and $V = V(0)$. The number of positive roots of (5.1) is the number of roots in $(0, \infty)$ and the number of variations V of $f(x)$ is $V = V(0) - V(\infty)$.

For example, the number of the roots of the equation

$$f(x) = x^4 - 5x^2 + 4 = 0 \qquad (5.3)$$

in the intervals $(-\infty, 0), (0, 1.5), (1.5, 3), (3, \infty)$ are determined as follows:

	$-\infty$	0	1.5	3	∞
$f(x) = x^4 - 5x^2 + 4$	+	+	−	+	+
$f'(x) = 4x^3 - 10x$	−	0	+	+	+
$f''(x) = 12x^2 - 10$	+	−	+	+	+
$f'''(x) = 24x$	−	0	+	+	+
$f^{(4)}(x) = 24$	+	+	+	+	+
$V(x)$	4	2	1	0	0

It is seen that two roots lies in $(-\infty, 0)$, each of the intervals $(0, 1.5)$ and $(1.5, 3)$ contain one root and no root lies in $(3, \infty)$. The roots of (5.3) are $\pm 1, \pm 2$.

The theorem can, in fact, be slightly strengthened as follows. If the derivative $f^{(k)}(x)$ does not vanish in the interval (a,b), then it is sufficient to consider only the variations of sign in the sequence

$$f(x), f'(x), \ldots, f^{(k)}(x)$$

at a and b.

Another extension of Descartes' rule of signs are the following theorems by Laguerre.

THEOREM 5.7. *Let the series*

$$f(x) = a_0 + a_1 x + a_2 x^2 + \cdots$$

with real coefficients converge for $|x| < \alpha$. Then the number of zeros of $f(x)$ on the real interval $[0, \alpha)$ cannot exceed the number of variations of sign in the sequence of coefficients. If the number of variations is finite and the series diverges for $x = \alpha$, then the difference is an even integer.

THEOREM 5.8. *Let $f(x) = a_0 x^n + \cdots + a_n$ be a real polynomial, and let, for $\alpha > 0$,*

$$\frac{f(x)}{x - \alpha} = b_0 x^{n-1} + b_1 x^{n-2} + \cdots + b_{n-1} + \frac{f(\alpha)}{x - \alpha}.$$

Then the number of zeros of $f(x)$ greater than α is equal to the number of variations of sign in the sequence

$$b_0, b_1, \ldots, b_{n-1}, f(\alpha)$$

or is less by an even integer.

Let $f(x)$ be a polynomial for which Eq. (5.1) has simple zeros only. Applying the Euclidean algorithm (1.5) to $f(x)$ and $f'(x)$,

$$\begin{aligned}
f(x) &= f'(x) Q_1(x) - R_1(x), \\
f'(x) &= R_1(x) Q_2(x) - R_2(x), \\
R_1(x) &= R_2(x) Q_3(x) - R_3(x), \\
&\vdots \\
R_{k-2}(x) &= R_{k-1}(x) Q_k(x) - R_k(x),
\end{aligned}$$

and taking the residuals with opposite sign, the sequence

$$f, f', R_1, R_2, \ldots, R_k \tag{5.4}$$

is called a Sturm sequence. Since $f(x) = 0$ does not have multiple roots, the last residual R_k is a constant different from zero.

More generally, the Sturm sequence is every sequence of polynomials

$$f(x), f_1(x), \ldots, f_m(x), \tag{5.5}$$

that satisfies the following four properties:

(i) two consecutive terms of the sequence cannot vanish at the same time;
(ii) if for some x an intermediate function vanishes, then its neighboring functions have opposite signs;
(iii) the last function $f_m(x)$ does not vanish. The sequence (5.4) has one further property:
(iv) in a close neighborhood of a root of Eq. (5.1) $f(x)$ and $f'(x)$ have opposite signs in front of the root and equal signs following the root.

A well-known theorem which gives the exact number of the real roots of Eq. (5.1) is the following

THEOREM 5.9 (STURM [1829]). *Let Eq.* (5.1) *have simple zeros only. The number of its zeros lying in the interval* (a,b) *is equal to* $V(a) - V(b)$, *where* $V(a)$ *and* $V(b)$ *are the number of variations of sequence* (5.4) *for* $x = a$ *and* $x = b$.

In the case where Eq. (5.1) has multiple zeros, the Sturm theorem states the following.

THEOREM 5.10. *Equation* (5.1) *has* $V(a) - V(b)$ *different roots in the interval* (a,b) *under the condition that each root, simple or multiple, is counted as one.*

Sturm has shown that this theorem can be generalized using the sequence (5.5) as follows.

THEOREM 5.11. *The number of the roots of Eq.* (5.1) *in the interval* (a,b) *is at least equal to* $|V(a) - V(b)|$, *where* $V(a)$ *and* $V(b)$ *are the number of variations of the sequence* (5.5) *for* $x = a$ *and* $x = b$.

If the polynomial $f(x)$ is given, we can easily find a sequence (5.5) possessing the three properties mentioned, namely let $\phi(x)$ be any real polynomial whose degree is less than the degree of $f(x)$, and let us divide

$$f(x) = \phi(x)Q_1(x) - R_1(x),$$

$$\phi(x) = R_1(x)Q_2(x) - R_2(x),$$

$$R_1(x) = R_2(x)Q_3(x) - R_3(x),$$

$$\vdots$$

We stop at the polynomial R_m, which does not vanish in the interval (a,b). Then the sequence

$$f(x), \phi(x), R_1, R_2, \ldots, R_m,$$

has the three properties mentioned.

See OBRESHKOV [1963a] and HOUSEHOLDER [1970] for the proofs of these theorems.

OBRESHKOV [1928] simplified Theorem 5.6 by considering finite differences instead of derivatives of the polynomial. He proved the following.

THEOREM 5.12. *Let $f(x) = 0$ be an algebraic equation of nth degree with real coefficients and let $V(x)$ be the number of variations of the sequence*

$$f(x), \Delta_h f(x), \Delta_h^2 f(x), \ldots, \Delta_h^n f(x),$$

where $\Delta_h f(x) = f(x+h) - f(x)$, $\Delta_h^k f(x) = \Delta^{k-1} f(x+h) - \Delta^{k-1} f(x)$, $k = 1, 2, \ldots$. Then the number of roots in the interval (a, b) is not greater than $V(a_1) - V(b)$, where $b - a = mh$, m is an integer and $a_1 = a - (n-1)h$.

6. Number of roots in a domain

The well-known *argument principle* states that

$$N - P = \frac{1}{2\pi} \underset{C}{\mathrm{Var}}\, \mathrm{Arg}\, f(z),$$

where N and P are the numbers of zeros and poles of the function f in the domain D on the complex plane, C is a rectifiable Jordan curve which is a contour of D and $\underset{C}{\mathrm{Var}}\, \mathrm{Arg}\, f(z)$ is the variation of $\mathrm{Arg}\, f(z)$ at the by-pass of C in the positive direction.

For the first time, Cauchy applied the argument principle to determine the number of roots of a polynomial equation

$$f(z) = \sum_{i=0}^{n} a_i z^{n-i} = 0, \tag{6.1}$$

in a given complex domain. Because of lack of poles of polynomials, the argument principle can be simplified. Indeed, let us assume that on the closed curve C, Eq. (6.1) has no roots. Let the roots that are in C be $u_1, u_2, \ldots, u_k$ and those out of C be $v_1, v_2, \ldots, v_m$. Letting

$$z - u_p = r_p(\cos \varphi_p + i \sin \varphi_p), \quad p = 1, 2, \ldots, k,$$
$$z - v_p = t_p(\cos \psi_p + i \sin \psi_p), \quad p = 1, 2, \ldots, m,$$
$$f(z) = R(\cos \Phi + i \sin \Phi) = P + iQ,$$

from the equality

$$f(z) = a_0 \prod_{s=1}^{k}(z - u_s) \prod_{s=1}^{m}(z - v_s) = R(\cos \Phi + i \sin \Phi),$$

if $a_0 = r(\cos \varphi + i \sin \varphi)$, then we have

$$\Phi = \varphi_1 + \varphi_2 + \cdots + \varphi_k + \psi_1 + \psi_2 + \cdots + \psi_m + \varphi.$$

Since $R\cos\Phi = P$, $R\sin\Phi = Q$, it follows that $\tan\Phi = Q/P$.

When z rotates entirely on the curve C, the angles $\varphi_i, i = 1, 2, \ldots, k$ increase by 2π and the angles $\psi_i, i = 1, 2, \ldots, m$, do not change their values (see Fig. 6.1). This means that after one rotation of z on C, the argument of $f(z)$ increases with $2k\pi$.

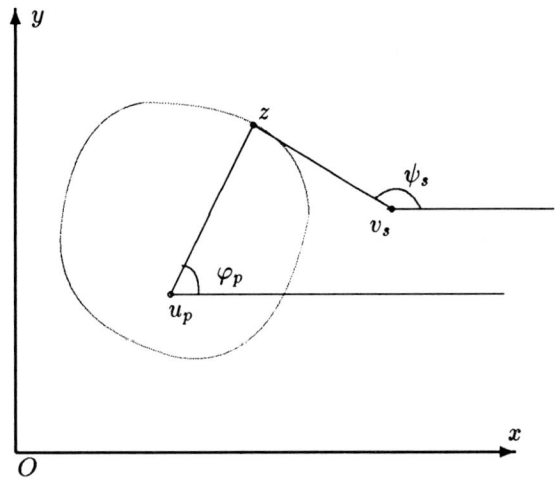

FIG. 6.1.

Let us note that for every change of Φ by 2π the quantity $\tan\Phi$ increases twice from negative to positive values. Therefore, after the complete rotation of z on C, Φ increases by $2k\pi$ and denoting by p the number of times $\tan\Phi$ vanishes when Φ passes from negative to positive, and by q nullification of $\tan\Phi$, when Φ passes from positive to negative, then $p - q = 2k$. The next theorem summarizes the above considerations.

THEOREM 6.1. *The number of roots of the equation $f(z) = P + iQ = 0$ that lie in a closed simple contour C is half of the difference of the number of nullifications of Q/P from negative to positive and from positive to negative when z rotates once on C.*

The basis of the proof of Theorem 6.1 lies in the variation of the argument and a series of results follow from this theorem:

RESULT 6.1. *If the polynomials f and g satisfy the inequality $|f(z)| > |g(z)|$ on the closed curve C, then the equations $f(z) = 0$ and $f(z) + g(z) = 0$ have an equal number of roots inside C.*

PROOF. Let $f(z) = 0$ have p roots inside C. Then $\operatorname{Arg} f(z)$ increases with $2\pi p$ after one rotation of z on C. The point

$$1 + \varphi(z)/f(z) = 1 + u$$

belongs to the disc with center $(1, 0)$ and radii < 1. Hence, $\mathrm{Arg}(1+u)$ does not change its value after a rotation of z on C. From

$$\mathrm{Arg}\, f(z)[1+u] = \mathrm{Arg}\, f(z) + \mathrm{Arg}[1+u]$$

by Theorem 6.1 it follows that the function $f(z) + \varphi(z) = f(z)[1+u]$ has p roots inside C. □

RESULT 6.2. *The roots of the algebraic equation $f(z) = 0$ are continuous functions of its coefficients.*

PROOF. Let $f(\alpha) = 0$ and in the disc $D_\rho = \{z\colon |z - \alpha| \leqslant \rho\}$ there are no other roots. Since $f(z) \neq 0$ on $C_\rho = \{z\colon |z - \alpha| = \rho\}$, there exists a polynomial g for which $|f - g| < |f|$ on C_ρ and the coefficients of g differ a little bit from these of f. By Theorem 6.1, the number of the roots of g inside C_ρ is equal to the multiplicity of α. As ρ can be taken arbitrary small the assertion follows. □

RESULT 6.3. *If $\lim_{m \to \infty} a_{im} = a_i, i = 0, 1, \ldots, n$, then the roots of the polynomials*

$$f_m(z) = a_{0m} z^n + a_{1m} z^{n-1} + \cdots + a_{nm},$$

converge to the roots of the polynomial

$$f(z) = a_0 z^n + a_1 z^{n-1} + \cdots + a_n,$$

and if the roots of f_m are real, so are the roots of f.

RESULT 6.4. *Let the coefficients of the equation*

$$f(z) = a_n z^n + a_{n-1} z^{n-1} + \cdots + a_0$$

satisfy $|a_p| > |a_0| + \cdots + |a_{p-1}| + |a_{p+1}| + \cdots + |a_n|$. Then in the disc $|z| < 1$, this equation has exactly p roots.

On the circle $|z| = 1$, we have

$$|f(z) - a_p z^p| \leqslant |a_0| + \cdots + |a_{p-1}| + |a_{p+1}| + \cdots + |a_n| < |a_p| = |a_p z^p|$$

and by Theorem 6.1, it follows that the number of roots of $f(z) = 0$ and $a_p z^p = 0$ in the disc $|z| < 1$ is equal, i.e. it is p.

RESULT 6.5. PELLET [1924] *proved that if, for the polynomial*

$$f(z) = a_n z^n + a_{n-1} z^{n-1} + \cdots + a_0,$$

the equation

$$F(z) = |a_0| + \cdots + |a_{p-1}| z^{p-1} - |a_p| z^p + |a_{p+1}| z^{p+1} + \cdots + |a_n| z^n = 0$$

has two positive roots $\alpha, \beta, \alpha < \beta$, then the polynomial f has exactly p roots in the disc $|z| \leqslant \alpha$ and has no roots in the domain $\alpha < |z| < \beta$.

PROOF. By Theorem 5.3, the equation $F(z) = 0$ has only α and β as positive roots. Let $\alpha < r < \beta$. Since $F(0) > 0, F(\infty) > 0$, it is clear that $F(z) < 0$ for $\alpha < z < \beta$ and from $F(r) < 0$, it follows that

$$|a_p| r^p > |a_0| + \cdots + |a_{p-1}| r^{p-1} + |a_{p+1}| r^{p+1} + \cdots + |a_n| r^n.$$

The last inequality shows that the polynomials
$$\varphi(z) = a_0 + \cdots + a_{p-1}z^{p-1} + a_{p+1}z^{p+1} + \cdots + a_n z^n, \qquad \psi(z) = a_p z^p,$$
satisfy the condition $|\varphi(z)| < |\psi(z)|$ on the circle $|z| = r$ and by Result 6.1, the polynomial $f(z) = \varphi(z) + \psi(z)$ and $\psi(z)$ have an equal number of roots in $|z| < r$. This number is p. Since r can be taken arbitrary close to α or β, the polynomial f has exactly p roots in $|z| \leqslant \alpha$ and has no roots in $\alpha < |z| < \beta$. $\square$

The idea for variation of the argument is used in the following.

THEOREM 6.2 (BIEHLER [1879], HERMITE [1879]). *If the equation $f(z) = U(z) + iV(z) = 0$ has roots only from one side of the real axis, where U and V are real polynomials, then the roots of the equations $U = 0$, $V = 0$ are real and mutually separated.*

If the real polynomials U and V have only real and mutually separated roots, then the roots of the polynomial $f(z) = U(z) + iV(z)$ lie on one side of the real axis.

7. Algebraic equations with a negative real part of the roots

Investigation of the stability of mechanical systems and other questions in mechanics leads to conditions which guarantee that all the roots of the equation
$$f(z) = a_0 z^n + a_1 z^{n-1} + \cdots + a_n, \quad a_0 > 0, \tag{7.1}$$
with real coefficients have a negative real part. Such polynomials are called Hurwitz polynomials (HURWITZ [1896]) or *stable* polynomials. We briefly present the basic results in this field without proofs. The proofs, with additional comments and history, can be found in OBRESHKOV [1963a].

THEOREM 7.1. *If Eq. (7.1) has roots only on the left-hand side of the imaginary axis, then all its coefficients are positive.*

The proof of the theorem is trivial.

Theorem 6.2 and the converse assertion also belong to the problem. ROUCHE [1862] proved the following.

THEOREM 7.2. *The necessary and sufficient condition that all the roots of the equation*
$$f(z) = a_0 z^n + a_1 z^{n-1} + \cdots + a_n = 0$$
lie on the left-hand side of the imaginary axis is that the elements of the first column in the table

a_0	a_2	a_4	a_6	a_8	$\cdots$
a_1	a_3	a_5	a_7	a_9	$\cdots$
α_0	α_2	α_4	α_6	α_8	$\cdots$
β_0	β_2	β_4	β_6	β_8	$\cdots$
$\vdots$					

are different from zero and have equal sign.

The table in Theorem 7.2 is built as follows: the element in the kth place in the third row is the product of the first element of the second row and the $(k+1)$th element of the first row minus the product of the first element in the first row and $(k+1)$th element of the second row and all this divided by the first element of the second row. In the same way, the elements in the fourth row can be obtained by the elements of the second and third rows, etc.

For example, for the equation $x^4 + 3x^3 + 4x^2 + 3x + 1 = 0$ we have

```
1  4  1
3  3  0
3  1
2
1
```

and by Theorem 7.2 this equation has only roots with a negative real part.

HURWITZ [1896] gave another solution of the problem as follows.

THEOREM 7.3. *The necessary and sufficient condition for the equation*

$$f(z) = a_n z^n + a_{n-1} z^{n-1} + \cdots + a_0 = 0, \quad a_0 > 0,$$

with real coefficients to have only roots with a negative real part is the positivity of the determinants

$$\Delta_s^{(n)} = \begin{vmatrix} a_1 & a_0 & 0 & 0 & 0 & 0 & \cdots \\ a_3 & a_2 & a_1 & a_0 & 0 & 0 & \cdots \\ a_5 & a_4 & a_3 & a_2 & a_1 & a_0 & \cdots \\ \vdots & & & & & & \\ a_{2s-1} & a_{2s-2} & & \cdots & & & a_s \end{vmatrix}, \quad s = 1, 2, \ldots, n,$$

where $a_s = 0$ for $s > n$.

Let us denote

$$f^*(z) \equiv \bar{a}_0(-z)^n + \bar{a}_1(-z)^{n-1} + \cdots + \bar{a}_n,$$

where $f(z) = a_0 z^n + a_1 z^{n-1} + \cdots + a_n$ and $\bar{a}$ means the conjugate value of a. The following theorems are due to SCHUR [1914, 1921, 1933] (see also OBRESHKOV [1963a]).

THEOREM 7.4. *If the complex numbers α and β satisfy $|\alpha| > |\beta|$, then the polynomials $f(z)$ and $\alpha f(z) - \beta f^*(z)$ are simultaneously either Hurwitz polynomials or not.*

THEOREM 7.5. *The polynomial $f(z)$ has all its roots with a negative real part if the same is true for the polynomial*

$$F(z, \xi) = \frac{f^*(\xi) f(z) - f(\xi) f^*(z)}{z - \xi}$$

and $|f(\xi)| < |f^*(\xi)|$, where ξ is an arbitrary number for which $\Re(\xi) < 0$.

Since $F(z,\xi)$ is a polynomial of degree $n-1$ with respect to ξ, then

$$F(z,\xi) = F_0(z) + \xi F_1(z) + \cdots + \xi^{n-1} F_{n-1}(z).$$

THEOREM 7.6. *Let ξ be an arbitrary number with a negative real part. The polynomial $f(z)$ is a Hurwitz polynomial if and only if $a_n \neq 0, \Re(a_{n-1}/a_n) > 0$ and such is the polynomial $F_0(z) + \xi F_1(z)$ of degree $n-1$.*

Suppose that the real polynomial

$$f(x) = a_0 x^n + a_1 x^{n-1} + \cdots + a_n, \quad a_0 > 0, \tag{7.2}$$

is stable. How much can the coefficients $\{a_i\}$ be perturbed while the polynomial (7.2) remains stable.

BIALAS and GARLOFF [1985] considered the problem as follows: let the real numbers $b_k \geqslant 0, c_k \geqslant 0$, $k = 0, 1, \ldots, n$, be given. Find the largest $t_0 \geqslant 0$ such that the polynomial $\alpha_0 x^n + \alpha_1 x^{n-1} + \cdots + \alpha_n$ is stable for

$$\alpha_k \in (a_k - b_k t_0, a_k + c_k t_0) \cup \{a_k\}, k = 0, 1, \ldots, n.$$

They give a simple determinant criterion and an approach for obtaining the largest t_0.

This problem was posed and solved for quartics by GUIVER and BOSE [1983] and for polynomials of arbitrary degree by BARMISH [1984].

THEOREM 7.7 (KHARITONOV [1978]). *The polynomial*

$$\alpha_0 x^n + \alpha_1 x^{n-1} + \cdots + \alpha_n$$

is stable for all $\alpha_k \in [\underline{a}_k, \bar{a}_k], k = 0, 1, \ldots, n$, if and only if the polynomials

$$f_1(x) = \underline{a}_0 x^n + \underline{a}_1 x^{n-1} + \bar{a}_2 x^{n-2} + \bar{a}_3 x^{n-3} + \underline{a}_4 x^{n-4} + \cdots$$

$$f_2(x) = \bar{a}_0 x^n + \underline{a}_1 x^{n-1} + \underline{a}_2 x^{n-2} + \bar{a}_3 x^{n-3} + \bar{a}_4 x^{n-4} + \cdots$$

$$f_3(x) = \bar{a}_0 x^n + \bar{a}_1 x^{n-1} + \underline{a}_2 x^{n-2} + \underline{a}_3 x^{n-3} + \bar{a}_4 x^{n-4} + \cdots$$

$$f_4(x) = \underline{a}_0 x^n + \bar{a}_1 x^{n-1} + \bar{a}_2 x^{n-2} + \underline{a}_3 x^{n-3} + \underline{a}_4 x^{n-4} + \cdots$$

are stable.

8. Number of roots in a disc

Let us consider the problem of determining the number of roots of the equation

$$f(z) = a_0 z^n + a_1 z^{n-1} + \cdots + a_n = 0, \quad a_0 \neq 0, \tag{8.1}$$

inside the circle C with center α and radius r. By the substitution $z = \alpha + ru$, the circle C transforms into the unit circle and therefore only the unit circle is considered.

THEOREM 8.1 (SCHUR [1921]). *All the roots of Eq.* (8.1) *lie inside the unit circle if and only if* $|a_0| > |a_n|$ *and all the roots of the polynomial of degree* $n - 1$,

$$\frac{1}{z}[\bar{a}_0 f(z) - a_n f^*(z)]$$

also lie inside the unit circle, where

$$f^*(z) = \bar{a}_n z^n + \bar{a}_{n-1} z^{n-1} + \cdots + \bar{a}_0.$$

COHN [1922] gives a method for determining the exact number of roots inside a given circle and on the circle. Cohn's rule is:

(1) if $|a_0| > |a_n|$, build the polynomial

$$z f_1(z) = \bar{a}_0 f(z) - a_n f^*(z),$$

where f_1 is a polynomial of degree $n - 1$. Then the polynomial f has one zero more inside C than f_1;

(2) if $|a_0| < |a_n|$, build the polynomial f_1 of degree $n - 1$,

$$f_1(z) = \bar{a}_n f(z) - a_0 f^*(z).$$

The polynomials f and f_1 have an equal number of roots inside C;

(3) if $a_0 = \varepsilon \bar{a}_n, a_1 = \varepsilon \bar{a}_{n-1}, \ldots, a_{k-1} = \varepsilon \bar{a}_{n-k+1}$, where $|\varepsilon| = 1, k \leqslant \left[\frac{1}{2}n\right], a_k \neq \bar{a}_{n-k}$, setting $b = (a_k - \varepsilon \bar{a}_{n-k})/a_0$, we can apply (2) for the polynomial of degree $n + k$, $G(z) = (z^k + 2b/|b|) f(z)$. Then we obtain a polynomial of degree n, which has the same number of roots as f;

(4) if there is no k, such that $a_k \neq \varepsilon \bar{a}_{n-k}$, then $a_k = \varepsilon \bar{a}_{n-k}, |\varepsilon| = 1, k = 0, 1, \ldots, n$. The polynomial $f_1(z) = z^{n-1} f'(1/z)$ and f have the same number of roots inside C;

(5) to determine the number of roots that lie on the unit circle, the rule is: after application of points (1)–(3), let the polynomial f_m be the first polynomial that is obtained by (4) and let the polynomial

$$f_{m+1}(z) = z^{s-1} f'_m(1/z)$$

have p zeros in the unit circle. Then f has $s - 2p$ zeros on the unit circle, where s is the degree of f_m.

THEOREM 8.2. *The necessary and sufficient condition for the roots of Eq.* (8.1) *to lie on the unit circle is* $a_k = \varepsilon \bar{a}_{n-k}, |\varepsilon| = 1, k = 0, \ldots, n$, *and the roots of the equation* $f'(z) = 0$ *must lie in the unit disc.*

9. The Gauss–Lucas theorem and Sendov's conjecture

Let us consider Gauss' mechanical interpretation of the zeros of polynomials (GAUSS [1850]). The point ν is called a critical point for the polynomial

$$f(z) = \sum_{i=0}^{n} a_i z^{n-i} = a_0 \prod_{i=1}^{n} (z - z_i) \qquad (9.1)$$

if $f'(\nu) = 0$. If $\nu \neq z_i, i = 1, 2, \ldots, n$, then from

$$\frac{f'(\nu)}{f(\nu)} = \sum_{i=1}^{n} \frac{1}{\nu - z_i} = 0, \qquad (9.2)$$

it follows that

$$\sum_{i=1}^{n} \frac{1}{\bar{\nu} - \bar{z}_i} = \sum_{i=1}^{n} \frac{1}{d_i} e_i = 0, \qquad (9.3)$$

where $\bar{z}$ is the conjugate value of z, $e_i = (\nu - z_i)/d_i$ is the unit vector from z_i to ν. At the points $\{z_i\}_{i=1}^{n}$ let equal power sources be located and these sources repulse every point of the complex plane with power inversely proportional to the distance to this point. The Eqs. (9.2), (9.3) show that the point ν is a point of equilibrium. Thus, the zeros of the derivative of (9.1) are points of equilibrium in this force field. Let the points $\{z_i\}_{i=1}^{n}$ lie in a convex domain D. From a mechanical point of view, every point $\xi \notin D$ can not be in stable equilibrium, because the resultant of the powers is different from zero, i.e. all the roots of the derivative lie in D. This is the contents of the following theorem.

THEOREM 9.1 (GAUSS [1850], LUCAS [1874]). *If all the roots of the polynomial (9.1) lie in a convex domain D, then D contains all the roots of its derivative.*

SENDOV'S CONJECTURE. Let all the roots of the polynomial

$$f(z) = z^n + a_1 z^{n-1} + \cdots + a_n = 0, \quad n > 0,$$

lie in the unit disc $U = \{z \colon |z| \leqslant 1\}$. Then if $f(\alpha) = 0$, there exists a ξ such that $f'(\xi) = 0$ and $|\alpha - \xi| \leqslant 1$.

Sendov's conjecture is evident for $n = 2$, because f has two roots z_1, z_2 and f' has one root $\xi = (z_1 + z_2)/2$. Sendov proved his conjecture for $n = 3, 4$. MEIR and SHARMA [1969] proved the case $n = 5$ under some restrictions. For the history of the problem, see MARDEN [1983].

A similar, but stronger conjecture was put forth by GOODMAN, RAHMAN and RATTI [1969] and independently by SCHMEISSER [1969]: if the roots of the polynomial f lie in U and β is a root of f, then the disc

$$\{z \colon |z - \beta/2| \leqslant 1 - |\beta|/2\}$$

contains at least one root of f'.

The connection between these two conjecture follows from

$$\{z \colon |z - \beta/2| \leqslant 1 - |\beta|/2\} \subseteq \{z \colon |z - \beta| \leqslant 1\}.$$

More than twenty papers have been published on these conjectures and for reference, see MILLER [1990].

Let us denote by $C(\alpha, r)$ the circle with center α and radius r. If $f(\nu) = 0$, the circle $C(\nu, 2)$ contains all the roots of f' by Theorem 9.1. On the other hand, all the roots of the polynomial $g(z) = z^n - 1$ lie on the unit circle and g' vanishes only at the origin. This means that the constant 1 in Sendov's conjecture can not be decreased and the minimal radius r^* for which the circle $C(\nu, r^*)$ contains the critical point satisfies $1 \leqslant r^* \leqslant 2$.

THEOREM 9.2 (DIMITROV [1983]). *If the roots of the polynomial* (9.1) *lie in* U *and α is an arbitrary root, then the circle*

$$C\left(\alpha, 1 + \frac{n-1}{n}|\alpha|\right)$$

contains at least one zero of the derivative, i.e. $r^* \leqslant 2 - 1/n$.

The formulas (1.4) give a better estimation $r^* \leqslant 2/n^{1/(n-1)}$.
Let P_n be the set of all polynomials whose roots lie in U. For

$$f \in P_n, \quad f(z) = \prod_{i=1}^{n}(z - z_i), \quad f'(z) = n\prod_{i=1}^{n-1}(z - \xi_i)$$

let

$$r(z_k) = \min_{1 \leqslant i \leqslant n-1} |z_k - \xi_i|,$$
$$r(f) = \max_{1 \leqslant k \leqslant n} |r(z_k)|,$$
$$r(P_n) = \sup_{f \in P_n} r(f).$$

The polynomial $f^* \in P_n$ that satisfies $r(f^*) = r(P_n)$ is called extremal. The existence of extremal polynomials is proved by PHELPS and RODRIGUEZS [1972]. They proved that if the root z_k of the extremal polynomial f^* lies inside U, then

$$[r(z_k)]^{n-1} = \frac{1}{n}\left(1 + |z_k|^2\right)\left(1 + |z_k|^2\right)^{n-3},$$

which leads to $r(z_k) < \sqrt{2/3}$ for $n = 3$ and $r(z_k) < 1$ for $n = 4$.

THEOREM 9.3 (GOODMAN, RAHMAN and RATTI [1969]). *Let all the roots of f lie in U and the root z_1 satisfy $|z_1| = 1$. Then at least one critical point of f lies in the disc $C(\frac{1}{2}z_1, \frac{1}{2})$.*

SCHMEISSER [1977] proved $r^* < 1.568$ and BOJANOV, RACHMAN and SZYNAL [1985] proved the following.

THEOREM 9.4. *If all the roots of the polynomial $\prod_{i=1}^{n}(z - z_i)$ lie in the disc $C(0, 1)$, then each of the discs*

$$C\left(z_\nu, (1 + |z_1 z_2 \cdots z_n|)^{1/n}\right), \quad \nu = 1, 2, \ldots, n,$$

contains at least one zero of f'.

As a corollary of this theorem, it follows that $r^* \leqslant 1.08331641\ldots$.
From Theorem 9.4, it follows that Sendov's conjecture holds for polynomials for which $f(0) = 0$ (see also SCHMEISSER [1969]).

10. Distribution of the roots on the plane

Rolle's theorem states that if the real polynomial f takes equal values at the points α and β, then f' has a zero ξ between α and β. The next theorem of GRACE [1902] and HEAWOOD [1907] is a generalization of Rolle's theorem for polynomials with complex coefficients.

THEOREM 10.1. *If the polynomial*

$$f(z) = a_0 z^n + a_1 z^{n-1} + \cdots + a_n = 0, \quad a_0 \neq 0, \tag{10.1}$$

satisfies $f(-1) = f(1)$, *then its derivative vanishes at the point in the disc with radius* $\cot(\pi/n)$ *and the center at the origin.*

The proof of the theorem is based on the following theorem by Grace.

THEOREM 10.2. *Suppose that for the equation*

$$\alpha(z) = \alpha_0 + \alpha_1 z + \cdots + \alpha_n z^n = 0, \quad \alpha_0 \beta_n + \alpha_1 \beta_{n-1} + \cdots + \alpha_n \beta_0 = 0,$$

not all the numbers $\beta_0, \beta_1, \ldots, \beta_n$ *are equal to zero. Then there exists at least one zero of* $\alpha(z)$ *in every circle, which contains all the zeros of the equation*

$$\beta_0 - \binom{n}{1}\beta_1 z + \binom{n}{2}\beta_2 z^2 + \cdots + (-1)^n \beta_n z^n = 0.$$

A useful generalization of Theorem 10.1 is the following.

THEOREM 10.3 (ALEXANDER [1915]). *If two zeros of the polynomial* f *of degree* n *lie in a circle with radius* R, *then the derivative* f' *has a root in a concentric circle with radius* $R \csc \pi/n$.

THEOREM 10.4. *If all the roots of Eq.* (10.1) *lie on one side of the straight* g, *then the roots of its derivative also lie on the same side of* g. *If not all the roots of Eq.* (10.1) *are on* g, *then the number* $\xi \in g$ *is the root of the derivative, if* ξ *is a root of Eq.* (10.1).

Theorem 9.1 states that if a convex polygon contains all the roots of a polynomial, then this polygon also contains all the roots of its derivative. In particular, if all the roots are real, then all the roots of the derivative are real. Theorem 9.1 can be considered as a consequence of Theorem 10.4.

THEOREM 10.5 (LAGER [1898]). *Let the polynomial* (10.1) *satisfy* $f(\alpha) \neq 0$ *and* $f'(\alpha) \neq 0$. *Then inside and outside every circle* C, *such that the points* α *and* $\alpha - nf(\alpha)/f'(\alpha)$ *lie on* C, *there exists at least one zero of* f *or all the roots of* f *lie on* C.

Other results that give the distribution of the zeros involving symmetric functions can be found in OBRESHKOV [1963a] and MARDEN [1949]. Let us mention only the generalizations of the Budan–Fourier Theorem 5.6 and Theorem 5.3.

THEOREM 10.6 (OBRESHKOV [1924]). *Let* $f(z) = 0$ *be an equation of degree* n *with real coefficients and let* $V(a)$ *be a number of variations of the sequence*

$f(a), f'(a), f''(a), \ldots, f^{(n)}(a)$. Then the number of roots that lie in a symmetric quadrangle according to the real axis, with two opposite vertices, points a and $b, a < b$, is $V(a) - V(b)$ or less by an even number. The angles at these vertices are $2\pi/[n - V(a)]$ and $2\pi/V(b)$, respectively.

In the particular case where $a = 0$ and $b = \infty$, we obtain the following.

THEOREM 10.7. *Let $f(z) = 0$ be an equation of degree n with real coefficients and let the number of variations of coefficients be V. Then the number of the roots that have arguments in the interval $(-\pi/(n-V), \pi/(n-V))$ is equal to V or less by an even number.*

CHAPTER II

Localization Bounds

In this chapter we consider improved Cauchy's bounds for the zeros of a given nth degree polynomial. It is shown, that these location bounds and other similar classical theorems can be established by using Gershgorin's estimate for the eigenvalues of a matrix and its improvement by Ballieu, known as theorems of Ballieu–Cauchy.

We give various estimations about the unique positive root of the algebraic equation $x^n - \sum_{i=1}^{n} a_i x^{n-i} = 0$, where $a_i \geq 0$. Such results play an important role for determination of the R-order of convergence of iterative processes in numerical analysis.

The problem for simultaneous approximate calculation of all positive roots of polynomial equation is also considered.

11. Elementary bounds

Since the zeros of $f(-x)$ are those of $f(x)$ with signs reversed and the zeros of $x^n f(1/x)$ are the reciprocals of those of $f(x)$, any technique that gives an upper bound for the positive real zeros can also be used for finding a lower bound for these zeros and for finding upper and lower bounds for the negative real zeros. There is one very simple device for this that is sometimes useful, based on the observation that a real polynomial with no negative coefficients can have no positive real zeros. Hence consider the polynomial

$$f(x) = a_0 x^n + a_1 x^{n-1} + \cdots + a_n, \quad a_0 > 0 \qquad (11.1)$$

and form

$$g(y) = f(y+h) = a_0 y^n + \cdots + y f'(h) + f(h).$$

If $f(h) \geq 0$, $f'(h) \geq 0, \ldots$, then $g(y)$ has no positive real zeros. But the zeros y of $g(y)$ and x of $f(x)$ are related by $x = y + h$. Hence $f(x)$ has no real zeros exceeding h. In fact if $h > 0$ and if in the division

$$\frac{f(x)}{x-h} = q(x) + \frac{r}{x-h},$$

the remainder $r > 0$ and $q(x)$ has no negative coefficient, then h is an upper bound to the positive real zeros of $f(x)$.

The following theorems are more readily applied.

THEOREM 11.1. *Let the polynomial $f(x)$ in (11.1) be real, and let $a_0 > 0$, $a_1 \geqslant 0$, $\ldots, a_{m-1} \geqslant 0$, $a_m < 0$. Then if $-a_0 \alpha$ is the value of the numerically largest negative coefficient, an upper bound for the real zeros of $f(x)$ is $1 + \alpha^{1/m}$.*

THEOREM 11.2. *Let the real polynomial $f(x)$ in (11.1) have the leading coefficient $a_0 = 1$ and the negative coefficients $-\alpha_i, -\alpha_j, -\alpha_k, \ldots$, there being m of these. Then*
$$\max\left[(m\alpha_i)^{1/i}, (m\alpha_j)^{1/j}, \ldots\right]$$
is an upper bound of the positive real zeros of $f(x)$.

THEOREM 11.3 (CAUCHY [1829]). *Let $f(z)$ in (11.1) be any polynomial, not necessarily real, with $a_0 \neq 0$. Then all its zeros lie in the circular disc whose center is the origin and whose radius is the single positive real root of the equation*
$$|a_0|r^n = |a_1|r^{n-1} + \cdots + |a_n|.$$

THEOREM 11.4 (CAUCHY [1829]). *If $f(z)$ in (11.1) is any polynomial, then any zero z satisfy*
$$|z| \leqslant 1 + \max\left|\frac{a_i}{a_0}\right|.$$

Let
$$a = \max\{|a_1|, \ldots, |a_n|\},$$
$$a' = \min\{|a_0|, \ldots, |a_{n-1}|\}.$$

THEOREM 11.5. *All zeros of the polynomial $f(z)$ satisfy*
$$\frac{|a_n|}{a' + |a_n|} \leqslant |z| \leqslant 1 + \frac{a}{|a_0|}.$$

THEOREM 11.6. *If $f(z)$ in (11.1) is any polynomial and $a_i > 0$, $i = 0, 1, \ldots, n$, then any zero z satisfies*
$$\alpha \leqslant |z| \leqslant \beta,$$
where
$$\alpha = \min\left[\frac{a_1}{a_0}, \frac{a_2}{a_1}, \ldots, \frac{a_n}{a_{n-1}}\right],$$
$$\beta = \max\left[\frac{a_1}{a_0}, \frac{a_2}{a_1}, \ldots, \frac{a_n}{a_{n-1}}\right].$$

THEOREM 11.7. *Let $d_i > 0$, $i = 0, 1, \ldots, n$, and*
$$d_n \geqslant |a_1|d_{n-1} + |a_2|d_{n-2} + \cdots + |a_n|d_0.$$
Then no zero of $f(z)$ ($a_0 = 1$) can be greater in modulus than
$$\max\left[\frac{d_n}{d_{n-1}}, \left(\frac{d_n}{d_{n-2}}\right)^{1/2}, \ldots, \left(\frac{d_n}{d_0}\right)^{1/n}\right].$$

THEOREM 11.8. *If $f(z)$ in (11.1) ($a_0 = 1$) is any polynomial, then no zero of $f(z)$ can be greater in modulus than*

$$\max \left[n|a_1|, (n|a_2|)^{1/2}, \ldots, (n|a_n|)^{1/n} \right]$$

and than

$$\max \left[|a_k| \frac{2^n - 1}{\binom{n}{k}} \right]^{1/k}, \quad k = 1, 2, \ldots, n.$$

THEOREM 11.9 (JOYAL, LABELLE and RAHMAN [1967]). *If*

$$B = \max \left(|a_j| : 0 \leqslant j < n - 1 \right),$$

then all the zeros of the polynomial

$$f(z) = z^n + a_{n-1} z^{n-1} + \cdots + a_0 \qquad (11.2)$$

are contained in the circle

$$|z| \leqslant \tfrac{1}{2} \left(1 + |a_{n-1}| + \sqrt{(1 - |a_{n-1}|)^2 + 4B} \right).$$

PROOF. If

$$|z| > \tfrac{1}{2} \left(1 + |a_{n-1}| + \sqrt{(1 - |a_{n-1}|)^2 + 4B} \right),$$

then $|z| > 1$ and

$$(|z| - 1)(|z| - |a_{n-1}|) - B > 0.$$

Multiplying by $|z|^{n-1}$ and dividing by $(|z| - 1)$, we obtain

$$|z|^n - |a_{n-1}||z|^{n-1} - \frac{B|z|^{n-1}}{|z| - 1} > 0.$$

But

$$\frac{B|z|^{n-1}}{|z| - 1} > B(1 + |z| + |z|^2 + \cdots + |z|^{n-2})$$

$$\geqslant \left| a_{n-2} z^{n-2} + a_{n-3} z^{n-3} + \cdots + a_0 \right|$$

and

$$|z|^n - |a_{n-1}||z|^{n-1} \leqslant |z^n + a_{n-1} z^{n-1}|.$$

Hence we have

$$|f(z)| > |z^n + a_{n-1} z^{n-1}| - |a_{n-2} z^{n-2} + a_{n-3} z^{n-3} + \cdots + a_0| > 0$$

and the proposition is proved. □

COROLLARY 11.1. *The polynomial* (11.2) *has all its zeros in the circle*

$$|z| \leq \tfrac{1}{2}\left(1 + \sqrt{1+4B'}\right),$$

where

$$B' = \max_{0<k\leq n-1} |a_{n-1}a_k - a_{k-1}|, \quad a_{-1} = 0.$$

COROLLARY 11.2. *The polynomial* (11.2) *has all its zeros in the circle*

$$|z| \leq 1 + (B'')^{1/2},$$

where

$$B'' = \max_{0<k\leq n-1} |(1-a_{n-1})a_k + a_{k-1}|, \quad a_{-1} = 0.$$

THEOREM 11.10 (JOYAL, LABELLE and RAHMAN [1967]). *Let*

$$B = \left(\sum_{j=0}^{n-2} |a_j|^p\right)^{1/p}, \quad p > 1.$$

Then all the roots of the polynomial (11.2) *are contained in the circle*

$$|z| \leq k,$$

where $k \geq \max(1, |a_{n-1}|)$ *is a root of the equation*

$$(|z| - |a_{n-1}|)^q(|z|^q - 1) - B^q = 0, \quad \frac{1}{p} + \frac{1}{q} = 1.$$

The theorem of ENESTRÖM [1920] and KAKEYA [1912] mentioned in the introduction states that if

$$a_n \geq a_{n-1} \geq \cdots \geq a_0 \geq 0,$$

then the polynomial

$$f(z) = a_n z^n + a_{n-1} z^{n-1} + \cdots + a_0 \tag{11.3}$$

has all its zeros in the unit circle. If we do not assume the coefficients to be non-negative, the conclusion does not hold.

THEOREM 11.11 (JOYAL, LABELLE and RAHMAN [1967]). *If*

$$a_n \geq a_{n-1} \geq \cdots \geq a_0,$$

then the polynomial (11.3) *has all its zeros in the circle*

$$|z| \leq \frac{a_n - a_0 + |a_0|}{|a_n|}.$$

If $a_0 \geq 0$, this result reduces to the theorem of Eneström and Kakeya.

WILF [1961] makes use of the Perron–Frobenius theorem to obtain certain known root location theorems for polynomial equations. As we shall show, these results and other classical theorems can be conveniently established by using the following easily proved theorem of GERSHGORIN [1931] (see also TAUSSKY [1949]).

THEOREM 11.12. *Let $A = [a_{ij}]$ be an $n \times n$ complex matrix, and let R_i be the sum of the moduli of the off-diagonal elements in the ith row. Then each eigenvalue of A lies in the union of the circles*

$$|z - a_{ii}| \leqslant R_i, \quad i = 1, \ldots, n.$$

The analogous result holds if columns of A are considered.

In most of our applications, we shall use the larger circles

$$|z| \leqslant |a_{ii}| + R_i, \quad i = 1, \ldots n.$$

Let us consider a theorem that generalizes a classical result by Cauchy, as given in a paper by BELL [1965].

THEOREM 11.13 (BALLIEU [1947]). *Let $A_1, A_2, \ldots, A_{n-1}$ be arbitrary positive numbers, $A_0 = 0$, $A_n = 1$. Then all the zeros of (11.3) satisfy the inequality*

$$|z| \leqslant \max_{0 \leqslant i \leqslant n-1} \left(\frac{A_i}{A_{i+1}} + \frac{|a_i|}{|a_n| A_{i+1}} \right). \tag{11.4}$$

We start with the matrix

$$C = \begin{pmatrix} 0 & 0 & \cdots & 0 & -a_0/a_n \\ 1 & 0 & \cdots & 0 & -a_1/a_n \\ \vdots & & & & \\ 0 & 0 & \cdots & 1 & -a_{n-1}/a_n \end{pmatrix}, \tag{11.5}$$

the companion matrix of f; and taking

$$P = \mathrm{diag}(A_1, A_2, \ldots, A_n), \tag{11.6}$$

we form the matrix

$$P^{-1}CP = \begin{pmatrix} 0 & 0 & \cdots & 0 & -a_0/a_n A_1 \\ A_1/A_2 & 0 & \cdots & 0 & -a_1/a_n A_2 \\ 0 & A_2/A_3 & \cdots & 0 & -a_2/a_n A_3 \\ \vdots & & & & \vdots \\ 0 & 0 & \cdots & A_{n-1}/A_n & -a_{n-1}/a_n A_n \end{pmatrix}. \tag{11.7}$$

Since the eigenvalues of (11.7) are the zeros of f, a direct application of Theorem 11.12 yields the conclusion of Theorem 11.13. We note that if $A_1 = A_2 = \cdots = A_{n-1} = 1$, the bound (11.4) is the classical one of Cauchy

$$|z| \leqslant \max \left(\left|\frac{a_0}{a_n}\right|, 1 + \left|\frac{a_1}{a_n}\right|, \ldots, 1 + \left|\frac{a_{n-1}}{a_n}\right| \right),$$

if

$$A_i = \left|\frac{a_i}{a_n}\right|, \quad i = 1, \ldots, n-1,$$

then (11.4) becomes
$$|z| \leq \max\left(\left|\frac{a_0}{a_1}\right|, 2\left|\frac{a_1}{a_2}\right|, \ldots, 2\left|\frac{a_{n-1}}{a_n}\right|\right),$$
a bound due to KOJIMA [1917].

The next theorems are due to Fujiwara, Walsh, Landau and Markovitch. We discuss three well-known theorems, which have similar proofs.

THEOREM 11.14 ((FUJIWARA [1916]). *If* $\lambda_1, \ldots, \lambda_n$ *are positive numbers with* $\lambda_1 + \cdots + \lambda_n = 1$, *then the zeros of* (11.3) *satisfy*
$$|z| \leq \max_j \left|\frac{1}{\lambda_j}\frac{a_{n-j}}{a_n}\right|^{1/j}.$$

THEOREM 11.15 (WALSH [1924]). *The zeros of* (11.3) *all lie in the circle*
$$\left|z + \frac{a_{n-1}}{2a_n}\right| \leq \left|\frac{a_{n-1}}{2a_n}\right| + \left|\frac{a_{n-2}}{a_n}\right|^{1/2} + \left|\frac{a_{n-3}}{a_n}\right|^{1/3} + \cdots + \left|\frac{a_0}{a_n}\right|^{1/n}. \qquad (11.8)$$

If in (11.6) we take
$$A_i = \rho^{n-i}, \quad i = 1, \ldots, n-1,$$
the matrix (11.7) takes the form
$$\begin{pmatrix} 0 & 0 & \cdots & 0 & -a_0/a_n\rho^{n-1} \\ \rho & 0 & \cdots & 0 & -a_1/a_n\rho^{n-2} \\ \vdots & & & & \\ 0 & 0 & \cdots & \rho & -a_{n-1}/a_n \end{pmatrix}.$$

To prove Theorem 11.14, we take
$$\rho = \max_j \left|\frac{1}{\lambda_j}\frac{a_{n-j}}{a_n}\right|^{1/j}, \quad j = 1, 2, \ldots, n,$$
and note that
$$\left|\frac{a_0}{a_n\rho^{n-1}}\right| + \left|\frac{a_1}{a_n\rho^{n-2}}\right| + \cdots + \left|\frac{a_{n-1}}{a_n}\right| \leq (\lambda_1 + \cdots + \lambda_n)\rho = \rho.$$

To prove Theorem 11.15, we let
$$\rho = \max_j \left|\frac{a_{n-j}}{a_n}\right|^{1/j}, \quad j = 2, 3, \ldots, n,$$
and note that the circles $|z - a_{ii}| \leq R_a$ are in this case all contained in the circle (11.8).

The following bound is due to RAHMAN [1970]. All the zeros of the polynomial (11.2) lie on the disc
$$D = \left\{z: |z + 0.5a_{n-1}| \leq \frac{|a_{n-1}|}{2} + \alpha M\right\},$$

where $M = \sum_{j=2}^{n} |a_{n-j}|^{1/j}$, $\alpha = 0$ if $f(z)$ is of the form $a_{n-1}z^{n-1} + z^n$, and

$$\alpha = \max_{2 \leq j \leq n} \left(M^{-1}|a_{n-j}|^{1/j} \right)^{(j-1)/j},$$

if $f(z)$ is not of the form $a_{n-1}z^{n-1} + z^n$.

THEOREM 11.16 (Landau and Markovitch, see MARDEN [1949]). *For a given positive number t let*

$$M = |a_i|t^i, \quad i = 1, 2, \ldots, n.$$

Then all the zeros of (11.3) *satisfy*

$$|z| > \frac{|a_0|t}{|a_0| + M},$$

i.e. all the zeros of

$$F(z) = z^n f(1/z)$$

lie in

$$|z| < \frac{|a_0| + M}{|a_0|t}.$$

For other bounds, see LANDAU [1906, 1907], VAN VLECK [1925], MONTEL [1935a], MARKOVITCH [1939].

Beginning with the inverse K of (11.5) and the matrix

$$R = \mathrm{diag}(1, t, \ldots, t^{n-1}),$$

we form the matrix

$$RKR^{-1} = \begin{pmatrix} -a_1/a_0 & 1/t & 0 & \cdots & 0 \\ -a_2/a_0 & 0 & 1/t & \cdots & 0 \\ \vdots & & & & \\ -a_{n-1}t^{n-2}/a_0 & 0 & 0 & \cdots & 1/t \\ -a_n t^{n-1}/a_0 & 0 & 0 & \cdots & 0 \end{pmatrix},$$

the eigenvalues of which are the reciprocals of the zeros of f.

By Theorem 11.12, these eigenvalues satisfy

$$|z| \leq \max \left(\frac{|a_0| + |a_i|t^i}{|a_0|t} \right) \leq \frac{|a_0| + M}{|a_0|t},$$

and the conclusion of Theorem 11.16 follows immediately.

Other bounds have been found by WERNER [1982, 1983].

THEOREM 11.17 (TIKOO [1967]). *All the zeros of the polynomial* (11.3) *lie in the circle*

$$|z| \leq \max_{0 \leq i \leq n-1} \left(\frac{K_i}{K_{i+1}}, \sum_{i=0}^{n-1} \frac{|a_i|}{|a_n|K_{i+1}} \right),$$

where K_i are positive numbers with $K_0 = 0$ and $K_n = 1$.

The estimation in Theorem 11.17 can be improved (see ASCHER [1970]).

THEOREM 11.18 (MOHAMMAD [1965a]). *For any given $t > 0$, all the zeros of*
$$F(z) = z^n f(1/z)$$
lie in
$$|z| < \frac{1}{t}\left[1 + \left(\frac{D_p}{|a_0|}\right)^q\right]^{1/q},$$
where
$$D_p = \left[\sum_{k=1}^n \left(|a_k|t^k\right)^p\right]^{1/p}, \quad p > 1, \quad q > 1, \quad 1/p + 1/q = 1.$$

THEOREM 11.19. (MOHAMMAD [1965a]). *Let*
$$G = \max_{1 \leqslant k \leqslant n} |a_k|^{1/k}.$$
Then all the zeros of $F(z)$ lie in
$$|z| < G\left(1 + \frac{1}{|a_0|}\right).$$

THEOREM 11.20 (MOHAMMAD [1965a]). *Let G be defined as in Theorem 11.19. Then all the zeros of $F(z)$ lie in*
$$|z| < \left[1 + \left(\frac{\delta_p}{|a_0|}\right)^q\right]^{1/q},$$
where
$$\delta_p = \left(\sum_{k=1}^n G^{kp}\right)^{1/p}.$$

THEOREM 11.21 (MOHAMMAD [1965a]). *Let*
$$S = \frac{\max |a_k|}{k}, \quad k = 1, \ldots, n.$$
Then all the zeros of
$$T(z) = Sz^n + a_1 z^{n-1} + \cdots + a_n$$
lie in
$$|z| < \frac{3 + \sqrt{5}}{2}.$$

In a recent paper, Mohammad makes use of Schwarz's lemma to obtain localization theorems for polynomial equations.

THEOREM 11.22. (MOHAMMAD [1965a]). *All the zeros of*
$$P(z) = a_0 z^n + a_1 z^{n-1} + \cdots + a_n$$
lie in
$$|z| \leqslant \frac{M}{|a_0|}$$
if $|a_0| \leqslant M$, *where*
$$M = \max_{|z|=1} |a_1 z^{n-1} + \cdots + a_n| = \max_{|z|=1} |a_n z^{n-1} + \cdots + a_1|.$$

The bound obtained in Theorem 11.22 is in general better than the traditional
$$\frac{|a_1| + |a_2| + \cdots + |a_n|}{|a_0|}.$$

COROLLARY 11.3. *If* $a_k \geqslant 0$, $k = 1, \ldots, n$, *and* $|a_0| \leqslant a_1 + a_2 + \cdots + a_n$, *then all the zeros of* $P(z)$ *lie in*
$$|z| < \frac{a_1 + a_2 + \cdots + a_n}{|a_0|}.$$

THEOREM 11.23 (MOHAMMAD [1965a]). *Let* r *be the modulus of the zeros of the largest modulus of* $P(z)$ *and*
$$M' = \max_{|z|=r} |a_0 z^{n-1} + \cdots + a_{n-1}|.$$
Then all the zeros of $P(z)$ *lie in the ring-shaped region*
$$\frac{r|a_n|}{M'} \leqslant |z| \leqslant r$$
if $|a_n| \leqslant M'$.

COROLLARY 11.4. *If* $a_k \geqslant 0$, $k = 1, \ldots, n-1$, $a_0 > 0$ *and if*
$$|a_n| \leqslant a_0 r^n + \cdots + a_{n-1} r,$$
then all the zeros of $P(z)$ *lie in*
$$\frac{r|a_n|}{a_0 r^n + a_1 r^{n-1} + \cdots + a_{n-1} r} \leqslant |z| \leqslant r.$$

With the help of Corollary 11.4, we can restate the Eneström–Kakeya theorem in the following form (see MOHAMMAD [1965b]).

If $a_0 \geqslant a_1 \geqslant \cdots \geqslant a_{n-1} \geqslant a_n > 0$, then all the zeros of $P(z)$ lie in the ring-shaped region
$$\frac{a_n}{a_0 + a_1 + \cdots + a_{n-1}} \leqslant |z| \leqslant 1.$$

THEOREM 11.24. *If* $a_0 \geqslant a_1 \geqslant \cdots \geqslant a_{n-1} \geqslant a_n > 0$, *then the number of zeros of* $P(z)$ *in* $|z| \leqslant 0.5$ *does not exceed*
$$1 + \frac{1}{\log 2} \log \frac{a_0}{a_n}.$$

The following theorem is due to MONTEL [1935] and MARTY [1932].

THEOREM 11.25. *All the zeros of the polynomial*
$$P(z) = a_0 + a_1 z + \cdots + a_{n-1} z^{n-1} + z^n$$
lie in
$$|z| \leq \max\left(L, L^{1/n}\right),$$
where L is the length of the polygonal line joining the points $0, a_0, a_1, \ldots, a_{n-1}, 1$ in succession; that is
$$L = |a_0| + |a_1 - a_0| + \cdots + |a_{n-1} - a_{n-2}| + |1 - a_{n-1}|.$$

THEOREM 11.26 (MOHAMMAD [1967]). *All the zeros of the polynomial of Theorem 11.25 lie in*
$$|z| \leq R = \max\left(L_p, L_p^{1/n}\right),$$
where
$$L_p = n^{1/q} \left(\sum_{i=0}^{n-1} |a_i|^p\right)^{1/p}, \quad 1/p + 1/q = 1.$$
The bound is sharp.

PROOF. We have
$$|P(z)| \geq |z|^n \left[1 - \sum_{i=1}^{n} \frac{|a_{n-i}|}{|z|^i}\right]$$
$$\geq |z|^n \left[1 - n^{1/q} \left(\sum_{i=1}^{n} \frac{|a_{n-i}|^p}{|z|^{ip}}\right)^{1/p}\right].$$

If $L_p \geq 1$, $\max\left(L_p, L_p^{1/n}\right) = L_p$. Let $|z| \geq 1$. Then
$$1/|z|^{ip} \leq 1/|z|^p, \quad i = 1, \ldots, n.$$
If $|z| > L_p$, then
$$|P(z)| \geq |z|^n \left[1 - \frac{n^{1/q}}{|z|} \left(\sum_{i=0}^{n-1} |a_i|^p\right)^{1/p}\right]$$
$$= |z|^n \left[1 - \frac{L_p}{|z|}\right] > 0.$$

Again if $L_p \leq 1$, $\max(L_p, L_p^{1/n}) = L_p^{1/n}$. Let $|z| \leq 1$. Then $1/|z|^{ip} \leq 1/|z|^{np}$, $i = 1, 2, \ldots, n$. Hence, if $|z| > L_p^{1/n}$, then

$$|P(z)| \geq |z|^n \left[1 - \frac{n^{1/q}}{|z|^n} \left(\sum_{i=1}^{n} |a_{n-i}|^p\right)^{1/p}\right]$$

$$= |z|^n \left(1 - \frac{L_p}{|z|^n}\right) > 0.$$

Hence $P(z)$ does not vanish for $|z| > \max(L_p, L_p^{1/n})$ and Theorem 11.26 follows. □

The limit in Theorem 11.26 is attained by

$$P(z) = z^n - \frac{1}{n}\left(z^{n-1} + \cdots + z + 1\right)$$

since

$$L_p = n^{1/q} \left(\sum_{p=0}^{n-1} \frac{1}{n^p}\right)^{1/p} = n^{1/q} \left(\frac{n}{n^p}\right)^{1/p} = 1$$

and 1 is a zero of $P(z)$.

Applying this result to $(1-z)P(z)$, we obtain the theorem of Montel and Marty mentioned above.

THEOREM 11.27 (MOHAMMAD [1967]). *If $0 < a_{i-1} \leq k a_i$, $k > 0$, then all the zeros of*

$$P(z) = a_0 + a_1 + \cdots + a_{n-1}z^{n-1} + a_n z^n$$

lie in

$$|z| \leq \max\left(M, M^{1/n}\right),$$

where

$$M = \frac{a_0 + a_1 + a_2 + \cdots + a_{n-1}}{a_n}(k-1) + k.$$

Putting $k = 1$ in Theorem 11.27, we obtain the following result due to Kakeya. If $0 < a_0 \leq a_1 \leq \ldots \leq a_n$, then all the zeros of the polynomial $P(z)$ lie in $|z| < 1$. This follows from the fact that $M = 1$, hence $\max(M, M^{1/n}) = 1$.

Let (11.3) be a polynomial with complex coefficients. Then (see KUNIEDA [1916], MONTEL [1935], TOYA [1933])

$$|z| < \left[1 + \left(\sum_{j=0}^{n-1} \left|\frac{a_j}{a_n}\right|^p\right)^{q/p}\right]^{1/q},$$

where $1/p + 1/q = 1$, $p > 1$, $q > 1$.

It is known see (FUJIWARA [1915], KELLEHER [1916]) that if z_1 is the zero of the largest modulus, then

$$|z_1| < \left(1 + \sum_{j=0}^{n-1} \left|\frac{a_j}{a_n}\right|^2\right)^{1/2}.$$

For other bounds, see WILIAMS [1922].

THEOREM 11.28 (REICH [1970a]). *If z_n is the zero of the smallest modulus, then*

$$|z_n| < \left(1 + \frac{1}{n}\sum_{j=0}^{n-1} \left|\frac{a_j}{a_n}\right|^2\right)^{1/2}.$$

PROOF (DEUTSCH [1971]). Denoting the zeros of $f(z)$ by $z_1, z_2, \ldots, z_n$, we have

$$|z_n|^n \leqslant |z_1 \cdots z_n| = |a_0/a_n|,$$

whence

$$|z_n| \leqslant |a_0/a_n|^{1/n}.$$

This inequality is stronger than that of the proposal. Indeed, denoting $\sum_{j=0}^{n-1} |a_j/a_n|^2$ by b, we have

$$|a_0/a_n|^{1/n} = \left(|a_0/a_n|^2\right)^{1/2n} \leqslant b^{1/2n} < ((1+b/n)^n)^{1/2n}$$

$$= (1+b/n)^{1/2}.$$

This completes the proof. □

Denote $(\max(|a_k/a_n|: 0 \leqslant k \leqslant n-1))^{1/n}$ by Q.

THEOREM 11.29 (REICH [1970b]). *Suppose that $a_{n-1} = 0$, and that $Q > 1$. Then the zeros of $f(x)$ (see (11.3)) lie in the circles*

$$|z| \leqslant Q + Q^2 + \cdots + Q^{n-1} \qquad (11.9)$$

and

$$|z| \leqslant \max_{\substack{0 \leqslant j,k \leqslant n-1 \\ j \neq k}} \left((1+|a_k/a_n|)(1+|a_j/a_n|)\right)^{1/2}.$$

The following bound is due to LOSSERS [1971]:

$$|z| < \tfrac{1}{2} + \sqrt{1/4 + Q^n}. \qquad (11.10)$$

Without loss of generality we may assume that $a_{n-1} = 1$. Let z be a zero such that $|z| > 1$. Since

$$-z^n = a_0 + a_1 z + \cdots + a_{n-2} z^{n-2},$$

we easily derive that

$$|z|^n = Q^n \frac{|z|^{n-1} - 1}{|z| - 1},$$

and from this inequality and the fact that

$$|z|^{n-1} > |z|^{n-1} - 1$$

it follows that

$$\frac{Q^n}{|z| - 1} > |z|,$$

which leads to inequality (11.10). Inequality (11.10) is stronger than (11.9) because

$$\tfrac{1}{2} + \sqrt{1/4 + Q^n} < 1 + Q^{n-2} < Q + Q^2 + \cdots + Q^{n-1}.$$

DATT and GOVIL [1978] improved Cauchy's bound and obtained the following result.

THEOREM 11.30. *All the zeros of the polynomial*

$$P(z) = z^n + \cdots + a_1 z + a_0$$

lie in the ring-shaped region

$$\frac{|a_0|}{2(1+A)^{n-1}(An+1)} \leq |z| \leq 1 + A\lambda_0,$$

where λ_0 is the unique root of the equation

$$(x - 1)(Ax + 1)^n + 1 = 0,$$

in the interval $(0, 1)$ and

$$A = \max_{0 \leq j \leq n-1} |a_j|.$$

The proof is based on the following lemma.

LEMMA 11.1. *Let*

$$f(x) = x - 1 + \frac{1}{(1 + Ax)^n},$$

where n is a positive integer and $A > 0$. Then if $nA \leq 1$, $f(x)$ is monotonically increasing for $x \geq 0$. If $nA > 1$, then there exists a $\delta > 0$ such that $f(x)$ is monotonically decreasing in the interval $[0, \delta]$ and $f(x)$ has a unique root in the interval $(0, 1)$.

PROOF OF THEOREM 11.30 (DATT and GOVIL [1978]). According to MARDEN [1949], we obtain

$$|p(z)| \geq |z|^n - A \sum_{j=0}^{n-1} |z|^j = |z|^n - A \frac{|z|^n - 1}{|z| - 1}.$$

Hence for every $\lambda > 0$, we have on $|z| = 1 + \lambda A$,

$$|p(z)| = (1 + \lambda A)^n - \frac{(1 + \lambda A)^n - 1}{\lambda} > 0, \tag{11.11}$$

if $\lambda > 1 - 1/(1 + A\lambda)^n$. Thus, if λ_0 is the unique root (Lemma 11.1) of the equation

$$x = 1 - \frac{1}{(1 + Ax)^n}$$

in $(0, 1)$, then every $\lambda > \lambda_0$ satisfies (11.11) and hence $|p(z)| > 0$ on $|z| = 1 + \lambda A$, which implies that $p(z)$ has all its zeros in

$$|z| \leqslant 1 + A\lambda_0.$$

If we denote the polynomial $(1 - z)p(z)$ by $g(z)$, then

$$g(z) = a_0 + \sum_{\nu=1}^{n-1}(a_\nu - a_{\nu-1})z^\nu + z^n - a_{n-1}z^{n-1} - z^{n+1} = a_0 + h(z),$$

say. If $R = 1 + A$, then

$$\max_{|z|=R}|h(z)| \leqslant R^{n+1} + R^n + |a_{n-1}|R^n + \sum_{\nu=1}^{n-1}|a_\nu - a_{\nu-1}|R^\nu$$

$$\leqslant R^n[R + 1 + A + (2n - 2)A] = 2(1 + A)^n(nA + 1). \tag{11.12}$$

Next we prove that $p(z)$ has no zero in

$$|z| < \frac{|a_0|}{2(1 + A)^{n-1}(1 + An)}.$$

Hence on $|z| \leqslant R$,

$$|g(z)| = |a_0 + h(z)| \geqslant |a_0| - |h(z)|$$

$$\geqslant |a_0| - \frac{|z|}{1 + A}\max_{|z|=1+A}|h(z)|,$$

by Schwarz's lemma,

$$|g(z)| \geqslant |a_0| - \frac{|z|}{1 + A}2(1 + A)^n(nA + 1),$$

and by (11.12), $|g(z)| > 0$ if

$$|z| < \frac{|a_0|}{2(1 + A)^{n-1}(1 + An)}.$$

The proof of Theorem 11.30 is complete. □

JAIN [1990] also improved Cauchy's bound and obtained the following results.

THEOREM 11.31. *All the zeros of $P(z)$ lie in the disc*

$$|z| < 1 + d_o r,$$

where d_0, the greatest root of the equation

$$(1 + xr)^{n-1}(x^2 r^2 + xrb - \beta) + \beta = 0$$

in the interval $[0,1]$, is always less than 1, except when $\beta = 0$, in which case it is 1, and

$$b = 1 - |a_{n-1}|,$$
$$\beta = \max(|a_j| : 0 \leq j \leq n-2),$$
$$r = \tfrac{1}{2}\left(-b + \sqrt{b^2 + 4\beta}\right).$$

The bound $1 + d_0 r$ is the best possible and is attained for the polynomial

$$P(z) = z^n - |a_{n-1}|z^{n-1} - \beta(z^{n-2} + \cdots + z + 1).$$

THEOREM 11.32. *All the zeros of $P(z)$ lie in the disc*

$$|z| \leq 1 + \frac{1}{2}\left(-b + \sqrt{b + 4\beta\left[1 - \frac{1}{(1+r)^{n-1}}\right]}\right),$$

where r, b and β are as in Theorem 11.31.

We consider the polynomial

$$P(z) = z^5 + a_4 z^4 + a_3 z^3 + a_2 z^2 + a_1 z + a_0,$$

where $|a_4| = 0.5$, $|a_3| = 0.3$, $|a_2| = 0.4$, $|a_1| = 0.4$, $|a_0| = 0.1$.
Table 11.1 gives various bounds (see JAIN [1990]).

TABLE 11.1.

Theorems	Bounds
Theorem 11.4 (Cauchy)	$\|z\| \leq 1.5$
Theorem 11.9	$\|z\| \leq 1.43$
Theorem 11.30	$R_1 \leq \|z\| \leq R,\ R > 1.43$
Theorem 11.31	$\|z\| \leq 1.344$

Theorems 11.31, 11.32 are based on the following lemma given by JAIN [1990].

LEMMA 11.2. *Let*

$$g(\lambda) = (1 + \lambda r)^{n-1}(\lambda^2 r^2 + \lambda rb - \beta) + \beta,$$

where $n \geq 2$ is a positive integer and $\beta > 0$. Then if $(n-1)\beta \leq b$, the equation $g(\lambda) = 0$ has only one root, namely zero, in $[0, \infty)$. If $(n-1)\beta > b$, then the equation $g(\lambda) = 0$ has an additional root (< 1) in $[0, \infty)$.

This lemma can be used to improve many classical estimations for the roots of algebraic equations.

The following result is due to Walsh (see MARDEN [1949]). If all the zeros of
$$f_1(z) = z^n + a_1 z^{n-1} + \cdots + a_n$$
lie in or on the circle C_1 with center c_1 and radius r_1 and if all the zeros of
$$f_2(z) = z^n + b_1 z^{n-1} + \cdots + b_n$$
lie in or on the circle C_2 with center c_2 and radius r_2, then each zero of the polynomial
$$h(z) = f_1(z) - \lambda f_2(z), \quad \lambda \neq 1,$$
lies in at least one of the circles T_k with center t_k and radius ρ_k, where
$$t_k = \frac{c_1 - \omega_k c_2}{1 - \omega_k}, \quad \rho_k = \frac{r_1 + |\omega_k| r_2}{|1 - \omega_k|}$$
and where $\omega_k, k = 1, 2, \ldots, n$, are the nth roots of λ.

As a very special case of this result we have the following.

COROLLARY 11.5. *For $j = 1, 2$, let*
$$f_j(z) = z^n + a_{1,j} z^{n-1} + a_{2,j} z^{n-2} + \cdots + a_{n,j}$$
be a polynomial of degree n having all its zeros in $|z| \leqslant 1$. If $|\arg \lambda_j| \leqslant \beta < \pi/2, j = 1, 2$, then the linear combination $\lambda_1 f_1(z) + \lambda_2 f_2(z)$ has all its zeros in
$$|z| \leqslant \frac{|\lambda_1|^{1/n} + |\lambda_2|^{1/n}}{\left(|\lambda_1|^{2/n} + |\lambda_2|^{2/n} - 2|\lambda_1 \lambda_2|^{1/n} \cos \frac{\pi - 2\beta}{n}\right)^{1/2}}.$$

Hence for every choice of numbers λ_1, λ_2 such that $|\arg \lambda_j| \leqslant \beta < \pi/2, j = 1, 2$, the polynomial $\lambda_1 f_1(z) + \lambda_2 f_2(z)$ has all its zeros in
$$|z| \leqslant \csc \frac{\pi - 2\beta}{2n}.$$

THEOREM 11.33 (RAHMAN [1972]). *For $j = 1, 2, \ldots, m$, let*
$$f_j(z) = z^n + a_{1,j} z^{n-1} + a_{2,j} z^{n-2} + \cdots + a_{n,j}$$
be a polynomial of degree n having all its zeros in $|z| \leqslant 1$. If $|\arg \lambda_j| \leqslant \beta < \pi/2, j = 1, 2, \ldots, m$, then the linear combination
$$\lambda_1 f_1(z) + \lambda_2 f_2(z) + \cdots + \lambda_m f_m(z)$$
has all its zeros in
$$|z| \leqslant \csc \frac{\pi - 2\beta}{2n}.$$

THEOREM 11.34 (RAHMAN [1972]). *If the polynomials*
$$f_1(z) = z^n + a_{1,1} z^{n-1} + a_{2,1} z^{n-2} + \cdots + a_{n,1},$$

$$f_2(z) = z^n + a_{1,2}z^{n-1} + a_{2,2}z^{n-2} + \cdots + a_{k,2}z^{n-k}$$

have all their zeros in $|z| \leqslant 1$, and $|\arg \lambda_j| \leqslant \beta < \pi/2$, $j = 1, 2$, then the linear combination $\lambda_1 f_1(z) + \lambda_2 f_2(z)$ has all its zeros in

$$|z| \leqslant \csc \frac{\pi - 2\beta}{n+k}.$$

12. Estimations of the unique positive root

In this section, we give a method for determining the upper and lower bounds of the unique positive root of the equation

$$x^n = \sum_{k=1}^{n} p_k x^{n-k}, \quad p_k \geqslant 0, \quad k = 1, 2, \ldots, n. \tag{12.1}$$

The knowledge of this root, or its upper bound, enables us to localize zeros of other polynomials with complex coefficients. This follows from Theorems 11.3 and 11.4 by Cauchy. The basic result is the following theorem.

THEOREM 12.1 (WESTERFIELD [1933]). *Let x_0 be the unique positive root of Eq. (12.1) and positive quantities*

$$(p_k)^{1/k}, \quad k = 1, \ldots, n,$$

after being arranged in order of decreasing magnitudes, form a sequence

$$q_1 \geqslant q_2 \geqslant \cdots \geqslant q_n.$$

Then x_0 satisfies the inequality

$$x_0 \leqslant \sum_{r=1}^{n} q_r g_r,$$

where

$$g_1 = y_1, \quad g_r = y_r - y_{r-1}, \quad r = 2, 3, \ldots, n,$$

and where y_k is the unique positive root of the equation

$$y^k = \sum_{r=1}^{k} y^{k-r}, \quad k = 1, 2, \ldots, n.$$

The following theorem by BOJANOV [1970] is more readily applied. Let x_0 be the unique root of Eq. (12.1), and let $c_1, c_2, \ldots, c_n$ be arbitrary positive numbers. We arrange the quantities

$$(c_k p_k)^{1/k}, \quad k = 1, 2, \ldots, n,$$

in order of decreasing magnitudes $q_1 \geqslant q_2 \geqslant \cdots \geqslant q_n$. Denote by $y(n; R_1, R_2, \ldots, R_m)$ the positive root of the equation

$$y^n = \sum_{j=1}^{m} \frac{1}{c_{R_j}} y^{n-R_j},$$

where $1 \leqslant R_1 < R_2 < \cdots < R_m \leqslant n$. Let
$$y_m = \max_{R_j}(n; R_1, R_2, \ldots, R_m).$$

THEOREM 12.2 (BOJANOV [1970]). *For any system of n positive numbers $c_1, c_2, \ldots, c_n$,*
$$x_0 \leqslant \sum_{r=1}^{n} q_r g_r,$$
where
$$g_1 = y_1, \qquad g_r = y_r - y_{r-1}, \quad r = 2, 3, \ldots, n.$$

The basic result of this section is the following.

THEOREM 12.3. *If x_j are positive roots of the equations*
$$x^n = a_{j1} x^{n-1} + a_{j2}^2 x^{n-2} + \cdots + a_{jn}^n, \quad a_{j1}, \ldots, a_{jn} \geqslant 0, \quad j = 1, 2, \ldots, m,$$
then the positive root z of the equation
$$x^n = \sum_{k=1}^{n} \left(\sum_{j=1}^{m} a_{jk} \right)^k x^{n-k}$$
satisfies the inequality
$$z < x_1 + x_2 + \cdots + x_m.$$

PROOF (BOJANOV [1970]). The proof is based on the following lemmas.

LEMMA 12.1. *If there is*
$$a_{jk} \geqslant 0, \quad j = 1, 2, \ldots, m, \ k = 1, 2, \ldots, n,$$
$$\sum_{k=1}^{n} a_{jk}^k \leqslant M, \quad M > 0, \ j = 1, 2, \ldots, m,$$
$$\omega_j \geqslant 0, \quad j = 1, 2, \ldots, m, \qquad \sum_{j=1}^{m} \omega_j = 1,$$
then
$$\sum_{k=1}^{n} \left(\sum_{j=1}^{m} \omega_j a_{jk} \right)^k \leqslant M.$$

LEMMA 12.2. *If $H > 0$ and*
$$H^n \geqslant \sum_{r=1}^{n} p_r H^{n-r},$$

then $H \geq x$, where x is the unique positive root of Eq. (12.1).

From the equality

$$x_j^n = \sum_{k=1}^{n} a_{jk}^k x_j^{n-k},$$

it follows that

$$\sum_{k=1}^{n} \left(\frac{a_{jk}}{x_j}\right)^k = 1.$$

From Lemma 12.1, with

$$\omega_j = \frac{x_j}{x_1 + x_2 + \cdots + x_m}$$

and $a_{jk} = a_{jk}/x_j$, we obtain

$$\sum_{k=1}^{n} \left(\sum_{j=1}^{m} \frac{x_j}{x_1 + x_2 + \cdots + x_m} \frac{a_{jk}}{x_j} \right)^k \leq 1,$$

$$\sum_{k=1}^{n} \frac{\left(\sum_{j=1}^{m} a_{jk}\right)^k}{\left(\sum_{j=1}^{m} x_j\right)^k} \leq 1,$$

$$\sum_{k=1}^{n} \left(\sum_{j=1}^{m} a_{jk}\right)^k \left(\sum_{j=1}^{m} x_j\right)^{n-k} \leq \left(\sum_{j=1}^{m} x_j\right)^n.$$

Now applying Lemma 12.2, we obtain

$$z \leq \sum_{j=1}^{m} x_j,$$

which ends the proof of Theorem 12.3. □

Another application of Theorem 12.3 gives a lower bound for the unique positive root of Eq. (12.1). Using the same notation as in Westerfield's theorem, we state the following.

THEOREM 12.4.

$$x_0 \geq \sum_{r=1}^{n} q_r g_{n+1-r}.$$

A generalization of Theorem 12.4 is as follows. Let x_0, q_r, g_r and c_r, $r = 1, 2, \ldots, n$, be defined as in Theorem 12.2. Then

$$x_0 \geq \sum_{r=1}^{n} q_r g_{n+1-r}.$$

OSTROVSKI [1966] and TRAUB [1964] obtained the following localization results about the unique positive root x_n of the algebraic equation:

$$f(x) = x^n - \sum_{k=1}^{n} x^{n-k} = 0, \qquad \frac{2n}{n+1} < x_n < 2$$

and

$$2 - \frac{1}{2^n}\left(1 + \frac{1}{n}\right)^n < x_n < 2 - \frac{1}{2^n}.$$

For other results, see PETKOV and KJURKCHIEV [1990]:

$$2 - \frac{a_n}{2^n} < x_n < 2 - \frac{b_n}{2^n},$$

where

$$a_n = \frac{2^{n+1}}{2^n + (2^{2n} - n2^{n+1})^{1/2}},$$

$$b_n = \left[1 + \frac{2}{2^{n+1} - n - 1 + \left((2^{n+1} - n - 1)^2 - 4n\right)^{1/2}}\right]^n.$$

Hence consider the polynomial equation

$$p_{n,p,q}(s) = s^n - (p+1)\sum_{i=0}^{n-1} q^i s^{n-i-1} = 0, \quad p \geq 0, \ q > 0, \ n \geq 2 \qquad (12.2)$$

THEOREM 12.5 (HERZBERGER [1986a]). *If $\sigma_{p,q}^{(n)}$ is a unique positive root of Eq. (12.2), then*

$$\sigma_{p,q}^{(n)} < \sigma_{p,q}^{(n+1)},$$

and

$$\frac{n}{n+1}(p+q+1) < \sigma_{p,q}^{(n)} < p+q+1, \qquad (12.3)$$

for $n > q/(p+1)$.

The case $p \geqslant 0, q = 1$ has been treated by TRAUB [1964].

TABLE 12.1. The roots $\sigma_{p,q}^{(n)}, q = 1$.

n	p			
	0	1	2	3
2	1.618	2.732	3.791	4.828
3	1.839	2.920	3.951	4.967
4	1.928	2.974	3.988	4.994
5	1.966	2.992	3.997	4.999
6	1.984	2.997	3.999	5.000
7	1.992	2.999	4.000	5.000

Using the same notation as in Herzberger's theorem, we state the following theorem (KJURKCHIEV [1992a]).

THEOREM 12.6.

$$p + q + 1 - \frac{(p+1)q^n}{(p+q+1)^n} e$$
$$< \sigma_{p,q}^{(n)} < p + q + 1 - \frac{(p+1)q^n}{(p+q+1)^n}. \tag{12.4}$$

PROOF. We define the polynomial

$$q_{n,p,q}(s) = (s - q)P_{n,p,q}(s) = s^{n+1} - (p + q + 1)s^n + (p + 1)q^n.$$

Hence

$$q'_{n,p,q}(s) = s^{n-1}[(n + 1)s - n(p + q + 1)]$$

and $q'_{n,p,q}(s)$ has only one nonzero root,

$$s^* = \frac{n}{n+1}(p + q + 1) > 0.$$

This ensures that the roots of $q_{n,p,q}(s)$ and of $P_{n,p,q}(s)$ are simple. Furthermore the relations

$$q_{n,p,q}(q) = 0,$$
$$q'_{n,p,q}(q) = q^{n-1}[q - n(p + 1)] < 0$$

are true which means that $\sigma_{p,q}^{(n)} > s^*$.

The second derivative of $q_{n,p,q}(s)$,

$$q''_{n,p,q}(s) = ns^{n-2}[(n + 1)s - (n - 1)(p + q + 1)],$$

has only one positive root

$$t = \frac{n-1}{n+1}(p + q + 1) = s^* - \frac{p+q+1}{n+1}$$

and $q''_{n,p,q}(s)$ has constant sign on $[s^*, p+q+1]$. Hence

$$q''_{n,p,q}(p+q+1) = 2n(p+q+1)^{n-1} > 0$$

and $q_{n,p,q}(s)$ is convex on $[s^*, p+q+1]$.

The straight line defined by the points $(s^*, q_{n,p,q}(s^*))$ and $(p+q+1, q_{n,p,q}(p+q+1))$ and the tangent to $q_{n,p,q}(s)$ at the point $(p+q+1, q_{n,p,q}(p+q+1))$ cross the abscissa, respectively, and the points

$$t' = p+q+1 - \frac{(p+1)q^n}{(p+q+1)^n}(1+1/n)^n,$$

$$t'' = p+q+1 - \frac{(p+1)q^n}{(p+q+1)^n}.$$

We obtain

$$t' < \sigma^{(n)}_{p,q} < t''$$

which ends the proof of Theorem 12.6. □

This is an improvement of the bounds in the theorem by Herzberger and follows the ideas given by TRAUB [1964].

We consider the polynomial equation

$$P_{n,a,b,c}(t) = t^n - at^{n-1} - b\sum_{i=1}^{n-1} c^i t^{n-1-i} = 0, \quad a,b,c > 0. \tag{12.5}$$

The unique simple positive root of Eq. (12.5) will be labeled $\tau^{(n)}_{a,b,c}$.

The following theorem gives us upper and lower bounds for $\tau^{(n)}_{a,b,c}$ which are asymptotically sharp.

THEOREM 12.7 (HERZBERGER [1986b]). *Putting* $g^2 = (a+c)^2 - 4c(a-b)$, *we have*

$$\tau^{(n)}_{a,b,c} < \tfrac{1}{2}(a+c+g) = \tau_{a,b,c},$$

$$\tau_{a,b,c} > c,$$

$$\lim_{n \to \infty} \tau^{(n)}_{a,b,c} = \tau_{a,b,c}.$$

For $n \geq n_0(a,b,c)$ *we have the inequality*

$$\frac{1}{2(n+1)}\left[n(a+c) + \sqrt{g^2 n^2 + 4c(a-b)}\right] < \tau^{(n)}_{a,b,c}.$$

THEOREM 12.8 (PETKOVIC and PETKOVIC [1989]). *For each* $n \geq 2$, *we have*

$$\tau^{(n)}_{a,b,c} > \frac{a + b(S_1 + S_2)}{1 + bS_1}, \tag{12.6}$$

where

$$S_1 = \begin{cases} \dfrac{n(n-1)}{2}, & c = 1, \\ \dfrac{c[(n-1)c^n - nc^{n-1} + 1]}{(c-1)^2}, & c \neq 1, \end{cases}$$

$$S_2 = \begin{cases} n-1, & c=1, \\ \dfrac{c^n - c}{c-1}, & c \neq 1. \end{cases}$$

The proof is based on the following theorem.

THEOREM 12.9 (DEUTSCH [1982]). *Let $A = (a_{ij})$ be a nonnegative irreducible $n \times n$ matrix and let x and y be positive vectors satisfying*

$$Ax = Dx,$$
$$A^T y = Dy,$$

for some positive diagonal matrix

$$D = \mathrm{diag}(d_1, d_2, \ldots, d_n).$$

If x is not a Perron vector of A, then

$$\rho(A) > \frac{y^T D x}{y^T x}, \tag{12.7}$$

where $\rho(A)$ is the spectral radius of the matrix A.

We give a method for determining the lower bound for the unique positive root Z of the equation

$$x^n = \sum_{k=1}^{n} \left(\sum_{j=1}^{n} a_{jk} \right)^k x^{n-k},$$

$$a_{j1}, a_{j2}, \ldots, a_{jn} \geq 0, \quad j = 1, 2, \ldots, n.$$

Using the same notation as in Bojanov's Theorem 12.3, we state the following.

THEOREM 12.10 (KJURKCHIEV and HERZBERGER [1992]).

$$Z > \frac{t_1 + \sum_{k=1}^{n-1}(k+1)t_{k+1}}{1 + \sum_{k=1}^{n-1} k t_{k+1}},$$

where

$$t_k = \left(\sum_{j=1}^{n} a_{jk} \right)^k, \quad k = 1, 2, \ldots, n.$$

PROOF. Let us associate with the polynomial,

$$P_{n,t_1,\ldots,t_n}(x) = x^n - t_1 x^{n-1} - t_2 x^{n-2} - \cdots - t_{n-1} x - t_n,$$

the corresponding matrix

$$A^{(n)}_{t_1,\ldots,t_n} = \begin{pmatrix} t_1 & t_2 & t_3 & \cdots & t_{n-1} & t_n \\ 1 & 0 & 0 & \cdots & 0 & 0 \\ 0 & 1 & 0 & \cdots & 0 & 0 \\ \vdots & & & & & \\ 0 & 0 & 0 & \cdots & 1 & 0 \end{pmatrix}$$

with $\det(A^{(n)}_{t_1,\ldots,t_n} - xI) = (-1)^n P_{n,t_1,\ldots,t_n}(x)$, namely, $P_{n,t_1,\ldots,t_n}$ is the characteristic polynomial of the matrix $A^{(n)}_{t_1,\ldots,t_n}$. The matrix $A^{(n)}_{t_1,\ldots,t_n}$ is nonnegative and its directed graph is strongly connected, i.e. $A^{(n)}_{t_1,\ldots,t_n}$ is irreducible. By the Perron–Frobenius theorem, this implies that $A^{(n)}_{t_1,\ldots,t_n}$ has a positive eigenvalue Z equal to its spectral radius $\rho(A^{(n)}_{t_1,\ldots,t_n})$.

Using the estimation (12.7), we have

$$Z = \rho(A^{(n)}_{t_1,\ldots,t_n}) > \frac{y^T Dx}{y^T x}.$$

Taking $A = A^{(n)}_{t_1,\ldots,t_n}$ and $x = [1 \ 1 \ \cdots \ 1]^T$ from the relation

$$Ax = Dx,$$

we find

$$D = \text{diag}\left(\sum_{k=1}^n t_k, 1, \ldots, 1\right).$$

The system

$$(A^T - D)y = 0$$

yields

$$y = \alpha[1 \ t_2 + \cdots + t_n \ t_3 + \cdots + t_n \ \cdots \ t_n]^T,$$

where $\alpha > 0$ is arbitrary. Now, we have

$$y^T Dx = \alpha \left(t_1 + \sum_{k=1}^{n-1}(k+1)t_{k+1}\right),$$

$$y^T x = \alpha \left(1 + \sum_{k=1}^{n-1} k t_{k+1}\right)$$

which ends the proof of the theorem. □

The following theorem is due to DEUTSCH [1982].

THEOREM 12.11. *Using the same notation as in Theorem* 12.9, *then*

$$\rho(A) > t - \prod_i (t - d_i)^{x_i y_i / y^T x} > \frac{y^T Dx}{y^T x} \tag{12.8}$$

for all
$$t > \rho(A) + \max_i(d_i - a_{ii}).$$

REMARK 12.1. The function
$$g(t) = t - \prod_i (t - d_i)^{x_i y_i / y^T x},$$
is strictly decreasing from $\max_i d_i$ to $y^T Dx/y^T x$ as t increases from $\max_i d_i$ to $+\infty$.

By Theorem 12.11, the values of $g(t)$ for
$$t > \rho(A) + \max_i(d_i - a_{ii})$$
are strict lower bounds for $\rho(A)$. However, since $\rho(A)$ is not known, one should evaluate $g(t)$ at $t = \beta + \max_i(d_i - a_{ii})$, where β is an upper bound of $\rho(A)$. Thus, for each upper bound β of $\rho(A)$, the number
$$\alpha = t - \prod_i (t - d_i)^{x_i y_i / y^T x},$$
where
$$t = \beta + \max_i(d_i - a_{ii}),$$
is a lower bound for $\rho(A)$ and α is a strictly decreasing function of β, bounded from below by $y^T Dx/y^T x \, (= y^T Ax/y^T x)$.

Some of the possible values of β are: the largest row sum of A, the largest column sum of $A, \max_i d_i$.

Using the estimation (12.8), we may establish the following.

THEOREM 12.12 (KJURKCHIEV and HERZBERGER [1992]). *If* $\sum_{j=1}^n a_{jk} > 1, k = 1, 2, \ldots, n$, *then*
$$Z > t_1 + 2 \sum_{k=2}^n t_k - \left[\sum_{k=2}^n t_k \left(t_1 - 1 + 2 \sum_{k=2}^n t_k \right)^\beta \right]^{1/(1+\beta)},$$
where $\beta = \sum_k^{n-1} t_{k+1}$.

PROOF. In view of (12.8) and since
$$t = \max_i d_i + \max_i(d_i - a_{ii}) = t_1 + 2 \sum_{k=2}^n t_k > 1,$$
it follows that
$$z > t - \prod_i (t - d_i)^{x_i y_i / y^T x} = t_1 + 2 \sum_{k=2}^n t_k$$

$$-\left[\sum_{k=2}^{n} t_k \left(t_1 - 1 + 2\sum_{k=2}^{n} t_k\right)^{\sum_{k=2}^{n} t_k + \sum_{k=3}^{n} t_k + \cdots + t_n} \left(1 + \sum_{k=1}^{n-1} k t_{k+1}\right)^{-1}\right].$$

□

REMARK 12.2. From the bounds above, we obtain a new bound for $\sigma_{p,q}^{(n)}$:

$$\sigma_{p,q}^{(n)} > t - \left[(p+1)(q + q^2 + \cdots + q^{n-1})(t-1)^\gamma\right]^{1/(1+\gamma)}, \qquad (12.9)$$

$$t = (p+1)[1 + 2(q + q^2 + \cdots + q^{n-1})], \qquad \gamma = (p+1)\sum_{k=1}^{n-1} k q^k.$$

We give a numerical example. For the zero $\sigma_{p,q}^{(n)} = 5.1$ of the polynomial

$$x^6 = 5x^5 + 0.5x^4 + 0.05x^3 + 0.005x^2 + 0.0005x + 0.00005,$$

$$n = 6, \quad p = 4, \quad q = 0.1$$

we obtain the following bounds: from (12.3), $\sigma_{p,q}^{(6)} > 4.371$; from (12.6), $\sigma_{p,q}^{(6)} > 3.817$; from (12.9), $\sigma_{p,q}^{(6)} > 4.815$.

These theorems can be used to improve many classical estimations for the roots of algebraic equations.

Other bounds for $\rho(A)$ have been found by LEDERMANN [1950], OSTROWSKI [1952], BRAUER [1957], OSTROWSKI and SCHNEIDER [1960], HALL and PORSCHING [1969], BRAUER and GENTRY [1974, 1976], FRIEDLAND and KARLIN [1975], DEUTSCH [1979, 1981], COHEN [1979], and MERIKOSKI [1979].

REMARK 12.3. These results can be applied to the determination of the R-order of convergence of iterative numerical processes. Let IP denote a general iterative process that produces a sequence of approximations $\{t^{(k)}\}$ with the limit point t^*. For the errors

$$\varepsilon^{(k)} = \|t^* - t^{(k)}\| \geqslant 0,$$

it is often possibile to derive a difference inequality like

$$\varepsilon^{(k+1)} \leqslant \gamma \prod_{i=0}^{n} \left(\varepsilon^{(k-i)}\right)^{q^i(p+1)}, \qquad p, q, \gamma > 0. \qquad (12.10)$$

According to SCHMIDT [1981], the recurrence (12.10) has an R-order of convergence $O_R(\text{IP}, t^*)$ (see ORTEGA and RHEINBOLDT [1970]) of at least $\sigma_{p,q}^{(n+1)}$, where $\sigma_{p,q}^{(n+1)}$ is the unique positive root of the Eq. (12.2).

Using the estimation (12.4), we can establish

$$O_R(0, \{\varepsilon^{(k)}\}) \geqslant \sigma_{p,q}^{(n+1)} > p + q + 1 - \frac{(p+1)q^{n+1}}{(p+q+1)^{n+1}} e.$$

The R-order is one of the most important measures to characterize the speed of convergence of sequences obtained by iterative processes in normed spaces (see BURMEISTER and SCHMIDT [1982, 1983, 1988], HERZBERGER [1989, 1990], KJURKCHIEV [1991]).

The characterization of the best R-orders of sequences arising in iterative processes has been treated by BURMEISTER and SCHMIDT [1985].

13. Sendov's method for localization of all positive roots

In this section, we obtain upper and lower bounds for the positive roots of algebraic equations.

A method, originally due to SENDOV [1974] for simultaneous approximate calculation of all positive roots of the equation

$$f(x) = a_0 + a_1 x + \cdots + a_m x^m = 0 \tag{13.1}$$

is based on the following theorem given by POINCARÉ [1883].

THEOREM 13.1. *Let f be a polynomial with real coefficients. If k is a large enough natural number, then the number of positive roots of the Eq. (13.1) is equal to the number of variations in sign in the sequence of nonnegative coefficients of the polynomial*

$$g(x) = (1+x)^k f(x) \,.$$

Let $0 < x_1 \leqslant x_2 \leqslant \cdots \leqslant x_p$, $p \leqslant m$ be positive roots of Eq. (13.1) ($a_0 > 0, a_m \neq 0$) and

$$(1+x)^k f(x) = \sum_{\nu=0}^{m+k} b_k(\nu) x^\nu. \tag{13.2}$$

Let us denote the smallest integer number by $\nu_k(1)$, for which $b_k(\nu_k(1)) \geqslant 0$ and $b_k(\nu_k(1)+1) < 0, b_k(0) = a_0 > 0$. In general, $\nu_k(s)$ is the smallest integer number for which

$$(-1)^{s-1} b_k(\nu_k(s)) \geqslant 0,$$
$$(-1)^{s-1} b_k(\nu_k(s)+1) < 0,$$
$$\nu_k(s) > \nu_k(s-1).$$

Then we obtain the numbers

$$\nu_k(1), \nu_k(2), \ldots, \nu_k(s). \tag{13.3}$$

According to Poincaré, there exists a number $k_0 = k_0(f)$, such that for every $k \geqslant k_0$, we have $s_k = p$, where p is the number of positive roots of Eq. (13.1).

The numbers (13.3) satisfy (see SENDOV [1974])

$$\frac{\nu_k(s)}{k - \nu_k(s) + 1} \leqslant \xi(k, \nu, s) \leqslant \frac{\nu_k(s) + 1}{k - \nu_k(s)}, \tag{13.4}$$

$$\lim_{k \to \infty} \frac{\nu_k(s)}{k - \nu_k(s) + 1} = \lim_{k \to \infty} \xi(k, \nu, s) = x_s,$$
$$f(x_s) = 0, \quad s = 1, 2, \ldots, p \,. \tag{13.5}$$

As far as the asymptotic (13.5) is known, we can obtain more precise local estimations, which are necessary for investigating the order of convergence and computational efficiency of the classes of methods in numerical analysis.

THEOREM 13.2 (KJURKCHIEV [1992b]). *If $0 < \delta \leqslant \frac{1}{2}$ and $k\delta \leqslant \nu \leqslant (1-\delta)k$, then*

$$\frac{b_k(\nu)}{\binom{k}{\nu}} = f\left(\frac{\nu}{k-\nu+1} - \frac{\frac{\nu}{k-\nu+1} - 1}{\left(\frac{\nu}{k-\nu+1}\right)^k}(1+1/k)^k\right) + \frac{C\theta_{k,\nu}}{k+1}, \tag{13.6}$$

where $C = C(f)$ does not depend on k and ν and $|\theta_{k,\nu}| \leqslant 1$.

PROOF. According to SENDOV [1974], there exist such numbers $\delta = \delta(f), \delta \in (0,1)$ and $N = N(f)$ such that for $k > N$, we have

$$\begin{aligned}\operatorname{sgn} b_k(\nu) &= \operatorname{sgn} a_0, & 0 \leqslant \nu \leqslant \delta k, \\ \operatorname{sgn} b_k(\nu) &= \operatorname{sgn} a_m, & (1-\delta)k \leqslant \nu \leqslant m+k.\end{aligned} \tag{13.7}$$

From (13.2), we obtain

$$\begin{aligned}\frac{b_k(\nu)}{\binom{k}{\nu}} &= a_0 + \frac{\nu}{k-\nu+1}a_1 + \frac{\nu(\nu-1)}{(k-\nu+1)(k-\nu+2)}a_2 + \cdots \\ &+ \frac{\nu(\nu-1)\cdots(\nu-m+1)}{(k-\nu+1)(k-\nu+2)\cdots(k-\nu+m)}a_m.\end{aligned}$$

If $\nu \leqslant \delta k$ and $0 \leqslant i \leqslant \nu$, then

$$0 \leqslant \frac{\nu - i}{k - \nu + i + 1} \leqslant \frac{\delta k - i}{(1-\delta)k + i + 1} \leqslant \frac{\delta}{1-\delta}$$

and

$$\left| b_k(\nu)\binom{k}{\nu}^{-1} - a_0 \right| \leqslant \frac{\delta}{1-\delta}\left[|a_1| + \frac{\delta}{1-\delta}|a_2| + \cdots + \left(\frac{\delta}{1-\delta}\right)^{m-1}|a_m|\right]$$

which proves (13.7).

It is easy to find

$$\frac{b_k(\nu)}{\binom{k}{\nu}} = f\left(\frac{\nu}{k-\nu+1} - \frac{\frac{\nu}{k-\nu+1} - 1}{\left(\frac{\nu}{k-\nu+1}\right)^k}\left(1+\frac{1}{k}\right)^k\right) + \sum_{i=1}^{m} L(k,\nu,i)a_i, \tag{13.8}$$

where

$$L(k,\nu,i) = \frac{\nu}{k-\nu+1}\frac{\nu-1}{k-\nu+2}\cdots\frac{\nu-(i-1)}{k-\nu+i}$$

$$-\left(\frac{\nu}{k-\nu+1} - \frac{\frac{\nu}{k-\nu+1} - 1}{\left(\frac{\nu}{k-\nu+1}\right)^k}\left(1+\frac{1}{k}\right)^k\right)^i.$$

If $ak > 1$, then

$$\frac{a(1+1/k)^k}{(a+1)^k} < \frac{a+1}{k+1}. \tag{13.9}$$

For $k\delta \leqslant \nu \leqslant (1-\delta)k$, we obtain

$$\frac{\nu-i+1}{k-n+i} < \cdots < \frac{\nu-1}{k-n+2} < \frac{\nu}{k-n+1} \leqslant \frac{1-\delta}{\delta}. \tag{13.10}$$

Letting $a+1 = \nu/(k-\nu+1) \leqslant (1-\delta)/\delta$, from $ak > 1$, (13.9) and (13.10) we obtain $\delta < k/(1+2k)$ and

$$|L(k,\nu,i)| \leqslant \left|(a+1)^i - \left[a+1 - \frac{a}{(a+1)^k}(1+1/k)^k\right]^i\right|$$
$$\leqslant i(a+1)^i \frac{1}{k+1} \leqslant i\left(\frac{1-\delta}{\delta}\right)^i \frac{1}{k+1}. \tag{13.11}$$

Equality (13.6) follows from (13.8) and (13.11), setting

$$C = C(f) = \sum_{i=1}^m i\left(\frac{1-\delta}{\delta}\right)^i |a_i|.$$

The theorem is proved. □

The next theorem gives upper and lower bounds for the positive roots $\xi(k,\nu,s)$

THEOREM 13.3. *The following inequalities hold:*

$$\frac{\nu}{k-\nu+1} - \frac{\frac{\nu}{k-\nu+1} - 1}{\left(\frac{\nu}{k-\nu+1}\right)^k}\left(1+\frac{1}{k}\right)^k$$

$$\leqslant \xi(k,\nu,s) \leqslant \frac{\nu+1}{k-\nu} - \frac{\frac{\nu+1}{k-\nu} - 1}{\left(\frac{\nu+1}{k-\nu}\right)^k}\left(1+\frac{1}{k}\right)^k, \quad s = 1,2,\ldots,p. \tag{13.12}$$

PROOF. From (13.6) and $(-1)^{s-1}b_k(\nu_k(s)) \geqslant 0, (-1)^{s-1}b_k(\nu_k(s)+1) < 0$, we obtain

$$(-1)^{s-1}\left[f\left(\frac{\nu}{k-\nu+1} - \frac{\frac{\nu}{k-\nu+1} - 1}{\left(\frac{\nu}{k-\nu+1}\right)^k}(1+1/k)^k\right) + \frac{C\theta_1}{k+1}\right] \geqslant 0,$$

$$(-1)^{s-1}\left[f\left(\frac{\nu+1}{k-\nu} - \frac{\frac{\nu+1}{k-\nu} - 1}{\left(\frac{\nu+1}{k-\nu}\right)^k}(1+1/k)^k\right) + \frac{C\theta_2}{k+1}\right] < 0,$$

where $\theta_1, \theta_2 \in [-1, 1]$.

Hence, there is only one point $\xi = \xi(k, \nu, s)$ for which the inequalities (13.12) hold true and

$$f(\xi) + \frac{C\theta}{k+1} = 0, \quad |\theta| \leqslant 1.$$

The theorem is proved. □

REMARK 13.1. The estimations (13.4) and (13.12) are in some sense analogous to the classical Ostrowski–Traub estimations for localization of the unique positive root α of the equation

$$x^k = A \sum_{j=0}^{k-1} x^j, \quad kA > 0,$$

$$A + 1 - \frac{A}{(A+1)^k}(1+1/k)^k < \alpha < A + 1 - \frac{A}{(A+1)^k}.$$

In this connection the advantage of Sendov's method is the simultaneous localization of all positive roots of (13.1).

REMARK 13.2. The estimation obtained (see SENDOV [1974]),

$$\left|\frac{\nu_k(s)}{k - \nu_k(s) + 1} - x_s\right| \leqslant \omega k^{-1/q},$$

in the case where x_s is a q-multiple root, can be improved using the following estimation:

$$\left|\frac{\nu_k(s)}{k - \nu_k(s) + 1} - \frac{\frac{\nu_k(s)}{k - \nu_k(s) + 1} - 1}{\left(\frac{\nu_k(s)}{k - \nu_k(s) + 1}\right)^k}\left(1 + \frac{1}{k}\right)^k - x_s\right| \leqslant \omega_1(k+1)^{-1/q}.$$

CHAPTER III

Local and Global Methods

All numerical methods for determining the roots of a polynomial presented in this chapter can be considered classical ones. Based on the theoretical results established more than hundred years ago some of them are at the same time global convergence methods, i.e. they guarantee convergence to a root of a polynomial equation. This fact makes them a useful tool for practical computer application. Some difficulties that arise in special cases can be easily avoided. For example, the Lehmer–Schur method can be described as a simple algorithm that ensures global convergence.

As is pointed by RALSTON [1965] the methods of Lehmer–Schur, Bernoulli, Graeffe and Laguerre do not have only historical and theoretical interest.

14. Bernoulli's iteration

A method, originally due to Daniel Bernoulli, for obtaining the roots of the algebraic equation,

$$x^n + a_1 x^{n-1} + \cdots + a_{n-1} x + a_n = 0, \tag{14.1}$$

is based on the related recurrence formula

$$u_k + a_1 u_{k-1} + \cdots + a_{n-1} u_{k-n+1} + a_n u_{k-n} = 0. \tag{14.2}$$

If the roots of (14.1) are $\alpha_1, \alpha_2, \ldots, \alpha_n$, and if (14.2) is considered as a difference equation, its general solution is found to be

$$u_k = C_1 \alpha_1^k + C_2 \alpha_2^k + \cdots + C_n \alpha_n^k, \tag{14.3}$$

where $C_i, i = 1, 2, \ldots, n$ are constants, independent of k, which are determined by the values of $u_0, u_1, \ldots, u_{n-1}$ if no roots are repeated. Under this assumption, let the roots be numbered in decreasing order of magnitude, so that here α_1 denotes the largest root of (14.1). Then, since (14.3) can be written in the form

$$u_k = C_1 \alpha_1^k \left[1 + \frac{C_2}{C_1} \left(\frac{\alpha_2}{\alpha_1}\right)^k + \frac{C_3}{C_1} \left(\frac{\alpha_3}{\alpha_1}\right)^k + \cdots + \frac{C_n}{C_1} \left(\frac{\alpha_n}{\alpha_1}\right)^k \right]$$

if $C \neq 0$, it follows that in any sequence generated by (14.2), the kth term is approximated by $C_1 \alpha_1^k$ as $k \to \infty$ and, indeed, that the ratio

$$r_k = \frac{u_k}{u_{k-1}}$$

tends to α_1 as $k \to \infty$ if the largest root α_1 is real and unrepeated and if no other root has equal magnitude, unless $u_0, u_1, \ldots, u_{n-1}$ are so chosen that the coefficient C_1 of α_1^k in (14.3) is zero.

The following is taken from HILDEBRAND [1956].

If the largest root α_1 is complex, and the coefficients of (14.1) are real, then α_2 is the complex conjugate of α_1 and is of equal magnitude. If we write

$$\alpha_1 = \xi_1 + i\eta_1 = \beta_1 e^{i\phi_1},$$
$$\alpha_2 = \xi_1 - i\eta_1 = \beta_1 e^{-i\phi_1},$$

where $\beta_1 > 0$ and $\xi_1, \eta_1, \beta_1, \phi_1$ are real numbers. The terms corresponding to α_1 and α_2 in (14.3) can be expressed in the real form

$$\beta_1^k (C_1 \cos \phi_1 + C_2 \sin k\phi_1),$$

if C_1 and C_2 are replaced by $(C_1 - iC_2)/2$ and $(C_1 + iC_2)/2$, respectively, in (14.3).

Thus, if α_1 and $\overline{\alpha}_1$ are not repeated and if all other roots are smaller in magnitude than β_1, it follows that

$$u_k \simeq \beta_1^k (C_1 \cos k\phi_1 + C_2 \sin k\phi_1), \quad k \to \infty. \tag{14.4}$$

But, if u_k were given exactly by the righ-hand side of (14.4), it would satisfy the recurrence relation

$$u_{k+1} - 2u_k \beta_1 \cos \phi_1 + \beta_1^2 u_{k-1} = 0,$$

and conversely, as is easily verified. A second relation, involving the two real unknown quantities β_1 and ϕ_1, would then be obtained, by replacing k by $k-1$, in the form

$$u_k - 2u_{k-1} \beta_1 \cos \phi_1 + \beta_1^2 u_{k-2} = 0.$$

The result of eliminating $\cos \phi_1$ from these two relations is

$$(u_{k-1}^2 - u_k u_{k-2}) \beta_1^2 = u_k^2 - u_{k+1} u_{k-1},$$

whereas the result of eliminating β_1^2 is

$$2(u_{k-1}^2 - u_k u_{k-2}) \beta_1 \cos \phi_1 = u_k u_{k-1} - u_{k+1} u_{k-2}.$$

Thus, if we introduce the definitions

$$s_k = u_k^2 - u_{k+1} u_{k-1},$$
$$t_k = u_k u_{k-1} - u_{k+1} u_{k-2},$$

these relations become

$$\beta_1^2 = \lim_{k \to \infty} \frac{s_k}{s_{k-1}},$$

$$2\beta_1 \cos \phi_1 = \lim_{k \to \infty} \frac{t_k}{s_{k-1}}.$$

Other exceptional cases, in which several roots have the same maximum absolute value, can be treated in a similar way.

If α_1 is real and unrepeated, the ideal situation would be that in which $u_0, u_1, \ldots, u_{n-1}$ were chosen so that $C_2 = \cdots = C_n = 0$ in (14.3), so that $u_0, u_1, \ldots, u_{n-1}$ would be proportional to $1, \alpha_1, \ldots, \alpha_1^{n-1}$, respectively.

The first calculated value of r, $r = u_n/u_{n-1}$, would then clearly be identical with α_1. In such cases, the starting values could be taken efficiently as successive powers of a previously determined approximation of α_1. If no information is easily available with regard to the nature of the largest root or roots, the starting values

$$u_0 = u_1 = \cdots = u_{n-2} = 0, \quad u_{n-1} = 1$$

are often convenient. For this set of values, it is easily seen that the undesirable case $C_1 = 0$ cannot occur.

A particularly notable set of n starting values, having the same property, is that determined from the formula

$$u_r = -(a_1 u_{r-1} + a_2 u_{r-2} + \cdots + a_{r-1} u_1 + r a_r), \quad r = 1, 2, \ldots, n \tag{14.5}$$

with $u_0 = u_{-1} = \cdots = 0$. For this set of starting values, it can be shown that all the C's in (14.3) are unity, and hence that u_k is then identified with the sum

$$\alpha_1^k + \alpha_2^k + \cdots + \alpha_n^k$$

for all $k \geq 1$. Thus, in particular, if $|\alpha_1| \gg |\alpha_2|, \ldots, |\alpha_n|$, then both $\alpha_1 \simeq u_k/u_{k-1}$ and $\alpha_1 \simeq u_k^{1/k}$ when k is sufficiently large. With the convention that $a_r = 0$ when $r > n$, it is seen that the recurrence formula (14.5) reduces to (14.2) when $r > n$. This special procedure is closely related to the Graeffe procedure described in the following section.

Bernoulli's procedure is analyzed by AITKEN [1926]. For other results, see MIGNOTTE [1976].

15. Graeffe's method

Many theoretical and technical questions lead to the problem of solving an algebraic equation with numerically given coefficients.

This section deals with the method of BERNOULLI [1728], DANDELIN [1826], LOBACHEVSKY [1834] and GRAEFFE [1837] devised for the approximative solution of algebraic equations. In eastern Europe, the method is usually called the method of Lobachevsky, whereas here and in western Europe it is usually called the method of Graeffe.

This method proceeds as follows. Let

$$f(z) = a_{0,0} + a_{1,0} z + \cdots + a_{n,0} z^n, \quad a_{n,0} = 1,$$

and we suppose its zeros $z_1, \ldots, z_n$ satisfy the inequality

$$|z_1| < |z_2| < \cdots < |z_n|. \tag{15.1}$$

We define the polynomials

$$f_\nu(z) = a_{0,\nu} + a_{1,\nu} z + \cdots + a_{n,\nu} z^n, \quad a_{n,\nu} = 1,$$

by
$$f_{\nu+1}(z) = (-1)^n f_\nu(\sqrt{z}) f_\nu(-\sqrt{z}), \quad \nu = 0, 1, 2, \ldots, \tag{15.2}$$

(so-called Graeffe-transforms), which is equivalent to the coefficient recursion

$$a_{n-m,\nu+1} = 2a_{n,\nu} a_{n-2m,\nu} - 2a_{n-1,\nu} a_{n-2m+1,\nu} + \cdots$$
$$+ (-1)^{m-1} a_{n-m+1,\nu} a_{n-m-1,\nu} + (-1)^m a_{n-m,\nu}^2,$$
$$m = 1, 2, \ldots, n.$$

Hence the coefficients $a_{k,\nu}$ can be easily computed. It follows from (15.2) that the zeros of $f_\nu(z)$ are exactly the numbers

$$z_1^{2^\nu}, z_2^{2^\nu}, \ldots, z_n^{2^\nu}.$$

Hence

$$\sum_{j=1}^n z_j^{2^\nu} = -a_{n-1,\nu}, \qquad \sum_{1 \leqslant j_1 < j_2 \leqslant n} (z_{j_1} z_{j_2})^{2^\nu} = a_{n-2,\nu},$$

etc.; i.e. from (15.1), we have

$$|z_n| = \lim_{\nu \to \infty} |a_{n-1,\nu}|^{2^{-\nu}}, \qquad |z_{n-1} z_n| = \lim_{\nu \to \infty} |a_{n-2,\nu}|^{2^{-\nu}},$$

or

$$|z_{n-1}| = \lim_{\nu \to \infty} \left| \frac{a_{n-2,\nu}}{a_{n-1,\nu}} \right|^{2^{-\nu}}.$$

Then the method asserts that

$$|z_k| = \lim_{\nu \to \infty} \left| \frac{a_{k-1,\nu}}{a_{k,\nu}} \right|^{2^{-\nu}} = r_k \tag{15.3}$$

for $k = 1, 2, \ldots, n$, i.e. the absolute values of the zeros are determined.

If we want the zeros themselves, we have only to expand $f_0(z)$ into a Taylor series around $z = h$, where h is so small that

$$|z_1 - h| < |z_2 - h| < \cdots < |z_n - h|$$

and apply the rule (15.3). Denoting the corresponding r_k-values $r_k(h)$, the points of intersection of the circles,

$$|z| = r_k, \ |z - h| = r_k(h),$$

leave only two possibilities for z_k, the wrong one of which can be easily removed.

The first theoretical disadvantage is that if $|z_1| = |z_2|$, this is no longer true. If, for example (α to be determined),

$$f_0(z) = (z-1)(z - e^{i\alpha})(z - e^{-i\alpha}), \tag{15.4}$$

then we have obviously

$$-a_{2,\nu} = 1 + e^{2^\nu i\alpha} + e^{-2^\nu i\alpha} = 1 + 2\cos 2^\nu \alpha.$$

Choosing $\nu = 2t + 1$, $\alpha = \pi/3$, we have

$$2^{2t+1} \equiv 2 \pmod{6},$$

$$\cos\frac{2^\nu \pi}{3} = \cos\frac{(6\nu + 2)\pi}{3} = \cos\frac{2\pi}{3} = -\frac{1}{2}$$

and

$$a_{2,2t+1} = 0, \quad t = 0, 1, 2, \ldots,$$

i.e. if the limes for $|z_n|$ exists, then it is 0 that does not give the right value of $|z_n|$ which is 1.

A practical disadvantage is presented by the fact that there is no method to decide whether (15.1) is satisfied. This means a further practical disadvantage that even if (15.1) is fulfilled, we have no rule to decide whether, for a certain $\nu = \nu_0$, the quantity

$$\left|\frac{a_{k-1,\nu_0}}{a_{k,\nu_0}}\right|^{2-\nu_0}$$

is 'near enough' to the right value r_k. For a given arbitrary large positive ω and arbitrary small positive ε, one can easily modify the example (15.4) replacing $e^{\pm i\alpha}$ by $(1 - \delta)e^{i\alpha}$ and $(1 - 2\delta)e^{-i\alpha}$ with a suitable positive δ ($< \frac{1}{10}$), so that there is a $\nu > \omega$ such that

$$|a_{2,\nu}| \leqslant \varepsilon$$

which is 'far' from the right value 1.

Hence the practical value of the method seemed to be very small in spite of all the effort and even the theoretical basis was clarified only by POLYA [1915]. The first real progress was made after the results of PASTOR [1932] were incorporated with the results of SAN JUAN [1935]. This idea was found independently by OSTROWSKI [1940] who resumed the question in 1940 in a paper of fundamental importance. He succeeded in getting rid of all of the above-mentioned defects by a modification of the method.

Instead of the coefficients $a_{j,\nu}$ (ν fixed, $j = 0, \ldots, n$) he introduced in this theory, as a new element, the notion of the Newton majorant of the polynomial $f_\nu(z)$ (which occurred previously in a disguised form in the quoted paper of San Juan), i.e. the polynom

$$M(z, f_\nu) = \sum_{j=0}^{n} T_{j,\nu} z^j,$$

which is uniquely determined by the following three postulates:

(a) $|a_{j,\nu}| \leqslant T_{j,\nu}$, $j = 0, 1, \ldots, n$;

(b) putting

$$R_{j,\nu} = \frac{T_{j-1,\nu}}{T_{j,\nu}},$$

we require

$$R_{j,\nu} \leqslant R_{j+1,\nu}, \quad j = 1, \ldots, n;$$

(c) if a polynomial

$$M^*(z, f_\nu) = \sum_{j=0}^n T^*_{j,\nu} z^j$$

satisfies (a) and (b), then

$$T_{j,\nu} \leqslant T^*_{j,\nu}, \quad j = 0, 1, \ldots, n.$$

Let

$$|z_1| \leqslant |z_2| \leqslant \cdots \leqslant |z_n|.$$

Then

$$\left(1 - 2^{-1/k}\right)^{2^{-\nu}} \leqslant \frac{|z_k|}{R_{k,\nu}^{2^{-\nu}}} \leqslant \left(1 - 2^{-1/(n-k+1)}\right)^{-2^{-\nu}}, \quad k = 1, 2, \ldots, n.$$

More precisely, for $k = n$ (see OSTROWSKI [1940])

$$n^{-2^{-\nu}} < \frac{|z_n|}{(T_{n-1,\nu})^{2^{-\nu}}} < 2^{2^{-\nu}}.$$

We give two procedures for obtaining approximating values for the case $k = n$ (see TURAN [1951], RENY and TURAN [1952]).

First rule. Denoting

$$f_\nu(z) = \sum_{j=0}^n a_{j,\nu} z^j, \quad a_{n,\nu} = 1,$$

and the jth power-sum of its zeros by $s_{j,\nu}$, we compute further the quantities $s_{1,\nu}, s_{2,\nu}, \ldots, s_{2n,\nu}$ by the Newton–Girard formulas

$$\begin{aligned}
s_{1,\nu} + a_{n-1,\nu} &= 0, \\
s_{2,\nu} + a_{n-1,\nu} s_{1,\nu} + 2a_{n-2,\nu} &= 0, \\
&\vdots \\
s_{n,\nu} + a_{n-1,\nu} s_{n-1,\nu} + \cdots + n a_{0,\nu} &= 0, \\
s_{n+1,\nu} + a_{n-1,\nu} s_{n,\nu} + \cdots + a_{0,\nu} s_{1,\nu} &= 0, \\
&\vdots \\
s_{2n,\nu} + a_{n-1,\nu} s_{2n-1,\nu} + \cdots + a_{0,\nu} s_{n,\nu} &= 0.
\end{aligned}$$

Then we have

$$n^{-2^{-\nu}} \leqslant \frac{|z_n|}{\left(\max |s_{j,\nu}|^{1/j}\right)^{2^{-\nu}}} \leqslant 2^{2^{-\nu}}.$$

Second rule. With an integer $m \leqslant n$ and the notation of the first rule, from the quantities $s_{m,\nu}, s_{m+1,\nu}, \ldots, s_{m+n,\nu}$, we have

$$n^{-1/m} < \frac{|z_n|}{\left(\max_{m \leqslant j \leqslant m+n} |s_{j,n}|^{1/j}\right)^{1/m}} < \left(\frac{e^6 m}{n}\right)^{n/m}.$$

If $m \to \infty$, then both tails tend to 1, though slowly.

Graeffe's method has many possible variants (see BRODETSKY and SMEAL [1924]).

This method inspired a number of other contributions (see, for instance, SEBASTIAO E SILVA [1941, 1946], GASKELL [1958], BAREISS [1960], RUTISHAUSER [1963], GRAU [1963], HOUSEHOLDER [1971] and CHUNG [1972, 1976]).

16. The method of Laguerre

Let

$$f(x) = (x - \alpha_1)(x - \alpha_2) \cdots (x - \alpha_n) \tag{16.1}$$

be a polynomial with real zeros α_k. Suppose, that

$$\alpha_1 \leqslant \alpha_2 \leqslant \cdots \leqslant \alpha_n.$$

A method originally due to LAGUERRE [1880] for obtaining the root of the Equation (16.1) is based on the fact that if $\alpha_k < x < \alpha_{k+1}$, then the equation,

$$\left((n-2)f'^2 - (n-1)ff''\right)(Z - x)^2 - 2ff'(Z - x) - nf^2 = 0,$$

has two real roots in the intervals (α_k, x) and (x, α_{k+1}).

The Laguerre iteration for the numerical solution of algebraic equations with simple real roots is defined by

$$Z(x) = x - \phi(x), \tag{16.2}$$

where

$$\phi(x) = \frac{nf(x)}{f'(x) \pm \sqrt{(n-1)[(n-1)f'^2(x) - nf(x)f''(x)]}}.$$

The sign of the root is selected in order to maximize the modulus of ϕ.

Other elaborate results have been obtained by HERMITE [1898], VAN DER CORPUT [1946] and OBRESHKOV [1952].

THEOREM 16.1. *Even in the complex case, the Laguerre iteration defined by (16.2) converges cubically to a simple zero of $f(z)$ provided z_0 is sufficiently close to 1.*

THEOREM 16.2 (KAHAN [1967]). *If $f(z)$ is a polynomial of degree n, then in the Laguerre iteration there is at least one zero α satisfying*

$$|\alpha - z_\nu| \leqslant n^{1/2} |z_{\nu+1} - z_\nu|.$$

THEOREM 16.3 (OBRESHKOV [1963b]). *The Laguerre method converges only linearly to a root α of multiplicity p.*

PROOF. Define the following computation scheme:
$$a_{n+1} = a_n + \frac{nf(a_n)}{-f'(a_n) + \varepsilon\sqrt{(n-1)[(n-1)f'^2(a_n) - nf(a_n)f''(a_n)]}},$$
$$\varepsilon = \pm 1, \quad n = 0, 1, 2, \ldots . \tag{16.3}$$

Let $f(x) = (x-\alpha)^p g(x)$. We will assume that $g(\alpha) \neq 0$. If we denote by $X = a_n - \alpha$, we have
$$f(a_n) = X^p g(a_n), \quad f'(a_n) = X^{p-1} A_n, \quad f''(a_n) = X^{p-2} B_n,$$
where
$$A_n = pg(a_n) + Xg'(a_n),$$
$$B_n = p(p-1)g(a_n) + 2pXg'(a_n) + X^2 g''(a_n).$$

Then (16.3) implies
$$\frac{a_{n+1} - \alpha}{a_n - \alpha} = 1 + \frac{ng(a_n)}{-A_n + \varepsilon\sqrt{(n-1)[(n-1)A_n^2 - ng(a_n)B_n]}}.$$

Hence,
$$\lim_{n\to\infty} \frac{a_{n+1} - \alpha}{a_n - \alpha} = 1 + \frac{n}{-p + \varepsilon\sqrt{p(n-1)(n-p)}}.$$

This completes the proof. □

VAN DER CORPUT [1946] and OBRESHKOV [1963b] consider the following generalization of the method (16.3):
$$a_{n+1} = a_n + \frac{nf(a_n)}{-f'(a_n) + \varepsilon\sqrt{(n/p - 1)[(n-1)f'^2(a_n) - nf(a_n)f''(a_n)]}},$$
$$\varepsilon = \pm 1, \quad n = 0, 1, 2, \ldots . \tag{16.4}$$

THEOREM 16.4. *The sequence a_n generated by (16.4) will converge cubically to the multiple root.*

PROOF BY OBRESHKOV. Denote by
$$\Delta = \left(\frac{n}{p} - 1\right)[(n-1)f'^2(a_n) - nf(a_n)f''(a_n)], \quad h = a_n - \alpha,$$
it follows that
$$a_{n+1} - \alpha = \frac{nf(a_n) - (a_n - \alpha)f'(a_n) + \varepsilon(a_n - \alpha)\Delta^{1/2}}{-f'(a_n) + \varepsilon\Delta^{1/2}}$$
$$= \frac{[nf(a_n) - (a_n - \alpha)f'(a_n)]^2 - (a_n - \alpha)^2 \Delta}{[-f'(a_n) + \varepsilon\Delta^{1/2}][nf(a_n) - (a_n - \alpha)f'(a_n) - \varepsilon(a_n - \alpha)\Delta^{1/2}]},$$
$$\tag{16.5}$$

$$\Delta = h^{2p-2}\Big[(n-p)^2 g^2(a_n) - 2(n-p)hg(a_n)g'(a_n)$$
$$+ \frac{n-p}{p}(n-1)h^2 g'^2(a_n) - \frac{n(n-p)}{p}h^2 g(a_n)g''(a_n)\Big]$$
$$= h^{2p-2}\eta(a_n),$$

$$[nf(a_n) - hf'(a_n)]^2 - h^2\Delta = \frac{h^{2p+2}}{p}[n(p-n+1)g'^2(a_n)$$
$$+ n(n-p)g(a_n)g''(a_n)],$$

$$[-f'(a_n) + \varepsilon\Delta^{1/2}][nf(a_n) - (a_n-\alpha)f'(a_n) - \varepsilon(a_n-\alpha)\Delta^{1/2}]$$
$$= h^{2p-1}[-pg(a_n) - hg'(a_n) + \varepsilon\eta^{1/2}(a_n)]$$
$$\times [(n-p)g(a_n) - hg'(a_n) - \varepsilon\eta^{1/2}(a_n)].$$

For $\varepsilon = -1$, letting $n \to \infty$ in (16.5), we find
$$\lim_{n\to\infty} \frac{a_{n+1} - \alpha}{(a_n - \alpha)^3} = \frac{n(p-n+1)g'^2(\alpha) + n(n-p)g(\alpha)g''(\alpha)}{2np(p-n)g^2(\alpha)}.$$

This completes the proof of the theorem. □

REMARK 16.1 (OBRESHKOV [1963a]). Let $a_1, a_2, \ldots, a_n$ be real numbers and $a_1 = a_2 = \cdots = a_p = a$ $(p < n)$. Let

$$A = pa + a_{p+1} + \cdots + a_n,$$
$$B = pa^2 + a_{p+1}^2 + \cdots + a_n^2.$$

By Cauchy's inequality, we obtain
$$(A - pa)^2 = (a_{p+1} + a_{p+2} + \cdots + a_n)^2$$
$$\leqslant (n-p)(a_{p+1}^2 + \cdots + a_n^2) = (n-p)(B - pa^2),$$
$$npa^2 - 2pAa + A^2 - (n-p)B \leqslant 0.$$

Then
$$\frac{A - \sqrt{\frac{n-p}{p}(nB - A^2)}}{n} \leqslant a \leqslant \frac{A + \sqrt{\frac{n-p}{p}(nB - A^2)}}{n}. \tag{16.6}$$

If $f(x)$ is a polynomial of degree n with roots $x_1, \ldots, x_n$ and if we denote
$$a_k = \frac{1}{x - x_k}, \quad k = 1, 2, \ldots, n,$$

$$A = \frac{f'(x)}{f(x)}, \qquad B = \left(\frac{f'(x)}{f(x)}\right)^2 - \frac{f''(x)}{f(x)}$$

in (16.6), then method (16.6) turns into method (16.4).

Various methods and their modification have been considered by HANSEN and PATRICK [1976,1977], DEKKER [1968], PARLETT [1964], DAVIES and DAWSON [1978]. HANSEN and PATRICK [1976] suggest a method for the determination of the multiplicities of the roots of a given algebraic polynomial with real coefficients.

Thus, for instance, the iteration scheme depends on parameter α:

$$a_{n+1} = a_n - p(p\alpha + 1)f(a_n)$$
$$\times \left[p\alpha f'(a_n) \pm \sqrt{p(p\alpha - \alpha + 1)f'^2(a_n) - p(p\alpha + 1)f(a_n)f''(a_n)}\right]^{-1},$$
$$n = 0, 1, 2, \ldots . \qquad (16.7)$$

The sequence $\{a_n\}$ generated by (16.7) converges cubically to a root of multiplicity p for finite constant α. Letting $\alpha = 1/(n-p)$ in (16.7), we obtain (16.4) directly.

The family of methods (16.7) includes the Laguerre, Halley, Ostrowski and Euler methods and as a limiting case, Newton's method.

DOCHEV, BURNEV and RUSSEV [1969] consider a method for approximate calculation of the roots of entire functions of the form

$$f(z) = \prod_{n=1}^{\infty}\left(1 - \frac{z}{a_n}\right),$$

which can be viewed as an analogue of the well-known Laguerre method.

Let $f(z)$ be an entire function of order ρ, $0 < \rho \leqslant 1$, possessing only real and positive zeros $0 < a_1 < \cdots < a_n < \cdots$. Put

$$L(x) = f'^2(x)(1 - \sigma x) + \sigma f(x)\{f'(x) + xf''(x)\},$$
$$M(x) = xf'^2(x)(2 - \sigma x)$$
$$\qquad + f(x)\{f'(x) + \sigma f(x) + \sigma x[f'(x) + xf''(x)] - xf''(x)\},$$
$$N(x) = 2xf(x)\{f'(x) + \sigma f(x)\},$$
$$P(x) = \sigma x^2 f^2(x),$$
$$\sigma = \sum_{n=1}^{\infty} \frac{1}{a_n} = -\frac{f'(0)}{f(0)} = -f'(0).$$

The following theorem holds.

THEOREM 16.5. *If $f(a) = 0$, then $F(a - x; x) \leqslant 0$ for every real x, where*

$$F(\xi; x) = L(x)\xi^3 + M(x)\xi^2 + N(x)\xi + P(x).$$

For $x > a_1$ and $f(x) \neq 0$, the third degree equation $F(\xi; x) = 0$ has three different real roots $\xi_1(x) < \xi_2(x) < \xi_3(x)$ for ξ. In addition, the inequalities

$$-x < \xi_1(x) < a_s - x < \xi_2(x) < 0 < \xi_3(x)$$

hold, where a_s is the largest zero of $f(x)$ that is smaller than x. In order to calculate some zero $a = a_s$ of $f(z)$, we start from an arbitrary initial approximation x_0 from the interval (a_s, a_{s+1}) and construct the sequence $\{x_n\}_{n=0}^{\infty}$, where $x_{n+1} = x_n + \xi_2(x_n)$.

This sequence is convergent and

$$\lim_{n \to \infty} \frac{x_n - a}{(x_{n-1} - a)^3} = H(a),$$

$$H(a) = \frac{\sigma a - 2}{8(\sigma a - 1)} \left(\frac{f''(a)}{f'(a)} \right)^2 - \frac{3f''(a) + 2af'''(a)}{12af'(a)},$$

i.e. the convergence of the process has a cubic rate.

For entire functions of the form

$$\varphi(z) = \prod_{n=-\infty}^{\infty} \left(1 - \frac{z}{b_n}\right) e^{z/b_n}$$

with real and simple zeros for which

$$s = \sum_{n=-\infty}^{\infty} \frac{1}{b_n^2} < +\infty,$$

the following theorem can be established in an analogous way.

THEOREM 16.6. *If $\varphi(b) = 0$, then $F(b - x; x) \leq 0$, where*

$$F(\xi; x) = \{(x + \xi)\xi f'(x) + xf(x)\}^2$$
$$+ x^2\{s(x + \xi)^2 - 1\}\{[f''(x)f(x) - f'^2(x)]\xi^2 + f^2(x)\},$$

and for any real x, the polynomial $F(\xi; x)$ has real roots only.

This theorem allows us to construct an iteration process for the calculation of the roots of $\varphi(z)$.

A detailed discussion on the problem can be found in the monograph by ILIEV [1987].

17. The Lehmer–Schur method

For the equation

$$f(z) = a_n z^n + a_{n-1} z^{n-1} + \cdots + a_1 z + a_0,$$

let us define

$$f^*(z) = z^n \overline{f}(1/z) = \bar{a}_n + \bar{a}_{n-1} z + \cdots + \bar{a}_1 z^{n-1} + \bar{a}_0 z^n,$$

where $\bar{a}$ is a conjugate number of a.

THEOREM 17.1 (RALSTON [1965]). *Let $f(0) \neq 0$. If for some $h, 0 < h < k$, $T^h[f(0)] < 0$, then f has one zero inside the unit circle. If $T^i[f(0)] > 0$*

for $1 \leq i < k$ and $T^{k-1}[f(z)]$ is a constant, then f has no zeros inside the unit circle. Here

$$T[f(z)] = \bar{a}_0 f(z) - a_n f^*(z), \quad T^i[f(z)] = T\{T^{i-1}[f(z)]\}.$$

Note that $T[f(0)] = a_0 \bar{a}_0 - a_n \bar{a}_n = |a_0| - |a_n|$.

Using this theorem, it is possible to determine whether f has a zero inside the unit circle by the following algorithm.

(a) If $f(0) = 0$, then $z = 0$ is a zero; else go to (b).

(b) If $T[f(0)] < 0$, then f has a zero inside the unit circle; else go to (c).

(c) Compute $T^j[f(z)]$, $j = 1, 2, \ldots$, until $T^j[f(0)] < 0$, $j < k$, or $T^k[f(0)] = 0$. Note that $\deg\left(T^j[f(z)]\right) < \deg\left(T^{j-1}[f(z)]\right)$. If $T^j[f(0)] < 0$, then f has a zero inside the unit circle. If $T^k[f(0)] = 0$ and $T^{k-1}[f(z)]$ is a constant, then f has no roots inside the unit circle. The case where

$$T^k[f(0)] = 0, \qquad T^{k-1}[f(z)]$$

is not a constant can easily be avoided by the following considerations.

If f has a zero inside the unit circle $|z - c| \leq \rho$, then $g(z) = f(\rho z + c)$ has a zero inside the unit circle and therefore we present the following algorithm for determining the root of f in the unit circle, using the notation $D(c, r) = \{z: |z - c| < r\}$.

(i) Let j be the smallest integer such that $f(2^{j+1} z)$ has a zero in $D(0, 1)$ and $f(2^j z)$ does not have zeros in $D(0, 1)$. This means that $f(z)$ has a zero in the domain

$$U = \{z: 2^j \leq |z| < 2^{j+1}\}.$$

Vice versa, if f has a zero in $D(0, 1)$ we can find a similar domain U dividing the radius. Setting $R = 2^j$, domain D can be covered by the discs

$$W_k = \{z: |z - \frac{3R}{2\cos \pi/8} e^{2\pi k i/8}| \leq 4R/5\}, \quad k = 0, 1, \ldots, 7, \; i^2 = -1.$$

(ii) In the discs W_k, we can find one that contains the root and applying the procedure from point (i), let the domain

$$U^1 = \{z: (4R/5)2^{-j_1} \leq |z - c_1| < (4R/5)2^{-(j_1-1)}\}$$

contain a zero of $f(z)$. Let $R_1 = (4R/5)2^{-j_1}$.

(iii) Continuing this process, on the kth step the root will be in the disc with radius $2R_k$, where $R_k \leq \left(\frac{2}{5}\right)^k R$.

If at step (a), $T^k[f(0)] = 0$ but $T^{k-1}[f(z)]$ is not a constant, then choose a new radius, for example βR, $\beta = \frac{3}{4}$. If this case arises at step (c), then use $\beta \in (1, 2)$.

CHAPTER IV

Iterative Methods for Computation of All Roots

This chapter is concerned with iterative solutions of algebraic equations. The first step for simultaneous determination of all roots of a polynomial was made in 1891 by Weierstrass and more than 50 years later this approach was discovered again by many authors. Many attempts were made for accelerating the quadratic rate of convergence of Weierstrass' method and for obtaining different modifications in the case of multiple roots.

The methods for factorization of a polynomial into linear and quadratic factors are a convenient tool for determining all the roots. Factorization methods of BAIRSTOW [1914], HITCHKOCK [1944], are widely used. Here we present DVORCUK's [1969] method.

The investigation on interval methods for polynomial root determining increased rapidly after the basic book of ALEFELD and HERZBERGER [1983] devoted to interval arithmetic. Interval approach ensures high accuracy of the results and as a rule an interval version can be given for all known numerical methods. Numerical experiments show satisfactory numerical properties of interval methods with respect to initial approximations, stability and rate of convergence.

18. Iterative methods without derivatives

Consider a monic polynomial of degree $n \geq 3$,

$$f(x) = x^n + a_{n-1}x^{n-1} + \cdots + a_1 x + a_0, \tag{18.1}$$

with simple real or complex zeros $x_1, x_2, \ldots, x_n$. Let $x_1^k, x_2^k, \ldots, x_n^k$ be distinct reasonably close approximations of these zeros and let

$$Q(x) = \prod_{j=1}^{n}(x - x_j^k).$$

Then, for $x = x_i^k$, $i = 1, 2, \ldots, n$, we have

$$Q'(x_i^k) = \prod_{\substack{j=1 \\ j \neq i}}^{n}(x_i^k - x_j^k).$$

Introducing the abbreviation $\Delta_i = -f(x_i^k)/Q'(x_i^k)$, the following second-order method to simultaneously find polynomial zeros has been the subject of many papers:

$$x_i^{k+1} = x_i^k + \Delta_i, \quad i = 1, 2, \ldots, n,$$

or, in the form

$$x_i^{k+1} = x_i^k - \frac{f(x_i^k)}{\prod_{j \neq i}^{n}(x_i^k - x_j^k)}, \quad i = 1, 2, \ldots, n, \quad k = 0, 1, \ldots, \tag{18.2}$$

where x_i^{k+1} is a new approximation to the zero x_i. The iterative formula (18.2) is a classical result introduced by WEIERSTRASS [1903] in connection with a proof of the fundamental theorem of algebra.

In 1960–1962, this method was rediscovered by DURAND [1960] and DOCHEV [1962a,b] and the theorem for the quadratic convergence of the method was given. Thus this method is called the Weierstrass method, the Durand–Kerner method or the Weierstrass–Dochev method.

For the first time, conditions for the choice of initial approximations that guarantee the convergence of the Newton type methods and of the methods of the type (18.2) appeared in the papers of ILIEV [1949] and ILIEV and DOCHEV [1963].

Different derivations of this formula were given later by BORSCH-SUPAN [1963], DOCHEV and BYRNEV [1964], KERNER [1966a,b], PRESIC [1966], SENDOV and POPOV [1976], PRESIC [1980] and others (see WERNER [1982] for some history).

Here we discuss the approach of KJURKCHIEV and MARKOV [1983].

THEOREM 18.1. *Let $0 < q < 1$, $d = \min_{i \neq j}|x_i - x_j|$ and $0 < c \leqslant d/(1 + \alpha n)$, where $\alpha = 1.7632283\ldots$ is determined from the equality $\alpha = e^{1/\alpha}$. If the initial approximations $\{x_i^0\}_{i=1}^{n}$ of the roots $\{x_i\}_{i=1}^{n}$ of Eq. (18.1) satisfy the inequalities*

$$|x_i^0 - x_i| \leqslant cq, \quad i = 1, 2, \ldots, n, \tag{18.3}$$

then for the approximations given by (18.2), the inequalities

$$|x_i^k - x_i| \leqslant cq^{2^k}, \quad i = 1, 2, \ldots, n, \tag{18.4}$$

hold true for all $k = 1, 2, \ldots$.

PROOF. By induction, the assumption (18.3) shows that (18.4) holds true for $k = 0$. Let (18.4) be satisfied for some $k = m$, i.e.

$$|x_i^m - x_i| \leqslant cq^{2^m}, \quad i = 1, 2, \ldots, n. \tag{18.5}$$

This implies, in view of $q < 1$,

$$|x_i^m - x_i| \leqslant c, \quad i = 1, 2, \ldots, n. \tag{18.6}$$

From (18.6) and the choice of c, it follows that $x_i^m \neq x_j^m$ for $i \neq j$. Moreover, for $i \neq j$, we have

$$|x_i^m - x_j^m| \geq |x_i - x_j| - |x_i^m - x_i| - |x_j^m - x_j| \geq d - 2c \geq c\alpha(n-1). \quad (18.7)$$

Using (18.2), we obtain for the difference $x_i^{m+1} - x_i$,

$$x_i^{m+1} - x_i = (x_i^m - x_i)\left(1 - \prod_{j \neq i}^n \frac{x_i^m - x_j}{x_i^m - x_j^m}\right).$$

We shall transform the last expression by means of the identity (see TASCHEV and KJURKCHIEV [1983])

$$\prod_{j \neq i}^n \frac{u_i - z_j}{u_i - u_j} - 1 = \sum_{s \neq i}^n \frac{u_s - z_s}{u_i - u_s} \prod_{j \neq i}^{s-1} \frac{u_i - z_j}{u_i - u_j}, \quad (18.8)$$

which holds true for arbitrary $2n$ numbers $z_1, \ldots, z_n, u_1, \ldots, u_n$, such that $u_i \neq u_j$ for $i \neq j$.

Using this identity with $u_i = x_i^m$ (which can be done as $x_i^m \neq x_j^m$ for $i \neq j$) and $z_j = x_j$, we obtain

$$|x_i^{m+1} - x_i| \leq |x_i^m - x_i| \left| \sum_{s \neq i}^n \frac{x_s^m - x_s}{x_i^m - x_s^m} \prod_{j \neq i}^{s-1} \frac{x_i^m - x_j}{x_i^m - x_j^m} \right|$$

$$\leq |x_i^m - x_i| \sum_{s \neq i}^n \frac{|x_s^m - x_s|}{|x_i^m - x_s^m|} \prod_{j \neq i}^{s-1}\left(1 + \frac{|x_j^m - x_j|}{|x_i^m - x_j^m|}\right).$$

Using Eqs. (18.5)–(18.8) in the above expression, we obtain

$$|x_i^{m+1} - x_i| \leq cq^{2^m} \sum_{s \neq i}^n \frac{cq^{2^m}}{|x_i^m - x_s^m|} \prod_{j \neq i}^{s-1}\left(1 + \frac{c}{|x_i^m - x_j^m|}\right)$$

$$< cq^{2^m}(n-1)\frac{cq^{2^m}}{c\alpha(n-1)}\left(1 + \frac{c}{c\alpha(n-1)}\right)^{n-1}$$

$$= \frac{cq^{2^{m+1}}}{\alpha}\left(1 + \frac{1}{\alpha(n-1)}\right)^{n-1} < \frac{cq^{2^{m+1}}e^{1/\alpha}}{\alpha} = cq^{2^{m+1}},$$

since α is such that $\alpha = e^{1/\alpha}$. This implies that (18.4) holds true for $k = m+1$, which proves the theorem. □

The convergence speed strongly depends on the choice of the starting point, $x_i^0 = r_0 e^{2\pi i t/n}, i = 1, 2, \ldots, n$ (see GUGGENHEIMER [1986]).

REMARK 18.1. The equality

$$\sum_{i=1}^n x_i^k = \sum_{i=1}^n x_i = -a_{n-1}, \quad k = 1, 2, \ldots,$$

holds true independently of the initial approximations x_i^0, $i = 1, 2, \ldots, n$. This can be used as a control over the computations (see also KJELLBERG [1984]).

REMARK 18.2. In a number of cases, the calculation of $f(x_\nu^k)$ in (18.2) is quite difficult. That is why DOCHEV and BYRNEV [1964], make use of the following recurrent formula relating three systems of consecutive approximations $x_\nu^{k+2}, x_\nu^{k+1}, x_\nu^k$, $\nu = 1, 2, \ldots, n$, obtained from (18.2):

$$x_\nu^{k+2} = x_\nu^{k+1} - D_\nu^k \prod_{\mu \neq \nu}^n \frac{x_\nu^{k+1} - x_\mu^k}{x_\nu^{k+1} - x_\mu^{k+1}}, \quad \nu = 1, 2, \ldots, n, \ k = 0, 1, 2, \ldots, \quad (18.9)$$

where

$$D_\nu^k = x_\nu^{k+1} - x_\nu^k + s^k + \sum_{\mu \neq \nu}^n \frac{x_\nu^k - x_\mu^k}{x_\nu^{k+1} - x_\mu^k} \left(x_\mu^{k+1} - x_\mu^k \right),$$

$$s^k = a_{n-1} + \sum_{\nu=1}^n x_\nu^k = \begin{cases} 0 & \text{for } k \geq 1, \\ a_{n-1} + \sum_{\nu=1}^n x_\nu^0 & \text{for } k = 0. \end{cases}$$

Equation (18.9) is verified by means of elementary though not very brief calculations. The process (18.9) is called the Dochev–Byrnev method.

The iteration procedure (18.2), where $Q(x)$ is a generalized polynomial for a given system of base functions has been discussed by MAKRELOV and SEMERDZHIEV [1985a]. It can be proved that the iteration (18.2) is the same as the Newton method applied, in the n-dimensional space C^n, to the function $F(X) = (F_1(X), \ldots, F_n(X))$, where

$$F_1(X) = x_1 + \cdots + x_n + a_{n-1},$$

$$\vdots$$

$$F_k(X) = \sum_{i_1 < \cdots < i_k} x_{i_1} \ldots x_{i_k} + (-1)^{k-1} a_k = S_k^{(n)}(X) + (-1)^{k-1} a_k,$$

$$\vdots$$

$$F_n(X) = \prod_{i=1}^n x_i + (-1)^{n-1} a_0,$$

and $S_k^{(n)}(X)$, $k = 1, 2, \ldots, n$, are the Viete symmetric functions. This Newton approach in the n-dimensional space allows us to define other methods as the Pasquini–Trigiante algorithm (see PASQUINI and TRIGIANTE [1981, 1985]), where $F(X) = (F_1(X), \ldots, F_n(X))$ is the following function: $F_k(X) = f[x_1, \ldots, x_k]$, $k = 1, 2, \ldots, n$, and $f[x_1, \ldots, x_k]$ is the divided difference of f with respect to the arguments $x_1, \ldots, x_k$. Note that this method is globally convergent when applied to polynomials with real roots. Moreover, as (18.2) always converges in practice, many authors conjecture that this scheme converges for almost any starting point

$\{x_i^0\}$, but no proof (except for $n = 2$) has been analysed by GREEN, KORSAK and PEASE [1976]. Asynchronous root finding methods on a distributed memory multicomputer can be found in BAUDET [1978], HOXHA [1988], FRAIGNIAUD [1989a], COSNARD and FRAIGNIAUD [1989].

Using the Gauss–Seidel approach, (18.2) can be accelerated. In such way, one obtains the single-step method

$$x_i^{k+1} = x_i^k - \frac{f(x_i^k)}{\prod_{j=1}^{i-1}\left(x_i^k - x_j^{k+1}\right) \prod_{j=i+1}^{n}\left(x_i^k - x_j^k\right)}, \qquad (18.10)$$

$i = 1, 2, \ldots, n, \ k = 0, 1, \ldots$.

Let $h_i^k = x_i^k - x_i$, $i = 1, 2, \ldots, n, k = 0, 1, \ldots$. Then

$$|h_i^{k+1}| \leqslant c|h_i^k| \left(\sum_{j=1}^{i-1} |h_j^{k+1}| + \sum_{j=i+1}^{n} |h_j^k| \right).$$

Thus, it follows that the R-order of convergence of procedure (18.10) is at least $1+\sigma_n$, where $\sigma_n > 1$ is the unique positive solution of the equation $\sigma^n - \sigma - 1 = 0$. The iterative method of the form (18.10) for real zeros has been analysed by ALEFELD and HERZBERGER [1974a,b] (see also KJURKCHIEV [1982]).

We use the following definition of the R-order of convergence (see ORTEGA and RHEINBOLDT [1970]). Let I be an iterative process with limit point x^*. Then the quantity

$$O_R(I, x^*) = \begin{cases} \infty, & \text{if } R_p(I, x^*) = 0 \\ & \text{for all } p \in [1, \infty], \\ \inf \{p \in [1, \infty) | R_p(I, x^*) = 1\}, & \text{otherwise,} \end{cases}$$

is called the R-order of I at x^*. $R_p(I, x^*)$ is called the R-factor of I at x^* and is defined by

$$R_p(I, x^*) = \sup \left\{ R_p\{x^k\} | x^k \in C(I, x^*) \right\}, \quad 1 \leqslant p < \infty,$$

where

$$R_p\{x^k\} = \begin{cases} \limsup_{k \to \infty} |x^k - x^*|^{1/k}, & \text{if } p = 1, \\ \limsup_{k \to \infty} |x^k - x^*|^{1/p^k}, & \text{if } p > 1, \end{cases}$$

and $C(I, x^*)$ is the set of all sequences generated by I and converging to x^*.

Using the Weierstrass correction $\Delta_j^k = -f(x_j^k)/Q'(x_j^k)$, NOUREIN [1977a] suggested the following improvement of the method (18.2) (called the improved Durand–Kerner method):

$$x_i^{k+1} = x_i^k - \frac{f(x_i^k)}{\prod_{j \neq i}^{n}\left(x_i^k - x_j^k - \Delta_j^k\right)}, \quad i = 1, 2, \ldots, n, \ k = 0, 1, \ldots . \qquad (18.11)$$

The convergence order of this method is three. Further acceleration of convergence can be attained combining the formulas (18.10) and (18.11) (see PETKOVIC and MILOVANOVIC [1983]):

$$x_i^{k+1} = x_i^k - \frac{f(x_i^k)}{\prod_{j=1}^{i-1}\left(x_i^k - x_j^{k+1}\right)\prod_{j=i+1}^{n}\left(x_i^k - x_j^{k+1} - \Delta_j^k\right)},$$

$i = 1, 2, \ldots, n, \quad k = 0, 1, \ldots$.

The R-order of convergence of this iterative process is at least $1 + \sigma_n$, where $\sigma_n > 1$ is the unique positive solution of the equation

$$\sigma^n - \sigma - \sum_{p=0}^{n-1} \sigma^p = 0.$$

Let us put $\Delta = \max_{1 \leq i \leq n} |\Delta_i^k|$. Assuming that Δ is small enough (in other words, all starting approximations are taken to be sufficiently close to the zeros), we have the development,

$$\prod_{j \neq i}^{n}\left(x_i^k - x_j^k - \Delta_j^k\right) = \prod_{j \neq i}^{n}\left(x_i^k - x_j^k\right)\left(1 - \frac{\Delta_j^k}{x_i^k - x_j^k}\right)$$

$$= Q'(x_i^k)\left(1 - \sum_{j \neq i}^{n} \frac{\Delta_j^k}{x_i^k - x_j^k} + O(\Delta^2)\right). \quad (18.12)$$

Taking only the linear terms of Δ_j^k in (18.12), it follows from (18.11) that (see BORSCH-SUPAN [1970]):

$$x_i^{k+1} = x_i^k + \frac{\Delta_i^k}{1 - \sum_{j \neq i}^{n} \frac{\Delta_j^k}{x_i^k - x_j^k}}, \quad i = 1, 2, \ldots, n, \quad k = 0, 1, \ldots, \quad (18.13)$$

or, in the form,

$$x_i^{k+1} = x_i^k - \frac{f(x_i^k)}{\prod_{j \neq i}^{n}\left(x_i^k - x_j^k\right) + \sum_{j \neq i}^{n} \frac{f(x_j^k)}{x_j^k - x_i^k}\prod_{s \neq j, i}^{n} \frac{x_i^k - x_s^k}{x_j^k - x_s^k}}, \quad (18.14)$$

$i = 1, 2, \ldots, n, \quad k = 0, 1, \ldots$.

The convergence of method (18.14) remains cubic (see NOUREIN [1975], KJURKCHIEV and TASCHEV [1981]).

Similar to constructing formula (18.11), the following method of the fourth order can be obtained from (18.13) (see NOUREIN [1977b]):

$$x_i^{k+1} = x_i^k + \frac{\Delta_i^k}{1 - \sum_{j \neq i}^n \frac{\Delta_j^k}{x_i^k - x_j^k - \Delta_j^k}}, \quad i = 1, 2, \ldots, n, \quad k = 0, 1, \ldots$$

REMARK 18.3. An interesting problem is to find weaker conditions imposed on the system of initial approximations $x_i^0, i = 1, 2, \ldots, n$, the iteration methods keeping their convergence. Thus, for instance, the condition for the method (18.14) is (see KJURKCHIEV [1983b]) $|x_i^0 - x_i| \leqslant cq$, $0 < q < 1$, where $0 < cnA/(d - 2c) < 1$, and A is a root of the equation $A^2 = e^{1/A}(2 + A)$. The computation shows that $A = 2.599\ldots$.

In this case, when we have a trigonometrical polynomial of the kind

$$T_n(x) = a_0 + \sum_{k=1}^n (a_k \cos kx + b_k \sin kx), \tag{18.15}$$

whose zeros $x_1, x_2, \ldots, x_{2n}$ are simple, ANGELOVA and SEMERDZHIEV [1982] give an iterative method for the simultaneous approximation of all zeros of the polynomial (18.15), between the lines $x = \pm \pi$,

$$x_i^{k+1} = x_i^k - 2B_k \frac{T_n(x_i^k)}{\prod_{j \neq i}^{2n} \sin \frac{x_i^k - x_j^k}{2}}, \quad i = 1, 2, \ldots, 2n, \quad k = 0, 1, \ldots,$$

where

$$B_k = \prod_{j=1}^{2n} \frac{\sin \frac{y - x_j^k}{2}}{T_n(y)},$$

(y is an arbitrary number in the interval $[-\pi, \pi]$, $y \neq x_i$, $i = 1, 2, \ldots, 2n$).
In this case, when we have an exponential polynomial of the kind

$$E_n(x) = a_0 + \sum_{k=1}^n (a_k e^{-kx} + b_k e^{kx}),$$

MAKRELOV and SEMERDZHIEV [1985b] proposed the following method (see also ZHIDKOV, MAKRELOV and SEMERDZHIEV [1983]):

$$x_i^{k+1} = x_i^k - 2C_k \frac{E_n(x_i^k)}{\prod_{j \neq i}^{2n} \sinh \frac{x_i^k - x_j^k}{2}}, \quad i = 1, 2, \ldots, 2n, \quad k = 0, 1, \ldots,$$

where

$$C_k = \prod_{j=1}^{2n} \frac{\sinh \frac{y - x_j^k}{2}}{E_n(y)},$$

(y is an arbitrary number in the interval $[-\pi, \pi]$, $y \neq x_i$, $i = 1, 2, \ldots, 2n$).

Various methods and their modification have been found by MAKRELOV and SEMERDZHIEV [1984a,b], WEIDNER [1988].

Let us consider some iterative methods on the basis of the Weierstrass–Dochev algorithm with rate of convergence $R + 2$. If the algebraic equation (18.1) has only simple roots then we suggest the following method (KJURKCHIEV and ANDREEV [1985]):

$$x_i^{k+1} = x_i^k + \Delta_i^{R+1,k}, \qquad \Delta_i^{p,k} = -f(x_i^k) \prod_{s \neq i}^{n} \left(x_i^k - x_s^k - \Delta_s^{p-1,k} \right)^{-1},$$

$$\Delta_i^{0,k} = 0, \quad i = 1, 2, \ldots, n, \; p = 1, 2, \ldots, R+2, \; k = 0, 1, \ldots. \tag{18.16}$$

The rate of convergence is equal to $R + 2$.

THEOREM 18.2 (ANDREEV and KJURKCHIEV [1989]). *Let* $0 < q < 1$, $d = \min_{i \neq j} |x_i - x_j|$ *and* $c > 0$ *is a number such that*

$$\frac{cq(1 + e^2)}{(d - c)} \leq 1, \qquad 0 < cne^2/(d - cq(2 + e^2)) < 1.$$

If the initial approximations $\{x_i^0\}_{i=1}^n$ *of the roots* $\{x_i\}_{i=1}^n$ *of Eq.* (18.1) *satisfy the inequalities* $|x_i - x_i^0| \leq cq$, $i = 1, 2, \ldots, n$, *then the estimate* $|x_i^k - x_i| \leq cq^{(R+2)^k}$, $i = 1, 2, \ldots, n$, $k = 0, 1, \ldots$, *holds true.*

PROOF. We prove the theorem by induction. When $k = 0$, the statement is true. Let us assume that the inequalities

$$|x_i^k - x_i| \leq cq^{(R+2)^k}, \quad i = 1, 2, \ldots, n, \tag{18.17}$$

hold true. We consider the $(k+1)$th approximations

$$x_i^{k+1} - x_i = x_i^k - x_i - \prod_{j=1}^{n} \left(x_i^k - x_j \right) \prod_{j \neq i}^{n} \frac{1}{x_i^k - x_j^k - \Delta_j^{R,k}}$$

$$= (x_i^k - x_i) \left(1 - \prod_{\beta_0 \neq i}^{n} \frac{x_i^k - x_{\beta_0}}{x_i^k - x_{\beta_0}^k - \Delta_{\beta_0}^{R,k}} \right). \tag{18.18}$$

For the expression in parentheses, we obtain

$$1 - \prod_{\beta_0 \neq i}^{n} \frac{x_i^k - x_{\beta_0}}{x_i^k - x_{\beta_0}^k - \Delta_{\beta_0}^{R,k}}$$

$$= 1 - \frac{x_i^k - x_n}{x_i^k - x_n^k - \Delta_n^{R,k}} \prod_{\beta_0 \neq i}^{n-1} \frac{x_i^k - x_{\beta_0}}{x_i^k - x_{\beta_0}^k - \Delta_{\beta_0}^{R,k}}$$

$$+ \prod_{\beta_0 \neq i}^{n-1} \frac{x_i^k - x_{\beta_0}}{x_i^k - x_{\beta_0}^k - \Delta_{\beta_0}^{R,k}} - \prod_{\beta_0 \neq i}^{n-1} \frac{x_i^k - x_{\beta_0}}{x_i^k - x_{\beta_0}^k - \Delta_{\beta_0}^{R,k}}$$

$$= 1 - \prod_{\beta_0 \neq i}^{n-1} \frac{x_i^k - x_{\beta_0}}{x_i^k - x_{\beta_0}^k - \Delta_{\beta_0}^{R,k}}$$

$$+ \left(1 - \frac{x_i^k - x_n}{x_i^k - x_n^k - \Delta_n^{R,k}}\right) \prod_{\beta_0 \neq i}^{n-1} \frac{x_i^k - x_{\beta_0}}{x_i^k - x_{\beta_0}^k - \Delta_{\beta_0}^{R,k}}$$

$$= 1 - \prod_{\beta_0 \neq i}^{n} \frac{x_i^k - x_{\beta_0}}{x_i^k - x_{\beta_0}^k - \Delta_{\beta_0}^{R,k}} + \frac{x_n - x_n^k - \Delta_n^{R,k}}{x_i^k - x_n^k - \Delta_n^{R,k}} \prod_{\beta_0 \neq i}^{n-1} \frac{x_i^k - x_{\beta_0}}{x_i^k - x_{\beta_0}^k - \Delta_{\beta_0}^{R,k}}$$

and in view of the fact that the term in the last parentheses is similar to the initial expression, we obtain recursively

$$1 - \prod_{\beta_0 \neq i}^{n} \frac{x_i^k - x_{\beta_0}}{x_i^k - x_{\beta_0}^k - \Delta_{\beta_0}^{R,k}} = \sum_{\alpha_0 \neq i}^{n} \frac{x_{\alpha_0} - x_{\alpha_0}^k - \Delta_{\alpha_0}^{R,k}}{x_i^k - x_{\alpha_0}^k - \Delta_{\alpha_0}^{R,k}} \prod_{\beta_0 \neq i}^{\alpha_0 - 1} \frac{x_i^k - x_{\beta_0}}{x_i^k - x_{\beta_0}^k - \Delta_{\beta_0}^{R,k}}$$

$$= \sum_{\alpha_0 \neq i}^{n} \frac{1}{x_i^k - x_{\alpha_0}^k - \Delta_{\alpha_0}^{R,k}}$$

$$\times \left(x_{\alpha_0} - x_{\alpha_0}^k + (x_{\alpha_0}^k - x_{\alpha_0}) \prod_{\beta_1 \neq \alpha_0}^{n} \frac{x_{\alpha_0}^k - x_{\beta_1}}{x_{\alpha_0}^k - x_{\beta_1}^k - \Delta_{\beta_1}^{R-1,k}} \right)$$

$$\times \prod_{\beta_0 \neq i}^{\alpha_0 - 1} \frac{x_i^k - x_{\beta_0}}{x_i^k - x_{\beta_0}^k - \Delta_{\beta_0}^{R,k}}$$

$$= \sum_{\alpha_0 \neq i}^{n} \frac{x_{\alpha_0} - x_{\alpha_0}^k}{x_i^k - x_{\alpha_0}^k - \Delta_{\alpha_0}^{R,k}} \left(1 - \prod_{\beta_1 \neq \alpha_0}^{n} \frac{x_{\alpha_0}^k - x_{\beta_1}}{x_{\alpha_0}^k - x_{\beta_1}^k - \Delta_{\beta_1}^{R-1,k}} \right)$$

$$\times \prod_{\beta_0 \neq i}^{\alpha_0 - 1} \frac{x_i^k - x_{\beta_0}}{x_i^k - x_{\beta_0}^k - \Delta_{\beta_0}^{R,k}}.$$

The expression in the last parentheses is again similar to the initial expression with the only difference that instead of R, we have $R-1$. Using this dependency, we can obtain successively

$$1 - \prod_{\beta_0 \neq i}^{n} \frac{x_i^k - x_{\beta_0}}{x_i^k - x_{\beta_0}^k - \Delta_{\beta_0}^{R,k}} = \sum_{\alpha_0 \neq i}^{n} \frac{x_{\alpha_0} - x_{\alpha_0}^k}{x_i^k - x_{\alpha_0}^k - \Delta_{\alpha_0}^{R,k}}$$

$$\times \left(1 - \prod_{\beta_1 \neq \alpha_0}^{n} \frac{x_{\alpha_0}^k - x_{\beta_1}}{x_{\alpha_0}^k - x_{\beta_1}^k - \Delta_{\beta_1}^{R-1,k}}\right) \prod_{\beta_0 \neq i}^{\alpha_0 - 1} \frac{x_i^k - x_{\beta_0}}{x_i^k - x_{\beta_0}^k - \Delta_{\beta_0}^{R,k}}$$

$$= \sum_{\alpha_0 \neq i}^{n} \frac{x_{\alpha_0} - x_{\alpha_0}^k}{x_i^k - x_{\alpha_0}^k - \Delta_{\alpha_0}^{R,k}} \left[\sum_{\alpha_1 \neq \alpha_0}^{n} \frac{x_{\alpha_1} - x_{\alpha_1}^k}{x_{\alpha_0}^k - x_{\alpha_1}^k - \Delta_{\alpha_1}^{R-1,k}} \right.$$

$$\left. \times \left(1 - \prod_{\beta_2 \neq \alpha_1}^{n} \frac{x_{\alpha_1}^k - x_{\beta_2}}{x_{\alpha_1}^k - x_{\beta_2}^k - \Delta_{\beta_2}^{R-2,k}}\right) \right]$$

$$\times \prod_{\beta_1 \neq \alpha_0}^{\alpha_1 - 1} \frac{x_{\alpha_0}^k - x_{\beta_1}}{x_{\alpha_0}^k - x_{\beta_1}^k - \Delta_{\beta_1}^{R-1,k}} \prod_{\beta_0 \neq i}^{\alpha_0 - 1} \frac{x_i^k - x_{\beta_0}}{x_i^k - x_{\beta_0}^k - \Delta_{\beta_0}^{R,k}}$$

$$= \sum_{\alpha_0 \neq i}^{n} \frac{x_{\alpha_0} - x_{\alpha_0}^k}{x_i^k - x_{\alpha_0}^k - \Delta_{\alpha_0}^{R,k}} \sum_{\alpha_1 \neq \alpha_0}^{n} \frac{x_{\alpha_1} - x_{\alpha_1}^k}{x_{\alpha_0}^k - x_{\alpha_1}^k - \Delta_{\alpha_1}^{R-1,k}}$$

$$\cdots \sum_{\alpha_R \neq \alpha_{R-1}}^{n} \frac{x_{\alpha_R} - x_{\alpha_R}^k}{x_{\alpha_{R-1}}^k - x_{\alpha_R}^k} \prod_{\beta_R \neq \alpha_{R-1}}^{\alpha_R - 1} \frac{x_{\alpha_{R-1}}^k - x_{\beta_R}}{x_{\alpha_{R-1}}^k - x_{\beta_R}^k}$$

$$\cdots \prod_{\beta_1 \neq \alpha_0}^{\alpha_1 - 1} \frac{x_{\alpha_0}^k - x_{\beta_1}}{x_{\alpha_0}^k - x_{\beta_1}^k - \Delta_{\beta_1}^{R-1,k}} \prod_{\beta_0 \neq i}^{\alpha_0 - 1} \frac{x_i^k - x_{\beta_0}}{x_i^k - x_{\beta_0}^k - \Delta_{\beta_0}^{R,k}} . \tag{18.19}$$

We estimate the products in (18.19). First, when $p \geq 1$,

$$|\Delta_\mu^{P,k}| = \left| f(x_\mu^k) \left(\prod_{\mu_1 \neq \mu}^{n} \left(x_\mu^k - x_{\mu_1}^k - \Delta_{\mu_1}^{P-1,k} \right) \right)^{-1} \right|$$

$$= \left| x_\mu^k - x_\mu \right| \prod_{\mu_1 \neq \mu}^{n} \frac{|x_\mu^k - x_{\mu_1}|}{\left| x_\mu^k - x_{\mu_1} + x_{\mu_1} - x_{\mu_1}^k - \Delta_{\mu_1}^{P-1,k} \right|}$$

$$= \left| x_\mu^k - x_\mu \right| \prod_{\mu_1 \neq \mu}^{n} \left| 1 - \frac{x_{\mu_1}^k - x_{\mu_1} + \Delta_{\mu_1}^{P-1,k}}{x_\mu^k - x_{\mu_1}} \right|^{-1}$$

$$= \left| x_\mu^k - x_\mu \right| \prod_{\mu_1 \neq \mu}^{n} \left| 1 - \frac{\left| x_{\mu_1}^k - x_{\mu_1} + \Delta_{\mu_1}^{P-1,k} \right|}{|x_\mu^k - x_{\mu_1}|} \right|^{-1} . \tag{18.20}$$

On the other hand,

$$|x_\mu^k - x_\mu| \leq cq, \quad |x_\mu^k - x_{\mu_1}| \geq |x_\mu - x_{\mu_1}| - |x_\mu^k - x_\mu| \geq d - c . \tag{18.21}$$

It follows from (18.20), (18.21) and the conditions of the theorem that $|\Delta_\nu^{s,k}| \leq cqe^2$ for $\nu = 1, 2, \ldots, n$ and $s = 0, 1, \ldots, R$. Indeed

$$|\Delta_\mu^{P,k}| \leq cq \prod_{\mu_1 \neq \mu}^n \left(1 - \frac{cq}{d-c}\right)^{-1} \leq cq \prod_{\mu_1 \neq \mu}^n \left(1 - \frac{1}{n}\right)^{-1}$$

$$\leq cq \left(1 + \frac{2}{n}\right)^n \leq cqe^2$$

and if we permit $\left|\Delta_\mu^{s-1,k}\right| \leq cqe^2$, $\mu = 1, 2, \ldots, n$, then

$$\left|\Delta_\mu^{s,k}\right| < cq \prod_{\mu_1 \neq \mu}^n \left|1 - \frac{\left|x_{\mu_1}^k - x_{\mu_1} + \Delta_{\mu_1}^{s-1,k}\right|}{d-c}\right|^{-1}$$

$$< cq \prod_{\mu_1 \neq \mu}^n \left(1 - \frac{cq(1+e^2)}{d-c}\right)^{-1} \leq cq \prod_{\mu_1 \neq \mu}^n \left(1 - \frac{1}{n}\right)^{-1}$$

$$\leq cq \prod_{\mu_1 \neq \mu}^n \left(1 + \frac{2}{n}\right) \leq cqe^2 .$$

Thus, we obtain

$$\left|\Delta_\mu^{s,k}\right| \leq cqe^2, \quad s = 0, 1, \ldots, R, \quad \mu = 1, 2, \ldots, n. \tag{18.22}$$

The estimates (18.21) and (18.22) allow us to find an upper bound of the products in (18.19),

$$\left|\prod_{s \neq p}^{t-1} \frac{x_p^k - x_s}{x_p^k - x_s^k - \Delta_s^{l,k}}\right| = \left|\prod_{s \neq p}^{t-1} \left(1 - \frac{x_s^k - x_s + \Delta_s^{l,k}}{x_p^k - x_s}\right)^{-1}\right|$$

$$\leq \prod_{s \neq p}^{t-1} \left(1 - \frac{\left|x_s^k - x_s\right| + \left|\Delta_s^{l,k}\right|}{\left|x_p^k - x_s\right|}\right)^{-1}$$

$$< \prod_{s=1}^{t-1} \left(1 - \frac{cq(1+e^2)}{d-c}\right)^{-1}$$

$$\leq \prod_{s=1}^n \left(1 - \frac{1}{n}\right)^{-1} \leq e^2 . \tag{18.23}$$

Finally, we have to estimate the denominators in (18.19). It follows from $p \neq 1$ and (18.21), (18.22) that

$$\left|x_p^k - x_l^k - \Delta_l^{s,k}\right| \geq \left|x_p^k - x_l^k\right| - \left|\Delta_l^{s,k}\right|$$

$$\geq |x_p - x_l| - \left|x_p^k - x_p\right| - \left|x_l^k - x_l\right| - cqe^2$$

$$\geq d - 2cq - cqe^2 = d - cq(2+e^2) > 0. \qquad (18.24)$$

Combining (18.17)–(18.19), (18.23) and (18.24), it is easy to obtain

$$\left|x_i^{k+1} - x_i\right| \leq cq^{(R+2)^k} \left(cq^{(R+2)^k}\right)^{R+1} n^{R+1} e^{2(R+1)} \left(d - cq(2+e^2)\right)^{-(R+1)}$$

$$\leq cq^{(R+2)^k + (R+2)^k(R+1)} \left(\frac{cne^2}{d - cq(2+e^2)}\right)^{R+1} \leq cq^{(R+2)^{k+1}}.$$

The theorem is proved. □

Numerical experiments. To illustrate the computing properties of this method, we carried out several numerical experiments.

The polynomial

$$x^9 + 3x^8 - 3x^7 - 9x^6 + 3x^5 + 9x^4 + 99x^3 + 297x^2 - 100x - 300 = 0$$

has the following different roots:

$$x_1 = -3, \quad x_{2,3} = \pm 1, \quad x_{4,5} = \pm 2i, \quad x_{6,7} = 2 \pm i, \quad x_{8,9} = -2 \pm i.$$

For numerical determination of these roots, we apply method (18.16) using the initial approximations:

$x_1^0 = -3.2 + 0.2i,$ $x_2^0 = -1.2 - 0.2i,$ $x_3^0 = 0.1 + 1.7i,$
$x_4^0 = -1.9 + 1.3i,$ $x_5^0 = -1.8 - 0.8i,$ $x_6^0 = 2.3 + 1.1i,$
$x_7^0 = 1.9 - 0.7i,$ $x_8^0 = 1.2 + 0.2i,$ $x_9^0 = 0.2 - 2.2i,$

when $R = 0, 1, 3, 6$ and 9.

Let us denote by $\sigma(R,k) = \sum_{i=1}^{9} |x_i^{k,R} - x_i^{k-1,R}|$, the error between two consistent approximations on step $k-1$ and k, $\{x_i^{k-1,R}\}_{i=1}^{9}$, $\{x_i^{k,R}\}_{i=1}^{9}$ by fixed R equal to $0, 1, 3, 6, 9$. Table 18.1 shows the $\sigma(R,k)$ obtained for different R and k.

19. Iterative methods with derivatives

Let the equation

$$f(x) = x^n + a_{n-1}x^{n-1} + \cdots + a_0 = 0 \qquad (19.1)$$

have different roots $x_1, \ldots, x_n$ and let $x_1^k, \ldots, x_n^k$ be distinct reasonably close approximations of these zeros. A class of iterative methods with derivatives for simultaneous calculations of the roots of a given algebraic equation is considered.

Contrary to the classical Chebyshev method, DOCHEV and BYRNEV [1964] proposed the following method:

$$x_i^{k+1} = x_i^k - f(x_i^k) \frac{2 \prod_{\substack{j=1 \\ j \neq i}}^{n}(x_i^k - x_j^k) - f'(x_i^k) + f(x_i^k) \sum_{\substack{j=1 \\ j \neq i}}^{n}(x_i^k - x_j^k)^{-1}}{\prod_{\substack{j \neq i}}(x_i^k - x_j^k)^2},$$

TABLE 18.1.

k	R				
	0	1	3	6	9
	Weierstrass –Dochev	Nourein			
1	0.3×10	0.3×10	0.3×10	0.3×10	0.3×10
2	0.6	0.2	0.2×10^{-1}	0.6×10^{-3}	0.2×10^{-4}
3	0.3×10^{-1}	0.9×10^{-4}	0.1×10^{-11}	0.3×10^{-14}	0.2×10^{-14}
4	0.1×10^{-3}	0.4×10^{-13}	0.5×10^{-14}		
5	0.3×10^{-8}	0.6×10^{-15}			
6	0.4×10^{-15}				

$$i = 1, \ldots, n, \quad k = 0, 1, \ldots . \tag{19.2}$$

SEMERDZHIEV [1985] (see also SEMERDZHIEV and PATEVA [1978]) proved the cubic rate of convergence of the above method. The cubic rate of convergence under weaker initial conditions was obtained by KJURKCHIEV [1982].

THEOREM 19.1. *Let $0 < q < 1$, $d = \min_{i \neq j} |x_i - x_j|$ and c satisfy the inequalities $d - 2c > 0$, $0 < cnA_1/(d - 2c) < 1$, where A_1 is a root of the equation*

$$A_1 = e^{1/A_1} \sqrt{1 + \frac{1}{n}} .$$

If the initial approximations satisfy the inequalities

$$|x_i^0 - x_i| \leqslant cq, \quad i = 1, \ldots, n,$$

then the estimate,

$$|x_i^k - x_i| \leqslant cq^{3^k}, \quad i = 1, \ldots, n, \quad k = 0, 1, \ldots$$

holds, i.e. the method (19.2) has a cubic rate of convergence.

The Dochev–Byrnev method inspired a number of other contributions (see MAKRELOV [1979], ZHIDKOV, MAKRELOV and SEMERDZHIEV [1983]).

Using the logarithmic derivative of the polynomial f, MAEHLY [1954] (and later, BORSCH-SUPAN [1963], EHRLICH [1967], ABERTH [1973], SAVENKO [1964] and others) derived the total-step method (TSM):

$$x_i^{k+1} = x_i^k - \frac{f(x_i^k)}{f'(x_i^k) - f(x_i^k) \sum_{j \neq i}^{n} \frac{1}{x_i^k - x_j^k}}, \quad i = 1, \ldots, n, \quad k = 0, 1, \ldots, \tag{19.3}$$

which has cubic convergence.

The single-step modification (SSM) of (19.3),

$$x_i^{k+1} = x_i^k - \frac{f(x_i^k)}{f'(x_i^k) - f(x_i^k)\left(\sum_{j=1}^{i-1} \frac{1}{x_i^k - x_j^{k+1}} + \sum_{j=i+1}^{n} \frac{1}{x_i^k - x_j^k}\right)}, \quad (19.4)$$

$$i = 1, \ldots, n, \quad k = 0, 1, \ldots,$$

has R-order of convergence $O_R((19.4), 0) > 3$.

Here we discuss a paper by ALEFELD and HERZBERGER [1974a,b]. Defining

$$\gamma_i^k = \sum_{j \neq i}^{n} \frac{(x_i^k - x_i)(x_j^k - x_j)}{(x_i^k - x_j)(x_i^k - x_j^k)}, \quad i = 1, \ldots, n, \quad k = 0, 1, \ldots$$

for TSM and

$$\gamma_i^k = \sum_{j=1}^{i-1} \frac{(x_i^k - x_i)(x_j^k - x_j)}{(x_i^k - x_j)(x_i^k - x_j^{k+1})} + \sum_{j=i+1}^{n} \frac{(x_i^k - x_i)(x_j^k - x_j)}{(x_i^k - x_j)(x_i^k - x_j^k)}$$

for SSM, both methods can be written in the form

$$x_i^{k+1} = x_i^k + \frac{\gamma_i^k}{1 + \gamma_i^k}(x_i^k - x_i), \quad i = 1, \ldots, n, \quad k = 0, 1, \ldots.$$

If we take

$$h_i^k = x_i^k - x_i, \quad i = 1, \ldots, n, \quad k = 0, 1, \ldots,$$

this may be written as

$$h_i^{k+1} = \frac{\gamma_i}{1 + \gamma_i^k} h_i^k, \quad i = 1, \ldots, n \quad (19.5)$$

and

$$|h_i^k| \leq \tfrac{1}{4} \min_{1 \leq j \leq n} |x_i - x_j| = \tfrac{1}{4} d_i, \quad i = 1, \ldots, n,$$

and we further assume, for $i = 1, \ldots, n$, $j \neq i$,

$$|x_i - x_j^k| \geq \tfrac{1}{2} d_i.$$

Then we obtain

$$|\gamma_i^k| \leq \frac{16}{3 d_i^2} |h_i^k| \sum_{j \neq i}^{n} |h_j^k|$$

for TSM and

$$|\gamma_i^k| \leq \frac{16}{3 d_i^2} |h_i^k| \left(\sum_{j=1}^{i-1} |h_j^{k+1}| + \sum_{j=i+1}^{n} |h_j^k|\right) \quad (19.6)$$

for SSM.

In addition, if the inequalities
$$|h_i^k| \leqslant h \leqslant \tfrac{1}{4} d_i$$
hold, then
$$|h_i^{k+1}| \leqslant h^3 \delta_i (1 - O(h^2 \delta_i)),$$
where
$$\delta_i = \frac{16(n-1)}{3 d_i^2}$$
for TSM and
$$\delta_i = \frac{16}{3 d_i^2} \left(h^2 \sum_{j=1}^{i-1} \delta_j + n - i \right)$$
for SSM.

THEOREM 19.2. *Let $\sigma_n > 1$ be the unique positive root of*
$$\bar{p}_n(\sigma) = \sigma^n - \sigma - 2 = 0 .$$
Then for the R-order for SSM we have
$$O_R(\text{SSM}, 0) \geqslant 2 + \sigma_n .$$

PROOF. Using (19.6), it follows from (19.5) that
$$|h_i^{k+1}| \leqslant \frac{16}{3 d_i^2} \frac{1}{1 - |\gamma_i^k|} |h_i^k|^2 \left(\sum_{j=1}^{i-1} |h_j^{k+1}| + \sum_{j=i+1}^{n} |h_j^k| \right)$$
$$\leqslant c |h_i^k|^2 \left(\sum_{j=1}^{i-1} |h_j^{k+1}| + \sum_{j=i+1}^{n} |h_j^k| \right)$$
as soon as
$$\frac{16}{3 d_i^2} \frac{1}{1 - |\gamma_i^k|} \leqslant c, \quad i = 1, \ldots, n.$$
We now set
$$\gamma = \sqrt{(n-1)c}, \quad |h_i^k| = \frac{1}{\gamma} \eta_i^k, \quad i = 1, \ldots, n,$$
$$\varepsilon = \frac{c}{\gamma^2} = \frac{1}{n-1},$$
and obtain
$$\eta_i^{k+1} \leqslant \varepsilon \left(\eta_i^k \right)^2 \left(\sum_{j=1}^{i-1} \eta_j^{k+1} + \sum_{j=i+1}^{n} \eta_j^k \right) .$$

As $\lim_{k\to\infty} |h_i^k| = 0$, $i = 1,\ldots,n$, we may assume

$$\eta_i^0 \leqslant \eta < 1, \quad i = 1,\ldots,n.$$

Then, we obtain

$$\eta_i^{k+1} \leqslant \eta^{m_i^{k+1}}, \quad i = 1,\ldots,n, \ k = 0,1,\ldots.$$

Defining the matrix A by

$$A = \begin{pmatrix} 2 & 1 & & & 0 \\ & 2 & \ddots & & \\ & & \ddots & & \\ & 0 & & 2 & 1 \\ 2 & 1 & \cdots & 0 & 2 \end{pmatrix},$$

the vectors $m^k = (m_i^k)$ can be successively calculated by

$$m^{k+1} = Am^k, \quad k = 0,1,\ldots, \tag{19.7}$$

with initial values $m_i^0 = 1$, $i = 1,\ldots,n$. The proof is by induction and is omitted.

The matrix A is nonnegative and its directed graph (see VARGA [1962]) is strongly connected, i.e. A is irreducible. By the Perron–Frobenius theorem this implies that A has a positive eigenvalue λ_1 equal to its spectral radius. But, by a simple application of Theorem 2.9 (see VARGA [1962], p. 49) we find that A is also primitive. Thus, for the remaining eigenvalues $\lambda_2,\ldots,\lambda_n$ of A, we obtain

$$\lambda_1 = \rho(A) > |\lambda_2| \geqslant \cdots \geqslant |\lambda_n|. \tag{19.8}$$

Let $A^k = (a_{ij}^k)$, $k = 1,2,\ldots$ denote the kth power of A. Since A is a primitive matrix, we obtain

$$A^k > 0 \text{ for } k \geqslant k_0.$$

For an arbitrary matrix with property (19.8), it can be shown that

$$\lim_{k\to\infty} \frac{a_{ij}^{k+1}}{a_{ij}^k} = \lambda_1$$

(see GROBNER [1966]).

If $\varepsilon > 0$ is given, then

$$\frac{a_{ij}^{k+1}}{a_{ij}^k} \geqslant \rho(A) - \varepsilon \quad \text{for } k \geqslant k(\varepsilon) \geqslant k_0$$

or

$$a_{ij}^{k+1} \geqslant \alpha(\rho(A) - \varepsilon), \quad i,j = 1,\ldots,n,$$

where

$$\alpha = \min_{1 \leqslant i,j \leqslant n} a_{ij}^k > 0.$$

Therefore
$$a_{ij}^{k+2} \geqslant a_{ij}^{k+1}(\rho(A) - \varepsilon) \geqslant \alpha(\rho(A) - \varepsilon)^2 ,$$
and, in general,
$$a_{ij}^{k+r} > \alpha(\rho(A) - \varepsilon)^r, \quad i,j = 1,\ldots,n, \quad r = 1,2,\ldots . \tag{19.9}$$
Now, combining (19.7) and (19.9) into a single inequality,
$$m^{k+r} = A^{k+r} m^0 = \sum_{j=1}^{n} a_{ij}^{k+r} \geqslant (n\alpha(\rho(A) - \varepsilon)^r) e ,$$
where $e = (e_i)$, $e_i = 1$, $i = 1,\ldots,n$, we obtain
$$\eta_i^{k+r} \leqslant \eta^{m_i^{k+r}} \leqslant \eta^{n\alpha(\rho(A)-\varepsilon)^r}, \quad i = 1,\ldots,n, \quad r = 1,2,\ldots$$
or
$$|\eta_i^{k+r}| \leqslant \frac{1}{\gamma} \eta^{n\alpha(\rho(A)-\varepsilon)^r} .$$
For
$$h^k = \max_{1 \leqslant i \leqslant n} |h_i^k| ,$$
we also have
$$\eta_i^{k+r} \leqslant \frac{1}{\gamma} \eta^{n\alpha(\rho(A)-\varepsilon)^r} .$$
Thus, it follows that
$$R_{\rho(A)-\varepsilon}\{h^k\} = \lim_{r \to \infty} \left(h^{k+r}\right)^{1/(\rho(A)-\varepsilon)^r}$$
$$\leqslant \limsup_{r \to \infty} \left(\frac{1}{\gamma} \eta^{\alpha n(\rho(A)-\varepsilon)^r}\right)^{1/(\rho(A)-\varepsilon)^r}$$
$$= \eta^{\alpha n} < 1 ,$$
and therefore
$$O_R(\text{SSM}, 0) \geqslant \rho(A) - \varepsilon.$$
This inequality holds for all $\varepsilon > 0$ and we immediately have
$$O_R(\text{SSM}, 0) \geqslant \rho(A) . \tag{19.10}$$
We now consider the characteristic polynomial $P_n(\lambda)$ of A
$$P_n(\lambda) = (\lambda - 2)^n - (\lambda - 2) - 2 .$$
If we set $\sigma = \lambda - 2$, then simply substituting this in the polynomial above yields
$$\bar{P}_n(\sigma) = \sigma^n - \sigma - 2 .$$

Since $\bar{P}_n(1) = -2$ and $\bar{P}_n(2) \geq 0$ for $n \geq 2$, there is a root σ_n with $1 < \sigma_n \leq 2$ and by Descartes' rule of signs, there can be no other positive root of $\bar{P}_n(\sigma)$.

Thus, for the spectral radius $\rho(A)$ of A, we have

$$\rho(A) = 2 + \sigma_n,$$

and combining this with (19.10) gives

$$O_R(\text{SSM}, 0) \geq 2 + \sigma_n,$$

which completes the proof. □

Using Newton's correction, NOUREIN [1977a] obtained the following modification of (19.3) (called the improved Ehrlich method):

$$x_i^{k+1} = x_i^k + \delta_i^k \left(1 + \delta_i^k \sum_{j \neq i}^n \frac{1}{x_i^k - x_j^k - \delta_j^k} \right)^{-1},$$

$i = 1, 2, \ldots, n, \quad k = 0, 1, \ldots.$

MILOVANOVIC and PETKOVIC [1983] obtained the following modified method:

$$x_i^{k+1} = x_i^k + \delta_i^k \left[1 + \delta_i^k \left(\sum_{j=1}^{i-1} \frac{1}{x_i^k - x_j^{k+1}} + \sum_{j=i+1}^n \frac{1}{x_i^k - x_j^k - \delta_j^k} \right) \right]^{-1},$$

$i = 1, \ldots, n, \quad k = 0, 1, \ldots.$

KJURKCHIEV [1983a] proposed the method

$$x_i^{k+1} = x_i^k - \frac{f(x_i^k)}{f'(x_i^k) - f(x_i^k) \sum_{j \neq i}^n \frac{1}{x_i^k - x_j^k} - f(x_i^k) \sum_{j \neq i}^n \frac{f(x_j^k)}{(x_i^k - x_j^k)^3} \prod_{s \neq i, j}^n \frac{1}{x_j^k - x_s^k}},$$

$i = 1, 2, \ldots, n, \quad k = 0, 1, \ldots.$

Various methods and their modification have been considered by MAKRELOV and SEMERDZHIEV [1983], MAKRELOV, SEMERDZHIEV and TAMBUROV [1986a,b], JENKINS and TRAUB [1970], FORD [1977], BROYDEN and FORD [1975], ATANASSOVA, DJUKANOVA and KJURKCHIEV [1985], KJURKCHIEV and ANDREEV [1987], SIMEUNOVIC [1989], PETKOVIC [1981], PETKOVIC and STEFANOVIC [1984, 1986].

We present an iterative method based on Ehrlich's algorithm with rate of convergence $2R + 3$.

Let the algebraic equation (19.1) have only simple roots. In this section, we suggest the following method

$$x_i^{k+1} = x_i^k - \frac{1}{H(x_i^k) - \sum_{\beta_0 \neq i}^n \frac{1}{x_i^k - x_{\beta_0}^k - \Delta_{\beta_0}^{R,k}}},$$

$$H(x_i^k) = \frac{f'(x_i^k)}{f(x_i^k)}, \quad i = 1, \ldots, n, \quad k = 0, 1, \ldots, \tag{19.11}$$

where

$$\Delta_s^{R,k} = -\frac{1}{H(x_s^k) - \sum_{l \neq s}^{n} \frac{1}{x_s^k - x_l^k - \Delta_l^{R-1,k}}}, \quad s = 1, \ldots, n, \quad k = 0, 1, \ldots,$$

$$\Delta_j^{0,k} = 0, \quad j = 1, \ldots, n, \quad k = 0, 1, \ldots.$$

The rate of convergence of (19.11) is equal to $2R + 3$.

THEOREM 19.3 (KJURKCHIEV and ANDREEV [1987]). *Let $0 < q < 1$, $d = \min_{i \neq j} |x_i - x_j|$ and $c > 0$ be a number such that*

$$d > 2c(1 + q(2n-1)),$$
$$c^2 n \left[(d-c)(d-2c-2cq) \left(1 - cq(n-1) \frac{3cq}{(d-c)(d-2c-2cq)} \right) \right]^{-1} \leqslant 1. \tag{19.12}$$

If the initial approximations $\{x_i^0\}_{i=1}^n$ of the roots $\{x_i\}_{i=1}^n$ of (19.1) satisfy the inequalities

$$|x_i^0 - x_i| \leqslant cq, \quad i = 1, \ldots, n,$$

then the estimate,

$$|x_i^k - x_i| \leqslant cq^{(2R+3)^k}, \quad i = 1, \ldots, n, \quad k = 0, 1, \ldots$$

holds true.

PROOF. The proof proceeds by induction on k. For $k = 0$, the theorem is evidently true. Let us assume that the inequalities

$$|x_i^k - x_i| \leqslant cq^{(2R+3)^k}, \quad i = 1, \ldots, n \tag{19.13}$$

hold. We consider the $(k+1)$th approximations,

$$x_i^{k+1} - x_i = x_i^k - x_i - \frac{f(x_i^k)}{f'(x_i^k) - f(x_i^k) \sum_{\beta_0 \neq i}^{n} \frac{1}{x_i^k - x_{\beta_0}^k - \Delta_{\beta_0}^{R,k}}}$$

$$= x_i^k - x_i - \left[\frac{1}{x_i^k - x_i} + \sum_{\beta_0 \neq i}^{n} \frac{1}{x_i^k - x_{\beta_0}} - \sum_{\beta_0 \neq i}^{n} \frac{1}{x_i^k - x_{\beta_0}^k - \Delta_{\beta_0}^{R,k}} \right]^{-1}$$

$$= (x_i^k - x_i) \left[1 - \left(1 + (x_i^k - x_i) \sum_{\beta_0 \neq i}^{n} \frac{x_{\beta_0} - x_{\beta_0}^k - \Delta_{\beta_0}^{R,k}}{(x_i^k - x_{\beta_0})(x_i^k - x_{\beta_0}^k - \Delta_{\beta_0}^{R,k})} \right)^{-1} \right]$$

$$= \frac{(x_i^k - x_i)^2}{1 + (x_i^k - x_i) \sum_{\beta_0 \neq i}^{n} \frac{x_{\beta_0} - x_{\beta_0}^k - \Delta_{\beta_0}^{R,k}}{(x_i^k - x_{\beta_0})(x_i^k - x_{\beta_0}^k - \Delta_{\beta_0}^{R,k})}}$$

$$\times \sum_{\beta_0 \neq i}^{n} \frac{x_{\beta_0} - x_{\beta_0}^k - \Delta_{\beta_0}^{R,k}}{(x_i^k - x_{\beta_0})(x_i^k - x_{\beta_0}^k - \Delta_{\beta_0}^{R,k})} \, . \quad (19.14)$$

The last sum can be rewritten in the form

$$\sum_{\beta_0 \neq i}^{n} \frac{x_{\beta_0} - x_{\beta_0}^k - \Delta_{\beta_0}^{R,k}}{(x_i^k - x_{\beta_0})(x_i^k - x_{\beta_0}^k - \Delta_{\beta_0}^{R,k})}$$

$$= \sum_{\beta_0 \neq i}^{n} \frac{x_{\beta_0} - x_{\beta_0}^k + \left[H(x_{\beta_0}^k) - \sum_{\beta_1 \neq \beta_0}^{n} \left[x_{\beta_0}^k - x_{\beta_1}^k - \Delta_{\beta_1}^{R-1,k} \right]^{-1} \right]^{-1}}{(x_i^k - x_{\beta_0})(x_i^k - x_{\beta_0}^k - \Delta_{\beta_0}^{R,k})}$$

$$= \sum_{\beta_0 \neq i}^{n} \frac{x_{\beta_0} - x_{\beta_0}^k + \left[\frac{1}{x_{\beta_0}^k - x_{\beta_0}} + \sum_{\beta_1 \neq \beta_0}^{n} \frac{1}{x_{\beta_0}^k - x_{\beta_1}} - \sum_{\beta_1 \neq \beta_0}^{n} \frac{1}{x_{\beta_0}^k - x_{\beta_1}^k - \Delta_{\beta_1}^{R-1,k}} \right]^{-1}}{(x_i^k - x_{\beta_0})(x_i^k - x_{\beta_0}^k - \Delta_{\beta_0}^{R,k})}$$

$$= \sum_{\beta_0 \neq i}^{n} (x_{\beta_0} - x_{\beta_0}^k)$$

$$\times \frac{1 - \left[1 + (x_{\beta_0}^k - x_{\beta_0}) \sum_{\beta_1 \neq \beta_0}^{n} \frac{x_{\beta_1} - x_{\beta_1}^k - \Delta_{\beta_1}^{R-1,k}}{(x_{\beta_0}^k - x_{\beta_1})(x_{\beta_0}^k - x_{\beta_1}^k - \Delta_{\beta_1}^{R-1,k})} \right]^{-1}}{(x_i^k - x_{\beta_0})(x_i^k - x_{\beta_0}^k - \Delta_{\beta_0}^{R,k})}$$

$$= \sum_{\beta_0 \neq i}^{n} \left[(x_{\beta_0} - x_i^k)(x_i^k - x_{\beta_0}^k - \Delta_{\beta_0}^{R,k}) \right]^{-1} (x_{\beta_0}^k - x_{\beta_0})^2$$

$$\times \frac{\sum_{\beta_1 \neq \beta_0}^{n} \frac{x_{\beta_1} - x_{\beta_1}^k - \Delta_{\beta_1}^{R-1,k}}{(x_{\beta_0}^k - x_{\beta_1})(x_{\beta_0}^k - x_{\beta_1}^k - \Delta_{\beta_1}^{R-1,k})}}{1 + (x_{\beta_0}^k - x_{\beta_0}) \sum_{\beta_1 \neq \beta_0}^{n} \frac{x_{\beta_1} - x_{\beta_1}^k - \Delta_{\beta_1}^{R-1,k}}{(x_{\beta_0}^k - x_{\beta_1})(x_{\beta_0}^k - x_{\beta_1}^k - \Delta_{\beta_1}^{R-1,k})}} \, .$$

It should be noted that the sum in the numerator in the last expression is similar to the initial sum with the only difference that we have $R-1$ instead of k. Using that dependence recursively, we obtain successively

$$\sum_{\beta_0 \neq i}^{n} \frac{x_{\beta_0} - x_{\beta_0}^k - \Delta_{\beta_0}^{R,k}}{(x_i^k - x_{\beta_0})(x_i^k - x_{\beta_0}^k - \Delta_{\beta_0}^{R,k})}$$

$$= \sum_{\beta_0 \neq i}^{n} \frac{(x_{\beta_0}^k - x_{\beta_0})^2 \left[(x_{\beta_0} - x_i^k)(x_i^k - x_{\beta_0}^k - \Delta_{\beta_0}^{R,k})\right]^{-1}}{1 + (x_{\beta_0}^k - x_{\beta_0}) \sum_{\beta_1 \neq \beta_0}^{n} \frac{x_{\beta_1} - x_{\beta_1}^k - \Delta_{\beta_1}^{R-1,k}}{(x_{\beta_0}^k - x_{\beta_1})(x_{\beta_0}^k - x_{\beta_1}^k - \Delta_{\beta_1}^{R-1,k})}}$$

$$\times \sum_{\beta_1 \neq \beta_0}^{n} \frac{(x_{\beta_1}^k - x_{\beta_1})^2 \left[(x_{\beta_1} - x_{\beta_0}^k)(x_{\beta_0}^k - x_{\beta_1}^k - \Delta_{\beta_1}^{R-1,k})\right]^{-1}}{1 + (x_{\beta_1}^k - x_{\beta_1}) \sum_{\beta_2 \neq \beta_1}^{n} \frac{x_{\beta_2} - x_{\beta_2}^k - \Delta_{\beta_2}^{R-2,k}}{(x_{\beta_1}^k - x_{\beta_2})(x_{\beta_1}^k - x_{\beta_2}^k - \Delta_{\beta_2}^{R-2,k})}} \times \cdots$$

$$\times \sum_{\beta_{R-1} \neq \beta_{R-2}}^{n} (x_{\beta_{R-1}}^k - x_{\beta_{R-1}})^2$$

$$\times \frac{\left[(x_{\beta_{R-1}} - x_{\beta_{R-2}}^k)(x_{\beta_{R-2}}^k - x_{\beta_{R-1}}^k - \Delta_{\beta_{R-1}}^{1,k})\right]^{-1}}{1 + (x_{\beta_{R-1}}^k - x_{\beta_{R-1}}) \sum_{\beta_R \neq \beta_{R-1}}^{n} \frac{x_{\beta_R} - x_{\beta_R}^k}{(x_{\beta_{R-1}}^k - x_{\beta_R})(x_{\beta_{R-1}}^k - x_{\beta_R}^k)}}$$

$$\times \sum_{\beta_R \neq \beta_{R-1}}^{n} \frac{x_{\beta_R} - x_{\beta_R}^k}{(x_{\beta_{R-1}}^k - x_{\beta_R})(x_{\beta_{R-1}}^k - x_{\beta_R}^k)}. \tag{19.15}$$

Let us estimate from the above the absolute value of the items in (19.15). We first show that the estimates,

$$|\Delta_s^{p,k}| \leqslant 2cq, \quad s = 1, \ldots, n, \quad p = 0, 1, \ldots, R, \tag{19.16}$$

hold. The proof can be done by induction on p. When $p = 0$, the inequalities (19.16) are satisfied since $\Delta_s^{0,k} = 0$ for $s = 1, \ldots, n$. Let us assume that $|\Delta_s^{m-1,k}| \leqslant 2cq$, $s = 1, \ldots, n$. Then we obtain for $\Delta_s^{m,k}$, $s = 1, \ldots, n$

$$\Delta_s^{m,k} = -\frac{f(x_s^k)}{f'(x_s^k) - f(x_s^k) \sum_{t \neq s}^{n} \frac{1}{x_s^k - x_t^k - \Delta_t^{m-1,k}}}$$

$$= -\frac{x_s^k - x_s}{\sum_{t=1}^{n} \frac{x_s^k - x_s}{x_s^k - x_t} - (x_s^k - x_s) \sum_{t \neq s}^{n} \frac{1}{x_s^k - x_t^k - \Delta_t^{m-1,k}}}.$$

It follows from the last equality and (19.13) that

$$|\Delta_s^{m,k}| \leqslant \frac{cq}{1 - cq \sum_{t \neq s}^{n} \left(\frac{1}{|x_s^k - x_t|} + \frac{1}{|x_s^k - x_t^k| - |\Delta_t^{m-1,k}|}\right)}.$$

From

$$|x_s^k - x_t^k| = |x_s^k - x_s + x_s - x_t + x_t - x_t^k|$$

$$\geq |x_s - x_t| - |x_s - x_s^k| - |x_t - x_t^k| > d - 2cq, \tag{19.17}$$
$$|x_s^k - x_t| \geq d - cq,$$

we finally obtain

$$|\Delta_s^{m,k}| \leq \frac{cq}{1 - cq(n-1)\left(\frac{1}{d-c} + \frac{1}{d-2c-2cq}\right)} \leq \frac{cq}{1 - \frac{2cq(n-1)}{d - 2c(1+q)}},$$

and for the validity of the inequality $|\Delta_s^{m,k}| \leq 2cq$, the following conditions are sufficient:

$$\left(1 - \frac{2cq(n-1)}{d - 2c(1+q)}\right)^{-1} \leq 2, \quad 1 - \frac{2cq(n-1)}{d - 2c(1+q)} > 0.$$

These two conditions are satisfied if $d > 2c(1 + q(2n - 1))$. Now we are able to estimate the sums in (19.15). In view of (19.13), (19.16) and (19.17), for an arbitrary item in (19.15), we obtain

$$\left[|x_\mu - x_\nu^k||x_\nu^k - x_\mu^k - \Delta_\mu^{s,k}|\left|1 + (x_\mu^k - x_\mu)\sum_{\lambda \neq \mu}^{n} \frac{x_\lambda - x_\lambda^k - \Delta_\lambda^{s-1,k}}{(x_\mu^k - x_\lambda)(x_\mu^k - x_\lambda^k - \Delta_\lambda^{s-1,k})}\right|\right]^{-1}$$

$$\leq \left[|x_\mu - x_\nu^k|(|x_\nu^k - x_\mu^k| - |\Delta_\mu^{s,k}|)\right.$$

$$\times \left.\left(1 - |x_\mu^k - x_\mu|\sum_{\lambda \neq \mu}^{n} \frac{|x_\lambda - x_\lambda^k| + |\Delta_\lambda^{s-1,k}|}{(d-c)(d-2c-2cq)}\right)\right]^{-1}$$

$$\leq \left[(d-c)(d-2c-2cq)\left(1 - cq(n-1)\frac{3cq}{(d-c)(d-2c-2cq)}\right)\right]^{-1} = A.$$

It follows from the last inequality, and (19.13)–(19.15) that

$$|x_i^{k+1} - x_i| \leq \left(cq^{(2R+3)^k}\right)^{2+2R+1}(nA)^{R+1} = cq^{(2R+3)^{k+1}}\left(c^2 nA\right)^{R+1}$$
$$\leq cq^{(2R+3)^{k+1}},$$

since $c^2 nA \leq 1$, according to the assumptions. Thus, the theorem is proved. □

Numerical results. In order to show the computation properties of the method, we carried out a series of numerical experiments.

The polynomial

$$x^9 + 3x^8 - 3x^7 - 9x^6 + 3x^5 + 9x^4 + 99x^3 + 297x^2 - 100x - 300$$

has the following different roots:

$$x_1 = -3, \quad x_2 = -1, \quad x_3 = 1, \quad x_4 = 2i, \quad x_5 = -2i,$$
$$x_6 = 2 + i, \quad x_7 = 2 - i, \quad x_8 = -2 + i, \quad x_9 = -2 - i.$$

TABLE 19.1.

k	$R=0$	1	3	6	9
	Ehrlich				
1	0.27×10	0.27×10	0.27×10	0.27×10	0.27×10
2	0.14	0.93×10^{-2}	0.45×10^{-4}	0.15×10^{-7}	0.47×10^{-11}
3	0.31×10^{-4}	0.60×10^{-14}	0.17×10^{-14}	0.28×10^{-15}	0.24×10^{-14}
4	0.17×10^{-14}				

For numerical determination of these roots we apply the method (19.11) using the initial approximations,

$$x_1^0 = -3.2 + 0.2i, \quad x_2^0 = -1.2 - 0.2i, \quad x_3^0 = 0.1 + 1.7i,$$
$$x_4^0 = -1.9 + 1.3i, \quad x_5^0 = -1.8 - 0.8i, \quad x_6^0 = 2.3 + 1.1i,$$
$$x_7^0 = 1.9 - 0.7i, \quad x_8^0 = 1.2 + 0.2i, \quad x_9^0 = 0.2 - 2.2i,$$

when $R = 0, 1, 3, 6$ and 9.

Let us denote by $\sigma(R, k) = \sum_{i=1}^{9} \|x_i^{k,R} - x_i^{k-1,R}\|$, the error between two consistent approximations on the step $k - 1$ and k, $\{x_i^{k-1,R}\}_{i=1}^{9}, \{x_i^{k,R}\}_{i=1}^{9}$ by fixed R equal to $0, 1, 3, 6, 9$. Table 19.1 shows $\sigma(R, k)$, obtained for different R and k.

Thus, we have a family for the following iteration method for finding all roots of $f(x)$ simultaneously (see WANG and ZHENG [1984a]):

$$x_i^{k+1} = x_i^k - \frac{\Delta_{p-1}(x_i^k)}{\Delta_p(x_i^k) - B_p\left(\sum_{j \neq i}^{n} \frac{1}{x_i^k - x_j^k}, \ldots, \sum_{j \neq i}^{n} \frac{1}{(x_i^k - x_j^k)^p}\right)}, \quad i = 1, \ldots, n \quad (19.18)$$

where

$$\Delta_p(f_i; x) = B_p(s_{1,i}, s_{2,i}, \ldots, s_{p,i}), \quad f(x) = (x - x_i)f_i(x), \quad i = 1, \ldots, n,$$

$$s_{\nu,i} = \sum_{j \neq i}^{n} \frac{1}{(x - x_j)^\nu}.$$

For Bell's polynomials, see RIORDAN [1958].

Specifically, letting $p = 1$, the iteration method of Ehrlich is obtained, which is of order 3 if the zeros are simple. Letting $p = 2$, we have a new method,

$$x_i^{k+1} = x_i^k - \frac{2\dfrac{f'(x_i^k)}{f(x_i^k)}}{\dfrac{2f'^2(x_i^k) - f(x_i^k)f'''(x_i^k)}{f^2(x_i^k)} - \left(\sum_{j \neq i}^{n} \frac{1}{x_i^k - x_j^k}\right)^2 - \sum_{j \neq i}^{n} \frac{1}{(x_i^k - x_j^k)^2}}$$

$i = 1, \ldots, n$, $k = 0, 1, \ldots$,

which is of order 4 if the zeros are simple. The method (19.18) is of order $p+2$.

Let

$$\nabla_j^{p,k} = \nabla_j^{p,k}(f; x_j^k) = \begin{vmatrix} \sigma_j^{1,k}(x_j^k) & 1 & & & 0 \\ \sigma_j^{2,k}(x_j^k) & \sigma_j^{1,k}(x_j^k) & 1 & & \\ \vdots & & \ddots & \ddots & \\ \sigma_j^{p-1,k}(x_j^k) & & \cdots & \sigma_j^{1,k}(x_j^k) & 1 \\ \sigma_j^{p,k}(x_j^k) & & \cdots & & \sigma_j^{1,k}(x_j^k) \end{vmatrix},$$

where

$$\sigma_j^{\nu,k}(x_j) = \sigma_j^{\nu,k}(x_j^k) = \frac{1}{\nu!}f^{(\nu)}(x_j^k)/f(x_j^k), \qquad \nabla_j^{0,k} = 1.$$

We suggest the following method (see ATANASSOVA, KJURKCHIEV and ANDREEV [1988]):

$$x_i^{k+1} = x_i^k + \Delta_i^{R+1,k},$$

$$\Delta_i^{s,k} = -\frac{f(x_i^k)}{\prod\limits_{j \neq i}^{n}(x_i^k - x_j^k + \nabla_j^{s-1,k}/\nabla_j^{s,k})}, \qquad (19.19)$$

$i = 1, 2, \ldots, n$, $s = 1, 2, \ldots, R+1$, $k = 0, 1, 2, \ldots$.

The rate of convergence of (19.19) is equal to $R + 3$.

Using Nourein's correction, we have

$$x_i^{k+1} = x_i^k + \Delta_i^{R+1,k},$$

$$\Delta_i^{s,k} = -\frac{f(x_i^k)}{\prod\limits_{j \neq i}^{n}(x_i^k - x_j^k)\left[1 - \sum\limits_{j \neq i}^{n}(\nabla_j^{s-1,k}/\nabla_j^{s,k})(x_i^k - x_j^k)^{-1}\right]},$$

$i = 1, \ldots, n$, $s = 1, 2, \ldots, R+1$, $k = 0, 1, 2, \ldots$.

Using Chebyshev's correction, we have

$$x_i^{k+1} = x_i^k + \Delta_i^{R+1,k},$$

$$\Delta_i^{s,k} = -\frac{f(x_i^k)}{\prod_{\substack{j=1 \\ j\neq i}}^{n}(x_i^k - x_j^k + \nabla_j^{s-1,k})},$$

$$i = 1,\ldots,n, \quad s = 1,2,\ldots,R+1, \quad k = 0,1,2,\ldots,$$

where

$$\nabla_j^{s,k} = \frac{f(x_j^k)}{f'(x_j^k)} \sum_{t=0}^{s}\left(\frac{f(x_j^k)}{f'(x_j^k)}\right)^t Y_{t,j}^k,$$

$$Y_{0,j}^k = 1, \quad Y_{t,j}^k = \frac{1}{t+1}(tD_{2,j}^k Y_{t-1,j}^k - (Y_{t-1,j}^k)'), \quad t > 0,$$

$$D_{t,j}^k = D_{t,j}^k(x_j^k) = \frac{f^{(t)}(x_j^k)}{f'(x_j^k)},$$

$$D_{1,j}^k = 1, \quad D_{t,j}^k = D_{2,j}^k D_{t-1,j}^k + (D_{t-1,j}^k)', \quad t > 1.$$

Let us discuss a generalization of Alefeld–Herzberger's method (KJURKCHIEV and ANDREEV [1992]).

For numerical solution of Eq. (19.1), we consider the following single-step method (SSM):

$$x_i^{k+1} = x_i^k - \left[H(x_i^k) - \left(\sum_{\beta_0=1}^{i-1}\frac{1}{x_i^k - x_{\beta_0}^{k+1} - \Delta_{\beta_0}^{R,k+1}} \right.\right.$$

$$\left.\left. + \sum_{\beta_0=i+1}^{n}\frac{1}{x_i^k - x_{\beta_0}^k - \nabla_{\beta_0}^{R,k}}\right)\right]^{-1},$$

$$i = 1,\ldots,n, \quad k = 0,1,\ldots, \quad R = 0,1,2,\ldots,$$

where

$$\Delta_s^{R,k+1} = -\left[H(x_s^{k+1}) - \left(\sum_{t=1}^{s-1}\frac{1}{x_s^{k+1} - x_t^{k+1} - \Delta_t^{R-1,k+1}} \right.\right.$$

$$\left.\left. + \sum_{t=s+1}^{n}\frac{1}{x_s^{k+1} - x_t^k - \nabla_t^{R-1,k}}\right)\right]^{-1},$$

$$\nabla_s^{R,k} = -\frac{1}{H(x_s^k) - \sum_{t\neq s}^{n}\frac{1}{x_s^k - x_t^k - \nabla_t^{R-1,k}}},$$

$$\nabla_t^{0,k} = \Delta_t^{0,k} = 0, \quad t = 1, \ldots, n, \quad k = 0, 1, \ldots.$$

THEOREM 19.4. *Under the conditions* (19.12), *the R-order of convergence from the above method is greater than*

$$2R + 3 + \frac{8(R+1)^2(2R-1)}{8(R+1)(2R-1) + 2(2R+1)(6R+5)((R+0.5)^{n-2} - 1)}.$$

20. Simultaneous approximation of multiple roots

Numerical methods for the determination of all roots of a given algebraic polynomial are considered in the case where the multiplicity of the roots is preassigned.

First we present iterative methods based on Weierstrass–Dochev's algorithm. Consider a monic polynomial f of degree n,

$$f(x) = x^n + a_{n-1}x^{n-1} + \cdots + a_0 = \prod_{j=1}^{m}(x - x_j)^{s_j}, \tag{20.1}$$

with complex zeros $x_1, x_2, \ldots, x_m$ having the multiplicities $s_1, s_2, \ldots, s_m$, where $s_1 + s_2 + \cdots + s_m = n$.

The following method is due to FARMER and LOIZOU [1977]:

$$x_i^{k+1} = x_i^k - \left(\frac{f(x_i^k)}{\prod_{j \neq i}^{m}(x_i^k - x_j^k)^{s_j}} \right)^{1/s_i}, \quad i = 1, \ldots, m, \quad k = 0, 1, \ldots. \tag{20.2}$$

The iterative formula (20.2) has quadratic convergence (see also LOIZOU [1982]). The method (20.2) is often used in practice because of its perfect computing properties, and attempts at modification were made with regard to the rate of convergence.

Let $x_1^k, \ldots, x_m^k$ be distinct, reasonably good approximations to the zeros $x_1, \ldots, x_m$ and let x_t^{k+1} be the next approximation to x_t, obtained by some iteration scheme. We now introduce the quantities

$$u_t^k = x_t^k - x_t, \quad u_t^{k+1} = x_t^{k+1} - x_t, \quad t = 1, \ldots, m, \quad u = \max_{1 \leqslant t \leqslant m} |u_t^k|.$$

Expanding the right-hand side of the appropriate iterative function using Taylor's series about x_j^k, we obtain

$$x_j = x_j^k - C(x_j^k) + U_j(u_j^k), \tag{20.3}$$

where $C(x_j^k)$ is a correction term and $U_j(u_j^k)$ is a 'remainder' in the development. From (20.1), we find

$$x_i = x - \left(\frac{f(x)}{\prod_{j \neq i}^{m}(x - x_j)^{s_j}} \right)^{1/s_i}, \quad i = 1, \ldots, m. \tag{20.4}$$

Letting $x = x_i^k$ in (20.4) and using (20.3) for $j \neq i$, we find

$$x_i^{k+1} = x_i^k - \left(\frac{f(x_i^k)}{\prod_{\substack{j\neq i}}^{m}(x_i^k - x_j^k + C(x_j^k) - U_j(u_j^k))^{s_j}} \right)^{1/s_i}. \tag{20.5}$$

Dropping $U_j(u_j^k)$ in (20.5), we obtain the following iterative method for the simultaneous approximation of multiple complex zeros of a polynomial f:

$$x_i^{k+1} = x_i^k - \left(\frac{f(x_i^k)}{\prod_{\substack{j\neq i}}^{m}(x_i^k - x_j^k + C(x_j^k))^{s_j}} \right)^{1/s_i}, \tag{20.6}$$

$$i = 1, 2, \ldots, m, \quad k = 0, 1, \ldots,$$

where the order of convergence of the iterative method (20.6) depends on the form of $C(x_j^k)$. If $C(x_j^k) = 0$, then (20.6) reduces to (20.2). The following total-step method is due to PETKOVIC and STEFANOVIC [1987a]:

$$x_i^{k+1} = x_i^k - \left(\frac{f(x_i^k)}{\prod_{\substack{j\neq i}}^{m}(x_i^k - x_j^k + N_j)^{s_j}} \right)^{1/s_i}, \tag{20.7}$$

where $N_j = s_j f(x_j^k)/f'(x_j^k)$. The iterative formula (20.7) has cubic convergence. The iterative process (20.7) can be accelerated by approximating all zeros in a serial fashion, i.e., using new approximations as soon as they become available (the so-called Gauss–Seidel approach). In this way, substituting $x_j := x_j^{k+1}$, ($j < i$), $x_j := x_j^k - N_j$ ($j > i$) in (18.4), we obtain the single-step method (see also LOIZOU [1983]):

$$x_i^{k+1} = x_i^k - \left[f(x_i^k) \left(\prod_{j<i}^{m}(x_i^k - x_j^{k+1})^{s_j} \prod_{j>i}^{m}(x_i^k - x_j^k + N_j)^{s_j} \right)^{-1} \right]^{1/s_i},$$

$$i = 1, 2, \ldots, m, \quad k = 0, 1, \ldots, \tag{20.8}$$

In the case of the single-step method (20.8), we use the definition of the R-order of convergence, introduced by Ortega and Rheinboldt. The R-order of convergence of an iterative process IP with the limit point $x = [x_1, \ldots, x_m]^T$ is denoted by $O_R(\text{IP}, x)$. The following theorem holds.

THEOREM 20.1 (PETKOVIC and STEFANOVIC [1987a]). *Suppose that the starting approximations $x_1^0, \ldots, x_m^0$ are chosen sufficiently close to the zeros $x_1, \ldots, x_m$ so that $|x_i^0 - x_i| \leq q < 1$, $i = 1, \ldots, m$. Then, for the method (20.8), the following estimate is true*

$$O_R((20.8), x) > \lambda_i \in (3, 4),$$

where λ_i is the unique positive root of the equation

$$g_i(\lambda) = (\lambda - 1)^i - (\lambda - 1)2^{i-1} - 2^{i-1} = 0.$$

REMARK 20.1. By (20.7) we obtain

$$x_i^{k+1} - x_i = -s_i^{-1}(x_i^k - x_i) \sum_{j \neq i} \frac{C_2(x_j)}{x_i - x_j}(x_j^k - x_j)^2 + O(u^4),$$

$$C_2(x_j) = \frac{s_j f^{(s_j + 1)}(x_j)}{(s_j + 1) f^{(s_j)}(x_j)}.$$

Numerical experiments. The efficiency of the iteration schemes (20.7) and (20.8) was illustrated numerically in the example of the polynomial,

$$f(x) = x^{13} + 5x^{12} + 8x^{11} + 40x^{10} + 133x^9 + 153x^8 + 496x^7 + 944x^6$$
$$+ 755x^5 + 2239x^4 + 520x^3 + 2088x^2 + 135x + 675.$$

The exact zeros of this polynomial are $x_1 = -3$, $x_{2,3} = \pm i$, $x_{4,5} = 1 \pm 2i$ with the multiplicities: $s_1 = 3, s_2 = 3, s_3 = 3, s_4 = 2, s_5 = 2$. As initial approximations to these zeros the following complex numbers were taken:

$$x_1^0 = -2.5 + 0.5i,$$
$$x_2^0 = 0.5 + 1.5i,$$
$$x_3^0 = 0.5 - 1.5i,$$
$$x_4^0 = 1.5 + 2.5i,$$
$$x_5^0 = 1.5 - 2.5i.$$

Applying the total-step method (20.7), after the third iteration, the following results were obtained:

$$x_1^3 = -2.9999999962637 + 1.72 \ldots 10^{-8} i,$$
$$x_2^3 = 3.44 \ldots 10^{-7} + 1.0000000768597i,$$
$$x_3^3 = 3.66 \ldots 10^{-8} - 1.0000000539716i,$$
$$x_4^3 = 1.0000001906934 + 2.00000026663385i,$$
$$x_5^3 = 1.0000000207791 - 1.99999993455011i.$$

Starting from the same initial approximations, the single-step method (20.8) has produced more improved approximations to the exact zeros:

$$x_1^3 = -3.0000000008301 - 2.45 \ldots 10^{-10} i$$

$$x_2^3 = 3.12\ldots 10^{-9} + 0.9999999983808i$$
$$x_3^3 = 1.46\ldots 10^{-10} - 1.0000000000997i$$
$$x_4^3 = 1.0000000000141 + 1.9999999999943i$$
$$x_5^3 = 0.9999999999995 - 2.0000000000002i$$

The following modification is based on the Weierstrass–Dochev's algorithm (see SEMERDZHIEV [1982], MAKRELOV and SEMERDZHIEV [1984b]):

$$x_i^{k+1} = x_i^k - s_i^{-1} \sum_{j=0}^{s_i-1} \frac{f^{(j)}(x_i^k)}{j!(s_j-1-j)!} \left(\frac{(x-x_i^k)^{s_i}}{X_{m,f}^k(x)} \right)^{(s_i-1-j)}_{x=x_i^k}, \qquad (20.9)$$

$$i = 1,\ldots,m, \quad k = 0,1,\ldots,$$

where

$$X_{m,f}^k(x) = \prod_{j=1}^{m} (x - x_j)^{s_j}.$$

THEOREM 20.2. *Let the numbers* $x_1,\ldots,x_m$ *be the roots of equation* (20.1) *with corresponding multiplicities* $s_1,\ldots,s_m$; $s_i > 1$, $i = 1,\ldots,m$, $s_1 + \cdots + s_m = n$. *Let* $d = \min_{i\neq s} |x_s - x_i|$ *and* $b = \min_{i\neq s} |x_s - x_i|$. *Assume that there are numbers* q *and* c *such that* $c > 0$, $0 < q < 1$, $d - 2c > 0$ *and*

$$c \left(\frac{2^n}{d-2c} + \max_{i=1,\ldots,m} \frac{1}{s_i} \sum_{\substack{u+t=s_i-1 \\ u>0,\ t>0}} \binom{s_i}{u} (d-2c)^{s_i-t-n} \right.$$

$$\left. \times \sum_{\substack{\nu_1+\cdots+\nu_{i-1}+\nu_{i+1}+\cdots+\nu_m=t \\ \nu_k \geq 0,\ k=1,\ldots,i-1,i+1,\ldots,m}} \prod_{\beta\neq i}^{m} \sum_{p=0}^{s-\nu_\beta} \sum_{r=0}^{p} \binom{s_\beta}{p} \binom{p}{r} b^r (cq)^{s_\beta - r} \right) < 1.$$

If the initial approximations $x_1^0,\ldots,x_m^0$ *of the roots* $x_1,\ldots,x_m$ *are such that*

$$|x_i^0 - x_i| < cq, \quad i = 1,\ldots,m,$$

then for every $k = 0,1,\ldots$ *and* $i = 1,\ldots,m$, *the inequalities*

$$|x_i^k - x_i| \leq cq^{2^k}$$

hold, i.e. the method (20.9) *has a quadratic convergence rate.*

REMARK 20.2. SEMERDZHIEV and TAMBUROV [1984] obtained a method to determine the multiplicities of the roots of a given algebraic polynomial with real coefficients. The method is based on the algorithm of Euclid and is reduced to the solution of an integer triangle system of linear algebraic equations. The iterative formula (20.2) in the case of multiple roots has only linear convergence (see RALL [1966]).

Other methods are given in CASCIO, PASQUINI and TRIGIANTE [1983, 1984], FARMER and LOIZOU [1975], STEFANOVIC [1986], PETKOVIC and CVETKOVIC [1990], PETKOVIC and HERZBERGER [1990].

Let us now consider iterative methods based on Ehrlich's algorithm. Using Ehrlich's approach, many authors have presented algorithms for the simultaneous determination of the roots of Eq. (20.1) in the case where their multiplicity is prescribed in advance (see GARGANTINI [1978, 1980, 1981], PETKOVIC [1982], MILOVANOVIC and PETKOVIC [1984], KJURKCHIEV, ANDREEV and POPOV [1984], KJURKCHIEV and ANDREEV [1989], ATANASSOVA, KJURKCHIEV and ANDREEV [1988]).

From

$$\frac{f'(x_i^k)}{f(x_i^k)} = \sum_{j=1}^{m} \frac{s_j}{x_i^k - x_j} = \frac{s_i}{x_i^k - x_i} + \sum_{j \neq i}^{m} \frac{s_j}{x_i^k - x_j},$$

we have

$$x_i = x_i^k - s_i \left(\frac{f'(x_i^k)}{f(x_i^k)} - \sum_{j \neq i} \frac{s_j}{x_i^k - x_j} \right)^{-1}. \qquad (20.10)$$

Letting $x_i = x_i^{k+1}$, $x_j = x_j^k$ ($j \neq i$) in (20.10), we find

$$x_i^{k+1} = x_i^k - s_i \left(\frac{f'(x_i^k)}{f(x_i^k)} - \sum_{j \neq i} \frac{s_j}{x_i^k - x_j^k} \right)^{-1}, \quad i = 1, \ldots, m, \; k = 0, 1, \ldots. \qquad (20.11)$$

The convergence order of this method is 3.

For $x_j = x_j^{k+1}$ ($j < i$) and $x_j = x_j^k$ ($j > i$), we obtain the total-step iteration

$$x_i^{k+1} = x_i^k - s_i \left(\frac{f'(x_i^k)}{f(x_i^k)} - \sum_{j=1}^{i-1} \frac{s_j}{x_i^k - x_j^{k+1}} - \sum_{j=i+1}^{m} \frac{s_j}{x_i^k - x_j^k} \right)^{-1},$$

$$i = 1, \ldots, m, \; k = 0, 1, \ldots. \qquad (20.12)$$

If the initial approximation $x^0 = (x_1^0, \ldots, x_m^0)$ of the roots $x = (x_1, \ldots, x_m)$ of Eq. (20.1) is chosen sufficiently close to $\{x_i\}_{i=1}^m$, then the following theorem holds (see MILOVANOVIC and PETKOVIC [1984]).

THEOREM 20.3. *Method (20.12) is convergent with the order of convergence*

$$O_R((20.12), x) \geq 2 + \lambda_m > 3,$$

where λ_m is the unique positive root of the equation

$$g_m(\lambda) = \lambda^m - \lambda - 2 = 0.$$

Let $x_j = x_j^k + \Delta_j^k$ and $\Delta_j^k = -s_j f(x_j^k)/f'(x_j^k)$ be Schroder's correction.
For the simultaneous determination of all multiple zeros, the following modified Nourein method is well known:

$$x_i^{k+1} = x_i^k - s_i \left(\frac{f'(x_i^k)}{f(x_i^k)} - \sum_{j \neq i} \frac{s_j}{x_i^k - x_j^k - \Delta_j^k} \right)^{-1}, \qquad (20.13)$$

$i = 1, \ldots, m, \quad k = 0, 1, \ldots$.

The convergence order of this method is 4.
For $x_j = x_j^{k+1}$ ($j < i$) and $x_j = x_j^k + \Delta_j^k$ ($j > i$), we obtain the method

$$x_i^{k+1} = x_i^k - s_i \left(\frac{f'(x_i^k)}{f(x_i^k)} - \sum_{j=1}^{i-1} \frac{s_j}{x_i^k - x_j^{k+1}} - \sum_{j=i+1}^{m} \frac{s_j}{x_i^k - x_j^k - \Delta_j^k} \right)^{-1},$$

$i = 1, 2, \ldots, m, \quad k = 0, 1, \ldots$. $\qquad (20.14)$

The next theorem gives the order of convergence of the proposed method (see MILOVANOVIC and PETKOVIC [1984]).

THEOREM 20.4. *Suppose that the starting approximations $x_1^0, \ldots, x_m^0$ are chosen sufficiently close to the zeros $x_1, \ldots, x_m$ so that $|x_i^0 - x_i| \leq q < 1$, $i = 1, \ldots, m$. Then, for the method (20.14), we have*

$$O_R((20.14), x) \geq 2(1 + \lambda_m) > 4,$$

where λ_m is the unique positive root of the equation

$$g_m(\lambda) = \lambda^m - \lambda - 1 = 0.$$

We propose a variant of (20.13):

$$x_i^{k+1} = x_i^k + \Delta_i^{R+1,k}, \quad i = 1, \ldots, m, \quad k = 0, 1, \ldots,$$

$$\Delta_i^{s,k} = -s_i \left(\frac{f'(x_i^k)}{f(x_i^k)} - \sum_{j \neq i} \frac{s_j}{x_i^k - x_j^k + \nabla_j^{s-1,k}} \right)^{-1}, \qquad (20.15)$$

$$\nabla_j^{s,k} = \sum_{q=1}^{s} \rho_{s,q}(s_j) Z_{q,j}, \quad \nabla_j^{0,k} = 0, \qquad j = 1, 2, \ldots,$$

where $\nabla_j^{s,k}$ is Chebyshev's correction and R is a nonnegative integer. For $\rho_{s,q}$ and $Z_{q,j}$, we obtain the relations

$$pZ_{p,j} - (p-1)Z_{p-1,j} + \frac{f(x_j^k)}{f'(x_j^k)} Z'_{p-1,j} = 0,$$

$$t\rho_{t,q} + (s_j q - t)\rho_{t-1,q} - s_j q \rho_{t-1,q-1} = 0, \qquad (20.16)$$

where $Z_{1,j} = f(x_j^k)/f'(x_j^k)$, $\rho_{t,0} = 1$ if $t \geq 0$, $\rho_{t,q} = 0$ if $t < q$.
The values $\rho_{t,q}(s_j)$ for different t and q are given in Table 20.1.

TABLE 20.1.

t	q			
	1	2	3	4
1	s_j			
2	$\frac{1}{2}s_j(3-s_j)$	s_j^2		
3	$\frac{1}{6}s_j(s_j^2-6s_j+11)$	$s_j^2(2-s_j)$	s_j^3	
4	$-\frac{1}{24}s_j(s_j^3-10s_j^2+35s_j-50)$	$\frac{1}{12}s_j^2(7s_j^2-30s_j+35)$	$\frac{1}{2}s_j^3(5-s_j)$	s_j^4

KJURKCHIEV, ANDREEV and POPOV [1984] proposed the following method for the simultaneous approximation of multiple zeros of Eq. (20.1):

$$x_i^{k+1} = x_i^k - s_i \left(H(x_i^k) - \sum_{\beta_0 \neq i}^{m} \frac{s_{\beta_0}}{x_i^k - x_{\beta_0}^k - \Delta_{\beta_0}^{R,k}} \right)^{-1}, \quad (20.17)$$

$$i = 1, \ldots, m, \quad k = 0, 1, \ldots,$$

where

$$H(x_i^k) = \frac{f'(x_i^k)}{f(x_i^k)},$$

$$\Delta_t^{R,k} = -s_t \left(H(x_t^k) - \sum_{q \neq t}^{m} \frac{s_q}{x_t^k - x_q^k - \Delta_q^{R-1,k}} \right)^{-1}, \quad t = 1, \ldots, m,$$

$$\Delta_t^{0,k} = 0, \quad t = 1, \ldots, m, \quad k = 0, 1, \ldots.$$

It is clear that when $R = 0$ the method (20.17) coincides with (20.11). The rate of convergence of (20.17) is $2R + 3$.

Here we prove the following theorem.

THEOREM 20.5. *Let* $0 < q < 1$, $d = \min_{i \neq j} |x_i - x_j|$ *and let* $c > 0$ *be a number such that*

$$d > c(2 + 3qn/s),$$

$$c^2(n-s') \left[(d-c)(d-2c-cqn/s) \left(1 - \frac{(n/s+1)(n/s'-1)c^2q^2}{(d-c)(d-2c-cqn/s)} \right) \right]^{-1} \leqslant 1,$$

$$s = \max_{1 \leqslant j \leqslant m} s_j, \quad s' = \min_{1 \leqslant j \leqslant m} s_j.$$

(20.18)

If the initial approximations $\{x_i^0\}_{i=1}^m$ *of the roots* $\{x_i\}_{i=1}^m$ *of Eq.* (20.1) *satisfy the*

inequalities
$$|x_i^0 - x_i| \leqslant cq, \quad i = 1, \ldots, m,$$
then the estimate
$$|x_i^k - x_i| \leqslant cq^{(2R+3)^k}, \quad i = 1, \ldots, m, \quad k = 0, 1, \ldots$$
holds true.

The next iterative methods are based on Halley's algorithm. Let $q_k(x)$ be defined as
$$q_k(x) = \frac{1}{f(x)} \frac{d^k}{dx^k}(f(x)), \quad k = 1, 2.$$
Then
$$q_1(x) = \frac{f'(x)}{f(x)} = \sum_{j=1}^{m} \frac{s_j}{x - x_j}. \tag{20.19}$$
Differentiating (20.19), we obtain
$$q_1'(x) = \frac{f(x)f''(x) - f'^2(x)}{f^2(x)} = -\sum_{j=1}^{m} \frac{s_j}{(x - x_j)^2}.$$
Since
$$q_2(x) = q_1^2(x) + q_1'(x),$$
we have
$$s_i^{-1} \left(\sum_{j \neq i}^{m} \frac{s_j}{x - x_j} \right)^2 + \sum_{j \neq i}^{m} \frac{s_j}{(x - x_j)^2}$$
$$= s_i^{-1} \left(q_1 - \frac{s_i}{x - x_i} \right)^2 - \left(q_1' + \frac{s_i}{(x - x_i)^2} \right)$$
$$= q_1^2 \left(1 + \frac{1}{s_i} \right) - q_2 - \frac{2q_1}{x - x_i},$$
i.e.
$$q_1^2 \left(1 + \frac{1}{s_i}\right) - q_2 - s_i^{-1} \left(\sum_{j \neq i}^{m} \frac{s_j}{x - x_j}\right)^2 - \sum_{j \neq i}^{m} \frac{s_j}{(x - x_j)^2} = \frac{2q_1}{x - x_i}. \tag{20.20}$$

Solving (20.20) for x, we find
$$x_i = x - \left\{ 0.5 q_1 (1 + s_i^{-1}) - 0.5 q_2 / q_1 \right.$$

$$-0.5q_1^{-1}\left[s_i^{-1}\left(\sum_{j\neq i}^m \frac{s_j}{x-x_j}\right)^2 + \sum_{j\neq i}^m \frac{s_j}{(x-x_j)^2}\right]^{-1}.$$

Using Halley's approach (see HALLEY [1809], HANSEN and PATRIC [1977]) many authors have given algorithms for simultaneous determination of the multiple roots of Eq. (20.1). The following modification of Halley's method has rate of convergence $\tau = 4$ (see PETKOVIC [1989a]):

$$x_i^{k+1} = x_i^k - \left\{h(x_i^k) - 0.5\frac{f(x_i^k)}{f'(x_i^k)}\right.$$

$$\left.\times\left[s_i^{-1}\left(\sum_{j\neq i}^m \frac{s_j}{x_i^k-x_j^k}\right)^2 + \sum_{j\neq i}^m \frac{s_j}{(x_i^k-x_j^k)^2}\right]^{-1}\right\}, \quad (20.21)$$

$$h(x_i^k) = (1+s_i^{-1})0.5\frac{f'(x_i^k)}{f(x_i^k)} - \frac{f''(x_i^k)}{2f'(x_i^k)}, \quad i=1,\ldots,m, \quad k=0,1,\ldots.$$

We define the following analogue of Halley's method (see KJURKCHIEV and ANDREEV [1990]):

$$x_i^{k+1} = x_i^k + \nabla_i^{R+1,k}, \quad (20.22)$$

where

$$\nabla_i^{p,k} = -\left\{h(x_i^k) - \frac{f(x_i^k)}{2f'(x_i^k)}\left[s_i^{-1}\left(\sum_{\beta_0\neq i}^m \frac{s_{\beta_0}}{x_i^k-x_{\beta_0}^k-\nabla_{\beta_0}^{p-1,k}}\right)^2\right.\right.$$

$$\left.\left.+\sum_{\beta_0\neq i}^m \frac{s_{\beta_0}}{\left(x_i^k-x_{\beta_0}^k-\nabla_{\beta_0}^{p-1,k}\right)^2}\right]^{-1}\right\},$$

$$h(x_i^k) = (1+s_i^{-1}0.5)\frac{f'(x_i^k)}{f(x_i^k)} - \frac{f''(x_i^k)}{2f'(x_i^k)}, \quad \nabla_i^{0,k} = 0,$$

$$i=1,2,\ldots,m, \quad p=1,2,\ldots,R+1, \quad k=0,1,\ldots.$$

The following theorem holds.

THEOREM 20.6. *Let* $0 < q < 1$, $d = \min_{i\neq j}|x_i - x_j|$ *and let* $c > 0$ *be a number such that*

(a) $d - 4cq > 0$;

(b) $2cqn(d-4cq)^{-2} \leqslant (d-cq)^{-1}$;

(c) $4cqn < d - cq$;

(d) $c^3n^2(2+4cq/(d-cq))(1-2cqn/(d-cq))^{-1}(d-4cq)^{-3} \leqslant 1$.

If the initial approximation $\{x_i^0\}_{i=1}^m$ of the roots $\{x_i\}_{i=1}^m$ of Eq. (20.1) satisfies the inequalities

$$|x_i - x_i^0| \leqslant cq, \quad i = 1, \ldots, m,$$

then the estimate

$$|x_i - x_i^k| \leqslant cq^{(3R+4)^k}, \quad i = 1, \ldots, m, \quad k = 0, 1, 2, \ldots$$

holds.

For other results see LAGUANELLE [1966], HANSEN and PATRIC [1976], WANG and ZHENG [1985], MAKRELOV, SEMERDZHIEV and TAMBUROV [1985], SEMERDZHIEV and TAMBUROV [1985], PETKOVIC, MILOVANOVIC and SEFANOVIC [1986], WANG and WU [1987], PETKOVIC [1987], PETKOVIC and STEFANOVIC [1987a,b], FRAIGNIAUD [1989a,b], RICE and JAMIESON [1989].

21. Multi-point methods for simultaneous approximation

A class of multi-stage methods for simultaneous calculations of the roots of a given algebraic equation is considered. It is shown that these schemes have a superlinear rate of convergence with respect to the multi-stage degree.

We propose a multi-point variant based on the Weierstrass–Dochev's algorithm:

$$x_i^{k+1} = x_i^k - \frac{f(x_i^k)}{\prod_{j \neq i}^n (x_i^k - x_j^{k-1})}, \quad i = 1, \ldots, n, \quad k = 1, 2, \ldots. \tag{21.1}$$

The following theorem gives the rate of convergence of the proposed method.

THEOREM 21.1. *Let $0 < q < 1$, $d = \min_{i \neq j} |x_i - x_j|$ and let the constant $c > 0$ satisfy*

$$0 < \frac{cnA}{d-2c} < 1. \tag{21.2}$$

Let A be a root of the equation

$$A = e^{1/A}. \tag{21.3}$$

If the initial approximations $\{x_i^0\}_{i=1}^n$, $\{x_i^1\}_{i=1}^n$ satisfy the inequalities

$$\begin{aligned} |x_i^0 - x_i| &\leqslant cq, \\ |x_i^1 - x_i| &\leqslant cq^r, \quad i = 1, \ldots, m \end{aligned} \tag{21.4}$$

then for every k

$$|x_i^k - x_i| \leqslant cq^{r^k}, \quad i = 1, \ldots, n \tag{21.5}$$

holds, where $r = (1 + \sqrt{5})/2$ is the unique positive root of the equation
$$r^2 - r - 1 = 0.$$

In the cases where the multiplicity of the roots is not known, it is suitable to modify the calculation procedures and to consider their multi-point analogues, because the multiple roots cause rapid growth of some quantities in a series of one-stage methods.

Let us note that changing the one-stage Weierstrass–Dochev method, results in a lower speed of convergence and at the same time, the existence of multiple roots ensures that the scheme (21.1) has a better stability than the one-stage iteration.

KJURKCHIEV and IVANOV [1984] proposed the following multi-point method:

$$x_i^{k+1} = x_i^k - \frac{f(x_i^k)}{\prod_{\substack{\beta_0=1 \\ \beta_0 \neq i}}^{n} (x_i^k - x_{\beta_0}^k - \Delta_{\beta_0}^{R,k-1})}, \quad i = 1, 2, \ldots, n, \quad k = R+1, \ldots, n, \tag{21.6}$$

where

$$\Delta_s^{R,k-1} = -\frac{f(x_s^{k-1})}{\prod_{\substack{l=1 \\ l \neq s}}^{n} (x_s^{k-1} - x_l^{k-2} - \Delta_l^{R-1,k-2})},$$

$$\Delta_j^{0,t} = 0, \quad j, t = 1, 2, \ldots, n.$$

Here we prove the following.

THEOREM 21.2. *Let $0 < q < 1$, $d = \min_{i \neq j} |x_i - x_j|$ and let $c > 0$ be a number such that*

$$0 < \frac{cnA}{d - 2c} < 1.$$

Let A be a root of the equation

$$A = e^{1/A} \quad (A = 1.763222894\ldots).$$

If the initial approximations $\{x_i^j\}_{i=1}^n$, $j = 0, 1, \ldots, R+1$ satisfy the inequalities

$$|x_i^j - x_i| \leq cq^{r^j}, \quad i = 1, \ldots, n, \quad j = 0, 1, \ldots, R+1,$$

then the estimate

$$|x_i^k - x_i| \leq cq^{r^k}, \quad i = 1, \ldots, n, \quad k = R+2, \ldots,$$

holds true, where r is the unique positive root of the equation

$$r^{R+2} - r^{R+1} - \cdots - r - 1 = 0. \tag{21.7}$$

PROOF. By induction

$$x_i^{k+1} - x_i = (x_i^k - x_i) \sum_{\alpha_0 \neq i}^{n} \frac{x_{\alpha_0} - x_{\alpha_0}^{k-1} - \Delta_{\alpha_0}^{R,k-1}}{x_i^k - x_{\alpha_0}^{k-1} - \Delta_{\alpha_0}^{R,k-1}}$$

$$\times \prod_{\beta_0 \neq i}^{\alpha_0 - 1} \frac{x_i^k - x_{\beta_0}}{x_i^k - x_{\beta_0}^{k-1} - \Delta_{\beta_0}^{R,k-1}}$$

$$= (x_i^k - x_i) \sum_{\alpha_0 \neq i}^{n} \frac{x_{\alpha_0} - x_{\alpha_0}^{k-1}}{x_i^k - x_{\alpha_0}^{k-1} - \Delta_{\alpha_0}^{R,k-1}}$$

$$\times \sum_{\alpha_1 \neq \alpha_0}^{n} \frac{x_{\alpha_1} - x_{\alpha_1}^{k-2}}{x_{\alpha_0}^{k-1} - x_{\alpha_1}^{k-2} - \Delta_{\alpha_1}^{R-1,k-2}}$$

$$\cdots \sum_{\alpha_R \neq \alpha_{R-1}}^{n} \frac{x_{\alpha_R} - x_{\alpha_R}^{k-R-1}}{x_{\alpha_{R-1}}^{k-R} - x_{\alpha_R}^{k-R-1}} \prod_{\beta_R \neq \alpha_{R-1}}^{\alpha_R - 1} \frac{x_{\alpha_{R-1}}^{k-R} - x_{\beta_R}}{x_{\alpha_{R-1}}^{k-R} - x_{\beta_R}^{k-R-1}}$$

$$\cdots \prod_{\beta_1 \neq \alpha_0}^{\alpha_1 - 1} \frac{x_{\alpha_0}^{k-1} - x_{\beta_1}}{x_{\alpha_0}^{k-1} - x_{\beta_1}^{k-2} - \Delta_{\beta_1}^{R-1,k-2}} \prod_{\beta_0 \neq i}^{\alpha_0 - 1} \frac{x_i^k - x_{\beta_0}}{x_i^k - x_{\beta_0}^{k-1} - \Delta_{\beta_0}^{R,k-1}}.$$

Then for $x_i^{k+1} - x_i$, we obtain

$$|x_i^{k+1} - x_i| \leqslant cq^{r^{k-R-1}(1+r+\cdots+r^{R+1})} \left(\frac{e^{1/A}}{A}\right)^{R+1}.$$

From $A^{-1}e^{1/A} = 1$ and (21.7), we finally obtain

$$|x_i^{k+1} - x_i| \leqslant cq^{r^{k-R-1}r^{R+2}} = cq^{r^{k+1}}.$$

Thus the theorem is proved. □

If $R = 0$, then $r = 1.618\ldots$. If $R = 1$, we obtain

$$r = \tfrac{1}{3}\left(\sqrt[3]{19 + 3\sqrt{33}} + \sqrt[3]{19 - 3\sqrt{33}} + 1\right) = 1.839\ldots .$$

Table 21.1 shows the values of $r = r(R)$ obtained.

22. Factorization of a polynomial

The problem of factorizing $f(z)$ is also quite intriguing. The method performs the factorization of the polynomial

$$f(z) = z^n + a_1 z^{n-1} + \cdots + a_n$$

into quadratic factors, i.e.

$$f(z) = \prod_{j=1}^{m}(z^2 + p_j z + q_j), \qquad (22.1)$$

TABLE 21.1.

R	r
0	1.618...
1	1.839...
2	1.927...
3	1.965...
8	1.999...

where a_i are real and n is even, i.e. $n = 2m$.

The factorization (22.1) with real coefficients $p_j, q_j, j = 1, \ldots, m$ exists for real $a_i, i = 1, \ldots, n$. Hence for polynomials with real coefficients, we can perform the calculation in real arithmetic only.

Denote by $\lambda_i^0, \lambda_{i+m}^0$, the roots of the polynomial

$$z^2 + p_i^0 z + q_i^0, \quad i = 1, 2, \ldots, m,$$

and by $\lambda_i^k, \lambda_{i+m}^k$, denote the roots of

$$z^2 + p_i^k z + q_i^k, \quad i = 1, 2, \ldots, m.$$

The method is based on the formulas (see DVORCUK [1967, 1969])

$$p_i^{k+1} = p_i^k + \frac{f(\lambda_i^k)}{\prod_{j \neq i}(\lambda_i^k - \lambda_j^k)} + \frac{f(\lambda_{i+m}^k)}{\prod_{j \neq i+m}(\lambda_{i+m}^k - \lambda_j^k)},$$

$$q_i^{k+1} = q_i^k - \lambda_{i+m}^k \frac{f(\lambda_i^k)}{\prod_{j \neq i}(\lambda_i^k - \lambda_j^k)} - \lambda_i^k \frac{f(\lambda_{i+m}^k)}{\prod_{j \neq i+m}(\lambda_{i+m}^k - \lambda_j^k)}, \quad (22.2)$$

$$i = 1, \ldots, m, \quad k = 0, 1, \ldots .$$

The following theorem holds.

THEOREM 22.1 (DVORCUK [1969]). *Let the polynomial $f(z)$ have distinct roots $z_1, z_2, \ldots, z_n$. Let $d = \min_{i \neq j} |z_i - z_j|$. Let the approximations $p_i^0, q_i^0, i = 1, \ldots, m$, of the coefficients in the factorization (22.1) be given such that the roots $\lambda_1^0, \lambda_2^0, \ldots, \lambda_n^0$ of the polynomials*

$$z^2 + p_i^0 z + q_i^0, \quad i = 1, 2, \ldots, m$$

satisfy the inequalities

$$|\lambda_i^0 - z_i| < \frac{1 - (1+q)^{1/(n-1)}}{1 - 2(1+q)^{1/(n-1)}} d, \quad (22.3)$$

where

$$0 < q < \frac{1}{8 \cdot 2^{1/(n-1)} - 7}. \tag{22.4}$$

Then the sequences $\{p_i^k\}_{k=0}^\infty$, $\{q_i^k\}_{k=0}^\infty$, $i = 1,\ldots,m$, determined by (22.2) are quadratically convergent.

PROOF. We denote

$$F_i^k = \frac{f(\lambda_i^k)}{\prod_{j \neq i}(\lambda_i^k - \lambda_j^k)}$$

and

$$z_i^k = \lambda_i^{k-1} - F_i^{k-1}.$$

Thus

$$z_i^k + z_{i+m}^k = -p_i^k = \lambda_i^k + \lambda_{i+m}^k,$$
$$z_i^k z_{i+m}^k - F_i^{k-1} F_{i+m}^{k-1} = q_i^k = \lambda_i^k \lambda_{i+m}^k$$

and

$$\lambda_i^k = 0.5\left(z_i^k + z_{i+m}^k + \sqrt{(z_i^k - z_{i+m}^k)^2 + 4F_i^{k-1} F_{i+m}^{k-1}}\right),$$

$$\lambda_{i+m}^k = 0.5\left(z_i^k + z_{i+m}^k - \sqrt{(z_i^k - z_{i+m}^k)^2 + 4F_i^{k-1} F_{i+m}^{k-1}}\right).$$

Hence if we choose the branch of the root such that

$$\sqrt{(z_i^k - z_{i+m}^k)^2} = z_i^k - z_{i+m}^k,$$

we obtain

$$|\lambda_i^k - z_i^k| = 0.5|z_i^k - z_{i+m}^k| \left|\left(1 + \frac{4F_i^{k-1} F_{i+m}^{k-1}}{(z_i^k - z_{i+m}^k)^2}\right)^{1/2} - 1\right|$$

$$\leq 2\frac{|F_i^{k-1} F_{i+m}^{k-1}|}{|z_i^k - z_{i+m}^k|}. \tag{22.5}$$

If we denote

$$b = \frac{1 - (1+q)^{1/(n-1)}}{1 - 2(1+q)^{1/(n-1)}}, \tag{22.6}$$

then it is proved in DOCHEV [1962a] that

$$|z_i^0 - z_i| \leq bqd,$$
$$|F_i^0| \leq (1+q)bd, \tag{22.7}$$
$$|z_i^1 - z_{i+m}^1| \geq (1 - 2bq)d.$$

According to (22.4) we have $(8 \cdot 2^{1/(n-1)} - 7)q < 1$; consequently
$$(1+q)^{1/(n-1)} 8q < 1 + 7q.$$
Hence
$$[(1+q)^{1/(n-1)} - 1]2(1+3q) < (2(1+q)^{1/(n-1)} - 1)(1-q)$$
gives
$$b < \frac{1-q}{2(1+3q)}.$$
Therefore, q_1 exists such that $0 < q < q_1 < 1$ and
$$b < 0.5 \frac{q_1 - q}{1 + 2q + qq_1}. \tag{22.8}$$

We perform the estimation using (22.5) and (22.8):
$$|z_i^1 - \lambda_i^1| \leqslant \frac{2b^2(1+q)^2}{1 - 2qb} d$$
$$< \frac{(q_1 - q)b(1+q)^2 d}{(1 + 2q + qq_1)[1 - q(q_1 - q)/(1 + 2q + qq_1)]} = (q_1 - q)bd,$$
and so
$$|\lambda_i^1 - z_i| \leqslant |z_i^1 - \lambda_i^1| + |z_i^1 - z_i| < q_1 bd.$$
Analogously, we estimate
$$|\lambda_{i+m}^1 - z_{i+m}| < q_1 bd.$$
Analogous considerations can be performed for k if we assume that
$$|\lambda_i^{k-1} - z_i| \leqslant bdq_1^{2^{k-1}}, \quad i = 1, \ldots, n,$$
because (22.7) assumes the following form for k:
$$|z_i^k - z_i| \leqslant bq_1^{2^{k-1}} d,$$
$$|F_i^{k-1}| \leqslant (1+q)bq_1^{2^{k-1}-1} d.$$
Further, we obtain
$$|z_i^k - \lambda_i^k| \leqslant \frac{2b^2(1+q)^2 q_1^{2^{k-2}}}{1 - 2bqq_1^{2^{k-2}}} d,$$
and using (22.8)
$$|z_i^k - \lambda_i^k| \leqslant \frac{(q_1 - q)b(1+q)^2 q_1^{2^{k-2}} d}{(1+q)^2 + q(1 - q_1^{2^{k-2}})(q_1 - q)},$$
hence
$$|z_i^k - \lambda_i^k| < (q_1 - q)bq_1^{2^{k-2}} d$$

TABLE 22.1. $f(z) = (z-1)^4(z-2)^3(z-3)^2(z-4)$.

j	p_j^0	q_j^0	p_j^{45}	q_j^{45}
1	6.24903434608	18.5911925932	−7.00121215639	12.0053638741
2	2.57087676919	17.9475448895	−2.92672894585	1.8112962497
3	0.89271919231	17.1336430938	−2.08416132007	1.0856580055
4	−1.78543838456	16.4482973701	−3.98890729233	2.9677317228
5	−4.46359596145	15.7903654752	−3.99999551239	3.9998973799

and

$$|\lambda_i^k - z_i| < bq_1^{2^k-2}d.$$

The quadratic convergence of the sequences $\{\lambda_i^k\}_{k=0}^\infty$, $\{p_i^k\}_{k=0}^\infty$, $\{q_i^k\}_{k=0}^\infty$, $i = 1, \ldots, m$, is proved. □

REMARK 22.1. For p_i^k determined by (22.2) and for $k = 1, 2, \ldots$, it holds that

$$p_1^k + p_2^k + \cdots + p_m^k = a_1.$$

Numerical experiment. The method is illustrated by the example in Table 22.1 (see DVORCUK [1969]).

For the application of Newton iteration to the determination of quadratic factors of polynomials, see BAIRSTOW [1914] and HITCHCOCK [1944]. Methods for factorization of a polynomial can be found also in LAWRENCE and LAWRENCE [1972], SEKULOVSKI [1972], KJURKCHIEV [1981].

23. Interval methods for polynomial root determining

Usually two kinds of interval arithmetic are used on the complex plane. For the following presentation we follow ALEFELD and HERZBERGER [1983]:

(i) Circular arithmetic deals with discs instead of complex numbers. Let $W = [x; r]$ denote a disc in the complex plane with center x and radius r, i.e. $W = \{z: |x - z| \leqslant r\}$. In this notation the complex number $z = \alpha + i\beta$ can be treated as a disc $W = [\alpha + i\beta; 0]$.

Let $* \in \{+, -, \cdot, :\}$ be a binary operation on the complex numbers. Unfortunately, if W_1, W_2 are discs on the plane then the set of points

$$W_1 * W_2 = \{z: z = z_1 * z_2, z_1 \in W_1, z_2 \in W_2\}$$

is not in general a disc, which is evident for multiplication. In order to remain within the realm of discs KRIER [1973], HAUENSCHILD [1974] give another definition of product of two discs, but the most convenient definition was given by GARGANTINI and HENRICI [1972] – see definition (b) below.

We use the following operation rules of circular arithmetic:

(a) $[x_1;r_1] \pm [x_2;r_2] = [x_1 \pm x_2; r_1 + r_2]$;
(b) $[x_1;r_1] \cdot [x_2;r_2] = [x_1 x_2; |x_1|r_2 + |x_2|r_1 + r_1 r_2]$;
(c) $1/[x_2;r_2] = [\bar{x}_2; r_2]/(|x_2|^2 - r_2^2)$, for $|x_2| \geq r_2$, where $\bar{x}_2$ denotes conjugate complex of x_2;
(d) $[x_1;r_1]/[x_2;r_2] = [x_1;r_1] \cdot (1/[x_2;r_2])$;
(e) $[x_1;r_1]^n = \left[x_1^n; \sum_{j=1}^{n} \binom{n}{j} |x_1|^{n-j} r_1^j \right] = [x_1^n; (|x_1|+r_1)^n - |x_1|^n]$;
(f) $[x_1;r_1] \subseteq [x_2;r_2] \Leftrightarrow |x_1 - x_2| \leq r_2 - r_1$;
(g) let W_1, W_2, U_1, U_2 be discs that satisfy $W_1 \subseteq U_1, W_2 \subseteq U_2$. Then

$$W_1 * W_2 \subseteq U_1 * U_2$$

holds for the operations $* \in \{+, -, \cdot, :\}$ defined above by (a)–(d).

(ii) Rectangular arithmetic deals with *complex intervals* instead of complex numbers. If

$$A = [a_1, a_2] = [x: a_1 \leq x \leq a_2]$$

denotes a real closed interval then the arithmetic operations with real intervals $A = [a_1, a_2]$ and $B = [b_1, b_2]$ are:

(a) $A \pm B = [a_1 \pm b_1, a_2 \pm b_2]$;
(b) $A \cdot B = [\min(a_1 b_1, a_1 b_2, a_2 b_1, a_2 b_2), \max(a_1 b_1, a_1 b_2, a_2 b_1, a_2 b_2)]$;
(c) $A : B = [a_1, a_2] \cdot [1/b_2, 1/b_1]$ for $0 \notin B$.

MOOR [1966] called (a)–(c) *exact interval arithmetic*. In computers the numbers are represented by a finite number of bits and to be sure that the computed interval contains the exact interval we must extend the computed interval, i.e. so called *rounded interval arithmetic* must be applied. More about *rounded interval arithmetic* and its computer realization can be found in ALEFELD and HERZBERGER [1983], YOHE [1977].

Let $A = [a_1, a_2], B = [b_1, b_2]$. The set

$$\Delta = \{a = a_1 + ia_2: a_1 \in A, a_2 \in B\}$$

of complex numbers is called a *complex interval*. Obviously Δ is a rectangle in the complex plane with sides parallel to the coordinate axes and the rectangle Δ can be written briefly in the form

$$\Delta = A + iB.$$

If $\Delta_1 = A_1 + iA_2$, $\Delta_2 = B_1 + iB_2$, the arithmetic operations of *rectangular arithmetic* are defined by

$$\Delta_1 \pm \Delta_2 = A_1 \pm B_1 + i(A_2 \pm iB_2),$$
$$\Delta_1 \cdot \Delta_2 = A_1 \cdot B_1 - A_2 \cdot B_2 + i(A_1 \cdot B_2 \pm A_2 \cdot B_1),$$

$$\Delta_1 : \Delta_2 = \frac{A_1 \cdot B_1 + A_2 \cdot B_2}{B_1^2 + B_2^2} + i\frac{A_2 \cdot B_1 - A_1 \cdot B_2}{B_1^2 + B_2^2}, \quad \text{if } 0 \notin B_1^2 + B_2^2.$$

The division $\Delta_1 : \Delta_2$ defined above yields a complex interval that is much larger than the range $\{z_1/z_2 : z_1 \in \Delta, z_2 \in \Delta\}$. The definition of ROKNE and LANCASTER [1971]

$$\Delta_1 : \Delta_2 = \Delta_1 \cdot \frac{1}{\Delta_2},$$

where $1/\Delta_2 = \inf\{C_1 + iC_2 : \{1/z : z \in \Delta_2\} \subseteq C_1 + iC_2\}$, gives a smaller rectangle but requires considerable computational effort.

Note that the intersection of two rectangles is again a rectangle, if the intersection is not empty.

The detailed investigation of the properties of rectangular and circular arithmetic are given in PETKOVIC [1989b].

Every method for numerical solution of the equation

$$f(x) \equiv x^n + a_1 x^{n-1} + a_{n-1} x + a_n = 0 \tag{23.1}$$

can be transformed into an interval version. For example, WANG and ZHENG [1984b] formulated the interval version of Weierstrass–Dochev method (18.2) for inclusion of zeros in the form:

$$W_i^{(k+1)} = x_i^{(k)} - f(x_i^{(k)}) \prod_{j \neq i}^{n} \frac{1}{x_i^{(k)} - W_j^{(k)}},$$

$$W_i^{(k)} = [x_i^{(k)}; r_i^{(k)}], \tag{23.2}$$

$$i = 1, 2, \ldots, n, \quad k = 0, 1, \ldots,$$

where $W_1^{(0)}, W_2^{(0)}, \ldots, W_n^{(0)}$ are isolated discs that contain the zeros of (23.1), $\xi_1, \xi_2, \ldots, \xi_n$ respectively, and let us mention that the slightly changed iteration formula (23.2)

$$W_i^{(k+1)} = x_i^{(k)} - \frac{f(x_i^{(k)})}{\prod_{j \neq i}^{n} \left(x_i^{(k)} - W_j^{(k)} \right)}, \quad i = 1, 2, \ldots, n, \quad k = 0, 1, \ldots, \tag{23.3}$$

gives almost the same numerical results. The difference between (23.2) and (23.3) is based on the fact that

$$\text{rad}\left(\frac{1}{W_1}\frac{1}{W_2}\right) \leqslant \text{rad}\left(\frac{1}{W_1 W_2}\right),$$

where rad W denotes the radius of the disc W.

Two Gauss–Seidel circular interval approaches of the Weierstrass–Dochev method (18.2)

$$W_i^{(k+1)} = x_i^{(k)} - f(x_i^{(k)}) \prod_{j<i} \frac{1}{x_i^{(k)} - W_j^{(k+1)}} \prod_{j>i} \frac{1}{x_i^{(k)} - W_j^{(k)}}, \tag{23.4}$$

$$W_i^{(k+1)} = x_i^{(k)} - f(x_i^{(k)}) \frac{1}{\prod_{j<i} x_i^{(k)} - W_j^{(k+1)} \prod_{j<i} x_i^{(k)} - W_j^{(k)}}, \quad (23.5)$$

are given in PETKOVIC [1989b] and ALEFELD and HERZBERGER [1983] respectively. Introducing the notations

$$\rho^{(k)} = \min_{1 \leq i,j \leq n, i \neq j} \min_{x \in W_j^{(k)}} |x - x_i^{(k)}|,$$

$$r^{(k)} = \max_{1 \leq i \leq n} r_i^{(k)}, \qquad \delta^{(k)} = \frac{r^{(k)}}{\rho^{(k)}},$$

the following theorem is true.

THEOREM 23.1 (WANG and ZHENG [1984b]). *Suppose that the initial discs* $W_1^{(0)}, \ldots, W_n^{(0)}$ *include the roots* $\xi_1, \ldots, \xi_n$ *of Eq.* (23.1) *respectively, and* $\delta^{(0)} \leq [3(n-1)]^{-1}$. *Then the sequences* $\{W_i^{(k)}\}_{k=0}^{\infty}$, $i = 1, 2, \ldots, n$ *produced by* (23.2) *satisfy* $\delta^{(k+1)} \leq 3(n-1) (\delta^{(k)})^2$, $k = 0, 1, \ldots$ *and contract to roots* $\xi_1, \ldots, \xi_n$ *of Eq.* (23.1) *respectively, i.e.*

$$\bigcap_{k=0}^{\infty} W_i^{(k)} = \xi_i, \quad i = 1, \ldots, n.$$

Similar to the (23.2) Nourein method (18.11) can be given in its circular interval version as

$$W_i^{(k+1)} = x_i^{(k)} - f(x_i^{(k)}) \prod_{j \neq i}^{n} \frac{1}{x_i^{(k)} - x_j^{(k)} + f(x_j^{(k)}) \prod_{s \neq j}^{n} \frac{1}{x_j^{(k)} - W_s^{(k)}}}, \quad (23.6)$$

$i = 1, 2, \ldots, n, \ k = 0, 1, \ldots$.

Under conditions similar to these in Theorem 23.1 the sequences $\{W_i^{(k)}\}_{k=0}^{\infty}$, $i = 1, 2, \ldots, n$, produced by (23.6) satisfy

$$r^{(k)} \leq C q^{3^k}, \quad k = 0, 1, \ldots$$

and contract to roots $\xi_1, \ldots, \xi_n$ of Eq. (23.1) respectively, i.e.

$$\bigcap_{k=0}^{\infty} W_i^{(k)} = \xi_i, \quad i = 1, \ldots, n.$$

A series of interval methods with accelerated order of convergence can be found in PETKOVIC [1989b].

As a numerical experiment let us consider the polynomial

$$f(z) = z^5 - (4+5i)z^4 + (6+20i)z^3 - (4+30i)z^2 + (15+20i)z + 75i \quad (23.7)$$

with zeros $\xi_{1,2} = 1 \pm 2i$, $\xi_3 = -1$, $\xi_4 = 3$, $\xi_5 = 5i$ (PETKOVIC [1989b]). Computer results with initial discs

$$W_1^{(0)} = [1.2 + 2.2i; 0.35], \qquad W_2^{(0)} = [0.8 - 2.2i; 0.35],$$
$$W_3^{(0)} = [-1.2 - 0.1i; 0.35], \qquad W_4^{(0)} = [1.2 + 2.2i; 0.35],$$
$$W_5^{(0)} = [1.2 + 2.2i; 0.35],$$

are:

(a) method (23.4)

$$W_1^{(3)} = [\ 1.000000036415\ldots + i2.000000007388895\ldots;$$
$$2.35\ldots 10^{-7}],$$
$$W_2^{(3)} = [\ 0.999999990517\ldots - i1.999999991647282\ldots;$$
$$5.59\ldots 10^{-8}],$$
$$W_3^{(3)} = [-1.000000000051\ldots - i2.06\ldots 10^{-10};$$
$$1.66\ldots 10^{-9}],$$
$$W_4^{(3)} = [\ 2.999999999998\ldots - i1.06\ldots 10^{-13};$$
$$1.20\ldots 10^{-11}],$$
$$W_5^{(3)} = [-6.46\ldots 10^{-15} + i5.000000000000001\ldots;$$
$$4.56\ldots 10^{-14}];$$

(b) method (23.5) gives slightly worse results

$$W_1^{(3)} = [\ 1.0000011175\ldots + i2.0000007006123\ldots;$$
$$4.63\ldots 10^{-6}],$$
$$W_2^{(3)} = [\ 0.9999998613\ldots - i1.9999997333866\ldots;$$
$$9.66\ldots 10^{-7}],$$
$$W_3^{(3)} = [-1.0000000036\ldots + i1.55\ldots 10^{-10};$$
$$3.65\ldots 10^{-8}],$$
$$W_4^{(3)} = [\ 2.9999999999\ldots + i5.20\ldots 10^{-11};$$
$$2.11\ldots 10^{-10}],$$
$$W_5^{(3)} = [-1.73\ldots 10^{-12} + i5.0000000000008\ldots;$$
$$7.45\ldots 10^{-12}].$$

Result 6.2 states that the roots of Eq. (23.1) are continuous functions of the coefficients $a_1, a_2, \ldots, a_n$. Quantitative estimation of this fact is given in Theorem 27.2. In this sense it is important to compute the discs that contain the zeros of

(23.1) if the coefficients $a_1, a_2, \ldots, a_n$ are not given exactly, i.e. it is known only that

$$a_1 \in A_1 = [\alpha_1; \beta_1], \quad a_2 \in A_2 = [\alpha_2; \beta_2], \ldots, \quad a_n \in A_n = [\alpha_n; \beta_n].$$

The Weierstrass–Dochev formula (18.2), except the interval versions (23.2), (23.3) can be written in the form

$$W_i^{(k+1)} = x_i^{(k)} - \left[\sum_{s=0}^{n} A_s \left(x_i^{(k)}\right)^{n-s}\right] \prod_{j \neq i}^{n} \frac{1}{x_i^{(k)} - W_j^{(k)}}, \qquad (23.8)$$
$$A_0 = [1;0], \quad i = 1, 2, \ldots, n, \quad k = 0, 1, \ldots .$$

Let us compare numerical experiments for root determining of the equation (23.7) applying methods (23.2) and (23.8). We start from the discs

$$W_1^{(0)} = [1.2 + 2.2i; 0.42], \qquad W_2^{(0)} = [0.8 - 2.3i; 0.42],$$
$$W_3^{(0)} = [-1.2 - 0.1i; 0.42], \qquad W_4^{(0)} = [2.8 + 0.1i; 0.42],$$
$$W_5^{(0)} = [0.2 + 4.9i; 0.42] :$$

(a) using the double precision arithmetic Weierstrass–Dochev method (23.2) gives on the fifth iteration the following discs

$$W_1^{(5)} = [\ 0.10000000000000\ldots 10^1 + i0.20000000000000\ldots 10^1;$$
$$0.2 \ldots 10^{-27}],$$
$$W_2^{(5)} = [\ 0.10000000000000\ldots 10^1 - i0.20000000000000\ldots 10^1;$$
$$0.4 \ldots 10^{-28}],$$
$$W_3^{(5)} = [\ -0.10000000000000\ldots 10^1 + i0.85179086418887\ldots 10^{-17};$$
$$0.6 \ldots 10^{-28}],$$
$$W_4^{(5)} = [\ 0.30000000000000\ldots 10^1 + i0.14793331544085\ldots 10^{-15};$$
$$0.3 \ldots 10^{-27}],$$
$$W_5^{(5)} = [\ -0.13425705666354\ldots 10^{-15} + i0.50000000000000\ldots 10^1;$$
$$0.1 \ldots 10^{-28}];$$

(b) method (23.8) with the following discs as coefficients

$$A_0 = [1; 0.0], \qquad A_1 = [-4 - 5i; 0.0001],$$
$$A_2 = [6 + 20i; 0.0001], \qquad A_3 = [-4 - 30i; 0.0001],$$
$$A_4 = [-15 + 20i; 0.0001], \qquad A_5 = [75i; 0.0001]$$

produces after four iterations the following discs

$$W_1^{(4)} = [\ 0.10000000003111\ldots 10^1 + i0.20000000001308\ldots 10^1;$$
$$0.438 \ldots 10^{-4}],$$
$$W_2^{(4)} = [\ 0.10000000006745\ldots 10^1 - i0.20000000000247\ldots 10^1;$$

$$0.196\ldots 10^{-4}],$$
$$W_3^{(4)} = [\ -0.10000000007468\ldots 10^1 - i0.17831245267697\ldots 10^{-15};$$
$$0.306\ldots 10^{-5}],$$
$$W_4^{(4)} = [\ 0.30000000000000\ldots 10^1 + i0.11505177715895\ldots 10^{-14};$$
$$0.648\ldots 10^{-4}],$$
$$W_5^{(4)} = [\ 0.52800545711190\ldots 10^{-16} + i0.50000000000000\ldots 10^1;$$
$$0.117\ldots 10^{-3}].$$

The next iterations do not contract the discs $\{W_i^{(k)}\}_{i=1}^n$, $k = 5, 6, \ldots$. Numerical experiments show stability of considered methods. For practical goals the conditions for the initial discs $\{W_i^{(0)}\}_{i=1}^n$ in Theorem 23.1 are not nessessery. For example, applying method (23.2) to the equation (23.7) with 'rough' initial discs

$$W_1^{(0)} = [1.2 + 2.2i; 101.42], \qquad W_2^{(0)} = [0.8 - 2.3i; 102.42],$$
$$W_3^{(0)} = [-1.2 - 0.1i; 103.42], \qquad W_4^{(0)} = [2.8 + 0.1i; 104.42],$$
$$W_5^{(0)} = [0.2 + 4.9i; 105.42],$$

after six iterations we have

$$W_1^{(6)} = [\ 0.10000000003111\ldots 10^1 + i0.20000000001308\ldots;$$
$$0.119\ldots 10^{-34}],$$
$$W_2^{(6)} = [\ 0.10000000006745\ldots 10^1 - i0.20000000000247\ldots 10^1;$$
$$0.198\ldots 10^{-34}],$$
$$W_3^{(6)} = [\ -0.10000000007468\ldots 10^1 - i0.20682405682722\ldots 10^{-16};$$
$$0.753\ldots 10^{-35}],$$
$$W_4^{(6)} = [\ 0.30000000000000\ldots 10^1 - i0.60893527797136\ldots 10^{-16};$$
$$0.148\ldots 10^{-34}],$$
$$W_5^{(6)} = [\ 0.11112781396401\ldots 10^{-15} + i0.50000000000000\ldots 10^1;$$
$$0.911\ldots 10^{-36}].$$

In the case when Eq. (23.1) has only real zeros, it is convenient to consider two-sided methods. The methods (18.2), (19.3), (18.11) are modified and their interval versions approximate the zeros of the polynomial from both sides. For details see ANDREEV and KJURKCHIEV [1987], MARKOV and KJURKCHIEV [1989].

CHAPTER V

Computational Complexity (Renegar and Neff Approach)

In this chapter we consider the computational complexity of polynomial root determining. The recent results of RENEGAR [1987] and NEFF [1990] are presented for the upper and lower bound of the number of arithmetic operations for approximating zeros with prescribed accuracy. PAN [1992] gives a useful detailed review about complexity of operations with polynomials (including root determining) in sequential and parallel case.

24. Definitions and notation

We use the notation $|z|$ for the usual norm of a complex number z, while $\|z\|$ is the number of digits required to represent the 'fractional part' of z using binary notation. That is, if β is a rational number of the form $a/2^m$, where a and $m \geqslant 0$ are integers, and a is odd, then $\|\beta\| = m$. If β is real and not of this form, then $\|\beta\| = \infty$; and for complex z, $\|z\| = \max\{\|\mathcal{R}(z)\|, \|\mathcal{I}(z)\|\}$.

Unless specifically stated otherwise, all logarithms are base 2.

Let $p(z) = a_n z^n + \cdots + a_0$ be a polynomial with complex coefficients. Define

$$\|p\| = \max_{0 \leqslant j \leqslant n} \|a_j\|, \qquad |p|_\infty = \max_{0 \leqslant j \leqslant n} |a_j|,$$

$$|p|_\alpha = \left(\sum_{j=0}^n |a_j|^\alpha\right)^{1/\alpha}, \quad \text{for every real } \alpha \geqslant 1.$$

If $p(z)$ is a polynomial of degree $n \geqslant 2$ and has roots $r_1, \ldots, r_n$, then the minimal root separation of p and the root radius of p are defined respectively by

$$\Delta(p) = \min_{j \neq k} |r_j - r_k|, \qquad \rho(p) = \max_{1 \leqslant j \leqslant n} |r_j|.$$

If z is a point in the complex plane, then

$$\Delta(z, p) = \min_{1 \leqslant j \leqslant n} |z - r_j|$$

is the distance from z to the set of roots of p. It is also convenient to define

$$\bar{\Delta}(p) = \min_{r_j \neq r_k} |r_j - r_k|$$

and call this the minimum distinct root separation of p. Notice that if p has multiple roots then $\Delta(p) = 0$, but that $\bar{\Delta}(p)$ is never equal to 0.

Suppose $q(z)$ is of degree k with roots $s_1, \ldots, s_k$. Define the root distance between polynomials p and q by

$$\Delta(p,q) = \begin{cases} \min_\sigma \left(\max_{1 \leq j \leq k} |s_j - r_{\sigma(j)}|\right), & \text{if } k < n, \\ \Delta(q,p), & \text{if } k > n, \end{cases}$$

where the minimum is taken over all permutations $\sigma = (\sigma(1), \sigma(2), \ldots, \sigma(n))$ of the integers $1, 2, \ldots, n$. Intuitively, $\Delta(p,q)$ is the furthest any root of the 'corresponding' root of q.

Let P_m^n denote the class of all polynomials $p(z)$ with integer coefficients, that satisfy $|p|_\infty \leq 2^m$ and $\deg p = n$.

Let MP_m^n denote the class of all monic polynomials $p(z)$ such that $|p|_\infty \leq 2^m$ and $\deg p = n$; and let $\mathrm{MP}_{M,m}^n$ denote the subclass of polynomials $p(z) \in \mathrm{MP}_m^n$ whose coefficients are rational and $\|p\| \leq M$. Given an n-degree polynomial $p(z)$, a μ-digit approximation to the roots of p is a set of complex numbers $r_1, r_2, \ldots, r_n$ such that, for all $1 \leq j \leq n$,

$$|r_j - \lambda_j| < 2^{-\mu},$$

where $\lambda_1, \lambda_2, \ldots, \lambda_n$ are the (unknown) roots of $p(z)$. We also require that r_j is real whenever λ_j is real.

25. The lower bound (Renegar approach)

In proving the lower bound, we consider all algorithms that can be modelled as a rooted tree (i.e. connected graph with no cycles and an end node specified as a root), with two types of nodes, arithmetic and branch nodes. Arithmetic nodes have at most one incoming edge and at most one outgoing edge. Branch nodes have at most one incoming edge and two outgoing edges. The algorithm is initiated at the root of the tree, the inputs being the coefficients, indexed in some manner, of the arbitrary polynomial $f \in \mathrm{MP}_m^n$, for which a zero is to be approximated within distance $2^{-\mu}$. (The parameter μ is assumed fixed; an algorithm need only handle the given μ).

At each arithmetic node encountered as the algorithm attempts to approximate a zero of f, a computational procedure specific to that node is carried out, the procedure involving numbers computed at previously encountered arithmetic nodes and/or the coefficients of f. At each branch node encountered as the algorithm attempts to approximate a zero of f, a decision (determinated by f) is made as to which of the two outgoing edges will be followed, i.e. a decision as to which computational procedures (arithmetic nodes) will be followed. Thus, for each $f \in \mathrm{MP}_m^n$, the algorithm follows a path, determinated by f, through the tree. We assume that the final node, i.e. leaf, in the path is an arithmetic node, and the number computed at that node is the desired $2^{-\mu}$-approximation to a zero of f. (In the case of approximating all zeros, it seems that a natural ploy to use would be to have n indices associated with the leaf, these indices indicating arithmetic nodes in the path where the numbers computed at those nodes are $2^{-\mu}$-approximations to the zeros of f. Such a tree could be easily altered to fit the single zero approximation framework.)

Now we describe the computational procedures allowed at arithmetic nodes. Each arithmetic node A is assigned one of the four operations $+, -, \cdot,$ div or the conjugation operation $z \mapsto \bar{z}$. If A is assigned $+, -, \cdot,$ div, respectively, then A is also assigned a pair (α, i) or a pair (i, j) where $\alpha \in \mathbb{C}$ and i (respectively j) is an index indicating either a preceding arithmetic node or an input coefficient. If assigned a pair (α, i), then the computational procedure to be carried out at A is $+, -, \cdot,$ div, respectively, on α and the number computed at the node indicated by i, or on α and the input coefficient indicated by i. (This is scalar arithmetic.) If assigned a pair (i, j), then $+, -, \cdot,$ div, respectively, is to be carried out on the number, computed at the node, or the coefficient, indicated by i and the number computed at the node, or the coefficient, indicated by j. (This is non-scalar arithmetic.)

Finally, if A is assigned the conjugate operation, then it is also assigned an index i. The operation to be carried out at A is then conjugation of the number computed at the preceding arithmetic node indicated by i, or conjugation of the input coefficient indicated by i.

Next we discuss restrictions on the decision-making procedures that occur at branch nodes. Any deterministic (i.e. determined by the input coefficients) decision-making procedure for deciding which of the two outgoing edges from a branch node will be followed can be represented by a function $G : \mathbb{C}^{n+1} \to \{0, 1\}$ representing some decision making procedure, and no restrictions are placed on G.

Now we discuss the cost of an algorithm fitting our model. For each $f \in \mathrm{MP}_m^n$, define the cost $C(f)$ of the algorithm in approximating a zero of f as the number of non-scalar arithmetic nodes involving multiplication and division encountered by the algorithm when applied to f, plus the number of branch nodes encountered by the algorithm when applied to f. The (worst case) cost of the algorithm is defined as $\sup_{f \in \mathrm{MP}_m^n} C(f)$.

THEOREM 25.1. *The cost of any algorithm (fitting our model) for obtaining a $2^{-\mu}$-approximation to a single zero of arbitrary $f \in \mathrm{MP}_m^n$ is at least $\Omega(\log(m + \mu)) - O(\log n)$, where $f(n) = \Omega g(n) \Leftrightarrow g(n) = O(f(n))$.*

REMARK 25.1. With a more complicated proof, the occurrence of $-O(\log n)$ can be eliminated.

PROOF. We prove that the stated lower bound is actually a lower bound for the simpler problem of approximating a single zero of an arbitrary polynomial of the form $z^n - s$, where $0 \leqslant s \leqslant m$. Thus, assume we have an algorithm fitting our model, but which need only be able to handle polynomials of this special form.

To each leaf of the tree which models the algorithm, is associated a rational function $p(z)/q(z)$. For any $s, p(z)/q(z)$ equals the number computed at the leaf if the sequence of computations (arithmetic nodes) corresponding to the path from the root to that leaf is carried out on the polynomial $z^n - s, s \in \mathbb{R}$. (Here, we have used the fact that s is a real number so that $\bar{s} = s$.) In particular, if the algorithm applied to $z^n - s$ terminates at that leaf, then there exists an nth root of s, say x ($x^n = s$), such that

$$\left|\frac{p(z)}{q(z)} - x\right| \leq \varepsilon, \quad \text{i.e.} \quad \left|\frac{p(x^n)}{q(x^n)} - x\right| \leq \varepsilon.$$

We may assume that for each leaf of the tree, the path from the root to that leaf is followed when the algorithm is applied to some polynomial $z^n - s$, since eliminating unused paths still gives an algorithm for the problem. Letting $C_A(s)$ denote the number of non-scalar arithmetic nodes involving multiplication and division encountered by the algorithm when applied to $z^n - s$, and defining $C_A = \max_{0 \leq s \leq m} C_A(s)$, it follows that rational function $p(z)/q(z)$ associated with a leaf satisfies

$$\deg p \leq 2^{C_A}, \quad \deg q \leq 2^{C_A}.$$

Defining C_B similarly with respect to branch nodes, it also follows that the number λ of leaves satisfies $\lambda \leq 2^{C_B}$.

Note that every zero ξ of the polynomial $z^n - s$ satisfies $|\xi| \leq 2^{m/n}$. Let p and q (q not identically zero) be any complex polynomials of degree not exceeding N, and let L be any line segment contained in $\{x : |x| \leq 2^{m/n}\}$. Define

$$l_m(p, q, L) = \text{length}\left\{x \in L : \left|\frac{p(x^n)}{q(x^n)} - x\right| \leq 2^{-\mu}\right\}$$

(length should of course be interpreted as the summation of lengths). We show that

$$l_\mu(p, q, L) \leq 2(Nn + 1)^3 2^{(Nm-\mu)/(Nn+1)} \tag{25.1}$$

unless

$$2^{m/n+\mu} < (Nn + 1)^{Nn+2}. \tag{25.2}$$

In particular, defining

$$L_j = \left\{re^{2\pi ij/n} : 0 \leq r \leq 2^{m/n}\right\}, \quad j = 0, 1, \ldots, n-1, \ i^2 = -1,$$

and assuming that $p(z)/q(z)$ is the rational function associated with some leaf (hence $N \leq 2^{C_A}$) and that

$$2^{m/n} \geq \left(2^{C_A} n + 1\right)^{2^{C_A} n + 2},$$

it follows that the set

$$\left\{x : x \in \bigcup_j L_j, \left|\frac{p(x^n)}{q(x^n)} - x\right| < 2^{-\mu}\right\},$$

is contained in a union of subintervals of $\bigcup_j L_j$, the summation of the lengths of which does not exceed

$$\sum_j l_\mu(p, q, L_j) \leqslant 2n \left(2^{C_A} n + 1\right)^3 2^{m/n} 2^{-(m/n+\mu)/(2^{C_A} n+1)}.$$

Since for each $0 \leqslant r \leqslant 2^{m/n}$ there exists some $j \in \{1, 2, \ldots, n-1\}$ such that the algorithm applied to $z^n - s$, $s = r^n$, results in a $2^{-\mu}$-approximation to $x = re^{2\pi i j/n}$, $i^2 = -1$, and since the number λ of leaves satisfies $\lambda \leqslant 2^{C_B}$, it follows that we must have

$$2^{C_B} 2n \left(2^{C_A} n + 1\right)^3 2^{m/n} 2^{-(m/n+\mu)/(2^{C_A} n+1)} \geqslant 2^{m/n}$$

unless

$$2^{m/n+\mu} < \left(2^{C_A} n + 1\right)^{2^{C_A} n+2}.$$

From this, the statement of the theorem is easily deduced.

Now we will show that for an arbitrary polynomial h of degree $E \geqslant 2$ and a real number $\varepsilon \leqslant 1/E^{E+1}$

$$\text{length}\{x \in L \colon |h(x)| \leqslant E|h|_\infty \varepsilon\} \leqslant 2E^3 \varepsilon^{1/E} \tag{25.3}$$

for every line segment L contained in $\{x \colon |x| \leqslant 1\}$. In proving (25.3) we may assume that h is monic.

Let $\xi_1, \ldots, \xi_E$ denote the zeros of h, counting multiplicities. Using the expressions for the coefficients of h as symmetric functions in the zeros of h, it is easily seen that for some subset $T \subseteq \{1, \ldots, E\}$, where $k = \#T$, $\#T$ is the number of elements in T, we have

$$|h|_\infty \leqslant \binom{E}{k} \prod_{i \in T} |\xi_i| \leqslant E^{E-k} \prod_{i \in T} |\xi_i|. \tag{25.4}$$

Let $T' = \{i \in T \colon |\xi_i| \geqslant 2\}$ and $k' = \#T'$. From (25.4), it is easily deduced that

$$|h|_\infty \leqslant E^{E-k} 2^{k-k'} \prod_{i \in T} |\xi_i| \leqslant E^{E-k'} \prod_{i \in T} |\xi_i|.$$

Since, for $|x| \leqslant 1$, we have

$$\left| \prod_{i \in T'} (x - \xi_i) \right| \geqslant \left(\tfrac{1}{2}\right)^{k'} \prod_{i \in T'} |\xi_i|,$$

it follows that $|x| \leqslant 1$ satisfies $|h(x)| \leqslant E|h|_\infty \varepsilon$ only if

$$\left| \prod_{i \notin T'} (x - \xi_i) \right| \leqslant E^{E-k'+1} 2^{k'} \varepsilon \leqslant E^{E+1} \varepsilon \leqslant E^{E+1} \varepsilon.$$

Hence, assuming $\varepsilon \leqslant 1/E^{E+1}$, we have that $|x| \leqslant 1$ satisfies $|h(x)| \leqslant E|h|_\infty \varepsilon$ only if x is within distance $(E^{E+1}\varepsilon)^{1/E} \leqslant E^2 \varepsilon^{1/E}$ of a zero of h. The inequality (25.3) follows.

TABLE 26.1. Lower and upper bounds of arithmetic operations for polynomial root determination.

Computing with	Order of sequential time		Order of parallel upper bound	
error $< 2^{-b}$	Lower bound	Upper bound	Time	Processors
One zero of a polynomial	$n + \log b$ RENEGAR [1987]	$n \log n \log b$ PAN [1987]	$\log^2 n \log(bn)$	$n \log b / [\log n \log(bn)]$ PAN [1987]
All zeros of a polynomial	$n + \log b$ RENEGAR [1987]	$n^2 \log b \log n$ PAN [1987]	$n \log n \log(bn)$ $\log^3(nb)$	$n \log b / \log(bn)$ PAN [1987] $(bn)^{O(1)}$ NEFF [1990]

Finally, we prove (25.1) and (25.2). Note that (25.1) is trivial if p and q are both constants since then $l_\mu(p,q,L) \leqslant 2 \min \{2^{-\mu}, 2^m\}$.

Let $\tilde{L}$ be the line segment $\tilde{L} = \{x/2^{m/n} : x \in L\}$ and let $\tilde{p}(z), \tilde{q}(z)$ be the polynomials $\tilde{p}(z) = p(2^{m/n} z), \tilde{q}(z) = 2^{m/n} q(2^{m/n} z)$. Then the inequality (25.1) is valid if and only if

$$\text{length} \left\{ x \in L : \left| \frac{\tilde{p}(x^n)}{\tilde{q}(x^n)} - x \right| \leqslant 2^{-\mu - m/n} \right\} \leqslant 2(Nn+1)^3 2^{-\mu/(Nn+1)}.$$

Consequently, in proving (25.1) we may assume that $m = 0$.

Let $h(z) = p(z^n) - zq(z^n)$. Because $n \geqslant 2, p$ and q are not both constants and $\deg p \leqslant N, \deg q \leqslant N$, the degree of the polynomial h satisfies $2 \leqslant \deg h \leqslant Nn+1$. Also, it is easily seen that for all $|x| \leqslant 1$, we have $|q(x^n)| \leqslant |h|_\infty (\deg q + 1)$. Consequently, applying (25.3) to $h, \varepsilon = 2^{-\mu}$ and $E \leqslant Nn+1$, the inequality (25.2) (for $m = 0$) follows. This completes the proof of the theorem. □

26. Algorithm for the upper bound (Neff approach)

In his review paper PAN [1992] summarized known results for lower and upper bounds of the number of arithmetic operations for approximating the roots of a polynomial of degree at most n with error less then 2^{-b}. Table 26.1 presents the sequential and parallel case. In the rest of the paper we concentrate on NEFF's [1990] estimation in Table 26.1. More in details, we show that there are positive constants C, D, α, β, such that, for any choice of integers n, m, μ, and a polynomial $p(z) \in P_m^n$, we can compute a μ-digit approximation to the roots of p in at most $C \log^\alpha(n + m + \mu)$ parallel steps, using at most $D(n + m + \mu)^\beta$ processors (NC polynomial root isolation).

Section 26 Computational complexity (Renegar and Neff approach)

We make the assumption that $2^{-\mu} \leqslant \frac{1}{4}\bar{\Delta}(p)$. Geometrically, this means that the precision specified in the input to the algorithm is fine enough so that the output will distinguish between all the distinct roots of p. This assumption is not essential to prove the results that follow, but it does simplify their justification.

We focus our attention on constructing what we call the basic algorithm, whose goal is only to approximate the real roots of the polynomial $p(z)$, rather than all the roots. While this may seem like a much less ambitious goal, it is in fact where most of the work lies, since the general problem can, by use of elementary computations, be reduced to a problem that is solvable by our basic algorithm.

The following is a broad outline of the basic algorithm for fixed n, m, μ.

ALGORITHM 26.1.

Input: A polynomial $p(z) \in P_m^n$.
Output: Rational numbers $p_1, \ldots, p_k$ ($k \leqslant n$) such that, for all $1 \leqslant j \leqslant k, |p_j - r_j| < 2^{-\mu}$, where $r_1, \ldots, r_k$ are the distinct, real roots of $p(z)$.

Step 26.1.1. Compute $\bar{p}(z) = p(z)/\mathrm{GCD}(p(z), p'(z))$, and set $m' = n + m$, where $\mathrm{GCD}(p, p')$ is the greatest common divisor of p and p'. Then $\bar{p}(z) \in P_{m'}^{n'}$ for some $n' \leqslant n$ (see Corollary 27.3). Moreover, $\bar{p}$ has the same distinct roots as p, but no multiple roots.

Step 26.1.2. Let $\bar{a}_{n'}$ be the leading coefficient of $\bar{p}$ and set $\bar{q}(z) := (1/a_{n'})\bar{p}(z)$. Compute $q(z) \in \mathrm{MP}_{M,m'}^{n'}$, where:

(a) $M = M(n', m', \mu)$ is a global constant for the entire computation which is given in detail later;

(b) $|q - \bar{q}|_\infty < 2^{-M}$.

Step 26.1.3. Set $k := \deg q$. If $k = 0$, then terminate this branch of the computation and return no value. If $k = 1$, then $q(z) = z + b_0$, so terminate and return the value $-b_0$.

Step 26.1.4. Compute relatively prime, monic polynomials $q_1(z)$ and $q_2(z)$, each having distinct roots, which are 'good' approximations to factors of $q(z)$. More precisely:

(a) There are (real) polynomials $\omega_1(z), \omega_2(z)$, and $w(z)$ such that

$$w(z), \quad q(z) = \omega_1(z)\omega_2(z)w(z),$$

has no real roots, and

$$|q_1 - \omega_1|_\infty < 2^{-M}, \quad |q_2 - \omega_2|_\infty < 2^{-M}.$$

(b) $q_1 \in \mathrm{MP}_{M,m'}^{\deg q_1}$ and $q_2 \in \mathrm{MP}_{M,m'}^{\deg q_2}$;

(c) $\max\{\deg q_1, \deg q_2\} \leqslant \lambda k$, where $\frac{5}{6} \leqslant \lambda < 1$ is a fixed positive constant that does not depend on any of the parameters n, m, μ (for example, $\lambda = \frac{23}{24}$ will work).

Step 26.1.5. Split the computation into two parallel branches. For one branch, set $q := q_1$ and return to Step 26.1.3; for the other branch, set $q := q_2$ and also return to Step 26.1.3.

As with most algorithms dealing with polynomials, the first Step 26.1.1 is to remove multiple factors. Several NC methods for doing this are already known. Obviously, Step 26.1.2 can also be done in parallel. For later reference, let both Steps 26.1.1 and 26.1.2 can be performed in time at most

$$C_0 \log^{\alpha_0}(n + m + M)$$

using at most

$$D_0(n + m + M)^{\beta_0}$$

processors.

Now, in order to better understand the global nature of Algorithm 26.1, let us call each pass through the Steps 26.1.3, 26.1.4 and 26.1.5, an S-node of the computation. It is clear from Step 26.1.4(c) that the number of S-nodes in any one branch of the algorithm is at most $-\log n'/\log \lambda$. If $F(k, M)$ is an upper bound for the parallel computation time of one S-node on a polynomial $q \in \mathrm{MP}^k_{M,m'}$, then the total parallel time $F(A)$ for Algorithm 26.1 is clearly bounded above by

$$F(A) < C_0 \log^{\alpha_0}(n + m + M) + F(n', M) + F(\lambda n', M) + \cdots + F(1, M). \tag{26.1}$$

In the following sections, it is shown that $F(k, M) \leq C_1 \log^{\alpha_1}(k + M)$ so that (26.1) becomes

$$F(A) < C_0 \log^{\alpha_0}(n + m + M) - C_1 \log n \log^{\alpha_1}(n + M)/\log \lambda.$$

Suppose also that $P(k, M)$ is an upper bound for the number of processors needed to compute one S-node on a polynomial $q \in \mathrm{MP}^k_{M,m'}$. If we can show that $P(k, M) \leq D_1(k+M)^{\beta_1}$, then an upper bound for the number of processors $P(A)$ needed in Algorithm 26.1 is given by

$$P(A) \leq \max\{D_0(n + m + M)^{\beta_0}, D_1 n(n + M)^{\beta_1}\}.$$

27. Approximate factorization

The following basic theorems are essential to the analysis in the remainder of the paper. As before let $p(z) = \sum_{j=0}^{n} a_j z^j$ be a polynomial of degree n.

LEMMA 27.1. $\rho(p) \leq |p|_\infty/|a_n|$.

An easy application of Minkowski's inequality gives the following.

LEMMA 27.2. *For all $1 \leqslant \gamma \leqslant \infty$ and polynomials p, q*

$$|pq| \leqslant |p|_\gamma |q|_1.$$

THEOREM 27.1. *If $p \in P_m^n, n \geqslant 2$ and p has no multiple roots, then*

$$\Delta(p) \geqslant \sqrt{3} n^{-(n+2)/2} |p|_1^{-(n-1)}.$$

COROLLARY 27.1. *For all $p \in P_m^n$*

$$\Delta(p) > 2^{-(n-1)m - (3/2n+1)\log n}.$$

THEOREM 27.2 ((OSTROWSKI [1966])). *Suppose $p(z) = z^n + a_{n-1} z^{n-1} + \cdots + a_0$ and $q(z) = z^n + b_{n-1} z^{n-1} + \cdots + b_0$ are monic polynomials of degree n. Let*

$$\gamma = 2 \max_{0 \leqslant j \leqslant n-1} \left\{ (\max\{|a_j|, |b_j|\})^{1/(n-j)} \right\}$$

and define $\delta \geqslant 0$ by $\delta^n = \sum_{j=0}^{n-1} |b_j - a_j| \gamma^j$. Then $\Delta(p,q) < 2n\delta$.

COROLLARY 27.2. *If p and q are monic polynomials of degree n, $|p|_\infty \leqslant 2^m - 1$, and $|p - q|_\infty \leqslant 2^{-k}$ for some $k > 0$, then*

$$\Delta(p, q) < 2^{m + \log n + 2 - k/n}.$$

THEOREM 27.3. *Suppose $p(z) = z^n + a_{n-1} z^{n-1} + \cdots + a_0$ is a monic (complex) polynomial and that $v(z) = z^k + v_{k-1} z^{k-1} + \cdots + v_0$ is a monic (complex) factor of $p(z)$ of degree k. That is, $p(z) = v(z) u(z)$, where $u(z)$ is a monic polynomial with complex coefficients. Then*

$$|v_j| \leqslant \binom{k-l}{j} |p|_2 + \binom{k-l}{j-l} \tag{27.1}$$

for all $1 \leqslant j \leqslant k-1$. Moreover, if we adopt the convention that

$$\binom{k-l}{-l} = \binom{k-l}{k} = 0,$$

then (27.1) remains true for $j = 0$ and $j = k$.

We can use a refinement of Stirling's formula to show that for all integers $0 \leqslant j \leqslant k, \binom{k}{j} \leqslant 2^k \sqrt{k+1}$. As a result, we have the following.

COROLLARY 27.3. *Suppose that $p(z)$ is a monic polynomial of degree n, and $v(z)$ is a monic polynomial factor of p of degree less than n. Then*

$$|v|_\infty < 2^n |p|_\infty.$$

Now, by combining these results, and using repeated applications of the triangle inequality, we prove the following.

THEOREM 27.4. *Suppose that p is a monic polynomial of degree n. Let m and M be real constants such that $|p|_\infty \leqslant 2^m - 1$, and $M > \log n$ and let $p_0, p_1, \ldots, p_{n-1}$ be a sequence of monic polynomials which satisfy the following conditions:*

$$|p - p_0|_\infty \leqslant 2^{-M}$$

and for each $0 \leqslant j \leqslant n-2$ there are monic polynomials $p_{j1}, p_{j2}, q_{j1}, q_{j2}$, and w_j, such that

$$p_j(z) = p_{j1}(z)q_{j1}(z)w_j(z),$$
$$p_{j+1}(z) = p_{j2}(z)q_{j2}(z)w_j(z),$$
$$\max\{|p_{j2} - p_{j1}|_\infty, |q_{j2} - q_{j1}|_\infty\} \leqslant 2^{-M}.$$

Then

$$|p - p_j|_\infty < 2^{-M} + 2^{2n+2m+\log n - M}$$

for all $1 \leqslant j \leqslant n-1$.

COROLLARY 27.4. *With the notation as in Theorem* 27.4, *if*

$$M \geqslant n(\mu + m + \log n + 4) + 2m + \log n + 1, \tag{27.2}$$

then $\Delta(p, p_j) \leqslant 2^{-\mu}$ *for all* $1 \leqslant j \leqslant n-1$.

The point of Corollary 27.4 is that if we take M in Step 26.1.2(a) to be the smallest integer greater than or equal to the quantity on the right in (27.2), then the rational numbers p_l available at the end of the Algorithm 26.1, will be within $2^{-\mu}$ of some root of p. Because of the condition in Step 26.1.4 that $w(z)$ has no real roots, it is easy to see that all of the real roots of p are approximated within $2^{-\mu}$ by some p_l. Thus, we know how accurately we must compute the approximate factors q_1 and q_2 in Step 26.1.4, so we are left with the problem of finding a fast parallel method for performing this computation.

28. q-Splittings of the complex plane

Approximating the factors $\omega_1(z)$ and $\omega_2(z)$ to the required accuracy, as discussed in the previous section, only assures that the values computed in the Algorithm 26.1 are accurate to the specified precision, $2^{-\mu}$. The key to making the algorithm run in polylog time however is condition 26.1.4(c). For example, we could easily use standard techniques to split the polynomial $q(z)$ of degree k into approximate factors $q_1(z)$ of degree 1 and $q_2(z)$ of degree $k-1$, but this would require n sequential passes through Steps 26.1.3, 26.1.4, and 26.1.5, which would ruin any hope of bounding the time complexity of the whole procedure by a power of $\log n$.

We begin with some notation. Let ζ be a complex number and $0 \leqslant \gamma < \infty$ be real and non-negative. The complex plane is partitioned into four disjoint open sectors, and their boundaries are given by

$$T_1(\zeta, \gamma) = \{z: -\gamma \mathcal{R}(z - \zeta) < \mathcal{I}(z - \zeta) < \gamma \mathcal{R}(z - \zeta)\},$$
$$T_{-1}(\zeta, \gamma) = \{z: \gamma \mathcal{R}(z - \zeta) < \mathcal{I}(z - \zeta) < -\gamma \mathcal{R}(z - \zeta)\},$$
$$T_i(\zeta, \gamma) = \{z: -\mathcal{I}(z - \zeta) < \gamma \mathcal{R}(z - \zeta) < \mathcal{I}(z - \zeta)\},$$
$$T_{-i}(\zeta, \gamma) = \{z: \mathcal{I}(z - \zeta) < \gamma \mathcal{R}(z - \zeta) < -\mathcal{I}(z - \zeta)\}.$$

Notice that for $\gamma = 0$, $T_1(\zeta, \gamma) = T_{-1}(\zeta, \gamma) = \emptyset$, and $T_i(\zeta, \gamma)$ and $T_{-i}(\zeta, \gamma)$ are the upper and lower half planes $\mathcal{I}(z) > \mathcal{I}(\zeta)$ and $\mathcal{I}(z) < \mathcal{I}(\zeta)$, respectively.

The solution of our problem is intimately tied to the computation of certain polynomial quotient and remainder sequences which are now discussed. Fast parallel methods for computing these polynomial sequences are already known, so, although we use them repeatedly in the construction of Algorithm 26.1, we do not discuss a specific method for computing them.

Let $s = (a_1, a_2, \ldots, a_l)$ be a sequence with real numbers. Denote by $V(s) = V(a_1, \ldots, a_l)$ the number of sign changes in s. A sign change is counted for each pair $j < k$ such that $a_j a_k < 0$, and $a_\nu = 0$ for all $j < \nu < k$.

Let $u(x)$ and $v(x)$ be polynomials with real coefficients. If $\deg u \geq \deg v$, let $t_0(x) = u(x), t_1(x) = v(x), t_2(x), \ldots, t_l(x)$ be the negative polynomial remainder sequence for the pair $u(x), v(x)$. That is, $t_{j-1}(x) = c_j(x) t_j(x) - t_{j+1}(x)$, where c_j is a polynomial, $\deg t_{j+1} < \deg t_j$, and $t_{l+1} = 0$. For each real number a, we set

$$V(u, v; a) = V(t_0(a), \ldots, t_l(a)).$$

If $\deg u < \deg v$, then write $v(x) = c(x) u(x) + v_1(x)$ where $\deg v_1 < \deg u$ and define $V(u, v; a) = V(u, v_1; a)$.

Sturm's Theorem 5.8 takes the following form.

THEOREM 28.1. *Let $u(x)$ be a polynomial with real coefficients and no multiple roots and let $[a, b]$ be an interval on the real line. If $u(a)u(b) \neq 0$, then the number of roots of u in the open interval (a, b) is equal to $V(u, u'; a) - V(u, u'; b)$.*

COROLLARY 28.1. *Let $u(x)$ and $v(x)$ be polynomials with real coefficients, neither of which has multiple roots. If*

$$u(a)u(b)v(a)v(b) \neq 0,$$

then the number of roots common to both u and v in the open interval (a, b) is exactly $V(w, w'; b) - V(w, w', a)$, where $w(x) = \text{GCD}(u, v)$.

If $z_0 \neq z_1$ are two complex numbers, let $\sigma(z_0, z_1; z)$ be the linear polynomial $z_0(1 - z) + z_1 z$.

If $q(z) = \sum_{j=0}^{k} \eta_j z^j$ is a polynomial, set $Rq(z) = \sum_{j=0}^{k} \mathcal{R}(\eta_j) z^j$ and $Iq(z) = \sum_{j=0}^{k} \mathcal{I}(\eta_j) z^j$. Then $q(z) = Rq(z) + iIq(z)$ and both Rq and Iq have only real coefficients. When z is real, then $Rq(z) = \mathcal{R}(q(z))$ and $Iq(z) = \mathcal{I}(q(z))$, but this need not be true for complex z.

THEOREM 28.2. *Let $q(z)$ be a polynomial with complex coefficients and no multiple roots. Let $\Gamma = [z_0, z_1, \cdots, z_{K-1}]$ be a positively oriented polygon in the complex plane, and for the sake of notation, set $z_K = z_0$. Suppose also that $q(z)$ has no roots on $\partial \Gamma$, the boundary of Γ. For $q_j(x) = q(\sigma(z_{j-1}, z_j; x))$,*

$$u_j(x) = Rq_j(x), \qquad v_j(x) = Iq_j(x).$$

Then the number of roots of q inside Γ is exactly

$$\tfrac{1}{2} \sum_{j=1}^{K} \left[V(u_j, v_j; 1) - V(u_j, v_j; 0) \right].$$

Notice that if $q \in \mathrm{MP}_{M,m}^k$, $|z_j| < T_1$ and $\|z_j\| \leqslant T_2$ for all $0 \leqslant j \leqslant K-1$, then $|q_j|_\infty < 2^k\sqrt{k+1}(2T_1)^k$ and $\|q_j\| \leqslant M + kT_2$ for all j. Combining this observation with Theorem 28.2 gives us the following corollary.

COROLLARY 28.2. *Suppose $q \in \mathrm{MP}_{M,m}^k$ has no multiple roots and Γ is a triangle in the complex plane with vertices $z_j = x_j + iy_j$, $j = 0, 1, 2$. If x_j and y_j are all rational numbers with*

$$|x_j| < k^2 2^{m+3}, \qquad |y_j| < k^2 2^{m+3}, \qquad \|x_j\| \leqslant M, \ \|y_j\| \leqslant M,$$

we can in at most $C_2 \log^{\alpha_2}(k+m+M)$ parallel steps using at most $D_2(k+m+M)^{\beta_2}$ processors:

(i) *determine the number of roots of q on $\partial\Gamma$;*

(ii) *if the answer to (i) is 0, determine the number of roots of q inside Γ.*

In particular we can decide if q has any roots in the closed triangle Γ.

Now let x be a point on the real line such that $|x| < 2^m$, $\|x\| \leqslant M$ and $q(x) \neq 0$. We can use x as the vertex of $4k + 2$ regions defined by

$$U_+(x, j) = T_1\left(x, \frac{j}{k(2k+1)}\right) - \overline{T_1\left(x, \frac{j-1}{k(2k+1)}\right)},$$

$$U_-(x, j) = T_{-1}\left(x, \frac{j}{k(2k+1)}\right) - \overline{T_{-1}\left(x, \frac{j-1}{k(2k+1)}\right)},$$

for $j = 1, 2, \ldots, 2k+1$. A polynomial with real coefficients has roots that are symmetric about the real axis and thus, by Lemma 27.1, if $q \in \mathrm{MP}_{M,m}^k$ and $|x| < 2^m$, then q has exactly twice as many roots in the closure of $U_+(x, j)$ as it does in the closure of the triangle $\Gamma_j(x) = [x, x+\xi_{j-1}, x+\xi_j]$, where $\xi_j = (k(2k+1)+ji)2^m$. Similarly, q has exactly twice as many roots in the closure of $U_-(x, j)$ as it does in the closure of the triangle $\Gamma_{-j}(x) = [x, x-\xi_{j-1}, x-\xi_j]$. Clearly, if x is not itself a root of q, there is at least one value of j, $1 \leqslant j \leqslant 2k+1$, such that both $\overline{U_+(x,j)}$ and $\overline{U_-(x,j)}$ contain no roots of q.

If $\|x\| \leqslant M$, then we can, using Corollary 28.2, find such a value of j in at most $C_2 \log^{\alpha_2}(k+m+M)$ parallel steps using at most $D_2(4k+2)(k+m+M)^{\beta_2}$ processors. This is precisely the construction we need in order to define the key idea of a splitting region.

Suppose $q \in \mathrm{MP}_{M,m}^k$ and $q(x) \neq 0$. Let $1 \leqslant j \leqslant 2k+1$ be an integer such that q has no roots in $\overline{U_+(x,j)} \cup \overline{U_-(x,j)}$ and set $\xi = k(2k+1)+(j-\frac{1}{2})i$. A *$q$-splitting at x* of the complex plane is the pair of (real) lines (L_+, L_-), where L_+ is the line passing through x and $x + \xi$ and L_- is the line passing through x and $x + \bar\xi$. Notice that we can represent any q-splitting by a pair (x, j), where x is a real number and j is an integer ($1 \leqslant j \leqslant 2k+1$).

Suppose that $S = (L_+, L_-)$ is a q-splitting at x and that γ is the slope of L_+. Then define

$$q_+(S; z) = \prod_{r_j \in T_1(x,y)} (z - r_j), \tag{28.1}$$

$$q_-(S;z) = \prod_{r_j \in T_{-1}(x,y)} (z-r_j), \tag{28.2}$$

$$w(S;z) = \prod_{r_j \in T_i(x,y)} (z-r_j).$$

All the roots of $q_+(S;z), q_-(S;z)$ and $w(S;z)$ lie in $T_1(x,y), T_{-1}(x,y)$ and $T_i(x,y)$, respectively, and

$$q(z) = q_+(S;z) q_-(s;z) w(S;z) \bar{w}(S;z).$$

We will write $q_+(z)$ and $q_-(z)$ as shorthand for $q_+(S;z)$ and $q_-(S;z)$.

29. Approximating the factors by contour integration

Let $Q(z)$ be a polynomial of degree k with roots $r_1, r_2, \ldots, r_k$. In this section, we use the notation $s_j(Q) = r_1^j + \cdots + r_k^j$. In BEN-OR, FEIG, KOZEN AND TIWARI [1988], it is shown that if $\rho(Q) < 2^{m+1}$ and if we have a collection of approximations $\tilde{s}_j$ ($1 \leqslant j \leqslant k-1$) satisfying

$$|\tilde{s}_j - s_j(Q)| < 2^{-M - 17mk^2}, \tag{29.1}$$

then we can, using only fast matrix operations, compute an approximation $\bar{Q}$ to Q satisfying $|\bar{Q} - Q|_\infty < 2^{-M}$. The method for doing this is a consequence of the Newton identities for polynomials. Thus, in order to find the good polynomial approximations q_1 and q_2 of the polynomials q_+ and q_- in (28.1), (28.2), we first find the degrees k_1 and k_2 of q_+ and q_-, respectively, and then compute approximations of the appropriate precision, $\tilde{s}_{1j}, j = 1, \ldots, k_1 - 1$, and $\tilde{s}_{2j}, j = 1, \ldots, k_2 - 1$, to $s_j(q_+)$ and $s_j(q_-)$, respectively. The $\tilde{s}_{1j}$ and $\tilde{s}_{2j}$ will be computed by evaluating, to high enough precision, the contour integrals

$$s_j(q_+) = \frac{1}{2\pi i} \int_{\partial \Gamma_+} \frac{z^j q'(z)}{q(z)} \, dz,$$

$$s_j(q_-) = \frac{1}{2\pi i} \int_{\partial \Gamma_-} \frac{z^j q'(z)}{q(z)} \, dz,$$

where Γ_+ and Γ_- are triangles determined by the splitting lines L_+ and L_- and certain vertical lines that are far away from the roots of q.

We now concentrate on computing the $\tilde{s}_{1j}$ approximations to the $s_j(q_+)$. The computation of $\tilde{s}_{1j}$ is nearly identical and can be performed in parallel. So, for the rest of this section, we write $\tilde{s}_j$ instead of $\tilde{s}_{1j}$, d instead of k_1, $k = \deg q$, and we assume that the splitting point x is given.

As before, we let g be the slope of the splitting line L_+. Notice that γ is a rational number of the form $(2l-1)/2k(2k+1)$ for some integer $1 \leqslant l \leqslant 2k+1$. We also fix ν, a positive integer such that $2^{-\nu+2}$ is less than $\Delta(x,q)$, the minimum distance from x to any root of q, and set $\delta = 2^{-\nu}$. Recall that $q(x) \neq 0$, so such an integer ν exists. In the context of our basic algorithm, we will be able to pick this constant in such a way that δ is not too small, but for now it will be left unspecified.

Let τ be the greatest integer less than or equal to $6 + 2\log k$, and set $\varepsilon = 2^{-\tau}$. We define a sequence of points ζ_k on L_+ by

$$\zeta_0 = x, \qquad \zeta_1 = x + \delta + \gamma\delta i,$$

$$\zeta_{h+1} = x + (1+\varepsilon)(\zeta_h - x) = x + (1+\varepsilon)^{h-1}(\delta + \gamma\delta i).$$

Let $Z = \zeta_K$ where K is the smallest integer larger than $64k^2(m+2+\nu)$, and define $\Gamma = \Gamma_+$ to be the triangle $[x, \bar{Z}, Z]$.

The following facts about this construction can be noticed, which hold for all $0 \leqslant h \leqslant K$:

$$|\Re(\zeta_h)| < 2^{2(m+2)+\nu+1}, \tag{29.2}$$

$$|\Im(\zeta_h)| < 2^{2(m+2)+\nu+1}, \tag{29.3}$$

$$\|\zeta_h\| \leqslant \max\{\|x\|, \|\delta\| + (64k^2(m+2+\nu))(6+2\log k)\}, \tag{29.4}$$

$$|\Re Z| > 2^{m+2}, \tag{29.5}$$

$$|\zeta_{h+1} - \zeta_h| < \tfrac{1}{4}\Delta(\zeta_h, q). \tag{29.6}$$

Notice that (29.2), (29.3) and (29.5) essentially follow from the inequalities $2 < (1 + 1/j)^j < 4$, which hold for all positive integers j, and that (29.4) is trivial. The last property (29.6) follows from the definition of q-splittings.

From (29.5) we see that the vertical side of Γ is well outside $\rho(q)$, the root radius of q, and hence all the roots of q that are in $T_1(x, y)$ are contained in the interior of Γ. Notice also that the theorems of Section 27 make it easy to find the number of roots of q inside Γ, which is exactly d (the degree of q_+). Thus we shall take it for granted that $d \leqslant k$ is known. We now concentrate on computing $\tilde{s}_j$ for some fixed but arbitrary j ($1 \leqslant j \leqslant d-1$). Again, the method used will allow the computation of all $\tilde{s}_j$ in parallel.

The integral around $\partial\Gamma$ will be split into three parts

$$\int_{\partial\Gamma} dz = \int_x^{x+\bar{Z}} dz + \int_{x+\bar{Z}}^{x+Z} dz + \int_{x+Z}^{x} dz = I_1^j + I_2^j + I_3^j.$$

If we can compute approximations $\tilde{I}_1^j, \tilde{I}_2^j, \tilde{I}_3^j$ such that for $l = 1, 2, 3$

$$|\tilde{I}_l^j - I_l^j| < 2^{-M - 17mk^2 - 2},$$

then by adding these approximations, we obtain an approximation $\tilde{I}^j = \tilde{s}_j$ that satisfies (29.1). We concentrate first on the approximate evaluation of I_3^j.

Let $f_j(z)$ be the meromorphic function $z^j q'(z)/q(z)$. At each ζ_k, we can expand a finite number of terms of the Taylor series of f, obtaining

$$f(z) = \alpha_{h0} + \alpha_{h1}(z - \zeta_h) + \cdots + \alpha_{ht}(z - \zeta_h)^t + R_{ht}(z)$$
$$= T_{ht}(z) + R_{ht}(z).$$

Let $d_k = |\zeta_{k+1} - \zeta_k|$, $B_k = \{z : |z - \zeta_k| < 2d_k\}$, and define
$$M_h = \max_{z \in B_k} |f(z)|.$$

It follows from the Cauchy estimates for f that for all z in the closed disc of radius d_k centred at ζ_k

$$|R_{ht}(z)| \leq M_h 2^{-t} \tag{29.7}$$

In particular, this estimate holds for all z on the closed line segment joining ζ_k and ζ_{k+1}.

Now from the definition of q-splittings and the definition of δ we see that for all z in the closed ball $|z - \zeta_k| \leq 2d_k$,

$$\Delta(z, q) > 2d_k > 2\varepsilon\delta.$$

Thus, for all h,

$$M_k = \max_{z \in B_k} \left| \sum_{j=1}^{k} \frac{z^j}{z - r_j} \right| \leq \max_{z \in B_k} \frac{k|z|^j}{\Delta(z, q)} < \frac{2^{j(2m+4) - \log \delta + 2} k}{2\varepsilon\delta}. \tag{29.8}$$

Combining (29.7) and (29.8), we obtain that for all z on the closed segment $[\zeta_k, \zeta_{k+1}] \subset L_+$,

$$|R_{ht}(z)| < 2^{j(2m+4+\nu)+5+3\log k+\nu-t}.$$

Suppose that we define $\tilde{I}_3^j$ by

$$\tilde{I}_3^j = -\sum_{h=1}^{K} \int_{\zeta_{k-1}}^{\zeta_k} T_{ht}(z)\, dz$$
$$= \sum_{h=1}^{K} \sum_{l=0}^{t} \frac{\alpha_{lh}}{l+1} \left(\zeta_{h-1}^{l+1} - \zeta_h^{l+1} \right). \tag{29.9}$$

If the arithmetic in this sum were carried out exactly, we would have

$$|\tilde{I}_3^j - I_3^j| = \left| \sum_{h=1}^{K} \int_{\zeta_{k-1}}^{\zeta_k} R_{ht}(z)\, dz \right|$$
$$< |Z - x| 2^{j(2m+4+\nu)+5+3\log k+\nu-t}$$
$$< 2^{(j+2)(2m+4+\nu)+5+3\log k+\nu-t}.$$

The arithmetic in (29.9) could be carried out exactly if we chose to calculate with rational numbers (we need to check that the integers involved do not become too large, but this is easy to do). Alternatively, we may choose to only approximate each term in the outer sum of (29.9) to within 2^{-t}. In this case, we have

$$|\tilde{I}_3^j - I_3^j| < 2^{(j+2)(2m+4+\nu)+5+3\log k+\nu-t} + 2^{-t} K$$
$$< 2^{(j+2)(2m+4+\nu)+7+3\log k+\nu-t}.$$

In either case, by picking t appropriately, we can compute I_3^j in at most $C_3 \log^{\alpha_3}(k+m+M+\nu+\|x\|)$ parallel steps using at most $D_3(k+m+M+\nu+\|x\|)^{\beta_3}$ processors, since we can use fast parallel methods to calculate the Taylor coefficients α_{lk} in (29.9).

Since the polynomial q has real coefficients, $I_1^j = -\bar{I}_3^j$. The calculation of $\tilde{I}_2^j$ is very similar, but actually much easier, because the whole segment $[Z,\bar{Z}]$ is 'far away' from the roots of q.

The net result of this section is as follows.

THEOREM 29.1. *Let $q(z)$ be the polynomial occurring in Step 26.1.3, x a real (rational) number with $q(x) \neq 0$ and ν a positive integer such that $\Delta(x,q) > 2^{-\nu+2}$. If $S = (L_+, L_-)$ is a q-splitting at x, then we can compute in at most $C_4 \log^{\alpha_4}(k+m+M+\nu+\|x\|)$ parallel steps using at most $D_4(k+m+M+\nu+\|x\|)^{\beta_4}$ processors the polynomials $q_1(z)$ and $q_2(z)$ that satisfy*

$$q_1 \in \mathrm{MP}_{M,m'}^{\deg q_1}, \qquad q_2 \in \mathrm{MP}_{M,m'}^{\deg q_2},$$

$$|q_1 - q_+|_\infty < 2^{-M}, \qquad |q_2 - q_-|_\infty < 2^{-M}.$$

30. Finding a balanced splitting point

For the rest of this paper let $q(z)$ be a polynomial of degree k and x a real number with $q(x) \neq 0$. Let $\gamma = 1/k$ and let k_1 and k_2 be the number of roots of q in $\overline{T_1(x,\gamma)}$ and $\overline{T_{-1}(x,\gamma)}$, respectively. We say that x is a *balanced splitting point* for q if $\max\{k_1, k_2\} \leq \lambda k$.

Our task in this section is to find a balanced splitting point x that also satisfies

$$\Delta(x,q) > 2^{-\mu-2}, \qquad \|x\| \leq \mu + 2,$$

when q is the polynomial occurring in Step 26.1.3. To simplify things, we are in need of still more geometric notation.

Let $\mathbb{C}_U = \{z \in \mathbb{C}: \mathfrak{I}z > 0\}$ and $\mathbb{C}_L = \{z \in \mathbb{C}: \mathfrak{I}z < 0\}$ be the open upper and lower half planes of the complex plane. If $\zeta \in \mathbb{C}_U$, we define

$$A(\zeta) = A_\gamma(\zeta) = \overline{T_{-i}(\zeta,\gamma) \cup \mathbb{C}_U},$$

and similarly, when $\zeta \in \mathbb{C}_L$, we define

$$A(\zeta) = A_\gamma(\zeta) = \overline{T_i(\zeta,\gamma) \cup \mathbb{C}_L}.$$

In both cases, we define

$$P(\zeta) = P_\gamma(\zeta) = A(\zeta) \cap \mathbb{R}.$$

and if $\zeta \in \mathbb{R}$ then

$$A(\zeta) = P(\zeta) = \{\zeta\}.$$

Let $f(x)$ be a continuous complex valued function of a real variable and let $[a,b] \subset \mathbb{R}$ be a closed interval. If f has no zeros in $[a,b]$, we denote by $\Delta_a^b \arg f$ the net change in the argument of f as x increases from a to b.

THEOREM 30.1. *Let $w(z)$ be a monic polynomial of degree $k \geq 21$ with complex coefficients and no multiple roots. Set $\lambda_0 = 15/16$, $u(x) = Rw(x)$, $v(x) = Iw(x)$ and $\gamma = 1/k$. Let*

$$t_0(x) = u(x), \qquad t_1(x) = v(x), \qquad t_{j-1}(x) = c_j(x)t_j(x) - t_{j+1}(x).$$

Let ζ be a complex number and suppose that the number of roots of w contained in the set $A_\gamma(\zeta) \setminus \mathbb{R}$ is at least $\lambda_0 k$. Then at least one of the quotient polynomials c_j is both linear and has its (one) root contained in $P_\gamma(\zeta)$.

PROOF. We will restrict the proof to the case $\mathcal{I}\zeta < 0$. Except for a few sign changes, the proof of the case $\mathcal{I}\zeta > 0$ is nearly identical, while the case $\mathcal{I}\zeta = 0$ is trivial since it can only happen when $\deg w = 1$.

We now have two cases to consider: w has no real roots and w has real roots.

Restricting our attention first to the case when w has no real roots, we consider the sequence $s_w = [t_0(x), t_1(x), \ldots, t_l(x)]$ as x varies on the real line. Since w has no real roots, u and v can have no real roots in common and hence $t_l(x)$ is of constant sign on $\mathbb{R}$. From this, we deduce that as x increases on the real line, the number of sign changes in the sequence s can change only at a root of u, and there the number of sign changes will increase if $\arg w(x)$ is increasing and decrease if $\arg w(x)$ is decreasing.

Let $P_\gamma(\zeta) = [a, b]$. Since

$$\Delta_a^b \arg w = \sum_{j=1}^{k} \Delta_a^b \arg(x - r_j),$$

we have

$$\Delta_a^b \arg w < -(\lambda_0 k)[\pi - 2/\tan\gamma] + \pi(1 - \lambda_0)k < -[(2\lambda_0 - 1)k - 1]\pi.$$

For $t \in \mathbb{R}$, let $I(t)$ denote the greatest integer less than or equal to t. Then it follows from the previous paragraph that

$$F = V(u, v; a) - V(u, v; b) \geq I((2\lambda_0 - 1)k - 1) \geq (2\lambda_0 - 1)k - 2.$$

We say that j ($1 \leq j \leq l-1$) is an *oscillation index* if

$$\text{sign}(t_{j-1}(a)) = \text{sign}(t_j(a)) = \text{sign}(t_{j+1}(a)),$$
$$\text{sign}(t_{j-1}(b)) = \text{sign}(t_j(b)) = \text{sign}(t_{j+1}(b)).$$

We want to show that there are many of these indices. Suppose that there are J of these indices. Then

$$2F < 2J + (l - 1 - J) + 2 = J + l + 1.$$

Since $l \leq k$,

$$J \geq (4\lambda_0 - 3)k - 5.$$

It is now easy to see that for $k \geq 21$, this can only happen if $J > k/2$ and this in turn implies that for at least one oscillation index l, c_l is linear. But

$$c_l(x)t_l(x) = t_{l-1}(x) + t_{l+1}(x)$$

and by definition of an oscillation index, the sign of the right-hand side is the same as the sign of $t_l(x)$ when they are evaluated at b, but opposite when they are evaluated at a. This can only happen if the sign of $c_l(a)$ is opposite to the sign of $c_l(b)$, and this implies that c_l must have a root in $[a,b] = P(\zeta)$. This completes the proof of this case.

The case when w has real roots can be reduced to the above case by the following simple argument. Let

$$\psi(z) = \prod_{r_j \in \mathbb{R}} (z - r_j).$$

Then the polynomial $w(z)/\psi(z)$ has no real roots but the c_j computed for it are exactly the same as the c_j computed for w. □

Now suppose that $w(z)$, instead of being an arbitrary polynomial with complex coefficients, is a polynomial of the form $w(z) = w_0(z + \alpha i)$ where $\alpha \in \mathbb{R}$ and w_0 is a polynomial with real coefficients, and suppose also that the ζ in the statement of Theorem 30.1 has the property that $|\Im \zeta| < 2|\alpha|$. Then

$$\Delta_a^b \arg w < -(\lambda_0 k)[\pi - 2/\tan\gamma] + \tfrac{1}{2}\pi(1 - \lambda_0)k.$$

If we then follow the same analysis as in the proof of Theorem 30.1, we are led to the following.

THEOREM 30.2. *Suppose that $w(z) = w_0(z + \alpha i)$, where $\alpha \in \mathbb{R}$ and w_0 has real coefficients. In the statement of Theorem 30.1, replace the value of λ_0 by $\lambda_0 = 11/12$ and, as before, assume that $\deg w \geqslant 21$. Also add the extra assumption that $|\Im \zeta| < 2|\alpha|$. Then the conclusion of Theorem 30.1 still holds.*

We now have the tool to compute a balanced splitting point x for our polynomial q in Step 26.1.3. We do this by computing several values of x in parallel and invoke Theorem 30.2 to conclude that at least one of them must be a balanced splitting point.

The set of points we construct will be called R_q. For each integer $j, -\mu \leqslant j \leqslant m + 2 - \log n$, we construct the negative polynomial remainder sequence for $u_j(x)$ and $v_j(x)$, where $w_j(x)$ is the polynomial

$$w_j(x) = q(z + 2^j i)$$

and u and v are as in the statement of Theorem 30.1. For each root r of a linear quotient $c_{lj}(x)$, we add to R_q the three rational numbers $r - 2^j/\gamma, r, r + 2^j/\gamma$. We also add to R_q the number q_{k-1}/k (rounded to precision 2^{-M}), where q_{k-1} is the coefficient of z^{k-1} in $q(z)$. Of course, all these computations are done in parallel. Theorem 30.2 guarantees that at least one of the points x in R_q is a balanced splitting point for q, except for the possibility that $q(x) = 0$. In fact

$$\max\{k_1, k_2\} \leqslant k - I(k/24) - 1, \tag{30.1}$$

where, as before, $I(t)$ is the greatest integer function. Notice that the quantity on the right is always less than $23k/24$.

In order to prove (30.1), we let K be the quantity on the right. For $\zeta \in \mathbb{C}_U$, we let

$$H_+(\zeta) = T_1(\zeta, \gamma) \cup T_i(\zeta, \gamma) \cup T_1(\bar{\zeta}, \gamma) \cup T_{-i}(\bar{\zeta}, \gamma),$$
$$H_-(\zeta) = T_{-1}(\zeta, \gamma) \cup T_i(\zeta, \gamma) \cup T_{-1}(\bar{\zeta}, \gamma) \cup T_{-i}(\bar{\zeta}, \gamma),$$

and let $h_+(\zeta)$ and $h_-(\zeta)$ be the number of roots of q in $\overline{H_+(\zeta)}$ and $\overline{H_-(\zeta)}$. We also let $a(\zeta)$ be the number of roots of q in $A_\gamma(\zeta) \cup A_\gamma(\bar{\zeta})$.

It is not difficult to see that there must be a $\zeta \in \mathbb{C}_U$ such that

$$h_+(\zeta) \geq k - K, \qquad h_-(\zeta) \geq k - K, \qquad a(\zeta) \geq \tfrac{11}{12}k.$$

For such a ζ, any point $x \in P_\gamma(\zeta)$ must split the roots of q according to (30.1). Let $P_\gamma(\zeta) = [a, b]$ and let j be an integer between $-\mu$ and $m + 2 - \log n$ which satisfies

$$2^{j-1} < \mathcal{I}\zeta \leq 2^j. \tag{30.2}$$

Then, applying Theorem 30.2 to $w_j(z)$, we see that at least one of the linear quotient polynomials c_{lj} corresponding to w_j must have its root in $[2a-b, 2b-a]$. Since (30.2) implies

$$2^j/\gamma < b - a \leq 2^{j+1}/\gamma,$$

the claim, (30.1), easily follows.

It is tedious but not difficult to verify that all these computations can be done in polylog time.

References

ABEL, N. (1826), Beweis der Unmoglichkeit, algebraische Gleichungen von hoheren Graden als dem vierten allgemein aufzulosen, *Grelles J.* **1**, S. 65.

ABERTH, O. (1973), Iteration method for finding all zeros of a polynomial simultaneously, *Math. Comput.* **27**, 339–344.

AITKEN, A. (1926), On Bernoulli's numerical solution of algebraic equations, *Proc. Roy. Soc. Edinburgh* **46**, 289–305.

ALEFELD, G. and J. HERZBERGER (1974a), On the convergence speed of some algorithms for the simultaneous approximation of polynomial roots, *SIAM J. Numer. Anal.* **11**, 237–243.

ALEFELD, G. and J. HERZBERGER (1974b), *Einfuhrung in die Intervallrechnung* (B. I. Wissenschaftsverlag, Zurich).

ALEFELD, G. and J. HERZBERGER (1983), *Introduction to interval computations* (Academic Press, New York).

ALEXANDER, J. (1915), Functions which map the interior of the unit circle upon simple regions, *Annals of Math.* **17**, 12–22.

ANDREEV, A. and N. KJURKCHIEV (1987), Two-sided methods for solvng the polynomial equation, *Math. Balkanica (New Series)* **1**, 72–82.

ANDREEV, A. and N. KJURKCHIEV (1989), Two-sided methods for solving equations, *IMACS Ann. Comput. Appl. Math.* **7**, 161–172.

ANGELOVA, E. and KH. SEMERDZHIEV (1982), Methods for the simultaneous approximate derivation of the roots of algebraic, trigonometric and exponential equations, *USSR Comput. Math. Math. Phys.* **22** (1), 226–232 (in Russian).

ASCHER, M. (1970), in: Problems and Solutions, *Amer. Math. Monthly* **77**, 380.

ATANASSOVA, L., N. KJURKCHIEV and A. ANDREEV (1988), Recursive generated iterative functions for approximate solution of algebraic equations, *Serdica* **14**, 271–277 (in Russian).

ATANASSOVA, L., T. DJUKANOVA and N. KJURKCHIEV (1985), Methods with $3R+4$ rate of convergence for computing the roots of an algebraic equation, *Annuaire Univ. Sofia Fac. Math. Mec.* **79** (1) (in Russian).

BALLIEU, R. (1947), Sur des limitations des recines d'une equation algebrique, *Acad. Roy. Belg. Bull. Cl. Sci.* **33**, 743–750.

BAREISS, E. (1960), Resultant procedure and the mechanization of the Graeffe Process, *J. ACM* **7**, 346–386.

BAIRSTOW, L. (1914), Investigations relating to the stability of the aeroplane, *Reports* and *Memoranda* **154**, Advisory Committee for Aeronautics.

BARMISH, B. (1984), Invariance of the strict Hurwitz property for polynomials with perturbed coefficients, *IEEE Trans. Automat. Contr.* **29** (10), 935–936.

BAUDET, G. (1978), Asynchronous iterative methods for multiprocessors, *J. ACM* **25** (2), 226–244.

BELL, H. (1965), Gershgorin's theorem and the zeros of polynomials, *Amer. Math. Monthly* **72**, 292–295.

BEN-OR, M., E. FEIG, D. KOZEN, P. TIWARI (1988), A fast parallel algorithm for determining all roots of a polynomial with real roots, *SIAM J. Comput.* **17**, 1081–1092.

BERNOULLI, D. (1728), *Comment. Petropolitanae* **3**.
BIALAS, S. and J. GARLOFF (1985), Stability of polynomials under coefficient perturbation, *IEEE Trans. Automat. Contr.* **30** (3), 310–312.
BIEHLER, C. (1879), Sur une classe d'equations algebriques dont toutes les racines sont reelles, *J. Reine Angew. Math.* **87**, 350–352.
BOJANOV, B. (1970), On an estimation of the roots of algebraic equations, *Appl. Math.* **11** (2), 195–205.
BOJANOV, B., Q. RAHMAN and J. SZYNAL (1985), On a conjecture of Sendov about the critical points of a polynomial, *Math. Z.* **190**, 281–285.
BORSCH-SUPAN, W. (1963), A posteriori error bounds for the zeros of polynomials, *Numer. Math.* **5**, 380–398.
BORSCH-SUPAN, W. (1970), Residuenabschatzung fur Polynom-Nullstellen mittels Lagrange-Interpolation, *Numer. Math.* **14**, 287–296.
BRAUER, A. (1957), The theorems of Ledermann and Ostrowski on positive matrices, *Duke Math. J.* **24**, 265–274.
BRAUER, A. and I. GENTRY (1974), Bounds for the greatest characteristic root of an irreducible nonnegative matrix, *Linear Algebra Appl.* **8**, 105–107.
BRAUER, A. and I. GENTRY (1976), Bounds for the greatest characteristic root of an irreducible nonnegative matrix II, *Linear Algebra Appl.* **13**, 109–114.
BRODETSKY, S. and G. SMEAL (1924), On Graeffe's method for complex roots of algebraic equations, *Math. Proc. Cambridge Philos. Soc.* **22**, 83–87.
BROYDEN, C. and J. FORD (1975), A new method of polynomial deflation, *J. Inst. Math. Appl.* **16**, 271–281.
BUDAN, J. (1826), *Nouvelle methode pour la resolution des equations numeriques* (Paris, 2nd ed.).
BURMEISTER, W. and J. SCHMIDT (1982), On the R-order of coupled sequences II, *Computing* **29**, 73–81.
BURMEISTER, W. and J. SCHMIDT (1983), On the R-order of coupled sequences III, *Computing* **30**, 157–169.
BURMEISTER, W. and J. SCHMIDT (1985), Characterization of the best R orders of coupled sequences arising in iterative processes, in: *Numerical Methods and Applications '84* (BAN, Sofia) 191–202.
BURMEISTER, W. and J. SCHMIDT (1988), On the R-order of coupled sequences arising in single-step type methods, *Numer. Math.* **53**, 653–661.
CASCIO, M., L. PASQUINI and D. TRIGIANTE (1983), Simultaneous determination of polynomial complex roots and multiplicities: Algorithm and problems involved, Tech. rep. Dip. di Metodi e Modelli Matematici per le scienze Applicate, Univ. Roma La Sapienza.
CASCIO, M., L. PASQUINI and D. TRIGIANTE (1984), Un polialgoritmo a convergenza rapida per la determinazione simultanea degli zeri reali di un polinomio e delle loro molteplicita, *Monografia di Soft. Matem.* N. **30**, Pubbl. dell'IAC.
CAUCHY, A. (1829), Sur la resolution des equations numeriques et sur la theory d'elieifation, *Oeuvres* **(12) 19**, 87–161.
CHUNG, S. (1972), An algorithm for the zeros of transcendental functions, *Numer. Math.* **32**, 351–371.
CHUNG, S. (1976), Generalization and acceleration of an algorithm of Sebastiao e Silva and its duales, *Numer. Math.* **25**, 365–377.
COHEN, J. (1979), Random evolutions and the spectral radius of a nonnegative matrix, *Math. Proc. Cambridge Philos. Soc.* **86**, 349–350.
COHN, A. (1922), Über die Anzahl der Wurzeln einer algebraischen Gleichung in einem Kreis, *Math. Z.* **14**, 110–138.
COSNARD, M. and P. FRAIGNIAUD (1989), Asynchronous Durand–Kerner and Aberth polynomial root finding methods on a distributed memory multi-computer, in: *Parallel Computing '89*, Leiden.
DANDELIN (1826), Recherches sur *la* resolution des equations numeriques, *Nouveaux Mem. de l'Acad. Roy. des Sci., et Belles Lettres de Bruxelles* **3**, 1–71.
DATT, B. and N. GOVIL (1978), On the location of zeros of a polynomial, *J. Approx. Theory* **24**, 78–82.

DAVIES, M. and B. DAWSON (1978), An automatic search procedure for finding real zeros, *Numer. Math.* **31**, 299–312.

DEKKER, T. (1968), Newton–Laguerre iteration, in: *Programmations en Mathematiques Numeriques*, Besanson, 7–14 September 1966 (Editions du Centre Nationale de la Recherche Scientifique, Paris) 189–200.

DEUTSCH, E. (1971), in: Problems and Solutions, *Amer. Math. Monthly* **78**, 799.

DEUTSCH, E. (1979), Nested bounds for the Perron root of a nonnegative irreducible matrix, manuscript; see *Notices Amer. Math. Soc.* **26**, A421–A422.

DEUTSCH, E. (1981), Bounds for the Perron root of a nonnegative irreducible partitioned matrix, *Pacific J. Math.* **92**, 49–56.

DEUTSCH, E. (1982), Lower bounds for the Perron root of a nonnegative irreducible matrix, *Math. Proc. Cambridge Philos. Soc.* **92**, 49–54.

DIMITROV, D. (1983), On a conjecture of Sendov, *C. R. Acad. Bulgare Sci.* **36** (5), 561–563.

DOCHEV, K. (1962a), A modified Newton method for simultaneous approximate calculation of all roots of a given equation, *Phys. Math. J.* **5**, 136–139.

DOCHEV, K. (1962b), Über Newtonsche Iterationen, *C. R. Acad. Bulgare Sci.* **15** (7), 695–701.

DOCHEV, K. and P. BYRNEV (1964), Certain modifications of Newton's method for the approximate solution of algebraic equations, *Z. Vycisl. Mat. i Mat. Fiz.* **4**, 915–920 (in Russian).

DOCHEV, K., P. BYRNEV, and P. RUSSEV (1969), On a method for calculation of the zeros of Laguerre entire functions, *Izv. Mat. Inst.* **10**, 155–160 (in Bulgarian).

DURAND, E. (1960), *Solution Numerique des Equations Algebraique* (Masson et Compagnie, Paris).

DVORCUK, J. (1967), Newton method for simultaneous finding of all roots of a polynomial, in: *Sb. Vykumnych praci, Ustav Vypoctove Techn. CSAV a CVUT*, 41–64.

DVORCUK, J. (1969), Factorization of a polynomial into quadratic factors by Newton method, *Apl. Mat.* **14**, 54–80.

EHRLICH, L. (1967), A modified Newton method for polynomials, *Comm. ACM* **10**, 107–108.

ENESTRÖM, G. (1920), Remarque sur un theoreme relatif aux racines de l'equation $a_n x^n + \cdots + a_0 = 0$. ou tous les coefficients sont reels et positifs, *Tôhoku Math. J.* **18**, 34–36.

FARMER, M. and G. LOIZOU (1975), A class of iteration functions for improving simultaneously, approximations to the roots of polynomials, *BIT* **15**, 250–252.

FARMER, M. and G. LOIZOU (1977), An algorithm for the total, or partial, factorization of a polynomial, *Math. Proc. Cambridge Philos. Soc.* **82**, 427–437.

FOURIER, J. (1831), Analyse des equations determines, Livre I, Paris.

FORD, J. (1977), A generalization of the Jenkins–Traub method, *Math. Comput.* **31** (137), 193–203.

FRAIGNIAUD, P. (1989a), Analytic and asynchronous root finding methods on a distributed memory multicomputer, Research Report LIP– IMAG.

FRAIGNIAUD, P. (1989b), The Durand–Kerner polynomials root finding method in case of multiple roots, Research Report LIP-IMAG.

FRIEDLAND, S. and S. KARLIN (1975), Some inequalities for the spectral radius of nonnegative matrices and applications, *Duke Math. J.* **42**, 459–490.

FUJIWARA, M. (1915), Über die Wurzeln der algebraischen Gleichungen, *Tôhoku Math. J.* **8**, 78–85.

FUJIWARA, M. (1916), Über die obere Schranke des absoluten Betrages der Wurzeln einer algebraischen Gleichung, *Tôhoku Math. J.* **10**, 167–171.

GARGANTINI, I. (1978), Further applications of circular arithmetic: Schroeder-like algorithms with error bounds for finding zeros of polynomials, *SIAM J. Numer. Anal.* **3**, 497–510.

GARGANTINI, I. (1980), Parallel square-root iterations for multiple roots, *Comput. Math. Appl.* **6**, 279–288.

GARGANTINI, I. (1981), An application of interval mathematics: A polynomial solver with degree four convergence, *Freiburger Intervall-Berichte* **7**, 15–25.

GARGANTINI, I. and P. HENRICI (1974), Circular arithmetic and the determination of polynomial zeros, *Numer. Math.* **18**, 305–320.

GASKELL, R. (1958), *Engineering Mathematics* (Dzyden Press, New York), 244–251.

GAUSS, K. (1850), Beitrage zur Theorie der algebraischen Gleichungen, *Abh. Ges. Wiss. Gottingen* **4**; *Ges. Werke* **3**, 73–102.

GERSHGORIN, S. (1931), Über die Abgrenzung der Eigenwerte einer Matrix, *Izv. Akad. Nauk SSSR* **7**, 749–754.

GOODMAN, A., RAHMAN, Q. and J. RATTI (1969), On the zeros of a polynomial and its derivative, *Proc. Am. Math. Soc.* **21**, 273–274.

GRACE, J. (1902), On the zeros of a polynomial, *Proc. Cambridge Philos. Soc.* **11**, 352–356.

GRAEFFE, C. (1837), *Die Auflösung der hoheren numerischen Gleichungen, als Beantwortung einer von der königlichen Akademie der Wissenschaften zu Berlin aufgestellten Preisfrage* (Friedrich Schulthess, Zurich).

GRAU, A. (1963), On the reduction of number range in the use of the Graeffe process, *J. ACM* **10**, 538–544.

GREEN, M., A. KORSAK and M. PEASE (1976), Simultaneous iteration to wards all roots of a complex polynomial, *SIAM Rev.* **18**, 501–502.

GROBNER, W. (1966), *Matrizenrechnung* (Bibliographisches Institut, Mannheim Vien–Zurich).

GUGGENHEIMER, H. (1986), Initial approximations in Durand–Kerner's root finding method, *BIT* **26** (4), 537–539.

GUIVER, J. and N. BOSE (1983), Strictly Hurwitz property invariance of quartics under coefficient perturbation, *IEEE Trans. Automat. Contr.* **28**, 106–107.

HALL, C. and T. POPSCHING (1969), Bounds for the maximal eigenvalue of a nonnegative irreducible matrix, *Duke Math. J.* **36**, 159–164.

HALLEY, E. (1809), A new, exact, and easy method of finding the roots of any equations generally, and that without any previous reduction (abridged by C. Hutton, G. Shaw and R. Pearson), *Philos. Trans. Roy. Soc. London* **3**.

HANSEN, E. and M. PATRICK (1976), Estimating the multiplicity of a root, *Numer. Math.* **27**, 121–131.

HANSEN, E. and M. PATRICK (1977), A family of root finding methods, *Numer. Math.* **27**, 257–269.

HAUENSCHILD, M. (1974), Arithmetiken fur komplexe Kreise, *Computing* **13**, 299–313.

HEAWOOD, P. (1907), Geometrical relations between the roots of $f(x) = 0, f'(x) = 0$, *Quart. J. Math.* **38**, 84–107.

HERMITE, C. (1866), Question 777, *Nouv. Ann. Math.* **5** (2), 432; Questions 778, 779, a. a. o., S. 479.

HERMITE, C. (1879), Sur l'indice des fractions rationelles, *Bull. Soc. Math. France* **7**, 128–131.

HERMITE, C. (1898), Sur un memoire de Laguerre concernant equations algebriques, *Oeuvres de Laguerre*, Paris, 461–468.

HERZBERGER, J. (1986a), On the R-order of some requrrences with applications to inclusion-methods, *Computing* **36**, 175–180.

HERZBERGER, J. (1986b), Bounds for the R-order of certain iterative numerical processes, *BIT* **26**, 259–262.

HERZBERGER, J. (1989), Iterationsferfahren hoherer Ordnung zur Einschliessung der Inversen einer Matrix, *Z. Angew. Math. Mech.* **69**, 115–120.

HERZBERGER, J. (1990), Using error-bounds for hyper-power methods to calculate inclusions for the Inverse of a matrix, *BIT* **30**, 508–515.

HILDEBRAND, F. (1956), *Introduction to Numerical Analysis* (McGraw–Hill, New York).

HITCHCOCK, F. (1944), An improvement on the G. C. D. method for complex roots, *J. Math. and Phys.* **23**, 69–74.

HOUSEHOLDER, A. S. (1970), *The Numerical Treatment of a Single Nonlinear Equation* (McGraw-Hill, New York).

HOUSEHOLDER, A. (1971), Generalizations of an algorithm of Sebastiao e Silva, *Numer. Math.* **16**, 375–382.

HOXHA, F. (1988), Calcul simultane des racines d'un polynome complexe: Contribution a l'algorithmique et mise *en* oeuvre sur un resean de processeur, These de l'Institut National Polytechnique de Toulouse.

HURWITZ, A. (1896), Über die Bedingungen, unter welchen eine Gleichung nur Wurzeln mit negativen reelen Teilen besitzt, *Math. Ann.* **46**, 273–284.

ILIEV, L. (1949), Über Newtonsche Iterationen, *Jahrb. Univ. Sofia*, **1**, 167–171 (in Bulgarian).

ILIEV, L. (1987), *Laguerre Entire Functions* (BAN, Sofia).

ILIEV, L. and K. DOCHEV (1963), Über Newtonsche Iterationen, *Wiss. Z. Tech. Univ. Dresden*, **12** (1), 117–118.

JAIN, V. (1990), On Cauchy's baund for zeros of a polynomial, *Approx. Theory Appl.* **6**, 18–24.

JENKINS, M. and J. TRAUB (1970), A three-stage algorithm for real polynomials using quadratic iteration, *SIAM J. Numer. Anal.* **7**, 545–566.

JOYAL, A., LABELLE, G. and Q. RAHMAN (1967), On the location of zeros of polynomials, *Canad. Math. Bull.* **10**, 53–63.

KAHAN, W. (1967), Laguerre's method and a circle which contains at least one zero of a polynomial, *SIAM J. Numer. Anal.* **4**, 474–482.

KAKEYA, S. (1912), On the limit of the roots of an algebraic equation with positive coefficients, *Tôhoku Math. J.* **2**, 140–142.

KELLEHER, S. B. (1916), Des limites des zeros d'un polynome, *J. Math. Pure Appl.* **2**, 169–171.

KERNER, I. (1966a), Ein Gesamtschrittverfahren zur Berechnung der Nullstellen von Polynomen, *Numer. Math.* **8**, 290–294.

KERNER, I. (1966b), Algorithm 283, *Comm. ACM* **9**, 273.

KHAPITONOV, V. (1978), On a generalization of a stability criterion, *Izv. Acad. Nauk Kazakh. SSR Ser. Fiz.-Mat.* **1**, 53–57 (in Russian).

KJELBERG, G. (1984), Two observation on Durand–Kerner's root finding method, *BIT* **24**, 556–559.

KJURKCHIEV, N. (1981), Some modifications of Dvorcuk's method for factorization of a polynomial into quadratic factors, *Annuaire Univ. Sofia Fac. Math. Mec.* **75**, 3–7.

KJURKCHIEV, N. (1982), On some iterational schemes of Dochev's type with increased rate of convergence, *Annuaire Univ. Sofia Fac. Math. Mec.* **76**, 3–10.

KJURKCHIEV, N. (1983a), Certain modification of Ehrlich's method for the approximate solution of algebraic equation, *Pliska* **5**, 43–50 (in Russian).

KJURKCHIEV, N. (1983b), Computational aspects and areas of application of the methods for simultaneous determination of all roots of an algebraic equation, *Annuaire Univ. Sofia Fac. Math. Mec.* **77**, 11–16 (in Russian).

KJURKCHIEV, N. (1991), Über die Konvergenzordnungen einiger Klassen Iterationsverfahren, *Serdica* **17**, 139–143.

KJURKCHIEV, N. (1992a), Note on the estimation of the order of convergence of some iterative methods, *BIT* **32**, 525–528.

KJURKCHIEV, N. (1992b), A note on a method for localization of the roots of algebraic equations, *C. R. Acad. Bulgare Sci.* **44** (9) (in print).

KJURKCHIEV, N. and A. ANDREEV (1985), A modification of Weierstrass Dochev's method with rate of convergence $R + 2$ for simultaneous determination of the zeros of a polynomial, *C. R. Acad. Bulgare Sci.* **38** (11), 1461–1463 (in Russian).

KJURKCHIEV, N. and A. ANDREEV (1987), Ehrlich's method with raised speed of convergence, *Serdica* **13**, 52–57.

KJURKCHIEV, N. and A. ANDREEV (1989), Two-sided method for computation of all multiple roots of an algebraic polynomial, *Serdica* **15** (4), 302–304 (in Russian).

KJURKCHIEV, N. and A. ANDREEV (1990), On Halley-like algorithms with high order of convergence for simultaneous approximation of multiple roots of polynomials, *C. R. Acad. Bulgare Sci.* **43** (9), 29–32

KJURKCHIEV, N. and A. ANDREEV (1992), A generalization of the Alefeld–Herzberger's method, *Computing* **47**, 355–360.

KJURKCHIEV, N. and J. HERZBERGER (1992), A new lower bound for the zeros of polynomials, *Serdica* (in print).

KJURKCHIEV, N. and R. IVANOV (1984), On some multi-stage schemes with a superlinear rate of convergence, *Annuaire Univ. Sofia Fac. Math. Mec.* **78**, 132–136 (in Russian).

KJURKCHIEV, N. and S. MARKOV (1983), Two interval methods for algebraic equations with real roots, *Pliska* **5**, 118–131.

KJURKCHIEV, N. and S. TASCHEV (1981), Method for simultaneous determination of the zeros of a polynomial, *C. R. Acad. Bulgaire Sci.* **34** (8), 1053–1055 (in Russian).

Kjurkchiev, N., A. Andreev and V. Popov (1984), Iterative methods for computation of all multiple roots of an algebraic polynomial, *Annuaire Univ. Sofia Fac. Math. Mec.* **78**, 178–185 (in Russian).

Kojima, T. (1917), On the limits of the roots of an algebraic equation, *Tôhoku Math. J.* **11**, 119–127.

Krier, N. (1973), *Komplexe Kreisarithmetik*, Ph. D. Thesis, Univ. Karlsruhe, Karlsruhe.

Kunieda, M. (1916), Note on the roots of algebraic equations, *Tôhoku Math. J.* **9**, 167–173.

Lagouanelle, J. L. (1966), Sur une method de calcul de l'ordre de multiplicite des zeros d'un polynome, *C. R. Acad. Sci. Paris* **262A**, 626–627.

Laguerre, E. (1880), Sur une methode pour obtenir par approximation les racines d'une equation algebrique qui a toutes ses racines reelles, *Nouv. Ann. Math.* 2s. **19**; *Oeuvres* **1**, 87–103.

Laguerre, E. (1898), *Oeuvres* **1**, Paris.

Landau, E. (1906), Über den Picardischen Satz, *Vierteljahrsschrift der Naturforschenden Geselschaft in Zurich* **51**, 252–318.

Landau, E. (1907), Sur quelques generalisations du theorème de M. Picard, *Ann. Sci. École Norm. Sup.* **24** (3), 179–201.

Lawrence, T. and E. Lawrence (1972), A new algorithm for factoring polynomials, *Proc. IEEE* **60** (6), 733–738.

Ledermann, W. (1950), Bounds for the greatest latent roots of a positive matrix, *J. London Math. Soc.* **25**, 265–268.

Lobacevsky, N. (1834), Algebra ili vycislenie konecnuh, *Polnoe Sobranie Socinenii* **4** (1948).

Loizou, G. (1982), Une note sur le procede iterativ de Marica Presic, *C. R. Acad. Sci. Paris* **295**, 707–710.

Loizou, G. (1983), Higher order iteration functions for simultaneously approximating polynomial zeros, *Internat. J. Comput. Math.* **14**, 45–58.

Lossers, O. (1971), *Amer. Math. Monthly* **78**, 681–683.

Lucas, F. (1874), Properietes geometriques des fractions rationelles, *C. R. Acad. Sci. Paris* **78**, 140–144, 180–183, 271–274.

Maehly, H. (1954), Zur iterativen Auflosung algebraischer Gleichungen, *Z. Angew. Math. Phys.* **5**, 260–263.

Makrelov, I. (1979), On a numerical method for simultaneous search of all zeroes of a given trigonometric polynomial, *Travaux Sci. Univ. Plovdiv* **17**, 205–217.

Makrelov, I. and Kh. Semerdzhiev (1983), A two analogue of a method of Ehrlich for simultaneous determination of all zeros of a trigonometric and exponential polynomials, *C. R. Acad. Bulgare Sci.* **36**, 879–882 (in Russian).

Makrelov, I. and Kh. Semerdzhiev (1984a), Methods for the simultaneous finding of all roots of an algebraic and exponential polynomials, with given multiplicity, *J. Comput. Math. Math. Phys.* **24** (10), 1443–1453 (in Russian).

Makrelov, I. and Kh. Semerdzhiev (1984b), Methods of finding simultaneously all the roots of algebraic, trigonometric and exponential equations, *J. Comput. Math. Math. Phys.* **24** (5), 99–105 (in Russian).

Makrelov, I. and Kh. Semerdzhiev (1985a), Dochev's method of a generalized polynomial over an arbitrary Chebyshev system, *C. R. Acad. Bulgare Sci.* **38** (10), 1323–1326 (in Russian).

Makrelov, I. and Kh. Semerdzhiev (1985b), On the convergence of two methods for the simultaneous finding of all roots of exponential equations, *IMA J. Numer. Anal.* **5**, 191–200.

Makrelov, I., Kh. Semerdzhiev and S. Tamburov (1985), Method for simultaneous finding of all zeros of a given generalized polynomial over Chebyshev system, Research Report JINR, Dubna P11-85-932 (in Russian).

Makrelov, I., Kh. Semerdzhiev and S. Tamburov (1986a), A modified Ehrlich's method, *C. R. Acad. Bulgare Sci.* **39** (5), 43–46 (in Russian).

Makrelov, I., Kh. Semerdzhiev and S. Tamburov (1986b), Method for simultaneous finding all roots of a generalized polynomial over an arbitrary Chebyshev system, *Serdica* **12**, 351–357 (in Russian).

Marden, M. (1949), *The Geometry of the Zeros of a Polynomial in a Complex Variable*, Math. Surveys **3** (Amer. Math. Soc., Providence, RI).

MARDEN, M. (1983), Conjectures on the critical points of a polynomial, *Amer. Math. Monthly* **90**, 267–276.
MARKOVITCH, D. (1939), Sur quelques limites superieures des modules des zeros d'un polynome, *Mathematica* **15**, 8–11.
MARKOV, S. and N. KJURKCHIEV (1989), A method for solving algebraic equations, *Z. Angew. Math. Mech.* **69** (4), 106–109.
MARTY, F. (1932), Sur une inegalite que verifient les zeros d'un polynome, *Bull. Sci. Math.* **56**, 276–281.
MEIR, A. and A. SHARMA (1969), On Ilyeff's conjecture, *Pac. J. Math.* **31**, 459–467.
MERIKOSKI, J. (1979), On a lower bound for the Perron eigenvalue, *BIT* **19**, 39–42.
MIGNOTTE, M. (1976), Note sur la methode de Bernoulli, *Numer. Math.* **26**, 325–326.
MILLER, M. (1990), Maximal polynomials and the Ilieff–Sendov conjecture, *Trans. of the Amer. Math. Soc.* **321** (1), 285–303.
MILOVANOVIC, G. and M. PETKOVIC (1983), On the convergence order of a modified method for simultaneous finding polynomial zeros, *Computing* **30**, 171–178.
MILOVANOVIC, G. and M. PETKOVIC (1984), The methods of high order for the simultaneous determination of multiple polynomials zeros, *Izv. Univ. Nis*, 95–100.
MOHAMMAD, Q. (1965a), On the zeros of polynomials, *Amer. Math. Monthly* **72**, 35–38.
MOHAMMAD, Q. (1965b), On the zeros of polynomials, *Amer. Math. Monthly* **72**, 631–633.
MOHAMMAD, Q. (1967), Location of the zeros of polynomials, *Amer. Math. Monthly* **74**, 290–292.
MONTEL, P. (1935), Sur quelques rapports nouveaux entre l'algebre et la theory des fonctions, *Mathematica (Cluj)* **9**, 47–55.
MONTEL, P. (1935a), Sur quelques limites pour les modules des zeros des polynomes, *Comment. Math. Helv.* **7**, 178–200.
MOORE, R. (1966), *Interval Analysis* (Prentice–Hall, Englewood Cliffs, New Jersey).
NEFF, A. (1990), Specified precision polynomial root isolation is in NC^4, Research Report, RC 15653 (69571), IBM Research Division, T. J. Watson Research Center, Yorktown Heights, NY 10598.
NOUREIN, A. W. (1975), An iteration formula for simultaneous determination of the zeroes of a polynomial, *J. Comput. Appl. Math.* **4**, 251–254.
NOUREIN, A. W. (1977a), An improvement on two iteration methods for simultaneous determination of the zeros of polynomial, *Internat. J. Comput. Math.* **6**, 241–252.
NOUREIN, A. W. (1977b), An improvement on Nourein's method for the simultaneous determination of the zeros of a polynomial (an algorithm), *J. Comput. Appl. Math.* **3**, 109–110.
OBRESHKOV, N. (1924), Über die Wurzeln von algebraischen Gleichungen, *Jahresber. Deutsch. Math. Ver.* **33**, 52–64.
OBRESHKOV, N. (1928), Über die Trennung der reellen Wurzeln von algebraischen Gleichungen, *Jahresber. Deutsch. Math. Ver.* **37**, 234–237.
OBRESHKOV, N. (1952), Sur les racines des equations algebriques, *Annuaire Univ. Sofia Fac. Math. Mec.* **47**, 67–83.
OBRESHKOV, N. (1962), *Advanced algebra* (Nauka i izkustvo, Sofia) (in Bulgarian).
OBRESHKOV, N. (1963a), *Verteilung und Berechnung der Nullstellen reeller Polynome* (VEB Deutscher Verlag der Wissenschafter, Berlin).
OBRESHKOV, N. (1963b), Sur la solution numerique des equations, *Annuaire Univ. Sofia Fac. Math. Mec.* **56**, 73–83.
ORTEGA, J. and W. RHEINBOLDT (1970), *Iterative Solution of Nonlinear Equations in Several Variables* (Academic Press, New York).
OSTROWSKI, A. (1940), Recherches sur la methode de Graeffe et les zeros des polynomes et des series de Laurent, *Acta Math.* **72**, 99–105.
OSTROWSKI, A. (1952), Bounds for the greatest latent root of a positive matrix, *J. London Math. Soc.* **27**, 253–256.
OSTROWSKI, A. (1966), *Solution of Equations* and *Systems of Eequations* (Academic Press, New York, 2nd ed.).
OSTROWSKI, A. and H. SCHNEIDER (1960), Bounds for the maximal characteristic root of a nonnegative irreducible matrix, *Duke Math. J.* **27**, 547–553.

PAN, V. (1987), Sequential and parallel complexity of approximate evaluation of polynomial zeros, *Comput. Math. Appl.* **14**, 591–622.

PAN, V. (1992), Complexity of computations with matrices and polynomials, *SIAM Rev.* **34**, 2, 225–262.

PARLETT, B. (1964), Laguerre's method applied to the matrix eigenvalue problem, *Math. Comp.* **18**, 464–485.

PASQUINI, L. and D. TRIGIANTE (1981), Il metodo di continuazione e l'approssimazione simultanea degli zeri di un polinomo, *Sem. Inst. Mat. Appl. Fac. Ing., Univ. Roma*, 128–146.

PASQUINI, L. and D. TRIGIANTE (1985), A globally convergent method for simultaneously finding polynomial roots, *Math. Comp.* **44**, 135–149.

PASTOR, R. (1932), *Lecciones de Algebra*, 2nd edition.

PELLET, M. (1924), Sur la racine de plus petit module des equations, *Bull. Sci. Math.* **48**, 265–267.

PETKOVIC, M. (1981), On a generalization of the root iterations for polynomial complex zeros in circular interval arithmetics, *Computing* **27**, 37–55.

PETKOVIC, M. (1982), Generalized root iterations for the simultaneous determinations of multiple complex zeros, *Z. Angew. Math. Mech.* **62**, 627–630.

PETKOVIC, M. (1987), Some interval iterations for finding a zero of a polynomial with error bounds, *Comput. Math. Appl.* **14** (6), 479–495.

PETKOVIC, M. (1989a), On Halley-like algorithms for simultaneous approximation of polynomial complex zeros, *SIAM J. Numer. Anal.* **26** (3), 740–763.

PETKOVIC, M. (1989b), *Iterative Methods for Simultaneous Inclusion of Polynomial Zeros* (Springer Verlag, Berlin).

PETKOVIC, M. and J. HERZBERGER (1990), Inclusion of multiple polynomial roots in complex rectangular arithmetic, *IMACS Ann. Comput. Appl. Math.* **12**.

PETKOVIC, M. and G. MILOVANOVIC (1983), A note on some improvements of the simultaneous methods for determination of polynomial zeros, *J. Comput. Appl. Math.* **9**, 65–69.

PETKOVIC, M., G. MILOVANOVIC and L. STEFANOVIC (1986), Some higher order methods for the simultaneous approximation of multiple polynomial zeros, *Comput. Math. Appl.* **9**, 951–962.

PETKOVIC, M. and L. CVETKOVIC (1990), On a hybrid method for a polynomial complex zero, in: *International Symposium on Computer Arithmetic, Scientific Computation and Mathematical Modelling*, Albena, Bulgaria, 23–27 September 1990 (Publishing House of the Bulgarian Academy of Sciences) 144–145.

PETKOVIC, M. S. and L. D. PETKOVIC (1989), On the bounds of the R-order of some iterative methods, *Z. Angew. Math. Mech.* **69**, T197–T198.

PETKOVIC, M. and L. STEFANOVIC (1984), On the convergence order of accelerated root iterations, *Numer. Math.* **44**, 463–476.

PETKOVIC, M. and L. STEFANOVIC (1986), On some improvements of square root iteration for polynomial complex zeros, *J. Comput. Appl. Math.* **15**, 13–25.

PETKOVIC, M. and L. STEFANOVIC (1987a), On some iteration functions for the simultaneous computation of multiple complex polynomial zeros, *BIT* **27**, 111–122.

PETKOVIC, M. and L. STEFANOVIC (1987b), On some parallel higher-order methods of Halley's type for finding multiple polynomial zeros, in: *Numerical Methods* and *Approximation Theory*, III (Faculty of Electronic Engineering, Niš), 329–337.

PETKOV, M. and N. KJURKCHIEV (1990), High accuracy localization estimates for roots of algebraic equations, *Math. Ed. Math.*, 388–391 (in Bulgarian).

PHELPS, D. and R. RODRIGUEZ (1972), Some properties of extremal polynomials for the Ilieff conjecture, *Kodai Math. Sem. Rep.* **24**, 172–175.

POINCARÉ, H. (1883), Sur les equations algebriques, *C. R. Acad. Sci. Paris* **97**, 1418–1419.

POLYA, G. (1915), Über das Graeffesche Verfahren, *Z. Math. Phys.* **63**, 275–290.

POULAIN, E. (1867), Theorems generaux–sur les equations algebraiques, *Nouv. Ann. Math.* **6** (2), 21–33.

PRESIC, M. (1980), A convergence theorem for a method for simultaneous determination of all zeros of a polynomial, *Publ. Inst. Math. Beograd* **28** (5), 159–165.

PRESIC, S. B. (1966), Un procédé iterative pour la factorisation des polynomes, *C. R. Acad. Sci. Paris* **262**, 862–863.
RAHMAN, Q. (1970), A bound for the moduli of the zeros of polynomials, *Canad. Math. Bull.* **13**, 541–542.
RAHMAN, Q. (1972), Zeros of linear combinations of polynomials, *Canad. Math. Bull.* **15**, 139–142.
RALL, L. (1966), Convergence of the Newton process to multiple solutions, *Numer. Math.* **9**, 23–37.
RALSTON, A. (1965), *A first Course in Numerical Analysis* (McGraw-Hill, New York).
REICH, S. (1970a), in: Problems and Solutions, *Amer. Math. Monthly* **77**, 655.
REICH, S. (1970b), in: Problems and Solutions, *Amer. Math. Monthly* **77**, 532.
RENEGAR, J. (1987), On the worst case arithmetic complexity of approximating zeros of polynomials, *J. of Complexity* **3**, 90–113.
RENYI, A. and P. TURAN (1952), On the zeros of polynomials, *Acta Math. Hungar.* **3**, 275–284.
RICE, T. and L. JAMIESON (1989), A highly parallel algorithm for root extraction, *IEEE Trans. Comput.* **28** (3), 443–449.
RIORDAN, J. (1958), *Introduction to Combinatorial Analysis* (Wiley, New York).
ROKNE, J. and P. LANCASTER (1971), Complex interval arithmetic, *Comm. ACM* **14**, 111–112.
ROUCHE, E. (1862), Memoire sur la serie de Lagrange, *J. Ecole Polyt.* **22**, 217–218.
RUTISHAUSER, H. (1963), On a modification of the Q. D. Algorithm with Graeffe–type convergence, in: *Inform. Proc.* 1962 (North-Holland Publishing, Amsterdam) 93–96.
SAN JUAN, R. (1935), Complements a la methode de Graffe pour la resulation des equations algebriques, *Bull. Sci. Math.* **59**, 104–109.
SAVENKO, S. (1964), Iteration method for solving algebraic equation, *Z. Vycisl. Mat. i Mat. Fiz.* **4**, 738–744 (in Russian).
SCHMEISSER, G. (1969), Bemerkungen zu einer Vermutung von Ilieff, *Math. Z.* **111**, 121–125.
SCHMEISSER, G. (1977), On Ilieff's conjecture, *Math. Z.* **156**, 165–173.
SCHMIDT, J. (1981), On the R-order of coupled sequences, *Computing* **26**, 333–342.
SCHUR, I. (1914), Zwei Satze uber algebraische Gleichungen mit lauter reellen Wurzeln, *J. Reine Angew. Math.* **144**, 75–88.
SCHUR, I. (1921), Über algebraischen Gleichungen, die nur Wurzeln mit negativen Realteilen besitzen, *Z. Angew. Math. Mech.* **1**, 307–311.
SCHUR, I. (1933), Untersuchungen uber algebraische Gleichungen I., Bemerkungen zu einem Satz von E. Schmidt, *Sitzungsber. Preuss. Acad. Wiss. Math.-Phys. Klasse*, 403–428.
SEBASTIAO E SILVA, J. (1941), Sur une methode d'approximation semblable a celle de Gräffe, *Portugal. Math.* **2**, 271–279.
SEBASTIAO E SILVA, J. (1946), Complementi al methodo di Gräffe per la risoluzione delle equazione algebriche, *Intit. Veneto Sci. Lett. Arti Atti Cl. Sci. Fis. Mat. Natur.* **8** (1), 335–343.
SEKULOVSKI, R. (1972), Uopstenje iterative metode S. Presica za faktorizaciju polynoma, *Mat. Vesnik* **9**, 257–264.
SEMERDZHIEV, KH. (1982), Method for the simultaneous computation of all multiple roots of an algebraic polynomial, *C. R. Acad. Bulgare Sci.* **35** (8), 1057–1060 (in Russian).
SEMERDZHIEV, KH. (1985), Methods of simultaneous deriving all roots of a given algebraic equation, Research Report JINR, Dubna (in Russian).
SEMERDZHIEV, KH. and S. PATEVA (1978), On a numerical method for simultaneous finding all roots of a given algebraic equation, *Travaux Sci. Univ. Plovdiv* **15**, 263–273, (in Bulgarian).
SEMERDZHIEV, KH. and S. TAMBUROV (1984), A method for the determination of the multiplicities of the roots of an algebraic polynomial, *C. R. Acad. Bulgare Sci.* **37** (9), 1143–1145 (in Russian).
SEMERDZHIEV, KH. and S. TAMBUROV (1985), Method for determining all zeros of a generalized polynomial over an arbitrary Chebyshev system, Research Report JINR, Dubna P11-85-931 (in Russian).
SENDOV, BL. (1974), A method for simultaneous approximate calculation of all positive roots of a polynomial, *Izv. Vyssh. Uchebn. Zaved. Mat.* **5**, 185–187 (in Russian).
SENDOV, BL. and V. POPOV (1976), *Numerical Methods,* I (Nauka i izkustwo, Sofia) (in Bulgarian).
SIMEINOVIC, D. (1989), On the convergence of an iterative procedure for the simultaneous determination of all zeros of a polynomial, *Z. Angew. Math. Mech.* **69** (4), 108–110.

STEFANOVIC, L. (1986), Some iterative methods for the simultaneous finding of polynomial zeros, Ph.D. Thesis, University of Niš (in Serbo-Croatian).

STURM, J. (1829), Memoire sur la resolution des equations numeriques, *Bull. Ferussac, Paris*.

TASCHEV, S. and N. KJURKCHIEV (1983), Certain modifications of Newton's method for the approximate solution of algebraic equations, *Serdica* **9**, 67–72 (in Russian).

TAUSSKY, O. (1949), A recurring theorem on determinants, *Amer. Math. Monthly* **56**, 672–676.

TIKOO, M. (1967), Location of the zeros of a polynomial, *Amer. Math. Monthly* **74**, 688–690.

TOYA, T. (1933), Some remarks on Montel's paper concerning upper limit of absolute values of roots of algebraic equations, *Sci. Reports Tokyo Bunrika Daigaku* **A1**, 275–282.

TRAUB, J. (1964), *Iterative Methods for the Solution of Equations* (Prentice–Hall, Englewood Cliffs, NJ).

TURAN, P. (1951), On approximative solution of algebraic equations, *Publ. Math. Debrecen* **2**, 26–42.

VAN DER CORPUT, J. (1946), Sur l'approximation de Laguerre des racines reelles, *Indag. Math.* **8**, 581–588.

VAN VLECK, E. (1925), On limits to the absolute values of the roots of a polynomial, *Bull. Soc. Math. France* **53**, 105–125.

VARGA, R. (1962), *Matrix Iterative Analysis* (Prentice–Hall, Englewood Cliffs, NJ).

WALSH, J. (1924), An inequality for the roots of an algebraic equation, *Ann. of Math.* **25**, 285–286.

WANG, D. and Y. WU (1987), Some modifications of the parallel Halley iteration method and their convergence, *Computing* **38**, 75–87

WANG, X. and S. ZHENG (1984a), A family of parallel and interval iterations for finding all roots of a polynomial simultaneously with rapid convergence (I), *J. Comput. Math.* **1**, 70–76.

WANG, X. and S. ZHENG (1984b), The quasi–Newton method in parallel circular iteration, *J. Comput. Math.* **4**, 305–309.

WANG, X. and S. ZHENG (1985), A family of parallel and interval iterations for finding all roots of a polynomial simultaneously with rapid convergence (II), *J. Comput. Math.* **4**, 433–444.

WEIDNER, P. (1988), The Durand–Kerner methods for trigonometric and exponential polynomials, *Computing* **40**, 175–179.

WEIERSTRASS, K. (1903), Neuer Beweis des Satzes, dass jede Ganze Rationale Funktion einer Veranderlichen dargestellt werden kann als ein Product aus Linearen Funktionen derselben Veranderlichen, *Ges. Werke* **3**, 251–269.

WERNER, W. (1982), *On the Simultaneous Determination of Polynomial Roots*, Lecture Notes in Mathematics **953** (Springer, Berlin).

WERNER, W. (1983), Über Abschatzungen von Polynomnullstellen mittels des Gerschgorinschen Kreisesatzes, *Z. Angew. Math. Mech.* **63**, T390–T391.

WESTERFIELD, E. (1933), A new bound for the zeros of polynomials, *Amer. Math. Monthly* **40**, 18–23.

WILF, H. (1961), Perron–Frobenius theory and the zeros of polynomials, *Proc. Amer. Math. Soc.* **12**, 247–250.

WILIAMS, K. P. (1922), Note concerning the roots of an equation, *Bull. Amer. Math. Soc.* **28**, 394–396.

YOHE, J. (1977), The interval arithmetic package, MRC Technical Summary Report 1755, Mathematics Research Center, Univ. of Wisconsin, Madison.

ZHIDKOV, E., I. MAKRELOV and KH. SEMERDZHIEV (1983), Two methods for a simultaneous search for all roots of exponential equations, Research Report JINR, Dubna P11-83-764 (in Russian).

Subject Index

Alefeld–Herzberger's method, 723
Argument principle, 645
Arithmetic node, 748

Basic theorem of algebra, 631
Bell's polynomial, 721
Bernoulli's iteration, 687
Branch node, 748

Cardano's formula, 639
Cauchy's bounds, 657
Characteristic polynomial, 680
Chebyshev's correction, 729
Chebyshev's method, 710
Circular arithmetic, 739
Cohn's rule, 651
Common divisor, 634
Contour integral, 759
Cost of an algorithm, 749
Critical point, 651

D'Alembert's lemma, 631
Descartes' rule of signs, 641, 643, 716
Discriminant of polynomials, 637, 638
Distribution of the roots, 654
Dochev–Byrnev method, 702
Durand–Kerner method, 700, 703

Ehrlich's method, 716
Euclidean algorithm, 634, 643
Exact interval arithmetic, 740
Extremal polynomial, 653

Factorization, 735
Fourier sequence, 642

Galoa's theory, 640

Gauss–Lucas theorem, 651
Gauss–Seidel approach, 725
Grace's theorem, 654
Graeffe transforms, 690
Graeffe's method, 689
Greatest common divisor, 634

Halley's algorithm, 731
Halley's method, 732
Hermite–Poulain theorem, 640
Homogeneous symmetric function, 635
Hurwitz polynomials, 648

Interval methods, 739

Jordan curve, 645

Laguerre iteration, 693
Laguerre theorems, 643
Lehmer–Schur method, 697
Lobachevsky's method, 689
Location theorems, 660
Lower bounds, 673, 683, 748

Minkowski's inequality, 754
μ-digit approximation, 748
Multi-point method, 734
Multiple roots, 724

Neff approach, 752
Newton majorant, 691
Newton type methods, 700
Newton–Girard formulas, 692
Newton's correction, 716
Newton's formula, 635
Nourein's correction, 722
Nourein's method, 729

Number of roots, 640, 645, 650
Number of variations, 641

Ostrowski–Traub estimations, 686

Parallel branches, 754
Parallel time, 754
Pasquini–Trigiante algorithm, 702
Perron vector, 679
Perron–Frobenius theorem, 714
Polylog time, 756

R-factor, 703
R-order of convergence, 682, 703
Rectangular arithmetic, 740
Renegar approach, 748
Resolvent of polynomials, 637
Rolle's theorem, 654
Root distance, 748
Rounded interval arithmetic, 740

Schwarz's lemma, 664

Sendov's conjecture, 652
Sendov's method, 686
Sequential time, 752
Simple symmetric function, 635
Single-step method, 703, 723, 725
Spectral radius, 679, 716
Stirling's formula, 755
Sturm sequence, 643
Symmetric functions, 635

Total-step method, 711, 726
Two-sided methods, 745

Upper bounds, 673, 683, 752

Viete symmetric functions, 702

Wandermond determinant, 638
Weierstrass correction, 703
Weierstrass method, 699
Weierstrass–Dochev method, 700, 734